KNIGHT'S
Forensic Pathology

Those who have dissected or inspected many bodies
have at least learned to doubt, while those who are ignorant of
anatomy and do not take the trouble to attend to it, are in no doubt at all.

Giovanni Morgagni 1682–1771
The Father of Morbid Anatomy

Taceant colloquia. Effugiat risus. Hic locus est
ubi mors gaudet succurrere vitae.
(Let conversation cease. Let laughter flee.
This is the place where death delights to help the living.)

Latin proverb

Seldom say never – seldom say always!

Forensic proverb

Third Edition

KNIGHT'S
Forensic Pathology

Pekka Saukko Dr.med.univ. (Vienna), Dr.Med.Sci., Specialist in Forensic Medicine, Dr.h.c.
Professor and Head, Department of Forensic Medicine, University of Turku, Finland

Bernard Knight CBE, MD, DM (Hon), BCh, MRCP, FRCPath, FHKCPath, DSc (Hon), LLD (Hon),
PhD (Hon), DMJ (Path), Barrister of Gray's Inn
Emeritus Professor of Forensic Pathology, University of Wales College of Medicine, UK
Formerly Consultant Forensic Pathologist to the Home Office, UK

ARNOLD

A member of the Hodder Headline Group
LONDON

First published in Great Britain in 2004 by
Arnold, a member of the Hodder Headline Group,
338 Euston Road, London NW1 3BH

http://www.arnoldpublishers.com

Distributed in the United States of America by
Oxford University Press Inc.,
198 Madison Avenue, New York, NY10016

Oxford is a registered trademark of Oxford University Press

Whilst the advice and information in this book are believed to be true and
accurate at the date of going to press, neither the author[s] nor the
publisher can accept any legal responsibility or liability for any errors or
omissions that may be made. In particular (but without limiting the
generality of the preceding disclaimer) every effort has been made to check
drug dosages; however it is still possible that errors have been missed.
Furthermore, dosage schedules are constantly being revised and new
side-effects recognized. For these reasons the reader is strongly urged to
consult the drug companies' printed instructions before administering any
of the drugs recommended in this book.

British Library Cataloguing in Publication Data
A catalogue record for this book is available from the British Library

Library of Congress Cataloging-in-Publication Data
A catalog record for this book is available from the Library of Congress

ISBN 0 340 76044 3

1 2 3 4 5 6 7 8 9 10

Commissioning Editor: Serena Bureau
Development Editor: Layla Vandenbergh
Project Editor: Anke Ueberberg
Production Controller: Deborah Smith
Cover Design: Stewart Larking

Typeset in 10/12.5 AGaramond by Charon Tec Pvt. Ltd, Chennai, India
Printed and bound in Italy

What do you think about this book? Or any other Arnold title?
Please send your comments to feedback.arnold@hodder.co.uk

Contents

Preface to the third edition

It is pleasant to record that the second edition of *Forensic Pathology* consolidated the international reputation of the original book as one of the foremost manuals of forensic pathology in the English language. This new third edition generally follows the same successful pattern, but there are some significant differences.

The editorship is being transferred to Professor Pekka Saukko and this volume is the product of the collaboration with the original author. As with previous editions, the text has undergone a complete revision to update where necessary and add new material where relevant. A major change is the extensive use of colour to replace original monochrome illustrations and in numerous new illustrations, including micrographs. More than 300 colour illustrations have been added, of which 175 are completely new from the archives of both the Cardiff and Finnish institutes, and others.

Another major improvement has been in the reference material where both corrections and numerous additions have been made. 'Further reading' is intended for those readers who do not have access to electronic libraries and to offer an overview of the literature on a particular topic.

The new edition maintains the philosophy of evidence-based forensic pathology with emphasis on the avoidance of over-interpretation, which regrettably still leads to instances of miscarriage of justice.

It is hoped that the new edition of this well-established textbook, with its emphasis on practical procedures and common-sense evaluation of autopsy findings, will continue to be of assistance to forensic pathologists all over the world.

Pekka Saukko
Bernard Knight

Preface to the second edition

The most gratifying reception accorded in many parts of the world to the first edition of this book has led to the need for an updated version less than five years later. No radical changes have been made in the format, but like an airliner during its periodic major service, every part has been scrutinised and replaced where it has become outdated or defective. In addition, new material has been added where appropriate.

Forensic pathology, unlike its sister discipline forensic science, does not change quickly or have dramatic developments such as the current DNA revolution. Indeed, because its base is the interpetation of autopsy findings, forensic pathology still rests largely on the principles of morbid anatomy founded in the nineteenth century and earlier. However, this is not to say that it remains fossilised in the era of Virchow – new findings and techniques appear constantly, albeit at a measured pace compared with other disciplines. The most useful of these advances have been incorporated into this new edition.

In particular, the sections on child abuse, head injuries and traumatic subarachnoid haemorrhage have been amended or supplemented. Sixty new illustrations have been incorporated, and another area of attention has been the references and recommended reading, as there were some textual citations not listed in the first edition – and very many more have been added. However, the literature is now so vast, both in forensic journals and scattered profusely throughout other specialist publications, that it is futile to try to capture all of even the most seminal papers, which now need computerised and other modern library techniques for their retrieval.

One of the many reviewers of the previous edition complained that many of the references were old, but I make no apology for this. The value of a publication is in its content, not in its date, as Harvey's *De Motu Cordis* and Morgagni's *De Sedibus* clearly demonstrate! Some of the most valuable papers in forensic pathology were written decades or even a century ago; the critical writings of Moritz, Shapiro, Adelson, Helpern, Gonzales, Polson – right back to Taylor and Tardieu in the nineteenth century – are examples of careful observation and logical thinking which some modern pathologists, given to overinterpretation, would benefit from studying.

The critical attitude to every autopsy finding has been maintained in this new edition. A number of recent criminal trials and Appeals have emphasised the vital need for expert medical witnesses to be totally objective in their interpretation of physical findings. To quote from the new (1996) *Practice Guidelines* of the Policy Advisory Board in Forensic Pathology of the British Home Office: 'The evidence should be objective: speculation should be avoided. Unwarranted conclusions can never be defended. The role of the expert witness is not to provide the evidence which supports the case for the Crown nor for the defence, unless that opinion is objectively reached and has scientific validity.' Perhaps, in the interests of justice, an additional new forensic aphorism should be on the frontispiece: 'If you can't prove it, don't claim it!'

Bernard Knight
1996

Preface to the first edition

This is a textbook of forensic *pathology*, not forensic *medicine*. Though there is a considerable overlap, forensic medicine includes medical jurisprudence, the legal aspects of medical practice and many ethical matters, none of which are found – nor are intended to be found – in these pages.

Such topics have marked geographical limitations, as a result of legal, ethnic, cultural, and even religious variations from place to place. Even within the British Isles it is almost impossible to write a single book on medical jurisprudence that can do equal justice to the different legal systems of England and Wales, Scotland and Ireland.

The subject matter of this volume has no such geographical constraints, as it is solely concerned with the examination of the dead body for medicolegal purposes. Even in this limited sphere, police procedures and the habits of pathologists will vary considerably with country and with resources, but it is hoped that the routines, techniques and philosophy offered in this book will offer a guide to good practice that can then be modified according to local circumstances.

The contents are intended to lead the pathologist – and in some countries, the non-pathologist – through the procedures that are needed in the examination of a body found under obscure, suspicious, or frankly criminal circumstances.

In developed countries with sophisticated medicolegal systems, such autopsies will be performed only by forensic pathologists or by histopathologists with considerable experience, but in many areas of the world – especially the developing countries – lack of manpower and resources as well as considerations of distance and facilities mean that almost any doctor may be called upon to perform medicolegal examinations. For both of these classes of medical men and women this book aims to act as a guide and a source of reference.

The subject matter follows a fairly conventional pattern, but the treatment of each topic is designed to offer practical advice linked with a philosophical approach that leads the doctor to analyse and question the interpretations drawn from physical findings.

All too often, dogmatic opinions are derived from an unsound factual base, learned from lectures or textbooks that repeat previous dogma with little sense of critical evaluation.

In some parts of the world forensic pathology is learned by rote from teachers who studied it themselves in the same fashion, and who have little or no practical experience in the hard schools of mortuary or witness-box. I hope that this book will at least stimulate trainee forensic pathologists to think twice, question and disagree – not least about some of the material in the following pages.

Some conventions have been discarded in the format of this book. The author feels that it is disruptive for ease of reading to have every line clogged with references to other authors, except where essential to the topic under discussion. Thus most references have been consolidated into groups, placed at the end of the appropriate sections in each chapter. In addition to actual references, there are many suggestions for further reading on the same topic. It is quite impossible to be comprehensive in offering relevant titles, as the amount published on forensic matters is now overwhelming, several hundred new titles appearing each month. A representative selection is offered, much of it quite recent – these papers themselves will then offer a relevant bibliography, so that the topic can be followed in almost geometric progression.

There is no discussion of forensic serology, as this is now a discipline of its own. Similarly, the toxicology is confined to a detailed consideration of the pathologist's role in obtaining samples and interpreting the results from the analytical laboratory. Though the most common poisons are discussed, this is purely from the autopsy aspect. Like serology, toxicology is now a vast subject that stands independently and it seems futile merely to scratch the surface in a text devoted to forensic morbid anatomy.

Another departure from the conventional text is that concise reminders of the forensic anatomy of important regions are given, adjacent to the topic under discussion. Many pathologists learned their anatomy a long time ago and it can be useful before an autopsy, or writing the report, or appearing in court, to have a quick refresher about the relations of the aortic arch to the second rib or the exact structure of the laryngeal cartilages. Illustrations in forensic textbooks are traditionally profuse and often spectacular. The only justification for a photograph is that it instructs, however, rather than entertains or shocks. This book uses photographs only where a relevant point is displayed, with a full caption that stands alone without having to refer to the text.

Many line drawings are used, as the author feels that they often get the message across better than a photograph, which of necessity contains irrelevant and perhaps distracting features. Similarly, many books are replete with anecdotal cases; these can be valuable, but often are more intriguing than useful. The space devoted to these can usually be put to better use and they are employed sparingly in this text.

Where the pronoun 'he' is used throughout this book, it is intended that the word 'she' is equally applicable, unless obviously inappropriate from the context.

Finally, an Appendix is offered with basic reference material on weights, sizes, temperatures, conversion tables and other useful facts. Histological and histochemical techniques relevant to forensic needs are given in detail.

Bernard Knight
1990

CHAPTER 1

The forensic autopsy

Though 'necropsy' is semantically the most accurate description of the investigative dissection of a dead body, the word 'autopsy' is used so extensively that there is now no ambiguity about its meaning.

The term 'post-mortem examination' is a common alternative, especially in Britain, where its meaning is never in doubt. Unfortunately, it suffers from a lack of precision about the extent of the examination, for in some countries many bodies are disposed of after external examination without dissection.

The forensic investigation of deaths was introduced relatively early from the requirements of the judicial system. The earliest known forensic dissections took place in Italy, probably in the middle of the thirteenth century, at the University of Bologna. The first one was recorded by William of Saliceto, a surgeon and a teacher on the medical faculty there. He lived from 1210 to 1277 and in his book *Surgery* he mentioned a case examined in about 1275. The principles of the modern medico-legal investigation were developed based on the codes of the sixteenth century Europe: the Bamberg Code in 1507, the Caroline Code in 1532 and later the Theresian Code in 1769. The hospital or clinical autopsy became meaningful first after the introduction of modern concepts of pathogenesis of diseases by Carl von Rokitansky (1804–1878) and cellular pathology by Rudolf Virchow (1821–1902). Further development of medico-legal autopsy has been greatly influenced by the judicial system adopted, the main emphasis in most countries being in the detection and investigation of criminal and other unnatural or unexpected deaths.

AUTOPSY STANDARDS

Discussions about the quality of the autopsy started at the beginning of the nineteenth century. The Austrian decree of 1855 included, in its 134 paragraphs, very detailed instructions as to the performance of medico-legal autopsies. The idea of quality control and quality assurance, first introduced into industrial production of goods in the twentieth century, found its way into medicine later via laboratory medicine. Although regional and national differences in this respect are huge and the pace of progress varies, there is need for standards in specialist education, continuing professional development, harmonization of investigative procedures and quality systems leading perhaps eventually to some form of accreditation of individuals and institutions.

In addition to the national measures to create guidelines and to harmonize the medico-legal autopsy, there has been an increasing international interest in achieving harmonized and internationally recognized rules on the way autopsies should be carried out. In 1991, the General Assembly of the United Nations endorsed the Model Autopsy Protocol of the United Nations. The European Council of Legal Medicine (ECLM) document 'Harmonisation of the Performance of the Medico-Legal Autopsy' was adopted by the General Assembly in London 1995. The latter document served largely as basis for the Pan-European Council of Europe – *Recommendation No. R (99) 3 On the Harmonisation of Medico-Legal Autopsy Rules and Its Explanatory Memorandum* – which was adopted by the Committee of Ministers in February 1999 (see Appendix 2, p. 610). Although the document is a 'recommendation' by nature, it has legal implications, because Council of Europe member countries have to implement these principles into their national legislation.

TYPES OF AUTOPSY

Though medical conventions and legal systems vary considerably from country to country, there are generally two main types of autopsy:

■ The **clinical** or **academic autopsy** is one in which the medical attendants, with the consent of relatives, seek to learn the extent of the disease for which they were treating the deceased patient. In most jurisdictions this type of autopsy should not be held to determine the nature of the fatal disease because, if this was unknown to the physicians, the death should have been reported for medico-legal investigation.

■ The **medico-legal** or **forensic autopsy**, which is performed on the instructions of the legal authority responsible for the investigation of sudden, suspicious, obscure, unnatural, litigious or criminal deaths. This legal authority may be a coroner, a medical examiner, a procurator fiscal, a magistrate, a judge, or the police, the systems varying considerably from country to country.

In most systems the permission of the relatives is not required, as the object of the legal investigation would be frustrated if the objections of possibly guilty persons could prevent the autopsy.

In many jurisdictions the medico-legal autopsy is often further subdivided into:

■ those held on apparently non-criminal deaths, such as accidents, suicides, deaths from sudden natural causes, or associated with medical and surgical treatment, industrial deaths, and so on

■ the truly forensic autopsy held on suspicious or frankly criminal deaths, usually at the instigation of the police. These deaths comprise murder, manslaughter, infanticide and other categories that vary in different jurisdictions.

The type of pathologist that deals with these categories also varies from place to place but, as the systems are so diverse, there is little point in discussing the details. What is much more important is that whichever pathologist tackles each type of case, he or she should be trained and experienced in that particular field. Unfortunately, either from lack of staff and resources or because the system is deficient, medico-legal autopsies – especially of major criminal cases – are frequently performed by pathologists inexperienced in forensic procedures.

Another serious defect in many countries is the separation of those who practise forensic pathology from those who profess to teach it in universities. It is impossible to be a credible and convincing teacher unless one has continuing practical experience of the subject.

Even more unfortunate is the performance of medicolegal autopsies by doctors who have no training in pathology at all. Though lack of resources make this a widespread and inevitable practice in many developing countries, the same regrettable practice is seen in some parts of Europe, the Americas and elsewhere. This is to the detriment of the high standard of expertise that is vital for the support of law enforcement and the administration of justice. A poor opinion is often worse than no opinion at all, as in the latter case, the legal authorities will at least be aware of the deficiency in their evidence, rather than be misled by the often dogmatic inaccuracies of an inexperienced doctor.

THE PROCEDURE FOR A FORENSIC AUTOPSY

Though the actual performance of an autopsy is fairly uniform whatever the nature of the death, there are a number of associated matters that vary according to the circumstances. For example, the procedural precautions required in a murder are not necessary in a sudden natural death, and the dissection in a criminal abortion or fatal rape is different from that upon a drowned body.

There are, however, many facets of the autopsy that are common to every death. These will be discussed in turn here, though the full significance of each item is discussed in detail in other chapters.

The objectives of an autopsy

- To make a positive identification of the body and to assess the size, physique and nourishment.
- To determine the cause of death or, in the newborn, whether live birth occurred.
- To determine the mode of dying and time of death, where necessary and possible.
- To demonstrate all external and internal abnormalities, malformations and diseases.
- To detect, describe and measure any external and internal injuries.
- To obtain samples for analysis, microbiological and histological examination, and any other necessary investigations.
- To retain relevant organs and tissues as evidence.
- To obtain photographs and video for evidential and teaching use.
- To provide a full written report of the autopsy findings.
- To offer an expert interpretation of those findings.
- To restore the body to the best possible cosmetic condition before release to the relatives.

Preliminaries to an autopsy

Before the body is even approached, a number of preliminaries are necessary.

AUTHORIZATION AND CONSENT

A medico-legal autopsy is carried out at the behest of the appropriate authority. The pathologist must not begin his examination until he is satisfied that such authority has been issued in respect of that particular death. The means of delivering such authority will vary from place to place: it may be a written document, a verbal or telephoned message, or a tacit standing arrangement.

Where two official organizations are involved, it must be clear who has the premier right to order an autopsy. For example, in England and Wales, the police may request a pathologist to examine a body externally at the scene of death, but the right to order an autopsy is the sole prerogative of the coroner. Though in serious incidents he or she should take the advice of the Chief of Police regarding the choice of a pathologist, the final decision remains that of the coroner.

As stated earlier, in a medico-legal autopsy the relatives are not consulted for their consent to autopsy, as such permission cannot be withheld. As a matter of courtesy it is usual to inform them before the autopsy is carried out unless the circumstances are too urgent. In most cases, however, a relative will have attended to identify the body before the examination begins. Pathologists should be cautious about performing autopsies where the authorization or consent aspects are not clear. It sometimes happens that a 'consent document' for a hospital death has been obtained but the case has later been reported for medico-legal investigation. The pathologist should not then proceed under the 'consent' authority until the coroner or other official has decided whether to order his own autopsy (perhaps using another pathologist). If that official decides not to proceed, then usually the consent document becomes valid once more.

Permission for the retention of material from an autopsy (ranging from small fluid samples to the entire body, if necessary) is usually covered in a medico-legal case by the original authority issued for the examination. There is, however, considerable variation in the legal aspects of tissue and organ retention in different countries, and each pathologist must become fully conversant with local regulations.

In the legislation controlling the English coroner, it is not only permissible, but also obligatory, for the pathologist to retain any tissue that may assist in the further investigation of the death.

However, the coroner (or procurator fiscal in Scotland) has only a negative power to forbid the use of tissues or organs for purposes other than the investigation of the death, and so cannot give positive consent for the use of these for transplantation, teaching or research; such permission must be obtained from the relatives, if the coroner does not object, under the Human Tissue Act 1961.

Who may be present at an autopsy

Once again, each nation or state has different legislation and regulations on the conduct of medico-legal examinations. Though it is pointless to try to survey these, it must be emphasized that every pathologist must learn and abide by the laws applicable to his or her position.

Often the relatives of the deceased person, or an accused person, must be informed of the place and time of the autopsy so that they may be represented by a lawyer or doctor acting on their behalf. In some jurisdictions, including Britain, there is nothing that specifically forbids the relatives attending in person and the authors have had several experiences of this nature. It is open to the pathologist to refuse to conduct the autopsy if he objects to their presence.

In many homicides, a second autopsy is performed by another pathologist acting on behalf of the defence lawyers representing the accused person. This usually takes place at a later date, after the accused has been charged and granted legal representation, but sometimes the second pathologist will attend the original autopsy. This is quite in order and is more valuable than a later exploration of extensively dissected and autolysed tissues.

The permission for such attendance is granted by the coroner, medical examiner, or equivalent legal authority. The first pathologist should grant his colleague every courtesy and facility in the expectation of similar behaviour when the roles are reversed.

Others entitled to be present naturally include the officials or deputies of the department ordering the autopsy – for example, a coroner, magistrate or judge. The police, including their technical teams, are also present if the death is criminal or suspicious. Whether other doctors and medical students are allowed depends upon the wishes of the official commissioning the examination. When the deceased has been under medical care before death, it is almost invariable practice to allow – and indeed encourage – the physician to be present, as he has the best knowledge of the medical history.

In a criminal or suspicious case, the pathologist should try to limit the number of those present to a minimum. Not only is there a greater risk of loss of confidentiality, but sheer physical numbers, especially of large policemen, can make the mortuary overcrowded. This hampers movement, causes distraction, and adds to the risk of infection and contamination, especially with the present concern about the various forms of hepatitis (B, C, D, E), tuberculosis and human immunodeficiency virus (HIV) infectivity. No one should be present merely as a casual observer, not even senior police officers not directly involved in the investigation. With the increased sophistication and complexity of forensic and police procedures, more and more people cram into the mortuary, cluttered with cameras, videos, recorders, scene-of-crime kits and so on, until there is hardly room for the pathologist to move.

Whoever is present at an autopsy on a criminal or suspicious death should be listed and named by the pathologist on the autopsy report.

EXAMINATION OF THE SCENE OF DEATH

In homicide, suspected homicide, and other suspicious or obscure cases, the pathologist should visit the scene of the death before the body is removed.

Once again, local practice varies but any doctor claiming to be a forensic pathologist should always make himself available to accompany the police to the locus of the death. This duty is often formalized and made part of a contract of service for those pathologists who are either full-time or substantially involved in assisting the police. In England

and Wales, the 'Home Office Pathologists' are permanently on call for such visits and in many other jurisdictions, such as the medical examiner systems in the USA, and the European State and University Institutes of Forensic Medicine, there is usually a prearranged duty roster for attendance at scenes of death. The function of an experienced forensic pathologist at the scene of death is generally to assess the environment, the local circumstances, and the position and the condition of the body. In a large proportion of instances crime can rapidly be excluded in favour of accident, suicide or even natural causes. This is a most useful and cost-effective function, as a spurious murder investigation involving perhaps scores of police, many vehicles and other expensive public facilities, may be disbanded promptly when the pathologist recognizes innocent circumstances.

The pathologist should always have appropriate equipment ready to take to a scene investigation at a moment's notice. Further equipment may be carried if autopsies have to be carried out in places where good mortuary facilities are not available. Most forensic pathologists carry a 'murder bag' in their car and though every expert has his own choice of equipment, the following is a reasonable inventory:

- waterproof apron and rubber gloves
- thermometer, syringes and needles, sterile swabs
- autopsy dissection set, including handsaw
- cutting needles and twine for body closure
- swabs and containers for blood and body fluids
- formalin jars for histological samples
- plastic bags, envelopes, paper, spare pen and pencil
- printed body charts for recording external injuries
- hand lens, electric torch, mini-tape recorder
- camera, usually 35 mm single-lens reflex with electronic flash. The recent advent of compact digital cameras or digital video cameras with the facility to take still pictures has made instant reviewing possible.

The thermometer can be either a long chemical mercury type, reading from 0 to 50°C, or the more modern electronic digital variety with a probe carrying a thermocouple. The amount of equipment varies with the facilities likely to be available. In developed countries there are likely to be good mortuary facilities available in a hospital or municipal mortuary and the police forces will have extensive scenes-of-crime expertise with photography, specimen containers and so on. In developing countries and the more remote areas of other states, the pathologist may have to be virtually self-sufficient in respect of both crime investigation and the subsequent autopsy.

In addition to medical kit, the experienced forensic pathologist will always have appropriate clothing such as rubber boots and rain- or snow-wear ready to hand for any call.

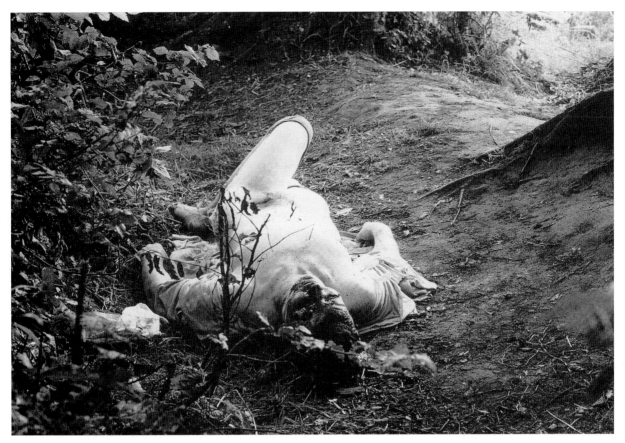

FIGURE 1.1 *The scene of a rape-homicide. The attending pathologist must record the posture, state of clothing and general relationship of the victim to the surroundings, but limit the examination at the scene to avoid any interference with the vital process of obtaining trace evidence. Rectal temperatures should not be taken until all swabs are completed, usually in the mortuary. Temperatures can be taken in the ear or deep nostrils, though with severe head injuries (as here) even this must be done with care.*

When at the scene of death, the pathologist's actions are dictated by the particular circumstances. Much will depend upon the availability or otherwise of police and forensic science assistance. In Britain, for example, several teams converge on a scene of crime, including photographers and video operators, and Scene of Crime Officers (SOCOs) whose function is to collect trace evidence. Scientists from the nearest forensic laboratory often attend with their police liaison officers, as well as fingerprint officers and, of course, the investigating officers from the Criminal Investigation Department.

Where no such backup is available, the pathologist must try to collect trace evidence himself, but he should remain within the limits of his own expertise.

The pathologist should accept the instructions of police officers in relation to the approach to the body so as to preserve the immediate environment as much as possible. Out-of-doors access is often limited to a single pathway marked by tapes, and in a building a track to the corpse is usually pointed out by the detective in charge.

The doctor should not touch anything unnecessarily and certainly not smoke or leave any object or debris of his or her own. Increasingly, those visiting the scene of a crime are given disposable overalls and overshoes to wear, so that fibres, hairs and so on from the visitor are not spuriously transferred to the scene.

If a forensic doctor has to act both as pathologist and clinical medico-legist or 'police surgeon' (that is, examining live victims or suspects), he or she must change clothing or wear a new set of protective garments to avoid transferring trace evidence, such as fibres or hairs, from victim to suspect.

The pathologist should observe a great deal, but do very little. He or she should note the position of the body in relation to nearby objects and establish the plan of the premises if indoors. A sketch or his own photograph is sometimes useful, and some pathologists use a Polaroid, digital or video camera for instant recording of the death scene.

Any obvious cause of death should be observed, and any blood pools or splashes noted in relation to the position of the corpse. The shape of such splashes should be observed,

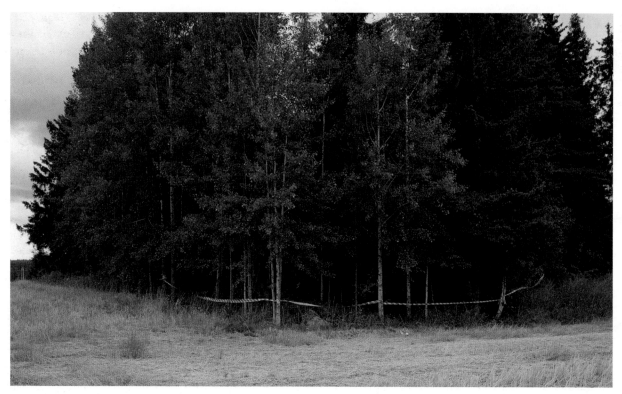

FIGURE 1.2 *Scene of a homicide-suicide where the locus of bodies should be widely marked off by tape to restrict access, and the actual body protected by a shelter from the weather and unauthorized onlookers.*

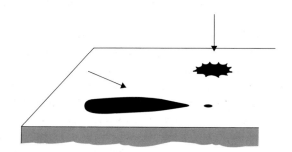

FIGURE 1.3 *At a scene of crime, the position of the body at the time of an assault can sometimes be clarified by observing the direction of blood splashing that may have been thrown off a weapon or blood-stained hands. Blood striking vertically causes round or crenellated circles, while blood hitting at an angle is lance-shaped with the narrow end facing the direction of travel. There is often a preceding drop of blood in advance of the major splash, forming an 'exclamation mark' stain.*

as blood striking perpendicularly to a surface leaves a circular mark, whilst that landing obliquely is pear-shaped, with the sharper end towards the direction of flight.

When photographs have been taken of the body in its original position, the pathologist then approaches it, after checking with the investigating officers that it is appropriate

for him to do so. Close examination can be made and the skin felt to assess temperature. The eyes, neck and hands can be examined and where necessary, clothing gently moved aside to look at the throat or upper chest. Any relevant findings should be photographed by the police before further disturbance.

If forensic scientists or scene of crime officers require any samples at this stage, their wishes must be respected. They may want to 'tape' the body, that is, press adhesive tape across the skin and clothing to capture any loose hairs and fibres. The body can then be moved to look at the sides and undersurface, again with caution so that no weapon, other object or trace evidence is disturbed. No set routine can be advised, as each case has its own individual aspects. The prime object is to assess the whole scene while causing the least disturbance to the body and clothing before the scientific teams have finished their tasks.

Estimating the post-mortem interval at the scene

The last sentence above raises the matter of estimating the time since death. The problem is fully discussed in Chapter 3, but has relevance here in relation to the pathologist's actions at the scene of death.

The general warmth or coolness of the hands and face can be assessed by touch, and the degree of rigor mortis felt by gently testing the limbs. The ambient (environmental) temperature must be taken as soon as possible after the discovery of the body, preferably by police scene of crime officers who usually arrive at the locus before the pathologist. The ambient temperature should be taken as near to the body as possible, as microenvironments can exist, even inside buildings or rooms. Information should be sought as to how much disturbance of the ambient temperature might have occurred, such as opening doors and windows, or turning fires or central heating on or off, so that some idea of post-discovery distortions of temperature can be estimated later. The insertion of a thermometer into the rectum at this stage in the investigation, as advocated by some textbooks, is controversial.

At a scene of death, this usually means either pulling down trousers or pants, and otherwise disturbing clothing, often in cramped and ill-lit places, frequently out in the open. It also risks contaminating the rectum and perineum, by introducing seminal fluid from the anal margin into the rectum, making subsequent examination of that area (and taking swabs for semen) of reduced value. As so many violent crimes now have sexual or homosexual overtones, the practice of taking rectal temperatures at the scene should be performed only if the forensic scientists or police scene of crime officers are satisfied that trace evidence from the clothing, swabs from the vulva, vagina and anus, etc., can be obtained satisfactorily before rectal thermometry is performed.

In other words, a cost–benefit analysis must be made at the scene, to decide if the difficulties of taking a rectal temperature are worth the small potential advantage of an earlier measurement. In many cases, where the body has obviously been there long enough for the core temperature to have reached ambient – or where other circumstantial evidence has indicated that the time of death is known to a greater degree of accuracy that can be hoped for by thermometry – then nothing is lost by postponing the procedure until the body arrives at the mortuary for autopsy, which, in British practice, is usually directly after the body is moved from the scene.

If the autopsy is to be delayed for many hours owing to difficulties with transport or lack of facilities, then much more must be done at the scene and temperature measurements are justified.

An alternative is to use a place other than the rectum. The axilla and mouth give low readings, which cannot reliably be correlated with the deep temperature because of variable exposure to the air temperature. More useful is the auditory meatus or nostril, the thermometer or thermocouple probe being inserted as deeply as possible. Reliable, reproducible readings can be obtained from these sites, which have the great advantage of being easily accessible without moving clothing, as well as not being required for swabbing to investigate possible sexual assaults. The use of temperatures to attempt to calculate the post-mortem interval is discussed fully in Chapter 3.

When the pathologist has made the best examination possible in the circumstances, his next function is to ensure that the corpse is removed to the mortuary for autopsy with the least disturbance and loss of evidence. He should supervise the removal himself or at least delegate the duty to another person whom he knows is careful and competent. Each hand should be enclosed in a bag, secured at the wrist by adhesive tape or string. A similar bag should be placed over the head. The packaging medium may vary, but generally paper bags are recommended.

The body should be placed gently in a 'body-bag', which has a zip closure, or moved on to a large, new plastic sheet, at least 2 metres square. If a sheet is used, the edges should be wrapped over the body and secured with adhesive tape. The object of the exercise is to retain any loose objects, hairs and fibres that may be adhering to the body or the clothing. The sheet or bag is taken by the forensic laboratory after the body is removed in the mortuary so that they may screen it for trace evidence. The transport of the body is the responsibility of the police or other agency such as the coroner or his officer. The body in its plastic wrapping should be placed in a rigid fibreglass 'shell' or ordinary coffin, and taken by hearse, van or police transport to the chosen mortuary.

Physical damage during the removal should be avoided as much as possible, though in difficult or inaccessible sites this is easier said than done. In fires, the body may be seriously damaged before or during recovery, sometimes because its presence is not suspected in the smoke-filled, often waterlogged, debris of a conflagration. The author (BK) has experience of such a scene where firemen walked over two bodies for several hours before it was realized that they were buried under burnt furniture and other debris. Handling brittle, charred, bodies can easily cause the splits at joints that may mimic ante-mortem injuries (see Chapter 12).

In summary, the function of a pathologist at any scene of suspicious death is to observe the situation, to conserve any fragile evidence, to supervise the removal of the body and offer an opinion, based on experience, about the nature of death where this can reasonably be done. He is not there to act as a latter-day Sherlock Holmes, voicing unsubstantiated theories on non-medical matters, nor attempting to overinterpret the situation from the flimsiest of facts. The pathologist is part of a team of specialists, all experts in their own field, and it is as a member of such a cooperative, coordinated group that his best contributions can be made.

PROPERTY, CLOTHING AND IDENTIFICATION

Whether or not the pathologist has been to the scene of a death, he should take notice of the clothing and other property of the body upon which he is to carry out an autopsy. This applies not only to every criminal or suspicious death, but also to many traffic and industrial accidents, as well as to the victims of falls from a height, drowning and so on.

In many instances, there will be no opportunity to examine the clothed body in the mortuary: if death has occurred in hospital or in an accident department, the clothing may have been removed before transfer to the mortuary. The pathologist should make a permanent request that a body from any traffic accident, or other case where trauma was the provisional cause of death, should be brought to the mortuary without having the clothing removed by police or nursing staff – unless of course the victim was still alive on arrival at hospital, and undressing was performed before attempted resuscitation or treatment. As a second best, the removed clothing should accompany the body to the mortuary so that it can be examined, if necessary, for damage, stains and other evidence. Unfortunately, such clothing is frequently destroyed before it can be seen.

The mortuary staff should be trained to regard clothing and property as important items of evidence, and a system should be established to retain, identify and store these, both from the evidential aspects and for the safety of valuables. The contents of the pockets, documents, keys and other items all assist in identification. Though primarily the task of the police, the pathologist will sometimes have an interest in this aspect. The clothes themselves, the style, fabric, colour and labels all assist in identity.

In trauma deaths, the injuries on the body should be matched up with damage on the clothing. Tears, slashes, stab wounds and especially firearm wounds in the clothes must be compared with the position of external lesions on the body, making allowance for movement and displacement during life. Some self-inflicted wounds may be confirmed by the non-alignment of the clothing damage with the injuries (see Chapter 8).

Blood, seminal, vaginal and other body secretions may be found on the clothing, and though this is primarily the responsibility of the forensic science laboratory, the pathologist may be the first or only person to detect their presence. In firearm deaths, gunshot residues on the clothing may be vital evidence about the range of the discharge and the identity of the ammunition.

In traffic fatalities, tearing of the clothes, grease marks, road dirt, broken lamp or windscreen glass, and even metallic or paint fragments from the vehicle may all assist in reconstructing the event and in identifying the unknown vehicle in a 'hit-and-run' tragedy.

Other objects associated with the body that may be helpful include medicines, which may assist in determining the nature of the disease from which the deceased had suffered, for example, amyl nitrite or insulin. In some suicides, empty drug or poison containers may be with the body. Other helpful artefacts include such items as hearing aids, syringes, external pacemakers and inhalers. The clothing must be removed carefully and, especially in criminal or suspicious cases, the pathologist should supervise and assist the mortuary technician, especially as some technicians are not always aware of the importance of clothing in the reconstruction of events.

If the body is not bleeding or otherwise fouled, it is best to remove clothing in the usual way by pulling over the head and limbs, unless this might interfere with any injuries or soiling. If rigor is intense or if there is blood on the face or hands, it may be advisable to cut off some or all of the clothing. This should be done after consultation with the forensic scientists, if they are present, so that the cuts will be made where they will least interfere with later laboratory examination. In any event, cuts should avoid passing through pre-existing damage or staining of the garments. Each item of the clothing should be placed separately into a paper bag to allow them to 'breathe'.

Identification of the body

The identification of an unknown body is a major forensic exercise, and is fully discussed in Chapter 4. Here, however, we are concerned with the formal recognition of the subject of an imminent autopsy. Before a pathologist makes any examination (and certainly before he begins any mutilating dissection), it is essential that he ensures that the corpse before him is indeed the correct person.

In every medico-legal case, some responsible person must have identified the body. This is usually a relative or close friend of the deceased person, who looks at the face of the body and verbally certifies to a police officer, mortuary attendant or doctor that it is indeed 'John Smith'. Where the body is burned beyond recognition, mutilated or putrefied, attempts at identification must be made by showing the relative documents, or items such as clothing or jewellery.

In non-criminal cases, such as sudden deaths and most accidents and suicides, the continuity of identity is carried on by a label or tag attached to the body by the police officer, nursing staff or mortuary attendant, which carries the name, address, serial number and other relevant details. This label may be tied firmly to a toe, or a durable wrist or ankle bracelet may be used. Some mortuaries write the name on the leg with an indelible marker, but this can be smudged or obscured during autopsy.

The pathologist should always satisfy himself of the identity by comparing the documents authorizing the autopsy with the toe label or bracelet. The details should agree and, if they do not, he should not proceed with the autopsy until the discrepancy is cleared up, if necessary by calling back the police officer or even the relative to make absolutely sure of the identity.

Many mistakes have been made in the past, with adverse publicity, embarrassing enquiries and even legal consequences. Autopsies on the wrong person, incorrect causes of death, relatives attending the wrong funeral and even cremation of the wrong body are regularly reported as a result of laxity in identification. To avoid confusion, the body should always be labelled as soon as it arrives in the mortuary. Labels on shrouds become detached and those on refrigerator doors are unreliable, as other parties (such as night porters) may shift occupants around without the knowledge of the pathologist or regular mortuary staff.

Some large mortuaries use special means of identity. One known to the authors has an automatic camera fitted in the ceiling of the mortuary entrance. Every new body wheeled in is photographed on its trolley with a serial number prominently displayed on a board placed across the upper chest, so that the face appears with the record number to resolve any later discrepancy.

In serious cases such as homicide, the pathologist must not rely on second-hand evidence of identity such as a toe label. Before the autopsy, someone must verbally confirm to him that the body they are both then viewing is 'John Smith'. This person must be either a relative or the police officer to whom a relative has already formally identified the corpse.

The pathologist must record in his autopsy report the date, time and particulars of the person identifying the body to him, so that 'continuity of evidence' is ensured for legal purposes, which cannot successfully be challenged by the defence at a subsequent trial.

THE USE OF THE HISTORY OF THE CASE

As in clinical medicine, the history of the deceased 'patient' or victim is a vital and indispensable part of the investigation. The extent to which it should influence the pathologist in coming to a decision as to the cause of death, however, is more controversial, as is discussed below.

In medico-legal autopsies – compared with hospital 'clinical' cases – the history is often scanty, absent or misleading.

If a person has been found dead, having had no previous medical attendant, there may be virtually no information at all. In criminal deaths, the person who knows most about the death may well be the perpetrator, who naturally may remain silent or give a distorted, misleading or totally false account of the circumstances. The forensic pathologist then often has to contend with a scanty or incorrect history.

Even when a story is given in good faith by relatives, the medical facts are often distorted because of incomplete knowledge and understanding. It may be further warped by transmission by a police officer or other non-medical person, so that only a garbled history reaches the pathologist. The latter should attempt to supplement deficiencies in information by further requests to the commissioning authority, such as the coroner or the police. Wherever possible, the pathologist should try to contact the doctor who may have treated the deceased in the recent past. In the urgency of forensic work, however, frequently at night or weekends, the autopsy may have to proceed without any additional history.

Though more detail may be obtained afterwards, the course of the autopsy might well have been different if such knowledge was available beforehand. For example, the author (BK) once performed an autopsy on a coal miner with no history other than a knowledge of his occupation and chronic chest disease. Autopsy revealed sufficient cardiopulmonary disease to account for death and the body was released for burial. It was not until the following day that the police in the rural area where the man had died, tardily produced the information that both an empty bottle of sleeping tablets and a suicide note had been found with the body. Paradoxically, the history is often less important in violent deaths where the wounds are self-evident, though a good description of the circumstances may assist in interpreting the direction of injuries, the nature of the weapon and other aspects.

In most autopsies the history directs the pathologist to the appropriate ancillary investigations, as should have happened in the case described above. Some pathologists have in the past advocated that the autopsy should be performed 'blind', so that the history does not prejudice the opinion of the pathologist. This is patently impracticable, for every autopsy would then have to be totally comprehensive, including such techniques as the removal of the spinal cord in every case, and all possible ancillary investigations, such as toxicology, microbiology, virology, radiology, diatoms, histology and so on, as there would be no means of knowing what was necessary and what was irrelevant. Apart from the intolerable burden of work, the expense of such an approach would be prohibitive, if applied to all autopsies.

A particular difficulty often arises in relation to bodies returned to a home country after death in a foreign state.

The problems vary greatly with the degree of both pathological and administrative sophistication of the foreign country. Where these are poor, then the problems of obtaining a good – or even any – history may be great, even after attempts at using international police or diplomatic channels.

Sometimes, a 'doctor-to-doctor' approach by telephone or fax may be the best way of obtaining information. Even a cause of death from the foreign country may be either unobtainable or so vague (such as 'heart failure') as to be useless. Previous autopsies may be incomplete, of poor quality, or even fraudulent, such as finding a stitched skin incision but no underlying dissection of organs. Several surveys of such problem autopsies have been published, with a plea for some kind of International Death Certificate (Green 1982; Leadbeatter 1991).

Difficulties arise when objective autopsy findings are scanty or even absent. The pathologist then has the dilemma of choosing between a cause of death based on a subjective knowledge of the alleged history (which may be wrong) or admitting that the cause of death is unascertained.

This problem, fully discussed by Leadbeatter and Knight (1987), is by no means uncommon. For example, sufferers from epilepsy or asthma are known to die suddenly and unexpectedly, an autopsy usually revealing no adequate morphological cause for their death. Another prime example is the sudden infant death syndrome, discussed in Chapter 21, where by definition there are no significant autopsy lesions and the history is usually essentially barren.

In hypothermia where the patient is warmed up in hospital but dies in a day or two, there may be nothing to find at autopsy, yet there is firm clinical history of a rectal temperature of 26°C. Moving to more forensic cases, a body may be recovered from a river after clothing and a suicide note have been found on the bank – yet at autopsy there may be no visible evidence of drowning whatsoever.

In these cases, should the pathologist – in the absence of objective evidence of hypothermia or drowning – decline to offer a cause of death and perhaps be accused of being obstructive or perverse? Or should he certify 'hypothermia' or 'drowning', and perhaps be challenged in court by a lawyer who claims that the pathologist relied only on hearsay and has no objective evidence to offer?

The best course is for the pathologist, if he feels that the history is sufficiently strong, to give the most likely and reasonable cause of death, but make it clear in his discussion in the autopsy report that this opinion is based on a consideration of the circumstances and is not a dogmatic statement of the kind that could be offered if the victim was shot through the brain. Where a summary of the history prefaces the autopsy report, the pathologist should be careful to indicate what is 'hearsay' as far as he is concerned. Thus he should not say 'The deceased was struck on the head by two men', but 'I was told that the deceased was struck on the head by two men'.

As is discussed later, the autopsy report should not be merely a bald recital of the anatomical findings, but should have a final commentary that includes a 'differential diagnosis' where the cause of death is not clear cut, as well as a justification for the eventual opinion or an admission that there is no way of deciding between alternative possibilities.

The main difficulty arises with the actual 'cause of death' phraseology, which will be entered into the legal and national records in the format required by the World Health Organization. This gives no opportunity to express preferences or give explanations but, on the 'best-guess' principle, the pathologist can do no more than enter his most reasoned choice or, with legitimate honesty, state that the cause is 'undetermined'.

PRECAUTIONS REGARDING POTENTIAL INFECTIVE CONDITIONS

Many forensic situations involve drug abusers and persons with promiscuous sexual behaviour, where the statistical risk of HIV and hepatitis infection is markedly greater than in the general autopsy population. This poses a risk to pathologists, mortuary staff, police and laboratory staff who may deal with post-autopsy samples. A great deal has been written about such risks but no consensus has yet been reached, though an excellent survey has been published by the Royal College of Pathologists (1995).

One school maintains that all autopsies should be carried out with total precautions against infective risks, so that it does not matter what case is handled. However, this is almost impossible to achieve in a busy coroner or medical examiner practice and does not solve the problem of possibly infected material being sent out to other laboratories.

A more common regime is to carry out pre-autopsy testing for HIV and hepatitis, using blood from a femoral needle puncture. The result can often be returned within hours, when a decision may be made as how to handle the autopsy – or even whether to abandon it, if the risk–benefit aspect is high. More usually, a positive result will result in the autopsy being carried out with special care, additional protective clothing, visors, masks and metal gloves, with restriction of access to observers, choice of more senior technicians and warnings sent to laboratories liable to handle samples.

In this respect, hepatitis is more of a risk than HIV infection. However, so far, about 100 health-care workers have acquired HIV infection from definite occupational exposure (Sidwell et al. 1999) and one pathologist is known to have become infected from autopsy work (Johnson *et al.* 1997). Also three morticians in the USA have possibly contracted occupation-related HIV positivity.

The time for which a corpse remains potentially contagious with HIV is variable. Infectious virus has been recovered from liquid blood held at room temperature for 2 months and virus in high concentrations has been found to remain viable for 3 weeks (Cao *et al.* 1993). Bankowski *et al.* (1992) found 51 per cent survival of virus in plasma and monocyte fractions from infected cadavers up to 21 hours post-mortem. Other series found survival in corpses from 18 hours to 11 days after death. Virus has been recovered from the spleen after 14 days post-mortem. Refrigeration seems to make little difference to viability. Douceron *et al.* (1993) cultured blood and effusions from refrigerated bodies and obtained viable virus up to 16 days post-mortem and concluded that there was no safe maximum time at which corpses ceased to be an infective risk. In industrialized countries, it has become standard to offer post-exposure prophylaxis after significant percutaneous exposure to blood or tissues of HIV patients.

Other infections, such as tuberculosis, hepatitis viruses, anthrax, plague, Creutzfeldt–Jakob, Marburg, Green Monkey diseases, etc., are usually the subject of specific health and safety regulations, which vary from country to country.

THE AUTOPSY: EXTERNAL EXAMINATION

In contrast to the 'clinical autopsy' performed to evaluate natural disease, the importance of the external examination is far greater in the forensic case, especially in deaths from trauma. In the latter, the medico-legal value of the external description may be paramount, as it is often from the outer evidence that inferences may be made about the nature of the weapon, the direction of attack and other vital aspects. Thus the forensic pathologist must spend all the time that is necessary in a careful evaluation of the body surface and not be too impatient to wield the knife mainly to seek material for histology, which is more justified in the purely clinical autopsy.

The routine for external examination will naturally vary according to the nature of the case but certain general principles apply. The following procedure is a useful baseline and may be adjusted according to personal preference. Variations in criminal cases to accommodate the needs of the investigating and scientific teams are mentioned later.

- After identification and removal of any clothing, the race and gender are noted. The apparent age is assessed in children by size and in adults by changes in skin and eyes, such as the loss of skin elasticity, senile hyperkeratosis, Campbell de Morgan spots, senile purpura and arcus senilis. Hair colour, tooth loss and arthritic changes are also obvious signs of ageing. The apparent age should be compared with the alleged age and enquiries made about any obvious discrepancy, in case it is the wrong body, an error which plagues most autopsy rooms from time to time.
- The body length is measured from heel to crown (in infants, more detailed measurements are described later). Ensure that the attendant does not take the 'undertaker's height' from toe to crown, as due to the plantar flexion of rigor, this can be a considerable number of centimetres more than the live standing height.

  It should also be appreciated that the post-mortem height may differ from the known living height by several centimetres. There are several opposing causes of variation, which do not necessarily cancel each other.

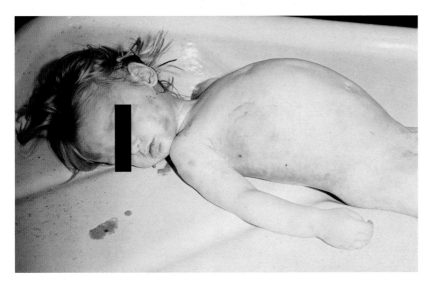

FIGURE 1.4 *External examination must note every feature; here there is obvious abdominal distension in a battered child with facial bruising. The intestine had been ruptured by a blow, and oxygen administered by the ambulance crew escaped to distend the peritoneal cavity.*

For example, muscle flaccidity allows joints to relax, unless rigor is present, but intervertebral discs appear to shrink, allowing shortening.

- The body weight in kilograms is measured if facilities are available; if not, it should be estimated. The weight of infants must always be measured. The general nutrition and physique is assessed in terms of obesity, leanness, dehydration, oedema, emaciation, and so on.

- The state of cleanliness, personal hygiene, hair and beard length, toenail and fingernail state, and urinary and faecal soiling is noted. Any parasitic infestation, such as fleas or lice, is combated before proceeding.

- The general skin colour is noted, especially hypostasis (discussed at length in Chapter 2). Congestion or cyanosis of the face, hands and feet is sought. Localized discoloration, especially unilateral in a limb, suggests arterial embolism or incipient gangrene. Pink or brownish pink patches over the large joints may indicate hypothermia (Chapter 17). Other abnormal colours include the brownish hue of methaemoglobinaemia in some poisonings, the bronze speckling of clostridial septicaemia and the dark red of cyanide that somewhat resembles the cherry-pink coloration of carboxyhaemoglobin. Naturally racial pigmentation will modify the ease with which abnormal skin coloration can be seen.

- Congenital deformities of any type are recorded, from talipes equinovarus to spina bifida, from a naevus to extra toes.

- Acquired external marks may be important for identification purposes or in relation to past injuries and disease. Tattoos, circumcision, amputations, surgical scars, old fracture deformities and scars of injuries, burns or suicidal attempts on the wrist and throat are noted. These are discussed further in Chapter 3. Increasingly, artefacts – both external and internal – arise from resuscitation attempts and must be carefully distinguished from original trauma. This emphasizes the importance of the history, to determine whether cardiopulmonary resuscitation was attempted by trained or untrained persons.

- The hands should be carefully examined for such signs as old and new injuries, defence wounds, bruised knuckles and electrical marks. The latter are often insignificant and difficult to see unless the rigor of flexed fingers is overcome, either by force or even cutting the flexor tendons at the wrist.

- Vomit, froth or blood may be present at the mouth and nostrils, and faeces and urine may have been voided. This must be correlated with the degree of post-mortem decomposition, which often leads to purging of fluids from orifices; most forensic pathologists have had the experience of being called by the police to the scene of 'a fatal haemorrhage', to discover only bloody fluid being purged by gases from a decomposing corpse.

Vaginal discharge or bleeding is noted and the ears examined for leakage of blood or cerebrospinal fluid. Post-mortem ejaculation of semen from the external

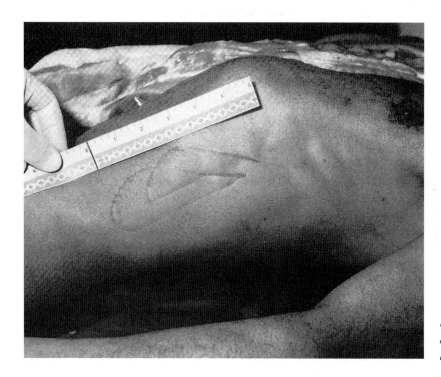

FIGURE 1.5 *Post-mortem artefacts on the body of a homicide victim. These are due to defibrillator paddles applied in a hospital casualty department.*

meatus is of no significance and can be seen in any type of death. It was shown by Mant (1984) not to be associated with sexual activity immediately before death. It is not particularly associated with asphyxial deaths, as sometimes stated.

- The degree of rigor mortis is assessed by flexing the arms and legs to test the resistance. The significance of this and hypostasis is discussed in Chapter 2.
- Recent injuries (other than scars already noted) are carefully examined. In fact this part of the autopsy is often the most significant element of forensic cases. Injuries may be conveniently recorded in the mortuary by marking them on printed body diagrams. The forms can be secured on a clipboard and the data later transcribed into a written description for the autopsy report. The original diagrams should be retained, as their production may be demanded in court if there is controversy about any particular injury.

All traumatic lesions should be clearly differentiated into abrasions, bruises, lacerations, incised wounds, burns and so on, according to the definitions given in Chapter 4. The shape and condition of the margins of each injury should be described where appropriate. It must be meticulously measured in terms of length, breadth, orientation to the axis of the body and the position with reference to surface anatomical landmarks. For example, a knife wound of the thorax might be described as follows, using ordinary language to explain any medical terms:

A stab wound was present on the left upper chest, placed obliquely, with the inner end lower than the upper outer end. The wound was 20 mm in length, which extended to 22 mm when the edges were opposed. The maximum width at the centre was 4 mm. The centre of the wound was just below the line joining the nipples, being 6 cm from the midline, 7 cm from the left nipple and 18 cm below the centre of the left clavicle (collar bone). The wound was 132 cm above heel level and was elliptical in shape, with the inner lower end slightly more sharply cut than the rather blunt upper end. The wound was shelved in a downwards direction, with subcutaneous tissue visible along the inside of the upper edge.

This description, along with police photographs, will convey an excellent impression of the wound at any future date, including at the trial, which may be many months later. The position of the injury is related to obvious anatomical points and the height above the ground may have relevance if the stature of the victim and assailant, and the angle of attack, become legal issues. On the scalp, the occiput and the tip of the ear can be used as reference points, together with the vertex and the centre line of the head. On the face, the obvious landmarks are the eyebrows, nasion, tip of nose, lips, point of chin and angle of jaw. Where large areas of abrasion or bruising are present, similar measurements of lesion size are needed, but more general descriptions of position may be sufficient, such as 'covering the external aspect of the left thigh' or 'extensive bruising 23 cm by 18 cm on the right side of the chest extending from axilla to costal margin'.

Where widespread burns are present, an estimate of the total area using the 'Rule of Nine' should be made, as described in Chapter 11.

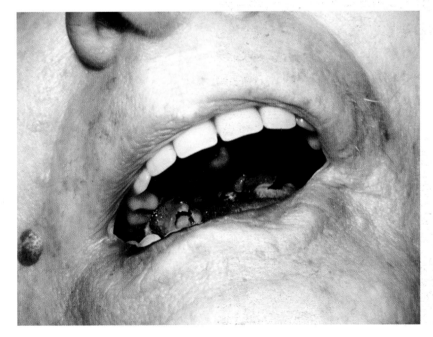

FIGURE 1.6 *Full external examination is vital, including the interior of the mouth. Here a large number of amylobarbitone capsules offer a presumptive cause of death, though analytical confirmation is still required.*

Other injuries, such as firearm wounds, are described in the same manner, being careful not to clean off any powder residues or other trace evidence before the forensic scientists have collected their samples.

With head injuries, the scalp is examined in its original condition first and any trace evidence collected. Then any clotted blood that frequently obscures the injuries can be gently removed, using a sponge and water. After this stage has been studied, it is usually necessary to shave off hair carefully around the wounds, so that the full extent of the lacerations and especially the state of their margins can be assessed and photographed. This shaving is best carried out with a scalpel fitted with a new blade, the blade being kept almost parallel with the surface to avoid making false cuts. The procedure should be carried out by the pathologist himself and not delegated to a mortuary technician. In this way any artefactual cuts can be recognized as such and not misinterpreted as part of the original wound.

The eyes must be examined carefully, especially to detect petechial haemorrhages on the outside of the eyelids, conjunctivae and sclera. Though these do not necessarily indicate an asphyxial process, such petechiae require an explanation. Petechiae should also be sought behind the ears and in the skin of the face, especially around the mouth, chin and forehead. Care must be taken to differentiate these fine petechiae from the more coarse intradermal blood spots often seen across the shoulders or upper chest, which are caused by post-mortem hypostasis in a body with marked agonal venous congestion – especially when that surface of the body has been dependent. Haemorrhages in postural hypostasis are of no diagnostic significance, as true ante-mortem bleedings can never be differentiated from those that commonly develop after death.

The size of the pupils is rarely useful, as rigor in the iris musculature can produce any degree of constriction, which may be unequal on either side (see Chapter 2). False eyes, contact lenses, lens opacity and other defects are to be noted. It is not possible to evaluate the degree of visual acuity during life from any type of post-mortem examination – though obviously a

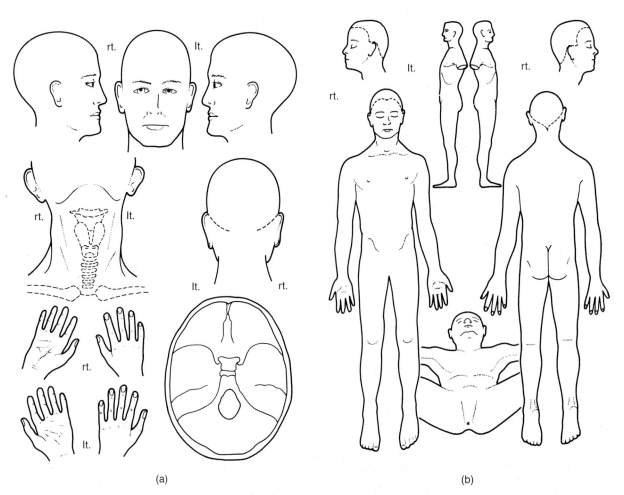

(a) (b)

FIGURE 1.7 *(a, b) Typical examples of the many anatomical diagrams available for the recording of external findings at autopsy.*

significant defect such as a cataract or a large vitreous haemorrhage is likely to affect vision.

- The mouth may reveal foreign bodies, drugs, damaged teeth, injured gums and lips (especially the ruptured frenulum of child abuse), and the bitten tongue of epilepsy or blows on the jaw. Dentures should be identified and removed before autopsy. Gastric contents in the mouth need not indicate ante-mortem regurgitation, as discussed in Chapter 14, but should be noted. Dried powder on the lips may suggest the recent taking of medicaments or poisons; corrosion of the mouth, lips and chin may be seen in irritant poisons. Bleeding from mouth, nostrils, or ears must be recorded, and later investigated as to source from internal examination. Frothy fluid, sometimes blood-tinged, may be seen issuing from the mouth or nostrils, or both, in drowning and from pulmonary oedema due to a variety of causes. Froth is sometimes pink or frankly blood-tinged. This has no particular significance unless gross, as in drowning, sudden infant death and other conditions with marked pulmonary oedema; rupture of small pulmonary or even pharyngeal vessels can add a little blood to colour the foam.

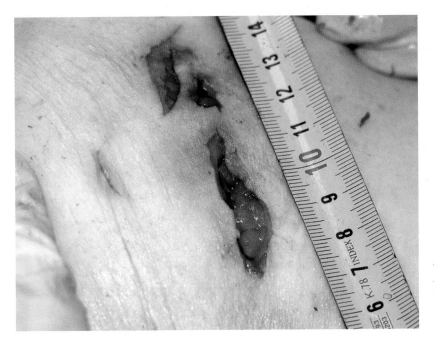

FIGURE 1.8 *Examination and photography of injuries; after full preliminary examination and forensic sampling, the area is cleaned, shaved if necessary, and photographed with a scale adjacent to the injuries.*

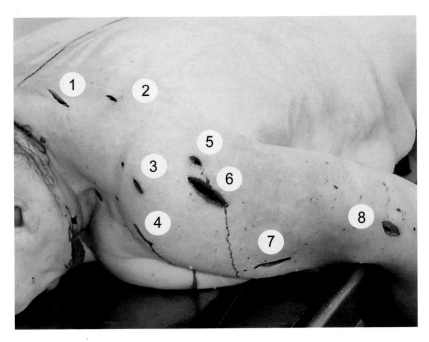

FIGURE 1.9 *Where there are numerous similar lesions, it assists the clarity of the autopsy report if numbers used during photography match those listed in the autopsy protocol.*

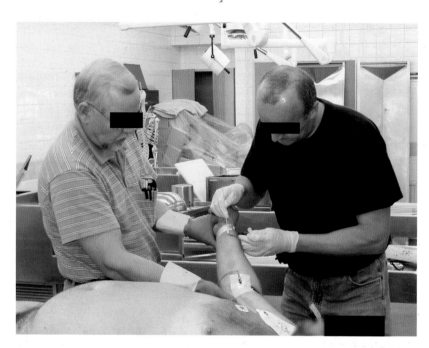

FIGURE 1.10 *Scene of crime officers recovering trace evidence from hands before a homicide autopsy. The pathologist must offer the rest of the team every facility to complete their work before he begins his dissection.*

The external genitals require careful examination, as does the anus. The state of the latter can be misleading, as a widely open, patulous anus is often seen post-mortem, due to flaccidity of the sphincter. The inner mucosa is often visible through the orifice. This is also the case in infants and children, and a diagnosis of sexual abuse must not be assumed without other corroborative evidence such as fresh mucosal tears or swabs positive for semen.

The 'funnel-shaped' anus, beloved of traditional textbooks as a sign of chronic homosexual activity, is such an extreme rarity that its true existence is doubtful. A funnel shape is a normal anatomical variant, the anus being set deeply between the buttocks, sometimes with a commissure of skin above it, making the approach seem even deeper. The alleged 'shiny, silvery hyperkeratinized skin of the habitual pederast' is also of little diagnostic value as scratching from chronic irritation, often associated with haemorrhoids, viral infections or threadworms, may lead to the same appearance. The only reliable criteria are fresh tears and old scars, as well as mucocutaneous eversion, though even these can arise from severe chronic constipation (see also Chapter 18).

Examination of the vulva and vagina is made to exclude obvious injury and disease, unless the nature of the case suggests some sexual interference, when a far more detailed examination and a special autopsy technique is carried out (Chapter 18). Routine examination of the male genitals usually need only extend to general inspection of the penis, glans and

scrotum, with palpation of the testes. Circumcision should be noted, as (rarely) it may assist in identification.

THE AUTOPSY: INTERNAL EXAMINATION

The dissection in a forensic case is basically similar to any other autopsy, with variations according to the nature of the death and the needs of the particular investigation, whether it be a criminal case, a civil dispute or an accident investigation.

There are a number of manuals devoted to the performance of an autopsy (see Ludwig 2002 or Knight 1996, for example) as well as one for the instruction of mortuary technicians (Knight 1984). Only an outline of the technique is offered here for those unaccustomed to examining the dead who may have autopsies thrust upon them by circumstances. In addition, special forensic procedures are described, though these are also discussed in each of the chapters devoted to the various types of injury and death. The autopsy on infants is dealt with in Chapters 20–22.

The usual incision is an almost straight line from laryngeal prominence to pubis, deviating to avoid the umbilicus. The upper end of this incision should not be prolonged above the larynx, as even a high-necked shroud will then fail to hide the subsequent suture line from relatives.

Another common method is to cut from behind each ear to a point above the manubrium and continue downwards in a 'Y-shape'. This is often done in infants and wherever it is desired to avoid disfiguring the front of the neck. In the USA in particular, the Y-incision is favoured or even a deep 'U-shape' carried across the upper chest.

In strangulation, hanging, and any condition where the larynx might be damaged, the Y-incision is to be preferred, as the skin of the upper neck can then be dissected off the mandible and raised clear to give a wide approach to the neck structures. Here, the incision should not be made until the skull-cap and brain have been removed, to avoid the congestive artefactual haemorrhages in the neck structures, described by Prinsloo and Gordon (1951), which can be confused with true ante-mortem trauma. Gordon *et al.* (1988) have further suggested that the brain be removed first in all autopsies so that abnormal odours can be detected before being swamped by the smell from the opened abdominal cavity.

The Y-incision is also required when dissection of the face is necessary, to look for deep bruising or bony damage. In fact the whole face can be dissected off completely from the skull and replaced with little effect upon the cosmetic result, if careful dissection is employed. The Y-incision in the neck is made continuous with the transverse scalp incision, joining these behind each ear, so that the anterior neck and facial skin can be removed in entirety.

Returning to the autopsy in general, the primary incision should be shallow over the neck to avoid cutting underlying structures, especially the trachea. The thorax can be cut down to the sternum, but care must be taken over the abdomen, where a light cut is made, sufficient to incise only skin and fat. A small puncture should then be made in the peritoneum and a finger inserted to lift it away from the intestines. The knife is then used to cut outwards along the length of the abdomen, to avoid penetrating the intestines.

The incision for access to the skull is made from behind each ear, meeting over the crown of the head. It is well to keep this posterior to the actual vertex, again to make the stitching less obvious, especially where the hair is scanty or absent. With abundant hair – and especially in children – the hair should be wetted and then combed backwards and forwards from a transverse parting made in the line of the prospective incision. Hair is not then severed and can be combed back later to cover the stitching.

Exposing the body cavities

The skin, subcutaneous tissues and fat are flayed off laterally from the main incision, taking care not to let the edge or point of the knife come through the skin, especially in the neck area, where repair can be unsightly. The tissues are taken back to the lateral edge of the neck and to the outer third of

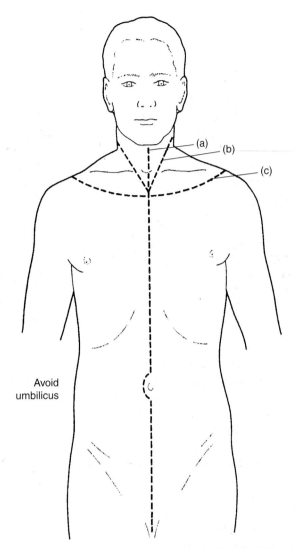

FIGURE 1.11 *Autopsy incisions: (a) standard midline, (b) 'V-shape' and (c) subclavicular.*

the clavicles. Over the thorax, the tissues, including pectoral muscles, are flayed off to the midaxillary line in the upper part and even further posteriorly towards the costal margin.

The anterior abdominal wall is similarly separated. This can be done either in two stages, first stripping back the skin and fat to expose the muscles – or the full thickness of skin, fat and muscle can be reflected together. The muscle must be cut from the costal margin and, if thick fat overlies, then some transverse relieving incisions can be made on the peritoneal surface of the lower abdominal wall, taking care not to come through to the skin.

Opening the thorax

The thorax is opened by first disarticulating both sternoclavicular joints. This is carried out by moving the shoulder tip with one hand, to identify the joint capsules. The point of a knife is then introduced vertically and cut laterally in a half-circle to separate the joints. If they are ankylosed, which often occurs in old age, then the clavicles can be cut through at the end of the next operation. This consists of the severing of the ribs and can be performed either with a handsaw or a rib shears. In children and many adults, the costal cartilages may be cut through with a knife, though this provides a rather narrow exposure of the chest contents. In infants, the soft cartilage can easily be divided with a scalpel: in older bodies, a stout knife should be kept for the purpose to save blunting the knife that is needed for organ dissection. Often the first rib has to be sawn through, even though the remainder are cut with a knife.

When a saw is used, the ribs are cut through lateral to the costochondral junctions from a point on the costal margin to the sternoclavicular joints or nearby. If a saw is used, it must be kept at a low angle to avoid the tip lacerating the underlying lung, especially if there are pleural adhesions. When the sternum and medial rib segments are free, the section is lifted and dissected away from the mediastinum, keeping the knife close to the bone to avoid cutting the pericardium. The sternal plate is examined for fractures or other lesions before it is put aside: damage caused by the considerable trauma of resuscitatory cardiac massage is frequently found at this point.

The whole of the thorax and abdomen is now open for inspection. The degree of inflation of the lungs should be assessed, noting complete or partial collapse, emphysema, overdistension and any asymmetry of inflation.

If a pneumothorax has been suspected beforehand, a post-mortem radiograph is the best confirmation. Alternatively, the chest wall can be punctured in the mid-axillary line after filling the reflected skin with water to observe if bubbles escape. This test is rarely successful and cannot succeed if there is a patent communication between the pleural cavity and the bronchial tree. If there is a marked tension pneumothorax, the hiss of escaping air may be heard when the tip of the knife penetrates the intercostal muscles and parietal pleura. The pleural cavities are inspected for adhesions, effusions, pus, blood, fibrin and even gastric contents.

Examining the abdomen

The abdomen is then inspected, though ascites, faeculent fluid, pus and blood may already have escaped on first opening the peritoneal cavity.

The omentum may show inflammation or fat necrosis. When moved aside, the loops of bowel are inspected for any abnormality, especially infarction, peritonitis and the distension of ileus. Beware of mistaking post-mortem hypostasis for the necrosis of mesenteric embolism or strangulated bowel. Though the dark colour may be similar, hypostasis usually has irregular segments when the gut is stretched out, whereas infarction occupies one continuous section – and if well established, the bowel wall will be lustreless and friable.

The bowel is gently moved aside to look at the posterior part of the abdomen: a retroperitoneal haemorrhage from a ruptured aorta may be visible, or an aneurysm itself.

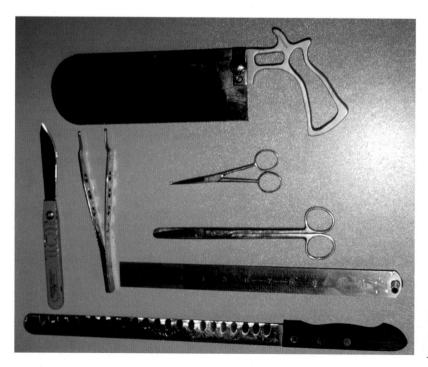

FIGURE 1.12 *The minimum instruments needed for performing an autopsy. Any further items may be useful but not essential.*

The collection of body fluid samples

In a large proportion of forensic autopsies and virtually every one with criminal connotations, samples of blood and other body fluids and tissues are needed for laboratory examination. In relation to sexual offences, the taking of swabs and other samples is described in Chapter 18. Where blood and other fluids are required for toxicological, biochemical, microbiological and serological investigations, they are usually collected at the early stages of the autopsy (see Chapter 27).

The site of collection depends on the nature of the test. When samples for toxicological analysis are required, considerable care should be employed in sampling; this is more fully discussed in Chapter 27.

It is not advisable to use visceral blood for sampling, especially for small molecule substances that can easily diffuse after death; these include alcohol and many pharmaceutical products. Though older textbooks advocate the use of heart blood as a convenient source of samples, it may be contaminated by post-mortem diffusion from the stomach and intestine. After death, the cellular barrier of mucosa and serous membranes breaks down, and substances in the stomach, intestine and air passages can migrate to other organs in the main thoracoabdominal cavity, causing a false rise of the true ante-mortem blood level.

Pounder (1985; see Chapter 27) found that a slurry containing alcohol and paracetamol, placed in the trachea after death to resemble gastric contents, gave rise to appreciable concentrations of those substances in blood samples taken from thoracic vessels, whereas femoral blood remained uncontaminated.

For substances such as carboxyhaemoglobin this does not matter, but alcohol is the prime example of a potential source of error if visceral blood is collected. The better choices for collection sites are:

- by needle and syringe puncture of the femoral vein before the autopsy dissection begins. This requires practice but, in adults, 20 ml can usually be aspirated without trouble. This is the method of choice if only an external examination is possible.
- from the subclavian or external iliac veins after the body has been eviscerated. By holding a small container under the cut end of a subclavian vein and raising the arm, blood can be collected directly. If the flow is slow, the arm can be massaged towards the shoulder. Similarly – and preferably if volume is required – by cutting across the iliac veins at the brim of the pelvis, a container can be dropped into the pelvis with its mouth under the vein and blood massaged into it by firm pressure moved up the inner thigh. As all these containers will be soiled externally, the blood should be decanted into a fresh tube for transmission to the laboratory.
- when the skin is dissected off the neck, the internal jugular vein is exposed, especially if a sternomastoid muscle is divided and pulled aside. When cut, a copious flow of blood is usually obtained, which can be collected directly into a container. The only disadvantage of this method is that if the blood wells

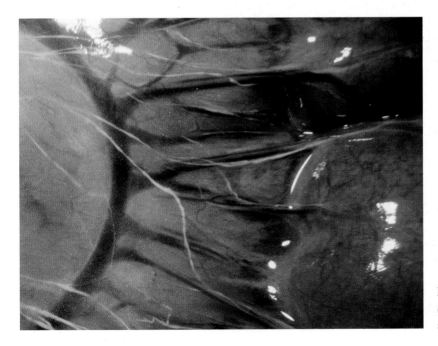

FIGURE 1.13 *White shining fat droplets (chylomicrons) in mesenteric lymphatic vessels suggesting postprandial state.*

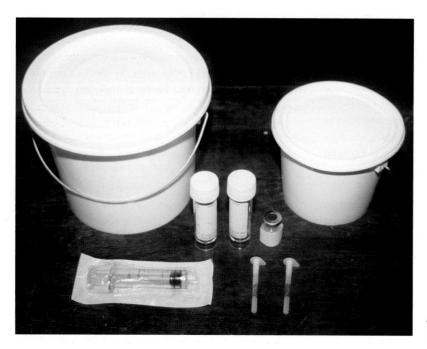

FIGURE 1.14 *Toxicology kit issued by the home office forensic science laboratories. Contained in a plastic bag are a large liver tub, a smaller stomach tub, two universal (30 ml) containers, one rubber-capped fluoride vial for blood alcohol, and a syringe and two needles.*

up from the thoracic inlet via the superior vena cava, heart blood is likely to be admixed, with the possible errors mentioned earlier. If the blood is collected from the upper segment of the jugular, then blood from the head is collected: this flow can usually be stimulated by raising and lowering the head during collection.

Samples for serology, microbiology and for analysis for substances such as carboxyhaemoglobin, which are not absorbed from the gastrointestinal tract, can be collected from any blood vessel, but blood should never be scooped up from the general body cavity after evisceration, as this can be contaminated with any leakage from other structures, such as gastric or bowel contents, mucus, urine, pus or serous fluids.

Blood for microbiological culture has traditionally been taken from the heart but there is no particular merit in this as opposed to peripheral blood. If an infective endocarditis is suspected, it is best to open the heart later with a sterile scalpel and excise the mitral or aortic valve cusps or vegetations for direct culture. Otherwise, blood for culture for a suspected septicaemia is taken from a peripheral vein.

Urine can be collected by catheter before autopsy or even by suprapubic puncture with a syringe and long needle. However, it is usually obtained after the abdomen is opened, but before the organs are removed. If the bladder is full, the fundus is penetrated, and urine collected either by syringe or directly into a container. If almost empty and contracted, the fundus is gripped and pulled upwards so that it stretches, then is incised and the contents removed by syringe. Care should be taken not to contaminate the urine with blood.

The removal of vitreous humour and cerebrospinal fluid may be required for toxicology or for attempts at estimating the time since death by the potassium content (see Chapter 2). Vitreous humour must be aspirated with care if any reliable results are to be attained. A fine hypodermic needle attached to a 5 ml syringe is inserted into the outer canthus of the globe after pulling the eyelid aside. When released, the lid will cover the small puncture mark, hiding any sign of interference. The needle should be entered into the centre of the globe to avoid aspirating material near the retina, which has a markedly different chemical composition due to shreds of detached retina entering the aspirate. The fluid should be sucked off slowly and gently, and as much taken as possible to obtain a mixed fluid: both eyes should be used, as they often differ somewhat in their chemical composition. After withdrawing vitreous, the globes can be re-inflated with water, to improve the cosmetic appearance of the eyes.

Cerebrospinal fluid may be obtained in the same way as in living patients, by passing a needle into the theca between the lumbar spines. A baby can be held upright by an assistant in a fully flexed position; an adult must be pulled into flexion whilst lying sideways on the autopsy table. An alternative technique is to perform a cisternal puncture through the atlanto-occipital membrane.

As there is no pressure within the theca in a cadaver, the fluid must be actively aspirated: sometimes all attempts at obtaining fluid by external puncture fail. The only course then is to try to puncture the ventricles through the exposed brain surface when the skull is opened. Attempting to obtain clear cerebrospinal fluid from the interior of the skull after removal of the brain is generally useless: though blood-stained fluid can be centrifuged to clarity, its chemical composition is then unreliable.

Removal of the viscera

After the body cavities have been inspected, the organs are removed *en bloc* by a modified Rokitansky procedure, more accurately described as Letulle's method. First, the intestine is removed, as follows.

The omentum is lifted upwards to expose the coils of small intestine. The uppermost part of the jejunum is identified, where it passes retroperitoneally to join the termination of the duodenum. Here the mesentery is perforated with the knife and the gut cut through. If it is essential to retain the duodenal/gastric contents or the small intestinal contents, two string sutures may be passed through the hole and tied before cutting the gut between them, but little contents are lost if this is not done. The intestine is stripped out by cutting along the mesentery near the attachment with the bowel until the ileocaecal valve is reached.

The caecum is then mobilized medially using manual traction with minimum use of the knife, to avoid puncturing the lumen. When the hepatic flexure is reached, the omentum is pulled downwards to draw the transverse colon tense against the mesocolon, which is cut through, taking care not to open the adjacent stomach. The splenic flexure is then pulled medially and downwards, and the descending and sigmoid colon separated from the posterior abdominal wall. The upper rectum is cut across, though some pathologists merely lay the gut outside the body, leaving the sigmoid and rectum attached.

Removing the neck structures

To make the removal of the neck structures easier, a block 10–15 cm high should be placed under the shoulders of the cadaver. This allows the head to fall back and thus extends the neck. This should be done gently, as with all handling of the body, to avoid the well-known 'undertaker's fracture', which is a subluxation of the lower cervical spine due to tearing of the intervertebral disc at about C6–C7. This can be misinterpreted as an ante-mortem injury, especially if the other common artefact of haemorrhage over the anterior longitudinal ligament of the cervical spine is present (Prinsloo and Gordon 1951). The neck structures are then freed by passing a knife under the skin of the upper neck until it enters the floor of the mouth. The knife is then run around the inside of the mandible to free the tongue. The tissues at the back and sides of the pharynx are divided, and the tonsillar area cut through. Fingers are then passed up behind the mandibular symphysis to grasp the tongue, which is then drawn down, the remaining tissues behind the larynx being divided to release the neck structures. This should be done as far lateral as possible, so that the carotids can be removed with the laryngeal structures. It is now advisable to look into the pharynx and glottis before any further disturbance, to see if any obstruction, bleeding or other abnormality is present in the upper airway.

Removal of the thoracic contents

The subclavian bundles of vessels and nerves are divided by passing the knife from inside the thorax around the medial ends of the clavicles and first ribs to release the trachea and oesophagus. With gentle traction, the neck structures are held up and pulled caudally, whilst carefully clearing all attachments to the thoracic spine with the knife, taking care to keep the blade on the bone and not stray anteriorly to damage oesophagus or aorta.

Traction should be minimal and, as soon as the thorax is entered, the hand should move from the neck structures to place two fingers under the upper lobes of the lungs, lifting them and the mediastinum as the knife clears the midline structures down to the diaphragm. If the neck structures are pulled too hard by using them as a handle to drag out the thoracic viscera, they may be ripped off. In addition, the descending aorta may suffer transverse intimal tears from traction, which resemble the genuine 'ladder tears' seen in many traffic accidents (Chapter 9).

Pleural adhesions may prevent clean removal of the lungs. If there are only a few, they can be cut through. If the whole pleural cavity is obliterated by adhesions, they may be pulled away by making a cleavage plane with the hand and stripping them off. Sometimes (especially in industrial chest disease and old tuberculosis) the adhesions are dense, tough or even calcified. Removal of the lung may then be achieved by running a knife down the whole length of the parietal pleura over the inner anterior aspect of the ribs, and forcing a hand through the slit to form a cleavage plane to force the parietal pleura off the intercostal muscles and ribs.

Removal of the abdominal organs

When the chest organs are free, they are laid back in the thorax and the diaphragm incised. One hand should pull the liver and spleen medially, putting the left leaf of the diaphragm on the stretch, while the knife cuts it through laterally, near the costal margin. The cut curves posteriorly under the organs to reach the spine, where it must cut through the cruciate ligaments, then passes caudally behind the kidney, which is mobilized forwards.

The knife cut then curves up over the psoas muscle and ends at the brim of the pelvis. The same is done on the opposite side, the operator moving around the body if necessary. The chest organs are then lifted and gently pulled forwards to carry the abdominal viscera towards the feet. Any resistance is usually due to incompletely severed cruciate ligaments, which must be transected.

Eventually the organs will lay inverted across the pubis, secured only by the iliac vessels and ureters, which are cut through and the whole pluck of viscera taken away to the dissecting bench where running water and good illumination must be available.

Removal of the pelvic organs

The treatment of the pelvic contents depends on the type of case. Where the presumed cause of death is unrelated to pelvic lesions, then in men the bladder may be opened widely and the mucosa and trigone inspected before the prostate is incised for examination. The testes are pushed upwards through the inguinal canals, which are widened with the knife. In women, the ovaries are incised and the tubes examined from above before the uterus is sliced in the midline from fundus to cervix.

A more thorough examination of either gender may be made by enucleating the pelvic contents. The knife is passed circumferentially around the pelvic bowl after pulling the bladder away from the pubis. When the walls are free, the knife cuts through below the prostate and then through the lower rectum to allow the pelvic organs to be lifted out. In women the ovaries and tubes are mobilized forwards and the knife passed around the wall of the pelvic bowl, then in front of and below the bladder. The vault of the vagina and rectum is transected, freeing the whole contents. In cases where sexual interference or abortion is suspected, a special technique described in Chapter 19 is employed.

Removing the brain

Attention is then turned to the head. The scalp is incised across the posterior vertex from a point behind the ear to the corresponding place on the other side. Where a Y-incision is used on the neck, the limbs of the Y may be continued right across the scalp, especially if a face dissection is necessary.

The tissues are reflected forwards to the lower forehead and back to the occiput. The deep scalp tissues may peel off by traction, but often require touches of the knife to free them. Bruising is sought and, where head injuries are present or suspected, the scalp should be reflected right back to the nape of the neck, paying particular attention to the tissue behind and below each ear where injuries causing vertebrobasilar artery

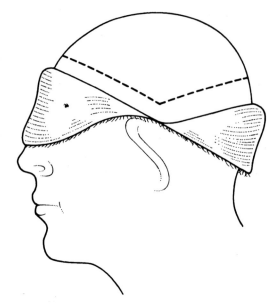

FIGURE 1.15 *Angled saw-cuts for removal of skull-cap to avoid slippage during reconstruction.*

damage occur. Where there are facial injuries, the skin of the face may be peeled back from the jaw line and downwards from the forehead, restoration being excellent if care is taken not to perforate the facial skin during removal.

The skull is sawn through, using either hand or power tools. The line of the cut should not be along a circumference, as it is then impossible to reconstitute the head without unsightly sliding of the calvarium. There should be an angled removal, with a horizontal cut from forehead to behind the ears joined by a second, which passes diagonally upwards at a shallow angle over the occipitoparietal area. Care must be taken not to place this posterior saw-cut too vertically (and thus anteriorly) on the skull, or the brain may be damaged by forcing its removal through too narrow an aperture.

The calvarium is then removed by leverage after complete cutting through. A mallet and chisel should not be used in forensic autopsies, even to ensure that the dura is kept intact. The risk of extending or even causing fractures by the use of excessive hammering is too great merely to justify an unmarked dural membrane. A cut dura is easily recognized as such by any competent pathologist. What is more important is to inspect the surface of the exposed dura and brain and assess any oedema, bleeding or inflammatory conditions that may be present. The skull-cap is carefully inspected for fractures and the dura peeled off the inside to study the inner skull surface.

To remove the brain, the dura is incised around the line of skull removal and two fingers slipped beneath each frontal lobe. With gentle traction the frontal lobes are lifted to expose the optic chiasma and anterior cranial nerves. The falx may have to be cut to free the brain, then a scalpel or blunt-pointed bistoury is passed along the floor of the skull to divide the cranial nerves, carotid arteries and pituitary stalk until the free edges of the tentorium are accessible. A cut is made along each side of the tentorium, following the line of the petrous temporal bones to the lateral wall of the skull. Continuing with traction on the brain, but being careful not to impact the upper surface against the posterior saw-cut, the knife severs the remaining posterior cranial nerves and then passes down into the foramen magnum to transect the spinal cord as far down as can be reached. The hand is now slid under the base of the brain, which is rotated backwards for removal, any attached dura being severed where necessary. The brain is taken into a scale pan and weighed before either fixation or dissection.

The floor of the skull is now examined and the basal dura stripped out with a strong forceps to reveal any basal fractures. Discarded dental forceps can be useful for this purpose. The venous sinuses are incised to search for thrombosis. Where appropriate – and always in infants – the petrous temporal bones are sawn, chiselled or cut with bone forceps to examine the middle and inner ears for infection.

Removal and examination of the spinal cord

It is not an invariable routine to remove the spinal cord at autopsy unless there are indications that some lesion may be present. Where there is the slightest possibility of damage to the vertebral column, its blood vessels or the contents of the spinal canal, however, there should never be any hesitation in extending the autopsy to include this area.

There are several methods of removing the cord and for full details, the texts of Ludwig (2002) or Knight (1983) should be consulted. Briefly, there are two main approaches to the spinal canal, the anterior and posterior.

In the anterior method, the vertebral bodies are removed after complete evisceration of the body, by sawing through the pedicles by a lateral cut down each side. The advantages are that the body need not be turned over on to its face and an extensive dorsal incision is avoided, which requires subsequent repair. The author finds this method more laborious, however, especially in the thoracic region where the heads of the ribs make the approach difficult.

The more usual posterior approach requires a midline incision from occiput to lumbar region, the paraspinal muscles being reflected along with subcutaneous tissues. Two parallel saw-cuts are then made down the length of the spine to divide the right and left laminae, and to give access to the spinal canal. This is best done with an electric oscillating saw, taking care not to cut so deeply that the spinal

dura is penetrated. The strip of bone may be dissected off from below upwards to expose the spinal canal.

The cuts should be placed sufficiently lateral to allow the cord to be removed without difficulty. When the canal is exposed, the dura is examined for haemorrhage, infection or other abnormalities, then removed – still within its dural sheath – by transecting the nerve roots and dural attachments, and peeling it out progressively from below upwards. The dura is then carefully opened with forceps and scissors to examine the cord itself. It can be fixed in formalin, as with the brain, before cutting, or dissected immediately and samples taken for histology. Crushing, infarction, infection, haemorrhage and degeneration are the main lesions in a forensic context. The empty spinal canal must be carefully examined for disc protrusions, tumours, fractures, haemorrhage dislocations and vertebral collapse.

Where in any autopsy spinal damage is suspected, a good preliminary test is to slide the hands under the back of the eviscerated body on the autopsy table and lift the dorso-lumbar spine upwards, whilst watching the interior vertebral bodies. If a fracture or dislocation is present, abnormally acute angulation will be seen, instead of smooth bending. The cervical spine can be tested by manual manipulation. If suspicious angulation is seen, a slice can be taken along with the anterior spine, through the vertebral bodies and discs, with an electric or handsaw. This will reveal the interior of the spine and exhibit any crushing, haemorrhage, or torn disc spaces: if one of these is found, the cord must always be removed.

EXAMINATION OF ORGANS

Examination of viscera

The thoracic and abdominal viscera are laid on a cutting bench at a convenient height and under good illumination. Ample washing water should be available from a flexible pipe, to flush the tissues as dissection proceeds. Some pathologists maintain that this should not be done, as the water can have an effect on the quality of subsequent histological sections, but this has recently been disproved (Cotton and Stephenson 1988). In any case, the vastly inferior naked-eye examination that results if blood is not removed at frequent intervals greatly outweighs any unsubstantiated objections about the more exquisite details of cell structure, especially as in most forensic autopsies the gross appearances are usually far more important.

The viscera should be laid so that the tongue faces the pathologist, with the aorta upwards. The same sequence of examination should be carried out whatever the nature of the case, so that a fixed routine will ensure that nothing is left undone.

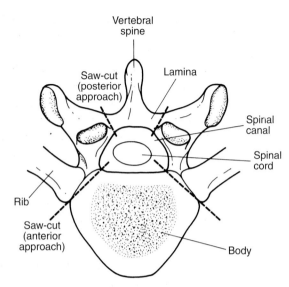

FIGURE 1.16 *The two approaches to the spinal canal for the removal of the spinal cord at autopsy.*

The neck structures

The tongue is examined for disease and injuries, including bites suggesting blows in the jaw or epilepsy. The tongue should be sliced to detect deep haemorrhages sometimes seen in strangulation. Such haemorrhage is seen mostly at the sides and centre of the mid-part of the tongue. Gross congestion, which may be due to either pressure on the neck or to other congestive modes of death, is usually in the posterior part of the tongue. The tonsils and pharyngeal walls are inspected.

The glottis is examined for mechanical or infective obstruction, and the hyoid and thyroid horns palpated for fractures. The oesophagus is opened with large (20 cm) blunt-nosed scissors, which along with a very sharp 10–15 cm bladed knife and a long-bladed 'brain knife', are the most useful tools for performing an autopsy.

The carotid arteries on each side are opened, including the bifurcations and sinuses. If necessary, the upper portions of the carotids are explored in the body itself and followed to the base of the skull. If thrombosis is suspected, the intracranial part should be examined in the cavernous sinus.

Returning to the neck structures, the thyroid should be sliced and inspected, then the oesophagus opened almost to the cardia of the stomach and any suspect material such as capsules, tablets or powder retained for analysis.

The scissors are then passed down the posterior line of the larynx and trachea to the carina. If pressure on the neck of any type, such as strangulation, is suspected, then special examination should be made, as described in Chapter 14.

The trachea and main bronchi should be inspected for disease and obstruction. Gastric contents are often found,

but the significance of this is discussed in Chapter 13 – it should not be assumed that ante-mortem aspiration has occurred merely from the presence of gastric contents in the air passages.

The lungs

The lungs are then removed, after careful examination of their external surfaces for patchy collapse, emphysema, petechiae and so on. Almost every autopsy will reveal a few petechiae, especially around the hilum and in the interlobar fissures. Their significance is also discussed in Chapter 13.

The lungs are removed from the thoracic pluck by passing a long-bladed knife (such as a brain knife) under the hilum with the blunt edge upwards. The knife is settled in the correct position before turning the sharp edge upwards to cut through the hilum. Before doing this it may be necessary to remove adhesions over the diaphragm and to cut through the pulmonary ligament, a thin sheet of tissue that ties the inferior medial edge of the lower lobe to the mediastinum.

As the hilum is being cut, the pathologist must notice if any embolism is visible within the pulmonary arteries. It has happened that such an embolism has slid out and been washed unnoticed down the sink. Some pathologists insist on opening the main pulmonary trunk and even right ventricle before removing the lungs, to seek a saddle embolus. This is not necessary, as any large embolus will be readily visible on examining the heart and the lungs in the usual sequence.

Both lungs are taken off and the hilum inspected before being laid aside for cutting. The lung should be weighed before cutting, as appreciable oedema fluid can run away during dissection. Then each is laid with the hilum down on the dissecting board, the opportunity being taken during handling to evaluate weight and oedema, as well as emphysema.

The lung is held on the upper surface by the left hand of the operator (or by an interposed sponge) and the organ cut across in the sagittal plane from apex to base with the large brain knife, held parallel to the board. This produces an anteroposterior slice, the lower medial part carrying the hilum. The cut surfaces can now be opened like a book and the surface examined for oedema, tumour, pneumonias, infarction, trauma and so on. The smaller bronchi must be inspected for such signs as mucosal thickening, infection and blockage. The smaller pulmonary arteries may reveal thrombosis or embolism that was not visible in the larger vessels.

INFLATING THE LUNGS WITH FORMALIN

In some medico-legal autopsies, especially in industrial lung disease such as pneumoconiosis or asbestosis, one or both lungs need to be inflated with formalin for fixation before cutting. This preserves the shape and histology in excellent condition, but delays examination for at least several days. It is carried out by holding or tying a cannula into the bronchus while 10 per cent formol saline is perfused through a tube from a reservoir held about 1 metre above the lung. The lung is then left in a bath of formalin covered with a formalin-soaked cloth to prevent drying.

The heart and great vessels

There are almost as many ways of examining the heart as there are pathologists, and each operator must decide upon the method that appeals most. In this summary there is no space for discussion of post-mortem angiography, which is moving from the field of research and special interest into routine use. A common and practical routine for examining the heart is described here.

First, the organ mass minus the lungs is rotated so that the lower end now faces the pathologist. The scissors are passed into the cut end of a common iliac artery and passed right up to the aortic arch and around to a few centimetres above the aortic valve, staying outside the reflection of the pericardium. The interior of the aorta is studied, especially for the degree of atheroma and for any aneurysms or

trauma. The inferior vena cava is opened from its lower end into the liver. The organ pluck is then turned over so that the heart is uppermost. The pericardium is inspected externally for fluid and blood tamponade, then opened widely with scissors. The heart is delivered through the incision and inspected externally for pericarditis, adhesions, discoloration of an underlying infarct and cardiac aneurysms, for example. In a child, the thymus would be inspected and dissected off at this stage.

The heart is then removed by holding it up with the left hand so that its attachment is tensed against the other organs. A long knife, such as a brain knife, is then passed horizontally across at the reflection of the pericardium, cutting through the root of the aorta and other great vessels just above the atria.

The now-detached heart is washed externally and placed in the anatomical position on the dissecting board, with the apex facing the operator and the anterior surface upwards. It should not be weighed until all the contained blood and clot is removed. The general size, shape and ventricular preponderance should be noted. Any dilatation or thickening of the pulmonary conus should be noted as an index of right ventricular hypertrophy, especially if striae of transverse muscle fibres are seen crossing the conus.

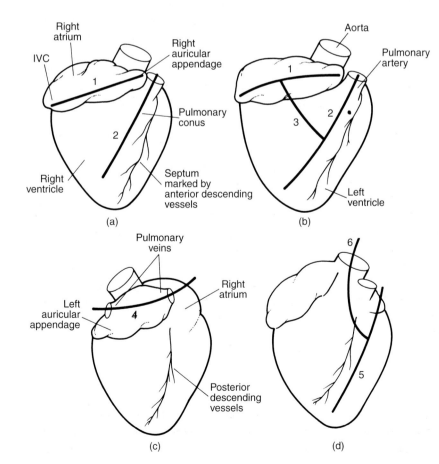

FIGURE 1.17 *Incisions for opening the heart at autopsy. (a) The right atrium is slit with an incision (1) to join the vena cava to the appendage; a cut parallel to the interventricular septum is made on the anterior wall of the right ventricle (2) passing up through the pulmonary conus. (b) These cuts are joined through the tricuspid valve (3). (c) The heart is reversed and the left atrium opened by a cut (4) joining pulmonary veins. (d) On the anterior wall a cut (5) is made parallel to the septum through the mitral valve and joined by (6) which passes through the aortic valve.*

The right atrium is then opened by introducing the scissors into the inferior vena cava and cutting across to the atrial appendage. The interior of the atrium is examined and the septum and tricuspid valve inspected.

The interventricular septum is then identified externally by the vessels running down the outside. With a knife a cut is made about 15 mm to the right of and parallel to the septum, over the right ventricle. This should be deep enough to enter the lumen, but not enough to cut the posterior wall. The scissors are now introduced into the cut and run up through the pulmonary conus and into the pulmonary artery until they meet the transected end. They are also extended downwards to the apex of the ventricle. The scissors are now put in midway down this linear cut and passed outwards at right angles, guided by the fingers of the left hand passed into the tricuspid valve from the opened atrium. The whole of the right side of heart is now open and displayed. It should be washed out and the endocardium and valve examined.

A similar routine is now employed on the left side. The scissors are introduced into a pulmonary vein and passed horizontally across to an opposite vein, thus opening the atrium. Fingers are introduced down through the mitral valve to estimate its size and detect any stenosis.

The heart is then restored to the anatomical position and a cut made again parallel to the septum, but on the left side, going deeper as the ventricle is thicker. Guided by the fingers still in the mitral valve, the cut is extended upwards through that valve and out at the top of the atrium.

A finger is now passed up the outflow tract to the aortic valve to estimate its size. Then the scissors are passed up at the side of the mitral valve, and the aortic valve and aortic stump opened. The whole heart is now open and can be washed out and weighed.

Various estimates of the normal heart weight exist and vary considerably (see the Appendix 1). It has been related to gender and body weight, though this is not altogether sound, as a fat person of moderate stature does not have a heart weight comparable with a large muscular person unless there is associated hypertension. This controversial matter cannot be pursued here, but as a rule of thumb the author (BK) accepts up to 380 g as normal in an adult man of average build.

After weighing, the endocardium and valves are examined, then the coronary arteries. Once again, controversy exists about methods of opening the coronary vessels, but the weight of opinion now lies almost universally with those who cut serial interrupted cross-sections with a knife, rather than open them longitudinally with small scissors. The disadvantages of lengthwise opening are that percentage assessment of stenosis or the recognition of total occlusion cannot be made once the vessel is flapped open, as restoring the cut edges can never reproduce the original conditions. In addition, the tip of the scissors may dislodge thrombus or an intimal flap. Cutting across the vessels allows an estimate of the percentage stenosis. It is admitted that this may not be the size of the lumen during life when normal blood pressure is operating, but the same disadvantage applies to longitudinal opening. An estimate of luminal size is relatively constant, however, in that the collapsed abnormal can still be compared with the collapsed normal.

The coronaries are therefore cut across at frequent intervals. Before the first cut, the ostia are examined for congenital variations (which are frequent) and for obstruction. The left coronary artery is then cut across from the epicardial surface, starting as close to the ostium as possible, as occlusion and severe stenosis can occur very near the origin. Serial cuts are then made at intervals of not more than 3 mm, first into the common trunk, then following the left circumflex laterally until the vessel becomes too small, usually when it dips down from the epicardium to become intramuscular. The anterior descending branch is then followed down the front of the septum almost to the apex.

Turning to the right coronary artery, the proximal segment is cut back from the point where the right ventricle was opened, transecting the artery in its mid-part. The cuts are made back to the aorta, then the distal segment is followed laterally until it becomes the posterior descending branch. During this process, the dominance of right versus left vessels is noted.

Difficulty arises where severe calcification exists, as the knife either fails to cut through the artery or shatters it because of the excessive force required. The lumen is crushed and the percentage stenosis is difficult or impossible to assess. Scissors may be used to exert more force than a knife, but the only real solution is to decalcify the vessels. Except for research purposes, it must be admitted that the days or even weeks of delay occasioned by decalcification provide a formidable deterrent for the busy coroner's pathologist unless the issues involved are important. Post-mortem angiography is the other alternative, though where autopsy caseloads are high, this can be difficult to arrange.

Once the coronary arteries have been examined, the myocardium can be studied more closely. One useful technique is the intramural or 'sandwich' cut through the thickness of the left ventricle. This is easier when there is some ventricular hypertrophy, but can be carried out in any heart. The heart is placed open on the cutting board, with the endocardium downwards. A long knife such as a brain knife is passed carefully into the cut edge of the left ventricle and sliced right through the muscle, keeping equidistant between endocardium and epicardium. The myocardium can then be opened out like a book, showing the interior with any infarcts or fibrotic plaques. If histological blocks through the entire wall are needed it is best to take these before slicing the heart as described, otherwise a full-thickness block will be hard to obtain. Some pathologists make a series of transverse heart slices about 8–10 mm thick, starting at the apex, before opening the heart. This displays the distal myocardium wall, but cannot expose the proximal part, as examination of the coronary arteries would then be compromised.

Examining the abdominal organs

The remaining organs are laid on the dissecting surface in the anatomical position, with the liver and stomach away from the pathologist, and the anterior surface upwards.

The stomach is opened and, if there is any question of requiring the contents for analysis, a suitable container should be ready. The stomach is washed externally with a stream of water and a small cut made in the greater curvature. If the contents are to be saved, this can best be done with the edge of the stomach projecting over the raised cutting board or over the edge of the sink, so that the container can be held underneath. The contents are allowed to run into the container, then the greater curvature is opened widely with scissors, and any remaining contents drained or scraped out. If powder or other substance is adherent to the mucosa, this can be scraped off and added to the container, or kept in a separate tube for analysis.

Some laboratories require the stomach wall to be retained for analysis as well as the contents. This can be

done after the organ has been fully opened and the lining examined. If the contents are not required – or when they have been collected – the organ is opened up from cardia to pylorus along the greater curvature. The lining is washed and inspected. The scissors are now passed through the pylorus around the duodenum until they meet the point where the gut was detached earlier. The gall bladder may be squeezed to demonstrate the patency of the bile ducts. In some few cases, bile may be required for analysis, as in morphine or chlorpromazine overdose.

The adrenals are examined next, the right one being on top of its kidney, the left being on the medial side. If the right kidney is taken in the left hand and lifted against the weight of the liver, a single cut into the stretched tissues between liver and kidney will transect the adrenal. The left is buried in the tissue between pancreas, spleen and kidney. The amount of cortical lipoid and the absence of bleeding or other abnormality is noted in each gland.

The spleen is removed by cutting through its pedicle and is sliced after weighing. The pancreas lies under the stomach and should be cut lengthwise from the curve of the duodenum to its tail lying against the splenic hilum.

The kidneys are exposed by incising their capsules, often after a thick layer of perirenal fat is traversed. The kidneys can usually be peeled out of their capsules unless these are adherent.

The renal vessels were examined when the aorta was opened, but can be re-examined at this stage and the ureters inspected. The organs can be detached at their hilum and weighed, then cut lengthwise to inspect the interior. The width of the cortex is important, being about 1 cm in a

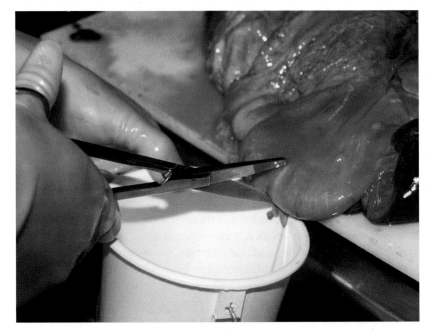

FIGURE 1.18 *Collecting stomach contents at autopsy. The exterior of the stomach is washed free from blood and the viscera moved to overhang the dissecting board. A chemically clean receptacle is held beneath the greater curvature while the latter is opened with scissors and the contents allowed to drain out. The stomach is then opened, the mucosa inspected and any adherent material scraped into the container. The stomach wall should then be dissected off and added to the contents if the laboratory is able to deal with tissue analysis.*

1: The forensic autopsy

healthy subject. The granularity of the surface and the clarity of the corticomedullary junctions is assessed, as well as the size of the renal pelvis.

The small intestine may have been examined at the earlier stage of removal, but can be inspected now. It is not usual to open the whole length of the gut in a forensic autopsy unless there is any particular indication to do so, though ideally this should always be carried out.

EXAMINATION OF THE BRAIN

After weighing, a decision has to be made whether to examine the brain immediately – the so-called 'wet-cutting' – or to suspend it in formalin until fixed, a process which takes at least several weeks. The advantage of fixation is, of course, that the firmness of the tissue allows thinner and more accurate knife-cut sections to be taken, as well as better histological preservation. Where neurological issues are involved, either traumatic or from natural disease, it is almost mandatory for the brain to be fixed before cutting. Even the impatience of the investigative authorities can usually be overcome if the advantages of a higher standard of opinion are explained.

The technique of brain fixation is well known, but to summarize briefly, the brain is suspended in a container of 10 per cent buffered formalin, the volume being at least 5 litres and preferably 8. The brain is removed with the dura leaving the parasagittal bridging veins and falx intact and suspending the brain in an upright position by the falx. An alternative method is to pass a thread or metal paperclip under the basilar artery and tie it to a support across the mouth of the container, so that the vertex is clear of the bottom.

In the majority of autopsies there is no real need for fixation if no cerebral lesions are either expected or apparent on external examination of the brain. Here, 'wet-cutting' is sufficient, though if any unexpected lesions are found, the process can be stopped and the slices of brain fixed by placing them in a large volume of formalin, on cotton wool pads, to prevent distortion.

One lesion is better examined in the unfixed state, though the brain may be suspended later; this is subarachnoid haemorrhage. It is easier to wash away fresh, unfixed blood with a stream of water and blunt dissection than the hardened blood that develops during formalin fixation. Further details are given in Chapters 5 and 25.

Whether the brain is examined 'wet' or fixed, the sequence is the same. The weight is first considered, the normal for a young male adult being between about 1300 and 1450 g, the female equivalent being around 100 g less. More details are given in Appendix 1. It should be noted that formalin fixation adds about 8 per cent to the original weight.

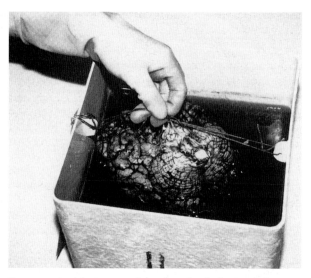

FIGURE 1.19 *A brain suspended in formalin for fixation before cutting. The tank is specially made of fibreglass, being cubical for stacking with a lid (not shown). There are lugs moulded into the sides to hold the suspensory strings, which support the brain by means of a paperclip hooked under the basilar artery. There should be sufficient fluid to allow the brain to float clear of the bottom of the receptacle.*

The brain is first examined for surface abnormalities, which in forensic practice usually means haemorrhage. This is dealt with in Chapter 5, but suffice to say here that meningeal bleeding is one of the most important lesions in forensic pathology, be it extradural, subdural or subarachnoid. This means that examination of the cerebral vessels, especially the arteries of the circle of Willis and the vertebral vessels, is vital – especially in the search for berry aneurysms. The general symmetry of the brain is then noted as well as any depression of the cortex from skull or meningeal masses. An estimate of cerebral oedema is made, partly from the weight, but mainly from flattening of the gyri, filling of the sulci and evidence of hippocampal herniation through the tentorial aperture. In lesser degree this may be seen as grooving of one or both unci, though a normal slight anatomical groove is often present. True uncal herniation is marked and often discoloured as a result of incipient infarction. Similarly, herniation or coning of the cerebellar tonsils through the foramen magnum must be distinguished from the common anatomical pouting of many tonsils: true pressure coning is often discoloured by local infarction. After careful inspection of the basal vessels and the exterior of the brain, and palpation for any fluctuant masses under the cortex such as internal haemorrhage, abscesses or cystic tumours, the organ is cut.

The first cut should be made through the cerebral peduncles using a long, broad-bladed knife to separate the cerebrum from the brainstem and cerebellum. The cerebellum is then held in one hand with the cut stem upwards.

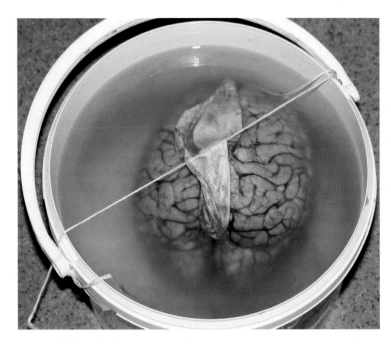

FIGURE 1.20 *An alternative method of suspension is to leave the falx intact and use it to suspend the brain base down in formalin.*

This is examined to assess the substantia nigra and aqueduct, as well as to note any primary or secondary haemorrhage, the latter often being due to raised intracranial pressure. The cerebellum and pons are then cut down vertically and opened like a book to display the fourth ventricle, dentate nuclei and the interior of the cerebellum. The lower pons and medulla can be further sectioned transversely or longitudinally.

The cerebral hemispheres are then placed base down on the cutting block and serial sections made in the coronal plane from the frontal lobes back to the occiput. The sections should be about 1 cm thick and each should be slid into a sequential place in rows along the cutting board so that orientation is preserved. Cuts should be made with careful but bold sweeps of the knife as erratic sawing motions will leave an irregular surface on each section, which obscures a good view. Cutting a fresh brain is less satisfactory than cutting a firmer fixed brain, especially if there is any post-mortem autolysis or softening as in a dead ischaemic brain after mechanical ventilation.

ANCILLARY INVESTIGATIONS

A wide range of samples may need to be taken either before, during or after the gross examination is completed. The nature of such ancillary investigations naturally depends upon the nature of the death, the history and the interests of the pathologist.

Microbiology

Though more common in clinical autopsies than forensic work, culture samples for 'bacteriology', virology and (rarely) fungi may be needed. Either plain swabs or swabs immersed in a transport medium can be employed for sampling a wide variety of sites at autopsy. Alternatively, tissue samples may be collected in sterile containers and this is the usual method for virological culture of lung and brain, for example. Blood cultures may be desired, and it is best to take blood with a sterile needle and syringe from a large vessel, such as the femoral vein, before starting the autopsy with its attendant inevitably widespread contamination with putrefactive organisms. Alternatively, blood can be taken from a freshly opened heart chamber using sterile instruments.

In all autopsy investigations, unless cultures are performed soon after death, there is often widespread contamination by organisms that travel rapidly through the dead tissues, especially from the gastrointestinal tract. It requires the expertise of an experienced microbiologist to advise on what is significant in the subsequent growth in the laboratory.

Toxicology

This has already been mentioned and is further discussed in the later chapters of this book but, as far as the collection of specimens is concerned, it may be repeated here that sampling is extremely important if reliable analytical results are expected. Blood, urine, stomach contents, organs (especially liver), intestinal contents, cerebrospinal fluid, bile and ocular fluid may be required.

The containers in which specimens are collected must be chemically clean to a very high standard. They are often supplied by the laboratory that will carry out the analyses. For example, the Home Office Forensic Science Service in Britain supply a kit containing two large plastic tubs with lids, several universal containers, fluoride tube, syringes and needles, together with instructions as to type and quantity of sample needed for various tests.

The pathologist should submit a form with the samples indicating the analyses required, the personal details of the deceased person, a brief history with details of suspected toxic substances, and a statement as to whether the subject was known to suffer from any infective condition, including hepatitis or HIV infection.

Histology

In most autopsies and inevitably in all criminal or litigious cases, the pathologist will need to carry out a histological examination on a range of tissues, even if only to exclude the possibility of some occult natural disease. The Royal College of Pathologists as well as the 1999 Council of Europe recommendation on the harmonization of medico-legal autopsy recommend that histology be taken from every autopsy. This advice should be followed wherever possible, even though in some medico-legal autopsies, the cost of such techniques may provide difficulty if the coroner or other commissioning authority declines to fund the procedure. It is customary to retain samples of liver, spleen, kidney, heart, lung, thyroid, adrenal, pancreas, muscle and brain as a minimum. Where there are indications to examine other parts of the body, these are retained in addition to the routine tissues. The tissues are either sampled by taking relatively large pieces at autopsy (which are later trimmed down to size) or by cutting blocks of a standard size (such as $20 \times 12 \times 5\,mm$) at the time of autopsy.

The tissue is placed in a large volume of buffered formol–saline and allowed to fix for at least several days before processing. The volume of fixative should be six times the total volume of tissue: it is all too common to see a mass of tissue squeezed into a small container, barely covered with formalin, half-fixed and even semi-dried. There are many specialized procedures also in use at present, such as histochemistry, fluorescent microscopy and immuno-histochemical examination; these are used especially in the pathology of sudden death where evidence of early myocardial infarction is sought. This is discussed in the chapter on sudden natural death (Chapter 25).

REQUEST FOR TOXICOLOGICAL ANALYSIS

Name _____ Age _____

Post Mortem No _____ Date of P.M. _____

Date of Death _____ Pathologist _____

SPECIMENS SUBMITTED: ___ Blood _____ Urine _____ Liver _____

Stomach contents _____ Kidney _____

Intestines _____ Brain _____

OTHER SPECIMENS _____

Any infective conditions suspected _____

ANALYSIS REQUIRED

BACKGROUND INFORMATION:

FIGURE 1.21 *Sample request form for toxicological analysis.*

AUTOPSY RADIOLOGY

The details of radiological findings are discussed in each appropriate chapter, particularly in relation to child abuse, gunshot wounds, identification and dentistry. In general, radiology is similar to photography in the autopsy room, though it requires more bulky apparatus, and someone to operate the equipment and process the films.

The quality of radiographic assistance available will vary widely from none to the most sophisticated techniques, even including computed tomography and even, in very few centres, magnetic resonance imaging (MRI).

The main difference is usually whether the autopsy is carried out in the mortuary of a well-equipped hospital where there is radiographic apparatus, radiographers to use it and radiologists to read the films – or whether the autopsy is performed in some remote public mortuary or in makeshift premises far from clinical facilities.

In many developing countries, radiography may be scarce for living patients let alone corpses, and the same standard of assistance for the pathologist cannot be expected. In larger, more affluent countries, remoteness may be the problem; here mobile equipment is available and sometimes used by forensic pathologists. There are small, portable X-ray kits that can be carried in two suitcases, and can function from an ordinary domestic power supply or from a portable petrol generator. In many instances a mortuary will have a small portable machine, sometimes one discarded from clinical use. This can be wheeled into position when needed, and films and technical assistance obtained from the nearest hospital, which is often adjacent.

For isolated organs and tissues, cabinet-type radiographic equipment is available, which can be used without the assistance of trained radiographers.

Where there is a large forensic institute, then full radiological facilities with the staff and equipment to operate and process plates will be available at all times. Where research projects involving radiology, such as post-mortem coronary angiography, are being carried out, there will usually also be ample facilities for routine use.

The stage at which radiology is employed in an autopsy will vary according to the individual circumstances, but is likely to be after the external examination is complete, but before dissection begins. Straight radiographs for bony injury are not often required, as the skeleton can be inspected directly by dissection in major trauma. The exception is child abuse, where, as fully described in Chapter 22, a full skeletal survey is needed before autopsy. Indeed, many forensic and paediatric pathologists would consider radiology essential in all infants who did not die of some obvious disease.

Suspected air embolism, pneumothorax, barotrauma, gunshot and explosive deaths should have radiological examination before the autopsy, and when a traumatic subarachnoid haemorrhage is suspected, vertebral artery angiography might be necessary, as described in Chapter 5.

Mutilated remains, especially those from mass disasters, may need to be X-rayed, as may victims from fires where the external damage makes dissection difficult. Where bombs or explosive devices are involved, it is essential to have radiographs to detect any parts of the mechanism that are embedded in the tissues.

Though the films are usually taken before the autopsy begins, some lesions may be better demonstrated on isolated

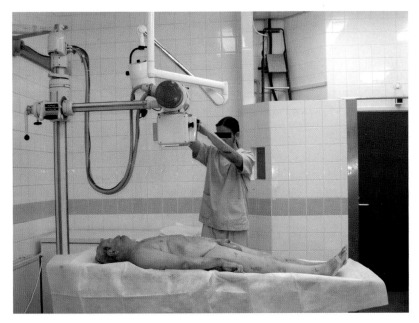

FIGURE 1.22 *Radiography is essential before some autopsies. Here it is being used to X-ray a gunshot wound of the chest.*

organs or structures. In child abuse, the callus of old fractures of posterior ribs may be better visualized on X-ray if the chest cage is dissected out, and radiographs taken without the soft tissues and the obscuring structures of sternum and anterior ribs. Similarly, a block of upper cervical spine may better reveal fractures of transverse processes carrying the vertebral artery, or a larynx may show fractures of the hyoid or thyroid cornuae more clearly when they are X-rayed outside the body.

FORENSIC PHOTOGRAPHY

Many forensic pathologists take their own photographs of both scenes of death and of autopsy appearances. Others rely on professional photographers such as the police and hospital medical photographers.

The standard of expertise amongst some doctor photographers is excellent, and their pictures grace many lectures and textbooks. It is to the more inexpert camera operators that these few general tips are offered.

The type of camera most favoured is the 35 mm single-lens reflex, of which there is now a vast range available, in all grades of sophistication and price. Some means of exact focusing is essential (either automatic or split-screen, for example) as picture sharpness is of prime importance.

The type of lens is a matter of personal choice, as some will prefer interchangeable lenses of various focal lengths. The standard 50 mm is most useful, but for scenes of crime or taking a full-length shot of a body in cramped conditions, a wide-angle lens of 28 or 30 mm is needed. A longer focal length of up to about 80 mm can be useful for close-up pictures of small lesions, but telephoto lenses of 100–200 mm are not required, though extension tubes, some with lenses, can be obtained for macrophotography.

Many pathologists, including the authors, prefer to combine lenses into a single variable-focus 'zoom' lens of 28–80 mm range. This saves time spent in changing lenses, and the image resolution of good-quality equipment is virtually indistinguishable from fixed focal length lenses.

Illumination is usually by electronic flash now often an integral part of the camera body, and the use of automatic thyristor control means that no complicated calculations about range are needed. For very close-range work, a flash attached to the camera may be unsatisfactory, so an extension cable is a useful and cheap accessory to keep the flashgun at a distance. Alternatively, the flash can be 'bounced' off the ceiling in the autopsy room or a 'ring-flash' around the lens used to avoid camera shadow.

Some will prefer tungsten light rather than flash, though this is more cumbersome unless a fixed station is installed in the autopsy room for taking photographs of organs. It is impracticable to use floodlights at the autopsy table or at a scene.

The type of film depends on the nature of the illumination. Speeds of 100 or 200 ASA are more than adequate for most flash work, though 400 ASA is now frequently used. Some keen medical photographers carry a separate camera body loaded with high-speed 1000 ASA film for special circumstances.

Ultraviolet (UV) and infrared sensitive film has been used to demonstrate surface lesions that are not visible to the human eye. It has been claimed that occult bruising can be revealed by UV photography, such as in child abuse, but care must be taken and experience gained to eliminate artefactual false positives.

Most doctors will want transparencies for projection at lectures, which can be made into prints, either colour or monochrome. If prints are specifically wanted for black and white publication in books or journals, it is better to take them originally on monochrome film, as colour negatives do not provide quite the same quality reproduction in black and white.

Some pathologists use Polaroid cameras either alone or together with conventional film. The advantage of instant prints is that a record of the scene of death can be obtained before the autopsy is carried out, and any findings checked back against the original surroundings. For example, if some linear mark is seen on the leg at autopsy, the pathologist can immediately refer to his Polaroid prints to check whether that leg had been resting on some object. Again, where multiple injuries exist, their number, position and size can be checked when writing the autopsy report, without waiting days or even longer for the police album to arrive. Correlation of wounds with blood splashes may also be useful. Such Polaroid pictures can be duplicated and even turned into transparencies, but it is preferable to have a conventional camera for these purposes.

Recent advances in electronics are revolutionizing photography, and have wide application and potential for forensic and autopsy work. Electronic cameras of varying grades of sophistication, resolution and cost, can now instantly store images on a small internal 'memory stick' or CD-ROM, which can then be viewed immediately on a computer VDU or printed on a colour laser printer. These images can be manipulated in many ways to enlarge sections or correct colour balance, sent via modems to distant locations, or incorporated within textual material and reports. At present, good resolution can still be obtained more cheaply with silver-based film stock but this situation is changing in favour of the digital photography. Alternatively, photographs and slides can be electronically scanned within minutes, the optical image being digitized into electronic storage for similar manipulation.

All electronic images can also be stored on CD-ROM or DVD equipment, which offers huge storage and retrieval capacities for record-keeping and educational display purposes. In addition, single frames from video camera recordings can be captured as still pictures and electronically stored.

In relation to the actual photography, a marked improvement in the pictorial quality can be achieved with a little care in composition. At scenes of death the viewpoint is often limited and the surroundings have to be photographed as they exist, without modification. The camera position can, however, usually be chosen to cut out as much extraneous background as possible. In the autopsy room, considerable improvement can be made by using the optimum viewpoint and by modifying the background. Many photographs are spoiled by having irrelevant and distracting objects in the background such as observers, buckets, boots and the other extraneous paraphernalia of the autopsy room. The picture frame should be filled as completely as possible with the object under display. A close shot should be taken to limit the irrelevant margins though, where necessary, anatomical landmarks should be included to orientate the viewer. The camera should be at right angles to the lesion being photographed, whenever possible. Tangential shots may foreshorten the required feature and, where size needs to be displayed, may distort both shape and length because of the foreshortening. A ruler or special white adhesive tape with centimetre markings should be placed very near the lesion or wound to provide a size reference.

Where a feature is obscured or insignificant, it may be pointed out by a probe or finger held in the appropriate position. Where part of the picture area consists of the metal or porcelain autopsy table or dissection bench, allowance should be made in exposure, as these very reflective areas may give a false reading in the light meter of the camera and thyristor of the flashgun.

If a full length or half shot of a body is required, an untidy background may be avoided by turning a mobile or rotatable table so that a blank wall forms the backdrop. If this is not possible, assistants can hold up a sheet behind the table to screen the distant confusion.

When photographing viscera, the camera should be near enough for the frame to be almost completely filled by the required object. The shot should be vertical to the lesion and it is often necessary either to place the dissecting board on the floor, or for the photographer to stand on a stool or some elevation to gain the required height.

Where isolated organs are being photographed, they should be placed on a green or blue cloth, such as a discarded operating gown. White can be used, though it may affect the exposure meter if much is visible around the periphery. The organ should be placed on the cloth in one movement and not moved thereafter, otherwise a wet dark stain will obtrude on the green or blue background. The organ should not be oozing blood onto its surface or onto the background. It should be dabbed with a dry cloth or sponge just before the photograph is taken to remove shiny wet highlights.

Ideally a special stage for organs should be used, such as a glass-topped table with a coloured (usually green) background set sufficiently far below the glass to be out of focus. Tungsten lights can be used to advantage on such a fixed stage.

THE AUTOPSY REPORT

Equally important as the autopsy itself is the report that the pathologist provides for whoever commissioned the examination. An autopsy is of little value if the findings and opinion of the forensic pathologist are not communicated in the most lucid and helpful way. The report is an integral part of the procedure and should receive as much attention as any physical procedure in the autopsy room. Unfortunately, some pathologists treat the process of making a report in a somewhat cavalier manner, which diminishes the expertise that they may otherwise possess.

The autopsy report is a permanent record of the findings and is especially vital for medico-legal purposes, when every word may be dissected in a court of law months or even years afterwards, and when all recollection of the examination has been driven from the mind of the pathologist by hundreds of subsequent autopsies. In a clinical autopsy in a hospital, the dissection may be demonstrated and discussed at the time with the interested physician. However, the report of a forensic autopsy becomes a legal document of possibly vital significance, and every effort must be made at the time to make it as comprehensive and useful as possible.

The form of the autopsy report

Reports fall into two main types described below, and local practice and indeed legislation may determine which is used, irrespective of the wishes of the pathologist. The choice is, however, often dictated by the nature of the case.

▪ A free-style 'essay', which usually adheres to a conventional sequence, but leaves the pathologist free to expand on various aspects according to his estimate of their importance. This type is usually used in criminal deaths and cases in which litigation is likely. It has the advantage that any part of the autopsy can be expanded without constraint; also the form of the report can be turned into a legal statement or a deposition for the court with little alteration.

- A printed proforma, in which the various sections of the examination and organ systems are already set out by title, leaving blank spaces for the insertion of the findings. The advantage includes the fact that this 'shopping list' acts as an *aide-mémoire* to those pathologists who do not conduct large numbers of autopsies – and also the non-medical recipient is more able to follow the set pattern of the report. One disadvantage is that the spacing prevents flexibility of description unless the proforma is large, when much of the space may be left blank. Also there is rarely enough space at the end of the form for an expansive discussion and opinion about the preceding factual findings. This type of form is commonly used for non-litigious autopsies – for example, the usual coroner's cases of sudden death and suicide.

Concentrating upon the more serious cases, the report, whatever the format, must contain certain information in some logical order. Consecutive numeration, computer codings and other administrative aspects are naturally conditioned by local practice, but the following matters must be catered for in all autopsy reports, though not necessarily in this sequence:

- Full personal details of the deceased subject, unless unidentified. This includes the name, gender, age, occupation and address.
- The place, date and time of the autopsy.
- The name, qualifications and status of the pathologist.
- Persons present at the examination.
- Usually, the authority commissioning the autopsy.
- A record of who identified the body.
- The name and address of the deceased subject's regular (or last) medical attendant.
- The date and time of death, where known.
- The history and circumstances of the death. The inclusion of this on the actual autopsy protocol may not be permitted in some jurisdictions as it is hearsay evidence, but unless expressly forbidden it should be included, as it remains a record for the pathologist's own files. It also justifies his eventual cause of death in those cases where the morphological findings are scanty or even absent, as his conclusions will be strongly influenced by his pre-knowledge of the mode of death. When the autopsy report is converted to a statement or deposition for legal use, this history may be omitted by those legal authorities responsible for transcribing the document.
- External examination.

- Internal examination.
- A list of specimens and samples retained for further examination. Those handed to other agencies, such as the forensic science laboratory, should be formally identified by means of serial numbers and the name of the person to whom they were handed.
- The results of further examinations such as histology, microbiology, toxicology and serology. When the main report is issued soon after the autopsy, these will not yet be available and a supplementary report will be necessary.
- A summary of the lesions displayed by the autopsy (often coded for departmental computer retrieval).
- Discussion of the findings, if necessary in the light of the known history.
- An opinion as to the definite or most likely sequence of events leading to the death.
- A formal cause of death, in the format recommended by the World Health Organization, suitable for the completion of a death certificate.
- The signature of the pathologist.

The 'external examination' should record those details described earlier in the chapter, the major items being:

- The height, weight and apparent state of nutrition.
- The presence of natural disease such as oedema, abdominal swelling, cutaneous disease, senile changes, etc.
- Identifying features such as skin colour, tattoos, scars, congenital or acquired deformities, dentures, eye colour and hair colour. When identity is an issue, naturally this section will be greatly expanded.
- The presence of rigor, hypostasis, decomposition and abnormal skin coloration. Body and ambient temperature should be recorded where appropriate, with calculations concerning the estimated range of times since death, though this aspect may well be deferred until the final 'Summary and Conclusions'.
- The condition of the eyes, including petechiae, arcus senilis, pupil size, and the condition of iris and lens.
- Condition of mouth and lips, including injuries, teeth and presence of foreign material.
- Condition of external genitals and anus.
- Listing and description of all external injuries, recent and old.

The internal examination records all abnormalities, usually in a conventional sequence such as:

- Cardiovascular system: heart weight, any dilatation, ventricular preponderance, congenital defects, the pericardium, epicardium, endocardium, valves, coronary arteries, myocardium, aorta, other great vessels and peripheral vessels.

- Respiratory system: external nares, glottis, larynx, trachea, bronchi, pleural cavities, pleura, lungs (including weight) and pulmonary arteries.
- Gastrointestinal system: mouth, pharynx, oesophagus, peritoneal cavity, omentum, stomach, duodenum, small and large intestine, liver (weight), pancreas, gall bladder and rectum.
- Endocrine system: pituitary, thyroid, thymus and adrenals.
- Reticuloendothelial system: spleen (weight) and lymph nodes.
- Genitourinary system: kidneys (weight), ureters, bladder, prostate, uterus, ovaries and testes.
- Musculoskeletal system: skull, spine, remaining skeleton and musculature where necessary.
- Central nervous system: scalp, skull, meninges, cerebral vessels, brain (weight), middle ears, venous sinuses and spinal cord (when examined).

The timing of the report

As with the format, there are two schools of practice in this respect. One advocates the issue of as full a report as possible on the gross findings as soon as the autopsy is completed, usually within a day or two. Obviously this can only be a preliminary, provisional report, as it may have to be modified (sometimes radically) by the results of ancillary investigations that may take days or weeks to return. Virological cultures, for instance, may take up to 6 weeks before a growth can be reported.

In a large proportion of forensic cases, however, especially those due to violence, the gross findings are unlikely to be substantially amended by ancillary investigations, though the possibility must always be left open until data have been gathered in.

The other philosophy will delay any report (except perhaps a provisional oral opinion) until everything is to hand, when a single final document is provided.

Whichever course is adopted, one aspect is vital to both. The descriptive facts must be recorded at or immediately after the completion of the autopsy. It is vital that no significant interval – certainly no more than few hours – be allowed between the physical performance of the examination and the setting down of the objective findings. The words 'setting down' are chosen carefully as the report may be handwritten or typed, or may be dictated to a secretary or into a tape recorder or other audio system. What is vital is that it is not consigned to the pathologists' memory for a few days, even reinforced by notes written on scraps of paper.

In Britain and many other jurisdictions, the court may demand to see any contemporaneous notes and even tapes from a tape recorder. Any diagrams, notes or rough drafts must be preserved for production on demand of the judge, coroner or advocates in court. Where the report is dictated (either to a secretary or into a tape recorder), then the first typed (or word-processed) draft constitutes the 'original report', along with any contemporaneous notes including body sketches.

The use of printed body sketches can be a very useful aid in the autopsy room. Many versions exist from the simple front and back views of the whole body used in clinical neurology to multiple sketches portraying every possible view of the body surface. Separate diagrams are available for the male and female perineum, and for the different body proportions of infants. Used on a clipboard these diagrams can be most useful, especially where there are multiple injuries, or large areas of burns or abrasions. Each lesion can be drawn in, with a measurement noted alongside each and distances from anatomical landmarks recorded. The data from the sketches can be transposed to written form at the end of the examination.

Discussion and conclusions in an autopsy report

Some pathologists, usually those not normally concerned with criminal and litigious cases, claim that an autopsy report should be a bare recitation of the physical findings, with no discussion or interpretation of the significance of those findings. In the authors' opinion, this is an abdication of the pathologist's responsibility because, especially in criminal deaths, it is these conclusions that are of most interest and use to the investigating officers, lawyers and courts.

After the detailed description of the external and internal appearances, a short resumé should be offered of the major positive findings and their relationship to the cause of death. In many cases this will be obvious, as in a gunshot wound of the head. Matters such as the probable type of weapon, the range, the direction and the likely rapidity of death, however, should also be discussed.

When the findings are less clear cut, or are multiple, then the alternatives should be discussed, giving a differential diagnosis of the cause of death and detailing the possible sequence of events. If it is possible, a ranking order of probability of the various alternatives can be offered. Time of death and the limitations of accuracy in this particular case should be set out when the issue is relevant to the investigation. What is really required is as full an interpretation as possible, without venturing into the undesirable fields of unwarranted speculation or Sherlock Holmes style of over-interpretation, which was the bane of forensic pathology in former years and is still practised too much even today, to the detriment of the good reputation of the speciality.

POST-MORTEM ARTEFACTS

Forensic pathology can only be learned by experience but no account would be complete without drawing attention to common artefacts found at autopsy, which can mislead the pathologist with insufficient forensic experience and even lead to a miscarriage of justice.

Some of the 'classic' mistakes were described many years ago by Shapiro (1954) and Moritz (1942), but each generation of pathologists discovers them a new – or what is worse, fails to discover them. Most artefacts are described in the various chapters dealing with specific lesions, but a reminder of some of the most important is given here:

- The pancreas is one of the first organs to undergo autolysis, because of the proteolytic enzymes within it. The autolysed tissue is often haemorrhagic and can easily be mistaken for acute pancreatitis, though histology will rapidly resolve the problem.
- Patches of haemorrhage, sometimes quite large and confluent, can occur in the tissues behind the oesophagus in the neck. These lie on the anterior surface of the cervical vertebrae and are caused by distension and leakage from the venous plexuses that lie in this area. They were described well by Prinsloo and Gordon (1951) and are sometimes known by this name. Their importance lies in confusion with deep neck bleeding in strangulation (and sometimes with spurious neck fractures), which is why the skull should be opened before the neck in any suspected strangulation or hanging, to release the pressure in the neck veins before handling the tissues.
- Autolytic rupture of the stomach can occur post-mortem in both child and adult, described by John Hunter in the eighteenth century. This so-called 'gastromalacia' appears as a slimy brownish black disintegration of the fundus with release of the stomach contents into the peritoneal cavity. Sometimes, the left leaf of the diaphragm is also perforated through a ragged fenestration, with escape of gastric contents into the chest.
- Heat fractures of the bones, either skull plates or long bones, may be seen in victims of severe fires, but are not evidence of ante-mortem violence. Also in conflagrations, the 'heat haematoma' within the burned skull can resemble an extradural haemorrhage of ante-mortem origin. The site is often at the vertex or occiput; however, unlike the usual parietal haemorrhage, there is no fracture line crossing the middle meningeal artery, the usual cause of a true extradural bleed. The frothy brown appearance of the false clot, together with heating effects in the adjacent brain, should indicate the true diagnosis. Shrinkage of the dura due to heat may cause it to split, with herniation of the brain tissue into the extradural space. Severe burns of the body surface may lead to heat contractures of the limbs with tears over joints such as the elbow. These must not be confused with ante-mortem lacerations or incised wounds.
- The bloating, discoloration and blistering of a putrefying body must not be misinterpreted as disease on injury. Blisters are quite unlike those of burns and dark blackish areas of discoloration must be distinguished from bruising. The latter can be difficult and incision into the tissues to seek blood in the dermis is advised. Histological sections may help but, where a body is badly decomposed, special stains for blood traces in the histological sections may assist, such as alpha-glycophorin to detect red cell envelopes. However, often it is quite impossible to differentiate the discoloration of decomposition from true bruising.
- Blood or bloody fluid issuing from the mouth may be due to putrefaction, even if the body surface is not overtly decomposed. If the lungs and air passages are discoloured and filled with sanguineous liquid, then this must be taken to be cause of the purging from the mouth and nostrils.
- Dark red discoloration of the posterior part of the myocardium is usually due to post-mortem gravitational hypostasis, not early infarction. Similarly, segmental patches of dark red or purple discoloration of the intestine is hypostasis, not infarction. The latter tends to be a single continuous length, the serosa being dull and the gut wall friable.
- Large petechiae or ecchymoses, sometimes with raised blood blisters, are often seen in the dependent skin of persons who have died a congestive death or where the upper part of the body has been hanging down after death. The usual place where these are seen is over the front of the upper chest and across the back of the shoulders, though in dependent heads the face may be shot with haemorrhages.
- Resuscitation artefacts are of increasing importance to the forensic pathologist and are discussed later.

EXHUMATION

Exhumation is the retrieval of a previously buried body for post-mortem examination. This is usually followed by a first autopsy or a re-autopsy following new information. The term 'exhumation' is usually applied to the removal of a body buried in a legitimate fashion in a cemetery or graveyard ('inhumation'), rather than the recovery of an uncoffined, clandestinely buried victim of a suspicious death. The latter is really a true 'scene of crime' and the pathologist should treat it as such.

Exhumations are required for one of the following reasons:

- Where all or part of a graveyard has to be moved for some development of the ground. Often no special examination of each body is made unless there is some historical or anthropological interest.
- Where some civil legal matter needs to be investigated, such as personal injuries for insurance or civil litigation for negligence – usually after a road, industrial or other accident.
- Where new information or substantiated allegations arise to suggest that a death was due to criminal action, either from injury or poison.
- In ancient or historical circumstances to investigate either the individual or a series of individuals for academic interest. A number of such investigations have been carried out on medieval and later inhumations in England, to study disease patterns and nutritional states in old populations – though many of these have been from dry vaults, rather than earth burials.

The legal procedures authorizing an exhumation do not concern us here, as they vary greatly from country to country. In all jurisdictions, however, there must be strict safeguards to identify the grave and the coffin, so that no mistake can be made. The grave must be positively identified by the cemetery authorities by reference to plans and records: an official must personally point out the grave to be opened.

Traditionally, exhumations are carried out at dawn but, except to avoid spectators and publicity, there is no real need to stumble about in a dark cemetery before first light. A better plan is for the grave to be dug down to just above coffin level by a mechanical digger or workmen on the previous day so that, the following morning, the police, coroner, pathologist and others can arrive in time to see the final exposure of the coffin. The coffin nameplate must be cleaned and read to confirm the identity, and, if possible, the funeral director who carried out the original burial should be present to identify the coffin and the plate.

If there is a suspicion of poisoning, samples of earth should have been taken from the surface of the grave, from other parts of the cemetery and from immediately above the coffin. When the coffin has been removed, further samples should be obtained from the sides and beneath the coffin, but these matters will usually be attended to by forensic scientists.

When the coffin is lifted to the graveside it is as well for the lid to be loosened a little by slackening the holding screws or prising the lid loose. This allows foul gases to escape into the open air, rather than in the mortuary. The coffin is then transported to the mortuary; if it is in a bad state of decay, it may have to be supported on a rigid base such as a trestle, or placed inside an extra large coffin or fibreglass shell. Excess earth and mud should be removed before transportation to avoid excessive fouling of the autopsy room. Where criminal action is suspected or has been alleged, a full photographic record must be kept (usually by the police) of every stage from identification of the grave to the findings during the autopsy.

At the mortuary, the coffin lid should be completely removed and the contents again identified, if possible by the funeral director who originally buried the body. He can again confirm the coffin plate, but also identify the internal coffin fittings, such as fabrics and shroud. When the body has not been buried for too long, he may be able to identify the features of the corpse from personal knowledge.

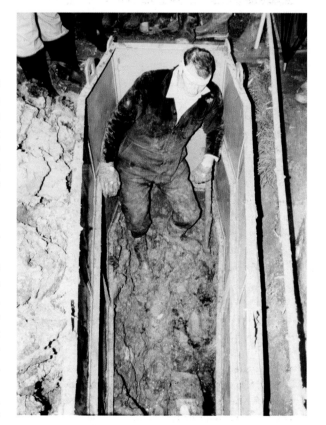

FIGURE 1.23 *Exhumation: a police officer making the final approach to the coffin. A metal cassion is lowered to protect the gravesides. The grave must be identified by the cemetery superintendent.*

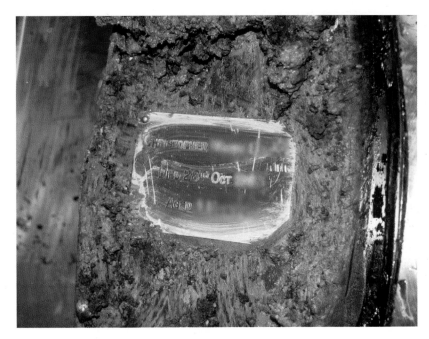

FIGURE 1.24 *Exhumation: when the coffin is exposed it must be identified by the funeral director and the coffin plate checked. If death from poisoning is suspected, samples of earth from above, below and the sides of the coffin as well as from a distant part of the cemetery must be taken, together with a sample of any grave water.*

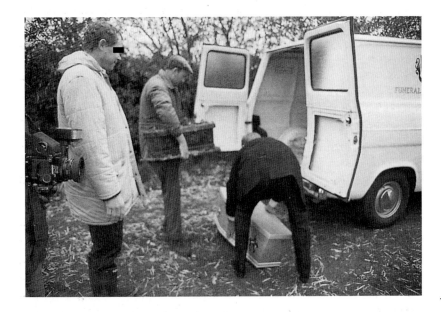

FIGURE 1.25 *Following exhumation, the body is transported to a mortuary for full autopsy. The former practice of autopsy in inadequate premises near the cemetery is no longer justified. Here the original rotted infant coffin is placed within a new coffin for transit.*

If poisoning is suspected, samples of the shroud, coffin trimming and any loose material such as packing or fluid should be retained for analysis. The body is then removed, undressed and a full autopsy carried out, as far as the condition of the body allows. Putrefaction, adipocere and mummification complicate the examination – sometimes, all three may be present in the same body.

The pathologist is sometimes asked by the authorities or by lawyers whether a proposed exhumation is worth carrying out, because of doubts about the usefulness of the result. Certainly the balance between the potential advantages must be weighed against the cost, publicity and distress to relatives that might be caused. In general, however, it is surprising how much information may be gained even when the body has been buried for many months or even a few years. Much will depend on the actual environment of the grave: a gravel or sandy soil, especially in an elevated position, will allow a body to remain in a much better state of preservation than one in the waterlogged loam of a valley. The author (BK) has seen burials only 20 years old with empty coffins containing silt, but no soft tissue or even bones (due to a constantly rising and falling water table) in an area of acidic peat.

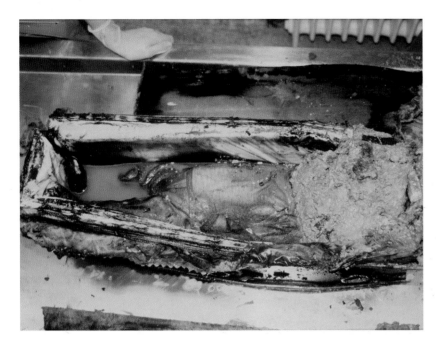

FIGURE 1.26 *When the coffin is first opened in the mortuary, the coffin fitting and fabrics should again be identified by the funeral director, as well as the body and its clothes, if they can be recollected. This infant has been buried for 3 years. The upper part of the coffin has leaked, allowing liquid mud to cover and substantially destroy the head.*

Even negative information gained at exhumation, such as the absence of alleged or suspected fractures, may be of considerable legal value. Some poisons, especially heavy metals, may persist for many years in a buried body and be detectable at exhumation. Even some organic chemicals may survive for a long time; barbiturates have been found after 7 years in a buried body. In all cases of suspected poisoning, it is vital that ample control samples are taken from the grave and its surroundings, to avoid the later accusation that any abnormal substances found were environmental artefacts or were unassociated with the corpse.

THE AUTOPSY ON THE PUTREFIED CORPSE

In forensic work, decomposed bodies are commonplace, especially in warm climates. Though the value of an autopsy is progressively reduced as the state of putrefaction advances, no short cuts should be taken by the pathologist merely because of the unpleasant nature of the examination. However bad the condition of the corpse, every effort should be made to carry out the autopsy as near to the usual routine as possible. It is often surprising – as with an exhumation – how much information can be gained. The interior of the body is often far better preserved than the outward appearances would suggest, so a policy of defeatism that leads to a skimped examination should never be adopted.

Externally, putrefaction hides bruising to a variable degree, the greenish black coloration of the skin masking the usual features of contusion. Abrasions, lacerations, incised wounds and gunshot wounds may, however, survive severe degrees of decomposition. Loss of bloody fluid from the mouth and nostrils (the so-called 'purging') is often mistaken by public, police and even some doctors as evidence of haemorrhage, but loss of serous, bloody or frothy fluid from any body orifice is common in the advanced stages of putrefaction.

Peeling and slippage of skin may hide some abrasions, though they may be visible when the desquamated epidermis is removed and the underlying skin examined. Marks around the neck from the tissues swelling with gas and becoming embedded in a collar have been mistaken for strangulation.

Where maggot or other insect infestation is present, some may be taken for expert entomological examination to help in assessing the post-mortem interval, as described in Chapter 2. As stated above, the external examination should be conducted as near as possible to the routine for a fresh body, and the back and perineum not neglected because of physical difficulties in handling the body.

Identity may be a problem when the facial features are too bloated for visual recognition. The usual procedures described in the next chapter may be employed where necessary. Fingerprints may be required by the police to assist in identity, but decomposition may seriously destroy the fingertips. These may become swollen and desquamate, or may shrivel and become leathery. Several methods of restoring the amputated tips have been described: some recommend a simple method of immersing the tips in 20 per cent acetic acid for 28–48 hours, when the shrivelling will swell to normal size. Others recommend immersion in glycerine.

Internally, much will depend on the state of decay. The abdominal and chest organs may be in a better state of preservation than the exterior. The subcutaneous tissues may be distended and crepitant with gas, as may be the swollen abdomen. Judicious penetration of the peritoneum with the tip of knife may be needed to release the pressure of gas. The technique of lighting the escaping methane with a burning newspaper may be spectacular and sometimes near explosive, but does little to reduce the smell and is not to be recommended.

Examination of the organs follows the usual pattern, modified according to state of putrefaction. The heart may be limp and discoloured, with haemolysis staining of the endocardium and vessels. The coronary arteries are often very well preserved, especially if atheromatous or calcified, or both. Ante-mortem thrombi may persist even after the muscle is semiglutinous. The larynx may be discoloured, but the hyoid and thyroid horns can be examined for fractures and may need to be X-rayed. It may be difficult to detect ante-mortem bleeding at the fracture sites. Fractures elsewhere in the skeleton naturally persist and may require radiography for their detection, as may foreign objects such as bullets.

The brain often decomposes early, and all too often is merely a pinkish-grey paste within the dura. Gross lesions like a large meningeal or intracranial haemorrhage may survive for examination, but the trauma of removing the calvarium and attached dura may seriously damage a semi-fluid brain. In Belgium, where exhumations are common due to the very low primary autopsy rate, a technique was developed in the University of Gent whereby the head of a decomposed body was removed from the body and deep frozen until solid. The head was then cut across in the coronal plane with a band-saw, leaving the brain in two halves within the cranium. These were then immersed in a large volume of formalin until fixed, when they could be removed in a relatively solid state for examination.

Internally, the detection of true subcutaneous bruising may be very difficult due to the discoloration of putrefaction. Histology is often highly unsatisfactory because of cellular lysis and degeneration; stains for haemoglobin may help in revealing focal collections of lysed blood, but are often diffusely positive even in control areas. Claims have been made for staining for glycophorin A to detect red cell envelopes, as opposed to diffuse haemolysis (Kibayashi *et al.* 1993).

RESUSCITATION ARTEFACTS AT AUTOPSY

In recent years, the advent of effective, but often aggressive and invasive, resuscitation procedures has made the task of the pathologist more difficult. At autopsy, injuries and abnormalities are now often found that could be due to terminal and even post-mortem resuscitatory measures. Where the pathologist is made aware of these, he can often exclude the damage being due to non-resuscitatory injury, though even when he is informed of the procedures they can still mask or mimic more sinister trauma. When he is not made aware – or such information cannot be made available – then the difficulties of interpretation are compounded.

There are now many publications describing resuscitation artefacts, including the review of Leadbeatter and Knight (1988). The following are the main categories of damage, for which the pathologist must always be alert:

- Bruising of the anterior chest wall, haemorrhage into the subcutaneous tissues and pectoral muscles, fractures of the sternum, fractures of the ribs, haemothorax, bruised lung, lacerated lung, pericardial haemorrhage, and even fractured dorsal spine, following energetic external cardiopulmonary resuscitation (CPR). Thoracic cage fractures are rare in children, however, because of the pliability of the ribs and costal cartilages, but it cannot be denied that they sometimes occur. The differentiation is naturally of vital interest where child abuse is being alleged.

  Internally all types of damage to the heart may occur, including ruptured atria and even ventricles, septal rupture and valve damage. The great vessels can suffer severe trauma, as described in the now extensive publications on resuscitation artefacts. Fat and bone marrow emboli in the pulmonary vessels have also been reported after cardiac massage (Mason 1993).

  Petechiae in the eyes and intra-ocular haemorrhages can occur after CPR, as well as after violent sneezing or coughing; they are well known to occur during whooping cough.

- Bruising of the face and neck, finger marks and nail marks on the face and neck, and damage to the lips and inner gums from mouth-to-mouth resuscitation, when the face and neck have been gripped by hands. Damage to lips, gums, teeth and pharynx can occur from the introduction of an artificial airway or endotracheal tube, especially in difficult, hurried emergency situations.

  Injuries to the larynx, even including fracture of the hyoid and thyroid cornuae, can occasionally occur from these procedures, which are difficult to distinguish from manual strangulation if the circumstances are obscure.

- Puncture marks for venepuncture may be confused with injection marks in drug dependence. The introduction of intravenous cannulae into veins in the neck may cause large haematomata and more diffuse bleeding into the tissues alongside the larynx.

Similar bruising may occur around puncture sites in the arms and groin. Intracardiac injections leave marks on the chest wall and may lead to a slight haemopericardium. The effects of injected noradrenaline and electrical defibrillation on the histological appearance of the myocardium are well recorded, with contraction bands being the most obvious artefacts which can be mistaken for pre-existing myocardial ischaemia.

- Damage to the mouth, palate, pharynx and larynx can occur from attempts to introduce a laryngoscope or airway. Even fracture of the mandible has been caused in this way. In infants, even digital clearance of the pharynx can cause mucosal damage. Damage to the pharyngeal mucosa may cause bleeding, which can seem sinister to police or relatives; this may be mixed with the fluid of pulmonary oedema to produce copious pink, bloody froth, seen in a number of cases, including sudden infant death syndrome.

- Electric defibrillator pads make marks on the chest, though these are usually easy to interpret, except where there is an unusual shape. Defibrillators and injected β-adrenergic catecholamines such as noradrenaline can, however, cause widespread histological damage to the myocardium, consisting of coagulation necrosis and contraction bands, which can be confused with infarction or electrocution. When both defibrillation and catecholamines have been used to resuscitate, the myocardial changes are even more marked (Karch 1987).

- During the Heimlich manoeuvre to clear an airway obstruction, rupture of the oesophagus, stomach and intestines have been reported. The oesophagus can be perforated by an incorrectly inserted airway. In the abdomen, external cardiac massage may cause ruptured stomach, ruptured liver, and damage to spleen and pancreas.

- Gastric contents in the air passages may have reached there by spontaneous agonal regurgitation or by pumping the chest and upper abdomen during resuscitation attempts. This makes the finding of vomit in the larynx and trachea of even less significance as a cause of death, as discussed in Chapter 14.

- The administration of oxygen by mask or tube may cause damage, as can overenergetic mouth-to-mouth resuscitation. Ruptures of oesophagus and lung have occurred, and other types of barotrauma include ruptured stomach and intestine. Where a pre-existing gut lesion exists, the administered gas may escape into the abdomen. The diagnosis of a pre-existing

pneumothorax may be impossible where forced ventilation has been administered.

- In the central nervous system, subarachnoid haemorrhage has been described after external cardiac massage, and from hyperextension of the neck to pass an airway or perform mouth-to-mouth resuscitation. The forced posture can tear the vertebral arteries, making another source of confusion for the forensic pathologist in this difficult area of potential trauma to the neck (Chapter 5).

- Myocardial and pulmonary bone marrow embolism has been reported following cardiac massage (Dziecol *et al.* 1992).

- Retinal haemorrhages, classically a sign of raised intracranial pressure and of head injury, have also been described in whooping cough and after CPR.

- Miscellaneous artefacts of which every pathologist should be aware include: skin maceration from a body lying in urine, kerosene, etc., post-mortem burns from adjacent radiant heat or hot-water bottles; and petechiae and larger haemorrhages in the face from postural hypostasis.

MASS DISASTERS – THE ROLE OF THE PATHOLOGIST

With the exception of the more dramatic murders, the activity which focuses most public attention on the work of forensic pathologists is the mass disaster. Unfortunately, such tragedies are becoming more common with the increase in terrorism, the expansion of travel facilities and the larger size of passenger aircraft. Recent years have seen a tragically frequent need for the expertise of mass disaster teams, following such events as the Zeebrugge and Estonian ferry capsizes, football tragedies like Ibrox Park, Heysel, Moscow and Hillsborough, crush tragedies at Mecca, and numerous massive aircraft crashes, such as Tenerife, Air India, Japan, Lockerbie and most recently the terror attacks in the USA. Mass disaster management is a discipline in itself and only the briefest summary can be offered here, together with useful references at the end of the section.

Forward planning

Many pathologists will thankfully spend their entire careers without having to participate in a major mass disaster; a commonly accepted definition is the death of more than 12 victims in a single event. No one can predict when such a tragedy might occur, however, as typified by the 1988

Pan Am sabotage, when almost 300 bodies fell out of the sky on a quiet and unsuspecting Scottish village. It is thus essential that every forensic institute, department and individual pathologist should make some forward provision for such an eventuality. In Britain, the Royal College of Pathologists (1990) have published a useful booklet on the role of the pathologist in these disasters.

In most advanced countries each region now has a Mass Casualty Plan covering medical and hospital services, fire service and police. This is often very detailed, covering every aspect of transfusion, drugs, casualty transport, emergency surgery and anaesthesia. The plans are clinically orientated, but often completely ignore provision for the dead – or they have some cursory statement at the end such as 'Mortuary accommodation will be provided' with obviously no thought given to how several hundred corpses are to be accommodated and examined. Though clinical planning is, of course, vital – especially in rail disasters, multiple motorway crashes and urban bomb outrages – it has to be appreciated that, in many air crashes, there are few if any survivors, and that all the clinical planning may be redundant, leaving a massive and unprepared crisis in relation to the dead.

It is therefore essential that forensic pathologists should ensure that, in the area for which they are responsible, there is cooperative preplanning that includes adequate provision for collection, accommodation, examination and disposal of large numbers of dead victims. Naturally the pathologist is usually in no position to do this alone, but he is often the person with the most foresight and professional knowledge to act as the stimulus and catalyst between the major agencies responsible for overall planning. These are usually the police and the local health administration. When a Mass Casualty Plan does exist, but has serious omissions in respect of dealing with the dead, or where no such plan exists, the forensic pathologist should energetically stimulate the responsible authorities into making a comprehensive plan. This entails a series of meetings to identify danger areas in the region (such as airports, motorways, railways and military installations), and to discuss potential buildings for temporary mortuaries, the provision of materials such as markers, plastic bags and labels, which may be needed in large quantities at a few hours' notice. Communications between such groups as police, pathologists, mortuary and laboratory technicians, radiographers, and dentists also need to be established in advance. The expertise of international funeral directors with experience in mass disaster fatalities is invaluable.

The objects of pathological investigation in mass disasters are:

- to retrieve and reconstruct bodies and fragmented bodies decently
- to establish personal identity
- to conduct autopsies on some or all of those bodies
- to establish the cause of death in some or all, especially air crew and drivers, and to assist in reconstructing the cause of the disaster
- to obtain material for toxicological analysis (especially alcohol and carbon monoxide) where appropriate
- to seek evidence of the cause of the disaster from autopsy examination, such as bomb or detonator fragments that may be embedded in the bodies.

Outline of necessities in mass disaster planning

PROVISION OF PATHOLOGISTS AND OTHER STAFF

Depending upon the scale of the tragedy, it may be necessary to recruit other pathologists to assist. In large cities, there may be sufficient persons with expert forensic knowledge, but elsewhere, hospital pathologists may be able to assist; forensic pathologists from a distance may also volunteer. It has to be remembered that a really large disaster may need many days or even weeks of work, and therefore personnel may be unavailable for the whole period. In addition, whatever the degree of willingness and unselfish devotion offered by doctors and all other staff, the physical and especially psychological stresses of this harrowing work mean that strictly limited periods of work should be imposed. Apart from the deleterious effect upon the doctor, the standard of work declines dramatically with fatigue and therefore it is in the interests of the investigation – as well as of the pathologists – that sufficient staff be recruited. This may, however, be easier said than done. One person must be in overall charge of the investigation. Usually a senior police officer has the ultimate responsibility, but the medical aspects should be firmly under the control of a senior pathologist, though he must delegate extensively to avoid being swamped by less important tasks and thereby being rendered totally inefficient. Again, all these aspects are modified by the scale of the disaster. Proper facilities for meals, rest and washing must be established, and again forward planning is essential for these mundane, but vital, features. Forensic dental and radiological expertise will be run independently by their own specialists, but there must still be a nominal chief in the form of the senior pathologist who acts as overall coordinator and arbiter of medical matters.

When a disaster, almost always an aircraft crash, occurs in some remote place or abroad where there are no satisfactory forensic or pathological services, it is the usual practice for a team from the country of origin of the aircraft – or a volunteer team arranged at governmental level – to fly to the scene and provide expertise to the local authorities.

In many advanced countries, especially Britain, the armed services have permanent aviation pathologists who deal with all service aircraft crashes anywhere in the world and who are often available to deal with, or attend as advisers, any civil air disaster.

PROVISION OF MORTUARY FACILITIES

Most hospital mortuaries and even larger public mortuaries have limited storage capacity for bodies, and even smaller provision for performing simultaneous autopsies. It must also be appreciated that the normal business of a mortuary has to continue even through a mass disaster, so the massive increase in work is an addition to, not a substitution for, the normal handling facilities. Where more than about ten bodies are involved, most mortuaries cannot cope with these problems, especially when it has to be remembered that some of the corpses may have to be retained for considerably longer periods than usual if identification cannot be made rapidly. Thus external facilities will have to be provided in some temporary accommodation. When the disaster is a long distance from the regular mortuary, transport and other logistic considerations may make it imperative to store and examine the bodies nearer to the crash site. Again forward planning is essential to identify hangars, storehouses, empty factories, halls and other buildings near potential danger spots such as airports. Whenever possible, all bodies should be taken to one site, as the separation of identification sites is a recipe for inconvenience, delay and mistakes. It is sometimes necessary, especially in remote regions, to set up tented mortuaries, but this is a last resort as facilities cannot be laid on with the same degree of efficiency. Where the crash is totally remote, it is usual for the authorities or the armed services to bring out the dead by helicopter or other transport to an urban site. A prime example was the Mount Erebus crash in Antarctica, where the dead were flown back to New Zealand. If a warehouse, or factory or building of similar size, can be used, certain minimum facilities are needed. Good electric lighting, portable lights for close inspection, and power points for radiographic equipment and electric instruments are required. Adequate piped water, and washing and toilet facilities are essential. If any of these is deficient, then portable generators and water tankers must be supplied by the armed services or the police. Telephone and, if possible, telex and fax facilities should be available for the input of identifying data.

In hot climates, or in the summer in temperate climates, body refrigeration is vital, not only for the decent preservation of the dead but for retention of tissues awaiting identification. If a disaster is too large to be handled in the usual mortuary, then some form of cooling is required. The renting of refrigerated trucks used for the transport of foodstuffs is the usual answer and, again, preplanning is necessary to discover sources of such facilities. Sometimes portable air-conditioning units can be installed in part of the mortuary, if this is sufficient to cool the storage area to an acceptable level. In disasters where there are both living and dead victims, the mortuary should be sited away from the clinical facilities or screened in some way to avoid the distressing sight of bodies arriving being visible to survivors or their relatives, and the press.

The temporary mortuary should be large enough for the expected load, and the area to be used for examinations and autopsies should not be too congested. No one should be allowed in who does not have direct business there, no matter of what eminence or rank. Security of admission should be tight, this being the responsibility of the police. Flooring should be waterproof and capable of being hosed down. It can be protected against blood, mud and burned fragments by covering with polythene from large rolls. Tables for examination can be wooden trestles, covered with polythene. These should be in rows one metre apart, with 2 metres between rows.

Retrieval of bodies

This is the task of the police or armed services, but must be carried out in a manner approved by the forensic identifying team. It is essential that every body is first certified as dead by a doctor at the scene. Often, volunteer casualty surgeons may be the first medical persons at the scene, whose primary duty is to rescue living survivors and to confirm death in the remainder.

Each body or fragment should be flagged with a sequential and unrepeatable serial number and marked on a grid plan, being photographed *in situ* wherever possible. It is then bagged and taken with its numbered label to the mortuary. Different teams will have different methods of dealing with the logistics of handling data and, increasingly, this is being performed on either microcomputers or on terminals linked to a central computer. The police have responsibility for these aspects, as they collect and record the clothing and personal belongings that play such an important part in personal identification.

Either the same serial number is used from the recovery stage or a different 'pathology' number is begun in the mortuary, which must be matched up with the previous serial number. Everything that has come from that body, including clothing, wallets, rings, teeth and jewellery, must carry the same number.

The pathologist and lay assistants undress the clothed bodies, and dictate a description of what is found as accompanying artefacts. The clothes are stored in strong paper

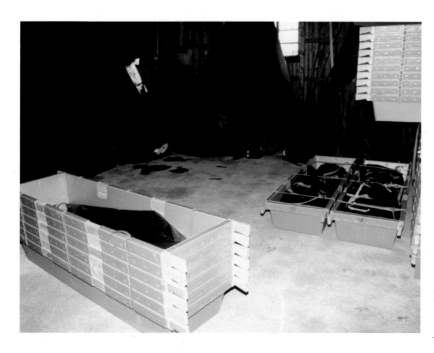

FIGURE 1.27 *Temporary coffins used to transport victims of the m/s Estonia disaster from the archipelago to the autopsy facility.*

bags to avoid the fungal growth that inevitably appears on damp fabric kept in plastic bags.

Many items will have been found loose at the site, but they must all be tagged and an attempt made to relate them to a nearby body, though this is obviously fraught with error. The objects found on a body are recorded on an inventory form and a separate form (usually the Interpol document) used for the purely medical and anatopathological aspects. The latter data are acquired by meticulous and systematic external examination, followed by an internal autopsy if this is to be carried out.

Whether or not an autopsy is to be performed on some or all of the victims will depend upon facilities, availability of pathologists, the legal direction and the system prevailing in the particular country. The wishes of the legal authority, such as coroner, judge, medical examiner or police, will be the deciding factor in determining how many victims are subjected to autopsy. The pathologist should exert his influence where there is reluctance to sanction any autopsies, emphasizing the benefit to the crash investigators of autopsy data on key victims. Pathology findings may often be of use – it has even been claimed that victims can be separated into smokers and non-smokers by finding 'smoker cells' in the lungs (Reiter and Risser 1994).

As mentioned, the aircrew or other persons in charge of a vehicle or train should always have a full examination and analysis of body fluids as part of the accident investigation. Full photography of the clothing and bodies should be taken, and then all physical features such as height, weight, gender, race, colouring, scars, tattoos and deformities must be recorded. The forensic dental examination is then carried

out on those bodies where obvious identity cannot be established by non-medical or dental means.

Radiological examination will almost always be required to assist in identification from osteological features and dental aspects – and perhaps also to seek foreign bodies that may assist in accident reconstruction, such as metal fragments blown upwards into the thighs and buttock in a hold explosion in an aircraft bomb – or even parts of the bomb or detonator itself, more especially in land-based terrorist attacks.

Toxicology should be taken as extensively as possible, even from some of those bodies that are not to have an autopsy. The data acquired from this painstaking work is then forwarded to the police bureau who have been collecting personal data from the records and relatives of the victims, and efforts are made to match the two sets of data. This is increasingly being performed by computer, and many efforts have been made by international agencies such as Interpol to set up universally compatible systems so that data can be acquired and exchanged electronically via telephone systems and modems from any part of the world.

In 1990, the Royal College of Pathologists published a definitive guide for pathologists to the problem of mass disasters, which is strongly recommended as a standard set of procedures.

THE OBSCURE AUTOPSY

Several surveys in various countries have shown that where a physician offers a cause of death without the benefit of autopsy findings, the error rate is of the order of 25–50 per cent, even in deaths in hospital. Thus the value of an autopsy in improving the value of death certificates is undoubted, but it still has to be conceded that the autopsy is by no means infallible in revealing the true cause of death. Estimates of the frequency with which autopsies fail to deliver an adequate or even any cause of death vary from pathologist to pathologist, as well as with definitions of what type of case a is included in such series. For example, the sudden infant death syndrome (SIDS) could be considered to provide 'negative autopsies', in that by definition, no significant findings are discovered.

Even excluding SIDS, there is probably at least a 5 per cent 'failure rate' in autopsy series from large medical centres and forensic pathology departments. This rate will also vary according to the habits, personality and seniority of the pathologists involved. Contrary to what might be expected, a higher rate of negative conclusions will originate from older and more experienced pathologists than from juniors. The younger pathologist is often uneasy about failing to provide a cause of death, feeling that it reflects upon his ability, whereas the more grizzled doctor, enjoying the security of tenure and equality with – or even seniority over – his clinical and legal colleagues, is less inhibited in his admissions of ignorance when the cause of death remains obscure.

These 'obscure autopsies' are more common in the younger age group. Even apart from SIDS, many autopsies on infants, especially neonates, are less than satisfactory in terms of definite morphological lesions discoverable in the autopsy room or the laboratory. The deaths often have a biochemical or hypoxic basis and, though inferences can be made from the clinical history, even expert paediatric pathologists have to make do with minimal or even absent findings in a significant proportion of cases. In teenagers and young adults, up to the age of about 35 years, there is a higher proportion of negative autopsies than in the older group, which provides the vast majority of the autopsy workload. An example is the obscure syndrome seen in East Asia, where Thai construction workers in Singapore suddenly die with no demonstrable pathological cause, similar cases occurring in China, Japan and Hong Kong.

This preponderance in the young may carry an inherent fallacy, even though there may be an absolute increase in the incidence of obscure fatal causes. The young adult does not have the almost universal overlay of degenerative cardiovascular disease that is seen in the older group. Thus it is probable that the same occult disease processes occur in that older group as in the young, but as the latter do not have other lesions that can be grasped (usually quite legitimately) as a valid cause of death, then nothing presents itself to the pathologist. For example, on one autopsy table might be the body of a man of 22 who dropped dead shortly after taking

part in a football match. There may be no adverse medical history, the gross examination revealed nothing abnormal and subsequently full histology with special stains, full toxicological screening, and microbiological and virological studies, were unrewarding. No cause of death can be extracted from these negative findings and the case must be recorded as 'unascertained' – or, as Professor Alan Usher of Sheffield points out, as 'unascertainable', if the pathologist is feeling particularly omnipotent!

On the next table in the autopsy room, however, may be a man of 60 who has been found dead with no available history. On examination he is found to have 60 per cent stenosis of the anterior descending branch of his left coronary artery, but no recent or old damage to the myocardium. Histology may well be performed, with no further information obtained. The cause of death is likely to be recorded as 'coronary artery disease' by most pathologists, yet he might well have died from the same obscure cause as the young man, but because he has just sufficient arterial degenerative disease to prove fatal, the latter is accepted as the most likely cause of death. This feeling of disillusion may be reinforced by the presence on the third autopsy table of another man of 60 who has been killed by a firearm, yet who has 80 per cent stenosis of all three coronary vessels, this obviously having played no part in the death.

Whatever the philosophical aspects of this problem, the practical difficulty remains of the pathologist's course of action when faced with negative findings in an autopsy.

At the end of the gross examination in the autopsy room, as the depressing realization increases that nothing significant has been found, further action will depend partly upon the facilities available to the pathologist, especially in relation to toxicological, biochemical, microbiological, virological and histological laboratory service.

Before proceeding further to review the dissection, attention must be paid to obtaining adequate samples for ancillary investigations. In many cases, especially where the history alerts the experienced pathologist that this might be a difficult case – and usually always in young people – samples of blood, urine and stomach contents will have been taken as routine during the removal and first dissection of the viscera.

If a blood sample has not already been taken, it should now be obtained, preferably from a peripheral vein such as the axillary or femoral to avoid contamination from the now empty trunk cavities. If urine was not retained from the bladder, a few drops may still be found in that opened organ by suction with a syringe. Stomach contents may well have been lost, but the liver can be retained for toxicological analysis. It might be useful to take vitreous humour if urine and stomach contents have been lost.

Some blood may be used for inoculation of blood culture bottles and swabs can still be taken for microbiological investigations. If a lung infection is possible, then either a few grams of lung tissue can be removed into a sterile jar, or swabs can be taken from peripheral bronchi or from the lung parenchyma itself. As the surface of all cut organs will have been contaminated during the first dissection, cuts should be made into the surface of the lung using a new sterile scalpel so that relatively fresh tissue is obtained for culture. At the same time, a cube of lung – or other organ if desired – should be taken into a sterile container for virus studies.

Before tissue for histology is taken, a full review of the more vital parts of the dissection should be reviewed. Even in younger victims the first area to be studied again is the coronary system, and in older obscure deaths it is essential to re-examine these vessels. Although the coronaries should have been transected at short intervals (not more than 3 mm apart) on the first examination, it is prudent to retrace each vessel carefully from the aortic origin distally, looking again at each cut segment and, where the interval appears too large, to make further intermediate cuts. In addition, it may be wise to join the segments longitudinally between cuts, in case a small isolated thrombus is lurking in the lumen. This should be done for common left trunk, anterior descending branch, left circumflex and right coronary artery.

This review of the coronary system sometimes pays dividends, especially in the middle-aged group that at first sight appears to have good coronary vessels. A tiny segment may be occluded or severely stenosed over a distance of only 2 or 3 mm, either by pure atheroma or by a subintimal haemorrhage, ruptured plaque or a localized thrombosis. If nothing is found, then after a quick review of the valves and great vessels, the myocardium can be sliced more extensively and a number of representative blocks taken for histology, to seek a myocarditis or some obscure cardiomyopathy.

The other organs should be examined again, the pulmonary arteries being scrutinized for pulmonary emboli in the smaller branches. This is rarely productive, but the author (BK) has on several occasions found multiple small emboli in more peripheral lung vessels, although whether these were a valid cause of death was debatable. The brain should be looked at once more, with special attention being paid to the basal arteries. These should be opened with coronary scissors and the dissection carried up into the middle cerebral arteries where they lie in the Sylvian fissures. It is also always worthwhile looking in the carotid arteries in the neck, though these should always be opened routinely at the first dissection from the aorta to a point just distal to the carotid sinuses; even the difficult area above this at the base of the skull has provided some surprises in the past. It is a place rarely examined, except by neuropathologists, but forensic pathologists should add it to their 'repertoire', as occasionally total thrombotic occlusion may be found, especially following some undisclosed neck injury.

When a complete review of the gross pathology has proved fruitless, then a full histological survey is required, especially of the myocardium. Special stains such as phosphotungstic acid-haematoxylin, dehydrogenase enzyme histochemistry (which requires unfixed, frozen sections), acridine-orange fluorescence stains and any other technique that the pathologist favours. Admittedly, where no cardiomegaly or coronary artery stenosis is present, the chances of finding an abnormality are slight, but an isolated myocarditis is an outside chance.

Toxicology may be difficult and expensive if there is no cause to suspect any particular drug or poison. A screen for unknown substances can be time consuming for the laboratory, which means a large expense to public funds. An alcohol estimation and a screen for acidic and basic substances, however, though not comprehensive, can at least exclude most common poisons. Microbiology and virology rarely point to a previously unsuspected fatal disease process unless the patient had clinical signs and symptoms before death.

When all the results are available, which may take several weeks (especially in the case of virus cultures), the case must be reviewed and an honest opinion offered as to whether any positive findings are sufficient to have caused death. In the experience of the authors, these ancillary investigations more often provide no help, than the times when they offer some assistance, but they must be carried out whenever possible in order to exclude such causes and to prevent allegations that the death was not investigated as fully as it should have been.

If at the end of the process no cause of death is apparent, then the appropriate investigating authority must be informed that no opinion can be offered in the present state of medical and scientific knowledge. It can be added, however, that the absence of injuries, evidence of poisoning, lethal infection or well-recognized natural disease is in itself significant negative evidence in that it confirms what the deceased did not die of, and the assumption is then that the balance of probabilities is that it was natural causes, rather than some unnatural external event.

There must be complete honesty on the part of the pathologist and a readiness to admit that the cause of death cannot be determined. The use of some meaningless euphemism such as 'heart failure' or 'cardiorespiratory arrest' is pointless and merely confuses the issue for non-medical persons such as police or magistrates. As mentioned above, there is a tendency on the part of some younger pathologists or histopathologists who rarely become involved in medico-legal cases to assume some unwarranted disease process or to attribute significance to insignificant findings. A **mode** of death is useless in lieu of a **cause** of death, so is the dangerous practice of using some agonal event such as 'inhalation of vomit' where there is no eyewitness confirmation of such an event taking place during life. It is also useless and positively dangerous to guess at some totally unprovable process, such as 'vagal inhibition', 'reflex cardiac arrest' or 'suffocation', just because these conditions are thought to leave no traces and therefore a death with no traces must be due to such a cause. This is illogical thinking and has led to several miscarriages of justice in the past, as well as to far more family anguish.

As the pathologist increases in experience and maturity, he or she is more ready to concede that he cannot find a cause of death, and this is far more satisfactory. In forensic work, this is not 'abrogating responsibilities' but being objective, sensible and just. There is no point in producing a speculative cause of death if that cannot be substantiated in later court evidence or legal statements. It is, of course, quite justifiable and indeed, part of the pathologist's responsibilities, to discuss the range of possible causes with the authorities responsible for investigating the death, but to be dogmatic about a single cause where the grounds for such a decision are tenuous does not help anyone and can lead to unfortunate consequences.

REFERENCES AND FURTHER READING

Adelson L. 1953. Possible neurological mechanisms for sudden death with minimal anatomical findings. *J Forensic Med* **1**:39–42.

Adelson L. 1974. *The pathology of homicide.* Thomas, Springfield.

Annegers JF, Coan SP. 1999. Sudep: overview of definitions and review of incidence data. *Seizure* **8**:347–52.

Asnaes S, Paaske F. 1980. Uncertainty of determining mode of death in medico-legal material without autopsy – a systematic autopsy study. *Forensic Sci Int* **15**:3–17.

Ball J, Desselberger U, Whitwell H. 1991. Long-lasting viability of HIV after patient's death. [letter] *Lancet* **6**:63.

Bankowski MJ, Landay AL, Staes B, *et al.* 1992. Postmortem recovery of human immunodeficiency virus type 1 from plasma and mononuclear cells. Implications for occupational exposure. *Arch Pathol Lab Med* **116**:1124–7.

Boukis D. 1986. Repeat autopsies on corpses from abroad. A futile effort? *Am J Forensic Med Pathol* **7**:216–18.

Bowen DA. 1966. The role of radiology and the identification of foreign bodies at postmortem examination. *J Forensic Sci Soc* **6**:28–34.

Braden G. 1975. Aircraft type crash injury investigation of a commuter train collision. *Aviat Space Environ Med* **46**:1157–60.

Brown T, Delaney R, Robinson W. 1952. Medical identification in the noronic disaster. *JAMA* **148**:621.

Buck N, Devlin HB, Lunn JN. 1988. *The report of a confidential enquiry into perioperative deaths. Perioperative deaths*, vol 39. Nuffield Provincial Hospitals Trust, London.

Cameron JM, Grant JH, Ruddick R. 1973. Ultra-violet photography in forensic medicine. *J Forensic Photogr* **2**:9–14.

Cameron HM, McGoogan E, Clarke J, Wilson BA. 1977. Trends in hospital necropsy rates. *Br Med J* **18**:1577–80.

Cameron HM, McGoogan E, Watson H. 1980. Necropsy: a yardstick for clinical diagnoses. *Br Med J* **11**:985–8.

Campling EA, Devlin HB, Lunn JN. 1990. *Gynaecology and the national confidential enquiry into perioperative deaths.* Royal College of Surgeons, London, pp. 466–7.

Camps FE. 1953. *Medical and scientific investigations in the Christie case.* Medical Publications, London.

Camps FE. 1972. Exhumation. *Criminologist* **7**:736.

Cao Y, Ngai H, Gu G, Ho DD. 1993. Decay of HIV-1 infectivity in whole blood, plasma and peripheral blood mononuclear cells. *AIDS* **7**:596–7.

Carpenter R, Dorn J, Hopkins B, *et al.* 1986. *Multiple death disaster response.* National Funeral Directors Association, Milwaukee, WI.

Clark DH. 1986. Dental identification problems in the Abu Dhabi air accident. *Am J Forensic Med Pathol* **7**:317–21.

Clark MA. 1981. The value of the hospital autopsy. Is it worth the cost? *Am J Forensic Med Pathol* **2**:231–7.

Clark MA. 1981. Applications of clinical laboratory tests to the autopsy: a practical guide for specimen collection. *Am J Forensic Med Pathol* **2**:75–81.

Claydon SM. 1993. The high risk autopsy. Recognition and protection. *Am J Forensic Med Pathol* **14**:253–6.

Copeland AR. 1986. Accidental non-commercial aircraft fatalities: the 7-year Metro-Dade county experience from 1977–1983. *Forensic Sci Int* **31**:13–20.

Cordner SM. 1985. The role of the second post-mortem examination. *Med Leg J* **53**:24–8.

Corwell WS. 1956. Radiography and photography in problems of identification. *Med Radiogr Photogr* **32**:34–40.

Cotton DW, Stephenson TJ. 1988. Impairment of autopsy histology by organ washing – a myth. *Med Sci Law* **28**:319–23.

Couch S, Noguchi TT, Wright J. 1981. Demonstrative evidence developed at the autopsy. *Am J Forensic Med Pathol* **2**:135–8.

de Craemer D. 1994. Postmortem viability of human immunodeficiency – implications for the teaching of anatomy. [letter] *N Engl J Med* **331**:1315.

Dodds JP, Nardone A, Mercey DE, *et al.* 2000. Increase in high risk sexual behaviour among homosexual men, London 1996–8:cross sectional, questionnaire study. *Br Med J* **320**:1510–11.

Donoghoe MC, Stimson GV, Dolan KA. 1989. Sexual behaviour of injecting drug users and associated risks of HIV infection for non-injecting sexual partners. *AIDS Care* **1**:51–8.

Douceron H, Deforges L, Gherardi R, *et al.* 1993. Long-lasting postmortem viability of human immunodeficiency virus: a potential risk in forensic medicine practice. *Forensic Sci Int* **60**:61–6.

Drake W, Lukash L. 1978. Reconstruction of mutilated victims for identification. *J Forensic Sci* **23**:218–30.

Durigon H. 1988. *Pathologie medico-legale*. Masson, Paris.

Durigon M, Ceccaldi PF, Renard J. 1983. Catastrophes et identifications: role des differentes structures. [Role of foreign physicians in the identification of catastrophy victims.] *Med-Armees* **3**:2524.

Dzieciol J, Kemona A, Gorska M, *et al.* 1992. Widespread myocardial and pulmonary bone marrow embolism following cardiac massage. *Forensic Sci Int* **56**:195–9.

Eckert WG. 1980. Catastrophes et morts collectives. Recent american experiences in mass deaths. *Am J Forensic Med Pathol* **1**:77–9.

Eckert WG. 1982. Fatal commercial air transport crashes, 1924–1981. Review of history and information on fatal crashes. *Am J Forensic Med Pathol* **3**:49–56.

Eckert WG. 1983. The untapped resource; the forensic and general autopsy. [editorial] *Am J Forensic Med Pathol* **4**:293.

Eckert WG. 1985. The disinterred body: do it right the first time. *Am J Forensic Med Pathol* **6**:5–6.

Enbom M, Sheldon J, Lennette E, *et al.* 2000. Antibodies to human herpesvirus 8 latent and lytic antigens in blood donors and potential high-risk groups in Sweden: variable frequencies found in a multicenter serological study. *J Med Virol* **62**:498–504.

Eriksson A, Krantz KP, Lowenhielm CG, *et al.* 1984. A device which allows dictation of the autopsy report during the autopsy. *Am J Forensic Med Pathol* **5**:279–82.

Evans KT, Knight B. 1986. Forensic radiology (see Notes). *Br J Hosp Med* **36**:14–20.

Fairburn G, McDonald K. 2000. Increased high risk sexual behaviour in homosexual men. Clarity may have been lost through including too much information. *Br Med J* **321**:1532.

Fatteh A. 1978. Exhumation, autopsy, second autopsy. *Leg Med Annu* 151–63.

Fatteh AV, Mann GT. 1969. The role of radiology in forensic pathology. *Med Sci Law* **9**:27–30.

Federal Emergency Management Agency. 1987. *Medical and emergency preparedness for disaster management: preventive medicine and public health aspects*. NATO-JCMMG, Study #4. Washington, DC.

Gee DJ. 1975. Radiology in forensic pathology. *Radiography* **41**:109–14.

Geller SA. 1990. HIV and the autopsy. [editorial] *Am J Clin Pathol* **94**:487–9.

Geller SA. 1990. The autopsy in acquired immunodeficiency syndrome. How and why [see comments]. *Arch Pathol Lab Med* **114**:324–9.

Gerber SR, Adelson L, Johnson L. 1956. The role of photography in the coroners office. *Med Radiogr Photogr* **32**:15–18.

Ghanem I. 1988. Permission for performing an autopsy: the pitfalls under Islamic law. *Med Sci Law* **28**:241–2.

Gilliland MG, McDonough ET, Fossum RM, *et al.* 1986. Disaster planning for air crashes. A retrospective analysis of delta airlines flight 191. *Am J Forensic Med Pathol* **7**:308–16.

Goldberg D, Scott G, Weir M, *et al.* 1998. HIV infection among homosexual/bisexual males attending genitourinary clinics in scotland. *Sex Transm Infect* **74**:185–8.

Goldman L. 1984. Diagnostic advances v the value of the autopsy. 1912–1980. *Arch Pathol Lab Med* **108**:501–5.

Goldman L, Sayson R, Robbins S, *et al.* 1983. The value of the autopsy in three medical eras. *N Engl J Med* **308**:1000–5.

Gonzales M, Halpern MH, Umberger CJ, Vance M. 1954. *Legal medicine and toxicology*, 2nd edn, vol. 64. Appleton Century Crofts, New York.

Gopinath C, Thuring J, Zayed I. 1978. Isoprenaline-induced myocardial necrosis in dogs. *Br J Exp Pathol* **59**:148–57.

Gordon I, Shapiro HA, Berson SD. 1988. *Forensic medicine; a guide to principles*, 3rd edn. Churchill Livingstone, Edinburgh.

Green MA. 1982. Sudden and suspicious deaths outside the deceased's own country – time for an international protocol. *Forensic Sci Int* **20**:71–5.

Gresham GA, Turner AF. 1979. *Post mortem procedures*. Wolfe Medical Publications, London.

Hartveit F, Karwinski B, Giertsen JC. 1987. Changes in autopsy profile – 1975 and 1984. *J Pathol* **153**:91–8.

Health Services Advisory Committee. 1991. *Safe working and prevention of infection in clinical labotories*. HMSO, London.

Heath Services Advisory Committee. 1991. *Safe working and the prevention of infection in the mortuary and postmortem room*. HMSO, London.

Hill IR. 1986. Toxicological findings in fatal aircraft accidents in the United Kingdom. *Am J Forensic Med Pathol* **7**:322–6.

Hirsch CS. 1971. The format of the medicolegal autopsy protocol. *Am J Clin Pathol* **55**:407–9.

Hollander N. 1987. Air crash disaster planning. [letter] *Am J Forensic Med Pathol* **8**:183–4.

Hunt AC. 1967. Instant photography in forensic medicine. *Med Sci Law* **7**:216–17.

Hunter J. 1772. *On the digestion of the stomach after death*. Philosophical Transactions of the Royal Society of London, Chapter 62, pp. 447–52. Royal Society of London, London.

Janssen W. 1984. *Forensic histopathology*. Springer Verlag, Berlin.

Jay GW, Leestma JE. 1981. Sudden death in epilepsy. A comprehensive review of the literature and proposed mechanisms. *Acta Neurol Scand Suppl* **82**:1–66.

Johnson HRM. 1969. The incidence of unnatural deaths which have been presumed to be natural in coroners' autopsies. *Med Sci Law* **9**:102–7.

Johnson MD, Schaffner W, Atkinson J, *et al.* 1997. Autopsy risk and acquisition of human immunodeficiency virus infection: a case report and reappraisal. *Arch Pathol Lab Med* **121**:64–6.

Kalichman SC. 1999. Psychological and social correlates of high-risk sexual behaviour among men and women living with HIV/AIDS. *AIDS Care* **11**:415–27.

Karch SB. 1987. Resuscitation-induced myocardial necrosis. Catecholamines and defibrillation. *Am J Forensic Med Pathol* **8**:3–8.

Kenyon CD. 1988. Identification and repatriation following major air disasters. *Forensic Sci Int* **36**:223–30.

Kibayashi K, Hamada K, Honjyo K, *et al.* 1993. Differentiation between bruises and putrefactive discolorations of the skin by immunological analysis of glycophorin A. *Forensic Sci Int* **61**:111–17.

Knight B. 1980. The obscure autopsy. *Forensic Sci Int* **16**:237–40.

Knight B. 1980. *Discovering the human body*. Lippincott & Crowell, New York.

Knight B. 1982. *Lawyer's guide to forensic medicine*. Heinemann Medical Books, London.

Knight B. 1983. *The coroner's autopsy*. Churchill Livingstone, London.

Knight B. 1984. *The post-mortem technician's handbook*. Blackwell Scientific Publications, Oxford.

Knight B. 1985. *Pocket picture guide to forensic medicine*. Gower Medical Publishing, London.

Knight B. 1988. A model medico-legal system. *Forensic Sci Int* **39**:1–4.

Knight B. 1996. *Simpson's forensic medicine*, 11th edn. Edward Arnold, London.

Koelmeyer TD, Beer B, Mullins PR. 1982. A computer-based analysis of injuries sustained by victims of a major air disaster. *Am J Forensic Med Pathol* **3**:11–16.

Kuller L, Lilienfeld A, Fisher R. 1966. Sudden and unexpected death in young adults: an epidemiological study. *JAMA* **198**:248–52.

Kunnen M, Thomas F, Van de Velde E. 1966. Proceedings of the British association in forensic medicine. Semi-microradiography of the larynx on post-mortem material. *Med Sci Law* **6**:218–19.

Landefeld CS, Chren MM, Myers A, *et al.* 1988. Diagnostic yield of the autopsy in a university hospital and a community hospital. *N Engl J Med* **318**:1249–54.

Langan Y, Nashef L, Sander JW. 2000. Sudden unexpected death in epilepsy: a series of witnessed deaths. *J Neurol Neurosurg Psychiatry* **68**:211–13.

Lawrence RD. 1985. Inaccuracy of measuring wounds on autopsy photographs. *Am J Forensic Med Pathol* **6**:17–18.

Leadbeatter S. 1986. Semantics of death certification. *J R Coll Physicians Lond* **20**:129–32.

Leadbeatter S. 1991. Deaths of British nationals abroad – a 10-year survey. *Forensic Sci Int* **49**:103–11.

Leadbeatter S, Knight B. 1987. The history and the cause of death. *Med Sci Law* **27**:132–5.

Leadbeatter S, Knight B. 1988. Resuscitation artefact. *Med Sci Law* **28**:200–4.

Lechat MF. 1976. The epidemiology of disasters. *Proc R Soc Med* **69**:421–6.

Leestma JE, Kalelkar MB, Teas SS, *et al.* 1984. Sudden unexpected death associated with seizures: analysis of 66 cases. *Epilepsia* **25**:84–8.

Leestma JE, Hughes JR, Teas SS, *et al.* 1985. Sudden epilepsy deaths and the forensic pathologist. *Am J Forensic Med Pathol* **6**:215–18.

Leestma JE, Annegers JF, Brodie MJ, *et al.* 1997. Sudden unexplained death in epilepsy: observations from a large clinical development program. *Epilepsia* **38**:47–55.

Li L, Zhang X, Constantine NT, *et al.* 1993. Seroprevalence of parenterally transmitted viruses (HIV-1, HBV, HCV, and HTLV-I/II) in forensic autopsy cases. *J Forensic Sci* **38**:1075–83.

Ludwig J. 2002. *Handbook of autopsy practice*, 3rd edn. Humana Press, Totowa, New Jersey.

Macdonald N, Evans B. 2000. Increased high risk sexual behaviour in homosexual men. There is no evidence for a decreased incidence of HIV infection. *Br Med J* **321**:1531–2; discussion 1532.

Mant AK. 1984. *Taylor's principles and practice of medical jurisprudence*, 13th edn. Churchill Livingstone, London.

Mason J. 1993. Resuscitation artefacts, including bone marrow. *Forensic medicine: an illustrated reference.* Chapman & Hall, London, pp. 39–42.

Mason JK. 1962. *Aviation accident pathology: a study of fatalities.* Butterworth, London.

Mason JK. 1962. The pathology of unsuccessful escape in flight. *Med Sci Law* **2**:124–30.

McCurdy WC. 1987. Postmortem specimen collection. *Forensic Sci Int* **35**:61–5.

McGarry P. 1967. A quick, simple method of removal of the spinal cord. *Arch Pathol* **83**:333–5.

Moritz A. 1942. *The pathology of trauma.* Lea & Febiger, Philadelphia.

Moritz AR. 1956. Classical mistakes in forensic pathology. *American Journal of Clinical Pathology* **26**:1383–92.

Morley AR. 1988. Value of the autopsy. *Assoc Clin Pathol News* **Spring issue**.

Nolte KB, Dasgupta A. 1996. Prevention of occupational cyanide exposure in autopsy prosectors. *J Forensic Sci* **41**:146–7.

Nolte KB, Taylor DG, Richmond JY. 2002. Biosafety considerations for autopsy. *Am J Forensic Med Pathol* **23**:107–22.

Peacock SJ, Machin D, Duboulay CE, *et al.* 1988. The autopsy: a useful tool or an old relic? *J Pathol* **156**:9–14.

Polson CJ, Marshall TK. 1975. *The disposal of the dead*, 3rd edn. English University Press, London.

Polson CJ, Gee D, Knight B. 1985. *Essentials of forensic medicine*, 4th edn. Pergamon Press, Oxford.

Pounder DJ. 1985. Natural disaster potential and counterdisaster planning in Australia. *Am J Forensic Med Pathol* **6**:347–57.

Prinsloo I, Gordon I. 1951. Post-mortem dissection artefacts of the neck and their differentiation from ante-mortem bruises. *S Afr Med J* **25**:358–61.

Puschel K, Lieske K, Hashimoto Y, *et al.* 1987. HIV infection in forensic autopsy cases. *Forensic Sci Int* **34**:169–74.

Puschel K, Lockemann U, Schneider V, *et al.* 1992. HIV-1 prevalence among drug deaths in major cities of central and northern europe. *Forensic Sci Int* **57**:57–62.

Reiter C, Risser D. 1994. Experience with the cytological demonstration of smoker cells in the identification of disaster victims illustrated by the findings concerning the Lauda Air airliner crash near Bangkok. *Forensic Sci Int* **66**:23–31.

Royal College of Pathologists. 1990. *Major disasters, the pathologist's role.* Royal College of Pathologists, London.

Royal College of Pathologists. 1993. *Guidelines for postmortem reports.* Royal Collage of Pathologists, London.

Royal College of Pathologists. 1995. *HIV and the practice of pathology; report of a working party of the Royal College of Pathologists.* Royal College of Pathologists, London.

Rutherford WH, de Boer J. 1983. The definition and classification of disasters. *Injury* **15**:10–12.

Saukko P. 1984. [Autopsy in Scandinavia.] *Beitr Gerichtl Med* **42**:339–41.

Saukko P, Pollak S. 2000. Postmortem examination: procedures and standards. In: Siegel JA, Saukko PJ, Knupfer GC (eds), *Encyclopedia of forensic sciences.* Academic Press, San Diego/San Francisco/New York/Boston/London/Sydney/Tokyo, Vol. 3, pp. 1272–5.

Schmidt G, Kallieris D. 1982. Use of radiographs in the forensic autopsy. *Forensic Sci Int* **19**:263–70.

Schultz TC. 1987. Simple method for demonstrating coronary arteries at postmortem examination. *Am J Forensic Med Pathol* **8**:313–16.

Shapiro H. 1954. Medicolegal mythology; some popular forensic fallacies. *J Forensic Med* **1**:144–69.

Sidwell RU, Green JS, Novelli V. 1999. Management of occupational exposure to HIV – what actually happens. *Commun Dis Public Health* **2**:287–90.

Simpson CK. 1965. *Taylor's principles and practice of medical jurisprudence*, 12th edn. J. & A. Churchill, London.

Skinner M. 1987. Planning the archaeological recovery of evidence from recent mass graves. *Forensic Sci Int* **34**:267–87.

Solheim T, van den Bos A. 1982. International disaster identification report. Investigative and dental aspects. *Am J Forensic Med Pathol* **3**:63–7.

Stevanovic G, Tucakovic G, Dotlic R, *et al.* 1986. Correlation of clinical diagnoses with autopsy findings: a retrospective study of 2,145 consecutive autopsies. *Hum Pathol* **17**:1225–30.

Stevens PJ. 1962. The medical investigation of fatal aircraft accidents. *Med Sci Law* **2**:101–9.

Stevens PJ. 1968. The pathology of fatal public transport aviation accidents. *Med Sci Law* **8**:41–8.

Stevens PJ, Tarlton S. 1963. Identification of mass casualties experience in four civil air disasters. *Med Sci Law* **3**:154–68.

Stewart TD (ed.). 1970. *Personal identification in mass disasters*. Smithsonian Museum. National Museum of Natural History, Washington, DC.

Sturt RH. 1988. Ver Heyden de Lancey lecture on a medico-legal matter. The role of the coroner with special reference to major disasters. *Med Sci Law* **28**:275–85.

Svendsen E, Hill RB. 1987. Autopsy legislation and practice in various countries. *Arch Pathol Lab Med* **111**:846–50.

Tedeschi LG. 1980. Future of the autopsy: a redelineation. *Am J Forensic Med Pathol* **1**:1034.

Titford M, Cumberland G. 1986. Forensic histotechnology: autopsy tissues and public issues. *J Histotechnol* **9**:263.

Tough SC, Green FH, Paul JE, *et al.* 1996. Sudden death from asthma in 108 children and young adults. *J Asthma* **33**:179–88.

Underwood JC, Slater DN, Parsons MA. 1983. The needle necropsy. *Br Med J Clin Res Ed* **286**:1632–4.

van den Bos A. 1980. Mass identification: a multidisciplinary operation. The Dutch experience. *Am J Forensic Med Pathol* **1**:265–70.

Vanezis P, Sims BG, Grant JH. 1978. Medical and scientific investigations of an exhumation in unhallowed ground. *Med Sci Law* **18**:209–21.

Waldron H, Vickerstaffe L. 1977. *Intimations of quality: antemortem and postmortem diagnoses*. Nuffield Provincial Hospitals Trust, London.

Wren C, O'Sullivan JJ, Wright C. 2000. Sudden death in children and adolescents. *Heart* **83**:410–13.

Wright RK, Tate LG. 1980. Forensic pathology. Last stronghold of the autopsy. *Am J Forensic Med Pathol* **1**:57–60.

CHAPTER 2

The pathophysiology of death

Most of the discussion concerning the definitions of death belongs to the field of legal medicine and even that of ethics, rather than forensic pathology. Notwithstanding this, a quick review of this complex problem is appropriate here, as when we come to describe the various post-mortem phenomena, some appreciation is necessary of the zero point from which such changes are timed.

TYPES OF DEATH

It is conventional to describe two types of death:

- somatic death, in which the person irreversibly loses its sentient personality, being unconscious, unable to be aware of (or to communicate with) its environment, and unable to appreciate any sensory stimuli or to initiate any voluntary movement. Reflex nervous activity may, however, persist, and circulatory and respiratory functions continue either spontaneously or with artificial support so that the tissues and cells of the body, other than those already damaged in the central nervous system, are alive and functioning.
- cellular death, in which the tissues and their constituent cells are dead – that is, they no longer function or have metabolic activity, primarily aerobic respiration.

Cellular death follows the ischaemia and anoxia inevitably consequent upon cardiorespiratory failure, but it is a process rather than an event, except in the exceptionally rare circumstance of almost instantaneous total bodily destruction, such as falling into molten metal or a nuclear explosion. Even fragmentation of a body by a bomb does not kill all cells instantly.

Different tissues die at different rates, the cerebral cortex being vulnerable to only a few minutes' anoxia, whereas connective tissues and even muscle survive for many hours, even days after the cessation of the circulation.

Brain death

Without trespassing too far into clinical medicine, it may be further noted that somatic death is virtually equated with brain death. When the higher levels of cerebral activity are selectively lost, either from a period of hypoxia, trauma, or toxic insult, the victim will exist in a 'vegetative state'. Here the survival of the brainstem ensures that spontaneous breathing will continue and therefore cardiac function is not compromised. The victim can remain in deep coma almost indefinitely – certainly for years – though debilitating complications such as postural skin necrosis, muscle contractures, and secondary chest infections may well shorten life. Such vegetative patients are not considered 'dead' by most standards, though there is a faction of the medical profession who claim that, because of the irreversible loss of their awareness of themselves and the world around them, they can no longer be considered 'human beings'.

As they are not on life-support machines, however, there is nothing short of euthanasia that can be done about their condition. Attitudes are changing, however, as evidenced by the case of Tony Bland, who declined into a persistent vegetative state, with functioning respiration, after hypoxia caused by crush asphyxia during the Sheffield Hillsborough football disaster. After several years in this persistent vegetative state, his family obtained the consent of the courts in 1993 to allow nutrition to be withdrawn and natural death to supervene.

It is another matter when brain death spreads below the tentorium. When the brainstem (specifically the midbrain, pons and upper medulla) suffers neuronal damage, the loss of the 'vital centres' that control respiration, and of the ascending reticular activating system that sustains consciousness, cause the victim not only to be irreversibly comatose, but also to be incapable of spontaneous breathing. Without medical intervention, hypoxic cardiac arrest inevitably follows within minutes and then the usual progression of 'cellular death' ensues. This invariably occurred in the past, before the advent of sophisticated devices that allowed the support of respiration after spontaneous function has ceased. Because of continued oxygenation, the heart continues to function, though it has been pointed out by Pallis (1983) that the vast majority of brainstem-dead patients suffer a cardiac arrest within 48–72 hours, even when adequately oxygenated.

This then is the state of 'brainstem death', and almost all doctors and most jurisdictions now accept that, once irreversible damage to the brainstem has been proved, the patient is 'dead' in the somatic sense. They are, however, not yet dead in the cellular sense and it is through this 'physiological window' that the spectacular advances in cadaver donor transplant surgery have been made.

MEDICO-LEGAL ASPECTS OF BRAIN DEATH

In relation to forensic pathology and criminal procedure, these matters have now a largely historical relevance in that several decades ago a number of fatal assaults were defended in court on the basis that the original head injuries led to the victims being placed on life-support machines that were later disconnected when brainstem death was diagnosed. The defence was that the assailant did not 'kill' the victim, because 'death' was caused by the action of the doctors switching off the machine. Several judicial decisions have disposed of this defence, however, as it was accepted, first, that death was diagnosed by the doctors before discontinuing artificial ventilation and, second, that the criminal act that initiated the train of events was not remote enough to avoid culpability for the death.

THE INDICATIONS OF DEATH

Here the signs of somatic death are considered, as those of cellular death are manifested by post-mortem changes, to be discussed in later sections. When cardiorespiratory arrest occurs, brain function ceases within seconds as a result of the collapse of cerebral blood pressure and consequent cortical ischaemia. Within minutes, this loss of brain function becomes irreversible. The actual number of minutes for which total anoxia will cause cortical damage is controversial; it was formerly held that 3 minutes was sufficient, but this time has been extended to 7 or 9 minutes. Even much longer times of total hypoxia, such as immersion under water, has been survived without brain damage. In these cases, an element of hypothermia is usual, which reduces the oxygen needs of the tissues. Thus 20 or even 40 minutes of hypoxia has been claimed as not leading to brain damage. All that can be said is that the period is very variable and that 3–4 minutes of cardiac arrest or failure of respiratory gas exchange carries the risk of cortical damage, even though three or four times this period may sometimes be survived without ill-effects.

- Unconsciousness and loss of all reflexes occurs, and there is no reaction to painful stimuli. Rarely, there may be post-mortem coordinated muscle group activity for up to one hour after death, possibly due to surviving cells in the spinal cord (Nokes *et al.* 1989).

- Muscular flaccidity occurs immediately upon failure of cerebral and cerebellar function. All muscle tone is lost, though the muscles are physically capable of contraction for many hours.

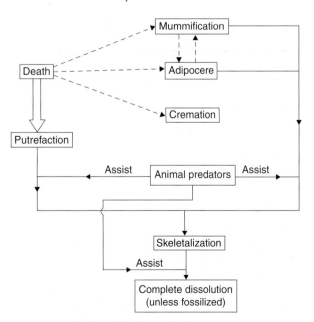

FIGURE 2.1 *The fate of a body after death.*

Eye signs include loss of the corneal and light reflexes leading to insensitive corneas and fixed, unreactive pupils. Though the iris responds to chemical stimulation for hours after somatic death, the light reflex is lost as soon as the brainstem nuclei suffer ischaemic failure. The pupils usually assume a mid-dilated position, which is the relaxed neutral position of the pupillary muscle, though they may later alter as a result of rigor. There may be a marked difference in the degree of dilatation of each pupil, but this has no significance as a diagnostic sign either of a brain lesion or of drug intoxication. In conditions such as morphine poisoning, where the pupils may be contracted during life, death may allow this to persist or the pupils may dilate to the 'cadaveric position'.

In addition to irregular size, the pupils may lose their circular shape after death as a result of uneven relaxation. This is usually easy to differentiate from the more obvious irregularity caused by ante-mortem abnormality of the iris. The eye globe tension decreases rapidly, as it is dependent upon arterial pressure for its maintenance. The eyeball feels progressively softer within minutes and the cornea soon loses its normal glistening reflectivity because of laxity and failure of lachrymal moistening. Normal tension was measured by Nicati in 1894, who found that it halved at death, fell to as low as an eighth in 30 minutes, and was nil by 2 hours after death. The eyelids usually close, but this is commonly incomplete, the flaccid muscles failing to produce the full occlusion that occurs in voluntary closure. Where the sclera remains exposed, two yellow triangles of desiccated discoloration appear on each side of the cornea within a few hours, becoming brown and then sometimes almost black, giving rise to the name 'tache noire'.

When viewed with an ophthalmoscope, the retina provides one of the earliest positive signs of death. This is the well known 'trucking' of blood in the retinal vessels, when loss of blood pressure allows the blood to break up into segments, similar to trucks in a railway train. This phenomenon occurs all over the body, but only in the retina is it accessible to direct viewing.

The test is not easy to carry out, as the retina of a corpse seems far more difficult to visualize than in a living person. Many observers have described the agonal and early post-mortem appearances of the retina, though some of their accounts are rather contradictory and of little practical value, especially when they attempt to use them to estimate the time since death. Most observers – for example, Kervorkian (1956, 1961) and Salisbury and Melvin (1936) – confirm that the blood flow slows and becomes irregular in density before breaking up into segments. This was apparent within 15 minutes of death as assessed by other means. Kervorkian claimed that colour changes in the retina were closely related to the post-mortem interval. Tomlin believed that segmentation was more indicative of cerebral death than cessation of the circulation, and agreed with others in accepting that 'trucking' was of grave prognostic significance.

One of the best investigations into the phenomenon was by Wroblewski and Ellis (1970), who studied retinal and corneal changes at death in 300 patients. About a third of the total exhibited trucking, most of them within an hour of death. Part of the difficulty in

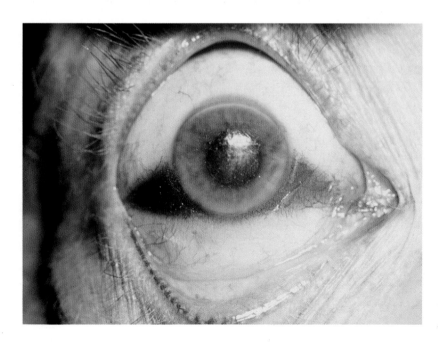

FIGURE 2.2 *Post-mortem change in the eye, the so-called 'tache noire'. These are brown areas of scleral drying caused by failure of the lids to close after death.*

examining the remainder was that clouding of the cornea occurred in 75 per cent of patients within 2 hours of death. They concluded that segmentation was a purely post-mortem change and any intravascular movement of blood, however irregular, was an indication for continued resuscitation.

■ Cessation of the heart beat and respiratory movements was the primary marker of death until the advent of mechanical cardiorespiratory support as it led to immediate ischaemia and anoxia of all other tissues. Determination of cardiac arrest may be made by prolonged auscultation of the chest to exclude heart sounds though, as in life, a feeble heartbeat may be muffled by a thick chest wall. The electrocardiograph is unchallengeable in confirming cardiac arrest.

Respiration is more difficult to confirm, especially in deep coma such as barbiturate poisoning, and prolonged listening with a stethoscope over the trachea or lung fields is necessary. All archaic procedures such as saucers of water on the chest, feathers before the nostrils and tourniquets around the fingers are only of historical interest.

The mode versus the cause of death

Confusion often arises, especially among students and younger doctors, about the distinction between the **mode** of death and its **cause**. This is particularly important in relation to the documentary certification of deaths, but the same confusion sometimes occurs among pathologists, especially those who are not habitually involved in medico-legal cases.

The mode of death refers to an abnormal physiological state that pertained at the time of death: for example, 'coma', 'congestive cardiac failure', 'cardiac arrest' and 'pulmonary oedema'. These offer no information as to the underlying pathological condition and should not be used as the definitive cause of death unless further qualified by the more fundamental aetiological process.

In most cases, the mode is unhelpful and immaterial in describing and understanding the cause of death, and some modal terms are quite useless, such as 'syncope' or 'cardiorespiratory failure'. Even 'bronchopneumonia' is such a common terminal event in numerous diseases that, used alone, it conveys no information about why the patient died. The British Registrar General has recently requested that it should be omitted from death certificates, the basic condition being preferable and sufficient for statistical purposes.

In addition to the mode and cause of death, here is also the **manner** of death, which is not really a medical decision. Manner refers to the circumstantial events, such as 'homicide, suicide, accident or natural cause' and is a legal or administrative categorization.

The recommendations of the World Health Organization, as given in its publication *The medical certification of death*, should be followed to improve both the comprehension and statistical accuracy of the cause of death. Even this booklet is inconsistent with the practice of certification in many advanced countries, in that it requests the doctor to enter the 'manner' of death (for example, homicide, accident or suicide) which, for example in the UK, is the prerogative of the legal authorities after full investigation (see Leadbeater and Knight 1987).

POST-MORTEM CHANGES OF FORENSIC IMPORTANCE

To the forensic pathologist a number of post-mortem changes are of interest and potential usefulness, mainly in relation to the estimation of the post-mortem interval, possible interference with the body, and an indication of the cause of death.

HYPOSTASIS

Post-mortem hypostasis is known under a variety of older names, such as 'lucidity', 'staining' or 'cogitation', but the current title is most suitable as it indicates the cause. Hypostasis occurs when the circulation ceases, as arterial propulsion and venous return then fail to keep blood moving through the capillary bed, and the associated small afferent and efferent vessels.

Gravity then acts upon the now stagnant blood and pulls it down to the lowest accessible areas. The red cells are most

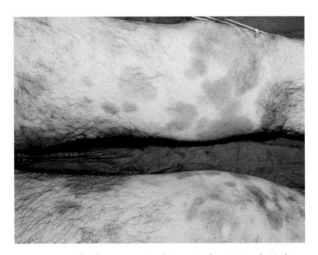

FIGURE 2.3 *Blotchy post-mortem hypostasis, forming in the early hours after death. The patchy disposition has no significance and this usually sinks down and becomes confluent in the most dependent areas within a few more hours.*

affected, sedimenting through the lax network, but plasma also drifts downwards to a lesser extent, causing an eventual post-mortem 'dependent oedema', which contributes to the skin blistering that is part of early post-mortem decay.

The arrival of erythrocytes in the lower areas is visible through the skin as a bluish red discoloration, 'hypostasis'. It often begins as blotchy patches on both lateral and dependent surfaces, but also on the upper surfaces of the legs, especially thighs. These soon coalesce and slide down to the lowest areas.

The distribution of hypostasis

The pattern of hypostasis depends on the posture of the body after death. It is most common when the deceased body is lying on its back, with the shoulders, buttocks and calves pressed against the supporting surface. This compresses the vascular channels in those areas, so that hypostasis is prevented from forming there, the skin remaining white. When the body lies for a sufficient time on the side or face, the hypostasis will distribute itself accordingly, again with white pressure areas at the zones of support.

If the body remains vertical after death, as in hanging, hypostasis will be most marked in the feet, legs and to lesser extent in the hands and distal part of the arms. In addition to pallor of the supporting areas, any local pressure can exclude hypostasis and produce a distinct pattern in contrast to the discoloured area. Examples include the irregular linear marks made by folds in rumpled bedlinen, the pattern of fabric from coarse cloth, the pressure of tight belts, brassière straps, pants' elastic and even socks. According to Bonte *et al.* (1986), when electrocution takes place in water (usually a bathtub), the hypostasis is sharply limited to a horizontal line corresponding to the water level.

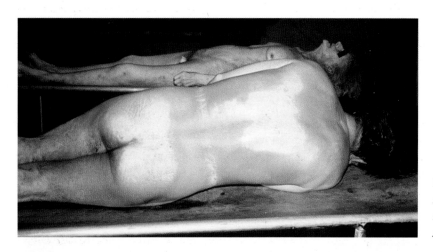

FIGURE 2.4 *Post-mortem hypostasis in the normal distribution. The pale areas are the result of pressure against a hard supporting surface.*

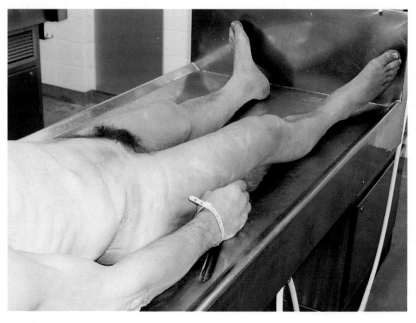

FIGURE 2.5 *Post-mortem hypostasis in a death from hanging. The discoloration of the skin is in the legs and hands, due to the vertical posture after death.*

The colour of hypostasis

The usual hue is a bluish red, but variation is wide. This depends partly on the state of oxygenation at death, those dying in a congested, hypoxic state having a darker tint as a result of reduced haemoglobin in the skin vessels. This is an unsure indicator of the mode of death, however, and no reliance can be placed on a cyanotic darkening of the hypostasis to indicate a hypoxic death in the sense of 'asphyxia'. Many natural deaths from coronary or other disease have markedly dark hypostasis. Often the colour of the hypostasis varies from area to area on the same body. Sometimes a rim of lighter colour may be seen along the margin of the lower darker area and sometimes there is a definite contrast between a bluish zone and a pink margin. This may appear and change as the post-mortem interval lengthens. Often the whole area of hypostasis is pink or bright red. When death has been due to hypothermia or exposure to cold in the agonal period, such as drowning, the colour may assist in confirming the cause of death; again this is relatively non-specific because bodies exposed to cold after death (especially in mortuary refrigeration) may turn pink after an initial stage of normal bluish-red tint.

The mechanism is not understood, but is obviously a result of oxyhaemoglobin forming at the expense of the darker reduced haemoglobin. This is understandable in hypothermia, where the reduced metabolism of the tissues fails to take up oxygen from the circulating blood, but its frequent formation in the post-mortem period is difficult to explain.

Several researchers have investigated the colour of hypostasis in relation to time since death. Schuller *et al.* (1987) noted an increasing paleness between 3 and 15 hours post-mortem, measuring this as a change in wavelength from 575 nm at 3 hours at an average rate of 2 nm per hour. Vanezis (1991) has used tristimulus colorimetry to study colour changes and secondary shifting of hypostasis, and claimed that there is a linear relationship between the fading colour and time during the first 2 hours after death, following which changes are unpredictable. Inoue *et al.* (1994) have also described measurement of hypostatic colour as a measure of time since death.

It may sometimes be noticed that originally bluish hypostasis becomes pink along the upper part of the horizontal margin, the lower parts remaining dark, so a quantitative change probably occurs, the haemoglobin being more easily re-oxygenated where the erythrocytes are packed less densely in the upper layers of hypostasis.

Other changes in the colour of hypostasis are more useful. The best known is the 'cherry-pink' of carboxyhaemoglobin, which is a unique colour and is often the first indication to the pathologist of carbon monoxide poisoning. Cyanide poisoning is said to have its own characteristic dark blue–pink hue,

but it is really an index of the congested, cyanotic, mode of death and, if the pathologist was not already aware of the potential cause from the history – and perhaps the odour of cyanide – it is doubtful whether hypostasis would be a primary indication of the nature of the death. The hypostasis may be a brownish red in methaemoglobinaemia and may be various shades in aniline and chlorate poisoning. In deaths from septic abortions where *Clostridium perfringens* is the infecting agent, a pale bronze mottling may sometimes be seen on the skin, though this is not confined to the areas of hypostasis.

Skin haemorrhages, varying in size from small petechiae to large blotches and even palpable blood blisters may develop in areas of hypostasis. The most common place is the back of the shoulders and neck, though they may appear on the front of the chest, even on a body lying on its back. They are more common in cyanotic, congestive types of death and become more pronounced as the post-mortem interval lengthens. Their importance is in not being mistaken for the so-called signs of 'asphyxia'. They appear in the most gross form when a body dies or is left with the head downwards: the confluent petechiae and ecchymoses may be so marked that they virtually blacken the face and neck.

The timing and permanence of hypostasis

Too much has been claimed in the past for the usefulness of hypostasis as an indicator of the time of death and post-mortem disturbance of the body. The phenomenon appears at a variable time after death – indeed, it may not appear at all, especially in infants, old people or those with anaemia. It may be so faint as almost to escape detection.

Hypostasis can appear within half an hour of death or it may be delayed for many hours. Its variability is such that it is useless for any estimation of the time since death. It is claimed that hypostasis can sometimes be observed in the living if the heart action is failing or if venous return is impaired by the immobility of deep coma. The latter is certainly associated with skin blistering caused by dependent oedema.

Once hypostasis is established, there is controversy about its ability to undergo subsequent gravitational shift. If the body is moved into a different posture, the primary hypostasis may either:

- remain fixed
- move completely to the newly dependent zones or
- be partly fixed and partly relocated.

Thus if a corpse is found with the hypostasis in an obviously inappropriate distribution related to the present posture, it must have been moved after death. This fact may

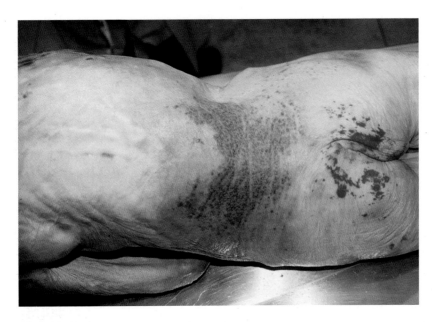

FIGURE 2.6 *Extensive confluent skin haemorrhages may occur within the dependent hypostasis. They worsen as the post-mortem interval lengthens and must not be taken to indicate so-called 'asphyxia'.*

have important significance in the investigation of criminal deaths, such as the return of the culprit or some other person to the scene. It may also migrate either partly or completely, however, thus negating its diagnostic usefulness. Older theories about 'fixation' of the staining after a certain time are not tenable, as there is no constant interval when this occurs.

Mallach (1964) analysed data including onset, confluence, maximum intensity, displacement and shifting, taken from publications between 1905 and 1963. These are summarized in Table 2.1, 'thumb pressure' meaning displacement by thumb pressure. Table 2.2 shows the variable opinions on hypostasis culled from standard textbooks.

A considerable amount of research has been devoted to the investigation of clotting of post-mortem blood, its subsequent lysis and inhibition of coagulation by fibrinolysins, but this cannot be translated into practice. Formerly, it was held that if a body had remained in its original posture for a certain minimum length of time, the blood would coagulate in the hypostatic areas, so that secondary shifting could not then occur if the body was moved. This is not true in the majority of instances, as there may be partial or complete secondary gravitation at any time – at least, until true staining of the tissues due to haemolysis begins as part of early decomposition, which is not until the second or third day in temperate conditions.

Suzutani *et al.* (1978) examined 430 bodies by pressure on hypostatic areas, finding that the colour could not be squeezed out in 30 per cent where death had occurred 6–12 hours previously. More than 50 per cent were fixed after 12–24 hours and no fading occurred in 70 per cent of those

TABLE 2.1 *Hypostasis related to the time of death (hpm) as derived from previous literature*

Stage	Mean	Standard deviation	Limits Lower	Limits Upper
Beginning	0.75	0.5	0.25	3
Confluence	2.50	1.0	1.00	4
Maximum	9.50	4.5	3.00	16
Thumb pressure	5.50	6.0	1.00	20
Complete shifting	3.75	1.0	2.00	6
Incomplete shifting	11.00	4.5	4.00	24

TABLE 2.2 *Time of onset of hypostasis as stated by previous authors*

Reference	Onset	Maximum
Adelson	30 min–4 h	8–12
Polson, Gee, Knight	30 min–2 h	6–12
Spitz and Fisher	2–4 h	8–12
Taylor (ed. Simpson)	0 h	12
Taylor (ed. Mant)	1 h	12
Gradwohl (ed. Camps)	20–30 min	6–12
Glaister, Brash	–	8–12
DiMaio	30 min–2 h	8–12
Sydney Smith	0 h	12
Mant	0 h	12
Gordon and Shapiro	'few' h	12

dead for more than 1–3 days. However, in a significant number, hypostasis was still mobile for at least 3 days.

Fechner *et al.* (1984) found no linear relationship between fixation and time of death and also observed variations in fixation according to storage temperatures.

Hypostasis in other organs

Just as blood settles in dependent skin, so it does in other tissues and organs. The importance in forensic autopsy work is the differentiation of organ hypostasis from ante-mortem lesions. In the intestine, dependent loops of jejunum and ileum may be markedly discoloured and mislead the inexperienced pathologist into suspecting mesenteric infarction or strangulation. This hypostasis is discontinuous, however, revealing interrupted segments when the gut is laid out. Often loops in the pelvis are worst affected, because of their lower position.

The lungs almost always show a marked difference in colour from front to back, the anterior margins being pale and the posterior edges lying in the paravertebral gutters being dark blue. This is often accompanied by an obvious difference in fluid content, congestion and oedema being more marked posteriorly. The myocardium often shows a dark patch in the posterior wall of the left ventricle that must not be mistaken for early infarction.

One of the most important hypostatic artefacts is haemorrhage behind the oesophagus at the level of the larynx. This has many times been confused with the trauma of strangulation, but the true nature was best investigated by Prinsloo and Gordon (1951). Areas of congestion developing into haemorrhage appear in the loose tissues on the back of the oesophagus lying on the anterior longitudinal ligament of the cervical spine. They may be prominent, sufficient to produce actual haematomas. They arise in the veins and venous plexus on the front of the spine, and can be avoided in cases of strangulation and suspected strangulation by draining the neck of blood before starting the dissection. This can be achieved either by removing the brain first or by opening the chest and incising the great veins in the superior mediastinum.

Differentiation between hypostasis and bruising

This is rarely a problem in fresh bodies, but when decomposition begins the two conditions become blurred. In fresh material the appearance of hypostasis is of a regular, diffuse engorgement of the surface vessels, the colour varying between purple–red and bright pink. The density varies from place to place but there are no sudden changes in colour nor any sharply circumscribed areas as occurs in bruising. As mentioned above, in the early stages of hypostasis there may be mottled blue areas, which later coalesce. This mottling is unlikely to be confused with bruising by any but the most inexperienced pathologist. The position in dependent areas is also characteristic, giving a generally horizontal orientation. Bruises may be anywhere on the body, are often discoid or have an irregular margin, but rarely cover a large area with

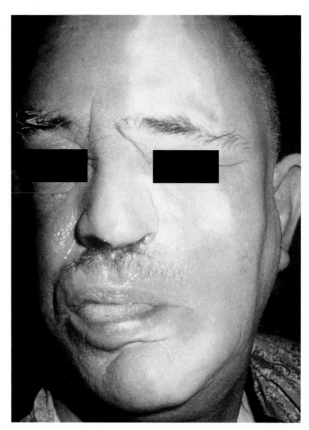

FIGURE 2.7 *White patches within the hypostasis on the face merely indicate pressure against the supporting surface after a face-down position. As in this case, they are usually post-mortem and are not indicators of suffocation.*

uniform density – and do not have a horizontal margin. Abrasions may be topographically associated with a bruise, but not with hypostasis. When there is difficulty in differentiating between the two – usually where there is racial pigmentation or really deep, cyanotic hypostasis that obscures possible bruises – the classic test is to incise the suspect area to see if the underlying blood is intravascular (hypostasis) or infiltrating the tissues outside the vessels (contusion).

Fresh bruises may also be swollen and slightly raised above the surface. If a post-mortem pressure mark (such as from a belt or tight clothing) crosses an area of hypostasis, there will be a pale bloodless zone, but a bruise will not be affected. Hypostasis is in the most superficial layer of the dermis and any exuded blood can be wiped or washed away from the incised surface. A bruise is often deeper in the skin or underlying tissues and is fixed, being infiltrated through the tissues outside the ruptured vessels. An exception is intradermal bruising, but this is usually patterned or linear and rarely can be confused with hypostasis. Histological examination may be necessary finally to decide the matter.

When post-mortem autolysis has developed, the diffusion of haemolysed blood from vessels makes the differentiation between hypostasis and bruising difficult and eventually impossible. Even histological examination may be of little help when the tissues become markedly degenerate.

RIGOR MORTIS

Unlike hypostasis, the stiffening of the muscles after death has some relevance in determining the post-mortem interval. It has been known since antiquity that immediately after death there is general muscular flaccidity, usually followed by a period of partial or total rigidity, which in turn passes off as the signs of decomposition appear. The timing of this sequence of events is so variable, however, that it is a poor indicator of the time since death. The usual range of times when rigor appears can be summarized as follows.

■ The flaccid period immediately after death is variable, but commonly extends to between 3 and 6 hours before stiffening is first detected, depending on environmental temperature and other factors. Rigor is first apparent in the smaller muscle groups, not because it begins there, but because the smaller joints, such as the jaw, are more easily immobilized. The sequence of spread of rigor is also variable but tends to affect the jaw, facial muscles and neck before being obvious in the wrists and ankles, then the knees, elbows and hips.

The usual method of testing is by attempting to flex or extend the joints, though the whole muscle mass itself becomes hard, and finger pressure on the quadriceps or pectorals can also detect the change. The onset of rigor may be markedly accelerated or retarded by the factors mentioned below, so that stiffness may develop within half an hour of death (even excluding cadaveric spasm) or may be postponed almost indefinitely. Some subjects, usually infants, the cachectic and the aged, may never develop recognizable rigor mortis, mainly because of the feebleness of their musculature.

■ Rigor spreads to involve the whole muscle mass, again within a variable period but in 'average' conditions it might be expected to reach a maximum within 6–12 hours. This state then remains constant until the muscle mass begins to undergo autolysis, which releases rigor gradually at a stage before overt post-mortem changes are visible externally, except perhaps for a commencing discoloration of the lower abdominal wall.

The duration of full rigor may be 18–36 hours, until it begins to fade in roughly the same order of muscle groups as it appeared. However, there are many exceptions to this rather misleading generalization.

Factors affecting the timing of rigor mortis

As a chemical process, the speed of onset and the duration of rigor is modified by temperature. The colder the environment the slower the process and vice versa. In near freezing conditions rigor will be suspended almost indefinitely. The author (BK) has attended a scene outdoors in winter where the body was quite flaccid one week after death, rigor developing rapidly as soon as the corpse was brought into the comparative warmth of the mortuary. Conversely, hot weather or tropical conditions can speed up the whole cycle so that rigor appears within an hour or even less. Total stiffness develops rapidly, then fades during the first day as decomposition supervenes.

The other modifier of the speed of onset of rigor is physical activity shortly before death. As will be seen when the

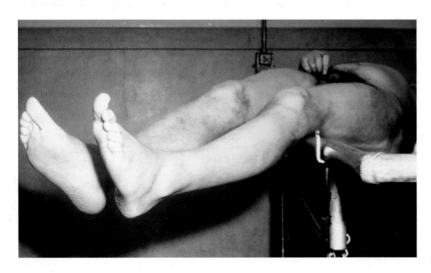

FIGURE 2.8 *Full rigor mortis 12 hours post-mortem.*

physicochemical basis of the phenomenon is discussed, the availability of glycogen and adenosine triphosphate in the muscle is a crucial element in rigor formation. Muscular exertion affects the interaction of these substances and hastens the onset of rigor. Cadaveric spasm, dealt with later, may well be an extreme variant of this accelerated rigor.

In view of the wide range of times at which the various stages of rigor appear and fade, it is a poor determinant of the time since death, compared with estimations of body temperature. Niderkorn's early work (1874) on 113 bodies showed a range of 2–13 hours for rigor to be complete, the main cluster being from 3 to 6 hours after death, a shorter period than would be accepted now. Mallach (1964) compiled a table from 150 years of published data, which suffered from gross variation in observer methodology (Table 2.3).

The following is a reasonable 'spot check' for use in average temperate conditions:

- If the body feels **warm** and is **flaccid**, it has been dead less than 3 hours.
- If the body feels **warm** and is **stiff**, it has been dead from 3 to 8 hours.
- If the body feels **cold** and is **stiff**, it has been dead from 8 to 36 hours.
- If the body feels **cold** and is **flaccid**, it has been dead more than 36 hours.

This crude estimate should never be used as a definitive statement in legal proceedings, as it is only meant as a rough guide 'on the spot'.

Rigor mortis in other tissues

Rigor occurs in all muscular tissues and organs, as well as the skeletal muscles. The iris is affected so that ante-mortem constriction or dilatation is modified. The rigor may be unequal in each eye, making the pupils unequal, confirming the fact that the post-mortem position is an unreliable indicator of toxic or neurological conditions during life.

In the heart, rigor causes the ventricles to contract, which may be mistaken by the inexperienced pathologist for left ventricular hypertrophy; this can be excluded by measuring the total weight, estimating the relative size of the left side, measuring the ventricular thickness (admittedly a rough guide) and – where the issue is important – by dissection and differential weighing of the two ventricles.

Rigor in the dartos muscle of the scrotum can compress the testes and epididymis which, together with the contraction of muscular fibres in the seminal vesicles and prostate, may lead to post-mortem extrusion of semen from the urethral meatus. This has been wrongly attributed to sexual activity and orgasm just before death in cases where a defence of provocation against a homosexual advance has been put forward. Mant showed that many corpses dying from a variety of causes have seminal fluid either at the meatus or in the penile urethra (Mant 1953, 1967; Mant and Furbank 1957). It is also said, without much foundation, that deaths from hanging and 'asphyxia' are commonly associated with post-mortem seminal emission.

Rigor in the erector pili muscles attached to the hair follicles can cause a pimpling or 'goose-flesh' appearance with elevation of the cutaneous hairs. This may have given rise to the persistent myth that the beard grows after death, though an additional explanation is that post-mortem desiccation and shrinkage of the skin allows the hair stubble to appear more prominent.

Studies by Krompecher and Bergerioux (1988) have shown that rigor also sets in more quickly in deaths from electrocution – and that it passes off more rapidly.

The biochemistry of rigor mortis

Though this has little direct forensic relevance apart from the association of the early onset of rigor with muscular

TABLE 2.3 *Time course of cadaveric rigidity as stated by previous literature*

| Rigor phase | Mean with standard deviation(s) | Hours post-mortem | | | | Number of publications evaluated |
| | | Limits of 95.5 per cent probability (2s) | | Variations | | |
		Lower limit	Upper limit	Lower limit	Upper limit	
Delay period	3 ± 2	–	7	< ½	7	26
Re-establishment possible	Up to 5	–	–	2	8	–
Complete rigidity	8 ± 1	6	10	2	20	28
Persistence	57 ± 14	29	85	24	96	27
Resolution	76 ± 32	12	140	24	192	27

exertion, the muscle chemistry of the phenomenon has been studied in great detail.

Szent-Gyorgi (1947) discovered that the essential contractile substances in muscle were the two proteins actin and myosin, arranged in interdigitating filaments. They form a loose physicochemical combination called 'actomyosin', which is physically shorter than the two substances uncombined (Hanson and Huxley 1955). If energy is supplied to the latter pair, the subsequent combination contracts. This energy is obtained by the splitting off of a phosphate complex from adenosine triphosphate (ATP) which then becomes adenosine diphosphate (ADP) (Erdos 1943). The free phosphate then engages in a phosphorylation reaction that converts glycogen to lactic acid, high energy being released in the process. Some is used to resynthesize the ATP from ADP, by the donation of a phosphate group from creatine phosphate; the remainder goes to activate the actin–myosin reaction.

In addition to supplying energy, ATP is responsible for the elasticity and plasticity of the muscle. The lactic acid is leached away back into the bloodstream and is returned to the liver for reconversion into glycogen. All these reactions are anaerobic and can continue after death, albeit in a distorted form.

In life there is a fairly constant concentration of ATP in the muscular tissues, there being a dynamic balance between utilization and resynthesis. At death, however, the ADP to ATP reaction ceases and the triphosphate is progressively diminished, with lactic acid accumulating. After a variable period, depending on temperature and the amount of ATP remaining, the actin and myosin become rigidly linked into a rigid, inextensible gel, with consequent stiffening of the muscle (see Bate-Smith and Bendall 1947; Forster 1964).

The resynthesis of ATP is dependent upon the supply of glycogen, which is depleted by vigorous activity before death; this explains the rapid onset of rigor in these circumstances. Normally there appears to be an initial period soon after death when the ATP level is maintained or even increased as a result of phosphate liberation by glycogenolysis.

Rigor is initiated when the ATP concentration falls to 85 per cent of normal, and the rigidity of the muscle is at maximum when the level declines to 15 per cent (see Bate-Smith and Bendall 1949).

Gross effects of rigor mortis

There has been some controversy over whether rigor only stiffens the muscles or actually shortens them. Sommer, as long ago as 1833, claimed that muscles contracted after death and the changes were actually known as 'Sommer's movements'. There have always been semi-apocryphal tales

of corpses moving in the mortuary and there seems little doubt that, if a limb happens to be poised in unstable equilibrium on the edge of a tray or table, the developing tension may occasionally cause it to spring off as rigor supervenes. The author (BK) has seen athetoid writhing of the foot of a corpse, which lasted for 40 minutes, more than an hour after death.

There seems to be no doubt that some shortening does occur, but the noticeable effects are slight because both flexor and extensor muscle groups oppose each other across most limb joints. Bate-Smith and Bendall (1949) decided that shortening only occurred when there had been marked depletion of glycogen by activity before death, but Forster (1964) was of the opinion that, when a muscle was under some tension, it did shorten. His experiments showed that when the muscle was unloaded there was no change in length when rigor set in. Forster further showed that a high environmental temperature and poisons that increase muscle tone, such as parathion, lead to more shortening during rigor.

When fully established, rigor is 'broken' by forcible movements of the limbs or neck, then it will not return, a phenomenon utilized daily by mortuary staff and undertakers when preparing a body for a coffin. If rigor is still developing, it will continue in the new posture of the limbs after they have been stretched. 'Breaking' fully established rigor is an accurate description, as the rigid, inelastic fibres are physically ruptured – sometimes tearing the muscle insertions from the bone. Rarely, rigor can assist in showing that a body has been moved between death and discovery. If an arm or leg is found projecting into free space without support, in a posture that obviously could not have been maintained during primary post-mortem flaccidity, then it must have been rolled over or otherwise moved. In these cases, a simple restorative movement (after the scene has been fully examined) can usually indicate the original attitude quite simply.

Conversely, it can never be assumed that the posture of rigor in which a body is found was that which obtained at the time of death, as any amount of movement during the period of primary flaccidity will not be mirrored in the subsequent rigor.

Cadaveric spasm

This topic has received a disproportionate amount of notice in textbooks compared with its practical importance. No doubt this is because of its curiosity value rather than its usefulness. Cadaveric spasm is a rare form of virtually instantaneous rigor that develops at the time of death with no period of post-mortem flaccidity.

Krompecher (1994), a major authority on rigor mortis, is extremely sceptical about the existence of true cadaveric

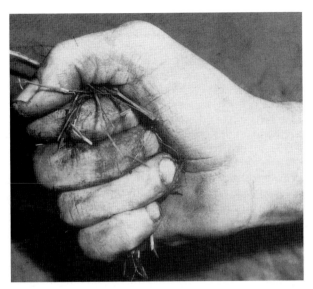

FIGURE 2.9 *Cadaveric spasm, an instantaneous form of rigor, in the victim of a fall into water. The victim was recovered within a short time (as can be seen from the absence of skin maceration) but had grass from the river bank firmly clutched in the hand.*

spasm, but many forensic pathologists claim to have seen such a phenomenon far too soon after death for it to be normal rigor mortis. The authors retain a healthy scepticism about the controversy, believing that most cases are misreported because of errors or uncertainties about the true time of death, so that early normal rigor could have supervened. However, one or two cases within BK's experience seem to be genuine enough to be remarkably early for true rigor.

It seems confined to those deaths that occur in the midst of intense physical and/or emotional activity, though how the latter can lead to instant post-mortem rigor is quite inexplicable. It presumably must be initiated by motor nerve action, but for some reason there is a failure of the normal relaxation. The phenomenon usually affects only one group of muscles, such as the flexors of one arm, rather than the whole body.

It was shown in the earlier section on the biochemistry of rigor that marked depletion of glycogen stores in the muscle by violent exertion immediately before death can hasten the onset of muscular rigidity. Most cases of cadaveric spasm occur in similar circumstances and it was said to be particularly common on the battlefield amongst soldiers slain in combat. In the civilian sphere it is most often seen in persons who fall into water or drop some distance down a precipitous slope such as a cliff. They may clutch at some nearby object, such as grass or shrubs, in an effort to break their fall and such material may be found held tightly in their fingers, even when the body is examined within a few minutes.

Another possibility, more common in detective fiction than in practice, is the gripping of a pistol with the finger still tightly flexed on the trigger, as evidence of true suicide rather than a 'planted' weapon in a homicide where an attempt has been made to simulate self-shooting. The chances of this actually being encountered by a pathologist are less than once in several professional lifetimes.

If found in the victim of drowning, or of a slide from a height, it has some value in confirming that the person was alive at the time of the fall, thus excluding the post-mortem disposal of an already dead body. Of course the body must be examined before ordinary rigor might be expected to have developed, or the presence of cadaveric spasm cannot then be assumed.

HEAT AND COLD STIFFENING

At extremes of temperature the muscles may undergo a false rigor. In extreme cold, well below zero, once the intrinsic body heat is lost, the muscles may harden because the body fluids may freeze solid – as in the commercial or domestic preservation of meat in a freezing cabinet. The temperature has to be below –5°C for cold stiffening to occur and is usually much lower. Part of the apparent stiffness is also due to solidification of the subcutaneous fat. When the body is warmed up, true rigor may supervene, though it may fail to appear as a result of intracellular damage caused by cell membranes being punctured by ice crystals.

Heat applied to the body also causes stiffness of the muscles, as the proteins of the tissues become denatured and coagulated as in cooking. The degree and depth of change depends on the intensity of the heat and the time for which it was applied. At autopsy the muscles may be shrivelled and desiccated, even carbonized on the surface. Beneath this there is a zone (which may be total) of brownish-pink 'cooked meat' and under that, if the process has not penetrated, normal red muscle. Marked shortening occurs, causing the well-known 'pugilistic attitude' of a burned body. This is because of the greater mass of flexor muscles compared with extensors, which forces the limbs into flexion and the spine into opisthotonus. These changes are purely post-mortem and are no indication of burning during life, as similar distortions occur during cremation.

POST-MORTEM DECOMPOSITION

Hypostasis and decomposition occur relatively soon after death when somatic death has occurred, but cellular death is incomplete. As discussed earlier, death is a process not an event and, while the cells of some tissues are still alive and even capable of movement (such as fibroblasts, leucocytes and muscle), others are dying or dead. The process of decomposition begin in some cells while others are still alive, and this overlap continues for several days in temperate climates.

Decomposition is a mixed process ranging from autolysis of individual cells by internal chemical breakdown to tissue autolysis from liberated enzymes, and external processes introduced by bacteria and fungi from the intestine and outer environment. Animal predators, from maggots to mammals, can be included in the range of destruction. Decomposition may differ from body to body, from environment to environment, and even from one part of the same corpse to another. Sometimes one portion of a corpse may show leathery, mummified preservation whilst the rest is in a state of liquefying putrefaction.

In addition, the time scale for decomposition may vary greatly in different circumstances and climates, and even in the same corpse: the head and arms may be skeletalized, whilst the legs and trunk, perhaps protected by clothing or other covering, may be moderately intact. All permutations may be found, making it even more difficult to estimate the probable time since death.

Within the general description of 'decomposition' there are several subclasses, which, as just stated, may merge into each other or may be uniform throughout the same cadaver. Most unembalmed bodies undergo putrefaction, in which the tissues become moist and gas-ridden, and eventually liquefy down to the skeleton.

Alternatives are dry decomposition, termed mummification, or a conversion to waxy substances, called adipocere; rarely, tannin occurs by the action of acid, protein-precipitating fluids in the anaerobic conditions of a peat bog. In some stillbirths an aseptic autolysis of a fetus dead *in utero* is known as maceration.

PUTREFACTION

The usual process of corruption of the dead body begins at a variable time after death, but in an average temperate climate may be expected to begin at about 3 days in the unrefrigerated corpse.

Even in temperate zones there can be a wide range of ambient temperatures, from below freezing to near blood heat. In the tropics, far higher temperatures are commonplace, but in high latitudes or elevations, deep-freeze conditions can keep decomposition at bay indefinitely, as in the case of modern discoveries of prehistoric mammoths and medieval Esquimaux. It is therefore futile to attempt to construct a timetable for the stages of decomposition, except to point out salient markers for an undisturbed body in an 'average' indoor environment of about 18°C in temperate climates. From this approximate baseline the pathologist must then extrapolate for local variations appropriate to his climatic and geographical conditions.

Sequence of putrefactive changes

Whatever the time scale, the general order of corruption is similar, though the degree of advancement may vary between different areas of even the same corpse.

Usually the first external naked-eye sign is discoloration of the lower abdominal wall, most often in the right iliac fossa where the bacteria-laden caecum lies fairly superficially. Direct spread of organisms from the bowel into the tissues of the abdominal wall breaks down haemoglobin into sulphaemoglobin and other pigmented substances. This discoloration spreads progressively over the abdomen, which in the later phase begins to become distended with gas.

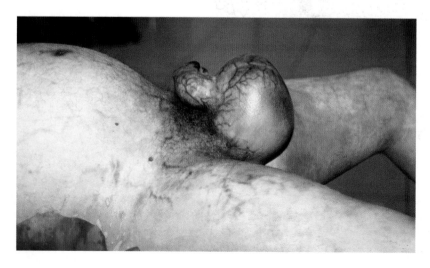

FIGURE 2.10 *Moderately early changes of decomposition, showing gaseous distension of scrotum and abdomen, and skin slippage and blistering in dependent areas. This was after about one week since death, but the changes vary greatly with environmental temperatures.*

At about this time, more generalized spread of bacteria begins to discolour the more moist tissues, which often comprise those dependent areas that show hypostatic coloration and oedema. The face and neck become reddish, and begin to swell. The putrefactive bacteria, which largely originate in the intestines and lungs, spread most easily in fluid so they tend to colonize the venous system, haemolysing the blood that stains the vessel walls and adjacent tissues. This gives rise to 'marbling', a branching outline of arborescent red, then greenish pattern in the skin, seen most clearly on the thighs, sides of the abdomen, and chest and shoulders. This stage may be about one week in the 'baseline' timetable, where the corpse is in air at 18–20°C.

At or even before the stage of marbling, skin blisters may appear, at first on the lower surfaces of trunk and thighs where hypostatic oedema has loaded the tissues with fluid. The upper epidermis becomes loosened, the so-called 'skin-slippage' giving rise to large, fragile sacs of clear, pink or red serous fluid. These may become so large that they are pendulous and soon burst, leaving areas of slimy, pink epidermis. Where this skin change occurs in hairy parts, such as scalp, axilla and pubis, the hair becomes detached and will slide off on slight pressure. Gas formation will now become marked, with increased tension in the abdomen.

The scrotum and penis may swell up to remarkable size and the neck and face will become grotesquely bloated, making visual identification difficult or impossible. The pressure may cause the eye globes and tongue to protrude.

Purging of urine and faeces may occur due to the intra-abdominal pressure and, occasionally, a uterine prolapse may be extruded. There are recorded instances of pregnant women having a macabre post-mortem 'delivery' of the fetus, from the same cause. Bloody fluid, which is tissue liquefaction stained by haemolysis, may leak from any orifice, especially the mouth, nostrils, rectum and vagina. By this stage, some 2–3 weeks may have elapsed since death.

To the inexperienced, this may suggest evidence of some lethal haemorrhage and many pathologists have been called to a scene of 'crime' because of the understandable concern of an investigating police officer that such bloody purging may be evidence of a violent mode of death. Pressure inside the chest due to gas formation in the abdomen may expel air, so that the fluids of decomposition in the trachea and bronchi may be blown into a bloody froth from the mouth and nostrils.

After several weeks, the reddish-green colour of the skin may deepen to a dark green or almost black, but there is marked variation in this aspect. Heavy maggot infestation will almost certainly have supervened except in winter conditions, and the destruction of skin by innumerable maggot holes and sinuses gives better access to other bacteria that may invade from the environment. The maggots secrete a proteolytic enzyme that speeds up the destruction of the tissues, in addition to the direct loss from the voracious appetites of these predators. Skin slippage causes shedding of the outer layers of the fingers and toes, making identification by fingerprints more difficult. Finger- and toenails last longer than the surrounding skin, but they too become loose and eventually fall out. Skin slippage may allow tattoos to become more visible and colourful for a time until the moist underlying dermis itself decomposes.

Internally, decomposition proceeds more slowly than at the surface. It is often quite surprising how valuable an

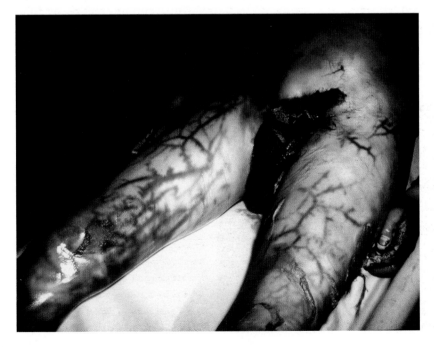

FIGURE 2.11 *Post-mortem decomposition of about 2 weeks' duration in water in a summer temperature. There is 'marbling' of the skin where breakdown products of haemoglobin have stained the venous channels.*

autopsy on a putrefying corpse can be, as the internal organs may be in far better condition than the exterior would suggest. Organs putrefy at markedly different rates. The lining of the intestine, the adrenal medulla and the pancreas autolyse within hours of death, yet the prostate and uterus may still be recognizable in a partially skeletalized body a year later. The brain soon becomes discoloured, being a soft pinkish-grey within a week and liquefying within a month.

Meningeal haemorrhage and haematomata persist well, but apart from some tumours, non-haemorrhagic lesions in the brain substance vanish quite early.

The heart is moderately resistant, and examination of the coronary arteries for the degree of atheromatous stenosis may be well worthwhile for many months, though staining of the vessel walls by haemolysis makes recognition of mural thrombosis difficult. Complete occlusion by firm ante-mortem

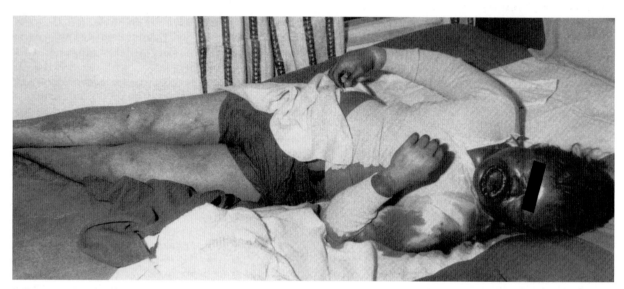

FIGURE 2.12 *Post-mortem decomposition showing putrefactive changes in the face, arms and trunk after one week in a warm room. The illustration shows the contrast sometimes seen between one part of the body and another, as the legs are hardly affected. The face, neck and hands are swollen with gas, and the clothing is stained by leaking skin blisters. The tongue is protruding because of gas pressure from the tissues below. Death was due to carbon monoxide poisoning caused by faulty installation of a room heater.*

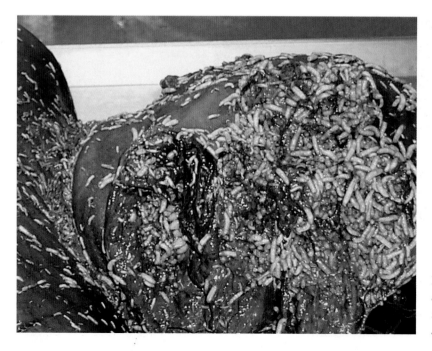

FIGURE 2.13 *Almost complete destruction of the facial soft tissues by maggots. Post-mortem time about 2 weeks in a centrally heated apartment.*

thrombus persists well. The heart may show a curious white granularity on the epicardial and endocardial surfaces, seen either during putrefaction or even on exhumation after a long interval. The nodules are a millimetre or less in size and are often called 'miliary plaques'. They were investigated by Gonzales *et al.* (1954) who found that microscopically they consisted of calcium and soapy material. The origin is obscure, but they seem to be confined to the heart and to be some degenerative product of the cardiac tissue.

In obese people, the body fat (especially perirenal, omental and mesenteric) may liquefy into a translucent, yellow fluid that fills the body cavities between the organs, and makes autopsy even more difficult and unpleasant.

Later putrefactive changes lead to the breakdown of the thoracic and abdominal walls, often hastened by the perforations of maggots and sometimes larger predators, such as rats and dogs. In some tropical countries, such as India and Sri Lanka, bodies left in the open are attacked by many animals, including monitor lizards, and in other parts of the world the indigenous fauna all contribute to the natural cycle that returns the body fats and proteins to the food chain.

After several months, the softer tissues and viscera progressively disintegrate, leaving the more solid organs, such as uterus, heart and prostate, together with the ligamentous and tendinous tissues attached to the skeleton. Often some areas of skin persist, especially where protected by clothing or under the body against the supporting surface. Much depends upon the environment, as a corpse in the open air will suffer far more from rain, wind and especially animal predators, compared with one in a locked room.

Eventually, the body will be reduced to a skeleton, but for some time, ligaments, cartilage and periosteal tags will survive. The season of year and the location will make a great difference to the time scale of skeletalization: a body dying outdoors in the late autumn will 'survive' longer through the cold winter and spring than one dying in the early summer. The effects of animal predators are profound in terms of removing soft tissues from the bones. In broad terms, a corpse outdoors in a temperate climate is likely to be converted to a skeleton carrying tendon tags within 12–18 months, and to a 'bare-bone' skeleton within 3 years; there are, of course, numerous exceptions, depending mainly on the local environment. In closed conditions indoors, a body may never skeletalize, often being converted to a dried, partly putrefied, partly mummified shell.

Decomposition in immersed bodies

The old rule-of-thumb that bodies decay twice as fast in air as in water is grossly inaccurate, but emphasizes the slower rate of decomposition of immersed corpses. Though in mortuary practice 'drowners' are generally regarded as being the major source of offensively rotten bodies, this is usually because discovery and recovery is far later than in deaths on dry land. Water, in fact, slows up putrefaction, mainly because of the lower ambient temperature, and protection from insect and small mammal predators.

The water also affects the usual processes of decay in that the epidermis becomes macerated and eventually detached, as described in the Chapter 16. Gas formation is the reason

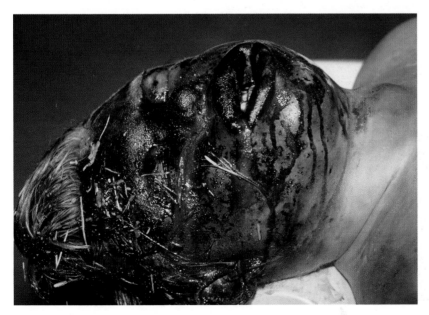

FIGURE 2.14 *Bloating of face and effusion of blood-tinged fluid from the nostrils and mouth. A body recovered from water, postmortem time approximately 11 days.*

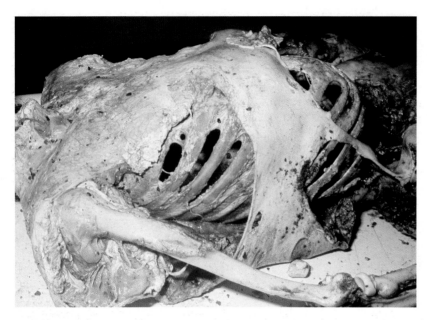

FIGURE 2.15 *Marine predation in a body after 3 months in the North Sea. The victim was from an oil rig and had floated on the surface in a life jacket. Much of the skin has been removed by crustaceans, and the arm muscles by larger fish who have cleaned out most of the body cavity.*

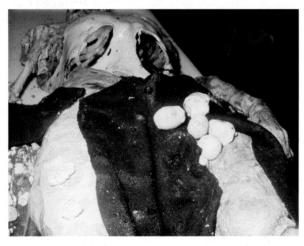

FIGURE 2.16 *Adipocere formation in a body after 3 months in the sea. Subcutaneous fat has been released from crustacean bites on the skin and has been converted into adipocere, which has been rolled by wave action within the clothing to form ovoid masses.*

for the inevitable flotation of an unweighted body, though the time of reappearance at the surface is extremely variable and certainly does not follow the speculative timetable of the older textbooks. The usual posture of a freely floating body is face down, as the head is relatively dense, and does not develop the early gas formation in the abdomen and thorax. This lower position favours fluid gravitation and hence more marked decomposition, so that the face is often badly putrefied in an immersed body, making visual recognition difficult or impossible at an early stage. As stated, temperature is the major determinant of the rate of putrefaction. Though it

is usually claimed that the nature of the water in respect of sewage, for instance, is important, it is a minor factor as most of the micro-organisms responsible for decay come from the alimentary canal and respiratory passages of the body itself.

Decomposition in buried bodies

The rate of decay of bodies buried in earth is much slower than of those in either air or water. In fact the process of putrefaction may be arrested to a remarkable degree in certain conditions, allowing exhumations several years later to be of considerable value. In this respect the prospect of an exhumation should never be dismissed on the grounds that because of the lapse of time, it is bound to be worthless. It may turn out to be of little value, but this cannot be anticipated, and not infrequently the condition of the body may be surprisingly good.

The speed and extent of decay in interred corpses depends on a number of factors. If the body is buried soon after death, before the usual process of decay in air begins, putrefaction is less and may never proceed to the liquefying corruption usually inevitable on the surface. A lower temperature, exclusion of animal and insect predators, and lack of oxygen are important factors. Although most bacteria originate in the intestine, there is less access for secondary invaders and the restriction of oxygen inhibits aerobic organisms. If the body is rotting before burial then, although the process slows down, it will still severely damage the corpse, as enzymatic and bacterial growth have had initial encouragement from a higher ambient temperature and free access of air, thereby producing conditions in which secondary

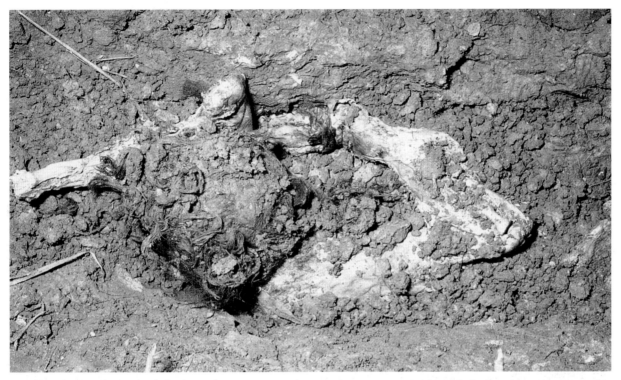

FIGURE 2.17 *Decomposition in a body buried in a shallow grave for 6 months (see Figure 1.2). The soil had collapsed into cavities around the corpse, partly due to the weight of tractors passing over it. This allowed access to flies and discovery by a dog. The body is partly putrefied, but has some adipocere.*

invaders (including anaerobes) can continue their work in a good culture medium that is already partly liquefied by the earlier stages.

Deep burial, as in the usual cemetery interment, preserves the corpse better than the shallow grave seen in some concealed homicides. The deep burial is colder (except in extremely cold weather), it excludes air better and, unless waterlogged, is not directly affected by rain.

The nature of the soil is not directly relevant except in its drainage and aeration properties. Heavy clay will exclude air and, if well above the water table, will exclude percolating surface water. By contrast, light sandy soil may allow access of both air and rainwater, but will drain more effectively. The soil factor is less important than the topography in which it lies – in a valley floor or below the water table, waterlogging is inevitable, but on a well-drained hillside the grave may remain relatively dry.

Another factor that aids the preservation of legitimately buried corpses is the coffin. Though modern coffins are often of wooden laminate or chipboard, which rapidly disintegrates when wet, any kind of coffin helps to exclude water and air for a time. A substantial, sound jointed coffin may last for years and the modern rarity of a sealed metal liner can keep a body in an excellent state of preservation for a long time.

A major factor that helps to slow decomposition is, of course, the absence of animal predation in burials. Again, if a corpse is buried before insect eggs are laid, the profound effect of maggot infestation is avoided. Rodents and larger mammals can only reach shallow burials, and in deep interments the coffin has to be breached before even the limited fauna of that stratum can gain access.

As in all putrefaction, it is unrealistic to try to construct a timetable for the stages of decay in burials. The permutations of factors mentioned above make it impossible, especially where adipocere formation takes place, as described below. The author (BK) has exhumed a chapel cemetery in the waterlogged peat of a Welsh valley and found not a trace of body, even skeleton, in graves with headstones confirming death only 20 years previously. By contrast, other bodies elsewhere were perfectly recognizable – and a standard autopsy could be carried out – one and a half years after death.

When bodies are buried in coffins in vaults, rather than in earth, then again there can be a variable rate of decay. Some bodies may develop adipocere, others may wholly or partly mummify.

There are many publications on this subject, mainly derived from the examination of historical sites or church crypts that have had to be cleared. The subject is of considerable interest but of limited forensic relevance.

FORMATION OF ADIPOCERE

An important and relatively common post-mortem change is the formation of adipocere, a waxy substance derived from the body fat. The name was given to it by Fourcroy in 1789, being derived from 'adipo' and 'cire', to indicate its affinity with both fat and wax. In most instances the change of adipocere is partial and irregular, though occasionally almost the whole body may be affected. In small amounts, adipocere is more common than usually thought in buried or concealed corpses. It is caused by hydrolysis and hydrogenation of adipose tissue, leading to the formation of a greasy or waxy substance if of recent origin. After months or years have passed, adipocere becomes brittle and chalky. The colour can vary from dead white, through pinkish, to a grey or greenish-grey. The substance itself is off-white, but staining with blood or products of decomposition can give it the red or greenish hues. The smell was accurately described by WED Evans (1962, 1963a, b) as being 'earthy, cheesy and ammoniacal'.

The chemistry of adipocere has been studied extensively. It contains palmitic, oleic and stearic fatty acids together with some glycerol, though the latter may have been leached out in older adipocere. These form a matrix for remnants of tissue fibres, nerves and muscles, which give some slight strength to the fats (see Mant and Furbank 1957). Crystals with radial markings can be found in the adipocere. Body fat at the time of death contains only about half of 1 per cent of fatty acids, but in adipocere, this may rise to 20 per cent within a month and more than 70 per cent in 3 months.

The formation of adipocere, as an alternative to total putrefaction, requires certain environmental conditions. A body left exposed in air, unless the conditions are conducive to mummification, will undergo moist putrefaction if the temperature remains above about 5–8°C. In burials, immersion in water, and in incarceration in vaults and crypts, adipocere often forms to a greater or lesser extent.

It is usually taught that moisture is necessary for the process, and it is undoubtedly a fact that most adipocere formation occurs in immersed bodies and those in wet graves and damp vaults. Numerous cases have been described, however, in which dry concealment also led to adipocere formation and here it must be assumed that the original internal body water was sufficient for the hydrolysis to proceed.

It is said that some warmth is necessary for adipocere formation, but the process seems to occur even in deep

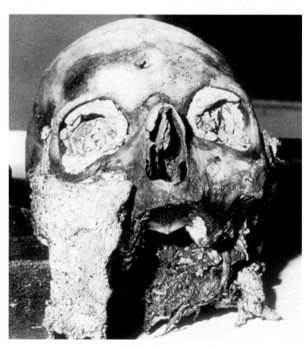

FIGURE 2.19 *Conversion of facial and orbital fat into adipocere after several months in water. There is also a penetrating wound on the forehead, obviously ante-mortem from the healing margins. The body was eventually identified by obtaining hospital radiographs of the person suspected of being the victim; these matched post-mortem radiographs in respect of the injury and frontal sinus outlines.*

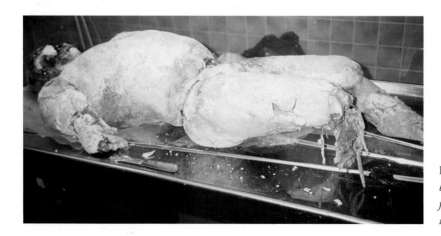

FIGURE 2.18 *Complete conversion of a body to adipocere. The body was recovered from a deep lake 8 years after disappearing in a boating accident during a heavy storm.*

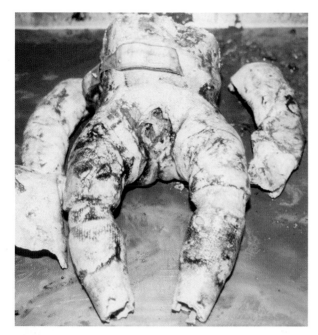

FIGURE 2.20 *Almost complete conversion of an infant's body to adipocere. The body was exhumed after 3 years' burial and was found to consist of a hollow shell of stiff adipocere with the skeletal elements loose within.*

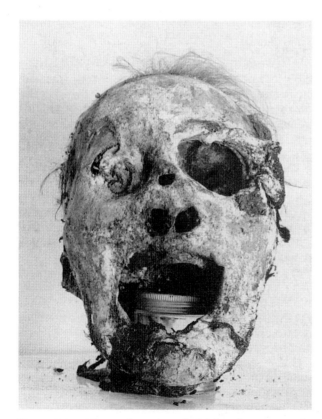

FIGURE 2.21 *Adipocere formation in body left in dry sewer tunnel for about 2 years. External water is not necessary for adipocere formation, as body fluids may be sufficient hydrolysis of fat.*

graves and in cold water. Early activity by anaerobes such as *Clostridium perfringens* assist in the reaction, as the bacteria produce lecithinase which facilitates hydrolysis and hydrogenation (see Mant 1967). Such bacteria need some warmth in the initial stages to reproduce and metabolize and Mant suggests that rapid cooling soon after death, such as by immersion in water, may actually retard the formation of adipocere.

The frequency with which adipocere forms may be gauged by the observations of those who have exhumed old cemeteries and vaults, as well as the victims of wartime slaughter (see Evans 1963a; Mant 1967; Polson *et al.* 1975; Evans 1963a). The latter found that over half the occupants of dry vaults had some adipocere. It was present in 63 per cent of women and 45 per cent of men.

The importance of adipocere formation

The process is more than a biochemical curiosity as, once it is formed, adipocere may persist for decades or even centuries. The usual dissolution of putrefaction is replaced by a permanent firm cast of the fatty tissues and, although distorted compared to the immediate post-mortem shape, it allows the form of the body and sometimes even of the facial features to be retained in recognizable form. Injuries, especially bullet holes, may be preserved in a remarkable fashion (Mant 1967). Though adipocere mainly affects the subcutaneous fat, it may also preserve the omental, mesenteric and perirenal adipose deposits; in addition, organs containing fat through pathological or degenerative processes may be preserved by adipocere forming in their parenchyma.

The time required for the production of adipocere has been a matter of controversy. The old authors claimed that 3–12 months were required, and Casper (1862) suggested 6 months, but it is obvious that the process can occur much faster than this.

There seems little reason to doubt that hydrolysis of body fat begins soon after death, as crystals of fatty acids have been found in infant bodies lying in water for only a week. This process is usually overtaken by liquefying putrefaction, however, which allows the fat, especially in obese persons, to collect as extracellular pools and pockets of triglycerides in the body cavities.

If the putrefactive process is slowed by burial or immersion, then hydrolysis and hydrogenation can outpace putrefaction. In addition, adipocere formation actually inhibits putrefaction, as the increasing acidity of tissues and the dehydration caused by the consumption of water in hydrolysis slow the growth and spread of the usual putrefactive organisms. The point at which adipocere becomes visible to the naked eye varies greatly, but it has been observed as early as 3 weeks, though 3 months is a more typical period. Adipocere is often mixed with the other forms of decomposition. Even within a coffin or other place of sequestration, there may be several different 'mini-environments'. One end of the body may be putrefied or skeletalized, whilst other parts may be mummified or in adipocere. Certain areas tend to develop adipocere, such as the cheeks, orbits, chest, abdominal wall and buttocks. Only rarely is the face preserved well enough by adipocere to be genuinely recognizable, as disintegration of the eye globes and shrinkage of the tissues around the nose and mouth obscure the most characteristic features.

MUMMIFICATION

The third type of long-term change after death is mummification, a drying of the tissues in place of liquefying putrefaction. Like the other modes of decomposition, this can be partial and can coexist with them in different areas of the same body. It is, however, more likely than the others to extend over the whole corpse.

Mummification can only occur in a dry environment, which is usually, but not exclusively, also a warm place. Mummification can occur in freezing conditions, partly because of the dryness of the air and partly because of the inhibition of bacterial growth. The most widely known forms of mummification are those in hot, desert zones. The process of artificial mummification practised for millennia in Egypt was an imitative process founded on the natural mummification of bodies in predynastic times. The essential requirement for mummification is a dry environment, preferably with a moving air current. If sterility of the tissues can be attained, as in a newborn baby, then putrefaction is held at bay whilst drying occurs. The appearances of mummification display desiccation and brittleness of the skin, which is stretched tightly across anatomical prominences such as the cheekbones, chin, costal margin and hips. The skin is discoloured (usually being brown), though secondary colonization by moulds may add patches of white, green or black.

The skin and underlying tissues are hard, making autopsy dissection difficult. The condition of the internal organs is variable, depending partly on the length of time since death. They may be partly dried, partly putrefied – and adipocere is not uncommon. In fact, slight adipocere formation is common in mummification, and perhaps the two are related in that the utilization of body water to hydrolyse fat in turn helps to dehydrate the tissues. The major factor, however, is evaporation from the surface in dry conditions.

Like adipocere, facial recognition may be possible in some instances, though the shrunken distortion and loss of eyes and full lips considerably alter the features. Mummification is likely to occur in temperate climates when the body is left undisturbed in a dry, warm place. These include closed rooms and cupboards, haylofts, attics and beneath floorboards. Because concealment favours mummification, a number of these bodies are hidden homicides – one of the best known being the 'Rhyl mummy' in North Wales, when a strangled woman was concealed in a cupboard for many years, whilst her pension continued to be claimed. Other instances are where a natural death has been concealed for some purpose. The author (BK) has also seen two deaths in hay barns, where the corpses were undisturbed for over a year.

Most experienced forensic pathologists are familiar with the mummified fetus or newborn infant, concealed in domestic circumstances, such as a house loft, where complete mummification has taken place. With small bodies such as these, evaporation is faster and more complete, and may extend

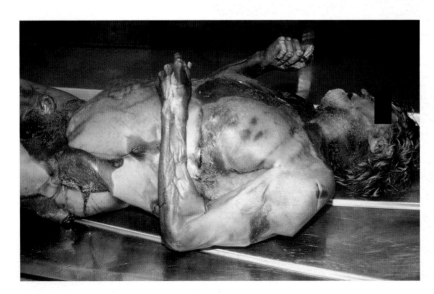

FIGURE 2.22 *Mummification in a man dead in a locked room for 10 weeks. The corpse is dry and leathery, with very little moist putrefaction.*

to all organs, especially as there would have been no invasion of putrefactive micro-organisms from the gut.

The timing of mummification is not well documented, as most mummified corpses have been concealed so well that discovery does not occur until long after the process has reached its maximum effect. It certainly takes some weeks and the early stages are often mixed with a degree of putrefactive change, especially in the internal organs.

After complete drying has taken place, the body may remain in that state for many years. Eventually, mould formation and physical deterioration progress, the dried tissues becoming split and powdery and gradually disintegrating. This process is usually hastened by animal predation. Even in the shelter of a barn or house, moths, beetles, mice and rats will wreak damage on the corpse. It will eventually skeletalize,

though tough, leathery shreds of skin, tendon and ligament may persist for many years. Mummification allows major injuries to be preserved, though as in the putrefied body, the detection of bruises and abrasion may be difficult or impossible to differentiate from discoloration, artefacts and fungal damage. The stiff tissues can be softened for better examination and histology, by soaking in a 15 per cent solution of glycerine for several days (see Evans 1962).

POST-MORTEM DAMAGE BY PREDATORS

Animal predation is part of the natural food chain, which returns the proteins, fats and carbohydrates of dead bodies

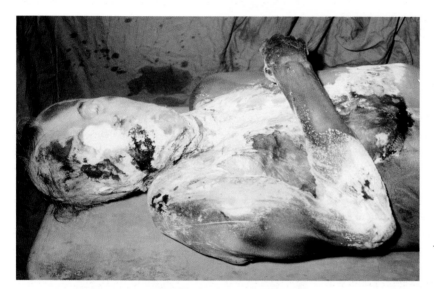

FIGURE 2.23 *The mummified body of an absconder from a mental hospital who was found a year later in a hay barn. The dry environment had inhibited wet decomposition.*

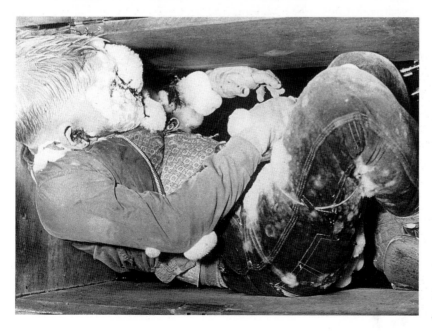

FIGURE 2.24 *Extensive mould formation and lack of putrefactive changes in a child who accidentally locked himself in a box and asphyxiated. The body was not found for 6 weeks.*

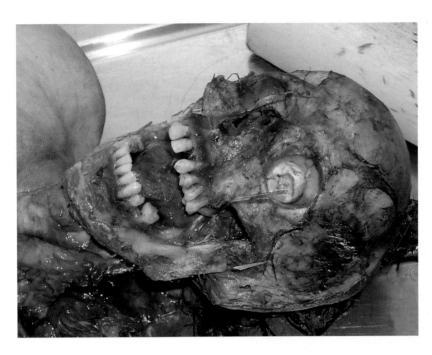

FIGURE 2.25 *Loss of all soft tissues of head and neck, in areas not covered by clothing, by post-mortem animal predation.*

to other animals, some of it passing back to the vegetable kingdom through soil nutrition. All types and sizes of animal are involved, the largest seen by the author (BK) being a 'near-miss' by a Malayan tiger, who dragged a sleeping soldier from his tent. Most animal damage is more mundane, the beasts varying from ants to foxes, and from bluebottles to monitor lizards. Foxes can drag parts of a body away to a distance of at least 2 miles.

The type of predation varies greatly with geography, season, and whether the dead body is indoors or out in the open. If it is lying in the countryside, large predators will cause prompt and severe damage, even complete destruction being possible in a short time. In temperate countries, foxes and dogs form the main agents, and the body may be dismembered and scattered over a wide area, especially if advancing putrefaction makes disarticulation easy. If corpses are in inland waters, damage from water rats and fish is possible, as well as attacks from dogs and foxes, if the body lies exposed on the bank of a river or a lake.

The type of damage from canine and rodent predators is usually obvious, as the local removal of large amounts of flesh is usually accompanied by evidence of teeth marks. Rats and cats leave a crenated edge to fairly clean-cut wounds, the post-mortem nature of which is obvious from the lack of bleeding or an inflamed marginal zone. Mice rarely attack bodies, but may help to remove the dried, crumbling tissue of a mummified corpse. The most active tissue removers are maggots, the larval stage of bluebottles (*Calliphora*) and flies (*Musca*). The use of the life cycle in timing death is dealt with elsewhere, but here we are concerned with their destructive effects on

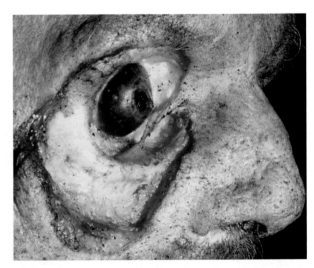

FIGURE 2.26 *Post-mortem rat bites of the orbit. Such injuries are – not unnaturally – often regarded with suspicion by the police. The complete absence of bleeding or reddening of the wound margins, as well as the unlikely shape and situation of the injury, make its post-mortem origin obvious.*

corpses. In temperate zones their activity is seasonal, but in hot countries their predatory work is ever present. The adult insects lay eggs on the fresh corpse (or even on a debilitated live victim), choosing wounds or moist areas such as the eyelids, lips, nostrils and genitalia. Once skin decomposition begins, the eggs can be deposited anywhere. The eggs hatch in a day or so, and several cycles of maggot develop, shedding their cases at intervals, depending on the species.

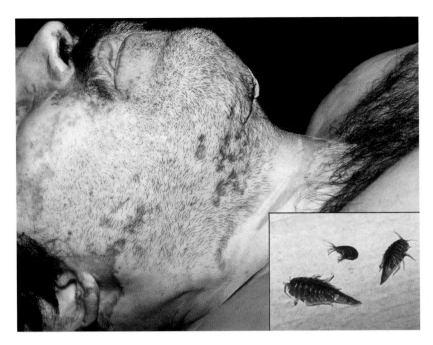

FIGURE 2.27 *A body recovered from the Baltic Sea with numerous superficial skin defects on the face and neck due to post-mortem predation, probably by the crustacean* Saduria entomon, *shown in the inserted picture with a smaller shrimp in the middle.*

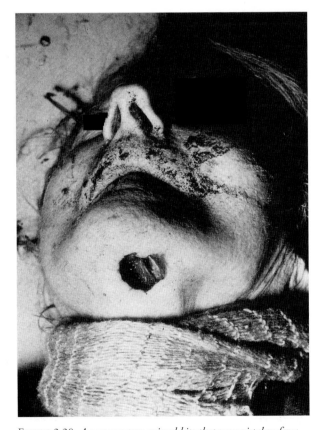

FIGURE 2.28 *A post-mortem animal bite that was mistaken for a criminal assault. The old lady was found locked in with a cat, having died from a gastric haemorrhage. The wound has not bled, the margins are not reddened and tooth crenations can be seen round its edge.*

The maggots are voracious and energetic, first exploring the natural passages, such as mouth and nostrils, then burrowing into the tissues. They secrete digestive fluids with proteolytic enzymes that help soften the tissues, burrowing beneath the skin, and making tunnels and sinuses that hasten putrefaction by admitting air and access to external micro-organisms. Successive waves of eggs are laid, producing new generations of maggots. Eventually, loss of tissue and drying make the host cadaver unattractive to egg-laying insects, and the later stages of decomposition become free from maggots.

Beetles and many other types of insect and arthropod join in the destruction, but one particular insect must be mentioned. This is the ant, which can attack the body soon after death before putrefaction begins. A common place for ant attack is around the eyelids, lips and on the knuckles. The lesions are superficial ulcers with scalloped, serpiginous margins. They can be mistaken for ante-mortem abrasions, but their position, margins and lack of bleeding or inflammatory changes usually make them easily recognizable. Shapiro, however, has documented cases where extensive linear ant lesions have resembled ligature abrasions around the neck (Shapiro *et al.* 1988).

Tropical ants can devour tissues to a considerable extent and, although stories of soldier ants reducing horses to skeletons within minutes are apocryphal, predation by large numbers of insects can be extensive.

In water, all manner of aquatic animals can mutilate immersed bodies, as well as land mammals if the corpse is in shallow water or grounded on a mudbank or the beach. Large fish can be totally destructive, especially in tropical waters, but even in temperate seas severe damage can occur. Some of the victims of the Air India aircraft disaster near Ireland in 1985 were ravaged by sharks. Large gouges from the wound edges, punctures from teeth and extensive tissue loss, even with fractures of large bones such as the femur, characterize shark attacks.

Smaller fish can wreak severe damage, the prime example being piranhas, though many species will devour both fresh and decomposing bodies. Crustaceans are also predatory and can remove circular areas of skin to expose the subcutaneous fat, which may detach inside the clothing to form masses of adipocere. Birds also cause damage, usually to the dead, though crows may mutilate live lambs. The habits of carrion birds, such as the vulture, are well known, but smaller birds will inflict injury on exposed bodies, especially when putrefaction softens the tissues.

All animal predation varies in appearance according to the size and shape of the teeth or jaws of the predator, but all such post-mortem injuries have features in common. There is no bleeding apart from the minute quantity actually in the vessels of the damaged part, and certainly no active haemorrhage into the wound margins. Naturally, there is no oedema or reddening of the edges as might be seen in an ante-mortem wound earlier than the perimortal period. Crenation of the edges is a useful guide where small rodents or other animals are involved, though large carnivores can make totally irregular tears in the tissue. Some animals, such as dogs and foxes, may leave punctured wounds adjacent to the damaged edge where sharp teeth have penetrated. On bones, the incisor teeth of rodents and larger carnivores can leave parallel gouges, which must not be mistaken for illicit human activities. In domestic surroundings, pets may inflict drastic post-mortem injuries if they are locked in with a dead person. Dogs and cats can cause injuries that puzzle those, such as the police, who are unaware of the possibility. Complete decapitation by Alsatian dogs has been seen by both of the authors, as well as genital injury.

THE ENTOMOLOGY OF THE DEAD AND POST-MORTEM INTERVAL

This is a highly specialized subject and, when the issue of time since death is important, such as a criminal investigation, it is essential that, wherever possible, the pathologist has the assistance of an entomologist with forensic experience. As in forensic toxicology and serology when serious medico-legal issues are at stake, there is no place in forensic entomology for the 'occasional expert' who dabbles in the subject when the opportunity arises. Having said this, it is

helpful to know sufficient about the topic to recognize when expert help is required, and to understand what information and specimens need to be obtained.

The rationale of forensic entomology is that after death invasion of an unprotected body by sarcosaprophagous insects and other small fauna comes in successive waves. Different species of arthropods colonize the corpse at different periods after death. In addition, some species (including the most common blowflies) pass through complex life cycles that can be used to determine at least the minimum time since death by studying the stage of maturation of the insects. The science is inexact and is modified by a number of factors, both climatic and geographical, but in expert hands can sometimes yield useful information about the date of death at a period when other indicators have ceased to function. These methods have been used since the middle of the eighteenth century, but Megnin placed forensic entomology on a sound basis with his publication of *La faune des cadavres* in 1894. There are now a substantial number of publications on the subject, though most of them need specialist zoological knowledge for the interpretation of the species involved and their complicated maturation cycles. It is essential that the entomologist has the fullest possible information about the nature of the environment in which the body was found and, if possible, he should visit the scene himself. It is also vital to have accurate data on the weather, especially the ambient temperature of the area during the period in which the body had been lying there, as the maturation times of insects (especially blowflies) are markedly altered by climatic conditions.

The most common insect found on relatively fresh corpses is the blowfly, a colloquial name for a group of flying insects of the order **Diptera**, with almost worldwide distribution. They mainly comprise the bluebottles, the greenbottles and the housefly. There are numerous species, with variations in life cycles that are altered by climatic conditions. The bluebottle (*Calliphora*) is the most common, especially *Calliphora vicina* Robineau–Desvoidy (*Calliphora erythrocephala* Meigen), the most frequent invader of dead flesh. These are large, bristly flies about 6–14 mm long, with iridescent blue abdomens.

They do not fly in the dark and thus eggs are laid only in daylight. This means that a corpse found at night or in the morning with eggs upon it, almost certainly died the previous day. Bluebottles rarely fly in winter, but may do on fine days, though when the temperature is below 12°C they are unlikely to lay eggs. Rain is also a marked deterrent to egg-laying, except in the case of the **Sarcophagidae**. Bluebottles prefer fresh rather than decayed carrion and lay their eggs soon after death, which may be of medico-legal significance. Indeed, they may lay eggs on the living, especially when the victim (man or animal) is debilitated or wounded. A single bluebottle may lay up to 300–2000 eggs in clusters of

30–150. The eggs are laid on moist areas, such as the eyelids, canthi of the eyes, nostrils, lips, mouth, genitals and anus. If there are any open wounds or weeping abrasions, these may also be colonized. The eggs are yellow and banana-shaped, about l.7 mm in length.

The many tables and diagrams available for the succession of sarcosaprophagous insects on corpses must be read in the knowledge that the environment, especially the temperature, makes a marked difference to the time span of the larval and pupal stages. As Nuorteva *et al.* (1967) state:

> Crimes do not occur under experimental conditions and standardized food supplies. Flies, as medico-legal indicators, must therefore be used in conjunction with the records of meteorological conditions existing at the time subsequent to the presumed crime.

Thus the following examples, mainly taken from Glaister and Brash's (1937) account of the notorious Ruxton murder, must be read with this caution firmly in mind – and wherever possible, the pathologist must enlist the aid of an experienced entomologist.

Adult bluebottles will begin to lay eggs about 4–5 days after emergence from pupation. Eggs will not hatch at temperatures below 4°C, but they will develop at 6–7°C. The time from laying to hatching is 8–14 hours, depending on the temperature.

The first maggot stage (first 'instar') tries to penetrate the tissues or enter any nearby body cavity such as the mouth or wounds. Maggots have powerful proteolytic enzymes that aid dissolution of the tissues and facilitate penetration. The first larval instar persists for another 8–14 hours, then the outer skin is shed and the second larger instar feeds for another 2–3 days.

After a final moult, the third instar spends about 6 days on the body before leaving it to migrate some distance to hide in the ground or under some other cover (even a carpet) to pupate. The pupa is a brown leathery capsule in which the insect metamorphoses into the winged fly after about 12 days. The new bluebottle emerges and leaves the empty pupa case behind, ready to begin the cycle over again, which thus lasts about 18–24 days from egg to adult. The greenbottle (*Lucilla caesar*) and the sheep maggot fly (*Lucilla sericata*) have life histories that are similar to that of the bluebottle.

The common house fly (*Musca domestica*) is different in that, unlike the bluebottles, it prefers to lay its eggs on already decomposed flesh, though it is more attracted to garbage and manure than to cadavers. The eggs are much smaller and white rather than yellow. Hatching time is 8–12 hours, the first instar at about 36 hours, the second instar at 1–2 days and the third at about 3–4 days. Pupation lasts up to 7 days, less in warm weather. The whole cycle

is thus about 14 days at about 22°C, though again it must be emphasized that variations in ambient temperature make considerable differences to the speed of maturation. A table by Busvine (1980) shows that the total cycle length varies from 9 days at 40°C to 32 days at 16°C.

Entomologists have constructed tables of variation in larval length according to age and temperature; expert knowledge and strict identification of the species is needed before definite opinions upon minimum times since cadaver death are offered. Some of the times quoted above were taken from the extensive entomological work performed on the Ruxton case in 1935, but do not correspond to the cycle periods published by Kamal in 1958. The total maturation times that he found in experimental conditions at 22°C are much longer, being 14–25 days (average 18) for *Calliphora vicina*.

In many of the published cases where *Calliphora* have assisted in the estimate of the time since death, it is an assessment of the age of larvae that is made from their size. Of course this can only be a minimum estimate, especially if mixed generations are present as a result of successive waves of flies laying eggs at different times. As already said, however, bluebottles do not favour decomposed tissue for oviposition, so egg-laying is likely to cease within a couple of days of death. If pupa cases are seen either on or near the body, then any larvae present may be from later waves – even second- or third-generation insects.

In addition to maggots on the body, other fauna in the soil beneath a corpse leave the area and a reduction in the number of species of normal soil insects may be a marker for the site of a body, even for some time after the latter has been removed. The minimum population of arthropods under a corpse is reached after about 2 months; it then revives, but with quite a different range of insects from the original inhabitants. The absence of eggs or maggots on a body may sometimes be of use, as it may indicate that a body has been in a sheltered place inaccessible to flies, even if it was later moved out. Where a body has been buried, even a shallow covering of soil may protect it from oviposition; where part of the body protrudes, this may well be the focus of maggot infestation.

Different types of insects invade the body after the moist, putrefaction stage that is associated with blowfly maggots has passed. At different seasons, different insects may be prevalent so that the finding of say, **Phoridae** and **Sphaerocerdiae** in Europe would suggest that the body had been there in the summer months. Larder beetles (*Dermestes*) may arrive 3–6 months after death; house moths may attack dried tissues such as mummies and can dispose of keratin such as hair and beard. Beetles (*Coleoptera*) are late arrivals and are usually found in dried or adipocerous corpses. These and many more are related more to season than time, so again the considered opinion of an expert is necessary. The absence of insects in certain climates may indicate that death took place in the winter months when no active colonization was occurring.

Collection of material for entomological study

To the practising forensic pathologist, the main concern in this context is the careful collection and dispatch of specimens to an entomologist with forensic experience.

First, the entomologist needs to know all available facts about the environment in which the body was found – preferably he should visit the locus himself if the matter is of legal importance. He should be told the temperature of the maggot mass and ambient temperature around the time the body was found. If no actual temperature measurements were taken by the pathologist at the scene – and even if they were – local records should be obtained from the nearest meteorological centre. Without this information the probable maturation rate cannot be estimated. The nature of the locus should be described, in terms of vegetation, trees and undergrowth if outdoors. Where maggots are present, some should be placed live in a tube and, if there is delay in transit to the entomology laboratory, a fragment of meat should be included for food. Any adult flies, other insects and eggs should also be collected without preservative.

In addition, some maggots, adults, pupae, empty pupa cases and eggs should be sent after fixation. They can be placed directly into 80 per cent alcohol, but preferably in three parts 80 per cent alcohol with one part glacial acetic acid. Even better is Pimple's fluid, which is six parts 35 per cent formalin, two parts glacial acetic acid, 15 parts 95 per cent alcohol and 30 parts water. Formol saline 10 per cent (as used for histological fixation) should not be used.

If there are different insects on the body, they should be placed in separate tubes – especially if they are alive – as some may devour the others before they reach the laboratory.

Whatever is sent should be labelled or numbered according to a key that records where on the body they were found. If outdoors, the soil beneath the body should be sampled and, where a full cycle has occurred, pupae or cases should be obtained by shallow trenching in radii around the body.

When the body has been recovered from water, any insects or crustaceans should be recovered. Body parasites may occasionally be useful. Fleas and lice can survive total immersion for some hours, but the advice of an entomologist should be sought if parasites are found on an immersed body to determine the minimum survival time of that particular species under the existing circumstances.

DETERMINATION OF TIME SINCE DEATH

ESTIMATION OF THE TIME SINCE DEATH BY BODY COOLING

Though the study of the rate of cooling of the dead human body is essentially an exercise in physiology, its potential use in determining the time since death have made it the most frequent topic for research in forensic medicine.

For more than one and a half centuries, papers have been published devoted to refining the problem further, which has obvious and important connotations in the investigation of criminal deaths. Unfortunately, the vast amount of labour in this direction has not been rewarded by comparable improvements in accuracy because of the permutations of factors that defeat exact calculation of the post-mortem interval. The history of this research is in itself extensive (Knight 1988) but a few cardinal points might be mentioned here to mark the various phases of investigation.

Though the fact that a dead body becomes progressively colder after death has naturally been known since earliest times, scientific measurements were first published in the nineteenth century. Dr John Davey in 1839 recounted experiments with dead soldiers in Malta and Britain, using a mercury thermometer. Though this pioneer made no practical contribution to the problem, some of his comments are remarkably pertinent across a gap of more than 150 years:

> Much judgement, however and nice discrimination may be requisite on the part of the medical man, in appreciating the circumstances likely to modify temperature, so as to enable him when called upon for his opinion (of the time of death), to give one which will be satisfactory to the legal officers – and to himself – on reflection.

These cautionary words are just as applicable nowadays when, unfortunately, some doctors offer a time of death with a confidence often inversely proportional to their experience. In 1863, Taylor and Wilkes wrote a classic paper which introduced many of the current concepts, such as the initial temperature plateau, the core temperature, heat gradient and the effect of insulation. Taylor was, of course, Alfred Swaine Taylor of Guy's Hospital, author of the textbook that remained the definitive work on forensic medicine for almost a century. Later in the nineteenth century, Rainy of Glasgow first applied mathematical concepts to the problem and produced a formula for calculating the time of death. He also pointed out that Newton's Law of Cooling did not apply to the human body. In 1887, Womack first used centigrade units, though his use of the now familiar temperature graphs was anticipated by Burman in 1880.

In this century, the most quoted papers were those by De Saram in Ceylon (De Saram *et al.* 1955; De Saram 1957), who published careful and detailed measurements of control cases obtained from executed prisoners. His data are still being studied and reworked. The names Fiddes and Patten are known to all those interested in this subject as, in 1958, they produced a paper that was a classic, as Taylor's had been in the previous century. Using repeated temperature measurements they devised a percentage cooling method and explored complex theoretical aspects, such as the 'infinite cylinder' model, for the human body.

Marshall and his collaborators dominated the publications in the 1960–1970 period, with papers that explored in depth the mathematical aspects and confirmed the double exponential or 'sigmoid' shape of the rectal cooling curve. In the last decade or so, many more papers and new techniques have been produced, with computer assistance increasingly used. Amongst these, Henssge and Madea in Germany have been predominant. Microwave and infrared thermography have been explored and the physics and mathematics of body cooling probed in such depth that often the scientist in the research group has difficulty in explaining the concepts to his medical collaborator. In spite of all this activity, practical methods of determining the time of death continue to lack accuracy. Though some recent publications offer firm advice and describe methods, they can do no more than provide a 'time bracket' of probability within which death is thought to have occurred.

Post-mortem cooling

Except where the environmental (ambient) temperature remains at or even above 37°C, the human body will cool after death. A uniform, homogeneous laboratory 'body' will cool according to Newton's Law of Cooling, which states that the rate of cooling is proportional to the difference in temperature between the body surface and its surroundings. Graphically represented, this will display the curve of a single exponential expression, not a straight line. A human body does not obey Newton's Law, though the size of the discrepancy varies according to several factors. When death occurs, heat transfer within the body through the circulation ceases. Metabolic heat production, occurring mainly in the muscles and liver, does not cease uniformly and some heat generation continues for a variable time. As soon as the supply of warmed blood ceases with cardiac arrest, the skin surface immediately begins to lose heat. The rate is variable because of clothing, posture and shielding against the supporting surface and, of course, the environmental temperature.

The centre or 'core' of the body cannot begin to cool until a 'temperature gradient' is set up by the cooling at the skin surface. As the tissues are poor heat conductors, this gradient takes a variable time to become established and therefore a thermometer placed near the core (usually in the rectum) will not register a fall for some time. This is the well-known 'plateau', which forms the upper flattened or slightly sloping part of the double exponential curve when

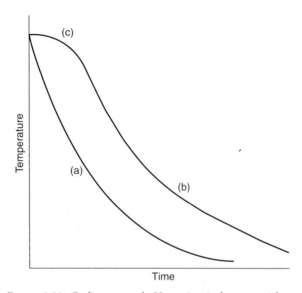

FIGURE 2.29 *Cooling curves: the Newtonian single exponential curve (a) does not occur in practice, except on the surface of the body. Because of the variable plateau (c), the true curve for deep core temperature (b) assumes a double exponential shape.*

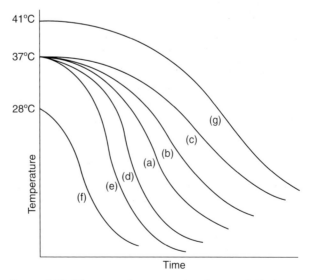

FIGURE 2.30 *Diagrammatic representation of some variables in body cooling curves: (a) average body, (b) obese body, (c) heavily clothed body, (d) thin body, (e) naked body, (f) hypothermic body and (g) febrile body.*

rectal temperatures are measured. If skin temperatures are used, as in some of the nineteenth century research, no plateau is found, and, using cranial temperatures taken through the nose, ear or skull, the plateau is less, as the core is nearer the surface.

The central part of the cooling curve approximates to Newtonian principles, being fairly straight or only a shallow curve. As the temperature differential between the body and environment approaches zero, the graph again flattens off into a lower shelf. Unlike the laboratory body, the human body rarely reaches the ambient temperature unless the latter is at or near freezing. This is probably because enzyme and bacterial action starts during early decomposition and, much as a compost heap warms up, the temperature may actually rise a few days after death.

The typical rectal cooling curve then, is a 'sigmoid' shape or 'double exponential' curve. The part that is of use in forensic medicine is the central section showing the steepest fall. Theoretically, if one assumes that the body temperature at the time of death was 37°C, then finding the point on this section corresponding to the measured rectal temperature should allow extrapolation back to the 37°C point which is at zero on the time scale, thus giving the postmortem interval.

Unfortunately, a number of variables make this attractive proposition impossible to attain in practice. Not only are there variables, but the variables themselves often vary during the period before the body is discovered and examined. For example, the ambient temperature may change markedly – perhaps several times – and often this may not be known to the examiner. Even opening doors and allowing draughts to play on the body will have profound effects on the cooling curve, which cannot be detected or corrected retrospectively.

Factors affecting the cooling curve

INITIAL BODY TEMPERATURE

This cannot be assumed to be 37°C and in fact is incapable of ever being measured in retrospect. Not only is there a difference between the rectal, liver, brain, axillary, mouth and skin temperatures in the living person, but the absolute values vary slightly from person to person and from time to time, even in health.

If the oral temperature is taken to be 37°C, then that in the axilla will be several degrees lower and that in the rectum at least one degree higher. There is a diurnal variation of almost 1°C, the temperature being lowest between 0200 and 0600 and highest between 1600 and 1800. Strenuous exercise raises the temperature by up to 3°C, which persists for up to 30 minutes after returning to rest.

When there is illness or trauma, much wider variations occur, which again are impossible to detect retrospectively. In febrile illness from micro-organisms or parasitic infections, the temperature may be 4 or 5°C higher. In the forensic context, infected wounds or a septic abortion are obvious examples. Cerebral (especially pontine) haemorrhage may also cause hyperthermia, as may some drug reactions. It is traditionally stated in many textbooks that asphyxia and strangulation cause agonal hyperthermia, but there is very little hard evidence for this, apart from anecdotal opinions passed from one author to another. One explanation may be that a homicide victim struggling desperately for life against strangulation will generate muscular heat as in any violent exercise, irrespective of an asphyxial mode of death.

At the other end of the scale, hypothermia is common even in temperate winters. Many victims of criminal assault may be left exposed before death and their temperature may be as much as 10°C lower than normal.

As virtually all methods and formulae for calculating the time of death depend upon the body temperature being 37°C, even a slight variation can introduce a fundamental error.

THE BODY DIMENSIONS

The temperature gradient, which drives cooling, varies with the mass of the body and the surface area as well as with the conducting properties of the tissues. Some more complex calculations correct for mass:surface area ratio by means of nomograms (for example, those served by Henssge), but these can only be an approximation. The height and weight of the body must be known, which is often impossible at the scene of discovery. The amount of subcutaneous and abdominal fat will affect the insulating properties and hence the temperature gradient, but there is no way of assessing or correcting accurately for obesity. Oedema and dehydration both have a marked effect because of the high specific heat of water (see James and Knight 1965). In general, a thin person cools more quickly because of both the mass:surface area ratio and the lack of fatty insulation. Children have a larger surface area for a given body weight.

POSTURE

The loss of heat from the skin that drives the temperature gradient is affected by the access of air to the skin and the opportunity for radiation and convection. A body curled into a fetal position will expose much less surface than one in an extended, spread-eagled posture. Another factor is the amount of skin resting on the supporting surface and the nature of that surface. A body lying full length on its back will lose heat by conduction faster than one resting semi-prone, though radiation and convection may be facilitated.

A body on a metal mortuary tray will cool more quickly than one lying on straw.

CLOTHING AND COVERINGS

All too obvious is the effect of external insulation by clothing or other coverings, even a hat. Radiation is a minor pathway for heat loss because of the low biological temperatures involved, but convection and conduction are markedly reduced by coverings. Even more confusion may be added when coverings actually contribute heat, such as an electric blanket left on after death. A duvet or 'continental quilt' will markedly retard cooling and in fact will accelerate decomposition to a considerable degree. Wet clothing will accelerate cooling, compared with dry coverings, because of the uptake of heat for evaporation.

THE AMBIENT TEMPERATURE

This is, of course, the major factor in cooling and, as was said at the outset, a body will not cool after death if the temperature of the environment is higher than the nominal 37°C, in fact, it may warm up. This may be climatic and seasonal, as in large areas of the world, not necessarily in the tropics. It may also be due to local heating, usually in dwellings or other buildings. This includes radiant heat from fires left burning near the body after death, electric blankets, or death in a house or vehicle fire. Where a victim dies in a warm bath then the whole cooling process is grossly distorted, the opposite of when immersion takes place in the cold water of baths, rivers, lakes or the sea.

AIR MOVEMENT AND HUMIDITY

Most skin cooling takes place by convection and conduction with the adjacent air as the transporting medium. In still conditions, a layer of warm air clings to the skin, especially if clothed or hairy, blocking the temperature differential. Any air movement brings fresh cooler air into contact with the skin and encourages the gradient from the core. The humidity is a less active factor, but damp air conducts heat more readily than dry. A body in a small space will cool more slowly than one exposed to the open air, as transfer of heat to the small volume of air will reduce the temperature differential.

THE MEDIUM AROUND THE BODY

This is usually air, but when it is water or (rarely) another fluid, skin cooling is far more effective. A body immersed in water, especially the moving water of a river or the sea, will rapidly lose heat, as is all too familiar during life when fatal hypothermia can occur within minutes in a cold sea. It is commonly stated that cooling is less rapid in contaminated water (such as sewage) than in clean water, but this is hard to believe, given the same temperature for each type of medium. As mentioned above, death in the warm water of a bathtub reduces the cooling rate – and may even elevate the temperature, making any attempt at estimating the time of death futile.

HAEMORRHAGE

It is traditional to say that severe haemorrhage shortly before death causes more rapid cooling. As the estimation of the time of death is fraught with such inaccuracy, it is difficult to see how this opinion can have been derived. The volume of blood lost will reduce the mass of the body, but only in a minimal fashion. It may be that terminal bleeding may cause a shutdown of cutaneous circulation in an effort to maintain blood pressure and that this might encourage the early formation of the temperature gradient – but such vasoconstriction would relax immediately at death and play no part in post-mortem cooling.

Methods of measuring body temperature

Estimation of temperature by touching with the hand is a useful first manoeuvre when at the scene of a death. A hand placed on the forehead, face or exposed hand may give a first impression of whether death occurred recently or not. Even if these exposed areas are cold, feeling inside the clothing to touch the chest, abdomen or axilla may detect some heat, as may sliding a hand under the body where it is in contact with the supporting surface. These crude methods are combined with an estimate of rigor mortis to provide a preliminary screening of a recent, as opposed to a remote, time of death. Though conditions vary enormously, a body indoors will feel cold on exposed areas in 2–4 hours and in protected areas after some 6–8 hours. The traditional method of taking the post-mortem temperature is by placing a mercury thermometer in the rectum. This must be a chemical thermometer (not a clinical instrument) or thermocouple, ideally reading from 0 to 50°C. The tip must be inserted to at least 10 cm above the anus, the instrument preferably having most of its gradations still visible when *in situ*. It should be left in place for several minutes for the reading to stabilize before being recorded. Where possible, it should be left *in situ* for multiple readings at intervals, though in operational circumstances (especially in criminal deaths) this may be difficult to arrange. There is considerable controversy about when such measurements should be carried out. It is often recommended that a doctor at the scene of death should measure the rectal temperature at once but logistic difficulties exist. Many cases where estimation of the time of death

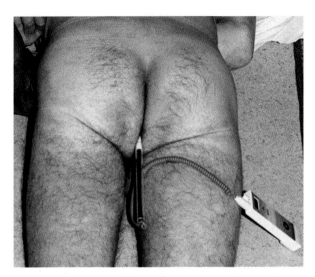

FIGURE 2.31 *Measuring the rectal temperature at the scene of a murder. This should be done only after forensic procedures such as rectal swabbing have been completed. Normally the temperature should be taken at the mortuary where removal of clothing can be carried out with full photographic and forensic science monitoring. In this case the body was unclothed at the scene and the circumstances did not warrant rectal swabbing.*

examinations are completed. Alternatives are to use the axilla, deep nasal passage or external ear for the insertion of a thermometer.

The technique of introducing a mercury or 'rototherm' thermometer through a stab wound in the abdomen to measure liver temperature is never justified. It inevitably leads to blood contamination of the skin and clothing and also leads to intraperitoneal bleeding that might be confused with existing internal injuries.

More modern measuring devices include thermocouples, which register temperature accurately with minimum stabilization time. They may be part of a compact electronic instrument, which has a digital readout, or they may be connected to a computerized recorder that can analyse several other sites at regular intervals (see Morgan *et al.* 1988). Microwave thermography of brain and liver (see Al-Alousi *et al.* 1986, 1994) and infrared monitoring of skin temperature are at present research tools that may lead to practical devices in the future.

The use of thermometry in estimating the post-mortem interval

In spite of the great volume of research and publications already mentioned, accuracy in estimating the time since death from temperature remains elusive. The old rule-of-thumb was that the temperature fell at about 1.5°F/hour, something under 1°C/hour. Another rule-of-thumb was that the fall in °C from 37°C, plus three (to arbitrarily allow for the plateau), was equal to the time since death in hours. For example, if a rectal temperature was found to be 32°C, then $37 - 32 + 3$ gave a post-mortem interval of 8 hours. The only confidence that one could place in these methods was that they were almost always wrong and that, if the answer happened to be correct, it was by chance rather than science! To hope for a linear fall was against all the principles of heat loss alluded to earlier. The first method took no account of the 'plateau' when rectal temperatures were used. This upper part of the double exponential curve is of variable length. If the body has been dead for some hours, serial temperature recordings fail to identify it, as the measurements begin on the steeper part of the curve, but where thermometry is begun soon after death, there is a variable flat area at the top of the sigmoid graph.

The length of the plateau has been discussed by several authors (see Shapiro 1965; Nokes *et al.*1985). Shapiro in particular has drawn attention to the invalidation of many formulae by the unknown length of the plateau. He claims that this can be as much as 4 hours 'and is possibly considerably longer'. Marshall and Hoare (1962) admit that the plateau may be as long as 5 hours. The plateau is the result

is important are criminal or suspicious deaths. These will often be associated with at least the possibility of sexual or homosexual assaults, and it may not be practicable to interfere with clothing in the perineal area or to contaminate the anal and vaginal region before full trace evidence procedures are carried out, usually by police scene of crime officers or forensic scientists, which may include adhesive taping of the clothing and skin, and the retention of underclothes for seminal stains, etc.

To wrestle with tight clothing, perhaps at night, in inclement weather and in confined spaces, and to try to introduce a thermometer into the rectum in these circumstances might ruin vital evidence of more importance than the admittedly uncertain calculations about time of death. However, many pathologists and police teams do carry out this manoeuvre as a routine, but each pathologist must decide in every individual case, whether it is preferable to wait until the body is taken to the mortuary where proper, controlled undressing is possible.

This applies where pathology and criminalistic expertise is readily available, but it is acknowledged that in less ideal circumstances, when no such expertise is likely to appear within a few hours (if at all), then some doctor at the scene should take a temperature. The procedure must be tailored to the individual circumstances but where there is a possibility of sexual interference, the rectum (and vagina) should be avoided until after full swabbing for semen and other of the lag in conducting heat from the core to the skin that is caused by the insulating properties of human tissue. This delays the establishment of the temperature gradient that must be in operation along the radius of the 'infinite cylinder', which is the model for the human body, before the core can begin to lose heat to the exterior. There may also be a small element of continuing heat production in the liver and musculature, as a number of investigators (including the first) noted that the body temperature could actually rise soon after death. As the length of the plateau is unknown in any particular case when there is a delay in starting measurements, most methods begin within this inbuilt inaccuracy.

At the lower end of the sigmoid curve, measurements again become almost useless, as when the temperature is within about 4°C of the environment, the rate of cooling becomes so slow that it provides no separation in time (see Fiddes and Patten 1958). Another empirical rule-of-thumb was devised by James and Knight (1965) to include variation in ambient temperature. The fall from 37°C was multiplied by a factor of 1, 1.25, 1.5, 1.75 or 2 for ambient temperatures of 0, 5, 10, 15 or 20°C, respectively, to give the time since death in hours. As another linear method, this was doomed to inaccuracy and was found to provide too short a post-mortem interval, though the authors emphasized that it was meant to be modified in each case by an appreciation of all other factors such as physique and clothing.

Nomogram method

At present one of the most useful practical guides is the nomogram published by Henssge. Based on conventional calculations such as those of De Saram and Marshall and backed up by a great volume of experimental data, Henssge has produced a method which can be carried out either by a simple computer program or by a nomogram. Adjustments are built in for body weight, ambient temperature, dry or wet clothing, still or moving air, or still or flowing water. The result is given within different ranges of error, with a 95 per cent probability of the true time of death falling within these ranges, which vary from 2.8 hours each side at the best estimate, down to 7 hours at worst. As with most methods, the difficulties arise in estimating the strength of the variable factors. It also cannot allow for variation of these factors over time, especially changes in ambient temperatures during the period before the body was examined. Henssge and Madea have recently refined their method to reduce the standard deviation of their nomograms so that the confidence range becomes smaller, by a whole battery of methods not dependent on temperature, such as electrical stimulation of muscle and the reaction of the eye pupils to drugs.

Another graphical method is that developed by Al-Alousi (1987) in Glasgow. In addition to his publications on microwave thermography, Al-Alousi has published a simple method based on rectal temperatures. He has constructed cooling curves for both naked and covered bodies, using the concept of 'temperature ratios'. The accompanying cooling curves may be used from a knowledge of the rectal temperature, ambient temperature and whether or not the body surface was covered. Again no correction is made for body size, posture or other variables, but the author claims that such factors made little difference to the standard errors, which he gives as shaded errors on each side of his graphs.

Multiple-site serial measurement methods

In an effort to reduce or eliminate the effect of the external variables when calculating the post-mortem interval, Morgan et al. (1988) have developed models using multiple sites in the body for temperature estimations. These are then taken serially at frequent intervals over a period using highly sensitive thermocouples and computerized data acquisition, and calculation, which is miniaturized sufficiently for use at scenes of crime.

The method also attempted to use the deep ear canal and nasal passages for temperature measurements, which avoids the problems of perineal contamination that occur when the rectum is used at scenes of death. The results were not encouraging, but recently French workers have revived the ear method, with claims of relative success. These methods have not been in routine use for sufficiently long to evaluate their operational accuracy.

STOMACH EMPTYING AS A MEASURE OF TIME SINCE A DEATH

With one exception, this controversial topic could be dismissed summarily as being quite irrelevant. For many years pathologists have argued over the reliability of the state of digestion of gastric contents as an indicator of the time between the last meal and death, the leading case in modern times being that of Truscott in Canada. There is now almost a consensus that with extremely circumscribed exceptions, the method is too uncertain to have much validity.

The original hypothesis was founded on the belief that food spent a fairly uniform time in the stomach before being released into the duodenum. In addition, it was claimed that its physical state was progressively altered by gastric juices and movements so that its appearance and volume was a measure of the time since it had been swallowed. Therefore, if the time of the last meal was known from circumstantial evidence, the time of death could be estimated.

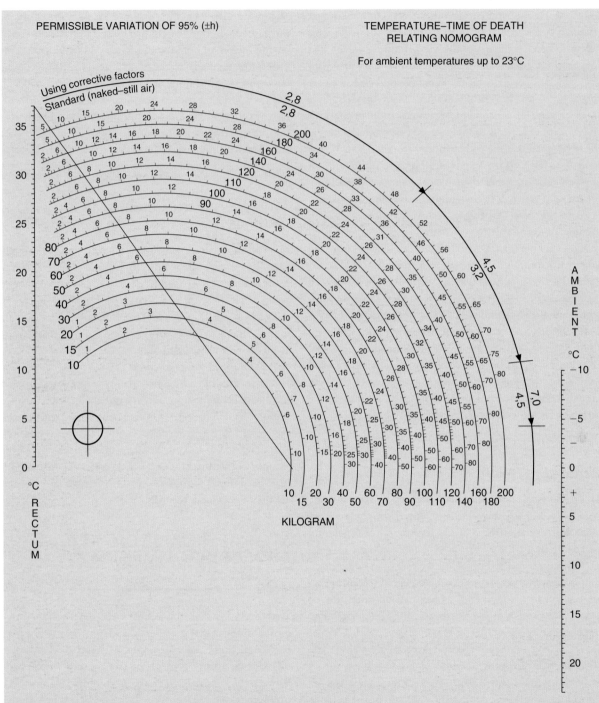

FIGURE 2.32 *Henssge's nomogram method for estimating the time since death from a single rectal temperature, where the environmental temperature is below 23°C. (From Henssge* et al. *2002.)*

The nomogram expresses the death time (*t*) by: $\dfrac{T_{rectum} - T_{ambient}}{37.2 - T_{ambient}} = 1.25 \exp(Bt) - 0.25 \exp(5Bt); \ B = -1.2815 \, (\mathrm{kg}^{-0.625}) + 0.0284$

The nomogram is related to the chosen standard, that is, naked body extended lying in still air. Cooling conditions differing from the chosen standard may be proportionally adjusted by corrective factors of the real body weight, giving the corrected body weight by which the death time is to be read off. Factors above 1.0 may correct thermal isolation conditions and factors below 1.0 may correct conditions accelerating the heat loss of a body.

How to read off the time of death

1 Connect the points of the scales by a straight line according to the rectal and ambient temperature. It crosses the diagonal of the nomogram at a special point.

2 Draw a second straight line going through the centre of the circle, below left of the nomogram and the intersection of the first line and the diagonal.

The second line crosses the semicircles, which represent the body weights. At the intersection of the semicircle of the body weight the time of death can be read off. The second line touches a segment of the outermost semicircle. Here can be seen the permissible variation of 95 per cent.

Example: temperature of the rectum 26.4°C; ambient temperature 12°C; body weight 90 kg. Result: time of death 16 ± 1.8 h. Statement: the death occurred within 13.2 and 18.8 (13 and 19) hours before the time of measurement (with a reliability of 95 per cent).

Note: if the values of the ambient temperature and/or the body weight (see 'corrective factors') are called into question, repeat the procedure with other values that might be possible. The range of death time can be seen in this way.

Empiric corrective factors of the body weight

Dry clothing/ covering	In air	Corrective factor	Wet through Clothing/covering wet body surface	In air/water
		0.35	Naked	Flowing water
		0.50	Naked	Still water
		0.70	Naked	Moving air
		0.70	1–2 thin layers clothing	Moving air
Naked	Moving	0.75		
1–2 thin layers clothing	Moving	0.90	2 or more thicker clothing	Moving air
Naked	Still	1.00		
1–2 thin layers clothing	Still	1.10	2 thicker layers clothing	Still air
2–3 thin layers clothing		1.20	More than 2 thicker layers clothing	Still air
1–2 thicker layers clothing	Moving or still	1.20		
3–4 thin layers clothing		1.30		
More thin/thicker layers clothing	Without influence	1.40		
		1.80		
Thick bedspread + clothing combined		2.40		

Note: for the selection of the corrective factor of any case, only the clothing or covering of the lower trunk is relevant.
Personal experience is needed; nevertheless, this is quickly achieved by consistent use of the method.

Requirements for use

- No strong radiation (for example, sun, heater, cooling system).
- No strong fever or general hypothermia.
- No uncertain* severe changes of the cooling conditions during the period between the time of death and examination (for example, the place of death must be the same as where the body was found).
- No high thermal conductivity of the surface beneath the body.[†]

---

* Known changes can be taken into account: a change of the ambient temperature can often be evaluation (for example, contact the weather station); use the mean ambient temperature of the period in question. Changes by the operations of the investigators (for example, take any cover off) since finding the body are negligible: take the conditions before into account!

[†] Measure the temperature of the surface beneath the body also. If there is a significant difference between the temperature of the air and the surface temperature, use the mean.

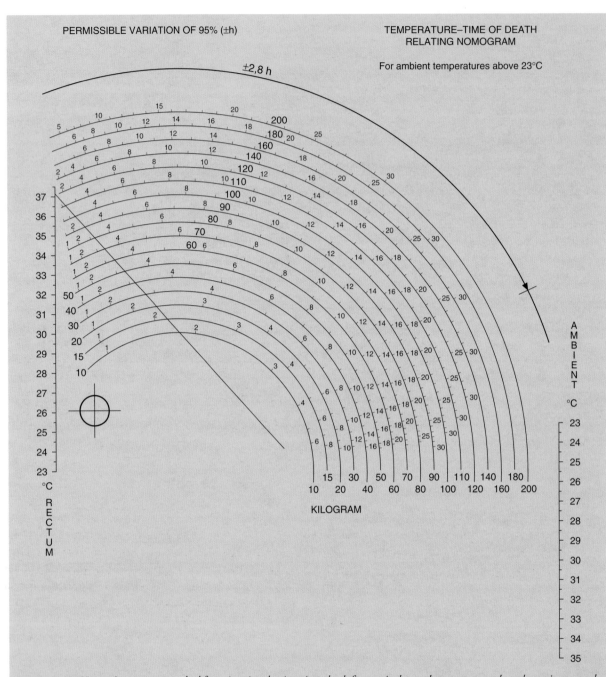

FIGURE 2.33 *Hennsge's nomogram method for estimating the time since death from a single rectal temperature, where the environmental temperature is above 23°C. (From Henssge et al. 2002.)*

The nomogram expresses the death time (*t*) by: $\dfrac{T_{rectum} - T_{ambient}}{37.2 - T_{ambient}} = 1.11 \exp(Bt) - 0.11 \exp(10Bt); \quad B = -1.2815 \, (\text{kg}^{-0.625}) + 0.0284$

The difference between this nomogram and that for ambient temperatures up to 23°C concerns only the relative length of the 'post-mortem plateau'. It is shorter in higher ambient temperatures (above 23°C) than in lower ones (that nomogram: up to 23°C). This nomogram for higher ambient temperatures was developed according to the data from De Saram, which were obtained in ambient temperatures between 27 and 32°C. These data show a relatively shorter length of the 'post-mortal plateau' than our own data of body cooling in lower ambient temperatures. Our own practical experience of the cooling of bodies in high ambient temperatures and therefore in using this nomogram, is small. It is recommended that the same permissible variation of 95 per cent as given in the nomogram for lower ambient temperatures is taken.

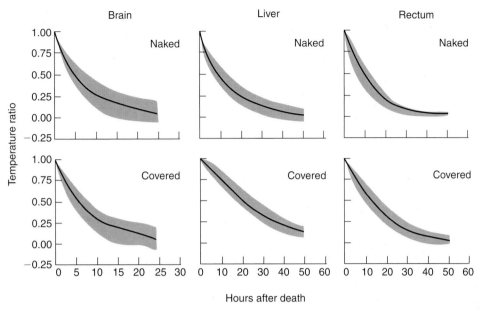

FIGURE 2.34 *Cooling curves for estimation of the post-mortem interval. In Al-Alousi's 'temperature ratio' method, the graphs above are used as follows. Assume that the body temperature (rectal) is 36.6°C at the time of death (T_b). Measure the environmental and rectal temperatures at the time of examination (T_r and T_e). Then the 'temperature ratio' is $T_r - T_e/T_b - T_e$. This ratio is then found on the vertical scale of the rectal graph, using either the graph for 'naked' or 'covered' as appropriate. The time since death is the point on the lower scale where a perpendicular falls from the point on the graph where a horizontal line meets it from the temperature ratio level. The shaded area indicates the limits of a 68 per cent probability at that particular point. For example, if the rectal temperature is 23.4°C and the air temperature 19°C, then the temperature ratio is 0.25. If the body is naked, then this gives 18 hours as the time since death, with a margin of plus 2.5 hours and minus 5 hours. (Reprinted with permission from Al-Alousi LM, Anderson RA. 1986. Microwave thermography in forensic medicine. Police Surgeon, **30**:30–42.)*

It was assumed that the physiological process of digestion of an 'average' meal lasted some 2–3 hours. This is based on the consumption of a test meal of gruel, however, hardly a representative example of a modern mixed diet. Moreover, the subjects of experimental work were healthy and presumably free from sudden stress during the experiments. More elaborate descriptions of digestion times of various foods have been drawn up, but they are of dubious value. As an example of the great variations offered, Modi (1957) gives 4–6 hours for a meat and vegetable meal and 6–7 hours for a farinaceous meal. Adelson (1974) stated that the stomach begins to empty within 10 minutes of swallowing, that a 'light' meal leaves the stomach by 2 hours, a 'medium' meal takes 3–4 hours and a large, heavy meal takes 4–6 hours. He noted that the head of an 'ordinary' meal usually reached the ileocaecal valve between 6 and 8 hours after ingestion. All these values, however, are subject to considerable variation.

More modern methods of investigation have used radioisotope techniques and have shown some interesting facts. When a solid meal is eaten and water drunk with it, the water leaves the stomach quickly irrespective of the nature or calorific content of the solid part. However,

calorific liquids stay longer in the stomach (Brophy *et al.* 1986). The emptying rate also increases with the weight of the meal, as long as the calorific content remains constant. If the latter is increased, then the pyloric opening is delayed. Further work by Moore *et al.* (1984) again emphasized the marked variability of emptying times, even in normal circumstances.

The following factors frustrate the use of gastric emptying as a measure of time since death:

■ Digestion may continue for some time after death.
■ The physical nature of a meal has a profound effect on emptying time: the more fluid the consistency, the faster the emptying. Liquids entering an empty stomach pass through without any appreciable pause.
■ The nature of the food modifies emptying time, notably fatty substances, which markedly delay the opening of the pylorus. Strong alcohol, such as spirits and liqueurs, also irritate the mucosa and tend to delay emptying.
■ Importantly, any nervous or systemic shock or stress, mediated through the parasympathetic (vagus) system, can slow or stop gastric motility and digestive juice secretion as well as holding the pylorus firmly closed.

The intestine, as opposed to the stomach, may increase its motility with psychogenic upsets, as noted by De Saram in his autopsies on hanged criminals.

The state of digestion, as opposed to the volume and exit of food from the stomach, is almost impossible to assess. Variations in the type of food eaten make vast differences to the dissolution rate. Hard objects, such as nuts and seeds, resist digestion and may even be voided intact *per rectum*, whereas soft carbohydrates can liquefy almost immediately. The size and dispersion of particles is crucial, including the amount of chewing and admixed saliva. The efficiency of the teeth and gastric acid, enzymes and motility are also of prime importance, as is the amount of liquid either in the original food or drunk during the meal. Fat and oil in the meal slow up pyloric opening, and all these variables make it impossible to time the rate of digestion.

One of the most important factors in the forensic context is the effect of a physical or mental shock or stress during the digestion process. As stated, this can completely inhibit digestion, gastric motility and pyloric opening. The author (BK) recalls a victim of a traffic accident who lived in a coma for a week after a mortal head injury. At eventual autopsy, the large volume of gastric contents looked as fresh as if it had just been swallowed.

Even if one accepts an 'average' gastric transit time of an 'average' meal as being of the order of 2–3 hours, the assumption that death took place within this time can only be valid if the death was quite sudden and unexpected, with no stressful prodromal event. For example, if an unsuspecting person was suddenly shot or run down without warning and died almost immediately, then one can assume that the undisturbed physiological processes of digestion – albeit with its many variables – had taken place. If, however, a domestic dispute or a developing altercation culminated in a strangling or stabbing, the antecedent stresses would almost certainly affect gastric function and render invalid any interpretation of the condition of stomach contents at autopsy.

What is valid is the nature of the last meal, which may be helpful in establishing the time of death. If it was known to the investigators that the deceased person ate a certain type of meal at a certain time, whether it be chicken curry or green beans, the identification of such food in the stomach would be persuasive evidence that he died after taking that food and that it was his final meal, before any other substantial food of a different type was taken.

THE USE OF VITREOUS HUMOUR CHEMISTRY IN TIMING DEATH

This topic has been the subject of considerable research in forensic medicine over the last 30 years. It has never gained

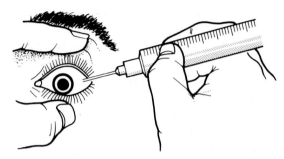

FIGURE 2.35 *Obtaining vitreous humour for analysis. The lids should be retracted and the needle introduced near the outer canthus, so that the hole will be covered when the lids are released. Fluid should be withdrawn slowly, keeping the tip of the needle in the centre of the globe to avoid dislodging the retina. Water can be reintroduced through the needle to restore the tension in the globe for cosmetic reasons.*

sufficient acceptance to become a routine tool, remaining a controversial procedure in spite of the large number of reports that now exists.

The most common chemical estimation performed on the vitreous fluid in the context of the post-mortem interval is that of potassium. There is a marked and progressive rise in the potassium concentration after death, the controversy revolving around whether this rise is simply linear or whether it is biphasic. The degree of confidence is also in dispute and the effect of variable factors is another contentious matter (see works by Coe, Sturner, Lange and Madea). First, the potassium values from either eye often differ, sometimes by a considerable amount. The sampling methods are then critical, as small or marginal samples vary greatly; if aspiration is forcible or from too near the retina, cellular fragments distort the values, because the potassium reaches the vitreous by leaching out from the retina. The effect of temperature changes post-mortem is also undoubtedly important. In addition, different analytical techniques used to estimate the potassium give different results, the older flame photometric methods producing a different range of values compared with modern selective-electrode procedures.

With all these variables, it is little wonder that different authors suggest widely different standard errors, varying from 1–7 hours to 26 hours either side of the true time of death. In addition, the errors seem much greater in persons dying of chronic illnesses, with nitrogen retention, compared with sudden deaths, presumably because of the premortal electrolyte disturbances in patients with metabolic disorders.

The rise in infants seems much faster than in adults – yet another variable – though in both adults and children the most potent influencing factor seems to be the post-mortem body temperature. The most popular calculation for estimating the time since death from vitreous potassium is that devised by Sturner, in which post-mortem interval =7.14 × potassium concentration (mEq/l) −39.1. This seems most satisfactory when the body has lain in an ambient temperature of not more than 10°C (50°F). The 95 per cent confidence limit during the first day is likely to be at least 4.7 hours either side of the true time and probably greater. Taking a sample from one eye at a later time than the first to attempt to calculate the rate of rise does not seem to add any accuracy to a single estimation method (see Adjutantis and Coutselenis 1972).

Hypoxanthine estimation in vitreous humour has also been used to attempt to time death, but more often as a marker of hypoxia. The results are not convincing, but there is an accumulating literature on the subject, more recent contributions being Madea *et al.* (1994) and also Rognum *et al.* (1991).

POST-MORTEM CHEMISTRY

The analysis of physiological chemical constituents of the body, as opposed to toxic substances, is often useful in investigating deaths from metabolic and biochemical disturbances.

Unfortunately, the concentration of many natural chemical substances in the dead body is rapidly distorted by post-mortem autolysis. Cell membranes become permeable to small molecules soon after the cells suffer ischaemic or anoxic damage, and agonal changes themselves may grossly alter the biochemical environment, even in the few minutes of the dying process. Thus both terminal and early post-mortem changes may render many of the analyses that are commonplace in clinical practice of little value – and indeed, quite misleading – when applied to body fluids obtained at autopsy. Some substances are more stable, however, and when results are carefully interpreted, considerable information can be obtained. Urea and creatinine are stable post-mortem, with little variation even up to 100 hours after death, so the diagnosis of ante-mortem nitrogen retention is quite reliable. The normal urea nitrogen range found in post-mortem serum is from 4.9 to 5.5 mmol/l, creatine being from about 70.7 to 212.2 μmol/l.

In the context of post-mortem chemistry the work of John Coe is best known in forensic pathology and his writings should be consulted for detailed information. Another very useful source is Madea, especially for vitreous fluid. The vitreous humour is much to be preferred to blood for post-mortem chemical analyses. Although still influenced by temperature changes, the vitreous is far less contaminated by body autolysis and is remote from the large organs and blood vessels of the abdominothoracic cavity.

There is a large body of literature on vitreous potassium, much of it centred around the controversy over the *in vivo* concentration of potassium, which can naturally rarely be measured directly in healthy persons, and the slope of the regression graph for relating potassium levels with post-mortem interval.

After death, intracellular potassium leaches from the retina through the now permeable cell membranes, into the vitreous body, naturally with an uneven distribution depending on the distance from the wall of eyeball (which is why all or a substantial proportion of the fluid should be withdrawn for analysis, to obtain a mean level). If fragments of retina are aspirated by the syringe, due to excessive suction, then a falsely elevated potassium measurement will be obtained.

Differences in the recommended regression gradient are observed between various workers: Madea states that 0.19 mmol/l/hour should be used, whereas Sturner claims 0.14 is preferable. The literature should be consulted for details (as in the 2002 book by Hennsge *et al.*); it is also pertinent to note that the methods of analysis can make a difference to the calculations. Generally speaking, the vitreous potassium method is of most use after the first 24–36 hours, when other methods have ceased to have application. Although the errors are great, some information can be derived for up to 100 hours post-mortem.

Caution must be used when interpreting results, as different analytical techniques provide different values. For instance, in relation to electrolytes, Coe and Apple (1985) state that flame photometric methods yield values about 5 mmol/l less for sodium, 7 mmol/l less for potassium and 10 mmol/l less for chloride, compared with more modern specific electrode methods. Electrolyte concentration differences between left and right vitreous humor samples were studied by Pounder *et al.* (1998) in 200 medico-legal autopsies using an ion-specific electrode system. Between-eye concentration differences of sodium and chloride were tolerable using this methodology, whereas differences in potassium, even in biochemically nonputrefied cases (potassium <15 mmol/l), were 0–2.34 mmol/l (0–21.8 per cent of mean) averaging 0.37 mmol/l (3.3 per cent), thus undermining the usefulness of vitreous potassium in estimation of time of death.

In relation to other vitreous electrolytes, the concentration of sodium and chlorides decrease after death, while potassium rises. The latter can be used as a check on the reliability of the others, as if potassium is <15 mmol/l, then the sodium and chloride concentrations may be acceptable. Chlorides decrease at less than 1 mmol/l/h and sodium by about 0.9 mmol/l/h, so the loss of this and sodium is insignificant in the first few hours, differing from potassium, which rises appreciably.

With the analysis of glucose in autopsy material, five different methods yielded five different results, presumably because interfering substances were included in varying amounts.

Returning to vitreous electrolytes, in mmol/l measured by flame photometry (in mmol/l), sodium >155, chloride > 135 and urea >40 is a reliable indication of ante-mortem dehydration. When sodium and chloride are normal but the urea exceeds 150, a diagnosis of uraemia is acceptable. These values can be distinguished from post-mortem decomposition, in which sodium is <130, chloride <105 and potassium >20.

In relation to glucose, a common problem is the autopsy diagnosis of uncontrolled diabetes and of hypoglycaemia. The vitreous glucose usually falls after death and can reach zero within a few hours. In 6000 analyses, Coe (1973) found that a vitreous glucose of more than 11.1 mmol/l was an invariable indicator of diabetes mellitus. The agonal or post-mortem rise in blood sugar is not reflected in the vitreous concentrations. In relation to hypoglycaemia, a vitreous glucose of less than 1.4 mmol/l was taken by Sturner et al. (1972) to be an indication of a low ante-mortem blood sugar, but others feel that whatever the concentration, no reliable interpretation can be made. In hypothermia there is also an elevated vitreous glucose, but never greater than 11.1 mmol/l.

REFERENCES AND FURTHER READING

Adelson L. 1974. *The pathology of homicide*. Thomas, Springfield.

Adelson L, Sunshine I, Rushforth NB, et al. 1963. Vitreous potassium concentration as an indicator of the post mortem interval. *J Forensic Sci* **8**:503–10.

Adjutantis G, Coutselinis A. 1972. Estimation of the time of death by potassium levels in the vitreous humour. *Forensic Sci* **1**:55–60.

Al-Alousi LM. 1987. *The post-mortem interval: a study of the postmortem cooling rate*. University of Glasgow, Glasgow.

Al-Alousi LM. 2002. A study of the shape of the post-mortem cooling curve in 117 forensic cases. *Forensic Sci Int* **125**:237–44.

Al-Alousi LM, Anderson RA. 1986. Microwave thermography in forensic medicine. *Police Surgeon* **30**:30–42.

Al-Alousi LM, Anderson RA, Land DV. 1994. A non-invasive method for postmortem temperature measurements using a microwave probe. *Forensic Sci Int* **64**:35–46.

Al-Alousi LM, Anderson RA, Worster DM, et al. 2002. Factors influencing the precision of estimating the postmortem interval using the triple-exponential formulae (TEF). Part I. A study of the effect of body variables and covering of the torso on the postmortem brain, liver and rectal cooling rates in 117 forensic cases. *Forensic Sci Int* **125**:223–30.

Ambrosi I, Carriero F. 1965. Hypostasis in the internal organs: histological aspects. *J Forensic Med* **12**:8–13.

Anonymous. 1963. Case of John David Potter (editorial). *J Forensic Med* **31**:195.

Balasooriya BA, St. Hill CA, Williams AR. 1984. The biochemistry of vitreous humour. A comparative study of the potassium, sodium and urate concentrations in the eyes at identical time intervals after death. *Forensic Sci Int* **26**:85–91.

Bate-Smith E, Bendall J. 1947. Rigor mortis and adenosine triphosphate. *J Physiol* **106**:177.

Bate-Smith E, Bendall J. 1949. Factors determining the time course of rigor mortis. *J Physiol* **110**:47.

Bendall J. 1960. *Post mortem changes in muscle*, vol. 3. Academic Press, London.

Benecke M. 1997. [Collecting insects, spiders and crustaceans for criminal forensic study.] *Arch Kriminol* **199**:167–76.

Betz P, Lignitz E, Eisenmenger W. 1995. The time-dependent appearance of black eyes. *Int J Legal Med* **108**:96–9.

Bohnert M, Weinmann W, Pollak S. 1999. Spectrophotometric evaluation of postmortem lividity. *Forensic Sci Int* **99**:149–58.

Bonte W, Sprung R, Huckenbeck W. 1986. [Problems in the evaluation of electrocution fatalities in the bathtub.] *Z Rechtsmed* **97**:7–19.

Borrman H, Du Chesne A, Brinkmann B. 1994. Medico-legal aspects of postmortem pink teeth. *Int J Legal Med* **106**:225–31.

Bray M. 1984. The effect of chilling, freezing, and rewarming on the postmortem chemistry of vitreous humor. *J Forensic Sci* **29**:404–11.

Brophy CM, Moore JG, Christian PE, et al. 1986. Variability of gastric emptying measurements in man employing standardized radiolabeled meals. *Dig Dis Sci* **31**:799–806.

Brown A, Marshall TK. 1974. Body temperature as a means of estimating the time of death. *Forensic Sci Int* **4**:125–33.

Brown A, Hicks B, Knight B, et al. 1985. Determination of time since death using the double exponential cooling model. *Med Sci Law* **25**:223–7.

Burton JF. 1974. Fallacies in the signs of death. *J Forensic Sci* **19**:529–34.

Busvine JR. 1980. *Insects and hygiene*, 3rd edn. Chapman & Hall, London.

Campobasso CP, Introna F. 2001. The forensic entomologist in the context of the forensic pathologist's role. *Forensic Sci Int* **120**:132–9.

Campobasso CP, Di Vella G, Introna F. 2001. Factors affecting decomposition and Diptera colonization. *Forensic Sci Int* **120**:18–27.

Camps FE. 1959. Establishment of time since death – a critical assessment. *J Forensic Sci* **4**:73–6.

Casper JL. 1862. *Handbook of forensic medicine*, 3rd edn. Engl transl. G W Balfour. New Sydenham Society, London.

Catts E, Goff M. 1992. Forensic entomology in criminal investigations. *Annu Rev Entomol* **37**:253–8.

Chowduri S, Chatterji PC, Banerjee SP. 1970. Histological study of liver tissue with regard to determining time of death. *J Indian Acad Forensic Sci* **9**:19–23.

Coe JI. 1969. Postmortem chemistries on human vitreous humor. *Am J Clin Pathol* **51**:741–50.

Coe JI. 1973. Further thoughts and observations on postmortem chemistry. *Forensic Sci Gaz* **5**:26.

Coe JI. 1974. Postmortem chemistry: practical considerations and a review of the literature. *J Forensic Sci* **19**:13–32.

Coe JI. 1974. Postmortem chemistries on blood with particular reference to urea nitrogen, electrolytes, and bilirubin. *J Forensic Sci* **19**:33–42.

Coe JI. 1977. Postmortem chemistry of blood, cerebrospinal fluid, and vitreous humor. *Leg Med Annu* **1976**:55–92.

Coe JI. 1989. Vitreous potassium as a measure of the postmortem interval: an historical review and critical evaluation. *Forensic Sci Int* **42**:201–13.

Coe JI. 1989. Postmortem chemistry of blood and vitreous humour in pediatric practice. In: Mason J (ed.), *Paediatric forensic medicine and pathology*. Chapman and Hall, London, pp. 191–203.

Coe JI. 1993. Postmortem chemistry update. Emphasis on forensic application. *Am J Forensic Med Pathol* **14**:91–117.

Coe JI, Apple FS. 1985. Variations in vitreous humor chemical values as a result of instrumentation. *J Forensic Sci* **30**:828–35.

Conference of Medical Royal Colleges and their Faculties in the United Kingdom. 1976. Diagnosis of brain death. *Br Med J* **2**:1187–8.

Contostavlos DL. 2001. Commentary on: Ely SF, Hirsch CS. Asphyxial deaths and petechiae. *J Forensic Sci* 2000; **45**(6):1274–7. *J Forensic Sci* **46**:1261.

De Letter EA, Piette MH. 1998. Can routinely combined analysis of glucose and lactate in vitreous humour be useful in current forensic practice? *Am J Forensic Med Pathol* **19**:335–42.

Department of Health and Social Security. 1983. *Code of practice on cadaveric organs for transplantation*. Her Majesty's Stationery Office, London.

Dervegie A. 1840. *Medicine-legale*. Baillière, Paris.

De Saram GS. 1957. Estimation of the time of death by medical criteria. *J Forensic Med* **4**:47–57.

De Saram GS, Webster G, Kathirgamatamby N. 1955. Postmortem temperature and the time of death. *J Crim Law Criminol Police Sci* **1**:562–77.

Devgun MS, Dunbar JA. 1986. Biochemical investigation of vitreus: applications in forensic medicine, especially in relation to alcohol. *Forensic Sci Int* **31**:27–34.

Eastham RD. 1971. *Biochemical values in clinical medicine*, 4th edn. John Wright, Bristol.

Easton AM, Smith KG. 1970. The entomology of the cadaver. *Med Sci Law* **10**:208–15.

Eliakis F. 1965. Determination of the hour of death by estimation of inorganic phosphorus content of the cerebro-spinal fluid. *Ann Med Leg* **45**:366–71.

Ely SF, Hirsch CS. 2000. Asphyxial deaths and petechiae: a review. *J Forensic Sci* **45**:1274–7.

Enticknap JB. 1960. Biochemical changes in cadaver sera in fatal acute heart attacks. *J Forensic Med* **7**:135–42.

Erdos T. 1943. Rigor, contracture and ATP. *Stud Ins Med Chem Univ Szeged* **3**:51–6.

Erzinclioglu YZ. 1983. The application of entomology to forensic medicine. *Med Sci Law* **23**:57–63.

Erzinclioglu YZ. 1989. Entomology, zoology and forensic science: the need for expansion. [editorial] *Forensic Sci Int* **43**:209–13.

Erzinclioglu YZ. 1989. Protocol for collecting entomological evidence. *Forensic Sci Int* **43**:211–13.

Evans WED. 1962. Some histological findings in spontaneously preserved bodies. *Med Sci Law* **2**:155–60.

Evans WED. 1963a. Adipocere formation in a relatively dry environment. *Med Sci Law* **3**:145–8.

Evans WED. 1963b. *The chemistry of death*. Thomas, Springfield.

Farmer JG, Benomran F, Watson AA, *et al.* 1985. Magnesium, potassium, sodium and calcium in post-mortem vitreous humour from humans. *Forensic Sci Int* **27**:1–13.

Fatteh A. 1966. *Estimation of time of death by chemical changes.* Commonwealth of Virginia, Office of Chief Medical Examiner, Virginia, pp. 163.

Fechner G, Koops E, Henssge C. 1984. [Cessation of livor in defined pressure conditions.] *Z Rechtsmed* **93**:283–7.

Fekete JF, Kerenyi NA. 1965. Postmortem blood sugar and blood urea nitrogen determinations. *Can Med Assoc Journal* **92**:970–74.

Fiddes F, Patten TA. 1958. Percentage method for representing the fall in body temperature after death. *J Forensic Med* **5**:2–15.

Findlay AB. 1976. Bone marrow changes in the post mortem interval. *J Forensic Sci Soc* **16**:213–18.

Fisher P. 1946. *Mechanism of death in the absence of postmortem evidence of disease or trauma. (seminar presentation)*, Department of Legal Medicine, University of Harvard, 22 October, 1946.

Foerch JS, Forman DT, Vye MV. 1979. Measurement of potassium in vitreous humor as an indicator of the postmortem interval. *Am J Clin Pathol* **72**:651–2.

Forman DT, Butts J. 1980. Electrolytes of the vitreous humor as a measure of the postmortem interval. *Clin Chem* **26**:1042–6.

Forster B. 1963. The plastic and elastic deformation of skeletal muscle in rigor mortis. *J Forensic Med* **10**:91–110.

Forster B. 1963. The contractile deformation of skeletal muscle in rigor mortis. *J Forensic Med* **10**:133–47.

Forster B. 1964. The plastic, elastic and contractile deformation of the heart muscle in rigor mortis. *J Forensic Med* **11**:148.

Gallois Montbrun FG, Barres DR, Durigon M. 1988. Postmortem interval estimation by biochemical determination in bird muscle. *Forensic Sci Int* **37**:189–92.

Gamero Lucas JJ, Romero JL, Ramos HM, *et al.* 1992. Precision of estimating time of death by vitreous potassium – comparison of various equations [see comments]. *Forensic Sci Int* **56**:137–45.

Gantner GE, Sturner W, Caffrey PR, *et al.* 1962. Ascorbic acid levels in the postmortem vitreous humor. *J Forensic Med* **9**:156–61.

Garrett G, Green MA, Murray LA. 1988. Technical method – rapid softening of adipocerous bodies. *Med Sci Law* **28**:98–9.

Glaister J, Brash J. 1937. *Medicolegal aspects of the Ruxton case.* Livingstone, Edinburgh.

Goff ML, Odom CB. 1987. Forensic entomology in the Hawaiian islands. Three case studies. *Am J Forensic Med Pathol* **8**:45–50.

Goff ML, Omori AI, Gunatilake K. 1988. Estimation of postmortem interval by arthropod succession. Three case studies from the Hawaiian Islands. *Am J Forensic Med Pathol* **9**:220–5.

Gonzales TA, Helpern M, Vance M. 1954. *Legal medicine and toxicology*, 2nd edn, vol. 64. Appleton Century Crofts, New York.

Gotouda H, Takatori T, Terazawa K, *et al.* 1988. The mechanism of experimental adipocere formation: hydration and dehydrogenation in microbial synthesis of hydroxy and oxo fatty acids. *Forensic Sci Int* **37**:249–57.

Grassberger M, Reiter C. 2002. Effect of temperature on development of the forensically important holarctic blow fly *Protophormia terraenovae* (Robineau-Desvoidy) (Diptera: Calliphoridae). *Forensic Sci Int* **128**:177–82.

Green MA, Wright JC. 1985. Postmortem interval estimation from body temperature data only. *Forensic Sci Int* **28**:35–46.

Green MA, Wright JC. 1985. The theoretical aspects of the time dependent Z equation as a means of postmortem interval estimation using body temperature data only. *Forensic Sci Int* **28**:53–62.

Haglund WD, Sperry K. 1993. The use of hydrogen peroxide to visualize tattoos obscured by decomposition and mummification. *J Forensic Sci* **38**:147–50.

Hanson J, Huxley H. 1955. The structural basis of contraction in striated muscle. *Symp Soc Exp Biol* **9**:228–64.

Hansson L, Uotila U, Lindfors R, *et al.* 1966. Potassium content of the vitreous body as an aid in determining the time of death. *J Forensic Sci* **11**:390–4.

Hellerich U, Bohnert M, Pollak S. 2001. [Hypostasis-induced changes in the breast area.] *Arch Kriminol* **207**:162–9.

Henry JB, Smith FA. 1980. Estimation of the postmortem interval by chemical means. *Am J Forensic Med Pathol* **1**:341–7.

Henssge C. 1988. Death time estimation in case work. I. The rectal temperature time of death nomogram. *Forensic Sci Int* **38**:209–36.

Henssge C, Madea B, Gallenkemper E. 1985. [Determination of the time of death – integration of various partial methods.] *Z Rechtsmed* **95**:185–96.

Henssge C, Madea B, Gallenkemper E. 1988. Death time estimation in case work. II. Integration of different methods. *Forensic Sci Int* **39**:77–87.

Henssge C, Knight B, Krompecher T, *et al.* 1995. *The estimation of the time since death in the early postmortem period.* Edward Arnold, London.

Henssge C, Althaus L, Bolt J, *et al.* 2000. Experiences with a compound method for estimating the time since death. II. Integration of non-temperature-based methods. *Int J Legal Med* **113**:320–31.

Henssge C, Knight B, Krompecher T, *et al.* 2002. *The estimation of the time since death in the early postmortem period*, 2nd edn. Arnold, London.

Henssge C, Wang H, Hoppe B. 2002. Light microscopical investigations on structural changes of skeletal muscle as artifacts after postmortem stimulation. *Forensic Sci Int* **125**:163–71.

Hill EV. 1941. Significance of dextrose and nondextrose reducing substances in postmortem blood. *Arch Pathol* **32**:452–6.

Hiraiwa K, Ohno Y, Kuroda F, *et al.* 1980. Estimation of postmortem interval from rectal temperature by use of computer. *Med Sci Law* **20**:115–25.

Hughes WM. 1965. Levels of potassium in the vitreous humour after death. *Med Sci Law* **5**:150–6.

Inoue M, Suyama A, Matuoka T, *et al.* 1994. Development of an instrument to measure postmortem lividity and its preliminary application to estimate the time since death. *Forensic Sci Int* **65**:185–93.

Introna F, Jr, Campobasso CP, Di Fazio A. 1998. Three case studies in forensic entomology from southern Italy. *J Forensic Sci* **43**:210–14.

Jaafar S, Nokes L. 1994. Examination of the eye as a means to determine the early postmortem period: a review of the literature. *Forensic Sci Int* **64**:185–9.

Jaffe F. 1962. Chemical postmortem changes in the intraocular fluid. *J Forensic Sci* **7**:231.

James RA, Hoadley PA, Sampson BG. 1997. Determination of postmortem interval by sampling vitreous humour. *Am J Forensic Med Pathol* **18**:158–62.

James WR, Knight B. 1965. Errors in estimating the time of death. *Med Sci Law* **5**:111–16.

Jit I, Sehgal S, Sahni D. 2001. An indian mummy: a case report. *Forensic Sci Int* **117**:57–63.

Johnston W, Villeneuve G. 1897. On the medicolegal applications of entomology. *Montreal Med* **26**:81–8.

Joseph AE, Schickele E. 1970. A general method for assessing factors controlling postmortem cooling. *J Forensic Sci* **15**:364–91.

Kamal AS. 1958. Comparative study of thirteen species of sacrosaprophagous Calliphoridae Sarcophagidae (Diptera). 1 Bionomics. *Ann Entomol Soc Am* **51**:261–71.

Kevorkian J. 1956. The fundus oculi and the determination of death. *Am J Pathol* **32**:1253–67.

Kevorkian J. 1961. *The eye in death.* Ciba Symposia, London.

Kevorkian J. 1961. The fundus oculi as a postmortem clock. *J Forensic Sci* **6**:261.

Knight B. 1968. Estimation of the time since death: a survey of practical methods. *J Forensic Sci Soc* **8**:91–6.

Knight B. 1979. The putrefied body. *Br Med J* **1**:1300–1.

Knight B. 1988. The evolution of methods for estimating the time of death from body temperature. *Forensic Sci Int* **36**:47–55.

Kominato Y, Harada S, Yamazaki K, *et al.* 1988. Estimation of postmortem interval based on the third component of complement (C3) cleavage. *J Forensic Sci* **33**:404–9.

Komura S, Oshiro S. 1977. Potassium levels in the aqueous and vitreous humor after death. *Tohoku J Exp Med* **122**:65–8.

Krompecher T. 1994. Experimental evaluation of rigor mortis. VIII. Estimation of time since death by repeated measurements of the intensity of rigor mortis on rats. *Forensic Sci Int* **68**:149–59.

Krompecher T, Bergerioux C. 1988. Experimental evaluation of rigor mortis. VII. Effect of ante- and post-mortem electrocution on the evolution of rigor mortis. *Forensic Sci Int* **38**:27–35.

Kuehn LA, Tikuisis P, Livingstone S, *et al.* 1979. Body cooling after death. *J Can Soc Forensic Sci* **12**:153–63.

Kuehn LA, Tikuisis P, Livingstone S, *et al.* 1980. Body cooling after death. *Aviat Space Environ Med* **51**:965–9.

Kulshrestha P, Chandra H. 1987. Time since death. An entomological study on corpses. *Am J Forensic Med Pathol* **8**:233–8.

Kulshrestha P, Satpathy DK. 2001. Use of beetles in forensic entomology. *Forensic Sci Int* **120**:15–7.

Lange N, Swearer S, Sturner WQ. 1994. Human postmortem interval estimation from vitreous potassium: an analysis of original data from six different studies. *Forensic Sci Int* **66**:159–74.

Langford AM, Pounder DJ. 1997. Possible markers for postmortem drug redistribution. *J Forensic Sci* **42**:88–92.

Langley RL. 1994. Fatal animal attacks in North Carolina over an 18-year period. *Am J Forensic Med Pathol* **15**:160–7.

Lasczkowski G, Riepert T, Rittner C. 1993. [Viewing the criminal site in unusual cadaver evidence: concealment, identification, determining time of death and reconstruction.] *Arch Kriminol* **192**:1–11.

Leadbeatter S, Knight B. 1987. The history and the cause of death. *Med Sci Law* **27**:132–5.

Leahy MS, Farber ER. 1967. Postmortem chemistry of human vitreous humor. *J Forensic Sci* **12**:214–22.

Leclercq M, Tinant-Dubois J. 1973. Entomologie et medicine legale. [Entomology and forensic medicine: dating of a death.] *Bull Med Legal Tox* **16**:251–5.

Lie JT. 1967. Changes of potassium concentration in the vitreous humor after death. *Am J Med Sci* **254**:136–43.

Lord WD, Burger JF. 1983. Collection and preservation of forensically important entomological materials. *J Forensic Sci* **28**:94–144.

Lorenzen GA, Lawson RL. 1971. A possible new approach for determining the postmortem interval by sperm motility. *J Crim Law Criminol* **62**:560–3.

Lothe F. 1964. The use of larval infestation in detemining time of death. *Med Sci Law* **4**:113–16.

Lucy D, Aykroyd R, Pollard M. 2001. Commentary on: Munoz JI, Suarez-Penaranda JM, Otero XL, Rodriguez-Calvo MS, Costas E, Miguens X, Concheiro L. A new perspective in the estimation of postmortem interval (PMI) based on vitreous. *J Forensic Sci* **46**:1527–8.

Lundquist F. 1956. Physical and chemical methods for estimating the time since death. *Acta Med Leg Soc* **9**:205–13.

Lyle H, Cleveland F. 1956. Determination of time since death by heat loss. *J Forensic Sci* **1**:11–24.

Madea B, Henssge C. 1990. Electrical excitability of skeletal muscle postmortem in casework. *Forensic Sci Int* **47**:207–27.

Madea B, Henssge C, Honig W, *et al.* 1989. References for determining the time of death by potassium in vitreous humor. *Forensic Sci Int* **40**:231–43.

Madea B, Herrmann N, Henssge C. 1990. Precision of estimating the time since death by vitreous potassium – comparison of two different equations. *Forensic Sci Int* **46**:277–84.

Madea B, Kaferstein H, Hermann N, *et al.* 1994. Hypoxanthine in vitreous humor and cerebrospinal fluid – a marker of postmortem interval and prolonged (vital) hypoxia? Remarks also on hypoxanthine in SIDS. *Forensic Sci Int* **65**:19–31.

Madea B, Kreuser C, Banaschak S. 2001. Postmortem biochemical examination of synovial fluid – a preliminary study. *Forensic Sci Int* **118**:29–35.

Mallach HJ. 1964. Zur Frage der Todeszeitbestimmung. [Definition of the time of death.] *Berlin Med* **18**:577–82.

Mant AK. 1953. Factors influencing changes after burial. In: Simpson K (ed.), *Modern trends in forensic medicine*. Butterworth, London.

Mant AK. 1967. Adipocere. In: Simpson K (ed.), *Modern trends in forensic medicine*, 2nd edn. Butterworth, London.

Mant AK, Furbank R. 1957. Adipocere – a review. *J Forensic Med* **4**:18–22.

Marshall TK. 1960. *The cooling of the body after death*. University of Leeds, Leeds.

Marshall TK. 1962. Estimating the time of death. *J Forensic Sci* **7**:210–21.

Marshall TK. 1965. Temperature methods of estimating the time of death. *Med Sci Law* **5**:224–32.

Marshall TK. 1969. The use of body temperature in estimating the time of death and its limitations. *Med Sci Law* **9**:178–82.

Marshall TK, Hoare F. 1962. Estimating the time of death – the rectal cooling after death and its mathematical representation. *J Forensic Sci* **7**:56–81.

Mason J, Klyne W, Lennox B. 1951. Potassium levels in the CSF after death. *J Clin Pathol* **4**:231.

Maxeiner H, Winklhofer A. 1999. [Eyelid petechiae and conjunctival hemorrhage after cardiopulmonary resuscitation] *Arch Kriminol* **204**:42–51.

Megnin P. 1894. *La faune des cadavres*. Gauthier-Villars, Paris.

Modi JP. 1957. *Medical jurisprudence and toxicology*. Tripathi, Bombay, India.

Mole RH. 1948. Fibrinolysin and the fluidity of blood postmortem. *J Pathol Bacteriol* **60**:413–19.

Moore JG, Christian PE, Brown JA, *et al.* 1984. Influence of meal weight and caloric content on gastric emptying of meals in man. *Dig Dis Sci* **29**:513–19.

Morgan C, Nokes LD, Williams JH, *et al.* 1988. Estimation of the post mortem period by multiple-site temperature measurements and the use of a new algorithm. *Forensic Sci Int* **39**:89–95.

Morovic-Buda KA. 1965. Experiences in the process of putrefaction in corpses buried in earth. *Med Sci Law* **5**:403.

Munoz JI, Suarez-Penaranda JM, Otero XL, *et al.* 2001. A new perspective in the estimation of postmortem interval (PMI) based on vitreous. *J Forensic Sci* **46**:209–14.

Munoz-Barus JI, Suarez-Penaranda J, Otero XL, *et al.* 2002. Improved estimation of postmortem interval based on differential behaviour of vitreous potassium and hypoxanthine in death by hanging. *Forensic Sci Int* **125**:67–74.

Myskowiak JB, Doums C. 2002. Effects of refrigeration on the biometry and development of *Protophormia terraenovae* (Robineau-Desvoidy) (Diptera: Calliphoridae) and its consequences in estimating post-mortem interval in forensic investigations. *Forensic Sci Int* **125**:254–61.

Nanikawa R, Tawa N, Saito K. 1961. Chemical studies on adipocere formation: revaluation of the saponification theory. *Jap J Legal Med* **15**:258–64.

Nauman HN. 1959. Postmortem chemistry of the vitreous body in man. *Arch Ophthalmol* **62**:356–63.

Nicati S. 1894. Loss of eye tension as a sign of death. *Med Rec* **45**:4801.

Niderkorn PF. 1874. Rigor mortis. *Br Med J* **1**:303–4.

Nokes LD, Brown A, Knight B. 1983. A self-contained method for determining time since death from temperature measurements. *Med Sci Law* **23**:166–70.

Nokes LD, Hicks B, Knight BH. 1985. The post-mortem temperature plateau – fact or fiction? *Med Sci Law* **25**:263–4.

Nokes LD, Hicks B, Knight B. 1986. The use of trachea temperature as a means of determining the post-mortem period. *Med Sci Law* **26**:199–202.

Nokes LD, Barasi S, Knight BH. 1989. Case report: co-ordinated motor movement of a lower limb after death. *Med Sci Law* **29**:265.

Nuorteva P. 1974. Age determination of a blood stain in a decaying shirt by entomological means. *Forensic Sci* **3**:89–94.

Nuorteva P. 1977. *Sarcosaprophagous insects as forensic indicators.* In: Tedeschi CG, Eckert WG (eds), *Forensic medicine.* W. B. Saunders, Philadelphia, vol. II.

Nuorteva P, Isokoski M, Laiho K. 1967. Forensic entomology. *Ann Entomol Fenn* **33**:217–20.

Ohya I. 1994. [Some findings of the lung in medicolegal autopsy cases.] *Nippon Hoigaku Zasshi* **48**:379–94.

Osuna E, Garcia-Villora A, Perez-Carceles MD, *et al.* 1999. Vitreous humor fructosamine concentrations in the autopsy diagnosis of diabetes mellitus. *Int J Legal Med* **112**:275–9.

Osuna E, Garcia-Villora A, Perez-Carceles M, *et al.* 2001. Glucose and lactate in vitreous humor compared with the determination of fructosamine for the postmortem diagnosis of diabetes mellitus. *Am J Forensic Med Pathol* **22**:244–9.

Pallis C. 1983. *ABC of brain death.* British Medical Association, London.

Polson CJ, Marshall TK. 1975. *The disposal of the dead,* 3rd edn. English Universities Press, London.

Polson CJ, Gee D, Knight B. 1975. *The essentials of forensic medicine,* 4th edn. Pergamon Press, Oxford.

Pounder DJ, Carson DO, Johnston K, *et al.* 1998. Electrolyte concentration differences between left and right vitreous humor samples. *J Forensic Sci* **43**:604–7.

Pounder DJ, Stevenson RJ, Taylor KK. 1998. Alcoholic ketoacidosis at autopsy. *J Forensic Sci* **43**:812–16.

Prinsloo I, Gordon I. 1951. Post-mortem dissection artefacts of the neck and their differentiation from ante-mortem bruises. *S Afr Med J* **25**:358–61.

Ramu M, Robinson AE, Camps FF. 1969. The evaluation of post-mortem blood sugar levels and their correlation with the glycogen content of the liver. *Med Sci Law* **9**:23–6.

Rognum TO, Hauge S, Oyasaeter S, *et al.* 1991. A new biochemical method for estimation of postmortem time. *Forensic Sci Int* **51**:139–46.

Roll P, Rous F. 1991. Injuries by chicken bills: characteristic wound morphology. *Forensic Sci Int* **52**:25–30.

Rossi ML, Shahrom AW, Chapman RC, *et al.* 1994. Postmortem injuries by indoor pets. *Am J Forensic Med Pathol* **15**:105–9.

Salisbury CR, Melvin GS. 1936. Ophthalmoscopic signs of death. *Br Med J* **1**:1249–51.

Schleyer F. 1963. Determination of the time of death in the early post-mortem interval. In: Lundquist F (ed.), *Methods of forensic science.* Interscience Publishers, John Wiley and Sons, New York, pp. 253–93.

Schleyer F. 1975. Leichenveränderungen. Todeszeitbestimmung im früh-postmortalen Intervall. In: Müller B (ed.), *Gerichtliche Medizin.* Springer-Verlag, Berlin.

Schuller E, Pankratz H, Liebhardt E. 1987. [Colorimetry of livor mortis.] *Beitr Gerichtl Med* **45**:169–73.

Scott KS, Oliver JS. 2001. The use of vitreous humor as an alternative to whole blood for the analysis of benzodiazepines. *J Forensic Sci* **46**:694–7.

Sellier K. 1958. Determination of the time of death by extrapolation of the temperature decrease curve. *Acta Med Leg Soc* **2**:279–301.

Shapiro HA. 1950. Rigor mortis. *Br Med J* **2**:304.

Shapiro HA. 1954. Medico-legal mythology; the time of death. *J Forensic Med* **1**:144–69.

Shapiro HA. 1965. The post-mortem temperature plateau. *J Forensic Med* **12**:137–41.

Shapiro HA, Gordon I, Benson SD. 1988. *Forensic medicine – a guide to principles*, 3rd edn. Churchill Livingstone, Edinburgh.

Shattock FM. 1968. Injuries caused by wild animals. *Lancet* **2**:412–14.

Shikata I. 1958. On the mortality of the leucocyte and the time lapse after death. *Jap J Legal Med* **12**:227–31.

Simonsen J, Voigt J, Jeppesen N. 1977. Determination of the time of death by continuous post-mortem temperature measurements. *Med Sci Law* **17**:112–22.

Smith KGV. 1973. *Forensic entomology*. In: Smith KGV (ed.), *Insects and other arthropods of medical importance*. British Museum of Natural History, London.

Smith KGV. 1986. *A manual of forensic entomology*. British Museum of Natural History, London.

Stephens RJ, Richards RG. 1987. Vitreous humor chemistry: the use of potassium concentration for the prediction of the postmortem interval. *J Forensic Sci* **32**:503–9.

Sturner WQ. 1963. The vitreous humour: postmortem potassium changes. *Lancet* **1**:807–8.

Sturner WQ, Ganter G. 1964. The postmortem interval. A study of potassium in the vitreous humor. *Am J Clin Pathol* **42**:137–41.

Sturner WQ, Dowdey AB, Putnam RS, *et al.* 1972. Osmolality and other chemical determinations in postmortem human vitreous humor. *J Forensic Sci* **17**:387–93.

Suzuki S. 1987. Experimental studies on the presumption of the time after food intake from stomach contents. *Forensic Sci Int* **35**:83–117.

Suzutani T, Ishibashi H, Takatori T. 1978. [Studies on the estimation of the postmortem interval. 2. The postmortem lividity (author's transl).] *Hokkaido Igaku Zasshi* **52**:259–67.

Szent-Gyorgyi A. 1947. *Chemistry of muscular contraction*. Academic Press, New York.

Tagliaro F, Bortolotti F, Manetto G, *et al.* 2001. Potassium concentration differences in the vitreous humour from the two eyes revisited by microanalysis with capillary electrophoresis. *J Chromatogr A* **924**:493–8.

Takatori T, Ishiguro N, Tarao H, *et al.* 1986. Microbial production of hydroxy and oxo fatty acids by several microorganisms as a model of adipocere formation. *Forensic Sci Int* **32**:5–11.

Takatori T, Gotouda H, Terazawa K, *et al.* 1987. The mechanism of experimental adipocere formation: substrate specificity on microbial production of hydroxy and oxo fatty acids. *Forensic Sci Int* **35**:277–81.

Takeichi S, Wakasugi C, Shikata I. 1984. Fluidity of cadaveric blood after sudden death: part I. Postmortem fibrinolysis and plasma catecholamine level. *Am J Forensic Med Pathol* **5**:223–7.

Takeichi S, Tokunaga I, Hayakumo K, *et al.* 1986. Fluidity of cadaveric blood after sudden death: Part III. Acid-base balance and fibrinolysis. *Am J Forensic Med Pathol* **7**:35–8.

Taylor A, Wilkes D. 1863. On cooling of the human body after death. *Guy's Hosp Rep* 180–211.

Tomlin PJ. 1967. 'Railroading' in retinal vessels. *Br Med J* **3**:722–3.

Tough SC, Butt JC. 1993. A review of fatal bear maulings in alberta, canada. *Am J Forensic Med Pathol* **14**:22–7.

Trujillo O, Vanezis P, Cermignani M. 1996. Photometric assessment of skin colour and lightness using a tristimulus colorimeter: reliability of inter- and intra-investigator observations in healthy adult volunteers. *Forensic Sci Int* **81**:1–10.

Tsunerari S, Oho S, Sasaki S, *et al.* 1975. Histopathological studies on the changes of the postmortem cornea. *Jpn J Legal Med* **29**:298–303.

Vain A, Kauppila R, Humal LH, *et al.* 1992. Grading rigor mortis with myotonometry – a new possibility to estimate time of death. *Forensic Sci Int* **56**:147–50.

Valenzuela A. 1988. Postmortem diagnosis of diabetes mellitus. Quantitation of fructosamine and glycated hemoglobin. *Forensic Sci Int* **38**:203–8.

Van den Oever R. 1976. A review of the literature as to the present possibilities and limitations in estimating the time of death. *Med Sci Law* **16**:269–76.

Vanezis P. 1991. Assessing hypostasis by colorimetry. *Forensic Sci Int* **52**:1–3.

Vass AA, Barshick SA, Sega G, *et al.* 2002. Decomposition chemistry of human remains: a new methodology for determining the postmortem interval. *J Forensic Sci* **47**:542–53.

Webb PA, Terry HJ, Gee DJ. 1986. A method for time of death determination using ultrasound – a preliminary report. *J Forensic Sci Soc* **26**:393–9.

Wroblewski B, Ellis M. 1970. Eye changes after death. *Br J Surg* **57**:69–71.

CHAPTER 3

The establishment of identity of human remains

The identity of the dead is an essential part of post-mortem examination, for various reasons. These include:

- the ethical and humanitarian need to know which individual has died, especially for the information of surviving relatives
- to establish the fact of death in respect of that individual, for official, statistical and legal purposes
- to record the identity for administrative and ceremonial purposes in respect of burial or cremation
- to discharge legal claims and obligations in relation to property, estate and debts
- to prove claims for life insurance contracts, survivor's pensions, and other financial matters
- to allow legal investigations, inquests and other tribunals, such as those held by coroners, procurators fiscal, medical examiners, judges and accident enquiries to proceed with a firm knowledge of the identity of the decedent
- to facilitate police enquiries into overtly criminal or suspicious deaths, as the identity of the deceased person is a vital factor in initiating investigations.

The establishment of identity has many facets, some of which have no medical content, such as the recognition of clothing, documents and personal property. Some aspects, though primarily the responsibility of the police, have a medical content, including identification of fingerprints and personal property such as hearing aids, spectacles, medicines, trusses and surgical prostheses. False dentures have such central importance that they will be considered in the section on odontology.

Identification from anatomical and medical features comprises two major aspects:

- The establishment of certain broad groupings, such as sex, stature, race and age. These may be determined solely from the available bodily remains, though corroboration may be obtained from other evidence. An obvious example would be sex determination from clothing and jewellery, though even this may no longer be absolutely reliable.
- Comparison of the remains with ante-mortem information and records from those thought to be the victims, which restricts the method by making it dependent upon the existence or availability of such comparable material.

The establishment of identity may be required upon:

- **Intact fresh corpses.** Here visual recognition, directly or by photography, may be made. Hair colour, skin pigmentation, scars and tattoos can be examined without difficulty.
- **Decomposed corpses.** Many surface features may be partially or wholly lost, but more information can be obtained than from a skeleton. Direct measurement of body height, for example, may be possible, as well as

serological investigations and organ abnormalities, such as past surgical intervention, may be found.

■ **Mutilated and dismembered corpses.** Depending on the degree of mutilation and the amount of tissue missing, identification may be hampered. If the remains are fresh, facts such as racial pigmentation may be determined, but direct measurement of stature may be impossible. Selective mutilation in some homicides may be deliberately directed at frustrating identification, such as the removal of teeth and finger-pads.

■ **Skeletalized material.** If all soft tissues are absent, identity depends solely on osteological examination and measurements and the recognition of any pathological or anatomical abnormalities in bone.

CHARACTERISTICS USEFUL IN IDENTIFYING THE DEAD

Facial appearance

Even in perfectly fresh bodies, recognition may be difficult because of alterations in the features caused by death. It is a common occurrence in mortuary viewing rooms for a close relative, even a parent or spouse, to have doubts about – or even to deny or mistakenly agree to – the identity of the deceased person. Though distress and emotion play a part, changes in the features may be profound. Hypostasis, contact flattening, oedema, muscle flaccidity and pallor may all combine to distort the face. Recognition in the living is partly a dynamic process, aided by facial muscle tone and especially eye contact and movement, all of which are absent in the corpse.

Eye colour

In the fresh corpse, eye colour corresponds with the living state, but it quickly deteriorates. Loss of intraocular tension and clouding of the cornea develops progressively within a few hours, making the iris harder to observe. Collapse of the front of the globe occurs within a day or two and, with developing decomposition, all irises tend to darken to brown. It is unsafe to depend on eye colour as a criterion of identity later than a few days following death – or even much sooner where environmental conditions hasten decomposition.

Skin pigmentation

In undamaged, unputrefied bodies, the major ethnic differences in skin pigmentation are obvious, though the slight melanin increase of the misnamed 'yellow' races of Asia may be impossible to differentiate from Mediterranean or Middle Eastern races. The onset of deathly pallor and post-mortem hypostasis is more profound than slight variations between sunburnt White people, northern Asians or Semitic races. When putrefaction sets in, skin slippage progressively removes the pigmented layers and eventually pigmentation becomes unavailable as a marker of identity, though histologically melanin may still be visible in the basal layer of any surviving epidermis.

Burnt bodies may also lose pigmented skin, either by heat destruction or by deposition of soot and other combustion products on the surface, though it is rare for this to be so complete as to obscure all evidence of pigmentation.

Hair colour

The head, pubic and axillary hair is one of the most resistant identifying features, sometimes lasting millennia in favourable environments. The original colour may, however, alter after burial, becoming a brownish-red or 'foxy' colour within as short a time as 3 months. The colour may be obscured by dirt or staining and expert treatment (usually by a biologist or museum technologist) may be required to restore the original colour. The possibility of deliberate chemical coloration or bleaching before death may have to be considered and again expert chemical analysis in a forensic science laboratory may be needed to confirm or eliminate this if the hair colour conflicts with other positive evidence of identity.

Hair structure

This is more the province of the forensic biologist or anthropologist, but factors such as whether the hair ends have been cut or are naturally pointed may sometimes have importance in identity. Racial features exist, Negroid head hair being dark and having a spiral twist with a flattened, elliptical cross-section. Mongoloid hair is less pigmented and is straight with a cylindrical cross-section. Caucasian hair is round or ovoid in cross-section, but shows great variation in colour and morphology compared with the other two major ethnic groups. Though head hair in Caucasians is round to ovoid in section, eyebrow hair tends to be triangular and pubic hair flattened. Where a hair root is present, blood grouping and other serological criteria can be determined. Grouping of the shafts of hairs has been repeatedly attempted and success claimed by some workers. The cells of the hair root can give a DNA profile and mitochondrial DNA (mtDNA) has been detected even in a sample from a single hair shaft.

Microscopic examination of the hair can assist in determining the species, if not human. Human hair has broad groupings when viewed microscopically. However, the topic of individual identity from hair is now the province of forensic biologists, and has a specialism and literature of its own.

Tattoos

Deliberate ornamentation of the skin by introducing pigments under the epidermis has been practised for millennia and in all parts of the world. The word 'tattoo' comes from the Polynesian '*ta tau*', meaning 'to mark'. Some races such as the Ibans of Sarawak may be tattooed over much of their body surface, but many men and some women in most countries have localized tattoos, which can be of considerable assistance in identification. Many different pigments are used, as well as more unusual substances such as soot or gunpowder. The colour is pricked into the upper dermis with a sharp instrument, usually a needle used manually, or by an electric vibrator.

Once under the outer skin, the material persists for a long time. Colours such as blue, green or red may be scavenged by tissue cells and leached into the lymphatic system after a number of years or decades. Black pigments, usually carbon particles in the form of Indian ink, are so resistant as to be virtually lifelong, though some may be transported to regional lymph nodes. Thus an original pattern of different colours may fade differentially over years, the black areas standing out in strong relief.

The patterns are so diverse as to defy classification, though much has been written on the subject. From the point of view of identity, tattoos may be useful in both a general sense and for comparison with potential victims.

The general applications require a knowledge of ethnic, national, cultural, religious and social practices, so that the tattoo can be assigned to some particular group of people. In Western society, the popularity of tattooing changes from time to time. Former statements that tattoos are seen mostly in the 'lower social classes' have little current validity, though it is obvious that bankers and parsons are less likely to sport tattoos than seamen and truck drivers. It is also now totally anachronistic to claim that most women with tattoos are prostitutes, though the nature and position of the tattoo is obviously relevant.

Certain tattoos have had particular significance such as a number, often '13', inscribed inside the lower lip of drug pushers or the bluebird on the extensor surface of the web of the thumb in homosexuals. The latter design is now so common as to be of little significance.

Tattoos are of most use when individual enough to be compared with known designs on a missing person. The design is often supplemented by actual names, though these are mostly forenames rather than family names. Designs are by no means unique and a professional tattooist may turn out hundreds of identical decorations, so names are a bonus when trying to achieve identity.

Initials may be used, but these can be misleading due to the use of nicknames and diminutives, such as 'B' for Bill, rather than William. In general, men have the names of girls on their tattoos, but initials are usually their own. Conversely, women with tattoos almost always display the names of sweethearts, rather than their own. Some tattoos may be numbers or unadorned names, the most tragic examples being those from Nazi concentration camps during the last war.

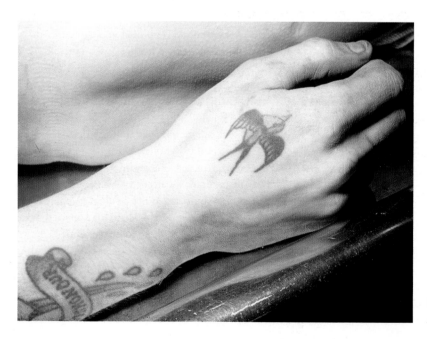

FIGURE 3.1 *Individualistic tattoos may assist the identification of unknown persons.*

The photography, distribution and matching of tattoos is police business, but the pathologist's duty is to make them accessible and clear to the police. Where decomposition has set in, tattoos may be obscured by wrinkled, peeling epidermis, but often this can be wiped off to reveal tattoos that are more vivid than on fresh skin. Once the tissues become green and slimy, then the pattern progressively vanishes, but early decomposition is no barrier to recognition. Where skin pigmentation may hide a design, skin slippage may actually enhance the clarity, especially of the weaker colours like blue, red and green. Attempts at the deliberate removal of tattoos are common, either from regret at having disfigured the body during youthful or drunken euphoria, or to remove evidence of identity. Many methods have been used, from surgical excision to scarification with sandpaper and from caustic soda to electrolysis. All methods depend upon damage to the epidermis and dermis, with consequent inflammation and scar formation. The tattoo can certainly be removed, but always by replacing it by a cicatrix to a greater or lesser extent, which will itself indicate that something pre-existed at that site.

It has been suggested (PA Edwards, personal communication) that the chemical nature of tattoo pigments might be used in identification. Although all manner of substances have been used to tattoo, most tattooists use black pigments containing carbon, green pigments containing potassium dichromate and red pigments containing mercuric chloride. Others use aniline-based dyes, so that microextraction and analysis in a forensic science laboratory might confirm or exclude the tattoo having been executed by a particular artist in the locality.

Finger, palm, foot and lip prints

The science of fingerprints, their classification, retrieval from records and methods of recording lie in the domain of police procedure, and, as with tattoos, the pathologist's role is merely to facilitate the taking of prints by police officers. Sometimes when a strange print is found at a scene of crime, the police may wish to take the fingerprints of doctors who visited the locus to eliminate them from their enquiries and there is obviously nothing objectionable about this. Indeed, some forensic pathologists who habitually assist the police leave their prints on file so that they are permanently available for exclusion. When called to a scene of death, the doctor should take care to avoid handling objects and furniture to reduce the need for such laborious screening of prints.

The doctor need know nothing about fingerprints except for his own interest, though it is as well to be prepared for the inevitable questions – no two fingerprints have ever been found to be identical and even identical twins have different prints. However, some recent claims point out that some prints are so similar that the criteria usually accepted as proof of congruence may not be sufficient. Police usually attend the mortuary to take full sets of fingerprints in the usual way by rolling ink on to the finger-pads and pressing the pulps against record cards.

The pathologist may help when there is strong rigor present, by either forcing the flexed fingers back or even by slitting the flexor tendons, though this has the danger of fouling the fingers with blood.

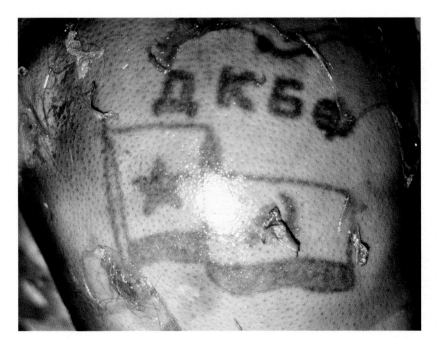

FIGURE 3.2 *Shoulder region of a decomposed body recovered from the sea showing a tattoo with Cyrillic letters (Д, К, Б, Ф) and a flag with a star and hammer and sickle suggesting a connection with the Russian Baltic Fleet.*

When the body is putrefied, the doctor can again assist by removing desquamated casts from the fingers for the police. These may need to be preserved or hardened up so that the decaying tissue does not lose further definition from the ridges that form the prints. The skin may be placed in formalin, alcohol or glycerine solution, especially where maceration in an immersed body has caused swelling and blurring of the epidermis. An alternative is immersion in 20 per cent aqueous acetic acid for 2–8 hours. Rarely, a criminal may attempt to obliterate his fingerprints by scarring the fingerpads. To be effective, this must be drastic enough to damage the underlying dermis and the consequent cicatrices will be more obvious than the original prints. Surgical grafting of skin from elsewhere on the body has been reported as a means of removing fingerprints, but again the result is self-evident proof of nefarious intent.

As with fingerprints, the skin pattern of palms, soles and even lips are said to be unique and have been used in identification, but again this is really police business. The pattern of veins on the back of hands is also said to be characteristic to one individual.

Identifying scars

These can be important in the identification of unknown bodies, even when some degree of putrefaction exists. The author (BK) used a cholecystectomy scar and scars of old surgical incisions on the legs to identify the body of a homicide victim submerged in a river for 6 weeks and many other cases are on record where scars provided similar vital information. Probably the best known instance is the Crippen case of 1910 in which much forensic controversy was generated over the distinction between a surgical scar and a skin crease on a piece of abdominal wall.

Scars on the skin may arise from any previous injury that has breached the epidermis, as superficial injuries to the upper layer of skin will heal without a trace. Where the dermis has been entered, healing occurs by organization of the plug of blood clot and/or granulation tissue, as described in Chapter 4. If the wound is narrow, such as that inflicted by a surgical instrument, sharp knife, razor or glass, then if the edges are kept together, especially by stitches or dressings, the resulting scar will be narrow and insignificant. Gaping or infection will widen the scar and obviously larger lacerations or burns will result in similarly greater scarring. In relation to identification, scars are of use only if those thought to be the victims are known to have similar scars, both in nature and position. The specificity of scars varies greatly, as many people may have appendicectomy scars, and many women have had hysterectomies or other gynaecological operations that leave lower abdominal scars. As always, scar evidence must be taken in conjunction with all other details of identity,

but where a cicatrix is unusual or even unique in nature or position, its value is greatly enhanced.

Turning to traumatic scars other than surgical, the pathologist may be able to recognize the cause, which can assist in identity. Naturally the vast majority of non-surgical scars are the result of accidental trauma and where family, friends, photographs or medical records indicate the existence of specific scarred sites on the body, then confirmation of identity may be greatly assisted or confirmed.

Some scars are deliberately produced as part of some ethnic or religious tradition, such as the facial scars in some African tribes, as well as deformed or perforated ear lobes or lips. Regrettably, another class of scars is becoming more common in many parts of the world, due to physical torture; this is dealt with in Chapter 10. Linear scars, cicatrices of burns, keloid overgrowth (especially in negroid races), hyperpigmentation or depigmentation and other persistent lesions may assist in identity in the appropriate circumstances. Much depends on the accuracy of the information concerning the person thought to be the victim; relatives are notoriously vague and inaccurate about medical matters and frequently confuse different surgical operations, thus misleading the investigators about scars. Sometimes surgical scars may be almost invisible. The author (PS) once worked as surgical assistant in a private hospital where one of the surgeons used to perform appendicectomy (in non-acute cases) through a 1 cm wide incision, closing the wound, for cosmetic reasons, with subcutaneous catgut sutures. Most of these wounds healed with virtually no scar whatsoever, unless the person had a tendency to keloid formation. Wherever possible, old hospital records or the notes of a family physician should be obtained.

The old scars of wrist- or throat-slashing indicate previous attempts at suicide. Large areas of scarring on the trunk or limbs that have parallel grooves and marginal extensions suggest severe brush lacerations, probably from a traffic accident. Knife stab wounds may scar in an elliptical fashion, sometimes even with a blunt and a sharp end indicating the position of a single-edged blade. Bullet wound scars may persist – and in 1989, became a matter of political controversy over the identity of Nazi war prisoner Rudolf Hess, who was alleged to have been an imposter because he had no scar from an old rifle bullet wound through the chest. Burns may provide good evidence of identity, especially if they are widespread cicatrices that may have been quite noticeable during life. Many scars on the fronts of the lower legs may indicate the repeated stumblings of a chronic alcoholic, who frequently walks into or falls over furniture.

The age of scars

The age of a scar is very difficult to assess and, once it becomes mature, no change will occur for the rest of the person's life. When a linear wound is inflicted, be it a surgical operation or a knife slash, the edges become mechanically strong within a week, assuming that no infection or haematoma develops. The wound is brownish red at this stage and remains vascular for several months, depending upon its width. The pinkness of contained blood vessels gradually fades and a narrow surgical incision may be white by 4–6 months. The avascular collagen tends to shrink for a year or so, but is white–silver after a year and remains in this state indefinitely. These times are variable depending on the nature of the skin, its pigmentation and the part of the body involved. Where a wound crosses a skin crease that is frequently flexed or extended, it tends to gape and widen, the subsequent scar following suit.

Histology does not contribute much to the examination of scars, except to confirm that a skin mark actually is a scar. Stains for collagen or elastin may confirm the discontinuity in the dermis. Scars do not carry hair follicles, sweat glands or sebaceous glands, though an occasional accessory skin structure may be present as a result of the inclusion of a viable fragment of original skin in an irregular wound – or where surgical repair has detached or invaginated a piece of the margin.

Occupational stigmata

Formerly given prominence in most textbooks, distinctive physical marks of occupation have decreased in incidence and importance. They are still of use in certain areas, but local knowledge of occupations and industries is required. The Victorian days of pen callosities in clerks and shoemaker's kyphosis have gone, but many other occupations have their stigmata, though most are relatively non-specific. The best known is the 'blue scar' of coal-miners, an involuntary tattoo caused by dust entering small lacerations on the hands and face. Some miners and quarrymen also have small facial scars due to rock splinters scattered during blasting. Steel workers and foundry men may have tiny burn scars on exposed areas from the spattering of hot metal. In more general terms, examination of the hands will indicate whether the deceased was a manual worker or involved in more sedentary occupations. Cuts, scars, callosities and hyperkeratosis of the hands are obvious indicators of rough work.

Internally, black, dust-laden lungs – with or without pneumoconiosis – points to mining, as coal trimmers no longer exist as dock workers. Thickened, pearly plaques on the parietal pleura and diaphragm are caused by exposure to asbestos, though in recent years the widespread use of this substance in so many industries makes it less helpful in identifying the occupation.

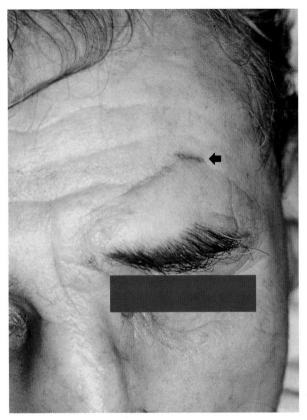

FIGURE 3.3 *Careful external examination may yield evidence that can assist identification. The small 'blue scar' on this forehead establishes that the deceased had been a coal-miner; coal dust enters small lacerations and remains visible after healing. Virtually every coal-worker has such marks on hands or face.*

The stature of an intact body

The stature of a corpse is not necessarily exactly that of the person measured during life. In the mortuary, care must be taken to measure the body from heel to crown, and not to accept the mortuary attendant's or funeral director's 'coffin measurement', which is made from toe to crown. Because of the usual plantar flexion of the foot, this latter height may be as much as 10 cm longer than the heel–crown length.

The height of a dead body may differ from the height during life in either direction, being slightly longer or shorter, though lengthening is much more common. In addition, the measured height may change a little at different periods after death. Because of the complete loss of muscle tone in the first stage of flaccidity, relaxation at large joints, such as the hip and knee, together with the lost tensioning effect of paraspinal muscles on intervertebral discs, the body may lengthen by up to 2–3 cm. Rigor mortis may then replace the muscle tone, shortening the body and tending to flex the legs a little. When rigor passes off and decomposition sets in, joints become lax. Loss of tension in the intervertebral discs tends to shorten the spinal column and hence the total height by a centimetre or so. According to Trotter and Gleser (1958, 1977), the average increase is about 2–5 cm. The errors in getting a really accurate post-mortem length include the difficulty of locating the measuring device exactly at the heel and the crown of the head, as well as fully extending the limbs, spine and neck of a body in rigor.

Determination of sex in non-skeletalized bodies

This is usually obvious and rarely presents problems. The issue of intersex and hermaphroditism is so rare as to be discounted in most forensic practice, except in some areas, such as South-east Asia, where deliberate transsexualism in men, aided by surgical intervention to feminize the genitalia and breasts occurs more frequently. Where this problem arises, expert advice must be sought. In general, the external genitalia remain recognizable until a late stage of putrefaction. In addition, breasts and general body shape, as well as the pattern of pubic hair, reveal the sex. Female pubic hair usually grows low on the abdomen, the upper margin being a horizontal or semicircular edge above the mons veneris. The male pattern rises more in the centre line, sometimes as far as the umbilicus. There are, however, always exceptions to these generalizations. The presence or absence of circumcision should be noted, as it may help in identification of certain ethnic and religious groups such as Jews and Muslims. Naturally it is of assistance here in eliminating only those where the prepuce is present, as many men of other religions are circumcised.

Clothing, hair length, hair style, hair coloration, earrings and other jewellery are no longer the reliable guide to sex that they once were. In certain cultures and religions there are obvious criteria that can assist in the determination of sex, but these are rarely needed as the more apparent anatomical differences can be used. Where putrefaction is advanced, examination of the internal pelvic organs may still reveal unequivocal evidence of sex. Internal viscera are often in better condition than the outside of the body. The uterus is the organ in the body most resistant to decomposition, though the prostate is also quite persistent.

Where almost total dissolution exists, then radiology of the pelvis or the criteria used in skeletal assessment can be used. Cytological examination of cell nuclei may indicate sex where only tiny fragments are available – such as tissue found on a road or rail vehicle where impact with a body is suspected. Usually it is the species rather than the sex that is the first consideration, and this is done by species-specific serology. When sex is to be determined, much depends on the state of preservation. When stained microscopic smears can be prepared or when tissue can be processed for histological sections, then sex-indicating nuclear chromatin may provide a definitive test. The 'drumsticks' of polymorphonuclear leucocytes, and the marginal chromatin masses or 'Barr bodies' in epithelial cells, such as the buccal mucosa, may indicate the sex, but in decomposed material this may be impossible.

The recent remarkable developments in cytogenetics and DNA analysis now give additional powerful tools in sexing and determining the human origin of sub-anatomical fragments, which will partly or wholly replace the older techniques mentioned above.

Other more recent techniques include counting the sex material within the nucleus stained with a fluorescent dye and viewed with ultraviolet light; this may be performed on neurones in a brain smear or in cells from the kidney.

Age of non-skeletalized bodies

Determining the personal age of a corpse is far harder than determining its sex. Ageing a living person can be difficult and a wide margin of error exists, especially as age advances, so the same exercise in a corpse can be expected to be even less exact. Where the body is relatively intact, the usual criteria known to the man in the street are applied to make a general estimate. Hair colour is of general applicability, though every one knows of someone whose hair is grey at 25 or someone who is dark haired at 70. The loss of elasticity in the skin, its thinness and hyperkeratosis and its red Campbell de Morgan spots are indicators of senility. These days teeth are less useful than in the past from the point of view of extractions, clearance, full dentures and oral hygiene, but the general impression remains. The objective determination of age from tooth attrition is a matter for a specialist forensic odontologist (see Chapter 26).

The eyes are useful, in that a grey or white ring around the pupil – the 'arcus senilis' – is rarely seen below 60 years. In infants and children, the height and weight may be compared with standard tables, but developmental defects, disease and malnourishment may introduce considerable errors. Internally, the evolution of degenerative changes such as arterial atherosclerosis and arthritis, may give a general impression, but personal variation is so great that it offers little more than a distinction between 'young' and 'old'. Where a distinction has to be made in a double death between two people of markedly different ages, however, then these generalities may be of considerable use. Up to the age of about 20–25, teeth, ossification centres and epiphyseal fusion are good indicators, but these are described in the section on skeletalized material.

Recent research, aimed mainly at skeletalized bodies but available for any corpse, is the determination of the racemization ratio of amino acids in teeth, as the preponderance of laevo- and dextro-compounds appears to be a function of personal age.

In addition, the Gustafson technique on teeth, described later, is also applicable to a non-skeletalized body, if ageing is important.

Racial and ethnic characteristics

Much of the identification of race depends on common knowledge and recognition of various ethnic traits, and is not primarily a medical problem. Everyone can recognize the deep pigmentation of a West African the epicanthic folds of the Mongoloid races, the red-haired Celt and the pale blond common in Scandinavia. There is a wide and almost continuous range of biological variability, however, not only because of extensive ethnic interbreeding, but also because of marked variations even within a coherent racial group.

In the intact or only partially decomposed body, the following factors may be used as pointers to ethnic classification, but the non-specificity of most of these must always be borne in mind:

- Clothing, ornaments and other associated objects. A vast catalogue can be assembled (such as the string around the wrist in Hindus), but it must be borne in mind that other races may adopt these through choice, marriage or deception.
- Hair texture, style and length and beards. Examples are the hair of the Sikh, the beard of the orthodox Jew, the crinkly hair or 'peppercorn' (clumped growth) of some Negroids, the multiplaiting of Rastafarian West Indians, the straight black hair of Asians and the ginger hair most common in Celtic people. With affected styles and convincing modern coloration and texture alteration, however, these features can be most misleading. Forensic science techniques may be needed to detect and identify bleaching and dyeing changes in hair.
- Physical artefacts include penile and vulval circumcision, nose and ear piercing, lip perforation, tribal facial scars, and earlobe distension in East Africans and some tribes in Sarawak. More bizarre forms, such as neck-stretching by rings, are now rare. Tattoos (mentioned elsewhere) may have an ethnic basis, as in the Ibans of Sarawak.
- Facial appearance is, of course, a major criterion with the high cheek bones and epicanthic folds of the

Mongoloid peoples, and the prognathism and nasal differences in Negroid peoples. So many intermediate forms exist, however, such as the Slav and the Polynesian, that only the classic groupings can be identified with confidence.

- Body size gives rise to the same uncertainty, especially as racial differences have lessened with better nutrition in some groups. It is obvious, however, that Japanese are generally smaller than northern Europeans and that in Negroid bone structure the femora are proportionately longer and less curved than those of other races. Teeth are discussed later, but the concave upper central incisors of the Mongoloid races can be helpful on occasions, though they are not absolutely specific.

Finally, skin pigmentation can obviously differentiate the Negroid races from the other main groups, though again there is a continuous range of skin colour. To a lesser extent the slighter melanin content of the skin of Mongoloid races is recognizable, but merges into the variable tints of Semitic, Asian and Mediterranean peoples.

It may well be that, in the near future, genetic DNA studies will revolutionize this aspect of identification. They are also likely to do the same for personal identification.

Identification by DNA characteristics

One of the most revolutionary advances in identification in recent years is the so-called 'DNA profiling or fingerprinting'. This is a technique devised by Alec Jeffreys of Leicester University, in which virtually unique sequences of bases in the DNA strands of chromosomes are used to compare one blood or tissue sample with another, and to investigate genetic relationships. The details of the technique are complex and require highly specialized reagents and apparatus. The method needs highly trained forensic scientists for its application to medico-legal problems. All that the pathologist needs is a basic knowledge of the principles of the technique and how it can be applied in a forensic context.

The deoxyribonucleic acid (DNA) that forms genetic material is composed of two strands of sugar and phosphate molecules that are twisted into a double helix, which is bound together by links formed from adenine and thymine and cytosine and guanine. Each helical twist has ten such links, like rungs on a twisted ladder. A single DNA molecule may have millions of such links and the permutations of the bases in each adjacent link create the genes, the segments of the DNA that carry genetic information. A gene consists of a segment containing some hundreds or thousands of links, but separating these discrete genes are segments that seem to have no genetic function, being redundant. There is about a metre of

DNA in each human nucleus, but only 10 per cent is used for genetic coding, the rest being redundant. Of these silent segments (sometimes called 'stutters'), there may be 200–14 000 repeats of each identical sequence on each DNA strand.

During investigations into a specific gene (that for synthesizing myoglobin), Jeffreys found that the adjacent redundant segments varied greatly in base sequence, but that they were constant for a given individual and that they were transmitted from parents in a regular fashion. In other words, they formed a 'signature' that was virtually unique for every individual person, except identical (uni-ovular) twins, in whom they must be the same as they share the same DNA in the fertilized ovum. The chance of two persons sharing the same sequence is, according to Jeffreys, about one in a million billion. Even among siblings, the chances are only one in ten thousand billion.

To identify the redundant segment (often called the 'minisatellite' or 'hypervariable regions'), a minute amount of human tissue containing nuclear material is required. A small volume of blood containing leucocytes is sufficient, or a semen sample, pulp from a tooth or a hair with some sheath cells at the root. The DNA from the contained nuclear material is broken up into fragments by enzymes called 'restriction endonucleases' that cleave the DNA strands at predetermined spots. The fragments are then separated by gel electrophoresis, which spreads the fragments into bands, transferred to nylon or nitrocellulose sheets and subjected to a 'DNA probe'. This is a single strand of DNA labelled with radioactive phosphorus-32. This latches on to the separated minisatellite fragments and – by microradiography – the position of each band is rendered visible on an X-ray plate.

The end result is a series of parallel bars, similar in appearance to the 'bar code' printed on goods in a supermarket. However, more recently the bar pattern from multilocus probes has been supplemented or replaced by simpler patterns from single-locus probes, though the principles remain the same. From the presence of different bars in given positions, comparisons can be made with other samples, so this is a classic forensic technique of comparison. The test is useless without something to be compared with, but the blood on a weapon in the possession of a suspect can be matched with virtually complete confidence against the blood of the victim. Seminal fluid in the vagina of a victim of a murder/rape can be matched against the blood DNA pattern of a suspect – there is no need to match semen against semen, as all the DNA in a given person must, by definition, be identical. A few hair roots found on a blunt instrument in the possession of a suspect from a murder can be matched against the autopsy blood sample. In sexual crime cases, a great advantage of DNA testing over conventional blood-group secretor tests is that DNA can distinguish between mixed semen and vaginal fluids from a swab, which can confuse or negate blood-group techniques.

Another wide medico-legal use is in paternity testing where, unlike blood group, haptoglobin and enzyme tests, a positive identity of parents can be made, rather than a mere exclusion. Every bar in the 'bar-code' must have come from either mother or father, half the number from each. In testing, the coding is made from child, mother and father. The bars in the child's code are first matched with those in the mother's pattern. The remaining bars then must correspond with those from the father – if not, he cannot be the father.

SAMPLES REQUIRED FOR DNA TESTING

Although amplification techniques, such as polymerase chain reaction (PCR), etc., now allow minute samples to be tested, the larger the sample, the better the chance of a successful DNA test.

Post-mortem material is inferior to live blood and tissue for DNA fingerprinting if any significant post-mortem change has proceeded enough to break down nuclear chromatin. Plain blood samples should be taken, however, though leucocytes may have already disintegrated. Some 5 ml of blood is taken into an EDTA tube, which extracts metallic ions and not only prevents clotting, but inhibits enzymes in blood or micro-organisms, which may break down DNA during storage. The best material is said to be muscle or the spleen and, if decomposition is advancing, the bone marrow is recommended. At least 0.5 g of tissue should be cut from the parenchyma of an organ and placed in a small plastic tube with no fixative or preservative. This should be frozen at −20°C if there is likely to be the slightest delay in transmission to the laboratory.

In sexual offences associated with homicide, as much material as can be obtained from the vagina should be collected, either fluid by pipette or multiple swabs from vagina, rectum and mouth. These again should be frozen if there is more than a few hours delay in transit to the laboratory (see also Appendix 1).

IDENTIFICATION OF SKELETALIZED REMAINS

One of the classic problems of forensic pathology, the identification of a whole or partial skeleton, involves techniques and expertise that span a number of disciplines from anatomy to radiology, from archaeology to dentistry. It often overshadows the equally important need to identify intact or decomposed corpses, but the disproportionate amount of space occupied by skeletal identification in most textbooks can be partly justified by the fact that bones can survive for decades, centuries or millennia, so that the cumulative reservoir of material is vast. As was observed in relation to intact bodies, the procedure for identifying bony remains falls into two distinct sections:

▪ allotting the bones to general categories based on absolute criteria concerning species, race, sex, stature, age and date
▪ comparative studies, where the remains are matched against ante-mortem data derived from those people who might be potential victims.

The general categorization of skeletal remains

When objects thought to be skeletal remains are found, the following questions need to be asked and, where possible, answered:

▪ Are they bones?
▪ Are they human bones?
▪ What is the sex?
▪ What is the stature?
▪ What is the race?
▪ What is the age?
▪ How long have they been dead and/or concealed?
▪ What was the cause of death?

Are the remains actually bones?

This question is not as facetious as it may seem, as untrained persons may provide objects that falsely resemble bones. The author (BK) has been offered shaped stones, plastic and even hard wood, which were thought to be bones. The mistake is even more common when these objects are mixed with undoubted bones, usually animal in origin, which may be found buried or mingled with rubble.

Recognition is usually easy, by the shape, texture and especially weight of the objects. Greater difficulty may be experienced when simulated human 'bones' are found, such as the 'radius' brought to the author (BK). This originated from a medical student's anatomical skeleton and was made from plaster coated with a plastic polymer. Visually it was indistinguishable from a real bone, but the abnormal lightness indicated the true nature.

Are the bones of human origin?

The recognition of species is important, but deciding on a human origin is usually easy, unless marked fragmentation

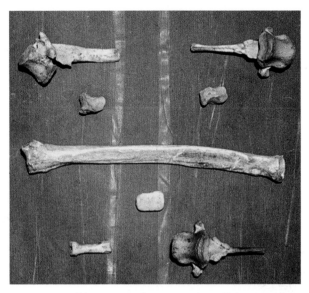

FIGURE 3.4 *All bones are not human – and not all 'bones' are bones. The smaller bones are animal, but the central 'radius' is from an ersatz student skeleton, made from plastic material, but thought by the police to be evidence of a criminal death.*

has occurred. Many animal bones are found by the general public and police who are not qualified to decide whether they are human. Extensive rebuilding programmes and the renovation and demolition of old sites reveal many caches of bones, but in the authors' experience the majority are of animal origin, often originating from butchers' debris.

First, the size is assessed and many small, slender bones excluded on obvious grounds. Even a turkey thigh cannot be mistaken for a metatarsal, nor a beef rib for human. The gross anatomy is then studied, and even if the pathologist makes no pretensions to being a comparative anatomist, the majority of intact animal bones can be recognized from their lack of correspondence to any human bone. Difficulties arise with smaller bones from some animals, especially the hands and feet, where digits, metatarsals and metacarpals require careful study to distinguish them from the human. Several errors have been made in respect of bear paws, which closely resemble the human hand.

When bones are incomplete or fragmentary, the problems escalate rapidly. If the ends of longer bones are present, then their non-human shape may be more readily determined, but cylindrical segments of the central shaft have little in the way of distinguishing features, apart from size. Burnt bone fragments offer similar problems, added to which is the possibility of heat distortion and shrinkage.

The advice of an anatomist is needed in such cases, preferably one with forensic experience and enthusiasm for the project. Unfortunately, every anatomist is not necessarily an osteologist and it may be more effective for the bone to be examined by a pathologist who has both enthusiasm and the relevant reference books.

Histological examination may offer a species differentiation – or at least to exclude a human origin. The Haversian architecture is different in many animals, but the few specialist papers on this subject must be consulted for details.

Where the animal species is relevant to the enquiry, then a veterinary or comparative anatomist must be consulted. If the bones are too fragmentary to provide any anatomical data, then serological investigations must be attempted. These depend on species-specific proteins being extracted from the bone into solution where they can be tested against specific antisera prepared by immunizing animals (usually rabbits) against a range of animal proteins, usually derived from blood. Thus the test is essentially seeking plasma constituents within the bone, the recognition being carried out by techniques such as electrophoresis or gel diffusion. DNA can now identify human tissue, if not the alternative species.

The drawback of such serological tests is that they cannot be applied to bones that no longer have extractable proteins, and these include burnt or cremated bone and bone that has been dead for some years. The length of time for which identifiable protein persists is variable, but a negative result is usually to be expected after 10 years following death, though DNA techniques may be more sensitive.

THE DETERMINATION OF SEX

The accuracy of determination of the sex of skeletal remains varies with the age of the subject, the degree of fragmentation of the bones and biological variability (Table 3.1).

Particularly when studying the skull and pelvis, a subjective impression by the experienced observer defies complete analysis, yet objective measurement may be no more accurate: in other words, the processes comprise morphological traits versus morphometry. The determination of sex is statistically the most important criterion, as it immediately excludes approximately half the population whereas age, stature and race each provide points within a wide range of variables. Obvious sex differences do not become apparent until after puberty,

usually in the 15–18-year period, though specialized measurements on the pelvis can indicate the sex even in fetal material. Sex and age are linked, especially where body size and weight are concerned. Similarly, race confuses sexing, for example, the size of the supraorbital ridges in a normal negroid female may exceed those in the average Caucasian male.

The accuracy of sexing is hard to estimate, as various loading factors exist. Krogman comments that he scored 100 per cent accuracy using the whole skeleton, 95 per cent on pelvis, 92 per cent on skull, 98 per cent on pelvis plus skull, 80 per cent on long bones and 98 per cent on long bones plus pelvis. He admitted, however, that, as most anatomy department material has a sex ratio of about 15:1 in favour of men, marked bias could be introduced by assigning all doubtful bones to the male category.

Stewart records that, for the whole skeleton, one can expect a 90–95 per cent success rate and for the skull alone only 80 per cent, but, if the mandible is also present, this rises to 90 per cent (Hrdlicka 1939). In general, adult female skeletal measurements are about 94 per cent that of the male of the same race, but different measurements may vary from 91 to 98 per cent.

The skull

The following features develop after puberty and are modified by senility, so are applicable only between about the 20th and the 55th year. Age as well as race has a profound effect.

- **General appearance.** The female skull is rounder and smoother than the rugged male.
- **Size.** Male skulls are larger, with an endocranial volume some 200 ml greater.
- **Muscle ridges** are more marked in male skulls, especially in occipital areas where larger muscles are

TABLE 3.1 *Pfitner's table of bodily dimensions in the female compared with the male (per cent of male dimensions). The common generalization that the female is 94 per cent of the male size varies in different areas of the body*

Stature	93.5	Arm length	91.5
Head breadth	98.0	Sitting height	94.5
Face breadth	94.0	Head circumference	96.0
Face height	90.0	Head height	96.0
Head length	95.5	Leg length	93.0

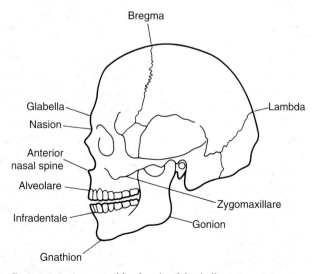

FIGURE 3.5 *Anatomical landmarks of the skull.*

attached to the nuchal crests and in temporal areas for larger masseter and temporalis muscles.

- **Supraorbital ridges** are more marked in male skulls and may be absent in female. The glabella (central forehead eminence above the nose) is small or absent in the female, and prominent in the male, though this is a poor discriminant.
- **Mastoid process.** This is larger in male skulls (see Hoshi).
- **Frontal and parietal eminences.** These are more prominent in female skulls, which resemble the shape in an infant more than in a male.
- **Palate.** This is larger and of a more regular U-shape in men. The smaller female palate tends to be parabolic.
- **Orbits** are set lower on the face in the male skull, with more square and less sharp edges (especially upper edge) than the female.

- **Nasal aperture.** This is higher and narrower in the male skull and has sharper edges. The nasal bones are larger and project further forward to meet at a more acute angle than in the female.
- **Forehead.** This is high and steep in the female skull, with a more rounded infantile contour than the male.
- **Teeth** are smaller in the female skull, molars usually having four cusps. The male often has a five-cusp lower first molar.
- **Zygomatic process.** The posterior ridge projects back beyond external auditory meatus in the male skull. The zygomatic arches bow outward more than the female, where they remain more medial.
- **Mandible.** This is large in the male skull, with a squarer symphysis region. Female jaws are more rounded and

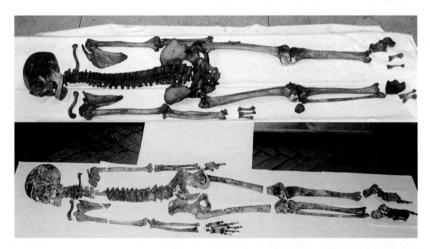

FIGURE 3.6 *Two recovered and reassembled skeletons. After cleaning, the bones should be laid out in correct anatomical position, to gain an approximate direct measure of the stature, allowing as well as possible for lost soft tissue. The upper skeleton, obviously male, shows the frequent loss of small hand and foot bones, but no injuries. The lower remains, from a hidden 40-year-old homicide, reveal that the body was sawn into six sections, there being cuts above the knees and through spine, scapula and humeri.*

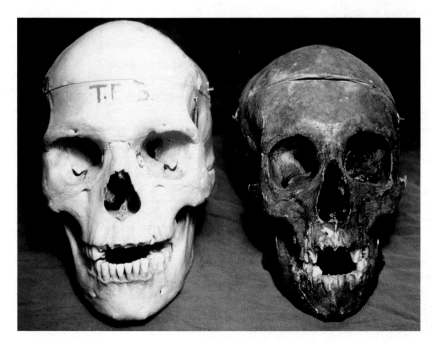

FIGURE 3.7 *Frontal view of male and female skull. The male (left) is larger, more massive and has heavier eyebrow ridges. The chin is squarer and the mandible heavier, The female has relatively larger height orbits, a smoother cranium, and fuller frontal and parietal eminences.*

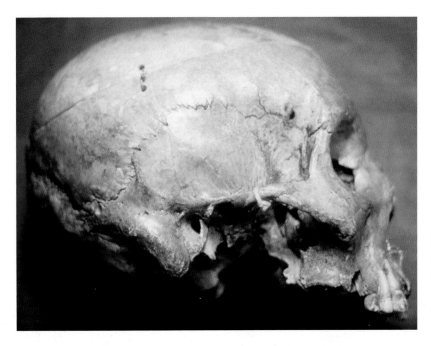

FIGURE 3.8 *A typical male skull, with a sloping forehead and prominent occipital ridges for large muscle attachment. Probably the best male feature is the large mastoid process; also, the zygomatic process extends well behind the auditory meatus.*

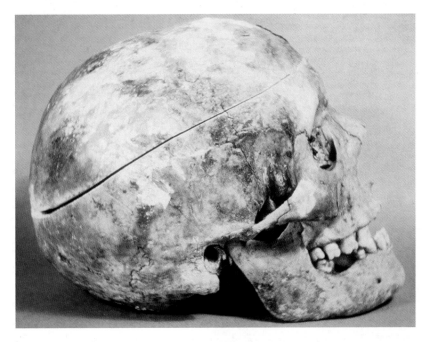

FIGURE 3.9 *A typical female skull, from a murder victim hidden for 40 years in a cave. The cranium is high, round and smooth with insignificant ridges for muscle attachment. The mastoid is tiny, one of the best discriminants. The post-zygomatic ridge does not continue behind the auditory meatus and there are no supraorbital ridges. The chin is round and smooth.*

project less at the anterior point. The vertical height at the symphysis is proportionately greater in the male. The angle formed by the body and the ramus is more upright in the male, being less than 125°. The condyles are larger in the male skull, as is the broader ascending ramus, and there is a more prominent coronoid process.

These sex variations represent the 'typical' White and, to a great extent, Asian skull. There is considerable overlap, especially in subjects from the Indian subcontinent, where osteological sex differences are much less marked. The criteria set out above exclude prepubertal and senile persons, and are less valid for those outside the 20–55 age group. For methods of sexing by discriminant function analysis, the work of Giles and Elliot (1963) should be consulted. In recent years craniometry has been applied to sexing the skull and multiple accurate measurements between discrete anatomical points have been used to produce discriminant function analysis. The papers of numerous authors must be consulted for details of this sophisticated and difficult technique that is accurate in 83–88 per cent of cases. The frequency of correct sexing is no greater than more subjective methods, but commands a greater degree of confidence level in respect to its accuracy.

Sex characteristics in the pelvis

The post-pubertal female pelvis is wider and shallower than the rather upright male girdle to allow for the passage of the fetus during childbirth. Though as always there is an overlap of the appearance and measurements in the least characteristic individuals, the usual variations are sufficient to allow sexing of the adult pelvis to be made with about a 95 per cent confidence rate (see work by Genovés). In the pelvis, unlike the skull, there are differences, albeit subtle, in immature (even fetal) pelves that allow sexual differentiation. The following features provide the most useful criteria. One must not be used in isolation, however; as many as possible must be assessed together. Sex features are independent of each other and one may even contradict the other in the same pelvis. It is often a first subjective impression by an experienced eye that determines the answer, though where the sex differences are slight, careful measurements may be needed to resolve the problem.

As in the skull, the male pelvis is more rugged because of the attachment of stronger muscles. It stands higher and more erect than the smoother, flatter, female pelvic girdle. The subpubic angle, measured at the medial intersection of two lines drawn along the best approximation of the lower border of both inferior pubic rami, approaches 90° in the female pelvis, but usually about 70° in the male.

This is often a subjective measurement, however and depends in turn upon the shape of the pubic bone itself. When the line of the inferior ramus is projected medially and intersected with a horizontal line laid across the upper border of the superior ramus, the reverse size of angle is seen, the male being wider than the female.

The body of the pubic bone, the block lateral to the symphysis, tends to be triangular in shape in the male, whilst the female pubis is more rectangular (Phenice 1969; Iscan and Derrick 1984). Certain sexual variations in the pubis have been used by Phenice. In the female these are:

- a bony ridge ('ventral arc') running down the ventral surface from the pubic crest
- a concavity of the lower margin of the inferior pubic ramus immediately lateral to the lower border of the symphysis

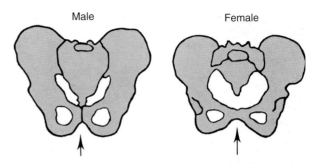

Male   Female

FIGURE 3.10 *Sex differences in the human pelvis. The most noticeable features are the narrower suprapubic angle and the higher iliac blades in the male pelvis.*

- a ridge of elevated bone on the medial aspect of the ischiopubic ramus, immediately lateral to the symphysis; in the male this area is broad and flat.

The 'ischiopubic index' devised by Washburn may be helpful, in which the pubic length (×100) is divided by the ischial length. The measurements must be carefully made, the pubic length being from the plane of the symphysis to the reference point in the acetabulum and the ischial length being from the same point to the most distal edge of the ischium. The reference point is the site of fusion of the three elements of the immature innominate bone, usually marked by a notch in the articular surface of the acetabulum (Schultz 1937). If the ischiopubic index (in White races) is less than 90, the pelvis is male; if over 95, it is female. The acetabulum is larger in the male, being an average of 52 mm in diameter, compared with 46 mm in the female. The male joint cup also faces more laterally than that of the female, which tends to look more forward. Naturally, acetabular size is related to that of the femoral head, which will be considered later. The greater sciatic notch is an important criterion, being deep and narrow in the male, wide and open in the female. The angle formed by the margins approaches closer to a right angle in the woman than it does in the man. Harrison (1968) and Hrdlicka (1939) both felt that the greater sciatic notch was one of the best discriminants for sex, the latter claiming a 75 per cent success rate using this criterion alone.

The obturator foramen is somewhat ovoid in the male, but triangular in the female. The pre-auricular sulcus, which marks the attachment of the anterior sacroiliac ligament, lies just lateral to the sacroiliac joint and is usually well marked in women but often absent in males. The pelvic inlet, looked at from above, is more circular in the female, the male being heart-shaped as a result of the protrusion of the sacrum into the posterior brim (Greulich and Thomas 1938). A number of other pelvic 'indices' have been devised by various authors (see, for example, the work of Turner, Greulich and Thomas, Caldwell and Molloy, Straus, and Derry).

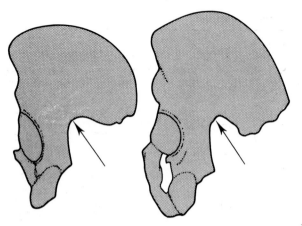

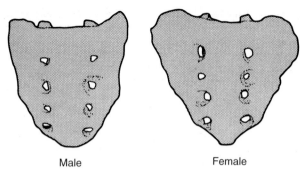

Male — Female

FIGURE 3.12 *The variation in shape of the male and female sacrum. The female is broader and more triangular.*

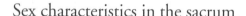

FIGURE 3.11 *The greater sciatic notch is narrower in the male innominate bone.*

Sex characteristics in the sacrum

The sacrum is functionally part of the pelvis and shares in its sex variations. The female sacrum is wide and has a shallow curve, again related to the larger pelvic canal for child-birth. It is shorter in the female and the curve is limited almost entirely to that distal part below the centre of the third sacral vertebra. The male sacrum may have more than five segments, which is rare in the female. The curve in the male is continuous down the whole bone and there may even be a slight forward projection of the coccyx. Fawcett (1938) compared the transverse diameter of the first sacral vertebra (CW) with that of the base of the sacrum (BW). The formula CW × 100/BW averaged 45 in the male and 40 in the female. Kimura (1982) has developed a 'base wing index', where the relative widths of the wing and base provide discriminant function coefficients for sex determination.

Sexing from the long bones

The femur is the most useful, its length and massiveness themselves being significant. There is, as usual, consider-able overlap of all long-bone sex characteristics, but Brash's series showed that the maximum (oblique) length in the male femur was around 459 mm, while that of the female was only 426 mm. Other figures from Pearson and Bell (1917) suggested mean values of 447 mm for men and 409 mm for women. Using the trochanteric oblique length, they suggested a range of 390–405 mm for women and 430–450 mm for men, though there was the usual overlap in the middle. Race and nutrition (which is related to the era and the place in which the samples were obtained) must be allowed for in such measurements.

TABLE 3.2 *Dwight's table for sexing from humeral and femoral head diameters (in mm)*

	Vertical humeral	Transverse humeral	Vertical femoral
Female	42.67	36.98	43.84
Male	48.76	44.66	49.68
Difference	6.09	5.68	5.84

TABLE 3.3 *Pearson and Bell's table for the 'mathematical sexing of the femur'. The area of uncertainty extends in increasing degrees of confidence outwards from the central column to the more definite limits on each side. Measurements are given in millimetres*

	Male	Male or female	Female
Vertical diameter of head	>45.5	43.5–41.5	<41.5
Popliteal length	>145	114–132	<106
Bicondylar width	>78	74–76	<72
Oblique trochanteric length	>450	405–430	<390

The size of the femoral heads is claimed to be a better dis-criminant of sex, the vertical diameter being said by Pearson and Bell to be greater than 45 mm in the male and less than 41 mm in the female, though again there is an overlap in the distribution curves around the 43 mm size (Table 3.2). Maltby (1917), however, measured 43–56 mm in the male and 37–46 mm in the female. Femoral head size is part of Pearson's 'mathematical sexing of the femur', which incor-porates several measurements (Table 3.3). Dwight (1904) studied the size of both femoral and humeral heads, claim-ing that they were more useful than bone length. Once again, discriminant function sexing has been carried out, using a number of measurements. Details should be sought in the work of Black and of Iscan and Miller-Shaivitz.

Another sex trait in the femur is the angle that the shaft makes with the vertical. Because the pelvis is relatively wider in the female, the shafts have to slope more to con-verge at knee level, so that the condyles at the lower end of

TABLE 3.4 *Long-bone lengths (mm) in White men and women of different stature*

Men							Women						
Humerus	Radius	Ulna	Stature	Femur	Tibia	Fibula	Humerus	Radius	Ulna	Stature	Femur	Tibia	Fibula
295	213	227	1530	392	319	318	263	193	203	1400	363	284	283
298	216	231	1552	398	324	323	266	195	206	1420	368	289	288
302	219	235	1571	404	330	328	270	197	209	1440	373	294	293
306	222	239	1590	410	335	333	273	199	212	1455	378	299	298
309	225	243	1605	416	340	338	276	201	215	1470	383	304	303
313	229	246	1625	422	346	344	279	203	217	1488	388	309	307
316	232	249	1634	428	351	349	282	205	219	1497	393	314	311
320	236	253	1644	434	357	353	285	207	222	1513	398	319	316
324	239	257	1654	440	362	358	289	209	225	1528	403	324	320
328	243	260	1666	446	368	363	292	211	228	1543	408	329	325
332	246	263	1677	453	373	368	297	214	231	1556	415	334	330
336	249	266	1686	460	378	373	302	218	235	1568	422	340	336
340	252	270	1697	467	383	378	307	222	239	1582	429	346	341
344	255	273	1716	475	389	383	313	226	243	1595	436	352	346
348	258	276	1730	482	394	388	318	230	247	1612	443	358	351
352	261	280	1755	490	400	393	324	234	251	1630	450	364	356
356	264	283	1767	497	405	398	329	238	254	1650	457	370	361
360	267	287	1785	504	410	403	334	242	258	1670	464	376	366
364	270	290	1812	512	415	408	339	246	261	1692	471	382	371
368	273	293	1830	519	420	413	344	250	264	1715	478	388	376

Modified by Krogman and Iscan (1986) from Hrdlicka (1939).

the femur sit horizontally on the tibial plateau. Thus when a female femur is seated on its condyles on a flat surface, the angle the shaft makes with that surface is of the order of 76°, while a male bone is more upright, the angle being around 80°. The angle of the neck on the shaft of the femur (the 'collodiaphyseal angle') was studied by Godycki (1957), the results suggesting that a bone with an angle of less than 40° had an 85 per cent chance of being male, while if the angle exceeded 50°, there was a 75 per cent chance of it being from a female (Table 3.4).

Most workers have worked with dry bone specimens; when methods using fresh bone are used, allowance must be made for articular cartilage where relevant. For example, the vertical diameter of a femoral head is 3 mm less in the dried specimen.

Sex determination from other bones

The sternum may be helpful in that the length of the manubrium in the female may equal or exceed half the length of the body, while the manubrium of the male is less than half the body length (Table 3.5). This was claimed in the nineteenth century by Hyrtl, but was denied by Krogman and by Dwight. The latter claimed that the ratio of manubrium: body was 52:100 in women and 49:100 in men, a poor discrimination. However, the method has been rehabilitated by Iordanidis (1961), who alleged a success rate of 80 per cent using the sternum alone. Stewart

TABLE 3.5 *Sex determination from the sternum. Mean (range) lengths of manubrium and sternal body (mm)*

	Male	Female
Manubrial length	51.7 (41–73)	48.4 (39–61)
Body length	95.4 (74–122)	78.6 (59–95)
Combined length	147 (131–180)	127 (107–140)

Taken from Jit *et al.* (1980) North Indian population.

and McCormick (1983) used a radiographic technique and claimed total accuracy in stating that a sternal length of less than 121 mm must be female and over 173 mm must be male.

The scapula has been studied extensively, but mostly in relation to age. There are relatively poor sex variations in the vertical diameter of the glenoid cavity: the threshold, according to Dwight, is 36 mm, those smaller being female. Iordanidis made an extensive study of scapular measurements and concluded that scapular height was the best discriminant, the male usually being greater than 157 mm, the female less than 144 mm.

The humerus, radius and ulna yield little helpful sexing evidence, apart from overall size. The presence of a perforated olecranon fossa at the lower end of the humerus occurs more often in females and more commonly on the left side, there being a 3.7:1 ratio compared with males. Godycki studied this and other characteristics of the arm bones as sex determinants, but their value is poor.

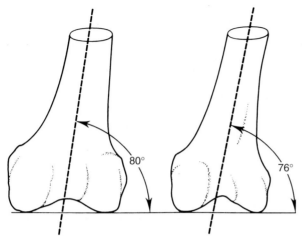

FIGURE 3.13 *Determination of sex of femur by angulation of the shaft. The condyles are set on a flat surface and the angle of the shaft measured. Because of the greater tilt caused by the relatively wider pelvis, the female angle is usually less than 80°.*

There are many reports on sexing from limb and girdle bones and the best approach seems to be a multiple assessment using the data for discriminant function analysis.

Evidence of pregnancy from the skeleton

More accurately, parturition causes some changes in the pelvis as a result of the local trauma of childbirth, which is reinforced by multiple pregnancies. These include 'pubic scars' from the tearing of tendon insertions and periosteum around the pubic bone. The dorsal pubic surface and the pre-auricular sulcus are best indicators, but most authorities agree that it is not possible to determine the number of births from osteological appearances. The papers of Angel and of Ullrich are most useful in this respect.

ESTIMATION OF STATURE FROM SKELETAL REMAINS

When a full skeleton is available, then obviously direct measurement of the correctly assembled bones will give the original height within a few centimetres. Allowance has to be made during assembly, however, for the loss of cartilage in joint spaces and especially for missing intervertebral discs. The accuracy achieved with direct measurement is not great, in that even with an intact body there can be a lengthening of up to 2.5 cm compared with the live height. The skeleton needs scalp and heel soft tissue thickness added – and with the obvious uncertainty about the cumulative allowances for disc thickness and joint cartilage, it is

unrealistic to expect accuracy of less than about 4–8 cm compared with the living height.

When incomplete skeletal material is available, calculations have to be made on the basis of one or more bones. Where possible, all available bones should be used and a consensus of results assessed, though the accuracy derived from different bones varies and the result from – say, a femur – is more reliable than that from an ulna. The descending order of usefulness is: femur, tibia, humerus, radius.

Many formulae have been constructed for the determination of stature from the length of long bones. The following cautions must be appreciated before they are used:

- The tables were constructed from differing ethnic groups and at different times, so that racial and nutritional factors introduce significant variations. The table most appropriate to the bones under investigation should be used, though by definition the exact provenance of these bones may be unknown, even including their ethnic origins.
- There is a marked sex difference in stature estimation and ageing of the person also reduces stature relative to long bone length. Trotter and Gleser (1958) found in 855 bodies that there was a 1.2 cm loss of height for each two decades of age over the age of 30, a loss of height equivalent to about 0.6 mm a year after the fourth decade. The same investigation showed that the length of the cadaver was about 2.5 cm longer than the known height during life. The maximum stature (at least in American men) was found in 1951 to be reached at the age of 23 years, a change from earlier estimates in which the peak was found to occur between 18–21 years of age.
- The bone lengths must be measured in exactly the same way as that used by the author of the tables.
- Old dry bones are slightly shorter than recent material, even when one excludes the loss of articular cartilage. Telkkä (1950) stated that 2 mm must be deducted from the length of fresh bone before the calculation is made, as most tables are based on dried skeletons. These differences, however, are slight compared with the greater errors likely if incorrect measuring methods are employed.
- There are inbuilt errors, which are expressed in the formulae. These standard errors are given as 'plus or minus' a certain figure, which applies only when the length of the bone is near the mean of the usual range of length for that particular bone. When the bone is near the extremes of the range (that is from a very tall or very short person), then the standard deviation must be doubled in order to stay within the same range of confidence of accuracy. The same holds good if the tables used are not from the same ethnic group as those

TABLE 3.6 *The stature tables of Trotter and Gleser. The upper table represents their original 1952 figures, the lower their modification of 1977, as quoted by Krogman and Iscan (1986)*

Male Whites	Male Negroes
Stature = 63.05 + 1.31 (femur + fibula) ± 3.63 cm	Stature = 67.77 + 1.20 (femur + fibula) ± 3.63 cm
Stature = 67.09 + 1.26 (femur + tibia) ± 3.74 cm	Stature = 71.75 + 1.15 (femur + tibia) ± 3.68 cm
Stature = 75.50 + 2.60 fibula ± 3.86 cm	Stature = 72.22 + 2.10 femur ± 3.91 cm
Stature = 65.53 + 2.32 femur ± 3.94 cm	Stature = 85.36 + 2.19 tibia ± 3.96 cm
Stature = 81.93 + 2.42 tibia ± 4.00 cm	Stature = 80.07 + 2.34 fibula ± 4.02 cm
Stature = 67.97 + 1.82 (humerus + radius) ± 4.31 cm	Stature = 73.08 + 1.66 (humerus + radius) ± 4.18 cm
Stature = 66.98 + (humerus + ulna) ± 4.37 cm	Stature = 70.67 + 1.65 (humerus + ulna) ± 4.23 cm
Stature = 78.10 + 2.89 humerus ± 4.57	Stature = 75.48 + 2.88 humerus ± 4.23 cm
Stature = 79.42 + 3.79 radius ± 4.66	Stature = 85.43 + 3.32 radius ± 4.57 cm
Stature = 75.55 + 3.76 ulna ± 4.72	Stature = 82.77 + 3.20 ulna ± 4.74 cm

Female Whites	Female Negroes
Stature = 50.12 + 0.68 humerus + 1.17 femur + 1.15 tibia ± 3.51 cm	Stature = 56.33 + 0.44 humerus − 0.20 radius + 1.46 femur + 0.86 tibia ± 3.22 cm
Stature = 53.20 + 1.39 (femur + tibia) ± 3.55 cm	Stature = 58.54 + 1.53 femur + 0.96 tibia ± 3.23 cm
Stature = 53.07 + 1.48 femur + 1.28 tibia ± 3.55 cm	Stature = 59.72 + 1.26 (femur + tibia) ± 3.28 cm
Stature = 59.61 + 2.93 fibula ± 3.57 cm	Stature = 59.76 + 2.28 femur ± 3.41 cm
Stature = 61.53 + 2.90 tibia ± 3.66 cm	Stature = 62.80 + 1.08 humerus + 1.79 tibia ± 3.58 cm
Stature = 52.77 + 1.35 humerus + 1.95 tibia ± 3.67 cm	Stature = 72.65 + 2.45 tibia ± 3.70 cm
Stature = 54.10 + 2.47 femur ± 3.72 cm	Stature = 70.90 + 2.49 fibula ± 3.80 cm
Stature = 54.93 + 4.74 radius ± 4.24 cm	Stature = 64.67 + 3.08 humerus ± 4.25 cm
Stature = 57.76 + 4.27 ulna ± 4.20 cm	Stature = 75.38 + 3.31 ulna ± 4.83 cm
Stature = 57.97 + 3.36 humerus ± 4.45 cm	Stature = 94.51 + 2.75 radius ± 5.05 cm

White males	SE	Black males	SE
3.08 Humerus + 70.45	4.05	3.26 Humerus + 62.10	4.43
3.78 Radius + 79.01	4.32	3.42 Radius + 81.56	4.30
3.70 Ulna + 74.05	4.32	3.26 Ulna + 79.29	4.42
2.38 Femur + 61.41	3.27	2.11 Femur + 70.35	3.94
2.52 Tibia + 78.62	3.37	2.19 Tibia + 86.02	3.78
2.68 Fibula + 71.78	3.29	2.19 Fibula + 85.65	4.08
1.30 (Femur + Tibia) + 63.29	2.99	1.15 (Femur + Tibia) + 71.04	3.53
1.42 Femur + 1.24 Tibia + 59.88	2.99	0.66 Femur + 1.62 Tibia + 76.13	3.49
0.93 Humerus + 1.94 Tibia + 69.30	3.26	0.90 Humerus + 1.78 Tibia + 71.29	3.49
0.27 Humerus + 1.32 Femur + 1.16 Tibia + 58.57	2.99	0.89 Humerus − 1.01 Radius + 0.38 Femur + 1.92 Tibia + 74.56	3.38

White females	SE	Black females	SE
3.36 Humerus + 57.97	4.45	3.08 Humerus + 64.67	4.25
4.74 Radius + 54.93	4.24	3.67 Radius + 71.79	4.59
4.27 Ulna + 57.76	4.30	3.31 Ulna + 75.38	4.83
2.47 Femur + 54.10	3.72	2.28 Femur + 59.76	3.41
2.90 Tibia + 61.53	3.66	2.45 Tibia + 72.65	3.70
2.93 Fibula + 59.61	3.57	2.49 Fibula + 70.90	3.80
1.39 (Femur + Tibia) + 53.20	3.55	1.26 (Femur + Tib) + 59.72	3.28
1.48 Femur + 1.28 Tibia + 53.07	3.55	1.53 Femur + 0.96 Tibia + 58.54	3.23
1.35 Humerus + 1.95 Tibia + 52.77	3.67	1.08 Humerus + 1.79 Tib	3.58
0.68 Humerus + 1.17 Femur + 1.15 Tibia + 50.122	3.51	0.44 Humerus − 0.20 Radius + 1.46 Femur + 0.86 Tibia + 56.33	3.22

All lengths are in centimetres, valid only for Americans between 18 and 30 years of age. Femur and tibia are maximum lengths. SE, standard error.

being estimated. Krogman indicated that a 95 per cent confidence rate applies only if twice the standard error is accepted each side of the favoured height – in an average man, this means a latitude of over 12 cm, which is too great to be of much use in identification.

Of the many available systems of calculation, those of Trotter and Gleser are most widely used, being based on Caucasian and Negroid Americans from the 1950s (Table 3.6). Older tables include those of Rollet whose measurements of French people were later reworked by Manouvrier and

TABLE 3.7 *Pearson's (1899) regression tables for calculating stature from dried long bones*

S = 81.306 + 1.880 Femur	S = 72.844 + 1.945 Femur
S = 70.651 + 2.894 Humerus	S = 71.475 + 2.754 Humerus
S = 78.664 + 3.378 Tibia	S = 74.774 + 2.352 Tibia
S = 85.925 + 3.271 Radius	S = 81.224 + 3.343 Radius
S = 71.272 + 1.159 (F + T)	S = 69.154 + 1.126 (F + T)
S = 71.441 + 1.220 F + 1.080 T	S = 69.561 + 1.117 F + 1.125 T
S = 66.855 + 1.730 (H + R)	S = 69.911 + 1.628 (H + R)
S = 69.788 + 2.769 H + 0.1958	S = 70.542 + 2.582 H + 0.2818
S = 68.397 + 1.030 F + 1.557 H	S = 67.435 + 1.339 F + 1.027 H
S = 67.049 + 0.913 F + 0.600 T	S = 67.467 + 0.782 F + 1.120 T

TABLE 3.9 *Telkkä's table for calculating stature of Finnish men and women*

Men	SE	Women	SE
169.4 + 2.8 (Humerus − 32.9)	5.0	156.8 + 2.7 (Humerus − 30.7)	3.9
169.4 + 3.4 (Radius − 22.7)	5.0	156.8 + 3.1 (Radius − 20.8)	4.5
169.4 + 3.2 (Ulna − 23.1)	5.2	156.8 + 3.3 (Ulna − 21.3)	4.4
169.4 + 2.1 (Femur − 45.5)	4.9	156.8 + 1.8 (Femur − 41.8)	4.0
169.4 + 2.1 (Tibia − 36.6)	4.6	156.8 + 1.9 (Tibia − 33.1)	4.6
169.4 + 2.5 (Fibula − 36.1)	4.4	156.8 + 2.3 (Fibula − 32.7)	4.5

by Pearson and quoted in a review by Hrdlicka (1939). Pearson allowed a standard addition of 2.5 cm to compensate for the difference between dead and living height (Table 3.7). More modern tables include those of Dupertuis and Hadden (1951) and Trotter and Gleser (1958), from American subjects. The latter used casualties from World War II and later from the Korean War to construct their tables (Table 3.8). Other calculation systems include Breitinger (1937; Germans), Telkkä (Finns) (Table 3.9), Allbrook (1961; African Negroids and English), Shiati (1983; Chinese), Mendes-Correa (1932; Portuguese) and Stevenson (1929; Chinese). Modern critics of the accuracy of the estimation of stature from long bones include Wells (1959), who suggested that even the preferred method of Trotter and Gleser has less accuracy than is generally acknowledged.

Estimation of stature from bones other than the major limb bones is far more inaccurate. Measuring the spinal column (from the tip of the odontoid to the bottom of the fifth lumbar vertebra) has been used by Krogman and by Dwight; Fully and Pineau (1960) used the spine plus a long bone. Tibbetts (1981), in his more modern study on the

spine, measured 23 individual vertebrae and produced a regression formula for both men and women. However, the results were far superior when long bones were used. Others have employed the clavicle (Jit and Singh 1956) and the scapula (Olivier 1969).

The use of fragmentary bones and those immature bones from which the epiphyses have been lost have been studied, the survey by Krogman and Iscan being the best account of the techniques employed by researchers such as Steele and McKern (1969) and Muller (1935). The estimation of the heights of infants and fetuses is even more difficult when working with skeletal material, as substantial parts of these bones may be detached and missing because of non-fusion of epiphyses and non-appearance of ossification centres. Mehta and Singh (1972) have specifically addressed this problem, as well as others summarized by Krogman and Iscan (1986).

ESTIMATING THE SUBJECT'S AGE FROM SKELETAL STRUCTURES

The age of the subject at death is usually more important than the stature and rivals the sex as the most vital indication

TABLE 3.8 *Dupertuis and Hadden's (1951) tables for estimating stature from bones. The length of the bones (measured in centimetres according to the authors' criteria) is multiplied by the factor in the table and added to the constant in the right hand column to give the body length (cm)*

Men	cm	Women	cm
2.238 (Femur)	+ 69.089	2.317 (Femur)	+ 61.412
2.392 (Tibia)	+ 81.688	2.533 (Tibia)	+ 72.572
2.970 (Humerus)	+ 73.570	3.144 (Humerus)	+ 64.977
3.650 (Radius)	+ 80.405	3.876 (Radius)	+ 73.502
1.225 (Femur + Tibia)	+ 69.294	1.233 (Femur + Tibia)	+ 65.213
1.728 (Humerus + Radius)	+ 71.429	1.984 (Humerus + Radius)	+ 55.729
1.422 (Femur) + 1.062 (Tibia)	+ 66.544	1.657 (Femur) + 0.879 (Tibia)	+ 59.259
1.789 (Humerus) + 1.841 (Radius)	+ 66.400	2.164 (Humerus) + 1.525 (Radius)	+ 60.344
1.928 (Femur) 0.568 (Humerus)	+ 64.505	2.009 (Femur) + 0.566 (Humerus)	+ 57.600
1.442 (Femur) + 0.931 (Tibia) + 0.083 (Humerus) + 0.480 (Radius)	+ 56.006	1.544 (Femur) + 0.764 (Tibia) + 0.126 (Humerus) + 0.295 (Radius)	+ 57.495

of identity. The estimation of skeletal age falls into various groups, which have marked differences in both method and accuracy. In general, the greater the personal age the less the confidence quotient. There are many publications on the subject, many of them arising from archaeological rather than forensic interest, as the age structure of a skeletal population is of great interest to social anthropologists and historians.

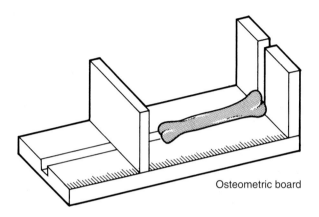

FIGURE 3.14 *Osteometric board for accurate measurement of bone length. There is a central slot in the headboard to accommodate the tibial head spines.*

The fetus and young infant

It is more usual to have to estimate fetal and neonatal age on the intact dead body, rather than the skeleton, as the immature bones are so easily dispersed, lost and destroyed compared to the more robust bones of older subjects. Both in archaeology and forensic pathology, however, such fetal and immature remains are sometimes present.

The major dating indices are the appearance of ossification centres in growing cartilage but, as stated above, these are rarely available in dried bones as the cartilage disintegrates within weeks or months and small ossification centres – both in diaphyses and epiphyses – rarely survive. The bones have to be examined with the cartilage still attached to offer much hope of ageing the remains. Radiology may provide more information than visual inspection.

Specialized books such as the classics by Fazekas and Kosa, Krogman and Iscan, and by Stewart and the numerous papers and monographs on the subject (a selection of which are listed at the end of this chapter) must be consulted where fetal issues are complex and important. Once again the help of interested anatomists and radiologists can be invaluable, especially as biological variation poses a constant trap for the inexperienced who slavishly follow printed tables without the knowledge to appreciate their limitations. Stewart has

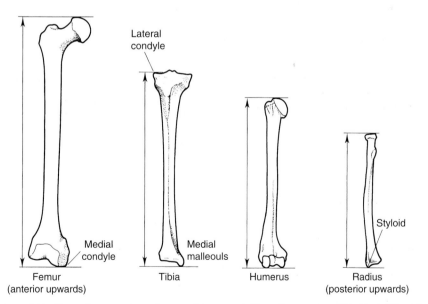

FIGURE 3.15 *Dimensions of dried bones for estimations of stature (Trotter and Gleser, Dupertuis and Hadden). The right side bone is used for preference. **Femur:** With the bone lying anterior surface upwards, the maximum length is measured from the medial condyle to the most proximal part of the head. **Tibia:** Maximum length between tip of medial malleolus and face of lateral condyle. The intercondylar eminence is not included. **Humerus:** Maximum overall length from the posterior margin of the trochlea to the upper edge of the head. **Radius:** From the tip of the styloid process to the head, lying with the posterior surface upwards. All bones should be measured either with an osteometric board or, if one is not available, on a flat bench with the maximum lengths taken between two vertical, parallel boards placed in contact with the bone ends. If the bones are not dry, but have articular cartilage in place, the following should be subtracted from the measured length before applying the formulae (Boyd and Trevor): radius and humerus 3 mm each, tibia 5 mm and femur 7 mm.*

produced a useful nomogram that relates fetal femoral length to crown–rump length and hence to approximate gestational age. Teeth are discussed in Chapter 26. Fazeka and Kosa's book is particularly useful to the pathologist (as bone lengths, etc. are directly related to fetal and infant age), as are the profuse illustrations.

Skeletal age in the child and young adult

There is no break in the methods used for the fetus and small infant and the older child and young adult. The appearance of ossification centres is complete by around 5 years and after this stage the fusion of epiphyses acts as a calendar up to the age of about 25, when the medial clavicular epiphysis is usually the last evidence of such fusion.

Lists and diagrams such as those shown here are the usual method of tracing the maturity of the skeleton. Several cautionary points must be appreciated and where possible the advice of a radiologist be obtained if there are important issues at stake. The paper by McKern and Stewart gives a valuable commentary on personal variation in skeletal age determination (Table 3.10).

- Maturity is not synonymous with calendar age. There are both sexual, racial, nutritional and other biological variations.
- Females are almost always in advance of males, and maturity tends to be accelerated in hotter climates, though the latter may be tempered by nutritional disadvantages.
- There is a marked range of closure dates in epiphyseal union, and the year suggested in some charts is merely the midpoint of that range.
- Union is a process, not an event. It may be different radiologically from gross inspection; it may also be slow in completion, so that it may be difficult to pinpoint a date that is needed to refer to published data. An example is the one that is usually the last to fuse, the medial end of the clavicle, which may slowly close during any period from about 18 to 31 years. Finally, as emphasized by Krogman and Iscan, multiple criteria of skeletal age should be used, dependence not being placed upon any single measurement.

Skeletal ageing in later years

The eruption of the third molar teeth and the fusion of the last epiphysis occurs approximately in the middle of the third decade. This is a watershed in skeletal dating, as the more objective markers of age are almost all on the younger side of this time. From around 25 years until old age, there are no dramatic events such as tooth eruption or the appearance of ossification centres. There are more subtle changes available for specialized interpretation, but the general decline through middle age to senility prevents assessment of age to within the nearest half-decade.

The major advances in this difficult period have been the use of the pubic symphysis and sternal ribs and the radiology of cancellous bone. However, dental technology may further refine the assessment of age.

Pubic symphysis and age

The opposing faces of the two pubic bones have been extensively studied by Todd (1920, 1921), by McKern and Stewart (1957) and by Gilbert and McKern (1973), who related the changing topography of the symphyseal faces to age. The technique is complex and requires bones that are free of cartilage, but not so eroded by drying and damage that the surface features are blurred.

ASSESSMENT OF AGE FROM THE MALE PUBIC SYMPHYSIS

As always, the details given in the original publications should be studied and practice gained by examining bones of known age. The method as originally devised by Todd has been radically modified by McKern and Stewart so that the technique is now the most useful in assessing the age of post-mature material. It must be noted that their method applies only to males and was not applied to female material until the work of Gilbert and McKern.

In summary, the face of the symphysis is analysed by reference to three 'components', each being scored on a scale of 6. In component I, the dorsal half of the face is assessed on a scale of 0–5; in component II, the ventral half is assessed; and in component III, the whole surface is considered in relation to different criteria to the preceding two stages.

Component I (the dorsal plateau) is scored as follows:

- 0: dorsal margin absent
- 1: slight margin formation appears in the middle third of the dorsal border
- 2: dorsal margin extends along whole dorsal border
- 3: grooves filled in with resorption of ridges to form an early plateau in the middle third of the dorsal demiface
- 4: te plateau, still with vestiges of billowing, extends over most of the dorsal demiface
- 5: billowing vanishes and the surface of the demiface becomes flat and slightly granular.

TABLE 3.10 *Time of appearance of major ossification centres*

(a) Healthy Caucasian boys

Birth
Calcaneus
Talus
Femur, distal
Tibia, proximal
Cuboid
Humerus, head

2 months
Capitate
Hamate
Lateral cuneiform

3 months
Femur, head
Capitulum
Tibia, distal

6 months
Fibula, distal

7 months
Humerus, greater tuberosity
Radius, distal

10 months
Triquetrum

11 months
Third finger–first phalanx
First toe–second phalanx

12 months
Second finger–first phalanx
Fourth finger–first phalanx
First finger–second phalanx

13 months
Third toe–first phalanx
Second metacarpal
Medial cuneiform

14 months
Fourth toe–first phalanx
Second toe–first phalanx
Fifth toe–second phalanx

15 months
Third metacarpal
Second toe–second phalanx
Fifth finger–first phalanx

16 months
Fourth toe second phalanx
Fourth metacarpal

18 months
Second finger–second phalanx
Third finger–second phalanx
Fourth finger–second phalanx
Fifth metacarpal

20 months
First toe–first phalanx
Middle cuneiform

21 months
Third finger–third phalanx
Fourth finger–third phalanx
Navicular of foot
Fifth toe–first phalanx

22 months
First metacarpal
First metatarsal

23 months
First finger–first phalanx

2 years
Fifth finger–second phalanx
Lunate

2 years, 2 months
Second metatarsal

2 years, 5 months
Second finger–third phalanx
Fifth finger–third phalanx

2 years, 11 months
Third metatarsal
Fibula, proximal

3 years, 1 month
Femur, great trochanter
Patella

3 years, 3 months
Fourth metatarsal

3 years, 4 months
Fifth toe–third phalanx

3 years, 7 months
Third toe–third phalanx
Fourth toe–third phalanx

3 years, 8 months
Fifth metatarsal
Second finger–third phalanx

3 years, 10 months
Radius, proximal

4 years, 2 months
Multangulate majus

4 years, 4 months
Navicular, hand

4 years, 8 months
Multangulate minus

5 years+
Humerus, medial epicond
Ulna, distal
Fifth toe–second phalanx

(b) Healthy Caucasian girls

Birth
Calcaneus
Talus
Femur, distal
Tibia, proximal
Cuboid
Humerus, head

2 months
Capitate
Hamate
Lateral cuneiform

3 months
Femur, head
Capitulum
Tibia, distal

4 months
Humerus, greater tuberosity

6 months
Fibula, distal
Radius, distal

7 months
First toe–second phalanx
Third finger–first phalanx
Fourth finger–first phalanx

8 months
Second finger–first phalanx
First finger–second phalanx
Third toe–first phalanx

9 months
Third toe–second phalanx
Fourth toe–first phalanx
Medial cuneiform

10 months
Second metacarpal
Second toe–second phalanx
Fourth toe–second phalanx
Third metacarpal
Second toe–first phalanx
Triquetrum

11 months
Fourth metacarpal
Fifth finger–first phalanx

12 months
Fourth finger–second phalanx
Third finger–second phalanx

13 months
Fifth metacarpal
Second finger–second phalanx

14 months
First metacarpal
First toe–first phalanx
Fifth finger–first phalanx
Third finger–third phalanx
Fourth finger–third phalanx
Navicular of foot
Middle cuneiform
First metatarsal

15 months
First finger–first phalanx
Fifth finger–second phalanx

17 months
Second finger–third phalanx
Fifth finger–third phalanx

19 months
Second metatarsal

21 months
Fifth toe–third phalanx

22 months
Third metatarsal

23 months
Patella

2 years
Lunate
Third toe–third phalanx
Fourth toe–third phalanx
Fibula, proximal
Femur, greater trochanter

2 years, 2 months
Second toe–third phalanx
Fourth metatarsal

2 years, 5 months
Fifth metatarsal

2 years, 8 months
Multangulate majus

2 years, 9 months
Humerus, medial epicon

3 years
Radius, proximal
Multangulate minus

3 years, 2 months
Navicular, hand

4 years, 6 months
Ulna, distal

5 years+
Fifth toe–second phalanx

After Francis and Werle (1939).

Component II (the ventral rampart) is scored as follows:

- 0: no ventral bevelling
- 1: ventral bevelling only at the superior end of the ventral border
- 2: bevelling extends along whole ventral border
- 3: ventral rampant starts as bony extensions from either or both extremities
- 4: extensive rampart, but still gaps, especially on the upper two thirds of the ventral border
- 5: complete ventral rampart.

Component III (symphyseal rim) is scored as follows:

- 0: no symphyseal rim
- 1: partial dorsal rim visible, usually at the upper end of the border; it is round, smooth and elevated above the surface
- 2: complete dorsal rim with beginnings of ventral rim, which starts at no particular site
- 3: complete circumferential symphyseal rim, enclosing a finely grained, slightly undulating surface
- 4: the rim begins to break down, no longer smooth but sharply defined. Some lipping on ventral edge
- 5: further breakdown of rim, especially along superior ventral edge. Rarefaction of symphyseal face. Disintegration and erratic ossification of ventral rim.

In practice, a three-figure score is made from evaluation of each component and added together. For example, component I = 3, component II = 4, component III = 1. Thus the score is 3 + 4 + 1 = 8 and by reference to the tables, the age suggested is between 24 and 28.

Since the work of Gilbert and McKern, a method has been offered to assess age in both males and females. Stewart has pointed out that, although Todd felt that the same criteria could be applied to females, there was risk of overestimation of age in women because pelvic trauma during parturition could deform the dorsal border of the symphysis in a manner likely to mimic age changes.

The other limitation of the method is that the upper limit is 50 years, so that a large segment of the range is not considered. Also the scoring is naturally subjective, depending on the experience and training of the observer. In spite of these drawbacks, the method remains the most useful ageing technique for post-mature males.

Gilbert and McKern established standards for females in 1973. The same three components are used, but the description of the symphyseal faces is different. Details must be sought in the original publications or in Krogman and Iscan's invaluable book. Gilbert concluded that, if the male criteria were used for females, the age assessment would be underestimated by about a decade, as the female pubis reaches full maturity about 10 years later than the male.

Several tests of the accuracy of this method have been made by Suchey (1979) and Meindl *et al.* (1985). There have been many reports on the subject, but it would seem that Todd's system remains the most accurate. Overall accuracy obtained by experienced observers lies in the range of 5–7 years around the true age.

The sternal rib methods

The costochondral junction has been studied by a number of physical anthropologists using different techniques. Michelson (1934) found that calcification in the first costal cartilage did not occur under 11 years and that after 16 years, males calcified much more quickly until 66, when the sexes again became uniform. Iscan and Loth (1986) made detailed studies of the shape of the rib end adjacent to the cartilage and constructed complex criteria for age-related changes. The original publications must be consulted for details as well as more recent developments such as those by Loth, Iscan and Sheuerman (1994).

Skull sutures and age

The use of skull suture fusion as an index of age has had a chequered history, beginning in the first century AD with a comment by Celsus. It is now generally discredited, except in the most broad terms.

It is common knowledge that most adults have at least part of their suture lines closed and that this tends to become more widespread as age increases. There are many exceptions and the rate of closure is not linear with time. This generality can be useful when skull fragments are found, as any visible fusion will at least indicate that the skull came from a mature individual, as it is unlikely below the age of 20 (Brothwell).

The claims of Dwight (1890), Parsons and Box (1905) and Todd and Lyon (1924, 1925) (who stated that sagittal fusion began at 22 and was complete by 35) for the use of fusion as an ageing tool, have been refuted by Singer (1953), Cobb (1952), McKern and Stewart (1957) and Genovés and Messmacher (1959). McKern and Stewart found that 25 per cent of 18-year-old males had begun closure of their sagittal sutures and that by 31–40 years, 90 per cent had some fusion. Yet many had no fusion at considerably older ages. Since these criticisms were made, much further work has been carried out, recorded by Krogman and Iscan's book in its 1986 edition. They concluded from the accumulated evidence of many publications that suture closure is not affected by sex, race or right/left differences. Only endocranial fusion must be studied, as that on the outer side is far more erratic. Even so, determination of age from suture closure is unsafe: they feel that in the 20–50 age range, it may be possible to

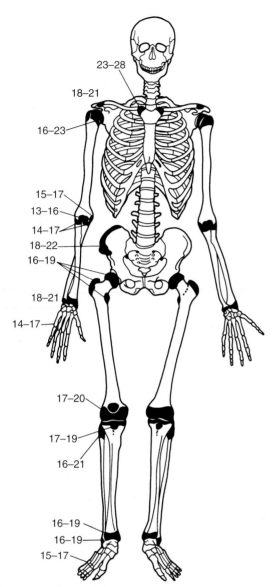

FIGURE 3.16 *A guide to the age of epiphyseal union in the major centres. The commencement and completion of union takes several years. The table is only a guide for male subjects (female slightly earlier) in non-tropical climates; the two dates are partial and complete union (years).*

Head of femur	16–19	Acromion	17–19
Greater trochanter	16–19	Distal femur	17–20
Lesser trochanter	16–19	Proximal tibia	17–19
Head of humerus	16–23	Proximal fibula	16–21
Distal humerus	13–16	Distal tibia	16–19
Medial epicondyle	16–17	Distal fibula	16–19
Proximal radius	14–17	Metatarsals	15–17
Proximal ulna	14–17	Iliac crest	18–22
Distal radius	18–21	Primary elements pelvis	14–16
Distal ulna	18–21	Sternal clavicle	23–28
Metacarpals	14–17	Acromial clavicle	18–21

place a skull within the correct decade only, older material being even more variable.

The basisphenoid synchondrosis cannot be included in this class, as its fusion is a relatively reliable indicator of a minimum age of about 20 years. The metopic suture, between the two halves of the frontal bone, usually closes at about 2 years of age, but occasionally persists into adult life.

Radiology can also assist in the determination of age, from the internal structure of the cancellous bone and cortical thickness of the head of the humerus, for example. Schranz (1959) developed a combination of external visual examination and radiographic features, indicating that the head of the humerus was a better determinator than the corresponding part of the femur. He produced a list of criteria that helped to age a skeleton from about 15 years of age up to one in excess of 75. This was pursued by Nemeskeri and later by him in conjunction with Acsadi (Acsadi and Nemeskeri 1970), to include the proximal parts of both humerus and femur, taking into account the radiological thinning of the cortex and the progressive rarefaction of the apex of the medullary cavity in the head of the bone. The original papers or their full synopsis in Krogman and Iscan's book must be consulted for details.

Histological structure has also received attention and remodelling of Haversion systems seem potentially useful

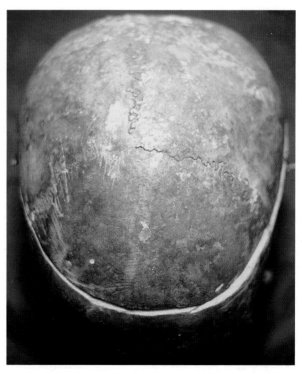

FIGURE 3.17 *The interpretation of cranial suture closure as an index of age is fraught with error. This person was 23 of age and, as would be generally expected, no segments of fusion are shown on the exterior of the skull.*

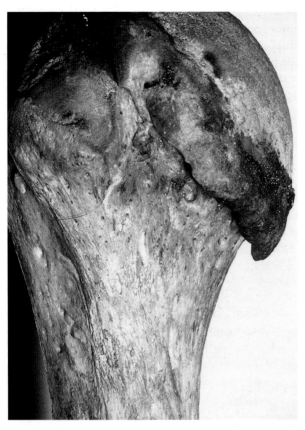

FIGURE 3.18 *Degenerative disease can assist in providing a general estimate of age, or at least exclusion of younger age groups. This grossly arthritic humerus assisted in distinguishing the near-skeletalized bodies of a 66-year-old man and his 22-year-old son.*

for the estimation of personal age. Eriksson and Westermark (1990) have claimed that amyloid inclusions in the choroid plexus can be used as a simple technique.

Chemical methods for assessing personal age lie partly within the field of forensic dentistry, such as the racemization of amino acids in teeth. This has also been applied to bone and depends upon the progressive conversion with advancing age of aspartic acid from the dextro- to the laevo-isomer (Ohtani 1994; Ritz *et al.* 1994).

DETERMINATION OF RACE FROM SKELETAL REMAINS

This is more difficult than any of the preceding investigations, partly because racial traits are not so marked and partly because so much ethnic mixing has taken place, especially in the large-scale immigrations into Europe and North America in recent years.

As usual, those at the extreme ends of the osteological range present little difficulty, as Brothwell (1972) remarks

when comparing Eskimos with Australian Aboriginals. Unfortunately, there is a large proportion of racially neutral skeletal material and also some that presents apparently classical racial features but turns out to be totally atypical, so providing a quite incorrect diagnosis. The following criteria are offered, but the usual warnings about dogmatic opinions are even more important in this field.

There are three main racial groups: Caucasian, Mongoloid and Negroid. All others are derived from these and skeletally cannot be distinguished, though when archaeologists and anthropologists are working within a major race, there may well be local criteria that can distinguish racial subgroups with varying degrees of confidence. Most work has been performed in North America and thus most available data are derived from Caucasian and Negroid Americans, and Native Americans.

The skull offers the best evidence on racial origins; Krogman and Iscan claimed that race can be determined in 90–95 per cent of cases. The mandible is excluded from this, apart from the teeth, which will be dealt with in another chapter. It may be mentioned here, however, that one of the most useful pointers to a Mongoloid skull is the present of posteriorly concave, 'shovel-shaped', upper incisors, which may be grooved on the rear surface. These were found by Hanihara (1967) to be present in up to 93 per cent of Japanese, 85 per cent of Chinese and 68 per cent of Eskimos, being absent in Caucasians and occurring in only up to 15 per cent in Negroid Americans.

The wide zygomatic arches that give the typical high-cheekboned features of the Mongoloid races can sometimes produce a skull in which, uniquely, the transverse facial width is greater than the width of any other part of the head. Krogman provides a useful table (Table 3.11), outlining the major racial differences in the skull. Elsewhere he subdivides the Caucasian group into its three main subgroups: Nordic, Alpine and Mediterranean. He points out once again that these describe the 'stereotypes' of each group and that there is an extensive grey zone of more neutral characteristics. Subjects in the Negroid group tend to be long headed (dolichocephalic) and broad headed (brachycephalic) in the Mongoloid group, with the whole range occuring in the Caucasian group. The Negroid orbit is lower and wider, compared with the higher, rounder eye socket of the Mongoloid. The Negroid nasal aperture is wide, and the prognathism of the lower face and jaw relatively marked.

There are racial differences in the pelvis, but specialized measurements as described by Todd and Lindala (1928) must be made in order to detect these. Iscan suggests that a 79–83 per cent success rate can be achieved in differentiating between Caucasian and Negroid subjects (see References and further reading). The long bones offer some assistance, especially the femur. This is straighter in Negroid groups, the anteroposterior bowing being less. Together with other long bones, especially those of the lower limb, Negroid bones are longer than those of Caucasian or Mongoloid skeletons, even for equal total body length, the leg proportions being greater. The radius and tibia are relatively longer (Table 3.12). Several writers offer various indices of relative bone lengths, such as those of Modi (1957), Munter (1936) and Schultz (1937). The scapula has been extensively studied, but seems a poor discriminator of race.

TABLE 3.11 *General racial features in the skull (after Krogman 1939)*

Feature	White ('Caucasoid') (excluding Alpine)	Negroid	Mongoloid
Height of skull	High	Low	Medium
Length of skull	Long	Long	Long
Breadth of skull	Narrow	Narrow	Broad
Breadth of face	Narrow	Narrow	Wide
Height of face	High	Low	High
Sagittal contour	Rounded	Flat	Arches
Nasal opening	Narrow	Wide	Narrow
Orbital opening	Angular	Rectangular	Rounded
Lower nasal margin	Sharp	Troughed	Sharp
Nasal profile	Straight	Slanted down	Straight
Palatal shape	Narrow	Wide	Medium

PERSONAL IDENTITY FROM SKELETAL MATERIAL

After the general groups of race, sex, stature and age have been investigated, the bones must be examined for any idiosyncratic features that give them a personal identity. This is invariably a matter of matching up such feature(s) with known pre-existing conditions, and depends upon a potential match being available. Circumstances are infinitely variable and the ways in which this suspected matter comes to the examiner's knowledge are legion. Sometimes there may be one 'good bet' and, indeed, the potential identity may be virtually certain from the circumstances, the anatomical confirmation being almost a formality. In

TABLE 3.12 *Selected anthropometric dimensions (mm) in White and Black* Americans*

	Men				Women			
	White		Black		White		Black	
	Mean	SD	Mean	SD	Mean	SD	Mean	SD
Body								
Stature	1706	60.5	1744	60.8	1597	78.1	1586	64.9
Total arm length	760	30.2	798	41.2	695	38.1	713	32.7
Upper arm length	333	16.4	340	21.9	302	22.8	303	15.6
Forearm length	249	12.4	269	15.0	225	16.7	237	14.7
Hand length	187	9.3	199	12.3	172	11.3	179	10.2
Leg length (anterior supine)	938	40.0	984	49.1	871	51.2	892	41.8
Thigh length	497	24.3	515	27.5	461	31.6	467	24.9
Lower leg length	376	19.8	401	23.7	352	25.8	365	19.8
Foot length	244	11.9	256	13.9	215	13.6	231	11.8
Bi-iliac breadth	292	16.9	270	16.5	287	22.5	267	24.7
Bi-spinous breadth	246	17.2	227	18.1	242	25.1	220	22.5
Head								
Maximum length	188	7.5	193	6.1	182	6.5	186	7.7
Maximum breadth	154	6.5	149	6.1	145	5.6	144	6.2
Auricular height	120	5.1	124	5.3	118	5.3	120	4.8
Face								
Bizygomatic breadth	139	6.7	139	6.1	130	7.0	132	8.7
Mandibular breadth	110	7.4	109	8.7	103	8.9	105	11.9
Interocular breadth	33	3.5	35	2.7	31	2.8	34	2.3
Total morphological height	122	9.7	125	7.6	113	9.5	116	11.6
Upper face height	69	6.3	71	5.6	66	6.2	67	4.5
Nasal height	54	4.7	52	4.8	52	3.8	50	4.4
Nasal breadth	35	3.7	43	3.7	32	4.9	40	4.1

*From Todd and Lindala (1928). Compiled by Krogman and Iscan (1986).

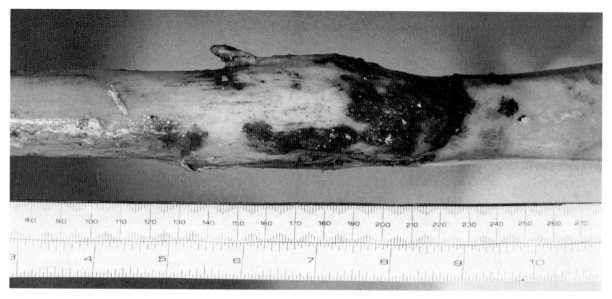

FIGURE 3.19 *Identification of a homicide victim, buried for almost 2 years in a garden, was achieved by matching this callus from a previous femoral fracture, with the medical notes and radiographs obtained from a hospital. The shape and size of the callus, together with the osseous spur due to muscle traction, was identical to follow-up films taken during life.*

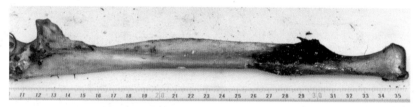

FIGURE 3.20 *Identification of a skeletalized body was achieved by matching this callus from a previous ulnar fracture, with the medical notes and radiographs obtained from a hospital. The shape and size of the callus, was identical to follow-up films taken during life.*

other cases there may be a list of hundreds of potential cases to search through in the hope of finding a match.

Individual characteristics may be of two main types.

- Anatomical shapes that can be matched by radiology, measurement or other means. Examples would be frontal sinus comparison, craniometry and radiological bone architecture.
- Discrete abnormalities such as healing fractures, metal prostheses, bone disease or congenital defects. Some artefacts, such as drill holes or wire, may immediately indicate that the bone is an anatomical specimen.

Anatomical matching depends upon accurate and detailed information about the living subject who is thought to correspond with the skeleton. Such information is usually radiographic and is derived from clinical records. The examples par excellence are dental charts and radiographs obtained from the dentist of the potential match; this is discussed in Chapter 26. Where skull films are available

from ante-mortem sources, identity can be almost assured. The lateral view of a head can be matched with similar views taken of the skull, and both obvious anatomical landmarks compared and cranial measurements taken. The matter is further discussed later in relation to radiology, but the profile of the pituitary fossa as well as various intracranial diameters can rapidly exclude a match. In fact, a cursory glance can often confirm that the two skulls are dissimilar; making a positive correlation takes more time and requires accurate orientation of the radiographs.

Frontal sinus identification

This has been extensively studied since Schuller suggested the technique in 1921, as it is particularly useful in mutilated or burnt bodies, such as those from mass disasters like air crashes. The sinuses are well protected from all but the most extreme damage and are unique in that – as first pointed out

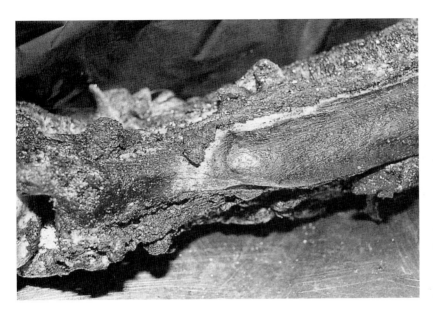

FIGURE 3.21 *Personal identity of this almost skeletalized fire victim was established from this healed callus on the tibia, the site of a well-documented fracture several years before death.*

by Poole in 1931 – no two persons (not even identical twins) have the same profile of these air spaces. They appear in the second year of life and increase in size for the first two decades. They are absent in about 5 per cent of persons and unilateral in another 1 per cent. For the sinuses to be used, an ante-mortem anteroposterior skull radiograph must be available, the most common source being from a previous hospital admission or examination, usually for a head injury. The cadaver skull or head must be X-rayed in exactly the same orientation and degree of enlargement, so that some superimposition technique can be employed. The 'forehead– nose' position was recommended by Schuller (1943), with the tube axis positioned level with the supraorbital margins. The scalloped upper margins of the sinuses are used for comparison, these being smaller and more numerous in the female. Asherson's thesis of 1965 recommends using the Caldwell occipitomental plane for the radiographs, used clinically for investigation of the nasal sinuses. This is prefer- able to the Wallers occipitofrontal view and the two projec- tions are not necessarily identical in terms of sinus profile. Asherson recommends outlining the sinus shape in black ink on the film or tracing it onto a sheet of paper. Turpin and Tisserand (1942) projected their films on to a cardboard screen and cut out a template, weighing these from both ante- and post-mortem films to determine whether they were identical. Computed tomography of the sinuses is recommended by Reichs (1993).

Other radiological methods of comparing identity include matching of hand and wrist films, matching the profile and structure of the first rib and clavicle, and the craniometric methods of Sassouni (1959) and of Voluter (1959). The methods must be sought in either the original papers or

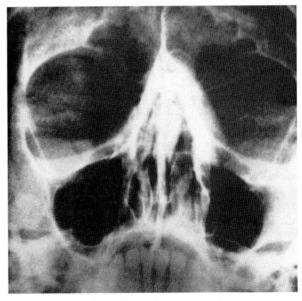

FIGURE 3.22 *The facial and cranial skeleton is unique to every person. If ante-mortem radiographs can be obtained for the person likely to be the victim, matching of the frontal sinus pattern can provide absolute identification. This body, which was washed up on the beach, was eventually matched with hospital radiographs through the sinus pattern seen at the top edge of the picture.*

surveys such as the textbook by Evans and Knight (1983). However, in general, it may be said that, wherever ante- mortem X-rays are available, especially of skull, thorax, hip or shoulder, then radiological comparisons of the dead material can almost always exclude an identity and, in many circumstances, can confirm it.

THE DATING OF SKELETAL REMAINS

One of the issues in identity, as well as in estimating the time since death, is the date (as opposed to the age) of human bones. A knowledge of the time of death, measured in years, decades or even centuries, can assist the investigating authorities considerably. In fact, where skeletal remains are shown to be of considerable antiquity, no investigation at all is required, as even if the death was criminal, the culprit may long since have died. This threshold of investigative interest lies at around 70 years and material older than this may be of concern only to historians and archaeologists.

It is the marginal cases that present difficulties, especially as the methods of dating in this period are so approximate. For example, the skeleton shown in Figure 3.6 was discovered 41 years after the woman had been murdered. When the police went searching for the suspected killer, they found that he had died peacefully 3 years before the discovery, of coronary disease – thus qualifying for the 'perfect murder'.

The major problem in dating bones is that the environment is far more potent than time in changing the state of the bone. In Wales, a historic country where a spectrum of skeletal material has been found dating back some 18 000 years, frequent opportunities present for examining bones from many periods and many conditions of environment. Some Roman or even Bronze Age material, which had been concealed in dry sand dunes or in well-drained ancient burial mounds, appeared almost as pristine as an anatomical demonstration skeleton. On the other hand, modern material buried in coffins in graves marked with headstones only 20 years old have completely vanished because acidic, peaty water repeatedly eluted the bone as the water table in marshy ground rose and fell. An even more striking demonstration of the effect of local conditions was the observation that some limb bones buried vertically in a rock fall in a cave were in excellent condition at the upper ends, yet the lower parts were totally eroded where they had been surrounded by damp rubble.

These facts emphasize that vast errors can be made in dating bone merely by the gross morphological appearances and – as is so often the case – the less experienced the examiner, the more dogmatic his incorrect opinions are likely to be. The following schedule can therefore be nothing more than a rough guide, which must be modified where possible, by a knowledge of the environment in which the bones lay. Certain physicochemical tests are of assistance, but even these are themselves dependent on the environment, with the exception of radiochemical tests that are of little value in the period of forensic concern.

Physical appearance

Recent bones will have soft tissue remnants adhering, in the form of tendon and ligament tags, especially around the joint ends. Periosteum may be visible as fibrous material closely adherent to the shaft surface. Cartilage may also be present on articular surfaces. The time for which these remnants persist is variable, according to the conditions in which the bone has been left. Animal predators may rapidly remove all soft tissue and cartilage, sometimes within days or weeks. If the body has been left in a protected place, such as a vault or closed building, then dried tissue can remain for many years. In temperate climates, bodies left out in the open usually become substantially skeletalized within the first year, though tendon tags and periosteum may survive for 5 or more years. If a body dies in the autumn, then the preservation is likely to be longer through the colder winter months than if it died in the spring or summer.

After all soft tissue has vanished, recent bones may still be differentiated from old material by the density and feel of the bone. For a variable period, depending on storage conditions, a bone will feel slightly greasy to the fingers for several years, sometimes up to a decade if kept indoors. It will also feel heavy compared with older skeletal material because of the preservation of the organic stroma. On sawing a recent bone, it will be hard (especially the shafts of limb bones such as the femur) and will be uniform through the whole thickness. A smell of burning organic tissue will be obvious if vigorous sawing produces heat. In an old bone, the loss of the collagenous stroma will lighten the bone and make it easier to cut. The outer cortex and – to a lesser extent – the zone around the marrow cavity, will lose the stroma first, so a 'sandwich' effect may be seen in which a central ring of hard collagenous bone is layered on each side by a zone of more porous, crumbling material. This is not seen in less than several decades – and sometimes centuries – unless the bone has been exposed to the sun and other elements. The fragile, brittle appearance of old bones is usually first apparent on the ends of long bones, adjacent to the joints, such as the tibial plateau or the greater trochanter of the femur. This is often because the outer layer of compact bone is thinner there than in the shaft, so that the soft cancellous bone of the extremities is more readily exposed. This occurs within a few decades if the bone has been outside, but may not develop for a century in protected material. The aged cortex will feel rough and porous and, in really old material, can be crumbled or pitted with a fingernail.

Another factor that markedly affects the rate of decay of bones is the size and type of the bone itself. Whilst thick, dense bone, such as femoral or humeral shaft, may last for centuries, smaller and thinner items may disintegrate rapidly. Skull plates, tarsal and carpal bones, digits and the thin bones of the facial skeleton will rot more quickly, as will the small bones of fetuses and infants.

Physical tests

In parallel with the physical appearance of the sawn bone, fluorescence in ultraviolet light can be a useful preliminary test. If a shaft is cut across and inspected in the dark under ultraviolet light, such as that from a Wood's lamp, recent bone will shine with a silvery-blue tint right across the whole section. As the bone ages, the outer rim will cease to fluoresce and this will progressively deepen towards the centre. As with visual and tactile examination, a similar zone will work its way outwards from the marrow cavity until only a thin sandwich-filling will survive. This then fragments and eventually vanishes so that all the cut surface is non-fluorescent. The time that this process takes is variable, but total loss of ultraviolet fluorescence takes somewhere of the order of at least 100–150 years to complete. Other physical tests have been described, including density and specific gravity measurements, ultrasonic conduction and thermal behaviour when heated under special conditions. All these criteria depend on the loss of organic stroma and the development of a calcified matrix with a porous structure.

Serological and chemical tests

Positive tests for the presence of haemoglobin may be obtained for a variable time on either the bone surface or powdered bone, this being partly dependent on the sensitivity

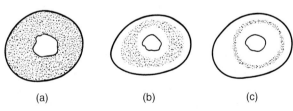

(a)   (b)   (c)

FIGURE 3.23 *Fluorescence of bone in ultraviolet light as a function of time since death. A freshly sawn cross-section of a dense bone such as femoral shaft is to be preferred. Up to several decades after death the whole cut surface fluoresces a bluish colour (a). From 3 to 80 years, greatly depending upon the environmental conditions, the outer zone and the zone around the marrow cavity progressively lose fluorescence (b). After a century or more, the residual fluorescence contracts to a narrowing central sandwich (c) before vanishing completely in the second century. Other methods of attempted dating include microscopic examination. Yoshino et al. (1991) claim that microradiography and electron microscopy reveal vacuoles in compact bone left in soil for 5 or 6 years.*

of the technique. Using the dye-peroxide methods (benzidine is most sensitive, but is now proscribed by Health and Safety regulations, so that the less satisfactory Kastel–Meyer test must be used), positive results may be obtained up to about 100 years.

Serological activity lasts only a short time in bones exposed to the weather. Bone powder eluted with weak ammonia and vacuum concentrated, may give a positive reaction with antihuman sera, such as Coombs reagent, for only about 5–10 years – again depending greatly on the environmental conditions.

The recent development of DNA techniques has led to both bone and bone marrow being used to produce profiles for identification. There seems to be a wide range of times during which this is successful. The author (BK) dealt with a case where DNA testing was successful after 8 years' burial, but other more recent skeletons did not yield such success. However, far older archaeological material has given DNA profiles, so, at present, the DNA criteria cannot be used for dating.

Chemical testing seeks to measure the degradation of the proteinous stroma, so knowing the total nitrogen and amino acid content can be useful. Fresh compact bone contains about 4.5 per cent nitrogen, which progressively diminishes with time. If a bone contains more than about 4 per cent nitrogen, it is unlikely to be older than 100 years, but if it has 2.5 per cent or less, it is likely to be older than 350 years.

Estimation of the racemization of amino acids in teeth (laevo/dextro proportions) is being used to determine age, and there is some evidence that it also changes linearly with post-mortem interval. Its use on skeletal structures other than teeth is being investigated.

Residual protein can be converted to its constituent amino acids by prolonged heating in 6M hydrochloric acid. The digest can then be analysed, either by autoanalytical methods or by two-dimensional chromatography. Fresh bone contains about 15 amino acids, mostly derived from collagen. Glycine and alanine are predominant, but proline and hydroxyproline are more specific markers for collagen. The latter two tend to vanish in about 50 years (as always, depending on the storage environment), so they are useful markers for the time threshold of forensic relevance. The other amino acids diminish over the succeeding scores and hundreds of years, so that a bone containing only four or five amino acids is likely to be relatively ancient. Glycine persists for millennia, being found in palaeolithic material.

Paradoxically, the methods available for archaeologists to use on ancient skeletal remains are proportionately more accurate, but of little or no use in forensic science. The radiocarbon test, which measures the loss of carbon-14 after death, cannot be applied to material less than a couple of centuries old, as the loss of radioactive carbon, which has a half-life of

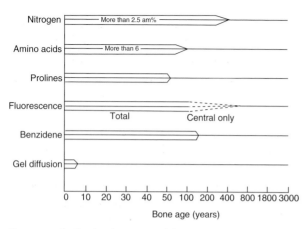

FIGURE 3.24 *Graphical summary of the criteria for estimating the approximate date of human skeletal remains.*

well over 5000 years, is too small to be measured in the half-century or so that interests the forensic pathologist.

Another radioisotope technique is the subject of current research at Aberdeen University, where Maclaughlin-Black *et al.* (1992) are measuring radiostrontium in skeletal remains, the principle being that pre-1945 bones should be free of endogenous strontium-90, derived from nuclear weapons and atmospheric tests, which was at a maximum in the environment in the early 1960s. The possibility exists that atmospheric contamination with other isotopes laid down in bone from dated tests and nuclear accidents may provide a profile that could bring forward the latest date during which the person must have been alive.

PHOTOSUPERIMPOSITION TECHNIQUES FOR IDENTIFICATION

Where potential candidate(s) for the identity of a skull are known to the investigating authority and photographs taken during life are available, a well established technique used for identification is 'photosuperimposition'. In this method, photographs of the skull are taken in exactly the same orientation in three planes as the available photograph. These are then enlarged to exactly the same dimensions as the photograph, and either the negative or a positive print is made on transparent film. This is then laid over the photograph and adjusted in an attempt to match up the major anatomical landmarks such as nasion, supraorbital ridges, angle of the jaw, nasal aperture, external auditory meatus and, especially, teeth. The actual anatomical markers will depend on what is visible, in frontal, lateral or oblique views. The test is mainly an exclusory one, in that, if the match cannot be made, then the skull is not that of the person in the photograph. If the

match is good, even excellent, then the two could be the same person, though the standard of proof is low unless some individualistic feature, such as a distinct dental character, is apparent.

The photofit method has been used for many years, one of the most familiar examples being that reproduced in many forensic textbooks, of the skull and face of the wife of Dr Buck Ruxton, a notorious murder in 1935 investigated by Glaister and Brash in Scotland.

A more modern variant of the photosuperimposition technique is with the use of video cameras where two images, one of the photograph and the other of the skull, are mixed on one video display unit. By altering the camera angles and the degree of magnification of the images, superimposition can be tested quickly without the need for laborious photographic processing. This method was used in 1994 to identify a number of the 12 victims of the notorious 'House of Horror' in Gloucester. This is a rapidly developing field of forensic interest, where even the relatively poor-quality images from security cameras can be matched with suspects.

RECONSTRUCTION OF THE FACIAL APPEARANCE FROM THE SKULL

The reconstitution of the visage from the skeletal base has been a goal for workers in many different fields in recent years. The advantages of such a technique are obvious as, when a skull is discovered one prime method of identification would be a reliable reconstruction of the face, so that direct recognition could be obtained from relatives, friends and photographic records.

The first methods were as much artistic as scientific and depended to a great extent on the sculpturing ability of the operator. Gerasimov (1971) was a Soviet pioneer of this method, though much of his work was archaeological and historical, rather than forensic.

The method depends on a pre-knowledge of the usual tissue thickness at a multitude of points on the normal skull, an anatomical exercise that now has quite a large database. Modelling clay is laid on to the unknown skull in layers corresponding to these standard thicknesses, then more imaginative modelling added to 'humanize' the basic shape. The obvious defects in this technique are the lack of knowledge about eyes, lips, nose, ears and head hair, all of which contribute greatly to individual characteristics. Similar methods have been used by graphic artists, rather than sculptors, who use their portraiture talents to create a face on the two-dimensional base provided by the skull profile, plus a knowledge of tissue thicknesses at many anatomical points. Additional information has been provided on tissue thicknesses by radiography of heads.

The method was used with success in the 1988 investigation of the murder of Karen Price in Cardiff. Skeletalized after being buried for 8 years in a carpet beneath a garden, medical artist Richard Neave rebuilt her face upon a skull with sufficient accuracy for its display on public television to be recognized by her parents.

Recently, considerable progress has been made by the use of computer graphic techniques, both in drawing reconstituted heads and in gathering tissue thickness data (Vanezis *et al.* 1989). Some devices are mechanical, measuring the profile of the skull with a device that converts angles and distances into digital data. More recently, a combination of video and laser equipment has allowed 20 000 measurements to be taken and stored within 30 seconds. The data from an unknown skull are then electronically 'clothed' with standard soft tissues from the memory bank and modified on screen to produce various images. These can be rotated electronically so that various profiles can be seen. A variety of stored eyes, ears and noses can be added, and any feature altered almost instantaneously to give a viewer a number of opportunities to recognize the missing person. As with so many techniques in forensic medicine and science, the technology is one for super-specialists at present, but the forensic pathologist should be aware that such methods exist and are increasing in availability and accuracy.

REFERENCES AND FURTHER READING

Acsadi G, Nemeskeri J. 1970. *History of human life span and mortality.* Akademiai Kiado, Budapest.

Allbrook D. 1961. The estimation of stature in British and East African males; based on tibial and ulnar bone lengths. *J Forensic Med* **8**:15–28.

Angel JL. 1919. The bases of paleodemography. *Anthropology* **30**:425–38.

Angel JL, Suchey JM, Iscan MY, *et al.* 1986. Age at death from the skeleton and viscera. In: Zimmerman MR, Angel JL (eds), *Dating and age determination in biological materials.* Croom Helm, London, pp. 179–220.

Asala SA. 2001. Sex determination from the head of the femur of South African whites and blacks. *Forensic Sci Int* **117**:15–22.

Asala SA. 2002. The efficiency of the demarking point of the femoral head as a sex determining parameter. *Forensic Sci Int* **127**:114–18.

Asherson N. 1965. *Identification by frontal sinus prints: a forensic medicine pilot survey.* HK Lewis, London.

Baccino E, Ubelaker DH, Hayek LA, *et al.* 1999. Evaluation of seven methods of estimating age at death from mature human skeletal remains. *J Forensic Sci* **44**:931–6.

Barbet JP, Houette A, Barres D, *et al.* 1988. Histological assessment of gestational age in human embryos and fetuses. *Am J Forensic Med Pathol* **9**:40–4.

Berg S. 1963. *The determination of bone age.* In: Lundquist F (ed.), *Methods in forensic science.* Interscience Publications, New York, pp. 231–52.

Black TK. 1978. A new method for assessing the sex of fragmentary skeletal remains: femoral shaft circumference. *Am J Phys Anthropol* **48**:227–31.

Boström K. 1973. Identification from roentgenograms of sinus frontalis and sella turcica. *Proceedings of Fifth Meeting Scandinavian Society of Forensic Medicine.*

Boucher BJ. 1957. Sex differences in the fetal pelvis. *Am J Phys Anthropol* **15**:581–600.

Boyd JD, Trevor J. 1953. Problems in reconstruction. In: Simpson CK (ed.), *Modern trends in forensic medicine.* Butterworth, London.

Breitinger E. 1937. Zur Berechnung der Körperhöhe aus den langen Gliedmassenknochen. *Anthropol Anz* **14**:249–74.

Brothwell D. 1972. *Digging up bones*, 2nd edn. British Museum, London.

Brown TC. 1950. Medical identification in the Noronic disaster. *Fingerprint Ident Mag* **6**:3–12.

Burnham JT, Preston Burnham J, Fontan CR. 1976. The state of the art of bone identification by chemical and microscopic methods. *J Forensic Sci* **21**:340–2.

Caldwell WE, Molloy HC. 1933. Anatomical variations in the female pelvis. *Am J Obstet Gynecol* **26**:479–505.

Castellano MA, Villanueva EC, von Frenckel R. 1984. Estimating the date of bone remains: a multivariate study. *J Forensic Sci* **29**:527–34.

Cattaneo C, Smillie DM, Gelsthorpe K, *et al.* 1995. A simple method for extracting DNA from old skeletal material. *Forensic Sci Int* **74**:167–74.

Cattaneo C, Craig OE, James NT, *et al.* 1997. Comparison of three DNA extraction methods on bone and blood stains up to 43 years old and amplification of three different gene sequences. *J Forensic Sci* **42**:1126–35.

Cattaneo C, DiMartino S, Scali S, *et al.* 1999. Determining the human origin of fragments of burnt bone: a comparative study of histological, immunological and DNA techniques. *Forensic Sci Int* **102**:181–91.

Cattaneo C, Ritz-Timme S, Schutz HW, *et al.* 2000. Unidentified cadavers and human remains in the EU: an unknown issue. *Int J Legal Med* **113**:N2–3.

Cheevers LS, Ascensio R. 1977. Identification by skull superimposition. *Int J Forensic Dent* **4**:14–16.

Christie AL. 1949. Prevalence and distribution of ossification centres in the newborn infant. *Am J Dis Child* **77**:355–61.

Cobb WM. 1952. Skeleton. In: Lansings AL (ed.), *Cowdry's problems of ageing*. Williams & Wilkins, Baltimore.

Colonna M, Pesce Delfino V, Introna F, Jr. 1980. [Identification by superimposition of the skull on face photography using television: experimental application of a new method.] *Boll Soc Ital Biol Sper* **56**:2271–7.

Colonna M, Introna F, Jr, Potente F, *et al.* 1984. Computer-aided skull-face superimposition by analytical procedures. *Acta Med Leg Soc Liege* **34**:139–49.

Culbert W, Law F. 1927. Identification by comparison of accessory nasal sinuses and mastoid processes. *J Am Dent Assoc* **88**:1634.

Davidson WM. 1960. Sex determination: diagnostic methods. *Br Med J* **4**:1901–7.

Derry DE. 1909. Note on the innominate bone in the determination of sex. *J Anthropol* **43**:266–76.

Derry DE. 1924. On the sexual and racial characters of the ilium. *J Anat* **4**:71–83.

Dixon AD. 1956. Postmortem persistence of sex chromatin. *J Forensic Med* **3**:161–8.

Dixon AD. 1957. Sex determination of human tissues from cell morphology. *J Forensic Med* **4**:11–17.

Dodd BE. 1985. DNA fingerprinting in matters of family and crime [news]. *Nature* **318**:506–7.

Dupertuis CW, Hadden JA. 1951. On the reconstruction of stature from long bones. *Am J Phys Anthropol* **9**:15–54.

Dutra F. 1944. Identification of person and determination of cause of death from skeletal remains. *Arch Pathol* **38**:339.

Dwight T. 1889. The sternum as an index of sex, height and age. *J Anat Physiol* **24**:527–35.

Dwight T. 1890. The closure of the sutures as a sign of age. *Boston Med Surg J* **122**:389–92.

Dwight T. 1904. The size of the articular surfaces of the long bones as characteristic of sex. *J Anat* **4**:19–32.

Earls J, Hester R. 1967. Tattooed sailors: Sociopsychological correlates. *Milit Med* **132**:48.

Eckert W. 1985. The forensic investigation of Josef Mengele [editorial]. *Am J Forensic Med Pathol* **6**:187.

Eckert WG, Teixeira WR. 1985. The identification of Josef Mengele. A triumph of international cooperation. *Am J Forensic Med Pathol* **6**:188–91.

Eckert WG, Willey LR, Blakeslee DJ. 1986. Identification by identi-kit composite from skull appearance. Combined efforts of the anthropologist, forensic pathologist, and criminal investigators. *Am J Forensic Med Pathol* **7**:213–15.

Eliakis C. 1967. Estimating height from the measurement of long bones. *Ann Med Leg* **212**:251–4.

Eliakis EC, Iordanidis PJ. 1963. Determination of sex from the medullary indices of long bones. *Am Med Leg* **43**:326–9.

Eriksson L, Westermark P. 1990. Amyloid inclusions in choroid plexus epithelial cells. A simple autopsy method to rapidly obtain information on the age of an unknown dead person. *Forensic Sci Int* **48**:97–102.

Evans KT, Knight B. 1983. *Forensic radiology*. Blackwell Scientific Publications, Oxford.

Ezra M, Cook SF. 1957. Amino-acids in fossil bone. *Science* **126**:8–86.

Facchini F, Pettener D. 1977. Chemical and physical methods in dating human skeletal remains. *Am J Phys Anthropol* **47**:65–70.

Fawcett E. 1938. Sexing of the human sternum. *J Anat* **72**:633–7.

Fazekas G, Kosa F. 1978. *Forensic foetal osteology*. Akademiai Kiado, Budapest.

Flecker H. 1942. Time of appearance and fusion of ossification centers as observed by roentgenographic methods. *Am J Roentgenol* **47**:97–105.

Francis GC, Werle PP. 1939. The appearance of centers of ossification from birth to 5 years. *Am J Phys Anthropol* **24**:273–86.

Fukushima H, Hasekura H, Nagai K. 1988. Identification of male bloodstains by dot hybridization of human Y chromosome-specific deoxyribonucleic acid (DNA) probe. *J Forensic Sci* **33**:621–7.

Fully G, Pineau H. 1960. Detemination de la stature an moyen du squelette. *Ann Med Leg* **40**:3–11.

Garn SM. 1958. The sex difference in tooth calcification. *J Dent Res* **37**:561–72.

Gatliff BP. 1984. Facial sculpture on the skull for identification. *Am J Forensic Med Pathol* **5**:327–32.

Gatliff BP, Snow CC. 1979. From skull to visage. *J Biocommun* **6**:27–30.

Genovés S. 1954. The problem of sex of fossil hominids. *J R Anthropol Inst* **84**:131–6.

Genovés ST, Messmacher M. 1959. *Valor de los patrones tradicionales para la determinación del edad por me las suturas craneos mexicanos. Serie anthropol. No. 7.* Cuadernos de Instit de Hist., Mexico City, Mexico, Vol. 7, pp. 7–53.

George RM. 1987. The lateral craniographic method of facial reconstruction. *J Forensic Sci* **32**:1305–30.

Gerasimov MM. 1971. *The face finder.* Lippincott, Philadelphia.

Gilbert BM, McKern TW. 1973. A method for aging the female os pubis. *Am J Phys Anthropol* **38**:31–8.

Giles E, Elliot O. 1963. Sex determination by discriminant function analysis of crania. *Am J Phys Anthropol* **21**:53–68.

Gill GW. 2001. Racial variation in the proximal and distal femur: heritability and forensic utility. *J Forensic Sci* **46**:791–9.

Glaister J, Brash J. 1937. *The medicolegal aspects of the Ruxton case.* Livingstone, Edinburgh.

Godycki M. 1957. Sur la certitude de determination se sexe après le femur, le cubitus et l'humerus. *Bull Mem Soc Anthrop Paris* Serie **10**:405–10.

Graves WW. 1922. Observations of age changes in the scapula: a preliminary note. *Am J Phys Anthropol* **5**:21–3.

Greulich WW. 1960. Value of X-ray films of hand in human identification. *Science* **1341**:155–62.

Greulich WW, Pye SI. 1959. *Radiographic atlas of the skeletal development of the hand and wrist,* 2nd edn. Stanford University Press, Stanford.

Greulich WW, Thomas H. 1938. The dimensions of the pelvic inlet of 789 white females. *Anat Rec* **72**:45–51.

Greulich WW, Thomas H. 1939. A X-ray study of the male pelvis. *Anat Rec* **75**:289–99.

Hanihara K. 1967. Racial characteristics in the dentition. *J Dent Res* **46**:923–6.

Harrison R. 1968. In: Camps F (ed.), *Gradwohl's legal medicine,* 2nd edn. John Wright, Bristol.

Hellman H. 1929. Racial characteristics in the human dentition. *Am Phil Soc* **67**:157–74.

Herrman L. 1953. Fingerprints and twins. *J Forensic Med* **1**:101–5.

Hill A. 1939. Fetal age assessment by centers of ossification. *Am J Phys Anthropol* **24**:251.

Hoshi, H. 1962. Sex differentiation in the shape of the mastoid process in norma occipalis and its importance to sex determination of the human skull. *Okajima's Folia Anat Jpn* **38**:309–17.

Howard JD, Reay DT, Haglund WD, *et al.* 1988. Processing of skeletal remains. A medical examiner's perspective. *Am J Forensic Med Pathol* **9**:258–64.

Hrdlicka A. 1920. Shovel-shaped teeth. *Am J Phys Anthropol* **3**:429.

Hrdlicka A. 1939. *Practical anthropometry.* Wistar Institute Press, Philadelphia.

Hunt EE, Gleiser I. 1955. The estimation of the age and sex of pre-adolescent children from bones and teeth. *Am J Phys Anthropol* **13**:479–87.

Iordanidis P. 1961. Determination du sexe par les os du squelette (atalas, axis, clavicle, omoplate, sternum). *Ann Med Leg* **41**:28–91.

Iscan MY, Derrick K. 1984. Determination of sex from the sacroiliac; a visual assessment technique. *Fla Sci* **47**:948.

Iscan MY, Loth SR. 1986. Determination of age from the sternal rib in white males: a test of the phase method. *J Forensic Sci* **31**:122–32.

Iscan MY, Miller-Shaivitz P. 1984. Discriminant function sexing of the tibia. *J Forensic Sci* **29**:1087–93.

Iscan MY, Miller-Shaivitz P. 1984. Determination of sex from the tibia. *Am J Phys Anthropol* **64**:53–7.

Iscan MY, Loth SR, King CA, *et al.* 1998. Sexual dimorphism in the humerus: a comparative analysis of Chinese, Japanese and Thais. *Forensic Sci Int* **98**: 17–29.

Iscan MY, Steyn M. 1999. Craniometric determination of population affinity in South Africans. *Int J Legal Med* **112**:91–7.

Iten PX. 1987. Identification of skulls by video superimposition. *J Forensic Sci* **32**:173–88.

Jantz RL. 2001. Cranial change in americans: 1850–1975. *J Forensic Sci* **46**:784–7.

Jedrzejowska ZK. 2001. Craniometry and mathematical calculations as a method for viscero-cranium profile determination. *Forensic Sci Int* **117**:145–51.

Jit I, Singh S. 1956. Estimation of stature from the clavicles. *Indian J Med Res* **44**:137–55.

Jit I, Jhingan V, Kulkarni M. 1980. Sexing the human sternum. *Am J Phys Anthropol* **53**:217–24.

Keen J. 1950. A study of the differences between male and female skulls. *Am J Phys Anthropol* **8**:65.

Keen JA. 1950. Sex differences in skulls. *Am J Phys Anthropol* **8**:479–87.

Kerley ER. 1965. The microscopic determination of age in human bone. *Am J Phys Anthropol* **23**:149–63.

Kerley ER. 1969. Age determination of bone fragments. *J Forensic Sci* **14**:59–67.

Kim MA, Bier L. 1972. Identification and location of the y body in interphase by quinacrine and giemsa. *Humangenetik* **16**:261–5.

Kimura K. 1982. Base wing index for sexing the sacrum. *J Anthropol Soc Nippon* **90**(Suppl):153–62.

Knight B. 1969. Methods of dating skeletal remains. *Med Sci Law* **9**:247–52.

Knight B. 1985. The examination of skeletal remains. In: Wecht C (ed.), *Legal Medicine Annual*, 1985 edn. Praeger Scientific, New York.

Knight B, Lauder I. 1967. Practical methods of dating skeletal remains: a preliminary study. *Med Sci Law* **7**:205–8.

Knight B, Lauder I. 1969. Methods of dating skeletal remains. *Hum Biol* **41**:322–41.

Kobayashi K. 1964. Estimation of age at death from pubic symphysis for prehistoric human remains in Japan. *Zinruig Zassi* **72**:1–16.

Kobayashi R, Nakauchi H, Nakahori Y, *et al.* 1988. Sex identification in fresh blood and dried bloodstains by a nonisotopic deoxyribonucleic acid (DNA) analyzing technique. *J Forensic Sci* **33**:613–20.

Koelmeyer TD. 1982. Videocamera superimposition and facial reconstruction as an aid to identification. *Am J Forensic Med Pathol* **3**:45–8.

Konigsberg LW, Hens SM, Jantz LM, *et al.* 1998. Stature estimation and calibration: Bayesian and maximum likelihood perspectives in physical anthropology. *Am J Phys Anthropol Suppl* **27**:65–92.

Krogman WCA. 1939. A guide to the identification of human skeletal material. *FBI Law Enforcement Bull* **8**:3.

Krogman WCA. 1946. The skeleton in forensic medicine. *Proc Inst Med* **16**:154.

Krogman WCA, Iscan MY. 1986. *The human skeleton in forensic medicine*, 2nd edn. Thomas, Springfield.

Loth SR, Iscan MY, Scheuerman EH. 1994. Intercostal variation at the sternal end of the rib. *Forensic Sci Int* **65**:135–43.

Lundy JK. 1985. The mathematical versus anatomical methods of stature estimate from long bones. *Am J Forensic Med Pathol* **6**:73–6.

Maclaughlin-Black SM, Herd RJ, Willson K, *et al.* 1992. Strontium-90 as an indicator of time since death: a pilot investigation. *Forensic Sci Int* **57**:51–6.

Mall G, Graw M, Gehring K, *et al.* 2000. Determination of sex from femora. *Forensic Sci Int* **113**:315–21.

Mall G, Hubig M, Buttner A, *et al.* 2001. Sex determination and estimation of stature from the long bones of the arm. *Forensic Sci Int* **117**:23–30.

Maltby J. 1917. Some indices and measurements of the modern femur. *J Anat* **52**:363–82.

Mann RW. 1998. Use of bone trabeculae to establish positive identification. *Forensic Sci Int* **98**:91–9.

Manouvrier L. 1893. Le determination de la taille après les grand os des membres. *Mem Soc Anthropol Paris* **4**:347–402.

Maresh MM. 1940. Paranasal sinuses from birth to adolescence. *Am J Dis Child* **60**:55–78.

Mayler J. 1935. Identification by sinus prints. *VA Med Mon* **62**:517–19.

McBride DG, Dietz MJ, Vennemeyer MT, *et al.* 2001. Bootstrap methods for sex determination from the os coxae using the ID3 algorithm. *J Forensic Sci* **46**:427–31.

McCormick WF. 1980. Mineralization of the costal cartilages as an indicator of age: preliminary observations. *J Forensic Sci* **25**:736–41.

McCormick WF. 1981. Sternal foramena in man. *Am J Forensic Med Pathol* **2**:249–52.

McCormick WF, Nichols MM. 1981. Formation and maturation of the human sternum. I. Fetal period. *Am J Forensic Med Pathol* **2**:323–8.

McKeehan HE. 1970. The restoration of desiccated cadaveric fingers for the purpose of identification. *J Forensic Sci Soc* **10**:115.

McKern TW, Stewart TD. 1957. *Skeletal age changes in young American males, analyzed from the standpoint of identification.* Headq. QM Res & Dev Command, Natick, MA.

Mehta L, Singh HM. 1972. Determination of crown-rump length from fetal long bones: humerus and femur. *Am J Phys Anthropol* **36**:165–8.

Meindl RS, Lovejoy CO, Mensforth RP, *et al.* 1985. A revised method of age determination using the os pubis, with a review and tests of accuracy of other current methods of pubic symphyseal aging. *Am J Phys Anthropol* **68**:29–45.

Mendes-Correa AA. 1932. La taille des portugais d'après des os longes. *Anthropology (Prague)* **10**:268–72.

Messmer JM, Fierro MF. 1986. Personal identification by radiographic comparison of vascular groove patterns of the calvarium. *Am J Forensic Med Pathol* **7**:159–62.

Michelson N. 1934. The calcification of the first costal cartilage in whites and negroes. *Hum Biol* **6**:543–57.

Miller KW, Budowle B. 2001. A compendium of human mitochondrial DNA control region: development of an international standard forensic database. *Croat Med J* **42**:315–27.

Modi JP. 1957. *Medical jurisprudence and toxicology.* Tripathi, Bombay.

Montanari GD, Viterbo B, Montanari GR. 1967. Sex determination of human hair. *Med Sci Law* **7**:208–10.

Moore KL, Barr ML. 1955. Smears from the oral mucosa in the detection of chromosomal sex. *Lancet* **2**:57–8.

Moss JP, Linney AD, Grindrod SR, *et al.* 1987. Three-dimensional visualization of the face and skull using computerized tomography and laser scanning techniques. *Eur J Orthod* **9**:247–53.

Müller G. 1935. Zur Bestimmung der Länge beschädigter Extremitätenknochen. *Anthropol Anz* **12**:70–2.

Munter AH. 1936. A study of the lengths of long bones of the arms and legs in man, with special reference to Anglo-Saxon skeletons. *Biometrika* **28**:84–122.

Myers JC, Okoye MI, Kiple D, *et al.* 1999. Three-dimensional (3-D) imaging in post-mortem examinations: elucidation and identification of cranial and facial fractures in victims of homicide utilizing 3-D computerized imaging reconstruction techniques. *Int J Legal Med* **113**:33–7.

Nagamori H, Ohno Y, Uchima E, *et al.* 1986. Sex determination from buccal mucosa and hair root by the combined treatment of quinacrine staining and the fluorescent feulgen reaction using a single specimen. *Forensic Sci Int* **31**:119–28.

Navani S, Shah JR, Levy PS. 1970. Determination of sex by costal cartilage calcification. *Am J Roentgenol Radium Ther Nucl Med* **108**:771–4.

Nemeskeri J, Harsanyi L, Acsadi G. 1960. Methoden zur Diagnose des Lebensalters von Skelettfunden. *Anthropol Anz* **24**:70–95.

Niyogi S. 1971. A study of human hairs in forensic work. *J Forensic Sci* **16**:176.

Norris SP. 2002. Mandibular ramus height as an indicator of human infant age. *J Forensic Sci* **47**:8–11.

Oettle AC, Steyn M. 2000. Age estimation from sternal ends of ribs by phase analysis in South African blacks. *J Forensic Sci* **45**:1071–9.

Ohtani S. 1994. Age estimation by aspartic acid racemization in dentin of deciduous teeth. *Forensic Sci Int* **68**:77–82.

Ohtani S, Matsushima Y, Kobayashi Y, *et al.* 2002. Age estimation by measuring the racemization of aspartic acid from total amino acid content of several types of bone and rib cartilage: a preliminary account. *J Forensic Sci* **47**:32–6.

Olivier G. 1969. *Practical anthropology.* Thomas, Springfield.

Olivier G, Pineau H. 1958. Determination de l'age du foetus et de l'embyon. *Arch Anat Pathol* **6**:21–8.

Parsons FG, Box CR. 1905. The relation of the cranial sutures to age. *J R Anthropol Inst* **35**:308.

Pearson FG. 1920. Sex differences in the skull. *J Anthropol* **54**:58–65.

Pearson K. 1914. On the problem of sexing osteometric material. *Biomedicine* **10**:479–87.

Pearson K. 1926. On the coefficient of racial likeness. *Biometrika* **18**:105.

Pearson K, Bell JA. 1917. A study of the long bones of the English skeleton. 1. The femur. In: *Drapers Co Res Mem.* Biomedicine, Series X. University of London, London, Chapter 14.

Perper JA, Patterson GT, Backner JS. 1988. Face imaging reconstructive morphography. A new method for physiognomic reconstruction. *Am J Forensic Med Pathol* **9**:126–38.

Pesce Delfino V, Colonna M, Vacca E, *et al.* 1986. Computer-aided skull/face superimposition. *Am J Forensic Med Pathol* **7**:201–12.

Phenice TW. 1969. A newly developed visual method of sexing the os pubis. *Am J Phys Anthropol* **30**:297–301.

Pounder DJ. 1984. Forensic aspects of aboriginal skeletal remains in Australia. *Am J Forensic Med Pathol* **5**:41–52.

Rao NG, Pai LM. 1988. Costal cartilage calcification pattern – a clue for establishing sex identity. *Forensic Sci Int* **38**:193–202.

Reichs KJ. 1993. Quantified comparison of frontal sinus patterns by means of computed tomography. *Forensic Sci Int* **61**:141–68.

Reynolds E. 1945. The boney pelvic girdle in early infancy: a roentgenometric study. *Am J Phys Anthropol* **3**:321–54.

Reynolds E. 1947. The boney pelvis in prepubertal childhood. *Am J Phys Anthropol* **5**:165–200.

Rhine JS, Campbell HR. 1980. Thickness of facial tissues in American blacks. *J Forensic Sci* **25**:847–58.

Rhine JS, Moore CE. 1982. *Facial reproduction tables of facial tissue thicknesses of American caucasoids in forensic anthropology.* Maxwell Museum, Albuquerque.

Rho YM. 1985. Importance of examination of the clothed victim. Fingerprint identification of assailant from skin fragment on knifing victim's clothing. *Am J Forensic Med Pathol* **6**:19–20.

Richardson L, Kade H. 1972. Readable fingerprints from mummified or putrefied specimens. *J Forensic Sci* **17**:325–8.

Ritz S, Turzynski A, Schutz HW. 1994. Estimation of age at death based on aspartic acid racemization in non-collagenous bone proteins. *Forensic Sci Int* **69**:149–59.

Ross AH, Konigsberg LW. 2002. New formulae for estimating stature in the balkans. *J Forensic Sci* **47**:165–7.

Ross AH, Jantz RL, McCormick WF. 1998. Cranial thickness in American females and males. *J Forensic Sci* **43**:267–72.

Sanders CF. 1966. Sexing by costal cartilage calcification. *Br J Radiol* **39**:233–7.

Sassouni V. 1959. Cephalometric identification: a proposed method of identification of war dead by means of roentgenographic cephalometry. *J Forensic Sci* **4**:1–10.

Scammon RE. 1937. Two simple nomograms for determining the age and some of the major external dimensions of the human foetus. *Anat Rec* **68**:221–32.

Scheuer L. 2002. Application of osteology to forensic medicine. *Clin Anat* **15**:297–312.

Schranz D. 1959. Age determination from the internal structure of the humerus. *Am J Phys Anthropol* **17**:273–8.

Schuller A. 1921. Das Röntgengramm der Stirnhöhle. *Monatsschr Ohrenheilkd* **55**:1617–20.

Schuller A. 1943. Note on the identification of skulls by X-ray pictures of the frontal sinuses. *Med J Aust* **1**:554–6.

Schultz A. 1937. Proportions, variability and asymmetry of the long bones of the limbs and clavicles in man and apes. *Hum Biol* **9**:281–328.

Sen NK. 1962. Identification by superimposed photographs. *Int Crim Police Rev* **162**:284–6.

Sharif R, Chandra H. 1972. Histological differentiation as to the origin of bones. *J Indian Acad Forensic Sci* **2**:23–30.

Shiati M. 1983. Estimation of stature by long bones of Chinese male adults in South China. *Acta Anthropol Sinica* **2**:80–5.

Simpson E, Henneberg M. 2002. Variation in soft-tissue thicknesses on the human face and their relation to craniometric dimensions. *Am J Phys Anthropol* **118**:121–33.

Singer R. 1953. Estimation of age from cranial suture closure; a report on its unreliability. *J Forensic Med* **1**:52–9.

Snow CC, Williams J. 1971. Variation in premortem statural measurements compared to statural estimates of skeletal remains. *J Forensic Sci* **16**:455–64.

Snow CC, Gatliff BP, McWilliams KR. 1970. Reconstruction of facial features from the skull: an evaluation of its usefulness in forensic anthropology. *Am J Phys Anthropol* **33**:221–8.

Snow CC, Hartman S, Giles E, *et al.* 1979. Sex and race determination of crania by calipers and computer: a test of the Giles and Elliot discriminant functions in 52 forensic science cases. *J Forensic Sci* **24**:448–60.

Steele D. 1970. *Estimation of stature from fragments of long limb bones.* In: Stewart T (ed.), *Personal identification in mass disasters.* National Museum of Nature History, Washington DC, pp. 85–7.

Steele DG, McKern TW. 1969. A method for assessment of maximum long bone length and living stature from fragmentary long bones. *Am J Phys Anthropol* **31**:215–27.

Stephan CN. 2002. Facial approximation: globe projection guideline falsified by exophthalmometry literature. *J Forensic Sci* **47**:730–5.

Stevenson PH. 1929. On racial differences in stature long bone regression formulae with special reference to stature reconstruction formulae for the Chinese. *Biometrika* **21**:303–18.

Stevenson PM. 1924. Age order of epiphyseal union in man. *Am J Phys Anthropol* **7**:53–93.

Stewart JH, McCormick WF. 1983. The gender predictive value of sternal length. *Am J Forensic Med Pathol* **4**:217–20.

Stewart TD. 1948. Medicolegal aspects of the skeleton. *Am J Phys Anthropol* **6**:315–21.

Stewart TD. 1952. *Hrdlicka's practical anthropometry,* 4th edn. Wistar Institute, Philadelphia.

Stewart TD. 1957. Distortion of the pubic symphyseal surface in females and its effect on a determination. *Am J Phys Anthropol* **15**:9.

Stewart TD. 1959. Bear paw remains closely resemble human bones. *FBI Law Enforcement Bull* **28**:18.

Stewart TD. 1962. Anterior femoral curvature; its utility for race determination. *Hum Biol* **34**:4–57.

Stewart TD. 1968. Evaluation of evidence from the skeleton. In: Camps F (ed.), *Gradwohl's legal medicine,* 2nd edn. John Wright, Bristol, p. 425.

Stewart TD. 1968. Subject: skull sutures and age. In: Camps F (ed.), *Gradwohl's legal medicine,* 2nd edn. John Wright, Bristol, p. 132.

Stewart TD. 1979. *Essentials of forensic anthropology: especially as developed in the United States.* Thomas, Springfield.

Stewart TD, Trotter M. 1954. *Basic readings on the identification of human skeletons: estimations of age.* Wenner-Gren Foundation for Anthropological Research, New York.

Steyn M, Iscan MY. 1998. Sexual dimorphism in the crania and mandibles of South African whites. *Forensic Sci Int* **98**:9–16.

Steyn M, Iscan MY. 1999. Osteometric variation in the humerus: sexual dimorphism in South Africans. *Forensic Sci Int* **106**:77–85.

Straus WL. 1927. The human ilium: sex and stock. *Am J Phys Anthropol* **11**:1–28.

Suchey JM. 1979. Problems in the aging of females using the os pubis. *Am J Phys Anthropol* **51**:467–70.

Suzuki K, Tsuchihashi Y. 1970. New attempt of personal identification by means of lip print. *J Indian Dent Assoc* **42**:8–9.

Swift B, Lauder I, Black S, *et al.* 2001. An estimation of the post-mortem interval in human skeletal remains: a radionuclide and trace element approach. *Forensic Sci Int* **117**:73–87.

Teixeira WR. 1982. Sex identification utilizing the size of the foramen magnum. *Am J Forensic Med Pathol* **3**:203–6.

Teixeira WR. 1985. The Mengele report. *Am J Forensic Med Pathol* **6**:279–83.

Telkkä A. 1950. On the prediction of human stature from long bones. *Acta Anat* **9**:103–17.

Thomas H, Greulich WA. 1940. A comparative study of male and female pelves. *Am J Obstet Gynecol* **39**:56–62.

Thompson DD, Galvin CA. 1983. Estimation of age at death by tibial osteon remodeling in an autopsy series. *Forensic Sci Int* **22**:203–11.

Thomsen JL. 1977. Sex determination of severely burned bodies. *Forensic Sci* **10**:235–42.

Thomsen JL. 1979. Y-chromosome bodies in brain and kidney: the normal variation and an unexpected finding in sudden infant death syndrome. *Med Sci Law* **19**:104–7.

Tibbets GL. 1981. Estimation of stature from the vertebral column in American blacks. *J Forensic Sci* **26**:715–23.

Tobias PV. 1953. The problem of race determination. *J Forensic Med* **1**:113–23.

Todd TW. 1920. Age changes in the pubic bone. *Am J Phys Anthropol* **3**:285–334.

Todd TW. 1921. Age changes in the pubic bone I–IV. *Am J Phys Anthropol* **4**:407.

Todd TW, Lindala A. 1928. Dimensions of the body; whites and American negroes of both sexes. *Am J Phys Anthropol* **12**:35–119.

Todd TW, Lyon DW. 1924. Endocranial suture closure; its progress and age relationship. Part I. *Am J Phys Anthropol* **7**:325–84.

Todd TW, Lyon DW. 1925. Cranial suture closure; its progress and age relationship. Part II. *Am J Phys Anthropol* **8**:23–5.

Todd TW, Lyon DW. 1925. Cranial suture closure; its progress and age relationship. Parts III–IV. *Am J Phys Anthropol* **8**:47–71, 149–68.

Trotter M, Gleser GC. 1958. A re-evaluation of the estimation of stature based on measurements of stature taken during life and on long bones after death. *Am J Phys Anthropol* **16**:79–88.

Trotter M, Gleser GC. 1977. Corrigenda to 'estimation of stature from long limb bones of American Whites and Negroes', American Journal Physical Anthropology (1952). *Am J Phys Anthropol* **47**:355–6.

Turner W. 1886. The index of the pelvic brim as a basis of classification. *J Anat Physiol* **20**:125–43.

Turpin R, Tisserand M. 1942. Etude correlative de sinus. *C R Soc Biol* **136**:203–10.

Tyler MG, Kirby LT, Wood S, *et al.* 1986. Human blood stain identification and sex determination in dried blood stains using recombinant DNA techniques. *Forensic Sci Int* **31**:267–72.

Ubelaker DH. 2001. Artificial radiocarbon as an indicator of recent origin of organic remains in forensic cases. *J Forensic Sci* **46**:1285–7.

Ubelaker DH, Volk CG. 2002. A test of the phenice method for the estimation of sex. *J Forensic Sci* **47**:19–24.

Ullrich H. 1975. Estimation of fertility by means of pregnancy and childbirth alterations at the pubis, ilium and sacrum. *Ossa* **2**:23–39.

Vanezis P, Blowes RW, Linney AD, *et al.* 1989. Application of 3-D computer graphics for facial reconstruction and comparison with sculpting techniques. *Forensic Sci Int* **42**:69–84.

Voluter G. 1959. The 'V' test. *Radiol Clin Basel* **28**:1–32.

Wahl J, Graw M. 2001. Metric sex differentiation of the pars petrosa ossis temporalis. *Int J Legal Med* **114**:215–23.

Walker GF. 1976. The computer and the law: coordinate analysis of skull shape and possible methods of postmortem identification. *J Forensic Sci* **21**:357–66.

Warren MW, Schultz JJ. 2002. Post-cremation taphonomy and artifact preservation. *J Forensic Sci* **47**:656–9.

Washburn S. 1948. Sex differences in the pubic bone. *Am J Phys Anthropol* **6**:199–298.

Wells LH. 1959. Estimation of stature from long bones; a reassessment. *J Forensic Med* **6**:171–7.

Wescott DJ. 2000. Sex variation in the second cervical vertebra. *J Forensic Sci* **45**:462–6.

Wescott DJ, Moore-Jansen PH. 2001. Metric variation in the human occipital bone: forensic anthropological applications. *J Forensic Sci* **46**:1159–63.

Williamson MA, Nawrocki SP, Rathbun TA. 2002. Variation in midfacial tissue thickness of African-American children. *J Forensic Sci* **47**:25–31.

Wiredu EK, Kumoji R, Seshadri R, *et al.* 1999. Osteometric analysis of sexual dimorphism in the sternal end of the rib in a West African population. *J Forensic Sci* **44**:921–5.

Yoder C, Ubelaker DH, Powell JF. 2001. Examination of variation in sternal rib end morphology relevant to age assessment. *J Forensic Sci* **46**:223–7.

Yoshino M, Kimijima T, Miyasaka S, *et al.* 1991. Microscopical study on estimation of time since death in skeletal remains. *Forensic Sci Int* **49**:143–58.

Yoshino M, Miyasaka S, Sato H, *et al.* 1987. Classification system of frontal sinus patterns by radiography. Its application to identification of unknown skeletal remains. *Forensic Sci Int* **34**:289–99.

CHAPTER 4

The pathology of wounds

DEFINITION OF A WOUND

A wound or injury can best be defined as 'damage to any part of the body due the application of mechanical force'. Some jurisdictions have a legal definition of a 'wound', which usually requires the integrity of the body surface to be breached. As this obviously excludes bruising and damage to deep organs, it is unrealistic in a medical sense, but there is always some legal alternative, such as 'causing serious bodily harm', which covers any injury to any tissue or organ. Other jurisdictions grade wounds not by their physical nature, but by the perceived risk to life or health of the victim; this can be an extremely difficult prognostic exercise.

MECHANISM OF WOUNDING

The human body is constantly subjected to mechanical forces during the normal course of life, varying from unceasing gravitational forces to the forceful impacts of a sporting contest. The body usually absorbs such forces either by the resilience and elasticity of its soft tissues or the rigid strength of its skeletal framework. It is only when the intensity of the applied force exceeds the capability of the tissues to adapt or resist that a wound or injury occurs.

The intensity of the force obeys the usual laws of physics, in that the force varies directly with the mass of the 'weapon' and directly with the **square** of velocity of impact.

Of course, the weapon can be anything, including the body itself, as is often seen in the violent deceleration of a fall or in a traffic accident.

The well-known formula: Force = ½ mass × velocity², means that a one kilogram brick pressed against the scalp will cause no injury, but the same brick thrown against the head at a velocity of 10 m/s may smash the skull. This principle is relevant not only in relation to blunt injury and firearm missiles, but also to stab wounds, as is discussed later.

Another factor of importance is the area over which the force acts. If a plank of wood is struck against the skin, the damage to the tissues will be far greater if the narrow edge is used, than if the impact is from the flat surface. Obviously, the force derived from the same mass and velocity is applied over a smaller area, thus delivering a greater impact to any given unit of tissue. This again is relevant to stab wounds, as all the kinetic energy of a moving knife is concentrated into the tiny area of the tip of the blade; the same energy delivered by the large surface area of a cricket bat might not even cause a bruise.

The effect of excessive mechanical forces on the tissues of the body can cause compression, traction, torsion, and tangential (shear) and leverage stresses. The resultant damage depends not only on the type of the mechanical insult but also on the nature of the target tissue. For instance, violent compression (as in an explosion) may do little harm to muscle, but may rupture lung or intestine, while torsion may leave adipose tissue unaffected, yet cause a spiral fracture in a femur.

The transfer of kinetic energy from the relative movements of the body and the weapon is the source of damage to the tissues. If the attacking object comes to rest in the tissues, then all its kinetic energy must have been transferred. A bullet which passes clean through the tissues thus fails to exchange all its energy into trauma production, which is the reason for the illegal 'dumdum' or more recent, explosive-tipped bullets, the object of which is to expand the missile and prevent its exit from the body, so increasing its 'stopping power' (see Chapter 8). If such energy transfer can be slowed down or spread over a wider area, then the intensity of force applied to the tissues per unit of time is less. This is part of the function of a seatbelt in a vehicle crash, where the stretching of the belt fabric extends the time of energy exchange and the considerable area of the belt surface is a preferable alternative to transferring all the kinetic energy via a few square centimetres of forehead against the windscreen.

Other ways in which the transfer of kinetic energy may be modified is in moving the body in the direction of the force. When a car strikes a pedestrian, that proportion of the momentum of the car that is used in projecting the victim along the road is not then available for damaging the tissues.

Similarly, if a boxer 'rides the punch', he is reducing the differential velocity between his head and his opponent's fist, as well as extending the time over which energy transfer occurs. With a high-speed impact, such as a bullet and – to a lesser extent a stab or violent blow – the inertia of the victim's body prevents any significant loss of energy transfer by movement. If the force does not strike in a linear fashion, but leads to a tangential impact – as in a glancing blow causing a 'graze' – then only part of the kinetic energy is transferred and the damage will be proportionately less.

CLASSIFICATION OF WOUNDS

This is quite arbitrary, but when writing medical reports (especially for legal purposes) it is essential that every doctor should use a standardized nomenclature when describing wounds. All too often reports are seen – especially from clinicians who are not used to medico-legal work – where 'laceration', 'incised wound' and 'abrasion' are used loosely, the accompanying descriptions making it obvious that no clear distinction between them was appreciated by the doctor.

Wounds may also be categorized by the motivation of their infliction, such as 'suicidal or accidental' (the 'manner' index of the WHO International Classification of Disease, ICD E-codes), but a pathologist should classify them by their appearance and the method of causation, such as 'laceration' or 'incised wound'. The most useful classification is:

- Abrasions – colloquially 'grazes or scratches'.
- Contusions – colloquially 'bruises'.
- Lacerations – colloquially 'cuts or tears'.
- Incised wounds – colloquially 'cuts', 'slashes' or 'stabs'.

FORENSIC ANATOMY OF THE SKIN

As most wounds involve the body surface, a reminder of the structure and nomenclature of the skin and subcutaneous tissues is appropriate. Most superficial is the keratinized dead layer of cells, the stratum corneum, which varies greatly in thickness from one part of the body to another. That on the soles and palms is the thickest, while that on protected areas such as the scrotum and eyelids measures

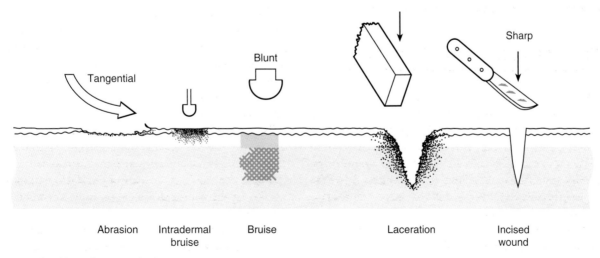

FIGURE 4.1 *Types of injury to the skin.*

only a fraction of a millimetre. This has forensic relevance in the amount of injury that is needed to penetrate the skin and allow bleeding from the underlying tissues.

The living layers of the skin combine with the horny layer to form the epidermis, which has no blood vessels in its thickness. The epidermis is generally corrugated, the under surface by papillae that dip into the dermis. The degree of undulation also varies greatly from place to place, the thinner skin tending to have a flatter junction between dermis and epidermis. The dermis (or 'corium') consists of mixed connective tissue carrying the skin adnexae, such as hair follicles, sweat glands and sebaceous glands. It has a rich network of blood vessels, nerves and lymphatics, and has numerous nerve endings of various types for tactile, pressure and heat sensing. The lower zone of the dermis has adipose tissue and – depending on the site in the body – deep fascia, fatty tissue and muscle will form strata below the skin itself.

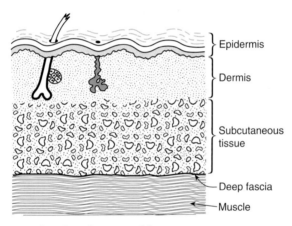

FIGURE 4.2 *General structure of skin.*

ABRASIONS

An abrasion is the most superficial of injuries and, in the most restrictive of definitions, is one that does not penetrate the full thickness of the epidermis. Thus the pure abrasion does not bleed, as blood vessels are confined to the dermis. Because of the corrugated nature of the dermal papillae, however, many abrasions enter the corium and bleeding commonly occurs.

Another definition (all of which are arbitrary) would describe an abrasion as a superficial injury to 'the skin', which would allow penetration of the upper dermis rather than only the epidermis, so that bleeding would fall within the definition.

Abrasions are known in lay terms as 'scratches' or 'grazes', though the former usually indicates a linear mark and the latter a 'brush' abrasion caused by wider tangential impact. Where these brush abrasions are the result of scraping contact with the ground, the lay term is a 'gravel rash'. There are many causes of abrasions, which are common everyday lesions, especially in children whose legs are rarely free from some scratches and bruises. Any contact that rubs across the epidermis and removes the keratinized layer and underlying cells will cause that area to become discoloured and moistened by exuded tissue fluid, even if bleeding does not occur from abraded dermal papillae.

When death ensues soon afterwards, the abrasion becomes stiff, leathery and of a parchment-like brown colour as a result of the drying of the moist exposed surface. This is classically seen, for example, in the ligature mark of hanging or strangulation. It is impossible to tell whether a superficial abrasion occurred immediately before or after

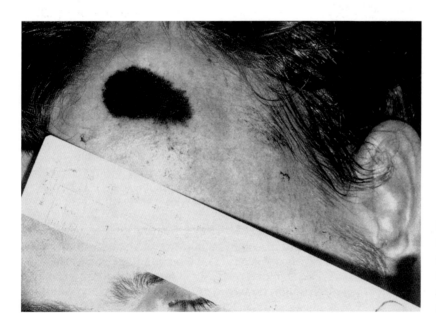

FIGURE 4.3 *Simple abrasion of the skin caused by an almost perpendicular impact of the head against the ground. There is only slight tangential scuffing though most abrasions have some element of sideways contact that damages the epidermis.*

death if there was insufficient time for any inflammatory reaction to occur at the margins. Post-mortem abrasions are common, especially after autopsy when the body is re-examined, because mortuary instruments and the moving of bodies into refrigerators and coffins can often make marks. These abrasions commonly appear yellow and translucent, and are absolutely devoid of any colour change at the edge.

Tangential or brush abrasions

Most abrasions are caused by a lateral rubbing action rather than vertical pressure. Where this tangential component is marked, the direction of the force can often be determined by tags of epidermis dragged to the terminal end of the abrasion. For example, in the 'brush abrasion', which is common in childhood falls and pedestrian accidents, the skidding of the body across a rough surface scrapes linear furrows across the skin. Strands and tags of epidermis may be peeled along these furrows to the further end where contact ceased. Visual examination, using a lens if necessary, can indicate the direction of movement of the body. Similarly, if a victim is struck a glancing blow with a rough object such as a stone or brick, similar epidermal tags may indicate the direction of the blow.

The same type of grooved abrasions can be caused when a victim is dragged along the ground, either in a vehicular accident or by an assailant. It may be important, though difficult, to attempt to differentiate such drag marks as being ante-mortem or post-mortem, a problem which is discussed in another chapter.

Crushing abrasions

Where the impact is vertical to the skin surface, no scraping or tangential marks occur. Instead the epidermis is crushed and an imprint of the impacting object is stamped on the surface. If the impact is substantial and the area of contact small,

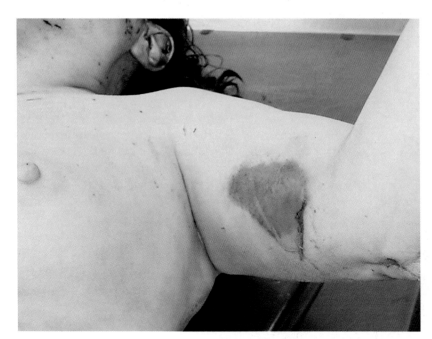

FIGURE 4.4 *A linear abrasion or 'graze', confined to the upper layers of the skin. The tangential direction of impact of the weapon was from above downwards (along the longitudinal axis of the upper arm), as can be determined by the shreds of epidermis peeled towards the lower end.*

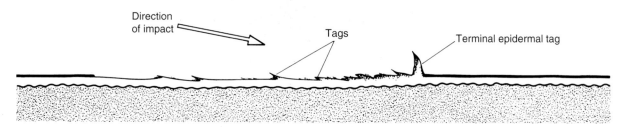

FIGURE 4.5 *Determination of the direction of impact in an abrasion caused by a tangential force. The epidermal tags raised by the impact tend to pile up at the distal end.*

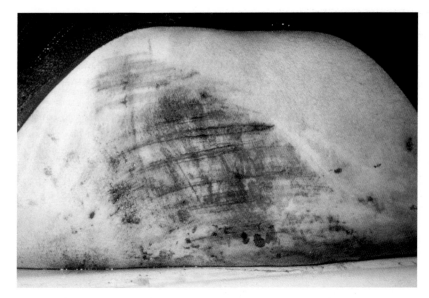

FIGURE 4.6 *'Brush abrasion' or 'grazes' caused by tangential contact of a moving body with a rough surface. Although most are seen in traffic accidents from contact with the road surface, this example is from a murdered woman dropped down a mine shaft. There are grazes running in two directions at right angles, indicating that she must have struck the wall twice, in different postures.*

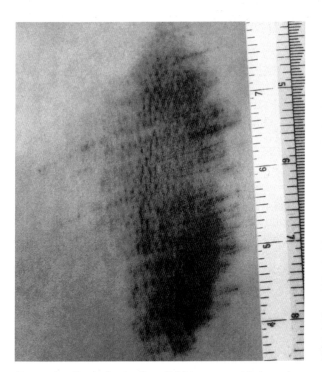

FIGURE 4.7 *Brush abrasion from skidding contact with the road surface during a drunken scuffle. The lesion is partly abraded and partly bruised. The direction of movement can be discerned, as the scratches begin more abruptly and deeply near the ruler, and tail off superficially at the opposite edge.*

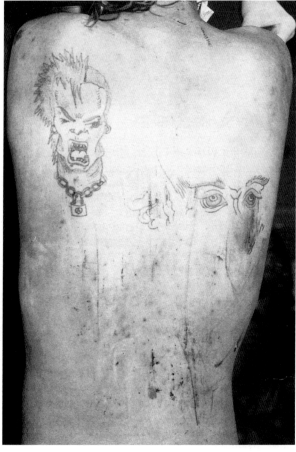

FIGURE 4.8 *Drag marks on the back of a murder victim. Death was caused by a stab wound of the front of the chest – the body was pulled along the ground for a short distance, obviously in the direction of the feet, as the scratch near the waist is deeper near the feet end and tails off at the opposite end.*

a punctured wound will be made, but otherwise a crushed abrasion will occur. The lesion is slightly depressed below the surface unless an underlying bruise or local oedema bulges the tissues. These abrasions are the ones that most clearly reproduce the pattern of the injuring object. An example

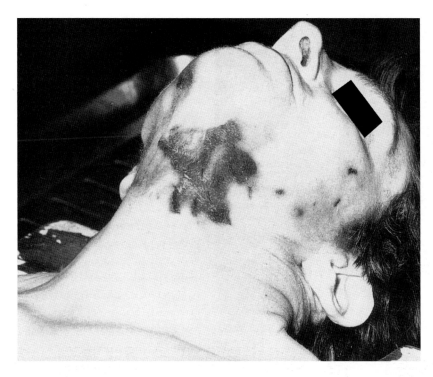

FIGURE 4.9 *Abrasions in manual strangulation. The area is more extensive than is usually seen in such circumstances. The large area of superficial damage to the epidermis is caused by sliding movements of the assailant's hands, the area having become dried and leathery during the post-mortem interval. The smaller marks are fingernail scratches.*

would be the marks of a vehicle radiator on a pedestrian victim or the pattern of a floor grid on to which a person has fallen. If the impact is forcible, then the dermis may also be injured: an area of bruising may underlie the abrasion.

Fingernail abrasions

These are important because of their frequency in assaults – especially child abuse, sexual attacks and strangulation. Often associated with focal bruises, fingernail abrasions are most often seen on the neck, the face, the upper arms and the forearms. They may be linear scratches if the fingers are dragged down the skin, or short, straight or curved marks when the skin is gripped in a static fashion. As women tend to have longer, sharper fingernails than men, they are naturally more often associated with causing such abrasions. A victim resisting a sexual or other attack may rake her nails down her assailant's face, causing linear, parallel scratches that may be several millimetres wide and placed a centimetre or two apart. The expected pattern may be fragmentary, however, as is often seen on the neck when a victim of either manual or ligature strangulation attempts to tear away the attacking fingers or cord. These marks are usually vertical, as opposed to the more random marks that may be inflicted by the nails of the assailant in manual strangulation.

The upper arms are a frequent site for gripping and restraint, both in adult assaults and child abuse. Bruising is most common, but fingernail marks may be superimposed. Static fingernail abrasions may be straight or curved, often

about half to one centimetre long. The direction of curvature must be interpreted with care if one wishes to decide which way the hand was held at the time of infliction.

Although it is natural to assume that the concavity of the mark indicates the orientation of the fingertip, experiments by Shapiro *et al.* (1962) have shown that this is often not the case. Because the skin is put under lateral tension when it is indented by the nails, it may distort, so that when the tension is released the elasticity of the skin causes it to return to its original position, carrying the nail mark with it. The curve may then reverse to form either a straight line or a convexity. The shape of the free edge of the fingernail also affects the mark, as pointed nails are more likely than those with straight edges to give these paradoxical results. Once again, the pathologist has to be wary of incorrect interpretation when, for instance, deciding if nail marks on a neck were made by hands approaching from the front or passing around the back of the neck. However, personal experiments with the Shapiro *et al.* contention have shown that it by no means always applies.

Patterned abrasions

Formerly it was often claimed that abrasions retained the pattern of the impacting object more accurately than other injuries such as bruises and lacerations. Though abrasions undoubtedly do preserve such patterns well, many of the examples were not in fact true abrasions, but were intra-dermal bruises, mentioned in the next section.

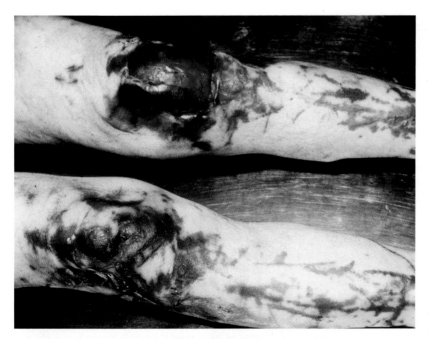

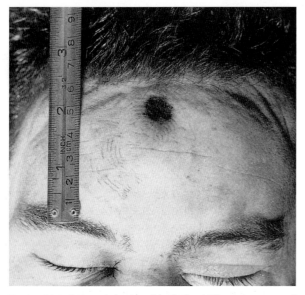

FIGURE 4.10 *Extensive abrasion of the knees and shins, in a drunk who stumbled amongst furniture before dying of a head injury. The damaged skin has exuded tissue fluid, which has dried post-mortem to produce the dark, leathery appearance.*

FIGURE 4.11 *Patterned abrasion of the forehead. The victim was struck on the head in a public house with a heavy glass ashtray, the bottom of which had embossed concentric circles moulded into the glass.*

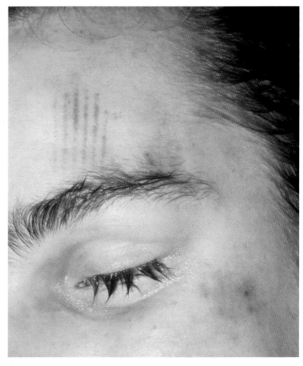

FIGURE 4.12 *Abrasions and intradermal bruising on the forehead of a swimming bath attendant. He was found drowned when there were no witnesses, but the spacing of the marks exactly matched the ridged tiles at the edge of the bath, so it was presumed that he had slipped and struck his head before falling unconscious into the water.*

Patterned injuries occur when the force is applied at or near a right angle to the skin surface, rather than with the skidding impact of a graze. If a weapon with a patterned surface strikes the skin – or the body falls against a patterned surface – the abrasion of the epidermis follows the ridges of the object if it has a profile of varying height. Not only may the epidermis be damaged, but the skin may be compressed into the cavities of the pattern, with consequent capillary damage leading to an intradermal bruise. Probably the best example of this is seen when a motor tyre passes over

the skin, leaving a pattern where the skin has been squeezed into the grooves of the rubber tread.

There is little point in trying to list all the possible patterns that can be distinguished in abrasions on a body, but a few

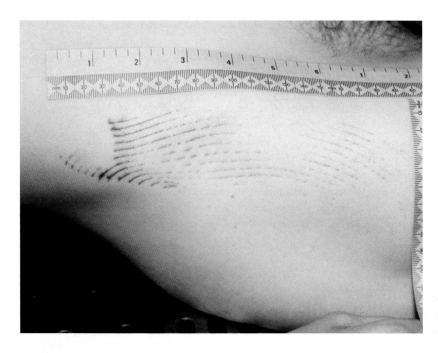

FIGURE 4.13 *Patterned abrasions from the back edge of a serrated 'Rambo' knife. Measurements and photographs with a scale should always be obtained to assist in the identification of the weapon.*

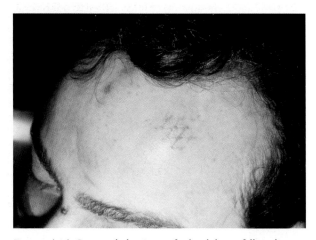

FIGURE 4.14 *Patterned abrasion on forehead due to falling down steps onto a metal grid. Here the abrasions are not produced by tangential force, but imprinted directly by impact at a right angle to the skin.*

have particular medico-legal significance. In former years the honeycomb grid of a motor-vehicle radiator provided many examples of patterned abrasions, but changes in vehicle design have relegated these to historical interest. There may still be projections on vehicles that cause damage, but these are more likely to inflict bruises and lacerations. The muzzle of a firearm can imprint an abrasion on the skin, which is of importance in that it confirms that the discharge was contact in nature. Impact against ribbed ceramic tiles in a bathroom or swimming bath may assist in reconstructing unwitnessed events. Blows from a weapon with a recognizable surface may

help to identify that weapon, such as a plaited rope or leather whip, or a solid object with an embossed pattern. Abrasions from objects with a recurring pattern, such as bicycle chain used in gang fights, or a serrated knife, can readily provide a clue to the nature of the weapon.

Post-mortem abrasions

Unlike post-mortem bruises, artefactual abrasions are common. They may have been inflicted after death from a variety of causes, including dragging a corpse or buffeting in moving water. Some post-mortem animal injuries also resemble abrasions such as insect bites, especially by ants.

Other damage may be caused following autopsy. As the post-mortem interval increases, so the skin becomes more fragile. Even the normal procedures of post-autopsy reconstruction and handling in the mortuary may cause dermal damage, especially after washing with hot water. If the pathologist returns for a later examination, or if he is retained to perform a second autopsy for the defence, the appearances should be checked with the original description or photographs, if some injuries suggest a post-mortem origin.

CONTUSIONS OR BRUISES

Although often combined with abrasions or lacerations, a pure bruise lies beneath an intact epidermis and consists of an extravascular collection of blood that has leaked from blood vessels damaged by mechanical impact. An extravasation of blood that is (arbitrarily) larger than a few millimetres in diameter, is usually termed a 'bruise' or 'contusion'. This size overlaps the older and now little used term 'ecchymosis', which is really a small bruise.

Even smaller is the 'petechial haemorrhage', which is the size of a pin head or less. Both ecchymoses and petechiae are not usually caused by direct mechanical trauma and are often seen on serous membranes and conjunctivae as well as on skin. However, moderate pressure, impact or, especially, suction on the skin can produce a patch of localized petechiae.

Bruises are caused by damage to veins, venules and small arteries. Capillary bleeding would be visible only under a microscope and even petechiae originate from a larger order of blood vessel than a capillary.

The word 'bruise' usually implies that the lesion is visible through the skin or present in the subcutaneous tissues, whilst a 'contusion' can be anywhere in the body, such as the spleen, mesentery or muscles. The two words are often interchanged at random, however, though 'bruise' is to be preferred when a doctor gives reports or evidence to a non-medical audience.

Intradermal bruises

These are important but rarely mentioned in most texts. The usual bruise from a blunt impact is situated in the subcutaneous tissues, often in the fat layer. When viewed through the overlying corium and epidermis, the bruise is somewhat blurred, especially at the edge. When a bruise is made by impact with a patterned object, however, the haemorrhage may be far more sharply defined, if it lies in the immediate subepidermal layer. The amount of blood is relatively small, but because of its superficial position and the translucency of the thin layer that overlies it, the pattern is distinct.

Such bruises are especially likely to occur when the impacting object has alternating ridges and grooves, as the skin will be forced into the grooves and be sharply distorted. Intradermal bleeding will occur here and the areas in contact with the raised ridges may remain pale, as the pressure forces the blood from the small vessels. A good example is that of a motor tyre running across the surface. Impacts from whips with patterned thongs may also show the same phenomenon, as do the ribbed rubber soles of 'trainer' shoes.

Factors affecting the prominence of a bruise

Several factors influence the apparent size and prominence of a bruise and, because of these, it is not possible to be dogmatic about the amount of force needed to produce any given bruise.

■ As it is a leakage of blood from a vessel, there must be sufficient space outside that vessel for free blood to accumulate. This explains the ease with which bruising appears in lax tissues such as the eye socket or scrotum and its rarity in the sole of the foot or palm of the hand, where dense fibrous tissue and restrictive fascial planes prevent accumulation of blood. Because of the greater volume of soft subcutaneous tissue in fat people, they

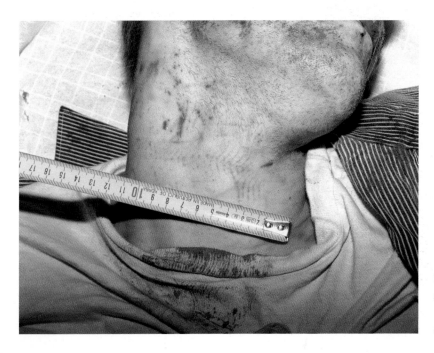

FIGURE 4.15 *Intradermal bruising showing the pattern of rubber soles of 'trainer' shoes on the neck and T-shirt of a homicide victim.*

tend to bruise more easily than thin ones, other factors being equal (such as vessel fragility and senile changes).

- The apparent prominence of a bruise beneath the skin varies with the amount of blood in the extravasation. The size of the haemorrhage depends partly, but not entirely, on the intensity of the injuring force. The size and density of the vascular network varies from place to place and the amount of damage that a given blow causes to local blood vessels is partly a matter of chance.

- Resilient areas, such as the abdominal wall and buttocks, bruise less with a given impact than a region where underlying bone acts an anvil with the skin between the bone and the inflicting force. The head, chest and shins are examples.

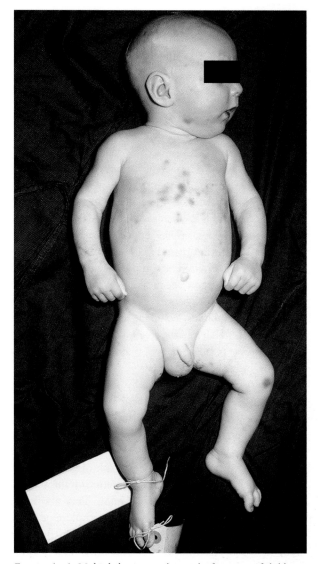

FIGURE 4.16 *Multiple bruises on the trunk of a victim of child abuse. The bruises are of the 'fingertip' type, caused by heavy prodding by adult fingers. The child died of a ruptured liver.*

- The depth at which the bruise is placed affects the apparent severity. A bruise may be placed superficially in the dermis to form the well-patterned intradermal bruise mentioned in the previous section; here, a minute amount of blood will be obvious. Most bruises are in the subcutaneous tissues above the deep fascia and will therefore be fairly obvious, but others can be confined below deeper fascial membranes so that the free blood has to be viewed through the skin and underlying adipose tissue. For a given size of extravasation, this bruise will be less prominent. Some bruises are confined to deep fascial compartments and never become visible without dissection.

- For a given impact, the volume of blood lost into the tissues can depend upon the fragility of the blood vessels and the coagulability of the blood. In old persons, vessel fragility may be extreme and a large bruise may develop from the slightest of knocks. Children tend to bruise more easily than adults, presumably because of the softer tissues and the smaller volume of protecting tissue that overlies the vessels. Any bleeding diathesis resulting from disease, a toxic condition, or certain medication, will also retard the normal clotting process that heals the breach in the bleeding vessels. Those with scurvy and chronic alcoholics bleed easily but, in contrast, certain people (such as boxers) seem able to avoid bruising from blows that would severely damage other people.

- It is common knowledge among lay people, as well as doctors, that a bruise may 'come out' – that is, become more prominent with the passage of hours or days. This is partly caused by continued bleeding from the ruptured vessels, but mainly by percolation of free blood from its origin deeper in the tissues upwards towards the epidermis. Another factor may be haemolysis, when the freed haemoglobin is able to stain the tissues in a more diffuse way and become more noticeable than intact red blood cells. This latter mechanism is certainly the reason not only for the well-known post-mortem phenomenon of bruises becoming more prominent after death, but of new bruises appearing later where none was visible at an autopsy performed soon after death. This is further considered in the chapter on post-mortem changes, but is repeated here because of the importance of recognizing the differences in appearance that can occur between two autopsy examinations spaced a few days apart. The second, usually for a defence opinion, may find new bruises not recorded by the first pathologist, but if the phenomenon of delayed appearance is appreciated, potential disputes may be avoided.

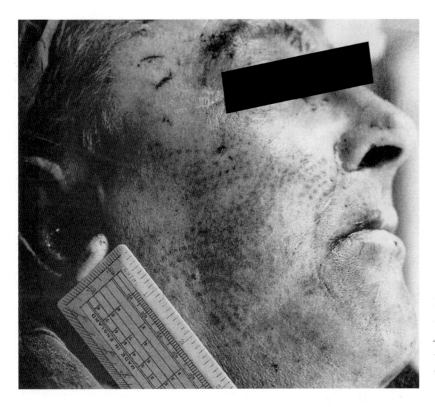

FIGURE 4.17 *Patterned abrasion and intradermal bruising of the face during a fatal armed robbery. The watchman was struck in the face by an assailant wearing a hard-corded driving glove with a coarse-weave pattern.*

Movement of bruises

A bruise may appear at a different place on the surface from the point of impact. When the bruise is superficial, especially intradermal bruising, the lesion appears immediately – or at least rapidly – and is at the point of infliction. When blood extravasates in the deep tissues, however, it may take time to reach the surface (if it ever does), and this may be some distance away because of deflection and obstruction by fascial planes and other anatomical structures.

In addition, bruises may move under gravity. The most frequent example is a bruise or a bleed under a laceration on the upper forehead. If the victim survives for at least some hours, then the subcutaneous haemorrhage can slide downwards over the eyebrow ridge and appear in the orbit, to give a 'black eye', which might be misinterpreted as direct trauma. Similarly a bruise of the upper arm or thigh may surface lower down around the elbow or knee.

Alteration of bruises with time

As already mentioned, bruises often become more prominent some hours or days after infliction because red cells or haemoglobin diffuse closer to the translucent epidermis. There is another temporal series of changes in bruises in the living person, this being part of the healing process. Fresh extravasation of blood is obviously dark red, though when viewed through the skin this may be purple or almost black in appearance. In racially pigmented victims, a bruise may sometimes be undetectable from the surface, apart from swelling caused by a haematoma and tissue oedema.

With the passage of time, the haematoma breaks down under the influence of tissue enzymes and cellular infiltration. The red-cell envelopes rupture and the contained haemoglobin undergoes chemical degradation, which causes a sequence of colour changes. The haemoglobin is broken down into compounds including haemosiderin, biliverdin and bilirubin, which lead the colour changes through a spectrum of purple to bluish brown, to greenish brown to green to yellow, before complete fading.

A small skin bruise in a healthy young adult might be expected to pass through all these stages and vanish in about a week, but there is a tendency to overestimate the length of time needed as shown by Roberts (1983), who observed that 'love bite' bruises in sexual offences could become yellow and vanish within a couple of days. Langlois and Gresham (1991) reviewed the literature on this subject, indicating the wide variation in opinion. They also made careful photographic records of the macroscopic appearance of bruising on 89 subjects, aged between 10 and 100 years. They concluded that the most significant change was the appearance of a yellow colour (in persons less than 65 years of age), which indicated that the bruise could not be less than 18 hours old. Blue, purple and red did not assist in

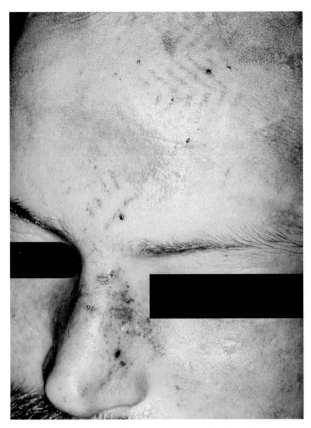

FIGURE 4.18 *Kicking and stamping injury to the face. The nose is bruised from a kick and the patterned rubber sole of the shoe has imprinted intradermal bruising on the forehead. It is essential to obtain accurate photographs and measurements of the shoe-tread pattern, to allow identification of the footwear.*

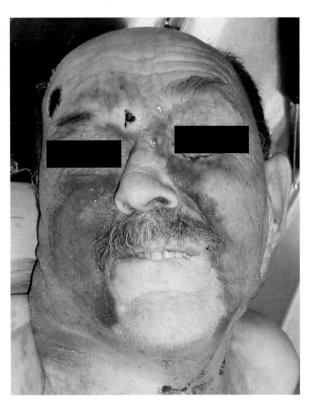

FIGURE 4.19 *Extensive bruising of the face due to hitting, kicking and stamping 6 days earlier. The victim had multiple fractures of the facial bones, bilateral serial rib fractures and a tension pneumothorax.*

dating bruises; brown was held to be a mixture of colours and was not considered as useful.

In the present authors' experience, it is impossible to comment on the age of a bruise less than 24 hours since infliction, except to say that it is 'fresh', as no visible changes occur in that time.

It is not practicable to construct an accurate calendar of these colour changes, as was done in older textbooks, as there are too many variables for this to be reliable. These include:

■ the size of the extravasation – changes begin at the margin and a larger bruise will take a longer time to be absorbed. A large old bruise may contain all the colours possible – from purple in the centre to yellow at the edges

■ the age and constitution of the victim. Aged persons may not heal their bruises at all and carry them for the remainder of their lives

■ a personal idiosyncrasy in the rapidity with which such changes occur in any one person, including coagulation defects.

Even histological examination is unreliable in the accurate dating of bruises, as is discussed later in this chapter. The appearance of stainable iron, in the form of haemosiderin, however, does not usually appear within the first 2 or 3 days, though Simpson suggests that it may be found as early as 24 hours. In meningeal haemorrhage, it seems to appear from around 36 hours.

Haematoidin, another breakdown product of blood pigment, can appear in old bruises and haematomas after the first week.

Though an absolute date cannot therefore be placed upon a bruise, the following observations are legitimate.

■ If a bruise appears fresh over all its area, with no observable colour change, it is unlikely to have been inflicted more than about 2 days before death, except in old persons.

■ If the bruise has any green discoloration, it was inflicted not later than 18 hours before death (Roberts 1983; Langlois and Gresham 1991).

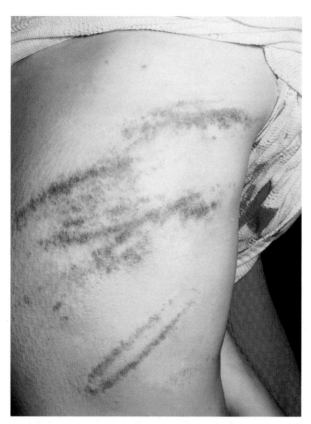

FIGURE 4.20 *Bruises from a beating with a broom handle. They are approximately parallel and several, especially the lowermost, show a double 'tram-line' appearance typical of the impact of a round or square-section rod. The pressure in the centre compresses the vessels so that they do not bleed.*

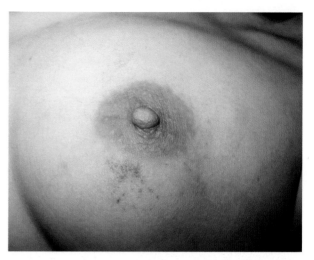

FIGURE 4.21 *Suction marks in the left breast of a 22-year-old homicide victim, who was killed by manual and ligature strangulation.*

■ If several bruises (of roughly comparable size and site) are present and are of markedly different colours, then they could not have been inflicted at the same time. This is particularly important in suspected child abuse, where intermittent episodes of injury have important diagnostic significance.

Bruising of special significance

Certain types of bruise and bruises at particular sites have a specific significance. Clusters of small discoid bruises of about a centimetre in diameter are characteristic of finger-tip pressure from either gripping or prodding. These groups are often seen in child abuse, when an adult hand grips the infant by a convenient 'handle'. Once called 'six-penny bruises' from their size, the lesions are commonly seen on the forearms or upper arms of the child, or sometimes around the wrist or ankle, though they can occur on the abdomen. Similar bruises from fingertips may be seen

on the neck of children or adults in manual strangulation, though there is often additional diffuse bruising caused by a sliding grip on the neck.

When the skin surface is struck by a rod or rectangular sectioned object such as a cane or lath, the consequent bruising may be of the 'tram-line' or 'railway line' type. This appears as two parallel lines of bruising with an undamaged zone in the centre. The mechanism of this double line is that the weapon sinks into the skin on impact so that the edges drag the skin downwards and the traction tears the marginal blood vessels. The centre compresses the skin, which, in the absence of underlying bone, causes little or no damage to the vessels. When the momentary impact is released, blood flows back into the injured marginal zones and leaks into the tissues. Impact from broom handles, narrow planks and wood or metal rods can all cause this characteristic lesion.

As with abrasions, bites can result in bruises; this is dealt with in Chapter 26. It might be noted here that the so-called 'love bites' are often bruises, with or without associated abrasions, being a shower of small petechial lesions caused by oral suction on the skin.

The common 'black eye' is dealt with under 'Head injuries' in Chapter 5, but again it is worth repeating that not all black eyes are true bruising from a blow in the orbit. Some are from fractured orbital roofs and others are the result of gravitational movement of a forehead injury.

A bruise below the ear in a death from subarachnoid haemorrhage needs careful examination of the upper cervical spine and basilo-vertebral arteries, again as discussed under 'Head injuries' in Chapter 5.

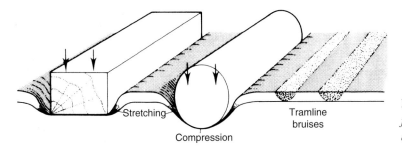

FIGURE 4.22 *Formation of 'tram-line' bruising from the application of a rectangular or cylindrical object.*

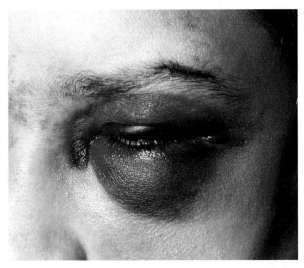

FIGURE 4.23 *A black eye (peri-orbital haematoma) of a live victim from a direct fist blow, which has also bruised the bridge of the nose and lacerated the corner of the eye (sutured).*

KICKING

The shod foot may leave a patterned bruise on the body, most often on the abdomen or chest, though it may be recognizable on the neck or face. A glancing kick is more likely to cause scuffed abrasions and bruising, and a kick from a toecap, a curved abrasion or even laceration. A vertical stamping action may imprint an intradermal bruise corresponding to the sole pattern, especially in these days of rubber 'trainer' shoes. As with a motor tyre, the skin can be forced into the slots in the sole, creating an accurate pattern of superficial bruising. There may also be more diffuse deep bruising if the impact is severe, but this is less useful in delineating an identifiable sole pattern.

Kicking has become increasingly common with the increase in violence and vicious hooliganism in society. The heavy footwear fashionable among some of the least responsible citizens adds to the severity of the lesions.

Though most kicking injuries end up in hospital casualty departments, an increasing number reach the pathologist.

Not all victims are drunken youths, as many assaults upon old people by intruders and muggers involve severe kicking.

Obviously, most kicks are delivered with the victim already lying or sitting on the ground, having been brought there by some other means of violence, including pushing, tripping and fist punches. Once prostrate, the 'boot is put in' towards the most convenient targets, which tend to be the concavities of the body. The loin, the groin, the neck and the face are often attacked, and – when the victim assumes a 'fetal position' on his side for protection – swings may be taken into the abdominal area. As an alternative to swinging kicks, the foot may be brought vertically down on the prone victim, the heel being the most damaging part, rather than the toecap. A grinding motion can also be added, which may tear the skin and cause ragged lacerations.

Yet another variant is standing on the body or actually jumping onto it with one or both feet. The chest is the most common target for this practice and fractured ribs or sternum, a flail chest and cardiac injuries can result.

The major characteristic of most kicking injuries is the severity of bruising and underlying damage. Even if the toecap does not cause lacerations, there may be large haematomata and intramuscular contusions from heavy kicks. Abdominal and thoracic viscera can be ruptured and the genitalia are also vulnerable, especially the scrotum and sometimes urethra.

A common danger with kicking to the face is fracture of either (or both) mandible and maxilla, nasal bones and zygoma, though the cranial vault is seldom fractured and kicks to the vertex of the head seem less common. With such facial injuries, death may occur from filling of the pharynx and air passages with blood. A kick on one side of the face can completely detach the lower maxilla – with the upper dental arch and palate – from the rest of the maxilla. A unilateral kick of the jaw can fracture both rami of the mandible, there being no necessity for kicks on either side.

Post-mortem bruising and other artefacts

It is possible to cause what appears to be a bruise by deliberate violence to a dead body, but the amount of force

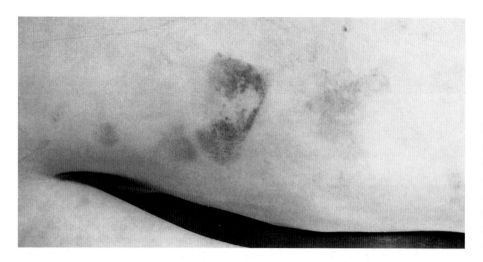

FIGURE 4.24 *A footmark imprinted in superficial bruising on the back. There is another partial mark at waist level, both being made by stamping with the flat of a foot through thin clothing, rather than by swinging kicks.*

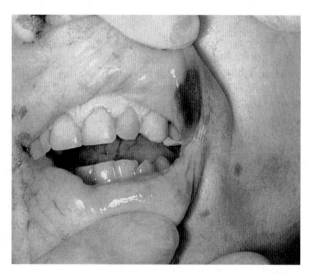

FIGURE 4.25 *Bruising of the interior of the lip from a blow in the mouth. The lip has been impacted on the underlying teeth, but not sufficiently hard to cause a laceration.*

as pressure on the neck, the venous system may be engorged at death and a number of artefactual haemorrhages may occur. One particularly important area described fully elsewhere is the neck, in which collections of blood between the oesophagus and cervical spine may simulate bruising from manual strangulation. These were fully investigated by Prinsloo and Gordon (1951) and, where neck trauma is suspected, it is advisable to remove the brain before dissecting the neck region to allow drainage of the engorged venous plexuses that give rise to the artefact. This phenomenon appears to be related to the post-mortem interval and is more likely to arise if there is a delay in autopsy.

LACERATIONS

The third major type of blunt injury is the laceration, in which the full thickness of the skin is penetrated.

Lacerations differ from incised wounds in that the continuity of the tissues is disrupted by tearing rather than clean slicing, but the distinction is often blurred because some lacerations are caused by jagged projections ripping into the skin in much the same manner as a blunt knife or axe.

Unless great force is used, most lacerations require a firm base to act as an anvil for the skin and underlying tissue to be pinned against. It is unusual for a blunt impact to lacerate the abdomen or buttock, but the scalp, shins, shoulder, face and – to a lesser extent – the thorax, are all prone to lacerated injury. Where a soft area such as buttock, thigh, calf or forearm is lacerated, the lacerating agent is either a projecting point or edge, or a completely blunt object is pulled obliquely against the tension of the skin until it tears. Because of the crushing and tearing components of a laceration, there is usually associated abrasion and bruising,

required is great. As there is no internal pressure in the small vessels that have to be ruptured, bleeding is a passive ooze rather than an active extravasation, so the size of the haemorrhage is slight in relation to the amount of effort expended. Thus, post-mortem skin bruising is of little practical significance to the pathologist – in most instances he can be reassured that new or more obvious bruising apparent when he returns several days later for a second examination of a body is genuine. Post-mortem abrasions are common, especially after a first autopsy and additional handling of the body in the mortuary, but these procedures rarely produce artefactual bruises.

More important than dermal artefacts are spurious bruises inside the body. Especially in congestive deaths, such

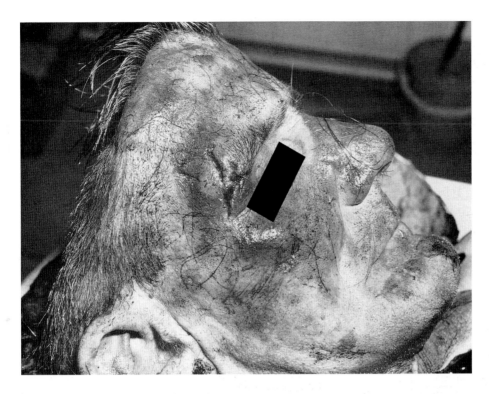

FIGURE 4.26 *Laceration of the eyebrow with surrounding bruising. The wound is stellate as a result of crushing against the underlying bone. The victim fell from a low cliff on to rocks. The sea has washed away the original bleeding.*

though these may be minimal if the lacerating force acts at right angles to the surface.

The scalp offers the best example of a laceration, as the skin and subcutaneous tissue lie over the bony platform of the skull and are crushed against it when the force impacts. In fact, scalp lacerations can resemble incised wounds, because this 'sandwich effect' is so pronounced that a blow from a blunt instrument can cleanly split the tissues against the skull, leaving a linear wound that appears to the inexperienced to be a knife or chopper cut.

A laceration can be distinguished from an incised wound by:

- the bruising and crushing of the margins, though this may be a very narrow zone, requiring inspection through a lens
- the persistence of tissue strands across the interior of the wound, including fascial bands, vessels and nerves. In a wound from a sharp weapon these are divided
- the absence of a sharply linear injury in the underlying bone, especially if it is the skull. A knife or axe is likely to chip or score the base of the wound
- if the area is covered with hair, as on the scalp, intact hairs will survive to cross the wound; an incised injury would divide them.

A flat impact may cause a laceration, especially on the scalp. If the head falls to the ground or is hit by a wide, flat weapon, the skin and subcutaneous tissues are compressed

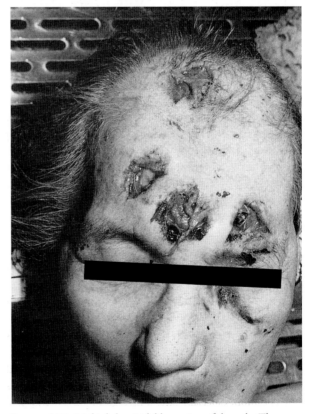

FIGURE 4.27 *Multiple homicidal lacerations of the scalp. The unusual shape is difficult to interpret, but they were caused by a claw hammer. Two are triangular, the upper and lower show tissue bridges because of the gap between the two claws.*

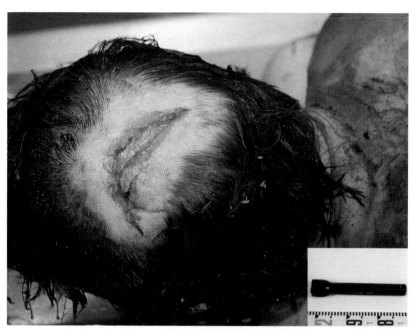

FIGURE 4.28 *Laceration of the scalp from a 30 cm long heavy torch (insert). The skin over the shoulders is reddish due to first- and second-degree burns. The victim was hit on the head while sleeping in bed, after which the husband poured petrol over the body and set it on fire.*

on the anvil of the skull and may split sideways, often with a zone of surrounding bruising.

Other lacerations are caused by the impact of an edged object, be this a rod, a brick, the edge of a kerbstone or the wing mirror of a vehicle. Though the impact may be virtually perpendicular to the skin surface, there is usually some tangential element and this can cause one edge of the wound to differ from the other. Where there is a glancing element, one edge will be relatively clean-cut, whereas the other will be ripped away from the first, suffering more tearing of the margin and often showing undercutting of the edge. If the impact is significantly asymmetrical, then this undercutting may be pronounced enough to form a flap of skin and underlying tissue, which is peeled off the underlying bone or deep fascia.

In extreme forms, this produces a 'flaying injury', where a large area of skin and subcutaneous tissue is rolled off a limb, almost always by the rotary action of a revolving motor wheel. A similar injury can occur on the scalp again from a rotating wheel – though a similar 'scalping' lesion can be caused by traction from hair being trapped in machinery. This was formerly a common industrial accident and was the reason for the 'snood' hairnet being worn by women factory workers during the last war.

Patterned lacerations

Lacerations do not reproduce the shape of the injuring agent nearly as well as do abrasions and intradermal bruises. As with

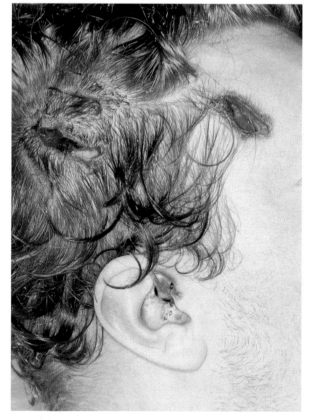

FIGURE 4.29 *Homicidal lacerations of the scalp penetrating the skull. Although some of the injuries resemble incised wounds, their margins are crushed, and hairs and tissue strands cross the injuries. The damage was probably inflicted with a metal rod with sharp edges.*

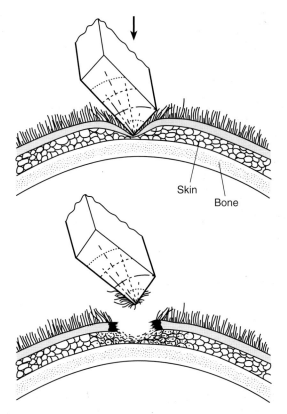

FIGURE 4.30 *Crushing impact of a blunt object on skin supported by bone, such as scalp on skull. The skin is sandwiched between weapon and bone and this causes a lacerated split that has bruised margins and bridges of hair and tissue in the wound.*

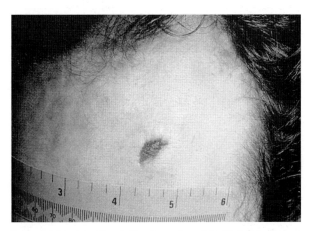

FIGURE 4.31 *A healing shallow laceration of the forehead, about one week after infliction. The base of the injury has filled with granulation tissue and the surrounding skin shows puckering due to contraction of the central scab.*

skull fractures, the magnitude of the force needed to cause a blunt tearing of skin leads to blurring of the impact shape, often with radiating or totally irregular tearing. Sometimes the shape is recognizable and probably the best example is a

hammer blow to the head. A circular face may punch out a circle or an arc of a circle, which may also be reproduced in an underlying depressed skull fracture. The exact size of the hammer face may not be accurately reproduced in the laceration, which may be slightly larger than the hammer.

Kicks may cause lacerations, especially if a heavy boot with a hard toecap is used. These tend to be tangential and may peel up a flange of tissue. They can be clean-cut and are sometimes mistaken for knife wounds. Stamping injuries are more likely to cause abrasions and bruises than lacerations, unless the violence is extreme. A heavy focal blow may cause a linear or a stellate laceration, the latter radiating out from the focus of impact. The surface may be abraded and the surrounding tissue deeply bruised, so the final lesion is complex.

Firearm wounds are a special form of laceration and will be dealt with separately.

BLUNT PENETRATING INJURIES

These 'puncture wounds' are a hybrid between lacerations and incised wounds, and have more of the features of the latter. Such injuries can occur from metal spikes, wooden stakes, garden or farm forks, and a variety of vehicular and industrial accidents. They are occasionally seen in homicides or suicides when weapons like screwdrivers are used as daggers. The interpretation of such skin wounds can be difficult, as in the 'Yorkshire Ripper' cases, when some small stellate stab wounds were thought to have been caused by a Phillips-type screwdriver. A number of fatal wounds, some of them homicidal, have been caused by chisels, usually very sharp woodworking tools with one face of the edge ground to a straight line. The edges of the chisel are squared off and the resulting skin defect may be rectangular.

When a blunt spike is driven through the skin, there will be inversion and abrasion of the edges, though the former may vanish if the weapon has been withdrawn. Foreign material such as rust, dirt or splinters may be left in the wound, and must be carefully preserved for forensic examination if the weapon has not been recovered.

INCISED WOUNDS

Injuries caused by sharp objects are classified as 'incised' wounds, though the nomenclature is again somewhat confused. Some authors make these a subcategory of lacerations and, when the weapon is relatively blunt (as in some axe or spike injuries), there may be sufficient crushing and bruising of the wound margins to make differentiation between incised and lacerated wounds difficult.

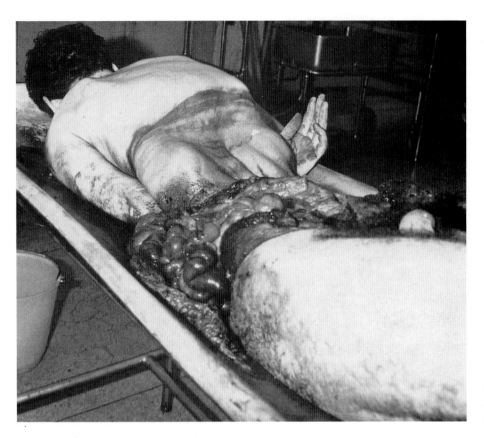

FIGURE 4.32 *Transection of a body into two halves at waist level. The victim jumped from a high-rise building and landed on a fence.*

The term 'incised wound' usually covers all types of injury from, for example, a knife, sword, razor, glass or sharp axe – though some writers would make stab wounds a separate category, reserving incised wounds for injuries that are longer than they are deep. These semantic variations are not important in themselves, but can lead to confusion in medical and autopsy reports, as well as in oral testimony if the doctor fails to clarify his meaning. The essential feature of all incised wounds is the clean division of the skin and underlying tissues so that the margins are almost free from any damage. Microscopically there is always a narrow zone of injury, but this is minimal compared with the tissue destruction caused by blunt injury. Healing is affected, as well as the extent of subsequent scarring.

Cuts or slashes

When an incised wound is longer than it is deep, it may be referred to as a 'cut' or 'slash', though a 'cut' may also be used by lay persons to describe a laceration. Such slashes when inflicted by knife, sword, razor, cleaver, parang, machete, panga, broken glass or bottle, are typical of a fight, when the assailant strikes out with a swiping action, rather than the thrust of a stabbing attack. They are common in gang fights and bar-room brawls and the weapon may be swung at arm's length in a horizontal arc so that if it contacts a body it will slice the skin and tissues as it passes by. They are also seen in suicidal injuries, usually on the wrist or throat. The characteristics of any given wound are a matter of a chance and relative positions. The slash may be deeper at the entry end or the exit point, though it seems true that many such injuries tend to dig in near the point of first contact and become progressively more shallow as the wound approaches the distal end. There may be a superficial 'tail', a shallow scratch, running out of the termination of the slash, as the weapon rises out of the wound and is drawn across the skin surface before leaving the body altogether.

There is a tendency among advocates to visualize a fight as a static confrontation and to attempt to reconstruct events as if the two participants were standing still, the assailant merely moving his arm. This is an unrealistic interpretation, as all fights are dynamic, with constant relative movement of the bodies and limbs of both parties. Therefore any relative angles and depths of contact between the victim and the weapon can occur and overinterpretation and simplification should be avoided.

Slashed wounds are less dangerous than stabs, as the relative shallowness of the wounds is less likely to affect vital organs – especially as the arms and face are the common targets. The rib cage and skull protects the chest organs and

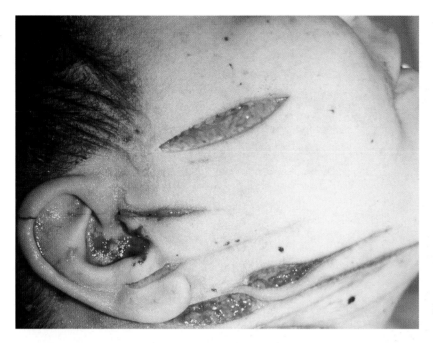

FIGURE 4.33 *Homicidal slashed wounds caused by knife; the length is greater than the depth, unlike stab wounds. The long tails are due to the knife rising from the skin, thus indicating the direction of the slash.*

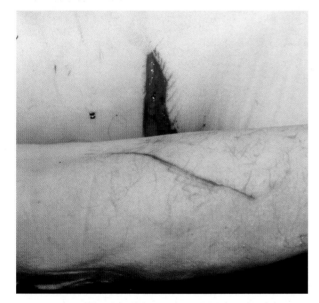

FIGURE 4.34 *A knife slash of the back showing regular scratches along the margin. This was inflicted with a 'Rambo' knife, which has deep serrations along the back edge that have somehow marked the skin on withdrawal.*

brain and the more vulnerable abdomen is seldom the target for a swung knife. Wounds of the neck are the most dangerous and are discussed below. Bleeding is the most serious complication of any slashed wound, though it will be external and more amenable to immediate treatment than the hidden internal bleeding of a stab wound.

A particular form of slashed wound arises from 'glassing', that is, the use of a broken drinking glass or bottle as a weapon. The glass may sometimes be broken prior to the attack, to produce edges that are exquisitely sharp. There may also be spikes of glass, which can inflict deep, almost stab wounds. Where, more commonly, a glass or bottle is used as a blunt instrument, it may shatter on impact with a victim's head, and the resulting injuries may both be blunt and incised.

Stab wounds and penetrating injuries

These are of major importance in forensic pathology, as they are extremely common in homicide. In Britain, stabbing with a knife is easily the most frequent mode of murder and manslaughter, primarily in domestic disputes and street violence. A stab wound is an incised wound that is deeper than it is wide. Though many penetrate only the skin and subcuta- neous tissues, those seen by forensic pathologists are most often fatal, having entered vital deep structures. Several aspects of this important topic need discussion.

THE NATURE OF STABBING WEAPONS

Knives are the weapons most frequently involved and their physical characteristics are important in shaping the wound. A pathologist called upon to examine a knife that may have been used in an assault should note and measure:

- the length, width and thickness of the blade
- whether it is single or double-edged
- the degree of taper from tip to hilt
- the nature of the back edge in a single-edged knife (for example, serrated or squared-off)

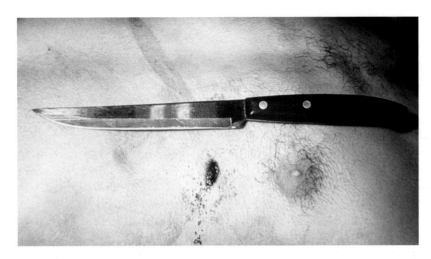

FIGURE 4.35 *A stab wound and the inflicting knife. The wound is slightly shorter than the width of the blade at the depth of penetration because of sideways gaping and the contractile elasticity of the skin.*

■ the face of the hilt guard adjacent to the blade
■ any grooving, serration or forking of the blade
■ most importantly, the sharpness of the edge and especially of the extreme tip of the blade.

Other knife-like weapons include scissors, chisels, swords, open razors and sharp tools of many kinds, including deliberately modified tools such as sharpened screwdrivers. Larger cutting instruments such as axes, choppers, parangs, machetes and pangas and agricultural implements such as shears, bill-hooks, hay-knives and many others have been used as stabbing weapons when used by the point rather the long edge.

Spiked instruments come in many forms, from icepicks to hay-forks, from case-openers to fire-irons. The appearances of their wounds vary with the physical nature of the implement. Some weapons are exquisitely sharp and the wounds made by them exhibit extremely fine division of the tissues. To razors and razorblades may be added surgical and craft knives, often with a disposable blade, together with carpet and general utility and hobby tools, such as the 'Stanley' knife. Equally sharp is broken glass and sometimes porcelain. Both sheet glass and smashed glass utensils can provide edges that equal or exceed surgical scalpels in their cutting ability.

A common weapon in a bar-room fight is a smashed beer tankard, which when held by the intact handle provides a formidable weapon for both slashing and stabbing. Smashed china, such as cups and mugs, can also provide sharp cutting edges. The external glaze can project, if the fracture line is oblique, producing a glass-like edge. From personal experiment, the author (BK) has shown that broken china can easily slice through the full thickness of skin and thus validate a defence that injuries were the result of falling on a broken mug.

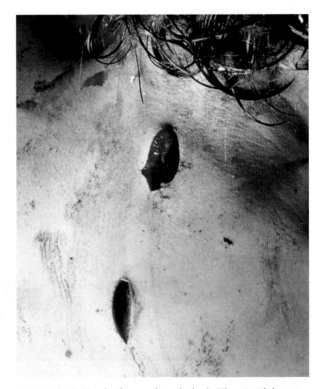

FIGURE 4.36 *Two knife wounds in the back. The wounds have a sharper lower edge compared to a rounder upper edge, due to a one-edged blade.*

THE CHARACTERISTICS OF A STAB WOUND

The surface and internal appearances of a stab wound allow the pathologist to offer an opinion upon:

■ the dimensions of the weapon
■ the type of weapon
■ the taper of the blade

- movement of the knife in the wound
- the depth of the thrust
- the direction of the thrust
- the amount of force used.

Dimensions of the weapon

The dimensions of the knife may be a vital part of the investigation of a homicide when the weapon has been removed from the scene by the assailant. The pathologist can sometimes assist the investigators by telling them, within limits, what size and type of knife to seek. When suspect weapons are recovered, his inspection of them may indicate whether or not they are consistent with having caused the wounds in question. As always in forensic medicine, however, caution must be employed and the cardinal sin of overinterpretation avoided.

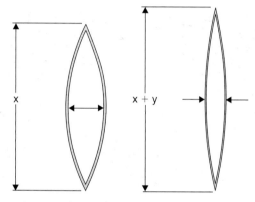

FIGURE 4.37 *A stab wound gapes across its width and shortens in length, especially when across skin or muscle planes.*

The length of the wound should be measured to the nearest millimetre as it lies undisturbed on the skin. In most instances the wound will have gaped across the centre, to form a long ellipse. The extent of gaping will depend on the anatomical situation, for example, over joints or in the axilla or groin, and whether the axis of the stab is in line with or across the tension of Langer's lines or underlying muscle bundles.

When the edges are gently opposed, the length of the wound may then extend slightly and should be measured again in this position, which more accurately approximates to the length when the blade was *in situ*.

An important additional factor, however, must always be taken into account because, when the knife is withdrawn the elasticity of the skin causes it to retract, making the wound smaller than when the blade was *in situ*. This mechanism may be amplified by contraction of the underlying muscles, which, if at right angles to the axis of the wound, may cause the wound to shorten from end to end, while gaping more widely at the centre. Using wound measurements to predict the size of the knife blade, one must take into account the other matters discussed below, such as movement of the blade in the wound, the taper of the blade and the depth of penetration.

Type of weapon

The type of blade usually refers to whether it had a single or double cutting edge. Most knifes have a single sharp edge, the back edge being blunt or otherwise machined. A few dagger-like weapons have both edges ground to sharpness,

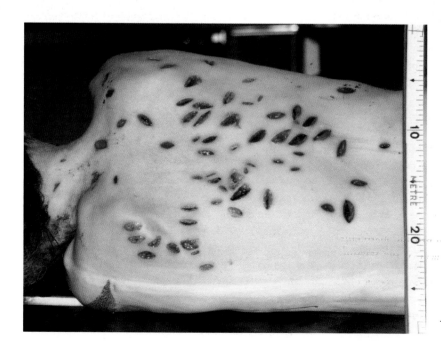

FIGURE 4.38 *Multiple stabs on the back from the same knife, showing differing shapes and sizes.*

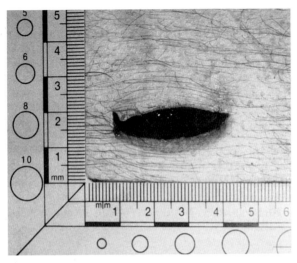

FIGURE 4.39 *A stab wound showing a unilateral 'fish-tail' split caused by the blunt back edge of the knife blade. This is sometimes bilateral due to tearing of the tissues. The other end of the wound is pointed due to the cutting edge of the blade.*

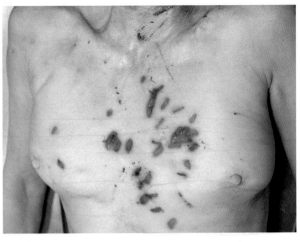

FIGURE 4.40 *Multiple stab wounds from the same knife, showing variations in the size and shape of the injuries. With multiple injuries, it is advisable to number each to facilitate easy reference in the autopsy report and when giving evidence in court.*

some have only the distal part of the back of the blade sharpened. On inspecting the skin wound, the pathologist frequently finds that both ends of the defect appear sharply cut, coming to a fine 'V-point' at the extremities. Unfortunately, this does not necessarily indicate that a knife with two sharp edges was used, as the skin often splits behind the blunt edge to produce a symmetrical appearance.

If, however, there is an obvious difference between one sharply pointed end and a rounded or even square-cut opposite extremity, then it can be said with some confidence that a single-edged knife was employed.

A knife with a thick blade that is squared off to a flat surface on the edge opposite the cutting edge, may sometimes be identified from the wound, where a definite double right-angled end to the skin defect is apparent. The skin may split back slightly from each of these corners, forming the so-called 'fish-tail' appearance.

Where a knife with a serrated back edge has been used, such as is found on some boy scout or other Bowie-type knives (or the recently fashionable 'Rambo' weapons), the back edge of the wound may be torn or ragged and – on some occasions where the knife has entered very obliquely – serrated abrasions may be seen on the skin adjacent to the end of the wound.

If the knife has been plunged into the full extent of the blade, then there may be a hilt bruise or abrasion on the skin surrounding the wound. This may even reproduce the pattern of the guard at the base of the hilt, if there is one. Careful photography, sketches and measurements are needed to capture the exact outline of such a mark, which are, admittedly, unusual.

Taper of the blade

The taper of the blade is naturally related to wound size. If a tapered blade is inserted to 4 cm, then the length of the wound (ignoring skin retraction for the moment) will be that of the width of the blade at that level. If the taper continues to the 8 cm level, then the wound will be correspondingly longer. Only when the blade edges become parallel will the wound size remain constant for further penetration of the knife.

Movement of the knife in the wound

Movement of the knife in the wound can result in loss of evidence as to the size of the blade, but can also add other information. Where a knife is stabbed directly into the body and withdrawn along the same track then, within the limits discussed above, the size of the wound will indicate the minimum width of the blade at the maximum depth of penetration.

If, however, the knife is 'rocked' in the wound, the skin defect will be enlarged, sometimes considerably. The term 'rocking' means a leverage or angulation in the plane of the wound, so that the cutting edge extends the incision. This rocking can occur either by the knife being actively moved in the wound by the assailant – or by the body moving relative to the knife – or by a combination of the two.

It is sometimes a misapprehension among both doctors and (especially) lawyers, that stabbings and other assaults occur in static circumstances, with the victim standing in the anatomical position. Directions of wounds are all too often interpreted as if the only movement came from the hand of the assailant, whereas in most fatal assaults the

This relative movement may extend the wound in a linear fashion, as described above or there may be twisting of the blade in the wound. In the latter case, the resulting skin incision may be V-shaped or totally irregular. Rarely, a single stab may produce multiple skin wounds, such as a tangential stab of the arm, which passes through the superficial tissues and then re-enters the chest wall. Another instance is a stab through a female breast where, especially if the breast is sagging, the knife can pass right through the edge before re-entering the thorax.

Depth of the thrust

The depth of a stab wound may be important in attempting to assess the length of a missing weapon. Again there are pitfalls to be avoided. First, if a knife is driven in up to the hilt, the depth of the wound as measured at autopsy may be greater than the true length of the blade. This is common in the abdomen and to a lesser extent in the chest, because the impact of a forceful stab may momentarily indent the abdominal or chest wall so that the tip of the knife penetrates tissues that apparently should have been out of reach. This is particularly so when the hilt guard of the weapon impinges on the skin. For example, the author (BK) has seen the tip of a broken knife embedded in a thoracic spine, where the distance from that tip to the anterior skin wound was less than the length of the blade when recovered.

As with direction, discussed below, the pathologist must also allow for differences in the position of internal organs as measured at autopsy in a supine body, compared with their position in the living body, often in the upright posture. Such variations in the *in vivo* distance from the skin wound to the organs penetrated must be taken into account when assessing the depth of a wound. In the chest and abdomen, visceral relationships vary with the stage of respiration. The lower ribs move upwards and laterally, and increase the distance between the skin and deeper structures.

Direction of the thrust

The direction of a stab wound is often a matter of contention in homicides, especially as trial lawyers (and their medical advisers) sometimes tend to overinterpret the facts when trying to reconstruct the scene of the fatal assault.

As mentioned above, a stabbing incident is often moving and dynamic, and the victim is rarely in a static, anatomical position. For example, a wound that enters the upper part of the left side of the chest and travels steeply downwards, is not inevitably the result of the killer being taller or situated above the victim, using a downward blow. The victim could equally well have been bending or crouching, the knife then entering on a horizontal plane relative to the floor. All that the pathologist can do is to determine the direction of the wound relative to the axis of the body – it is then a

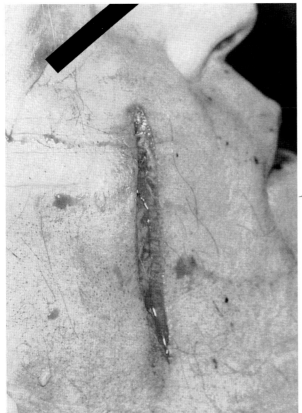

FIGURE 4.41 *A slashed facial wound from a knife, showing undercutting or 'shelving' on the edge nearest the mouth, indicating the angle of the knife relative to the surface. The tailed nature of the lower end also indicates that that knife was drawn downwards across the face.*

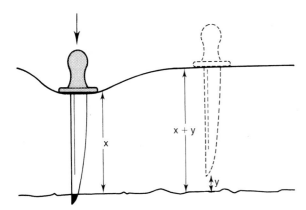

FIGURE 4.42 *Forcible stabbing can indent the body surface so that deep structures can be injured that appear to be beyond the reach of the knife.*

victim bends, turns and twists, and the assailant often follows with similar gyrations. Thus a knife that is thrust into the body may itself move or the body may move against it before it is withdrawn.

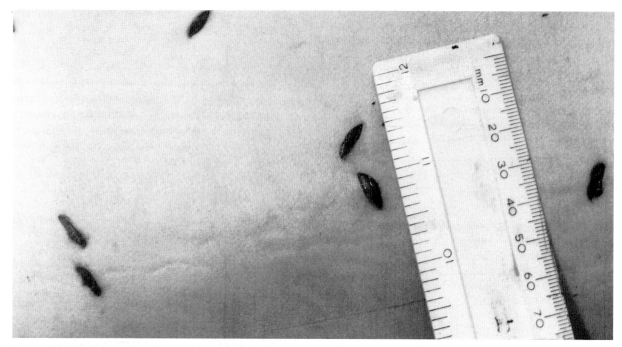

FIGURE 4.43 *Multiple stab wounds from the same knife. Although those at the bottom left are obviously square-ended, the more central ones are almost equally sharp at the extremities – illustrating the dangers of being too dogmatic about describing a missing knife to the investigators.*

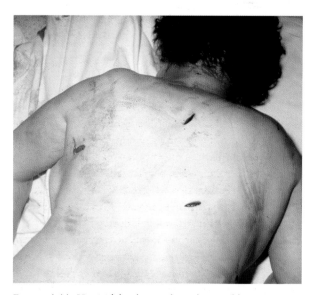

FIGURE 4.44 *Homicidal stab wounds misdiagnosed by an attending doctor as 'haematemesis or epistaxis'. The lower right wound clearly shows evidence of a single-edged blade. The wound in the left axilla is V-shaped because of the twisting knife.*

matter of non-medical evidence to relate that to the posture of the victim when struck.

Determination of the direction relies on both the appearance of the skin wound and the track in the deep tissues.

Where a knife penetrates the skin with the plane of the blade at appreciably less than a right angle to the surface, the wound is often 'undercut', being shelved so that subcutaneous tissue is visible below one edge of the wound. Where the knife is plunged in obliquely, but the plane of the blade remains perpendicular to the surface, no such shelving can be seen at the sides of the wound though it may just be visible at the end of the wound.

More information about direction comes from careful examination of the track of the stab wound. This is an anatomical exercise during autopsy, the layers of tissue being examined in sequence from the surface downwards and damage to deep structures and organs compared with the position of the surface wound. For example, a stab wound of the chest may lie below the left nipple. Dissection of the subcutaneous tissues and muscles may reveal that the defect in the chest wall lies in the sixth intercostal space and that, inside the thorax, the right ventricle of the heart has been transfixed, and that there is a wound in the diaphragm that terminates in the liver just to the right of the midline. This information obviously indicates that the direction of the wound was downwards and from left to right. Similar deductions can be made for all other sites, but caution must be exercised, as mentioned earlier, in allowing for the change in position of organs in the supine post-mortem posture compared with the erect, living state. A thorough knowledge of surface anatomy is required, especially of the thorax, as well

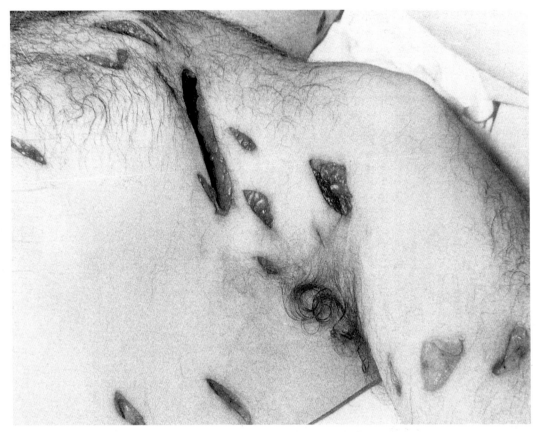

FIGURE 4.45 *Multiple homicidal knife wounds, all inflicted with the same weapon. This shows the marked variation in wound size from the same knife, caused by rocking and twisting movements of either weapon or victim.*

as diagrams of the position of internal organs mapped out in relation to surface markers; samples of such diagrams are given in this book.

Attempts have been made to delineate the track of a stab wound before dissection either by filling the defect with a radio-opaque fluid before taking X-rays, or by filling with a plastic or even metallic substance that will harden to form a cast. In practice, these methods appear to have little advantage over careful dissection. When radio-opaque liquids or pastes are used, there is often leakage from the stab wound into the thoracic or abdominal cavities, leading to a confusing radiological picture. Recently, magnetic resonance imaging (MRI) has been used to visualize the wound track, but such facilities are rarely available for dead victims.

Estimation of the degree of force used in stabbing
The amount of force required to inflict any given stab wound is often a matter of extensive debate in criminal trials. The prosecution naturally gains from showing that a stabbing was inflicted with 'considerable force', sometimes even using pejorative terms such as 'violent' or 'frenzied'. This tends to confirm the intention to stab, whereas the defence proposition is often that the victim inadvertently fell or was pressed against a weapon held passively by the accused. An expert medical witness has difficulty in replying to the almost inevitable question by counsel: 'What amount of force was necessary to cause this wound, doctor?'

Assessment of force is subjective and cannot be quantified in any satisfactory way that is meaningful to the court. Physical units such as dynes/cm^2, even if they can be measured, mean nothing to a judge and jury. The only measure that the medical witness can offer is a broad grading, based on common sense knowledge, such as 'slight pressure', 'moderate force', 'considerable force' and perhaps 'extreme force', the latter being reserved for exceptional cases where the knife has impacted in dense bone, penetrated the skull, or left a marked bruised impression of the hilt guard on the skin. A number of investigators, including the author (BK), have carried out measurements on the force needed to inflict stab wounds, both in animal, cadaver and surrogate tissues. The usual method is to attach some type of dynamometer or transducer to a knife, which records the maximum force applied during penetration, preferably with the duration of impact.

From this work, the following useful generalizations can be made.

- Apart from bone or calcified cartilage, the tissue most resistant to knife penetration is the skin (Knight 1975), followed by muscle where large muscle bundles underlay the fascia.
- The sharpness of the extreme tip of the knife is the most important factor in skin penetration. The cutting edge of the knife, once the tip has penetrated, is of relatively minor importance.
- The speed of approach of the knife is particularly important in achieving penetration. A knife held against the skin, then steadily pushed, requires far more force to penetrate than the same knife launched against the skin like a dart. As in blunt injury, this is an example of the physical law that requires that the force varies directly not with the mass of the weapon, but also with the square of the velocity.
- Stretched skin is easier to penetrate than lax skin. The chest wall, where skin tends to be intermittently supported by underlying ribs, is relatively easy to puncture with a sharp knife as the skin and tissues are stretched over intercostal spaces in the manner of a drum membrane.

- Though the thick skin of the palms and soles is much tougher than on the rest of the body, the variation in resistance of the rest of the skin to a sharp knife is of little importance compared with other factors. Similarly, the skin of the aged, or of women, is not appreciably less resistant to a sharp point than that of men or young persons.
- When a knife-point impacts against skin, the latter dimples and resists until penetration suddenly occurs. The tension developed in the stretched skin appears to act as an 'elastic reservoir' and, when the threshold of resistance is exceeded, the knife 'falls' through the subcutaneous tissues without any further force being imparted to it unless impeded by bone or cartilage. Thus no additional effort is needed by the assailant to achieve deep or even full penetration up to the hilt. It is sometimes incorrectly claimed by the prosecution that a deep stab wound must imply extreme force or continued pushing after penetration. This is not so and experiments have shown that once penetration occurs, it is difficult or even impossible to prevent deep penetration because of the suddenness of the breakthrough.
- When the knife penetrates the skin rapidly, for example, if the body falls or runs on to the blade, the knife does not need to be held rigidly in order to prevent it being pushed backwards. Its inertia, if the tip is sharp, is quite sufficient to hold it in place while the body spears itself on the blade.

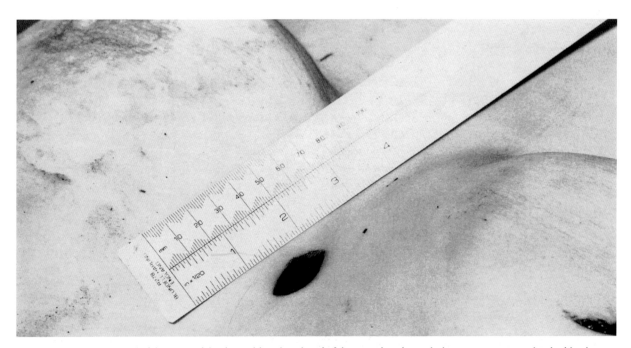

FIGURE 4.46 *A stab wound of the centre of the chest. Although each end of the wound is identical, the weapon was a single-edged kitchen knife. The end of the wound adjacent to the back of the blade has split making it impossible to say if a single- or double-edged knife was used. The sternum beneath was penetrated to reach the heart, so considerable force must have been used.*

It has been wrongly argued against a defence of falling or running onto a knife, that the hilt would have had to have been supported against, for example, the hip of the person holding the knife to immobilize it against the advancing body. Experiments have shown that this theory is invalid.

Uncalcified cartilage, especially that in the costal cartilages of young and middle-aged persons, is easily penetrated by a sharp knife, though naturally more force is required than if the blade passed through an intercostal space. Calcified rib and bone provide a much more resistant barrier, but a forceful stab from a strong, sharp knife can easily penetrate rib, sternum or skull. Firm tissues like myocardium, liver and kidney are easily traversed by all but the most blunt of weapons, and their resistance is far less than that of cartilage or skin.

INJURIES BY WEAPONS OTHER THAN KNIVES

The general features of injuries from knives apply equally to other sharp objects that cause incised and stab wounds. Razors and broken glass have extremely sharp edges so that, when applied tangentially or at a small angle to the skin, undercutting may be a marked feature. The wound may appear as a shallow slice which bleeds profusely and, in a hairy area such as the scalp, it will reveal cut hair bulbs on the shelved surface. Deliberate wounds with razors or sharp knives may exhibit patterns or even words; these may occur in gang fights or sadistic homicides.

Glass can be employed as a cutting weapon, again typically in bar fights or gang vendettas, where a broken bottle may be held by the neck or a smashed beer tankard by the handle.

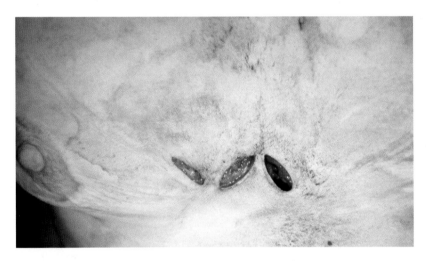

FIGURE 4.47 *Three wounds from a single stab with a knife, which was in place when the body was discovered. The knife had entered obliquely through the inner side of the right breast, emerged into the cleavage and re-entered the mid-line. If the knife had not been in situ, interpretation could have been more difficult.*

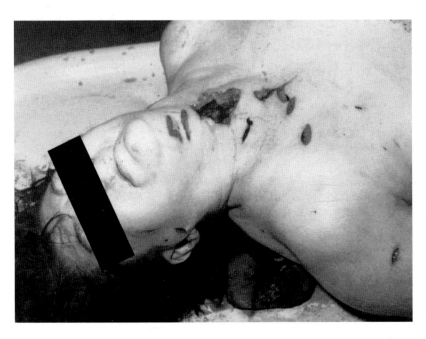

FIGURE 4.48 *Homicidal stab wounds of the throat and head showing the pleomorphism of injuries caused by the same knife. The wound under the chin is V-shaped caused by twisting of the weapon; the large throat wound consists of several superimposed thrusts and over the manubrium there is a 'tail' caused by the tip of the knife slipping out of the wound on withdrawal.*

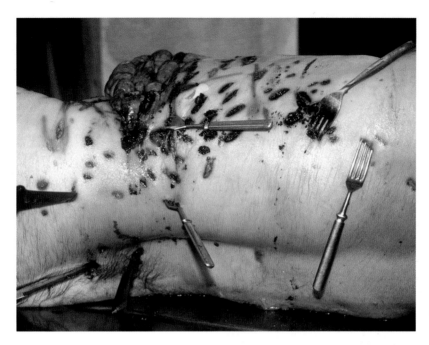

FIGURE 4.49 *Multiple homicidal stab and incised wounds inflicted with various kitchen utensils.*

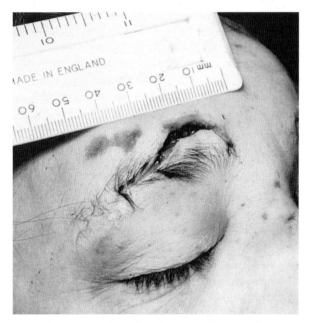

FIGURE 4.50 *A wound over the eyebrow caused by impact from a broken drinking glass. Although this location is commonly the site of laceration from blunt blows, this injury is sharp-edged and has unbruised margins, indicating that it is an incised wound. There is an associated abrasion from non-cutting contact and there is bleeding into the upper eyelid, probably from gravitational seepage from the wound.*

Official estimates in Britain suggest that between 3400 and 5400 offences occur annually in which glass is used as a weapon. Surveys in London and Bristol by Shepherd *et al.* (1990a) and Hocking (1989) showed that bar drinking glasses were the most common weapons, and that 75 per cent of these were from straight-sided pint glasses. Unexpectedly, this research showed that most of the glasses were intact until thrown or thrust at the victim – they had not been smashed prior to the assaults. Most of these non-fatal injuries were to the face. The fragility of these glasses varies greatly from manufacturer to manufacturer, so that there can be a sixfold difference in their propensity to smash on impact.

Though these formidable weapons are usually used for slashing, long slivers of glass can act – sometimes inadvertently – as stabbing agents. The sliver may break off and remain in a deep wound, which may be overlooked if the entry is small.

As many casualty surgeons have learned to their cost – or to the cost of their medical protection society or medical insurers – glass is almost invariably radio-opaque, even though this is either unknown or even denied by the doctor. Numerous civil actions for negligence have occurred – though usually in non-fatal circumstances – but, on occasion, the first person to find a deep fragment of glass in a vital position has been a forensic pathologist.

As mentioned earlier, broken china and porcelain, as from a smashed cup, mug or plate, may have a sharp edge on the exposed glaze and can easily cause a slashed wound.

INJURIES FROM SCISSORS

Stabbing by a pair of scissors is not uncommon and is seen most often in domestic circumstances where a woman uses a weapon upon her husband or consort which is both familiar and near to hand. The appearances of the wound will

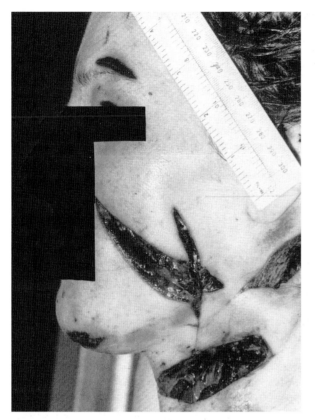

FIGURE 4.51 *Incised wounds, which in spite of their large size are typical of those inflicted by a sharp-edged weapon rather than a crushing laceration. The instrument was a butcher's cleaver.*

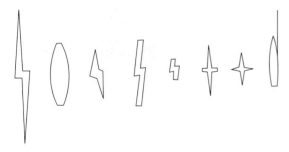

FIGURE 4.52 *Various profiles made by scissors stabbed through the skin. The cross shapes are caused by blade screws or rivets; the one on the right is a full penetration of one blade of an open pair of scissors, the other blade impinging flat on the skin.*

differ according to whether the scissors were used open or closed. If open and one blade is stabbed into the victim, then the appearances will be virtually indistinguishable from a knife wound. Some modern scissors, however, have a two-part blade in which a steel cutting edge is riveted to a carrier continuous with the handles. This may produce a stepped wound that may show a notch or variation in linearity in the margin of the stab wound.

More characteristic is the wound produced when both blades of a closed pair of scissors are plunged through the skin. Some scissors have a double-sharp point, but most domestic, tailors' or dressmaking scissors are fairly blunt at the tips when closed, so considerable force is needed to drive them through the skin – tending to work against a defence of an accidental movement against a passively held weapon.

The skin wound made by closed scissors is typically shaped like a flat 'Z' or the usual impressionist sign for a flash of lightning. The offset of the two blades gives this shallow zig-zag pattern, which is unmistakable when present. Some scissors, however, especially long narrow ones in which the blades close almost completely over one another, may not reproduce this appearance and the wound may look more like that from a thick knife. Sometimes, there are small lateral splits in the wound centre from a projecting hinge screw.

DEFENCE WOUNDS

In assaults of any kind, the natural reaction of the victims is to protect themselves. The limbs used for protection can themselves be injured and these defence wounds may be of considerable medico-legal significance, as they indicate that the victim was conscious, at least partly mobile and not taken completely by surprise. Defence wounds can be sustained from attacks by fists, feet and blunt or sharp instruments. The classic position for them is on the forearms and hands, which are instinctively raised to protect the eyes, face and head. Other defence injuries may be inflicted on the thighs, when attempts are made to shield the genitals.

With attacks from blunt instruments or fists, bruises are the hallmark of defence attempts. They are common on the outer sides of the forearms, the wrists, the backs of the hands and knuckles. The size and shape of the bruises naturally depends upon the attacking object. Abrasions may accompany the bruises but the latter are more common. Fractures of the carpal bones, metacarpals and digits may occur. If the arm is held in front of the face, the inner (palmar) side of the forearm may also receive blows. There may also be defence bruises and abrasions on the thigh, as blows or kicks aimed at the lower part of the body cause the victim, especially men, to protect the genitals. The leg may be brought across the other or the thigh raised, so that its outer side may receive blows or kicks.

The most obvious defence injuries are seen in knife attacks, as the victim often attempts to ward off the thrusts by seizing the weapon. When the fingers are closed around the blade, its withdrawal cuts across the flexures of the phalanges, slicing through the skin and perhaps tendons, or sometimes all four fingers. This may be seen in one, any, or even all of the three sets of flexures.

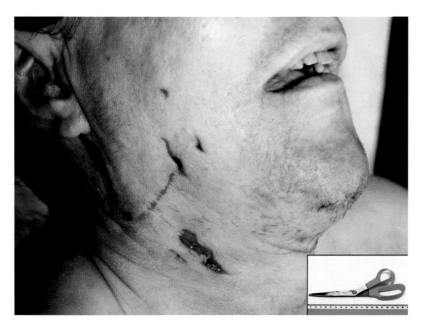

FIGURE 4.53 *Multiple homicidal stab wounds by closed scissors.*

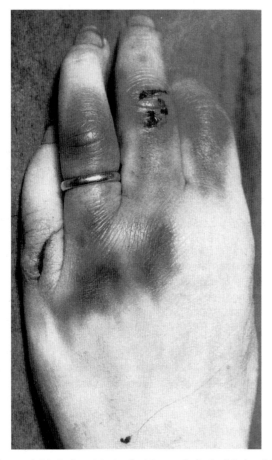

FIGURE 4.54 *Defence injuries: bruising on the back of the hand in an attempt to fend off a blunt instrument in this case a metal poker that was used to inflict fatal head injuries. Such injuries confirm that the victim was conscious and active during the attack, and that it was not made covertly while the victim was unaware.*

The other typical knife defence wound is in the web between the base of the thumb and index finger, when the blade is grabbed in an attempted pincer action. Other knife wounds can be on the backs of the hands or fingers from non-grasping movements trying to ward off the weapon. Defence wounds from knives are often sharply sliced, as the blade is drawn across the tightly applied skin. They are often markedly 'shelved', with loose flaps of skin and copious bleeding.

Defence wounds also occur in firearms injuries, where an arm is raised in a desperate attempt to shield the trunk or head from the blast. This accounts for some shooting deaths where there is an entrance and an exit wound in (often) the upper arm, the missile(s) then repenetrating the trunk.

DATING OF WOUNDS BY HISTOLOGY AND HISTOCHEMISTRY

There are many publications on this subject, as it is a favourite topic for research. As with time of death, it can be an important matter in forensic medical investigations to determine whether a wound found at autopsy was inflicted before or after death and, if inflicted ante-mortem, how long before death it was sustained.

Unfortunately, as with so many problems, biological variability introduces a wide margin of uncertainty, so that a range of probabilities can be offered, but never a definite time interval. Much of the experimental work has been performed on animals and the results are not transferable to man – a common defect in all animal work. The smaller

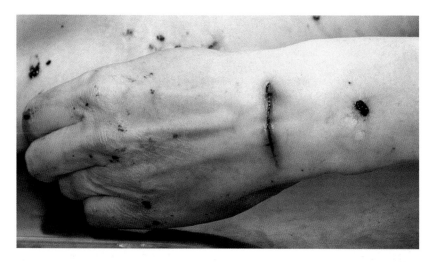

FIGURE 4.55 *Defence wound on the back of the hand from trying to ward off the knife.*

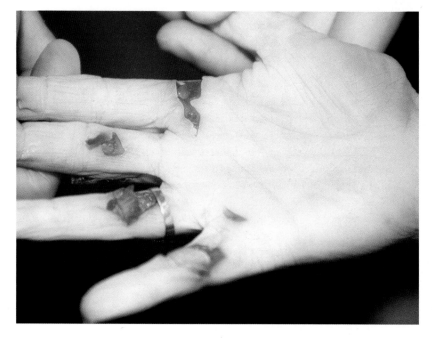

FIGURE 4.56 *Typical defence injuries in a victim of a knife attack. In grasping the blade to deflect it, there have been cuts across the palmar surfaces of the finger joints and a slash between the thumb and forefinger, together with a cut at the base of the thumb.*

the animal, the more rapid the tissue scavenging and reparative changes: more primitive animals have far greater powers of regeneration than man, both in wounds and in regrowing organs and even limbs.

The changes will also vary according to the size of a wound, the type of wound (bruise, abrasion, incision or laceration), the tissue (epidermal or mesodermal), whether there is infection and the age and health of the victim.

The subject is complex and often contradictory and the following schedule of events is offered only as a guideline. The original papers should be consulted if any particular criterion is to be followed; histological appearances, including fluorescence studies may be backed up by histochemical and biochemical assays. The sequence of changes in bruises is far less distinct than in abrasions or lacerations and histology is much less helpful. The most useful criterion

in a bruise is probably Perl's reaction for haemosiderin, which becomes positive about 3 days after infliction – though some workers claim an earlier appearance, even down to 12 hours. Haemolysis of red blood cells is irregular and patchy, many intact cells being seen in some bruises after many days, so their rupture and ghosting cannot be used as an index of age.

Chronological histological changes after wound infliction

30 MINUTES–4 HOURS

Margination of polymorph leucocytes in dilated small vessels may occur, a feature which is often completely absent. It is also not a reliable sign of ante-mortem infliction, as

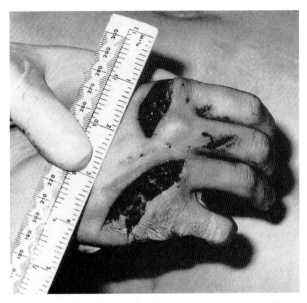

FIGURE 4.57 *Defence wounds of hand in attempts to ward off an assault with a meat cleaver.*

leucocytes may congregate for many hours after death, especially in skin and around aspirated material in the lung.

Some extravascular emigration may begin at the end of this period, but a significant number of polymorphs usually delay for many more hours. Polymorphs tend to appear earlier in the subcutaneous fat than in the upper dermal layers. Basophilic 'mast cells' lose their granules. Fibrin appears in the wound within a few minutes, but this also occurs in post-mortem injuries.

4–12 HOURS

Leucocyte infiltration is likely to be more definite, still mostly polymorphs, but some mononuclear cells as well. A scanty mixed population of lymphocytes and poorly differentiated 'monocytes' appears, usually after 12 hours. Tissue oedema and swelling of vascular endothelium occurs. In small wounds involving the skin, the start of epithelial regeneration may be seen at the sides at the level of the basal layer of epidermis.

12–24 HOURS

Leucocytes tend to demarcate the area of the wound by forming a marginal palisade. The polymorph response declines and the macrophage and mononuclear cell population increases from now on. Removal of necrosed tissue begins, with macrophages evident and a basophilic tinge to the ground substance. Mitoses are visible in fibroblasts from about 15 hours. The epidermis begins to spread across the surface of the scab and down the sides of a cut into the wound.

24–72 HOURS

Leucocyte infiltration reaches a peak at about 48 hours; repair begins concurrently with many fibroblasts appearing, but rarely before 72 hours. New capillaries then begin to bud from vessels, the vascular, infiltrated stroma becoming 'granulation tissue'.

3–6 DAYS

Repair is proceeding apace: collagen begins to form and giant cells may be visible around necrotic debris and foreign matter. The epidermis is actively growing if the wound involves the surface: in animals, it grows laterally at about 200 μm/day. Haemosiderin becomes stainable from about the third day onwards, if there is a bruise or any bleeding into the wound, but is often not obtainable by Perl's reaction until the fifth day even though some claim it can appear on the first or second day.

10–15 DAYS

Cellular reaction subsides in small wounds. Vascularity decreases and the cell population drops, especially leucocytes. Fibroblasts are most active, with collagen being laid down. The epidermis becomes thin and flat, but no papillae ('rete pegs') are reformed for many weeks. Elastic fibres are scarce for a long time and less than in adjacent undamaged tissue.

TWO WEEKS TO SEVERAL MONTHS, DEPENDING ON SIZE AND OTHER FACTORS

Consolidation of the healing tissue continues. The inflammatory response has vanished, unless the wound has become infected. Collagen and elastin increase and a vascular scar is formed, which gradually becomes more dense and avascular. The epithelium remodels and dermal papillae reappear unless the wound is wide and irregular. Skin adnexae do not reappear in the scar unless islands of viable skin survive within the wound area.

Histochemical changes in injured tissues

Histochemical and immunohistochemical methods have been studied widely in recent years, again mainly on animals, the transfer to the human situation being suspect in some cases. A wide variety of markers have been claimed as reliable for both the differentiation between ante-mortem and post-mortem injuries and for dating of ante-mortem wounds.

Electrolytes, such as sodium, zinc, magnesium and calcium, serotonin, esterases, glycophorin A and especially histamine have been used for this purpose.

Mainly as a result of the pioneering work of Jyrki Raekallio in Finland, the histochemical sequence of events in wounds has been actively pursued in recent years. Some techniques need frozen sections, others can be carried out on fixed tissue. Estimations of histamine or serotonin are usually 'tube' methods, rather than microscopic, though some fluorescent techniques have been developed. Betz and his co-workers have also published extensively on the immunohistochemistry of wound dating.

At the present time these methods still remain mainly in the realm of the research laboratory, apart from a few enthusiasts who employ them in casework. For the histochemical novice, it would be unwise to put such procedures into evidence without first gaining extensive experience of control material. Experience emphasizes that strictly standard conditions are required for the production of such histochemical sections, the end result depends largely on laboratory procedures – 'change your technician and you change the answer'.

A list of standard procedures for some of these reactions is given in Appendix 1.

The following are some of the histochemical wound changes described by Raekallio and others:

▪ In a wound through the skin surface there is a central zone 0.2–0.5 mm wide that will become necrotic and in which enzyme activity rapidly decreases. This may be termed 'negative vital reaction'. Immediately beyond this layer, is a 0.1–0.3 mm zone of reaction and eventual repair, where a number of enzymes and other substances become increased in concentration during the reparative process, compared to the normal level in the areas outside the wound. Enzymatically, this can be called 'positive vital reaction', as no such zone develops in a post-mortem wound.

▪ Within one hour after injury, esterases and adenosine triphosphatase increase in the positive zone. At around 2 hours, aminopeptidase activities increase and, at 4 hours, acid phosphatase activity increases. Alkaline phosphatase activity is delayed another hour or so though, of course, all these times are relative and subject to the usual biological variability.

▪ Where death occurs at some stage of this process, the enzyme pattern is 'frozen' at that point and post-mortem changes do not substantially alter the reactions within a few days after death, especially if autolysis is kept at bay by refrigeration. Senility, severe illness and cachexia, as well as widespread multiple injuries, may distort the usual pattern by reducing the ability to produce these reparative enzymes. In contused wounds, the reactions are less useful than in cutaneous injuries, as the damage is more diffuse and there are no definite 'zones'.

In all wounds, lack of reaction cannot be taken as indisputable proof of a post-mortem origin, though, if the opposite occurs, positive increase in the outer zone must only be the result of a vital reaction. Other enzymes have been used for wound dating: the review by Janssen (1984) in his authoritative book on forensic histology should be consulted for details, as well as the work of Betz.

▪ Tissue cathepsins are said to increase almost immediately if the stroma is damaged, being demonstrable within 5–10 minutes. Two other substances are of use in establishing that wounds are ante-mortem and giving some idea as to their age. Both are produced during the inflammatory response that accompanies tissue damage – histamine and serotonin (5-hydroxytryptamine). They tend to be complementary to the enzymes, as they appear soon after infliction, within the hour or so before adenosine triphosphatase and esterases become detectable.

These vasoactive amines appear in maximum concentration about 10 minutes (serotonin) and 20–30 minutes (histamine) after wounding. One of the first demonstrations of this forensic aid was by Fazekas and Varagos-Kis (1965), who showed that a ligature mark in hanging revealed increased serotonin; presumably the hanging was atypical and the victim took 10 minutes to die which is rather unusual. For the employment of the test in human autopsy work, about 2 grams of skin freed from subcutaneous fat are sampled, together with a similar control sample from a nearby normal area of skin from the same corpse. This is to allow for the markedly different amounts found in different people and, indeed, in the same persons at different times.

To establish that a wound was ante-mortem rather than inflicted after death, the level of histamine in the wound must be at least 50 per cent greater than the control sample – and, for serotonin at least, twice the concentration of the control skin.

SURVIVAL PERIOD AFTER WOUNDING

A pathologist is often asked either by police during an investigation, or by counsel at trial, what was the probable interval between the fatal injuries and death? A supplementary query is how long would the victim have been active, even if still alive?

These are extremely difficult questions to answer, as a number of variables enter the estimation. The doctor should never give a dogmatic answer, unless the nature and severity of injuries are obviously incompatible with continued life or activity.

A person who has his brainstem destroyed by a penetrating injury, or his aortic arch completely transected, will be inactive and clinically dead almost immediately. It would not necessarily be the case if his frontal lobes were damaged or his abdominal aorta was crushed by a railway wheel. Extraordinary instances of survival in both these latter instances are on record.

An opinion should always err on the side of caution in expressing opinions on this subject, as victims can do far more than might be expected after injury. The author (BK) once dealt with a homicide in which the victim was stabbed through the heart, yet ran more than a quarter of mile before collapsing. A wound in the left ventricle can partly seal itself by the contraction of the muscle around the defect and collapse may only occur when sufficient blood has leaked into the pericardium to form a tamponade. Wounds of the right ventricle are often more rapidly fatal as, although the pressure of contained blood is less, the thinner wall is not so effective in preventing the leak.

Head injuries can present many paradoxical instances of prolonged survival, depending partly on what part of the brain is injured. As mentioned, frontal lobes seem remarkably resistant to damage and it is often the generalized head impact, rather than focal damage to this area, that causes most harm. For example, a Finnish man who committed suicide made a home movie of himself firing a pistol into his brain. There was immediate collapse but, just at the end of the 4-minute film, the victim opened his eyes and raised his head, finally dying some uncertain time after the spool ran out.

In the more usual stabbing, head injury, cut throat or shooting, the pathologist must try to assess the nature and severity of the physical damage, and relate that to the age, health and environment of the victim. This is naturally an imprecise exercise. A senile old lady, or someone with severe cardiac or respiratory disease, is less likely to survive multiple injuries for as long as a robust young person – though if the nature of the injury is grossly life-threatening, these factors will make little difference.

A cut artery will lose blood faster than a vein of the same general size, especially if it is only partly severed so that it cannot retract. Other factors, such as the possibility of air embolism occurring in a cut jugular vein, might alter the usual pattern of expected events. The heart is less vulnerable than great thoracic vessels in many stab wounds, as mentioned above. Many wounds of the ventricles are survivable. The author (BK) has twice been warned by police of an imminent autopsy on victims admitted for emergency surgery – only to hear later that, thankfully, they had walked out of the hospital after a successful operation. One had a through-and-through stab wound of the left ventricle that transfixed the heart from front to back.

Where a wound has transected a major coronary artery, then prolonged survival is unlikely, as is one that interrupts a major branch of the conducting system. Other than injuries to the brain or to a large blood vessel, most other injuries can rarely be declared to have caused sudden death or rapid loss of function. In criminal cases, it may be a point of some importance to decide whether the victim could have continued fighting, have run away, have resisted, or even have inflicted injuries on someone else before collapsing and dying. It is difficult to swear that at least some activity was not possible in the great majority of instances. In the adrenaline response of 'fight or flight', the shock element of pain is greatly suppressed – many soldiers have been quite unaware of having sustained severe or lethal wounds until they notice the blood or the battle is over. Thus the usual 'shock' effect may be damped down considerably in an assault and only the sheer physical and haemodynamic sequelae of the injury will eventually lead to a slowing down, then collapse and death. In the interval, injured victims may be able to perform normal physical activity, sometimes to an astonishing degree, albeit followed by sudden deflation of their capacity for exercise.

As in most aspects of forensic medicine, it is unwise of the doctor to be too definite about these matters – the old forensic aphorism 'Seldom say never – seldom say always' is even more true here than usual.

Most issues of this nature revolve around periods of a few minutes, the perimortal or agonal time when few morphological signs are available. The more sophisticated enzyme and serotonin techniques mentioned elsewhere in this chapter may give some clue about the survival period, but are rarely unequivocal enough to be used as hard forensic evidence. If survival is longer, then both gross and histological changes of 'vital reaction', such as thrombosis, inflammation, infection and healing may be useful, but they usually require hours or even days of survival to appear.

The accepted wisdom of wound dating is that polymorph leucocytes begin to appear in wounded tissue within a few minutes, but it has been shown that this can happen even several hours after death, as all leucocytes do not become immobile with cardiac arrest. A good, conventional inflammatory response must be a vital reaction, however, though several hours survival is needed for it to be convincing. The author (BK) has seen a dramatic red flare caused by post-mortem burning at least 30 minutes after undoubted death from strangulation.

Another problem with differentiating 'ante-mortem' from 'post-mortem' injuries is the definition of the moment of death. Again, lawyers, judges and coroners tend to assume that death is an **event**, whereas, in reality, it is a **process** (Chapter 2). Though in most criminal or accidental deaths the moment of death is conventionally – and reasonably – taken to be the moment of cardiac arrest, and thus collapse of blood pressure and cerebral circulation, the cells of the body are still alive and remain so for a variable time – only minutes in the case of neurones, but leucocytes a[...] vive for many hours, and connective tiss[...] fibroblasts, for days. Thus, it is unreasonable [...] matic changes within minutes in skin wounds, etc[...] gressive hypoxia alters biochemical processes and [...] activity. Leucocytes may be motile for more than 12 h[...] and can aggregate around chemotactically active materia[...] such as gastric contents aspirated into the air passages. This makes the 'vital reaction' a dubiously valid phenomenon in the perimortal period. Much more research is needed into the histology, histochemistry and biochemistry of the perimortal period to clarify these issues, but in the mean time, less dogmatic reliance must be held upon the old criteria of 'ante-' and 'post-' mortem phenomena and the 'vital reaction'.

REFERENCES AND FURTHER READING

Adams VI, Hirsch CS. 1989. Venous air embolism from head and neck wounds. *Arch Pathol Lab Med* **113**:498–502.

Ali TT. 1988. The role of white blood cells in post-mortem wounds. *Med Sci Law* **28**:100–6.

Betz P. 1994. Histological and enzyme histochemical parameters for the age estimation of human skin wounds. *Int J Legal Med* **107**:60–8.

Betz P. 1995. Immunohistochemical parameters for the age estimation of human skin wounds. A review. *Am J Forensic Med Pathol* **16**:203–9.

Betz P, Nerlich A, Wilske J, *et al.* 1992. Comparison of the solophenyl-red polarization method and the immunohistochemical analysis for collagen type III. *Int J Legal Med* **105**:27–9.

Betz P, Nerlich A, Wilske J, *et al.* 1992. The time-dependent rearrangement of the epithelial basement membrane in human skin wounds – immunohistochemical localization of collagen IV and VII. *Int J Legal Med* **105**:93–7.

Betz P, Nerlich A, Wilske J, *et al.* 1992. Time-dependent appearance of myofibroblasts in granulation tissue of human skin wounds. *Int J Legal Med* **105**:99–103.

Betz P, Nerlich A, Wilske J, *et al.* 1992. Time-dependent pericellular expression of collagen type IV, laminin, and heparan sulfate proteoglycan in myofibroblasts. *Int J Legal Med* **105**:169–72.

Betz P, Nerlich A, Wilske J, *et al.* 1993. The immunohistochemical localization of alpha 1-antichymotrypsin and fibronectin and its meaning for the determination of the vitality of human skin wounds. *Int J Legal Med* **105**:223–7.

Betz P, Nerlich A, Tubel J, *et al.* 1993. The time-dependent expression of keratins 5 and 13 during the

Betz [...] histo[...] in huma[...]

Betz P, Nerlich [...] localization of k[...] wounds. *Int J Lega[...]*

Betz P, Lignitz E, Eisenme[...] ...pendent appearance of black eyes. [...] [...]6–9.

Biddinger PW. 1987. Postmortei. [...]uscence. A report of three cases. *Am J Fore. ...ed Pathol* **8**:120–2.

Bohnert M, Baumgartner R, Pollak S. 2000. Spectrophotometric evaluation of the colour of intra- and subcutaneous bruises. *Int J Legal Med* **113**:343–8.

Byard RW, Gilbert JD, Brown K. 2000. Pathologic features of fatal shark attacks. *Am J Forensic Med Pathol* **21**:225–9.

Camps FE. 1952. Interpretation of wounds. *Br Med J* **2**:770–4.

Fatteh A. 1966. Histochemical distinction between antemortem and postmortem skin wounds. *J Forensic Sci* **11**:17–27.

Fatteh A. 1971. Distinction between antemortem and postmortem wounds: A study of elastic fibers in human skin. *J Forensic Sci* **16**:393–6.

Fazekas IG, Viragos-Kis E. 1965. [Free histamine content in the groove caused by hanging as an *in vivo* reaction.] *Dtsch Z Gesamte Gerichtl Med* **56**:250–68.

Fernandez P, Bermejo AM, Lopez Rivadulla M, *et al.* 1994. Biochemical diagnosis of the intravital origin of skin wounds. *Forensic Sci Int* **68**:83–9.

Green MA. 1978. Stab wound dynamics – a recording technique for use in medico-legal investigations. *J Forensic Sci Soc* **18**:161–3.

Grellner W, Madea B, Kruppenbacher JP, *et al.* 1996. Interleukin-1 alpha (IL-1 alpha) and n-formyl-methionyl-leucyl-phenylalanine (FMLP) as potential inducers of supravital chemotaxis. *Int J Legal Med* **109**:130–3.

Gupta SM, Chandra J, Dogra TD. 1982. Blunt force lesions related to the heights of a fall. *Am J Forensic Med Pathol* **3**:35–43.

... *. 2000. [Morphology ... eath by kicking (II).] *Arch ... 4.

... Cueto C, Luna A, Lorente JA, *et al.* 1987. ... tudy of cathepsin A, B and D activities in the skin wound edges. Its application to the differential diagnosis between vital and postmortem wounds. *Forensic Sci Int* **35**:51–60.

Hernandez-Cueto C, Luna A, Villanueva E. 1987. Differential diagnosis between vital and postmortem wounds: ions as markers. *Adli Tip Derg* **3**:14.

Hiss J, Hirshberg A, Dayan DF, *et al.* 1988. Aging of wound healing in an experimental model in mice. *Am J Forensic Med Pathol* **9**:310–12.

Hocking MA. 1989. Assaults in south east London. *J R Soc Med* **82**:281–4.

Hou Jensen K. 1969. Some enzyme conditioned vital reactions in the initial phase of wound healing and their medico-legal significance. *Dan Med Bull* **16**:305–8.

Hunt AC, Cowling RJ. 1991. Murder by stabbing. *Forensic Sci Int* **52**:107–12.

Janssen W. 1984. *Forensic histopathology*. Springer Verlag, Berlin.

Kibayashi K, Hamada K, Honjyo K, *et al.* 1993. Differentiation between bruises and putrefactive discolorations of the skin by immunological analysis of glycophorin A. *Forensic Sci Int* **61**:111–7.

Knight B. 1975. The dynamics of stab wounds. *Forensic Sci* **6**:249–55.

Kosa F, Kurucz E. 1986. Immuno-histochemical reactions with monoclonal antileukocyte antibodies in vital injuries. *Acta Med Leg Soc (Liege)* **36**:176–90.

Laiho K. 1967. Immunohistochemical studies on fibrin in vital reactions. *Acta Med Leg Soc (Liege)* **20**:187–91.

Laiho K. 1998. Myeloperoxidase activity in skin lesions. I. Influence of the loss of blood, depth of excoriations and thickness of the skin. *Int J Legal Med* **111**:6–9.

Laiho K. 1998. Myeloperoxidase activity in skin lesions. II. Influence of alcohol and some medicines. *Int J Legal Med* **111**:10–2.

Langlois NE, Gresham GA. 1991. The ageing of bruises: a review and study of the colour changes with time. *Forensic Sci Int* **50**:227–38.

Logoida DM. 1959. Assessment of survival after trauma, by the leucocyte counts in the capillary network of internal organs. *Sud-Med Ekspert* **4**:5–13.

Maeno Y, Takabe F, Mori Y, *et al.* 1991. Simultaneous observation of catecholamine, serotonin and their metabolites in incised skin wounds of guinea pig. *Forensic Sci Int* **51**:51–63.

Mason JK. 1965. The importance of the histological examination in death from accidental trauma. *Med Serv J Can* **21**:316–25.

Maxeiner H. 1998. 'Hidden' laryngeal injuries in homicidal strangulation: how to detect and interpret these findings. *J Forensic Sci* **43**:784–91.

McCausland IP, Dougherty R. 1978. Histological ageing of bruises in lambs and calves. *Aust Vet J* **54**:525–7.

Muir R, Niven J. 1935. The dating of contusions. *J Pathol Bacteriol* **41**:183–8.

Niu WY, Hu JZ, Zhang XM. 1991. A new staining method for constriction marks in skin. *Forensic Sci Int* **50**:147–52.

Njau SN, Epivatianos P, Tsoukali Papadopoulou H, *et al.* 1991. Magnesium, calcium and zinc fluctuations on skin induced injuries in correlation with time of induction. *Forensic Sci Int* **50**:67–73.

Ohshima T. 2000. Forensic wound examination. *Forensic Sci Int* **113**:153–64.

Ojala K. 1967. Histochemical and morphological of vital reactions in muscle wounds. *Acta Med Leg Soc (Liege)* **20**:193–4.

Ortiz-Rey JA, Suarez-Penaranda JM, Da Silva EA, *et al.* 2002. Immunohistochemical detection of fibronectin and tenascin in incised human skin injuries. *Forensic Sci Int* **126**:118–22.

Presswalla FB. 1978. The pathophysics and pathomechanics of trauma. *Med Sci Law* **18**:239–46.

Prinsloo I, Gordon I. 1951. Postmortem dissection artefacts of the neck and their differentiation from ante-mortem bruises. *S Afr Med J* **25**:358–61.

Quan L, Fujita MQ, Zhu BL, *et al.* 2000. Immunohistochemical distribution of c-reactive protein in the hepatic tissue in forensic autopsy. *Forensic Sci Int* **113**:177–82.

Rabinovitz A. 1956. Medicolegal conclusions on the form of the knife used based on the shape of the stab wounds received. *J Forensic Med* **6**:160–5.

Raekallio J. 1960. Enzymes histochemically demonstrable in the earliest phase of wound healing. *Nature* **188**:235–45.

Raekallio J. 1963. Histochemical distinction between antemortem and postmortem skin wounds. *J Forensic Sci* **9**:107–10.

Raekallio J. 1966. Enzyme histochemistry of vital and postmortem skin wounds. *J Forensic Medicine* **13**:85–90.

Raekallio J. 1967. Application of histochemical methods to the study of traffic accidents. *Acta Med Leg Soc (Liege)* **20**:171–8.

Raekallio J. 1970. *Enzyme histochemistry of wound healing.* Gustave Fischer Verlag, Stuttgart, Germany.

Raekallio J. 1972. Determination of the age of wounds by histochemical and biochemical methods. *Forensic Sci* **1**:3–16.

Raekallio J. 1980. Estimation of time in forensic biology and pathology. An introductory review. *Am J Forensic Med Pathol* **1**:213–18.

Raekallio J, Makinen PL. 1966. Histamine content as a vital reaction: experimental investigation. *Zacchia* **41**:273–84.

Raekallio J, Makinen PL. 1969. Serotonin content as vital reaction. I. Experimental investigation. *Zacchia* **5**:587–94.

Raekallio J, Makinen PL. 1970. Serotonin and histamine contents as vital reactions. II. Autopsy studies. *Zacchia* **6**:403–14.

Ritz-Timme S, Eckelt N, Schmidtke E, *et al.* 1998. Genesis and diagnostic value of leukocyte and platelet accumulations around 'air bubbles' in blood after venous air embolism. *Int J Legal Med* **111**:22–6.

Roberts R. 1983. Sexual offences. In: *Rape – The new police surgeon supplement.* A. P. S. G. B., Northampton,UK.

Robertson I, Hodge PR. 1972. Histopathology of healing abrasions. *Forensic Sci* **1**:17–25.

Robertson I, Mansfield RA. 1957. Antemortem and postmortem bruises of the skin – their differentiation. *J Forensic Med* **4**:2–10.

Sato Y, Ohshima T. 2000. The expression of mrna of proinflammatory cytokines during skin wound healing in mice: a preliminary study for forensic wound age estimation (II). *Int J Legal Med* **113**:140–5.

Sevitt S. 1970. Reflections on some problems in the pathology of trauma. *J Trauma* **10**:962–73.

Shapiro HA, Gluckman J, Gordon I. 1962. The significance of the nail abrasion of the skin. *J Forensic Med* **9**:17–19.

Shepherd JP, Price M, Shenfine P. 1990. Glass abuse and urban licensed premises. [letter] *J R Soc Med* **83**:276–7.

Shepherd JP, Shapland M, Pearce NX, *et al.* 1990. Pattern, severity and aetiology of injuries in victims of assault. *J R Soc Med* **83**:75–8.

Shepherd JP, Huggett RH, Kidner G. 1993. Impact resistance of bar glasses. *J Trauma* **35**:936–8.

Simpson CK. 1979. *Forensic medicine,* 8th edn. Edward Arnold, London.

Spitz WU, Petty CS, Fisher RS. 1961. Physical activity until collapse following fatal injury by firearms and sharp pointed instruments. *J Forensic Sci* **6**:290–6.

Strauch H, Wirth I, Taymoorian U, *et al.* 2001. Kicking to death – forensic and criminological aspects. *Forensic Sci Int* **123**:165–71.

Takamiya M, Saigusa K, Aoki Y. 2002. Immunohistochemical study of basic fibroblast growth factor and vascular endothelial growth factor expression for age determination of cutaneous wounds. *Am J Forensic Med Pathol* **23**:264–7.

Teare RD. 1960. Blows with the shod foot. *Med Sci Law* **1**:429–36.

Thoresen SO, Rognum TO. 1986. Survival time and acting capability after fatal injury by sharp weapons. *Forensic Sci Int* **31**:181–7.

Thornton RN, Jolly RD. 1986. The objective interpretation of histopathological data: an application to the ageing of ovine bruises. *Forensic Sci Int* **31**:225–39.

Torre C, Varetto L. 1985. Sem study of dermal surface. A new approach to forensic traumatology. *Am J Forensic Med Pathol* **6**:256–70.

Torre C, Varetto L, Mattutino G. 1986. Dermal surface morphology in wound healing. An experimental scanning electron microscope study. *Am J Forensic Med Pathol* **7**:337–43.

Wang D, Zhu J. 1992. Localization and quantification of the nonspecific esterase in injured skin for timing of wounds. *Forensic Sci Int* **53**:203–13.

Watson AJ. 1978. *Kicking, karate and kung-fu.* In: Mason JK (ed.), *Pathology of violent injury.* Edward Arnold, London.

Wilson EF. 1977. Estimation of the age of cutaneous contusions in child abuse. *Pediatrics* **60**:750–2.

Zhong FC, Zhen ZJ. 1991. Localization and quantification of histamine in injured skin as parameters for the timing of wounds. *Forensic Sci Int* **51**:163–71.

CHAPTER 5

Head and spinal injuries

Of all regional injuries, those of the head and neck are the most common and most important in forensic practice. Adelson (1974) gives these sound reasons for this dominance of head injuries:

- The head is the target of choice in the great majority of assaults involving blunt trauma.
- When the victim is pushed or knocked to the ground, he often strikes his head.
- The brain and its coverings are vulnerable to degrees of blunt trauma that would rarely be lethal if applied to other areas.

A sound practical understanding of the neuropathology of trauma is more essential to the forensic pathologist than any other aspect of his subject, as head injuries provide the major contribution to death in assaults, falls and transportation accidents.

INJURY TO THE SCALP

The scalp is often, though by no means invariably, damaged in trauma that causes injury to the underlying skull and brain. The usual range of abrasions, contusions and lacerations may be inflicted, though a modifying factor is the presence of hair, which may deflect a tangential blow or partly cushion a direct impact.

When an injury is visible on the forehead, the back of the neck, the lower temple or on a bald area, the examination is no different from elsewhere on the body. In hair-covered areas, care must always be taken at autopsy to palpate the scalp in any case in which there is a possibility of injury, otherwise abrasions, swelling, bruising and even lacerations may be missed. When a lesion is found or suspected, the hair must be carefully shaved away to expose the scalp for further examination and photography.

Forensic anatomy of the scalp

Superficially, the skin carries hair follicles, sebaceous glands and sweat glands. The skin is attached to the aponeurosis (see below) by vertical strands of fibrous tissue that break up the subcutaneous layer into pockets filled with fat. The blood vessels and nerves lie in this layer, above the epicranial aponeurosis (formerly called the 'galea aponeurotica'). This is a dense sheet of fibrous tissue that lies in the deep layer of the scalp over the whole cranium. It is really a flattened tendon uniting the frontal and occipital bellies of the occipitofrontalis muscle.

Deep to the aponeurosis is a thin layer of loose connective tissue that separates it from the pericranium, which is the exterior periosteum of the skull, the dura being the internal counterpart. Some veins traverse all the layers from the superficial fascia to the pericranium, and go on to penetrate the skull and communicate with the intracranial venous sinuses, thus forming a route for meningitis and sinus thrombosis from infected injuries of the scalp.

Abrasion of the scalp

Brush abrasions are less common than in other sites because of the protective effect of the hair, which also tends to prevent or blur the patterned effect of less severe impacts. Impact abrasions from a perpendicular force are imprinted as usual on to the scalp, though again the intervening hair may reduce the severity. Unless the hair is carefully removed

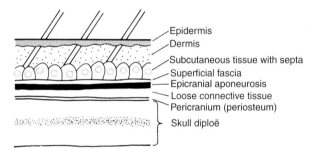

FIGURE 5.1 *Anatomy of the scalp.*

at autopsy, with a sharp scalpel or razor, and care taken not to cause artefactual cuts, lesser degrees of abrasion will inevitably be missed.

Bruising of the scalp

Bruising may be difficult to detect until the hair has been removed. Marked swelling is a common feature of extensive bruising, as the liberated blood cannot extend downward because of the rigidity of the underlying skull. However, this subsides, or at least diffuses, after death. Commonly, a severe head injury leads to a thick, swollen, indurated layer of blood beneath the scalp, which may extend over a wide area. The blood is sometimes below the aponeurosis, the tough fascial layer of the scalp, but is more often between this and the epidermis.

Blood may also be present beneath the pericranium, the periosteum that is closely applied to the outer surface of the skull. This is often seen in head injuries in infants, usually in association with skull fractures, as the source of the blood is from the fracture line itself. The close attachment of the pericranium to the suture lines in infants may sharply circumscribe the extent of the bleeding.

In addition to frank bleeding beneath the scalp, marked oedema may occur after injury and the layers of the scalp may be greatly swollen and thickened by a jelly-like infiltration of tissue fluid.

As will be discussed under 'black eye', bleeding under the scalp may be mobile, especially under gravity. Thus a bruise or haematoma under the anterior scalp may slide downwards within hours – even minutes – to appear in the orbit,

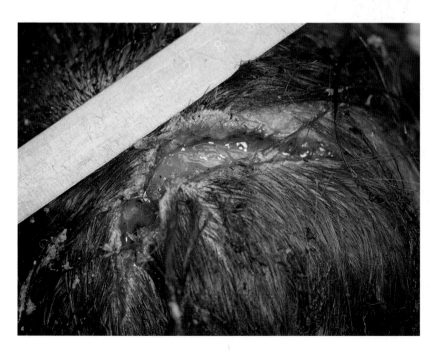

FIGURE 5.2 *A laceration of the scalp caused by a blow from an iron bar. The edges are crushed and bruised, with strands of connective tissue and hairs crossing the gap, indicating that it was not caused by a sharp-edged weapon.*

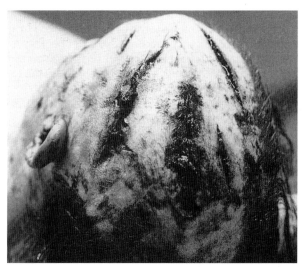

FIGURE 5.3 *Lacerations of the scalp from an iron bar. The margins are bruised and the scalp tissue is extruding in places. The generally parallel direction of the five wounds indicates that the assailant probably delivered the blows in rapid succession with little change of orientation between weapon and head.*

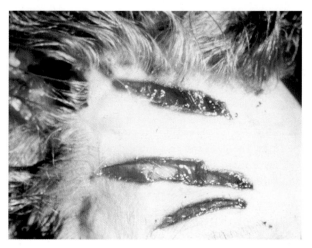

FIGURE 5.5 *Wounds from a metal poker superficially resembling incised cuts, but having edges and tissue bridges within the wounds.*

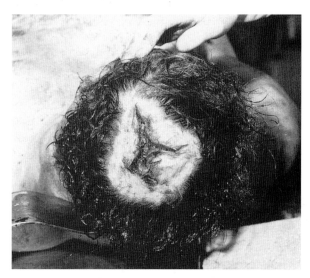

FIGURE 5.4 *Stellate laceration of the scalp caused by a heavy blow with a piece of timber. The support of the underlying skull has caused the tissues to split widely. At autopsy, full clearance of the hair must be made to allow detailed examination and photography.*

simulating a black eye from direct trauma. Similarly, a temporal bruise may later appear behind the ear, suggesting primary neck impact. As with bruises elsewhere, those under the scalp may be obvious immediately after infliction – or their appearance may be delayed, either during life or as a post-mortem phenomenon. They may first become evident, or much more prominent, some hours – or even a day or so – after death. This is caused either by movement of the

liberated blood through tissue planes or by haemolysis spreading outwards to stain the subcutaneous tissues, making it always advisable to return to examine the body a day or two following the autopsy.

The shape of an inflicting weapon or object is poorly reproduced on the scalp, again due to the padding effect of the hair. Where the scalp is free of hair, as in the upper forehead or bald areas, all traumatic lesions are similar to elsewhere on the body, with the exception that blunt impact may cause very sharply defined lacerations.

Laceration of the scalp

Lacerations of the scalp bleed profusely, and dangerous and even fatal blood loss can occur from an extensive scalp injury if it is not checked by treatment. The most gross injury is avulsion of a large area of scalp, which can be torn from the head, thereby exposing the aponeurosis or skull. This may happen if the hair becomes entangled in machinery, as was formerly not uncommon in women working in factories. A more common cause nowadays is a traffic accident, where a rotating vehicle tyre comes into contact with the head, causing a 'flaying' injury similar to that seen on limbs.

Scalp injuries may bleed profusely **even after death**, especially if the head is in a dependent position. A post-mortem injury to the head may bleed considerably if inflicted soon after death and these facts may sometimes cause confusion about the ante-mortem or post-mortem nature of the wound, or about the length of time of survival following the injury. There is no reliable way of resolving this difficulty.

Lacerations of the scalp may reproduce the pattern of the inflicting object, even though a random splitting is so common. Severe blows from shaped objects such as hammers or heavy tools may reproduce the profile of the weapon totally or in part. A circular-faced hammer may punch a circle in the scalp, but more often only an arc of a circle is seen. In such cases, the position of the edge that digs in most deeply may give an indication of the angle of the blow. There may be a depressed fracture of the underlying skull of the same shape and size, though the interposition of the dense scalp may cause the skull defect to be slightly larger than the weapon. A depressed fracture in these circumstances is not inevitable, however, and one or more linear fractures may radiate from the impact site.

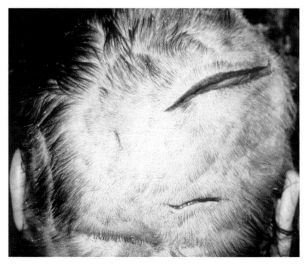

FIGURE 5.6 *Deep linear incised wounds due to a heavy, sharp cleaver. The depth of penetration varies, the large wound overlying extensive skull fractures. The wounds on the neck are due to light contact with the edge of the same blade.*

A major problem in scalp injuries is the differentiation between incised wounds and lacerations from blunt injury.

The scalp is the best example of a surface tissue lying over an unyielding bony support. Violent compression will crush the scalp against the underlying skull, so a blow from a blunt rod-like weapon may split the skin and underlying tissues in a sharply demarcated fashion, which may appear remarkably like a slash from a sharp instrument. Close examination, using a lens if necessary, will show that this blunt laceration has:

▪ bruised margins, even though this zone may be narrow
▪ head hairs crossing the wound, which have not been cut
▪ fascial strands, hair bulbs and perhaps small nerves and vessels in the depths of the wound.

Scalp injuries from falls

It is vital for the pathologist to appreciate that falls on to a flat surface, or a blow from a wide, flat object such as a plank or paving stone, may sometimes leave no external mark whatsoever on the exterior of the head, but commonly such an injury will cause a ragged split which may be linear, stellate or quite irregular.

Such injuries on the back point of the head are commonly caused by falling, especially in inebriated victims. Falls backwards against a ridge, such as a wall or pavement kerb, may cause a transverse laceration, which may be undercut and partly detached from the underlying bone so that a flap of scalp is loosened from the skull.

Falls usually injure the occipital protruberance, the forehead or the parietotemporal areas. Injuries on the vertex

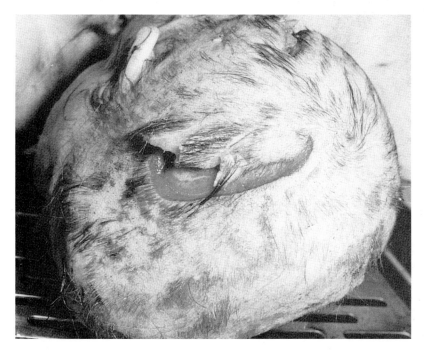

FIGURE 5.7 *Sliced incised wound of the scalp, from a large knife. The wound is markedly undercut, turning a wide flap of scalp. The clean edges, with a lack of any abrasion or bruising, indicate the sharpness of the weapon.*

should always raise the suspicion of assault, as it is unusual to fall upon the top of the head, even from a considerable height. Occasionally, a fall backwards that just happens to reach a vertical surface, such as a wall or piece of furniture, can cause damage to the top of the head, but there is then usually an obvious grazing component to the lesion.

FACIAL INJURIES

Damage to the face is common, but unless gross, with skeletal damage, is rarely fatal in itself unless it leads to bleeding into the air passages. It is often ancillary to fatal cranial damage, or it may be the route by which severe trauma reaches the brain.

The usual range of injuries may be present externally, but all degrees of underlying damage may also occur in the facial skeleton. Because of the complex contours of the face, the various prominences of chin, nose, cheekbones, eyebrows, ears and lips may intercept impacts, with consequent characteristic damage. The eyebrow is particularly vulnerable, being exposed during falls and blows. A blunt impact on the brow often splits the skin and may cause an underlying frontal fracture that can involve the orbital margin.

The distal part of the nose is flexible and often escapes serious damage, though abrasion is common. The bony bridge of the nose is often fractured, which may be detected by movement and crepitus during external palpation – and by dissection at autopsy. Bleeding in the nose is more important than structural damage, as profuse haemorrhage in an unconscious victim may pass back through the posterior nares into the throat and cause fatal airway obstruction.

The maxillae and mandible may be fractured by direct blows and again cause dangerous intra-oral bleeding from associated soft-tissue damage. A heavy blow or kick to one side of the jaw can cause ipsilateral, bilateral or even contralateral fractures. Gross injury to the face, seen in kicking and some transport accidents, may actually detach the facial skeleton from the base of the skull. The lower part of the maxilla, carrying the palate and upper teeth, may be completely separated from the rest of the skull. At autopsy, the best view of the facial skeleton may be gained by dissecting the whole facial skin upwards from the neck incision and reflecting it as far as the orbits, if necessary. Good restoration can be achieved as long as the skin is not penetrated by the knife.

Injuries to the mouth and lips are very common in 'beating-up' incidents, including child abuse. The lips may be bruised or lacerated, much of the damage arising from compression of the lips against the teeth or bony gums. Lacerations on the gingival aspect of the lips may often be exactly matched with the edges of teeth and, as discussed in

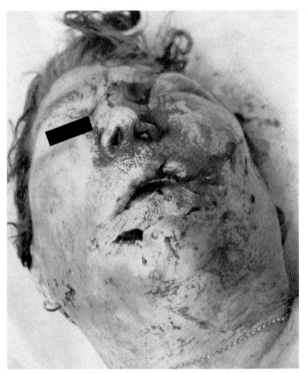

FIGURE 5.8 *Facial injuries caused by kicking. The upper lip is split and the maxilla fractured on that side. The face and orbital region is grossly swollen and bruised. Death was caused by blockage of the air passages by blood.*

Chapter 22, rupture of the frenulum inside the upper lip of a child is virtually pathognomonic of a sideswipe across the mouth, if damage from clumsy and forceful attempts at introducing a feeding bottle, dummy or airway can be excluded.

Kicking

Kicking of the face is regrettably common and again the prominences suffer most. Bruising, laceration and fractures may result from kicking under the side of the jaw: similar lesions occur on the maxillary area and the eyebrows. Patterned abrasions from boot soles may be seen or crescentic marks from toecaps. Brush abrasions from glancing kicks may be present on the cheeks or forehead as the sole of the shoe scrapes across the skin. It is uncommon to suffer a 'pure' black eye from a kick without other facial injuries, such as scuffed abrasion on the cheekbones, or marks on the brows or bridge of the nose. Teeth may be loosened, broken or detached by both kicks and heavy punches and black eyes and fractures of the nose are common. A kick on the side of the jaw may cause bilateral jaw fractures or even a single contralateral fracture.

It may be difficult or impossible to differentiate in every case, between injuries (especially to the face) caused by kicks

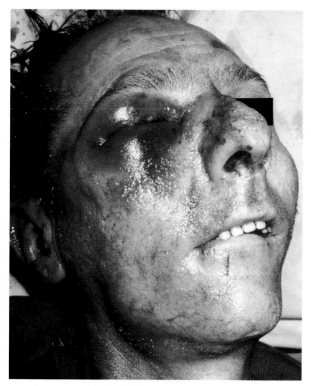

FIGURE 5.9 *Black eye from a direct impact into the orbit from a punch. This is the third mechanism of production of a periorbital haematoma, the others being a fracture of the anterior base of the skull and a frontal scalp wound.*

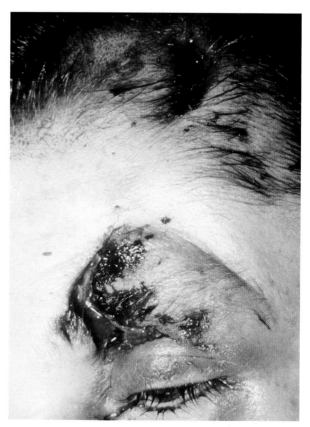

FIGURE 5.10 *Black eye as a result of gravitational seepage of blood downwards from a forehead injury. The woman was struck with a rock on the frontal area and eyebrow, blood then descending during the few hours of coma before death occurred.*

and those from blows from a blunt object. Toecap marks are not all that common, especially since the more flexible rubber 'trainer' shoes have become almost universal footwear.

In stamping, there is the chance that the sole pattern may leave an imprint, but a swing from a toe may leave a non-specific abrasion, bruise or laceration. It may be that the severity of the injury, including underlying bone damage, may be a better indication of a kick than the shape of the injuries, as the force delivered by a swinging foot at the end of a muscular leg is greater than that from a fist.

Black eyes

The usual periorbital haematoma or 'black eye' is usually caused by a direct punch or kick into the eye-socket, but the pathologist must always consider the several alternative explanations. A black eye may be the result of:

- direct violence, which may or may not be associated with abrasion or laceration on the upper cheek, eyebrow, nose or other part of the face
- gravitational seepage of blood beneath the scalp from a bruise or laceration on or above the eyebrow. Survival

and at least a partially upright posture of the head must have been maintained for at least some minutes, usually longer, between the time of injury and death. When the scalp lesion is high up on the frontal region, this time will probably be measured in hours

- percolation of blood into the orbit from a fracture of the anterior fossa of the skull. This is often from a contrecoup injury caused by a fall on to the back of the head, leading to secondary fracture of the paper-thin bone of the orbital roof. It is invariably associated with contrecoup contusion of the frontal lobes of the brain, as described later in this chapter.

A simple fall onto the face on a flat surface does not usually cause a black eye, as the prominences of the eyebrow, cheekbone and nose prevent damage to the orbit.

Damage to the ear

The external ear often suffers from blows to the head and is an obvious target in child abuse. Bruising and laceration of

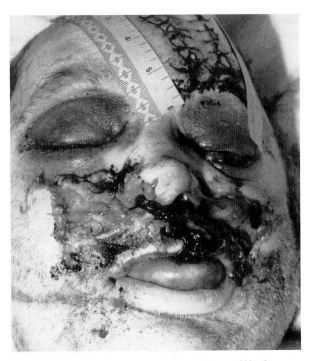

FIGURE 5.11 *Bilateral black eyes caused by leakage of blood into the orbits through comminuted fractures in the floor of the anterior fossa. This homicide victim was struck on the head with a shovel and survived for some days. Brain tissue is escaping from the nostrils through basal skull fractures.*

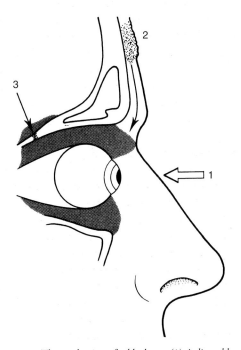

FIGURE 5.12 *The production of a black eye: (1) A direct blow into the orbit. (2) An injury to the front of the scalp, draining down over the supraorbital ridge. (3) A fracture of the base of the skull (direct or contrecoup) allowing meningeal haemorrhage to escape through the orbital roof.*

the pinna is obvious on examination and – in severe trauma – the root of the ear may be detached from the head, usually by a tear at the posterior margin where the ear joins the head. Where gross damage is present, especially with partial avulsion of the pinna, kicking must be considered.

The ear may be bitten and even partly detached, a fate which occasionally is suffered by the nose. In such cases the advice of a forensic odontologist may be invaluable, as teeth marks may form vital evidence.

FALLS

Falls are extremely common, the severity not necessarily being directly related to the distance that the person falls. Many people die after falling from a standing position, yet others sometimes survive a fall of many metres.

Falls from a standing position can occur if a person is drunk, from an assault, during illness (such as a fit or faint) and for many other reasons. Death can follow from a head injury, especially onto the back of the head. An occipital scalp laceration or a fracture of the skull is not necessary for cerebral damage (often frontal contrecoup) to occur. There may also be a subdural or (less often) an extradural haemorrhage, the latter more common from a fall on to the side of the head.

The vexed question of head injury from falls in children is discussed in Chapter 22, but here it may be stated that, although fatal head injury from a fall usually requires a drop of a number of feet, there are well-authenticated instances of skull fractures and brain damage from trivial falls, including some medically witnessed falls from tables and settees. The experimental work of Weber (see Chapter 22) showed that the skulls of small infants could be fractured against a variety of floor surfaces from passive falls of only 34 inches. It is thus invalid for medical witnesses to claim it **cannot** happen, as even one authenticated case creates a precedent. In adults, fractures have certainly occurred from falls onto very hard surfaces from only a foot or so. One such case was a drunk lying on concrete; equally drunken friends attempted to lift him but allowed his head and shoulders to fall back from about half-sitting position, causing occipital fracture.

Falls in old people very frequently cause fractures of the post-cranial skeleton – especially the neck of femur – though ribs, arms and pelvis may also suffer. Osteoporosis is the major reason for the large number of such injuries from falls. More than 47 000 fractured femora occur each year in Britain, with a 25 per cent mortality rate, mainly from subsequent pulmonary embolism or bronchopneumonia.

Falls from a height

Falls from a considerable height, usually from a building, are common in suicide and in some accidents, especially to children. Occasionally deaths from a high fall may be homicidal, again especially in children.

When a person falls or jumps from a height, the trajectory is downwards and outwards, and the distance that the body strikes the ground from the jumping point is variable. Goonetilleke (1980) has published some research on how far from the wall a body is likely to land. Much depends on whether the victims fell passively from near the wall or projected themselves outwards at the top. The body may fall whilst maintaining the same orientation to the ground, but usually turns and twists in an unpredictable manner, the amount of alteration of posture partly depending upon the height of the fall and so the time available for turning. This means that the body may strike the ground in a number of different attitudes – and may also strike some obstruction part of the way down, making interpretation of injuries difficult.

The primary impact is usually the site of the most severe injury, but this is not always the case, as it may strike two areas simultaneously, such as the head and shoulder – or it may bounce or ricochet so that two or more major impacts occur in quick succession. The amount of kinetic energy acquired during the fall has to be fully expended by the time the body comes to rest so that, if only one impact occurs, it is likely to be more damaging than a series of lesser impacts, such as a bouncing, rolling strike.

If the body falls on to the head, there is likely to be a massive fracture, often (but not always) a scalp laceration and possibly extrusion of brain. Both vault and base can fracture and sometimes the base is driven down over the cervical spine, the latter projecting into the posterior fossa. The latter injury is, however, more common with high falls onto the feet when the impact is transmitted up the spinal column and the upper vertebrae – together with a ring of bone around the foramen magnum – are intruded into the skull, causing the classic 'ring fracture' of the occipital bone. Where the fall is onto the feet, the deceleration stress can break the axial skeleton at a number of points. The legs can be broken at any point, at tibial or femoral level, often bilaterally. The femoral necks can be snapped off, the hip joints can dislocate and over-ride, or the pelvis may fracture. The latter is often through the sacroiliac joints, the upward force (or more accurately, downward force of the body on to the legs) driving the sacrum down as a wedge into the pelvis.

If the lower limbs and pelvic girdle remain intact, the transmitted force may then fracture the spine, often at mid- or upper thoracic level.

Where the fall occurs onto the side of the body, any combination of injuries can occur. Multiple rib fractures, shoulder girdle or arm fractures, lacerations of back, buttocks or limbs and severe abdominal injuries can occur, with consequent internal lesions, such as rupture of the liver, lungs, heart or spleen.

In falls from high-rise buildings, the injuries can be extreme, as in a suicide from the twentieth floor seen by the author (BK), where the victim fell onto a fence and was completely transected at waist level.

It must also be remembered that biological and circumstantial variability allows for some remarkable escapes from falls; some persons, including children, have fallen from great heights yet have virtually walked away unscathed. Once again, it is very unwise to over-interpret the relationship between observed injuries and the likely length of the fall.

FRACTURES OF THE SKULL

Forensic anatomy

The cranium and facial bones are laid down from membrane in fetal life. The anterior fontanelle closes functionally between 9 and 26 weeks after birth, though is not tightly sealed until about 18 months. The posterior fontanelle closes between birth and 8 weeks of age. Suture lines close by interdigitation during childhood and osseous fusion occurs irregularly at variable dates during adult life.

The adult cranium consists of two parallel tables of compact bone called the 'diploë', the outer being about twice the thickness of the inner. They are separated by a central zone of soft cancellous bone, which is often misnamed the diploë. This zone is interrupted at suture lines and vanishes where the bone becomes particularly thin, especially in the floor of the skull.

The cranium varies in thickness in adults and varies from place to place, thin plates being reinforced by stronger buttresses, such as the petrous temporal, the greater wing of the sphenoid, the sagittal ridge, the occipital protruberance and the glabella. This tensile architecture of the skull has been well described and illustrated by Rowbotham (1964). The more vulnerable thin areas lie in the parietotemporal, lateral frontal and lateral occipital zones.

The average frontal and parietal thickness in a young male is between 6 and 10 mm. The thinnest area is in the temporal bone, where it may be only 4 mm, while in the occipital bone in the midline it may be 15 mm or even more. The thickness of the skull is sometimes an issue in courtroom propositions about the special vulnerability of a victim but, unless it is abnormally thin, such theorizing has little forensic relevance as it is well known that fatal brain damage can often occur with an intact skull. It has even been claimed that a thin skull is less likely to fracture,

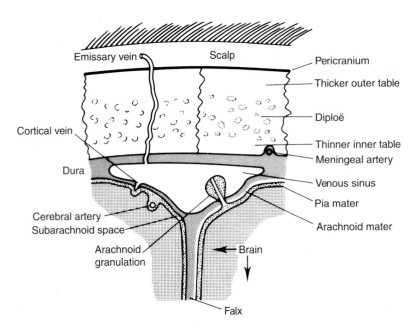

FIGURE 5.13 *Forensic anatomy of skull and meninges.*

as it is more flexible and can return to normal after distortion without cracking; this is certainly true of the skulls of infants. This may be irrelevant when assessing intracranial damage, however, which is the major issue in head injuries.

It is rarely the skull fracture itself that is a danger to life, but the concomitant effect of transmitted force upon the cranial contents. The presence of a skull fracture is, however, an indication of the severity of the force applied to the head and it is uncommon for a head injury that is sufficiently severe to crack the skull not to cause some intracranial effect, even if it is only transient concussion, though, once again, there are many remarkable exceptions to this generalization.

In skeletal material, fractures of the skull are often seen and the differentiation between ante-mortem injury and post-mortem damage can sometimes be difficult or even impossible in the absence of any soft tissues. Artefactual damage to a skull may be caused during recovery or exhumation, and even stones in the soil can cause erosion and even cracking of the softened, degenerate bone after long burial. Zuo and Zhu (1991) have described scanning electron microscopic details of microfractures and collagen damage, which can differentiate ante- from post-mortem injury, but these are unlikely to assist in old decayed material.

The mechanics of skull fracture

This subject has been extensively studied in living animals, isolated human heads and dried skulls. For details, the writings of Gurdjian, Webster and Lissner (1949, 1950), Weber (1984) and Rowbotham (1964) should be consulted;

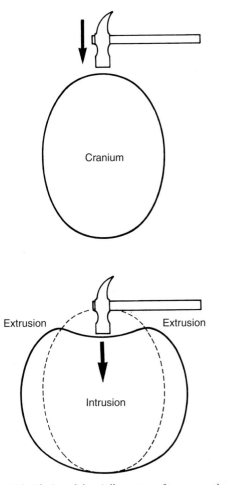

FIGURE 5.14 *The 'struck hoop' illustration of impact on the skull. There is a momentary deformation, with the area of impact bending inwards and compensatory bulging elsewhere. This sets up stresses in the inner and outer tables.*

a concise summary has also been provided by Shapiro *et al.* (1988). These and other workers have shown that:

- When the skull receives a focal impact there is momentary distortion of the shape of the cranium, the extent of which may be surprisingly large, though transient. Infant skulls, which are more pliable and have flexible junctions at suture lines, may distort much more than the more rigid skulls of adults. The area under the point of impact bends inwards and, as the contents of the skull are virtually incompressible, there must consequently be a compensatory distortion or bulging of other areas – the well-known 'struck hoop' analogy.

  Both these intruded and extruded areas can be the site of fracturing if the distortion of the bone exceeds the limits of its elasticity.

- When the skull is deformed, compression occurs on the concavity of the curved bone and tension (tearing) forces on the convexity. If the latter exceed the elastic threshold, then fracturing takes place. Thus the inner

table will fracture where the skull is indented and the outer table will fracture at the margins of the deformed area. If the forces are great enough, a depressed comminuted fracture will occur.

- In the more common circumstance of a wider impact from a blunt injury, the deformation of the skull is less localized but, where the force is sufficient, fractures can still occur from the same mechanism of exceeding the elastic limits. The fractures may be remote from the area of impact, following lines of structural weakness – or may extend from the area of impact, or even commence at a distance and run back to the impact site.

  By using skulls coated with a brittle varnish, Gurdjian showed that stress lines developed in the cranium when it was struck and that these corresponded with the fractures that occurred with heavier impacts.

  Blows in certain areas of the skull constantly give rise to fractures in specific localities – for instance, impact on the upper temporal or parietotemporal areas cause fissured fractures running obliquely downwards across the temporal area. If heavier, another fracture line tends to run obliquely contralaterally across the vault of the skull.

  A heavy impact on the side or top of the head often leads to the vault fracture running into the base of the skull, usually across the floor of the middle cranial fossa along the anterior margin of the petrous temporal bone, to enter the pituitary fossa. In major injuries, this fracture line may often cross the floor of the skull completely to form a 'hinge fracture', separating the base of the skull into two halves. These fractures do not start at the point of impact unless there is also local

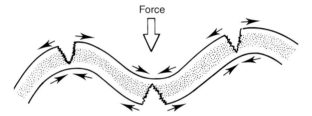

FIGURE 5.15 *The skull is more susceptible to traction forces than compression, so that convexities tend to fracture during the distortion of the 'struck hoop'.*

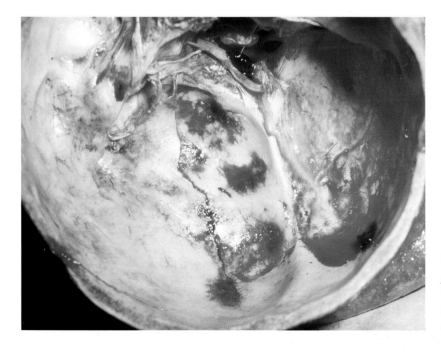

FIGURE 5.16 *Linear fracture of the posterior fossa, due to a fall on the occiput. The fracture typically crosses the thinner bone, avoiding the central buttress and ends near the foramen magnum.*

depressed fracturing; they are initiated at a distance due to the compensatory deformation, but usually run back towards the impact site.

When the frontal area is struck, the usual course for a linear fracture is vertically down the forehead, turning around the orbital margin to run backwards across the floor of the anterior fossa, perhaps into the cribiform plate or air sinuses, or both. A blow or fall onto the occiput may produce a fracture that typically passes vertically or obliquely downwards just to the side of the midline of the posterior fossa, commonly reaching the foramen magnum. In addition, the contrecoup element of an occipital fall may cause fractures of the orbital plates in the anterior fossa, as a result of transmitted force through the brain itself, though the mechanism is not fully understood.

▪ When severe local impact causes focal and general deformation, a combination of depressed fractures and radial fracture lines may form a 'spider's-web' pattern.

▪ When the focal impact is severe, the depressed fracture may follow the actual shape of the impacting object, such as a hammer-head. The shape may follow only that part of the object that drives into the skull – for example, the circular head of the hammer may strike at an acute angle, so only a semicircle of bone will be punched inwards, the opposite edge sloping downwards from an irregular crack.

The deepest part of the depression will indicate where the weapon first struck; there may be 'terracing' of the margins. The author (BK) has seen a recent instance where a victim was struck with a hammer through a thin plastic bag enveloping the head. Parallel terracing cracks had opened for a fraction of a second during the blow, sufficient to trap lines of plastic into the multiple defects in the outer table. Where the impact is from a narrow edge or ring, only the outer table may be fractured, being punched into the softer centre without depression of the inner table.

▪ The presence of hair and scalp markedly cushions the effects of a blow, so that a far heavier impact is required to cause the same damage, compared to a bare skull. The pattern and nature of the skull fractures are, however, the same. It should be noted that the interposition of scalp and hair may slightly alter the dimensions of the skull lesion from a focal blow. For example, the padding effect of the scalp may add a few millimetres in diameter to the depressed fracture caused by a hammer, compared with the actual measured diameter of the hammerhead.

▪ Where two or more separate fractures occur from successive impacts and meet each other, the sequence of injuries may be determined by 'Puppe's rule', which is

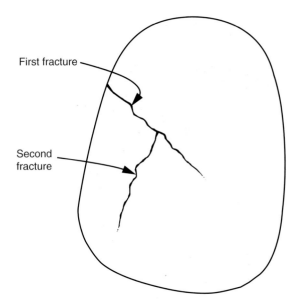

FIGURE 5.17 *Diagram to illustrate Puppe's rule for the sequence of fractures. The course of a later fracture will be interrupted by an earlier pre-existing fracture line.*

really eponymous common sense. The later fracture will terminate at (that is, not cross) the earlier fracture line, which naturally interrupts the cranial distortion which precedes fracturing (Figure 5.17).

Types of skull fracture

Arising from the mechanisms described above, it is conventional to classify skull fractures as follows.

LINEAR FRACTURES

These are straight or curved fracture lines, often of considerable length. They either radiate out from a depressed zone, or arise under or at a distance from the impact area, from bulging deformation. They may involve the inner or outer table, but commonly traverse both.

Depending on the stress contours of that part of the skull and the localization of the impact, they may occur anywhere in the skull, but are especially common in the weak unsupported plates. The temporal, frontal, parietal and occipital plates may all carry single or multiple linear fractures. They may extend downwards into the foramen magnum, across the supraorbital ridges, or into the floor of the skull. A common basal linear fracture is one that passes across the floor of the middle fossa, often following the petrous temporal or greater wing of the sphenoid bone into the pituitary fossa. This frequently continues symmetrically across the other middle fossa separating the base of the

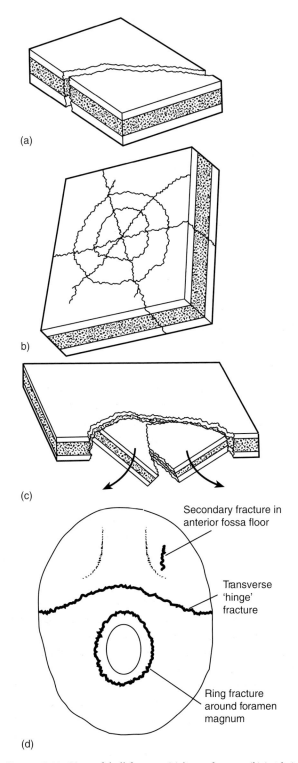

(a)

b)

(c)

Secondary fracture in
anterior fossa floor

Transverse
'hinge'
fracture

Ring fracture
around foramen
magnum

(d)

FIGURE 5.18 *Types of skull fracture: (a) linear fracture; (b) 'spider's-web' fracture; (c) depressed fracture; and (d) base fractures.*

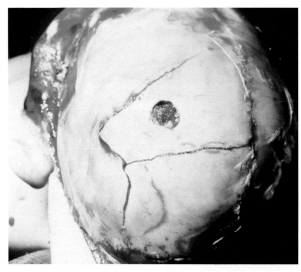

FIGURE 5.19 *Linear fractures of the skull in child abuse. Blunt impact near the vertex has caused a double fracture to run down the parietal bone and continue into the temporal area, the course of the fracture being determined by lines of stress and weakness in the skull. The central burr-hole was for the surgical evacuation of a subdural haemorrhage.*

from one temporal area to the other via the occiput rather than around the front.

In children and young adults, a linear fracture may pass into a suture line and cause a 'diastasis' or opening of the weaker seam between the bones. This is most often seen in the sagittal suture between the two parietal bones, but the interfrontal line of weakness left by the earlier fusion of the metopic suture can also reopen under mechanical stress. In infants, especially in the child abuse syndrome, a linear fracture of a parietal bone may reach the sagittal suture and continue across it into the opposite plate. The continuation may be direct or may be 'stepped', so that the two fractures are not in line. This appearance usually means a blow or fall onto the vertex, and the two fractures may be simultaneous but not continuous, explaining the 'stepping'.

RING FRACTURES

These occur in the posterior fossa around the foramen magnum and are most often caused by a fall from a height onto the feet. If the kinetic energy of the fall is not absorbed by fractures of the legs, pelvis or spine, the impact is transmitted up the cervical spine. This may be rammed into the skull, carrying a circle of occipital bone with it.

POND FRACTURES

This is merely a descriptive term for a shallow depressed fracture forming a concave 'pond'. It is more common in

skull into two halves, usually being caused by a heavy blow on the side of the head; this lesion was sometimes called the 'motorcyclist's fracture' for obvious reasons. Linear fractures may follow a horizontal course around the skull, usually

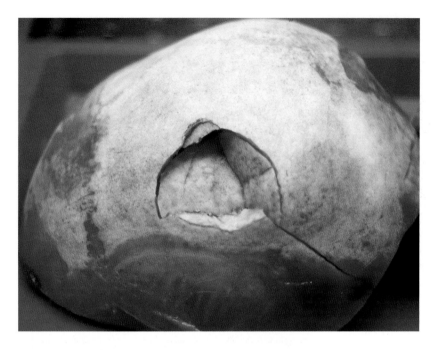

FIGURE 5.20 *Pond fracture.*

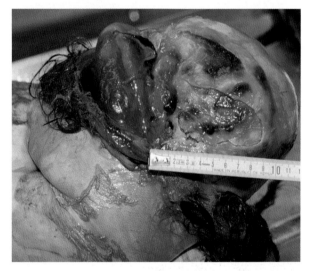

FIGURE 5.21 *Comminuted skull fracture with depression of the central area. This could also be termed a 'pond fracture' in that there is an ovoid depressed zone with radiating linear fractures. The head was struck with a heavy piece of wood along the line of the depressed area.*

the more pliable bones of infants and, indeed, a depression can occur in the absence of a fracture akin to the distortion produced by squeezing a table-tennis ball.

MOSAIC OR SPIDER'S-WEB FRACTURES

As already described, a comminuted depressed fracture may also have fissures radiating from it, forming a spider's-web or mosaic pattern. The degree of actual depression may be minimal or even absent.

DEPRESSED FRACTURES

Focal impact causes the outer table to be driven inwards and, unless absorbed in the diploë, the inner table will also usually be intruded into the cranial cavity with all the dangers of direct damage to the contents. Even sharp-edged weapons, such as heavy knives and axes, which may cause a clean-cut defect externally, usually split and deflect flaps downward from the inner table.

With axes and heavy cutting weapons such as swords, there is a characteristic lesion in the bones, whether skull or elsewhere. The initial impact slices cleanly through the bone on one edge, often burnishing the bone to an ivory-like gloss. The rebound removal of the weapon is at a slightly different angle, either from deliberate intent, or from relative movement between bone and blade. This cracks off an irregular fragment of bone of the opposite face so that the residual defect has one smooth and one rough edge. It is often seen in historical and archaeological material from battles or massacres.

The force required to cause fractures of the skull

Unlike less reliable subjective estimates of the force required to cause other injuries, objective quantitative measurements have obtained for adult skull fractures. Again, the publications of Gurdjian, Webster and Lissner should be consulted for detailed information. The following useful facts arise from their investigations:

■ The tensile strength of the adult skull is of the order of 100–150 p.s.i., the compressive strength varying from

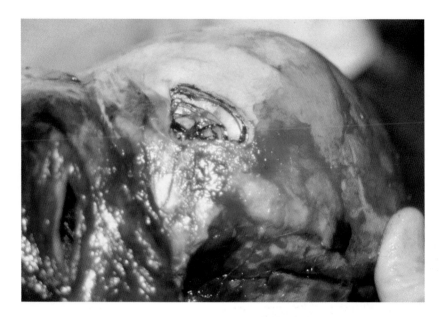

FIGURE 5.22 *A depressed fracture of the skull from a blow with a heavy club hammer. The defect is wedge shaped with a curved anterior border caused by the hammer striking at an angle. The depression is concentrically terraced, with the lowest fragments lacerating the surface of the brain.*

5000 to 31 000 p.s.i. (Gurdjian *et al.* 1949). A simple fissured fracture of the skull can be sustained by walking into a fixed obstruction (Kerr 1954). This requires a force of about 5 foot-pounds (73 N). Fast running into an obstruction produces about 70 ft-lb (1020 N). Falling to the ground from an erect posture also develops at least 60 ft-lb (873 N) and can easily produce skull fractures. A small stone or golf ball weighing about 100 g (4 oz) may also cause a linear fracture when thrown with moderate force against the temporal region (Graham and Lantos 2002).

- The adult head weighs between 3 and 6 kg (7–14 lb), averaging 4–5 kg (10 lb). When falling through about one metre (3 ft), so that the frontal area strikes a hard surface, impact energy of about 35 ft-lb (510 N) develops. This can cause one or two linear fractures or a mosaic fracture (Gurdjian *et al.* 1950).
- Only a small additional amount of energy above that needed to cause a single crack is required to produce multiple fractures.

In spite of these experimental data, it must never be forgotten that, like all biological phenomena, great variation is encountered and skull fractures, though they may be caused by as little as 5 ft-lb (73 N), may be absent when the impact exceeds 90 ft-lb (1314 N). The area of the skull struck, the thickness of the skull, scalp and hair, the direction of the impact and other imponderables, all affect the outcome.

As further discussed in Chapter 22, Weber carried out experiments in which he dropped the bodies of dead infants from a fixed height of only about 85 cm (34 inches) onto various hard and soft surfaces. A high proportion sustained skull fractures, both of the parietal and occipital areas, some of them crossing suture lines.

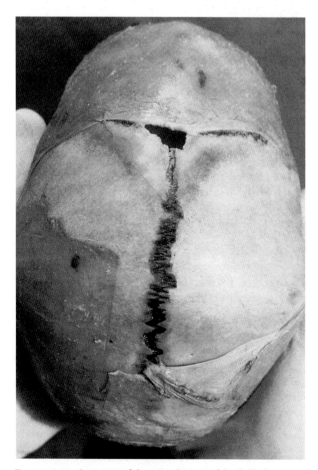

FIGURE 5.23 *Springing of the sagittal suture of the skull of an infant. Though there was no skull fracture, the suture line has widened after a fall that caused a subdural haemorrhage.*

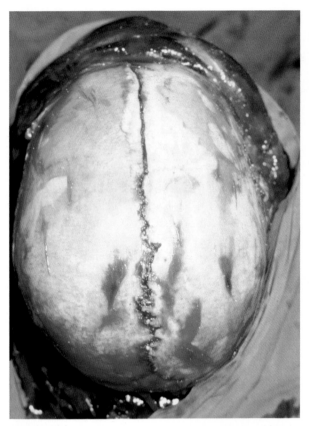

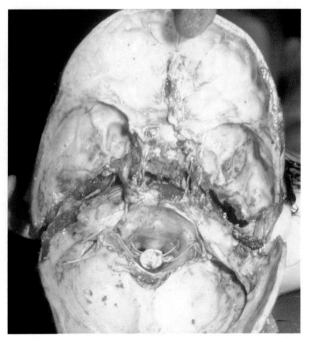

FIGURE 5.24 *Diastasis or 'springing' of the sagittal suture of a young adult who fell from a height onto the vertex of his head. The opening of the interparietal suture has extended anteriorly along the line of weakness of the fused metopic suture between the two halves of the frontal bone.*

FIGURE 5.26 *A 'hinge' fracture of the base of the skull where the fracture line runs from side to side across the floor of the middle cranial fossa, passing through the pituitary fossa in the midline, following the course of least structural resistance. The victim was a young pedestrian who was hit by a car and then sustained secondary injuries by striking the left side of the head on the ground. This injury is common in road accidents and is sometimes called the 'motorcyclist's fracture'.*

Dangers of fractures of the skull

It has been emphasized that, in the majority of cases, the significance of a fractured skull is an indicator of a substantial insult to the head, with possible injury to the vital contents, rather than the fracture itself being a danger to life.

There are occasions, however, when the fracture itself has dangerous sequelae. The most common is when the crack passes through an embedded meningeal artery, causing a meningeal haemorrhage, which is considered later. A depressed fracture may impinge upon the brain and its membranes, and bone fragments may lacerate or penetrate the brain tissue.

TRAUMATIC EPILEPSY

A late effect of a depressed skull fracture may be 'traumatic epilepsy'. This is of great medico-legal significance, especially in the field of civil litigation where an accident or assault may result in lifelong neurological disability for which very large monetary compensation may be awarded.

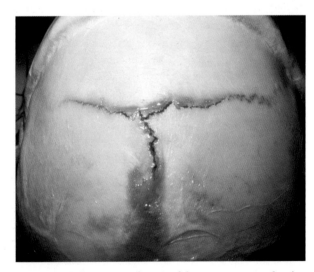

FIGURE 5.25 *Post-mortem diastasis of the sutures as an artefact due to freeze-up of the brain simulating intra-vital skull fracture.*

Traumatic epilepsy usually manifests as tonic and clonic fits, which may be difficult to differentiate from idiopathic epilepsy, if the injury occurred in early life. When fits begin within weeks, or a year or two of a major head injury in a mature person who had never had fits before, the diagnosis is easier, but all cases need expert neurological examination. There must have been a substantial head injury, usually with a depressed fracture impinging on the underlying cortex, often in the parietotemporal area. The epilepsy appears usually within a range of a few weeks to up to 2 years. It is more common in open head injuries when infection has occurred, or when a spicule of bone has penetrated the meninges, as the mesodermal scarring of the cortex that results is more likely to irritate the brain than the astrocytic reaction found in closed head injuries.

INFECTION FOLLOWING SKULL FRACTURE

Other complications may occur, even in the absence of depression or comminution. The most common is infection of the meninges, or the development of a brain abscess, or both. Infection can gain access via skull fractures:

- by direct spread through a compound fracture, especially where there is a contaminated scalp injury;
- by spread from the nasal cavity when a fracture of the cribriform plate has allowed communication with the anterior fossa. This fracture is not uncommon as part of 'contrecoup' lesions, described later. Sometimes the cribriform plate is ruptured by objects entering a nostril and carrying infected material into the cranium: the author (BK) has seen two such fatalities, one from an umbrella ferrule and another from a dirty bamboo garden cane. Another case was seen by PS where a suicide attempt was made with a small calibre pistol. The bullet penetrated the right temple and went through the skull just above the anterior cranial fossa, which was fractured and caused a leakage of the cerebrospinal fluid through the nose. The victim recovered well but, in spite of prophylactic treatment with antibiotics, died one year later from purulent meningitis.
- by spread from fractures that involve a paranasal sinus, such as the frontal or ethmoid, or from the mastoid air cells or middle ear cavity. Basal fractures may allow these spaces, which communicate with the infected outside environment, to reach the meninges, especially when the latter are torn by the traumatic event. A history of leakage of cerebrospinal fluid from the nose or ear must alert both clinician and pathologist to the possibility of communicating basal fractures. In any autopsy on a suspected head injury, however slight, care must be taken to remove the dura from the interior

of the vault and base so that a close inspection for fracture lines can be made.

INTRACRANIAL INJURIES

The contents of the skull are the most fragile of the vital organs, necessitating their enclosure in the strong bony box of the cranium. Damage may occur either to the neural tissues or to the rich vasculature that surrounds and penetrates those tissues.

FORENSIC ANATOMY OF THE BRAIN MEMBRANES

The pachymeninges consist of the dura mater and the leptomeninges, the arachnoid and the pia mater (see Figure 5.13). The **dura** is formed of two layers of tough collagenous tissue, the outer of which is firmly attached to the skull and acts as its internal periosteum. The inner layer merges with the arachnoid, so that in reality there is no true subdural space, only a potential cleavage plane.

The dura forms the falx and tentorium, and the cranial venous sinuses run within it. Branches of the meningeal arteries course over and through its substance. The dura is penetrated by bridging veins, especially along the vertex and at the tips of the temporal lobes, also to a lesser extent at the frontal and occipital poles, as well as by random vessels elsewhere. Polypoid invaginations of the dura penetrate the inner walls of the venous sinuses, especially the sagittal sinus, to form the 'arachnoid granulations'.

The **arachnoid** is a thin, vascular meshwork that is intimately applied to the inner surface of the dura by means of the 'boundary layer' so that no subdural space exists in normal conditions, though their junction is so tenuous that they are easily split apart. Sheaths of arachnoid follow vessels into the brain as they penetrate into the neural surface. These vessels and thin strands of connective tissue anchor the brain within the subarachnoid space. This is filled with cerebrospinal fluid and the width of the space varies from less than a millimetre in the young to a centimetre or more in the old, in whom cerebral atrophy has developed. This means that the anchoring strands and the bridging vessels are longer and more vulnerable to shearing and rotatory stresses. Even though anatomically in the subarachnoid space, rupture of these bridging vessels often manifests itself in the subdural space.

The **pia** is not a true membrane, but a surface feltwork of glial fibres that are inseparable from the underlying brain.

EXTRADURAL HAEMORRHAGE

Also known as 'epidural haemorrhage', bleeding between the inner surface of the skull and the dura mater is the least common of the three types of brain membrane haemorrhage. According to Rowbotham (1964), only about 3 per cent of head injuries have an epidural haemorrhage large enough to be of surgical significance; a similar figure of between 1 and 3 per cent was recorded by Tomlinson (1970). Of the 635 fatal head injuries investigated by Adams (see References and further reading) in Glasgow, 10 per cent had extradural haemorrhages. The mortality rate, even with surgical intervention, averages about 11 per cent under the age of 20 years, rising to between 18 and 40 per cent in later life.

The dura is closely applied to the interior of the skull, forming the endocranium or periosteum. It is so tightly applied to the base of the skull that, except in the posterior fossa, extradural bleeding does not occur over the skull floor. In the vault there is a potential space between the dura and the bone, which can be separated by both arterial and – less often – venous leakage. Most extradural haemorrhages are associated with fractures of the skull, but about 15 per cent occur in intact skulls (McKissock 1960). According to Harwood-Nash *et al.* (1971), the incidence in children without a fracture is only 1 per cent, though Adams found that half the children with extradural bleeds in his series of over 600 fatal head injuries had no fracture. About 10 per cent of extradural haemorrhages are associated with subdural haemorrhages. Bilateral epidural haemorrhages are rare, but have been recorded.

The usual site is unilateral in the parietotemporal area, caused by rupture of a branch of the middle meningeal artery where the latter is transected by a fracture line. The posterior branch of this vessel is most commonly involved as it courses diagonally backwards across the squamous temporal bone on the lateral wall of the cranium. The anterior (frontal) branch is rarely the source of bleeding, occurring only twice in Rowbotham's series of 33 cases. The vessel usually lies in a deep osseous groove in the first part of its course. It has been claimed that almost all ruptures occur where the artery is completely roofed over in a bony tunnel so that it is unable to escape damage from a fracture, but observation does not confirm this contention.

Leakage of the high-pressure arterial blood strips back the underlying dura with progressive accumulation of a haematoma, which can reach a volume of several hundred millilitres and cover an appreciable part of the hemicranium. Adams suggests that a minimum volume of 35 ml is needed before clinical signs are apparent, though other writers suggest 100 ml is usually the minimum associated with fatalities.

In the less common occipital and frontal sites, smaller branches of meningeal arteries may be involved or the bleeding may be from torn venous sinuses, in which case there need not be a fracture. When bleeding is venous, the haematomas rarely reach a large size as the pressure is insufficient to tear back much of the dura.

The clinical signs of an epidural haemorrhage are classically those of a 'lucid' or 'latent' interval, as there may be recovery from the initial phase of concussion (see below) before sufficient blood accumulates to cause raised intracranial pressure and consequent relapse into unconsciousness. This classic picture is so frequently absent, however, that no diagnostic reliance can be placed upon it. The coma from the increasing space-occupying lesion formed by the bleed may follow the period of concussion without a break so that there is no temporary phase of recovery. Only 27 per cent of McKissock's series showed the classic history.

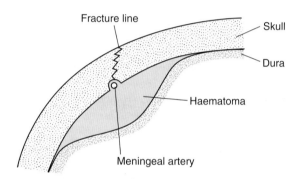

FIGURE 5.27 *Formation of an extradural haemorrhage.*

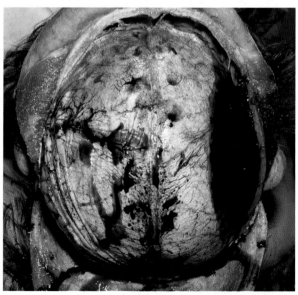

FIGURE 5.28 *A large temporoparietal extradural haemorrhage. The under surface of the scalp on the right shows bruising at the point of impact. There was a linear fracture of the skull passing through the right middle meningeal artery.*

The latent interval may be of variable duration and, as just noted, may not occur if either concussion is prolonged or other brain damage coexists. Half an hour may be enough for the formation of a significant arterial haematoma, though some slow bleeds have taken more than a day to become clinically apparent. In Rowbotham's series, the range was from 2 hours to 7 days, but most were apparent after 4 hours.

More recent investigations using computed tomography, quoted by Adams, suggest that the old concept of worsening clinical symptoms being caused by the progressive accumulation of blood is incorrect, as computed tomograms show that the major volume of blood may appear soon after the injury and that, as with many space-occupying lesions, clinical signs result from other factors, such as cerebral oedema or diffuse neuronal injury.

Medico-legal considerations of extradural haemorrhage

A medico-legal danger is that a victim may be discharged from the care of a doctor or hospital casualty department when he recovers from his transient concussion only to deteriorate and perhaps die at home; negligence may then be alleged against the unsuspecting doctor. Unfortunately, even when the diagnosis is made, the results of surgical intervention are not good, there being a fatal outcome in more than half the cases operated on. Part of the reason for this poor prognosis is that many victims of extradural haemorrhage also have other damage such as cerebral contusion.

When a victim of a head injury recovers from concussion and then lapses into coma within the first 24 hours, the differential diagnosis is between an extradural or subdural haemorrhage, or cerebral fat embolism, especially if there is other skeletal damage. At autopsy the lesion is self-evident, as most haematomas lie in the temporal or parietal areas, and are opened when the usual saw-cut is made to remove

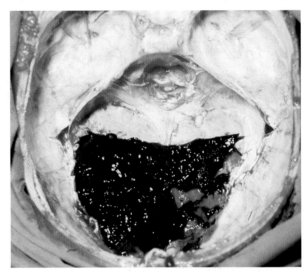

FIGURE 5.29 *An extradural haemorrhage in the posterior fossa. This is an unusual site for this type of lesion, as most occur in the temporal or parietal area as a result of tearing of the middle meningeal artery. In this case a fracture line passed down the posterior fossa towards the foramen magnum, but no bleeding point could be identified.*

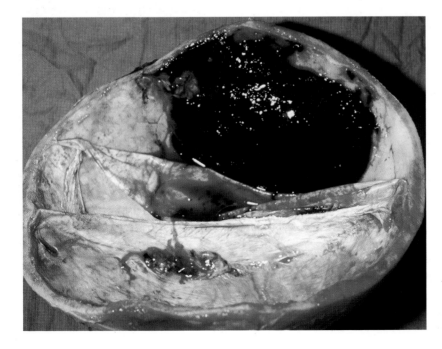

FIGURE 5.30 *A fresh extradural haemorrhage in the temporoparietal area from a fracture crossing the middle meningeal artery. About 85 per cent of such haemorrhages are associated with skull fractures.*

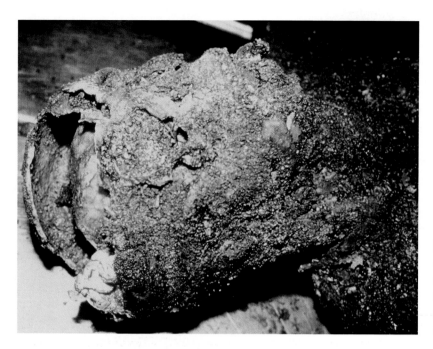

FIGURE 5.31 *Fire victim with extensive defect of the carbonized skull showing reddish-brown 'heat haematoma' on the inner surface of the skull and shrunken brain with brain tissue oozing out through a split in the dura.*

the calvarium. If in the posterior fossa, the dark blood is seen through the raised dura. Wherever it is situated the dimensions and approximate volume should be measured and an estimate made of the inward projection. The brain surface will be flattened or otherwise distorted if the haematoma is of significant size and may have given rise to the usual appearances of raised intracranial pressure, described later. The midline of the brain may be shifted laterally if the bleed is large.

Extradural haemorrhage is never a 'contrecoup' injury, this being purely a cerebral tissue lesion.

HEAT HAEMATOMA

One well-known artefact mimics an extradural haemorrhage. When a head has been exposed to severe external heat sufficient to burn the scalp and perhaps the skull, blood may be extruded from the diploë and venous sinuses into the extradural space to produce a 'heat haematoma'.

The mechanism is obscure, but may be the result of blood being 'boiled' from the diploic layer of bone through emissary veins, or shrinkage of the brain may aspirate blood from the skull. The false haematoma is brown and friable, and the adjacent brain shows hardening and discoloration from the heat.

The importance of the artefact is that it may be mistaken for a true epidural bleed from a head injury, and may mislead the pathologist and investigators into thinking that the fire was started criminally to cover up a fatal assault. As most instances are seen in conflagrations in buildings,

there is often a significant level of carboxyhaemoglobin in the body if the death occurred when the fire was in progress. This should be of the same concentration in the heat haematoma as in the peripheral blood; if the victim suffered a head injury before the fire started, then there should be little or no carboxyhaemoglobin in the haematoma.

SUBDURAL HAEMORRHAGE

Bleeding beneath the dura is much more common than extradural haemorrhage. It is also proportionately less often associated with a fractured skull, but in absolute numbers far more fractured skulls cover subdural than extradural haemorrhages. The Glasgow series of 635 fatal head injuries described by Adams included 18 per cent of subdural haematomata.

The lesion is traditionally classified into three types: the acute, the subacute and the chronic. It is unhelpful to subdivide the acute type, however, and only acute and chronic haemorrhage need be considered.

Subdural haemorrhage can occur at any age, but is common at both extremes of life. It is one of the major causes of fatal child abuse and the rediscovery of that syndrome by Caffey (1946) consisted of an association of subdural haemorrhage with long bone fractures. In old people they commonly exist in a chronic form and can be mistaken either for 'strokes' or for senile dementia. The condition is always due to trauma and there is probably no such entity as 'spontaneous subdural haematoma'. Even in states of vascular fragility, such as in senility and in bleeding diatheses, some minimal trauma must precipitate the bleeding even if it was too trivial to be recorded in the history. It is almost certain that minor subdural bleeds, insufficient to give rise to any neurological or clinical symptoms or signs other than a transient headache, occur with the trivial knocks of everyday life. Only when the bleeding is extensive enough to become either a cortical irritant or a space-occupying lesion (probably between 35 and 100 ml) does it become clinically apparent. Of course, many subdural haemorrhages exist in combination with both subarachnoid bleeding and with cerebral damage, making its contribution to the overall symptomatology impossible to assess.

As with the extradural haematoma, the position of a subdural can never be interpreted as a 'contrecoup' lesion and is thus of no use in differentiating a blow from a fall.

Acute subdural haemorrhage

This is a common sequel to any substantial head injury, and the presence or absence of a fracture is immaterial except as an indicator of trauma to the head. Unlike extradural bleeding, a fracture plays no part in the pathogenesis of the haemorrhage, which arises from torn communicating veins that traverse the subdural space between the cortical vessels and the dural sinuses. Less often the sinuses themselves give rise to the haemorrhage.

Naturally in an open head injury or when comminuted fractures penetrate the membranes and perhaps the brain itself, subdural bleeding is merely part of a complex that includes subarachnoid bleeding, and cerebral laceration and contusion.

The lesion is often pure, however, being associated with a closed head injury where the only other signs may be scalp bruising – or even nothing at all, as blunt impacts may leave no signs in the scalp, externally or internally, and no skull fracture.

The latter situation is probably the explanation in most of the cases formerly attributed to shaking of the infant. Many paediatricians and pathologists have enthusiastically adopted the shaking aetiology when there was no overt sign of impact (or sometimes even where there was such evidence!) to such an extent that it is frequently proffered as the favoured diagnosis. However, the concept of the shaken-baby subdural has been strongly challenged recently, as it has been shown that the shearing force (required to rupture subdural vessels) is of the order of 50 times less in shaking than in impact (Duhaime *et al.* 1987). Thus it is very probable that perhaps the majority of allegedly shaken babies have, in fact, had an occult head impact, which has not left any signs on the scalp, subscalp tissues or skull.

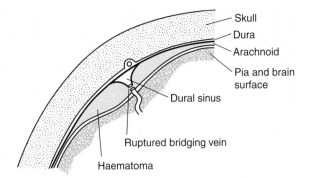

FIGURE 5.32 *Formation of a subdural haematoma.*

Subdural bleeding arises from shear stresses in the upper layers of the cerebrum, which moves the communicating veins laterally sufficiently to rupture their junctions at either the cortical veins or the sinus surfaces. It is very rarely possible to identify the bleeding points. Subdural bleeding is most often over the lateral surface of a cerebral hemisphere, high up in the parasagittal area.

As with most intracranial damage, the mechanical cause is a change of velocity of the head, either acceleration or deceleration, almost always with a rotational component. Where a blunt impact strikes the skull, the subdural bleed need not be situated directly under the impact area – it need not even be on the same side of the head. It is sometimes tempting to attribute a localized subdural to either a 'coup' or to a 'contrecoup' effect (see below), but this is an unsafe interpretation. In addition, a subdural haemorrhage – unlike an epidural – is quite mobile. Lesions that have obviously originated high on the parietal area commonly drain down under gravity and cover the whole hemisphere, with a large accumulation in the middle and anterior fossas, and even through the tentorial opening into the posterior fossa.

The haemorrhage may remain fluid or may clot into a firm mass: both modes are commonly present. If the bleeding is relatively slight, then a 'thin-film' subdural may be found. If the thickness of blood is less than a few millimetres, it cannot be claimed to be a space-occupying lesion, even if the area covered is quite large, as the cerebrospinal fluid in the adjacent subarachnoid compartment can be displaced sufficiently to accommodate an equivalent volume of blood.

Again, Adams suggests that, as in any intracranial space-occupying lesion, a minimum volume of about 35 ml is required to cause neurological signs, though other writers prefer a larger volume, such as 100 ml.

Whether this film of fresh blood is a sufficient irritant to cortical activity – as it undoubtedly is in a subarachnoid haemorrhage – to be a danger to life, is uncertain. It is difficult to claim that a thin layer of blood in the subdural

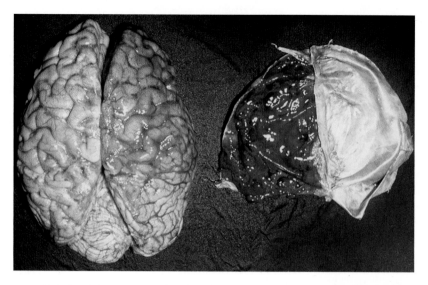

FIGURE 5.33 *Chronic subdural haemorrhage in an old person. Brown liquid escaped from the encapsulated lesion adherent to the meninges leaving a gelatinous outer membrane, as seen. The surface of the right cerebral hemisphere is stained brown from old altered blood and there is some compression of the hemisphere with a midline shift to the left. There was no history of a head injury and no significant neurological deficit.*

space is the sole cause of death, but almost inevitably the force that caused the bleeding will also have had a deleterious effect on the brain tissue, even if this is macroscopically occult such as diffuse axonal damage.

As with the extradural haemorrhage, there may be a latent interval before clinical signs and symptoms appear. After the almost inevitable concussion, which may be very brief, the victim may recover, then relapse into deepening stupor and coma when intracranial pressure rises as the subdural bleeding proceeds. Associated brain damage may, however, cause uninterrupted coma from the time of injury.

When there is a lucid interval, this may be longer than the average 4 hours of the faster arterial bleeding of the epidural haemorrhage. In fact, there is no upper limit to this interval, as the acute subdural haemorrhage merges into the chronic condition, which may recur after weeks or even months. In severe acute bleeds, as are commonly encountered in criminal cases, such intervals tend to be short or non-existent.

Chronic subdural haematoma

This lesion is most often found in old people, frequently as an incidental finding at autopsy where death was caused by some unrelated condition.

The gross appearance varies with age; recent lesions up to several weeks old are tan or red-brown with a gelatinous membrane covering the surface. The contents are thick but liquid and may have areas of redder, more recent bleeding. An older haematoma, up to months or even a year old, is firmer, with a tough membrane around both surfaces, resembling a rubber hot water bottle filled with jelly or oil. The contents are liquid and may be brown or even straw coloured. Sometimes the interior may be much firmer and

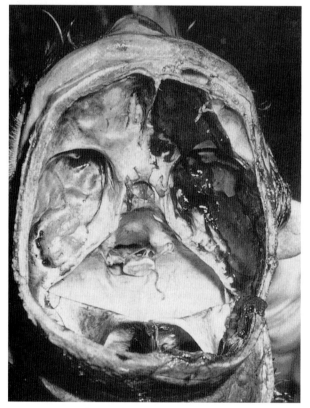

FIGURE 5.34 *A chronic subdural haemorrhage discovered as an incidental finding at an autopsy on an old person dying of an unrelated cause. The blood was brown and gelatinous, but there was no membrane.*

variegated in colour due to bleeds of different ages. Loculation is common, with different coloured fluids or ooze in each locule. The underlying brain will be depressed if the haematoma is large (more than 50–100 ml), and is often stained brown or yellow from altered haemoglobin.

Many such subdural bleeds in old people are small and obviously gave rise to no neurological abnormality; the mere finding of such a small lesion at autopsy should not be used to provide a cause of death, which should be sought elsewhere in the body. Some subdurals are substantial, however, reaching a volume of 100–150 ml. They may still have been asymptomatic, but others give rise to neurological symptoms that may have been ascribed to some other pathological cause. Examples are 'strokes', when unilateral signs were thought to be caused by a cerebral thrombosis or haemorrhage; disordered behaviour of the old person may have been blamed upon senile confusion or dementia, whereas in fact a space-occupying haematoma was really responsible.

The chronic haematoma may become large and press down on the cerebral hemisphere sufficiently to dent and distort the surface. This may progress, as does the large acute haemorrhage, to cause signs of hippocampal and cerebellar tonsillar herniation and all the attendant dangers to the vital centres in the brainstem. The chronic haematoma arises from the acute lesion, which, after an interval, becomes sheathed in a capsule of connective tissue. The haematoma may eventually absorb, it may remain dormant at the same size, or it may enlarge at any later date.

The mechanism of the enlargement is controversial. One common explanation, which seems the most reasonable, is that it occurs from repeated further bleeding, perhaps from new blood vessels that penetrate the mass as part of the healing process. The other theory involves osmosis, said to operate because the centre of the haemorrhage commonly liquefies, forming a haemorrhagic fluid that osmotically attracts into it the cerebrospinal fluid from outside the capsule, which acts as a semipermeable membrane.

The first mechanism seems more likely, as areas of fresh bleeding are often found inside a substantial haematoma but, whatever the cause, the final effect is a worsening of the space-occupying effect.

The dating of a subdural haemorrhage

An estimation of the date of onset of a subdural haematoma may have considerable forensic significance, especially if the lesion is obviously mature. There may have been one or more episodes of trauma on record, any of which may have criminal or civil connotations and the opinion of the pathologist will be sought to relate or to eliminate the lesion found from the potential causative event.

For example, in one of the author's cases an old lady was struck on the head by intruders and died several weeks later. At autopsy, a large chronic subdural haematoma was the main finding, but the defence sought to show that the haematoma must have been present before the assault by claiming that the woman's confused behaviour over the previous year was caused by the pre-existing intracerebral lesion. Furthermore, in accidents of any type, there may be doubt about whether the subdural haematoma arose as a result of the injury, or whether a pre-existing lesion caused unsteadiness that may have precipitated the accident.

Unfortunately, in spite of several claims to reliable methods of dating subdural haematomata, such estimations are of doubtful value, partly because repetitive bleeding results in varying ages within the same haematoma.

A subdural haematoma gradually changes from dark red to a brownish colour, first being apparent not before 5 days and sometimes not obvious for 10–12 days (Crompton 1971, 1985).

Reaction to subdural bleeding begins within a few hours of onset, when cellular infiltration begins from the dural surface. A delicate 'neomembrane', histologically composed of thin-walled capillaries and fibroblastic granulation tissue, grows from the periphery to cover the outer (dural) surface of the clot during the next few days and weeks. If no further enlargement occurs, this capsule becomes more and more fibrous, though rarely does it completely absorb the haematoma by fusing with the outer capsule. According to Crompton, the presence of a membrane firm enough to be picked off with forceps makes the subdural haemorrhage at least 12 days old.

Although claims have been made for accurate dating of subdural haematomas by histological criteria (Munro and Merritt 1936), these cannot be depended upon, especially after a few months, as there is considerable personal variation in healing rates. Also, because of the frequency of repeated subsequent fresh bleeding, attempts at estimating the date of the original bleed are unrealistic. As they are of some use as an approximate guide to age, Munro and Merrit's histological criteria are summarized briefly here:

- Fibroblasts appear at the margin of the clot within 36 hours and in 4 days the neomembrane adjacent to the dura is a few cells thick. From 5 to 8 days, the membrane becomes well established and fibroblasts migrate from it into the clot.
- By 8 days the membrane is 12–14 cells thick and is visible to the naked eye. From a few days after onset, there is progressive red-cell lysis and after 5 days haemosiderin-laden phagocytes are present, which may be stained by Perl's reaction.
- From 11 days the clot is subdivided by strands of fibroblasts. By 15 days a membrane is also present on the under surface of the clot and the outer neomembrane is half to one-third the thickness of the dura itself. By day 26 it equals the thickness of the dura, but the inner membrane is still only half as thick.

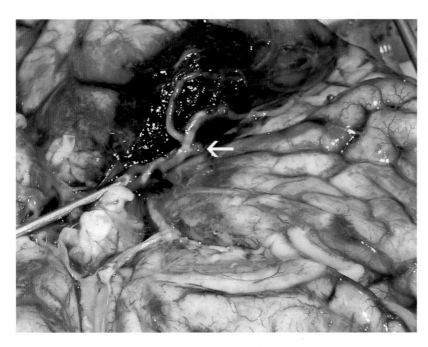

FIGURE 5.35 *Subarachnoid haemorrhage from a tiny berry aneurysm (arrow) of the right middle cerebral artery.*

■ Between 1 and 3 months the membrane has lost many fibroblast nuclei and is becoming hyaline. By 6–12 months the membrane becomes thick and fibrous, resembling the dura itself.

A number of later writers have pointed to marked variations in this chronological scheme. Within the first couple of months large sinusoidal vessels appear in the newly formed connective tissue.

From gross appearances, a rough guide is that brown colour changes occur between the first and second week, when a discrete surface membrane becomes obvious. After a month or so a firm capsule develops, forming a cystic cavity containing dark brown, watery fluid. According to Munro, liquefaction of the contents does not occur in less than 3 weeks. Some haematomas remain solid with an organizing blood clot within, often with areas of fresher haemorrhage of different ages.

When a substantial subdural bleed has occurred, the underlying cerebral cortex may be infarcted, caused by either a natural infarct having bled through the arachnoid into the adjacent subdural space or, more often when there has been a head injury, the pressure of the haematoma on cortical blood vessels (Crompton 1971, 1985).

SUBARACHNOID HAEMORRHAGE

The third type of brain membrane bleeding is even more common than subdural haemorrhage, but has a mixed aetiology. Whenever there is damage to the cortex, there will be some degree of subarachnoid bleeding, so all penetrating injuries of the brain, as well as many blunt injuries that give rise to extradural or subdural haemorrhage, will be associated with traumatic subarachnoid bleeding.

It is not common, though not unknown, for traumatic subarachnoid bleeding to occur as a pure lesion where there is no cortical contusion, no neck injury, no deep brain lesion and no other membrane haemorrhage. Slight subarachnoid bleeding probably occurs very frequently after a moderate impact upon the head (as with slight subdural bleeding), but as the vast majority of such victims survive, no autopsy evidence is forthcoming. The increased sensitivity of medical imaging techniques, especially nuclear magnetic resonance, can demonstrate such minor bleeds which hitherto went undetected.

The other complicating issue with subarachnoid bleeding is that it frequently occurs as a result of natural disease, especially rupture of vascular malformations of several types. When trauma is also present, the complex association of either the trauma precipitating the rupture or a rupture causing a fall or other accident leading to the trauma, has to be considered. This is discussed in a later paragraph.

Although the pathology of subarachnoid haemorrhage is of prime forensic importance, because of the relationship to ruptured berry aneurysm, much of the description is offered in the chapter on sudden natural death (Chapter 25), and only the interaction between trauma and this type of bleeding is discussed here.

Appearances and mechanism of formation

The appearance of subarachnoid haemorrhage caused by trauma varies greatly according the nature and extent of the

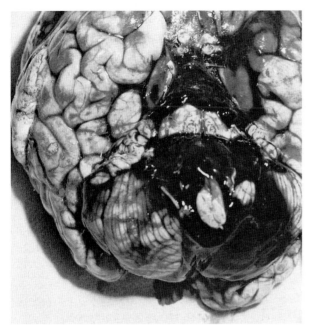

FIGURE 5.36 *An extensive basal subarachnoid haemorrhage arising from a traumatic tear of a basilovertebral artery caused by a blow on the side of the neck.*

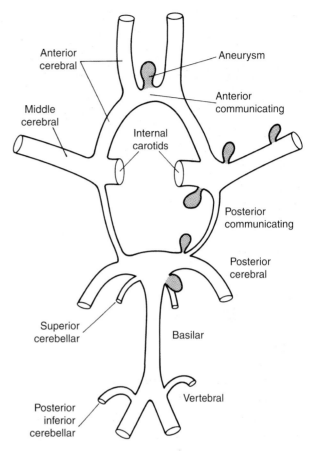

FIGURE 5.37 *Cerebral arteries ('circle of Willis') and common sites for aneurysms.*

injury. Where it is secondary to laceration of the brain or extensive cortical contusion, then its localization and severity depend upon the primary injury. Where it arises from a blunt impact, with or without other membrane bleeding or cortical bruising, its position is not a good localizing sign. Once again, its position cannot be interpreted in the same way as contrecoup contusion of the cortex, though some pathologists use its position to claim that a head injury was sustained either from a fall or from a blow to a mobile head; this is unjustified. Although where the circumstances are known, the meningeal bleeding may be seen in the correct location, this is fortuitous and is equally often sited elsewhere.

Blood in the subarachnoid space mixes with the cerebrospinal fluid, which dilutes it, makes it less ready to clot and allows more mobility. Thus bleeding high over the cerebral hemispheres readily slides down to cover the brain and enter the basal skull fossae, but usually not in a concentration sufficient to form a thick clot. The sulci tend to collect more blood, especially in the insula. Unlike those with subdural bleeding, survivors from subarachnoid haemorrhages rapidly dispose of the blood. Haemolysis turns the cerebrospinal fluid a xanthrochromic yellow and, within weeks, the blood is gone. There may be some residual brown or yellow staining of the pia or arachnoid, similar to that seen when a slight dural bleed leaves its signature on the inner surface of the dura. A positive Perl's reaction for haemosiderin can develop within 36 hours and may remain for months or even years, even after macroscopic discoloration of the membranes has vanished.

This forms a trap for those attempting to date both subdural and subarachnoid haemorrhage in infants, as the common bleeding arising from head-moulding during childbirth may leave a positive haemosiderin reaction for at least a year. Thus if a suspected child abuse head injury occurs in the first months of life, histological attempts to date the bleeding by Perl's reaction may be affected by residual haemosiderin from parturition.

Bleeding in the subarachnoid space is caused by the same mechanism as that in the subdural space, as shear stresses and rotational movements of the brain, described in a later section, shear or rupture the bridging veins that leave the cortex and penetrate the arachnoid en route for the large draining veins and sinuses that lie in the dura. In addition, small cortical arteries may contribute much of the leakage. Where laceration, contusion or infarction of the cortex is present, bleeding will come from cortical veins and small arteries directly into the subarachnoid space. It may also arise from intracerebral bleeding breaking out through the cortex. The subarachnoid haemorrhage allegedly caused by damage to the vertebral arteries near the foramen magnum will be discussed under spinal injuries.

The relevance of a subarachnoid haemorrhage in causing death may be difficult to decide, though this is of more importance in the natural variety caused by a ruptured aneurysm.

In head injuries, death is far more likely to be the result of the other concomitant associated injuries to the brain substance than to a moderate amount of blood in the subarachnoid space.

In the uncommon instances when a substantial subarachnoid haemorrhage seems to be the only sequel of a fatal head injury it must be accepted as the cause of death, though cerebral oedema and microscopic diffuse axonal injury should be excluded as competitors even though this exclusion may be difficult or impossible when death follows rapidly after injury. It is indisputable, however, that sudden death can occur from massive natural subarachnoid haemorrhage in the absence of any traumatic lesions so, by analogy, the pure traumatic bleed – if severe enough – cannot be excluded as a sole cause.

Death can be remarkably rapid when a profuse haemorrhage occurs into the subarachnoid space. The mechanism is not understood, but seems to be confined to those cases where the brainstem is suddenly exposed to a large volume of blood bathing the brainstem in the posterior fossa, usually from a ruptured aneurysm or from a torn basilar or vertebral artery. Numerous instances of victims virtually dropping dead are on record, though many more exhibit the familiar signs of headache, neck stiffness, vomiting and progressive failure of consciousness, before dying at a variable period after the haemorrhage.

FORENSIC IMPLICATIONS OF BRAIN MEMBRANE HAEMORRHAGE

Because of its common occurrence, certain medico-legal problems associated with bleeding into the brain membranes must be considered.

First, the latent or 'lucid' interval in both extradural and subdural haemorrhage may lead to civil suits for negligence where a doctor – usually in a hospital emergency department – discharges an apparently well patient who later dies at home or is readmitted **in extremis.** The clinical aspects cannot be considered here, but suffice to say that it is highly unlikely that such patients would not have suffered concussion, albeit transient. Radiology of the skull is not mandatory if the clinical indications are not present, but failure to X-ray can be a legal impediment for the defence. A subdural

haemorrhage is commonly present with an intact skull, though this is uncommon with extradural bleeding.

As already mentioned, the dating of subdural haematomas may be crucial in both criminal and civil cases when it is being either maintained or denied that a particular episode of head injury causes the haematoma. Dogmatic adherence to any accurate histological dating regimen is unjustified, though broad distinctions in terms of days, weeks or months may be justified.

The possibility of a previous bleed being the precipitating factor in some later accidental injury, which then caused further bleeding, must be kept in mind.

Using a membrane haemorrhage to localize an impact can be subject to over-interpretation. An extradural haematoma is almost invariably on the same side as the blow, but because of the distortion of the skull described earlier, the fracture that traverses the meningeal artery can be some distance from the point of impact. Using Gurdjian's work, however, a reasonable estimate of the zone can be offered.

Where subdural or subarachnoid bleeding is concerned, it can be misleading to offer dogmatic opinions about the nature and position of the impact, unless there is scalp or skull damage. Though sometimes it is clear from the presence of a scalp injury that the haemorrhage is either 'coup' or 'contrecoup', there are so many exceptions when the bleeding is unrelated to the site of the blow, that a firm opinion is not justified.

RUPTURED BERRY ANEURYSM AND TRAUMA

A major cause of medico-legal problems is the association of trauma and subarachnoid haemorrhage from a ruptured 'berry' aneurysm. The pathology of the latter is described in another chapter, but here we are concerned with the allegations that an injury led to rupture of a pre-existing aneurysm.

Several variations of this scenario exist. Most commonly, an assault is rapidly followed by the signs of subarachnoid bleeding and subsequently death. Occasionally death may be extremely rapid, as previously described. The question of causation then arises, the prosecution claiming that the head injury mechanically ruptured the aneurysm. Whether this is actually so is virtually beyond absolute proof. Aneurysms of the circle of Willis are remote from the skull surface and lie deeply protected under the buffer provided by the mass of the brain. However, it is hard to deny that a heavy blow to the head, jaw or neck could not rupture, split or weaken the fragile wall of a large, thin-walled aneurysm, but when the bleeding comes from a tiny sessile bulge the evidence is not so convincing.

The complicating factor is that most assaults occur in 'fight or flight' conditions in which both aggressor and victim are physically and emotionally active, so that the adrenal response is likely to be present. Muscle tone, heart rate and blood pressure are increased by catecholamines, and it is likely that raised internal blood pressure in a weak aneurysm is a far more potent reason for rupture than a blow on the head.

A second possibility is that a person with an already spontaneously leaking aneurysm may have a rapidly developing neurological or even behavioural abnormality that leads him into conflict with another person, or into a dangerous physical position, such as a fall or traffic accident. If all this occurs over a short period of time, autopsy may not be able to distinguish the sequence of events and the aneurysmal rupture may be blamed on the trauma instead of the reverse. This may have profound civil as well as criminal legal consequences.

SUBARACHNOID HAEMORRHAGE AND ALCOHOL

A factor that is often said to increase the chance of rupture is alcohol, though there is no objective proof of this claim. A high blood alcohol is said to facilitate bursting of an aneurysm because it dilates cerebral blood vessels, increases cerebral blood flow and raises blood pressure.

The latter is not true because alcohol does not raise systolic pressure, though the pulse pressure – the difference between systolic and diastolic – may widen. The fibrous wall of an aneurysm is incapable of dilating, neither can the major basal arteries do so to any appreciable degree, as they possess little muscle in their walls. The pharmacological evidence that alcohol has any significant effect on the cerebral circulation is extremely weak. There is no evidence that alcohol is associated with completely natural subarachnoid haemorrhage from a ruptured aneurysm, though intense physical activity, such as sport or coitus, certainly does predispose to rupture.

Where alcohol and ruptured berry aneurysm are concerned, a more likely explanation is that the association is coincidental – as most altercations resulting in 'flight, fight and fisticuffs' are catalysed by alcohol. Many of the cases of ruptured aneurysm and violence occur within and on the pavements outside bars and clubs, where a high blood alcohol is virtually inevitable – but not necessarily causative.

The other aspect of alcohol is that it may cause or contribute to unsteadiness, a fall or some other traumatic event, which itself might lead to rupture of a fragile aneurysm. Ataxia and hypotonia are a feature of acute

drunkenness and, together with the aggressive behaviour and alcoholic environment of most physical violence, seem sufficient to account for their circumstantial association.

THE RAPIDITY OF DEATH IN SUBARACHNOID HAEMORRHAGE

The immediacy of death is sometimes surprising, especially in association with trauma. It is general clinical experience that the victim of a spontaneous rupture of a berry aneurysm suffers a severe headache, neck stiffness and vomiting, which may resolve or which may progress over hours or days to coma and death. Sudden death is certainly the exception in these clinical cases – but these are from a hospital population, which, by definition, excludes the rapid deaths that reach the mortuary rather than the wards.

In forensic practice, much more rapid demise is not uncommon. For example, the author (BK) recollects that as two men involved in a violent argument in a public house emerged through the outer doors, one struck the other a heavy blow on the head. The victim fell to the ground and never moved again, being certified dead a few minutes later. At autopsy, a typical fresh subarachnoid bleed from a ruptured aneurysm was displayed.

The amount of blood present in most subarachnoid haemorrhages, from whatever cause, often seems insufficient to constitute a space-occupying lesion, especially as, unlike subdural bleeding, it is able to diffuse more widely over the brain and displace cerebrospinal fluid into the spinal theca. The total volume may be considerable, however, and where survival for some hours has occurred, then the typical appearances of raised intracranial pressure may be seen at autopsy, though some of this may be contributed by progressive cerebral oedema.

Most rapid deaths exhibit substantial bleeding into the basal cisterns at autopsy, the brainstem and cranial nerve roots being bathed in a thick layer of blood and clot. As blood in the subarachnoid space seems irritant even in small quantities, it seems possible that such sudden irrigation of the medulla may lead to a rapid cardiorespiratory failure. Where the haemorrhage appears less extensive, the mechanism of death is more obscure.

Crompton points out the sensitivity of cerebral arterioles during surgical operations, when a slight touch upon the cortex leads to blanching spasm of the vessels. Subarachnoid bleeding is undoubtedly irritant and a possible reason for the sudden collapse and death is a widespread vascular spasm, which may have an effect on vital centres in the brainstem.

ROTATIONAL TRAUMA TO THE HEAD AND UPPER NECK: BASILOVERTEBRAL ARTERY INJURY

During the last few years it has been recognized that blows to the side of the neck and/or head can give rise to fatal subarachnoid bleeding. This has been attributed to tearing or dissection of a vertebral artery, allowing blood to track along the upper part of the vessel and enter the cranial cavity where the artery penetrates the dural membrane at the foramen magnum.

The evolution of this concept of traumatic subarachnoid bleeding is interesting. Originally, it was thought that most cases had a fracture of the transverse process of the first cervical vertebra, thus damaging the artery contained in the tunnel-like foramen in this bone – indeed, it was often called the 'CV-One syndrome'.

The hypothesis was that a blow to the side of the neck caused deep injury, usually manifested by skin bruising and bleeding into the muscles deep in the upper neck. This same injury was considered to fracture the transverse process and lead to tearing or dissection of the wall of the contained vertebral artery; blood then tracked upwards and medially to penetrate the dura and emerge inside the subarachnoid space of the posterior cranial fossa to cause a fatal haemorrhage.

Soon cases were being described with no such atlas vertebra fracture, but it was still accepted that mechanical forces, especially of a tilting and rotational nature, could damage the vertebral artery within the foramina of the upper cervical spine and lead to the same dissecting lesion, and hence to fatal subarachnoid haemorrhage. Until very recently, this was the theory – which is still strongly held by many pathologists – that satisfied the aetiological needs of this injury.

However, though it is likely that this classical mechanism does account for some of the deaths, there are several problems with universal acceptance of the hypothesis:

- Many pathologists – including the authors – find it hard to believe that a tiny dissection of a small artery like the vertebral artery – a lesion which often needs serial microscopic sections to confirm – could allow the torrent of blood necessary to enter the cranial cavity and produce a massive haemorrhage (sometimes well in excess of 100 ml) which may cause death within minutes.
- Several instances of a damaged vertebral **vein** have been reported in association with subarachnoid haemorrhage. Because of the very much lower intravascular pressure in a vein compared with an artery, the possibility of this causing a massive intracranial bleed by percolation through the dural fenestration is even less credible than in the case of the artery.
- Increasing numbers of cases are being described with positive evidence of a blow on the side of the neck or head and a large fatal subarachnoid haemorrhage, but with completely intact vertebral arteries.

Thus, if sudden tilting and rotational forces acting on the upper spine and head can lead to subarachnoid haemorrhage without damage to the vertebral vessels, then the causative link is destroyed. Even where vertebral damage is demonstrable, this may be merely a **concomitant** event, the mechanical forces which primarily led to subarachnoid haemorrhage by direct injury to intracranial vessels also having caused the vertebral artery damage. In other words, the two lesions may in some cases – or for all we know, every case – be a **parallel** phenomenon, not a **cause-and-effect** situation. There may well be a further concomitant effect, in that direct occult brain damage, manifested later by diffuse axonal injury, is the major cause of cerebral dysfunction, both the subarachnoid haemorrhage and the vertebral artery lesion (if there is one) being merely markers of a heavy impact.

In these deaths – and certainly where no lesion at all is discernible in the upper spinal vessels – we need to look elsewhere for an explanation of the subarachnoid bleeding.

Occasionally, this is quite obvious and is situated in the intracranial vertebrobasilar vessels. For example, the author (BK) has seen a wide split in the wall of a vertebral artery **within** the posterior cranial fossa, and another where the vertebral artery was totally avulsed and transected at the internal side of the dural perforation. Both these cases arose as a result of trauma to the side of the neck, and both had a massive subarachnoid haemorrhage with no damage to vessels outside the cranium.

Bostrom, Helander and Lindgren (1992) published details of two cases of rupture of the posterior inferior cerebellar artery due to blunt basal head trauma, and proposed that the term 'traumatic subarachnoid haemorrhage' be abandoned and replaced by the nature and localization of the bleeding site.

The demonstration of intracranial bleeding from the vertebrobasilar system is difficult, as the very process of opening the skull at autopsy and removing the brain, however carefully performed, inevitably causes vascular damage. These artefacts cannot be distinguished from original bleeding points due to ante-mortem trauma.

The use of post-mortem angiography by the injection of radio-opaque contrast medium into the lower vertebral and carotid arteries has not lived up to its original claims. There is almost always diffuse leakage of contrast medium from apparently artefactual defects, and localization of true bleeding points is often obscured by a haze of contrast opacity. However, occasionally the method reveals a specific leak, usually within the posterior cranial fossa.

The original descriptions of and claims for vertebral artery damage as the cause of traumatic subarachnoid haemorrhage were published by Cameron and Mant (1972), Coast and Gee (1984), Contostavlos (1971, 1995), Simonsen (167, 1976) and others. Leadbeatter (1994) drew attention to the problems of a universal cause-and-effect relationship; Contostavlos (1995) refuted these claims, but did not satisfactorily dispose of the concomitant hypothesis. Pathologists, both from their dissection experience and reading of the literature must make up their own minds on the matter, but should make a critical evaluation of the practicality of a massive subarachnoid bleed appearing, sometimes within minutes, from a tiny dissection of a small artery outside the dural membrane.

As many pathologists still adhere to the original concept of a subcranial vertebral artery causation for traumatic subarachnoid haemorrhage (and in a small number of instances, the evidence is persuasive), the topic is further pursued here, with the over-riding qualification that most traumatic massive meningeal bleeds are due to intracranial causes consequent upon a tilting, rotatory impact upon the head and/or neck, with or without concomitant damage to a vertebral vessel.

Forensic anatomy

The two vertebral arteries arise from each subclavian artery in the region behind the sternoclavicular joints. Each artery ascends behind the common carotid to reach the transverse process of the sixth cervical vertebra. It enters the foramen in that process and passes upwards through each similar foramen until it emerges from the upper edge of the second (axis) vertebrae. The artery then bends laterally and enters the final foramen in the atlas vertebrae. Emerging on the upper surface, the artery bends back and medially around the superior articular process, and penetrates the postero-lateral aspect of the atlanto-occipital membrane and the underlying spinal dura and arachnoid, emerging on the lateral side of the spinal canal just below the foramen magnum. Both arteries then ascend and converge on the ventral surface of the medulla and pons to fuse in the midline to become the basilar artery. Each vertebral artery is often of markedly different size.

Autopsy appearances

With the caveats expressed earlier, the possibility of vertebral artery trauma, concomitant or otherwise, should always be borne in mind when an external bruise is seen on the

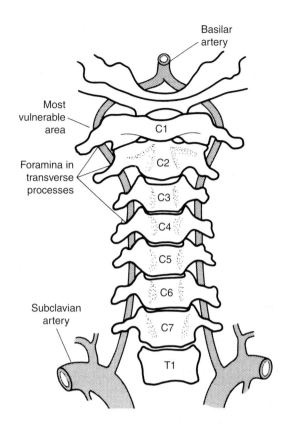

FIGURE 5.38 *The origin and course of the vertebral arteries. They arise from the subclavian arteries at the level of the sternoclavicular joints and ascent via the foramina in the transverse process.*

side of the neck of the victim of a fatal assault. A blow from a fist, foot or blunt weapon may land in the region between the angle of the jaw to the side of the back of the neck, the area below the ear being the most common place to find an injury.

There may be no external sign at all, but on dissection of the neck, a subcutaneous or deep bruise may be found. Unfortunately, this is an area that is not routinely dissected at autopsy, the usual incision for the removal of the neck organs being too far anterior to reveal many of these injuries, which usually lie in the strong neck muscles. This is probably why the syndrome was not recognized until a few years ago – and also an explanation why so many sub-arachnoid haemorrhages were said to be due to a berry aneurysm that could not be found because the bursting had destroyed it. No doubt a number of subarachnoid bleeds are due to rupture of non-aneurysmal vessels or to an aneurysm too small to find, but equally, unrecognized head trauma, with or without vertebral artery damage, must have accounted for some of the remainder.

In some autopsies, there is no external neck injury and the cause of death is unknown until the cranium is opened, and a fresh subarachnoid haemorrhage discovered. A decision then needs to be made whether to remove the brain to search for a ruptured berry aneurysm – or begin specialized techniques to seek a rupture of a vertebral artery (described below). If there is a history of assault or other trauma, as opposed to a presumed natural death, then particular methods should be employed. The two avenues are not mutually exclusive, as long as the pathologist is aware of his objectives. The vessels can be clamped off at the base of the brain and the brain removed for a search for an aneurysm or other bleeding-point without spoiling the other techniques.

Mechanism of vertebral artery trauma

When a head is rapidly rotated by a blow that lands at the junction of the head and the neck, there may be a sudden lateral rocking (tilting sideways) at the atlanto-occipital joint, accompanied by rotation of the head. There may also be an element of hyperextension or hyperflexion, the whole episode forming a complex pattern of sudden abnormal movement at the atlanto-occipital junction. It may be that the unexpected impact may allow more unrestrained rotation and angulation of the head, due to absence of anticipatory muscle tensing in the large paravertebral and sternomastoid musles; this may be exacerbated by alcoholic intoxication causing slow protective responses, as most of such episodes occur during altercations related to drinking sessions.

The mechanics are not fully understood and probably differ from case to case but, whatever the mechanism, the vertebral artery can become damaged either:

■ in the canal within the first cervical vertebra (whether or not the transverse process is fractured)
■ just below the axis, in the space between the transverse processes of the axis and atlas
■ as it emerges from the exit of the canal in the atlas to penetrate the spinal dura just below the foramen magnum
■ probably much more frequently within the subarachnoid space above the foramen magnum or even higher in its course towards the confluence with the basilar artery – and even the basilar itself. The type of damage is usually a tear or dissection of the wall of the vertebral artery.

Vertebral artery damage was originally said to allow blood to track under arterial pressure within the adventitia and to appear in the subarachnoid space after the vessel has penetrated the dura and arachnoid, though, as discussed above, the likelihood seems slight of these minute lesions

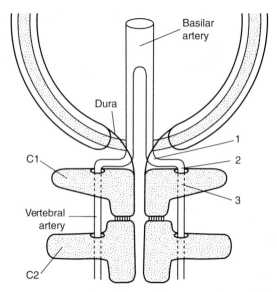

FIGURE 5.39 *Most vulnerable points for trauma to the vertebral arteries: (1) at penetration of dura; (2) at exit from atlas transverse process; (3) in osseous canal in atlas.*

allowing the large volume of blood seen in most subarachnoid haemorrhages to flow through the small periarterial window in the dura.

Autopsy demonstration of basilovertebral artery damage

When circumstantial evidence suggests a subarachnoid haemorrhage following trauma or where a bruise is seen on the side of the neck, vertebral artery damage should be suspected, then confirmed or eliminated. The first intimation that it may have occurred may be when the skull-cap is removed and a subarachnoid haemorrhage is discovered.

If the view is taken that most subarachnoid haemorrhage following upper neck trauma is due to intracranial vascular damage, then logically it is unnecessary to use time-consuming and laborious procedures which slow up the completion of the case. In many such deaths, there will be no lesion in the upper cervical spine or extracranial vertebral arteries and even if there is, it is likely to be a concomitant lesion, occurring synchronously, but with no cause–effect relationship with the intracranial vessel rupture.

However, there may be academic satisfaction in demonstrating the concomitant neck lesion, even if it played no role in producing the subarachnoid haemorrhage. In such a case, when the deceased has been in a fight or had some violence applied to the side of his neck, the same routine should be employed.

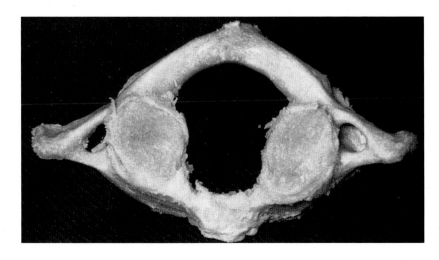

FIGURE 5.40 *The first cervical ('atlas') vertebra viewed from above to show the foramina in the transverse processes through which the vertebral arteries pass.*

Different pathologists have different procedures, but the following would be a reasonable method of investigation:

■ Radiographs of the upper cervical region, both anteroposterior and lateral, should be taken as these may (rarely) reveal a fracture of the transverse process of the atlas vertebra. Such a fracture is, however, present in only a minority of vertebral artery injuries – and even when present, straight X-rays may not reveal it.

■ Post-mortem angiograms should be taken if facilities exist. There are several methods of performing these. The lower neck is carefully dissected to reach the origins of the vertebral arteries. The best method is to open the subclavian vessels and identify the ostia of the vertebrals, which are the first (most medial) branches of the subclavian arteries. These can be cannulated and contrast media injected, one side at a time, while cervical and skull radiographs are taken. This method tends to fill many intracranial vessels and produce a confused, blurred picture.

More satisfactorily, the brain should be carefully lifted from the skull and, as soon as the basilar artery is accessible, it should be clamped off with surgical forceps and/or ligated and the brain completely removed as usual after the basilar artery has been transected just above the clamp. Alternatively, each vertebral artery can be clamped or ligated in its terminal course. The angiogram is now performed, either by perfusing up one vessel and forcing contrast medium back down the other via the clamped basilar, or by consecutive injections on either side. Only sufficient medium to fill the system should be introduced to avoid spillage from small branches which obscure the films. The object is to detect any significant leakage from a vertebral vessel in its upper course, usually within the foramen of the atlas or just outside the atlanto-occipital membrane or within the spinal theca.

■ As by definition, there will have been a substantial subarachnoid haemorrhage, this sometimes makes it difficult to identify and ligate the basilar or vertebral vessels. The brain should be minutely examined for berry aneurysms or other vascular malformations as, if they are present (and ruptured), then further investigation of vertebral artery damage is pointless. Assuming no such bleeding point is found, the upper cervical region is dissected to determine whether the vertebrals have been injured. When no X-ray or angiographic facilities exist, this is the only method available.

The upper cervical spine should be exposed by a posterior approach, which is continued up to meet the transverse scalp incision. The spine should be freed from the surrounding muscles, taking care to detect and record any muscular bruising in the vicinity. It should then be sawn through at about C4 level or lower.

The occipital bone should then be cut through on each side from the transverse skull saw-cut and prolonged down on each side of the foramen magnum, and then across the clivus to release the central part of the floor of the posterior fossa, carrying the foramen magnum and attached upper spine. Alternatively, using a power saw with a wedge-shaped blade, a square may be cut out of the floor of the posterior fossa to detach the spinal block. If possible, X-rays should be taken of the detached portion, as it may be possible to see a fracture of the transverse process of the atlas better than in the intact body.

The block of bone removed should then be decalcified by prolonged immersion in a large volume of 10 per cent formic acid.

After a week, the spine will be soft enough to slice with a scalpel, so that the lateral parts of the transverse processes can be shaved away, taking care not to get near the arterial foramina. The block is then returned to fresh decalcifying fluid for a further week.

Once the bone has been softened enough to be cut easily by a sharp knife, the transverse processes can be further shaved down on each side to the level of the foramina, so exposing the artery in its whole course. Both sides should be so dissected, the last stages being taken deeper and deeper with extreme care to remove the lateral walls of the canals without damaging the underlying vessel. Naturally, the crucial area is in the upper one or two vertebrae, but though laborious, this method provides the most elegant and convincing demonstration.

Specimens should be taken of any obvious or suspicious breach in the wall for histological examination. The usual type of damage is either a frank tear of the intima and media, or a dissection that allows blood to track through the adventitia.

The papers by Vanezis, Simonsen, and Cameron and Mant, among others, should be consulted for further details of the recommended procedures, but the above is a practical approach to demonstrating vertebral artery lesions. Once again, the relationship must be assessed of any tiny dissection, to the volume of blood found in the cranial meninges – and a decision made as whether this is more likely to be a concomitant injury to intracranial vessels rather than a solitary external vertebral artery lesion.

HEAD INJURIES IN BOXERS

It has become increasingly apparent in recent years that persons who indulge in boxing are at risk of both acute and chronic damage to their brains. In some countries, including parts of Scandinavia, both professional and amateur boxing is banned for this reason. The acute injuries are less common but occur during or soon after the fight itself. A number of boxers have died in the ring or after removal to hospital and, in these fatalities, by far the most common lesion is a subdural haemorrhage. Extradural bleeding almost never occurs, because boxing injuries rarely cause skull fractures. Occasionally a subarachnoid haemorrhage may occur in rare cases where a berry aneurysm is present.

Much attention has been paid to the chronic changes in boxers' brains, which are very common and give rise to what is generally known as the 'punch-drunk' syndrome. It appears that the length of time for which a boxer has been involved in fighting is more important than the number of serious traumatic events he has suffered. It is a cumulative process and many episodes of minor head injury add up to produce the typical lesions described in the now extensive publications on the subject.

There are both anatomical and microscopic lesions in such brains, both in professionals and amateurs exposed over a number of years. The clinical symptoms do not concern the pathologist, but they are explained by the morphological abnormalities. Grossly affected brains may show some cortical atrophy and slight hydrocephalus; the septum pellucidum is characteristically perforated with enlargement of the cavum and tearing of the septal leaves. The fornices and adjacent corpus callosum may be thinned or torn, and throughout the brain substance there may be scars and patches of gliosis. Neurones are lost from the cerebellum and the substantia nigra, the latter often losing pigment.

Another change that has intrigued neuropathologists is the development of an Alzheimer's-like condition, with neurofibrillary tangles throughout the cerebral cortex and brainstem, though no senile plaques are present.

CEREBRAL INJURIES

Though bleeding or infected scalp injuries, depressed fractures, meningitis and substantial meningeal haemorrhage can themselves cause death, in most fatal head injuries it is damage to the substance of the brain itself that is lethal.

In medico-legal practice it is sometimes difficult to convince lawyers that, in most instances, a victim does not die of a simple fractured skull, but that the fracture is evidence only of a substantial head injury, being a 'marker' for concomitant brain damage, which was the real lethal lesion. Similar problems of communication exist with a fracture of the hyoid bone in strangulation, lay persons often being under the misapprehension that a broken hyoid is a mortal injury, instead of merely being an inconstant marker of pressure on the neck.

The neuropathology of brain damage is a large and complex subject, the more subtle varieties requiring both specialist techniques for demonstration and expert knowledge for interpretation. The textbooks of Graham, Adams and Leestma are recommended for detailed description and discussion of cerebral trauma.

The mechanisms of production of some traumatic lesions are matters of conflicting theories, but the forensic pathologist still has to be aware of the general principles of causation in order to offer some interpretation of the injuries.

As always, caution has to be employed, as both the pathological and clinical manifestations of a head injury may appear to be at variance with the degree of force applied to the head. There is a wide range of lesions from a given insult to the head and it is dangerous to be too dogmatic in theorizing about the magnitude of an injury that gave rise to the demonstrable lesions.

It is similarly unwise to hypothesize too firmly about what clinical features must have occurred when the head injury was sustained – for example, quite severe head

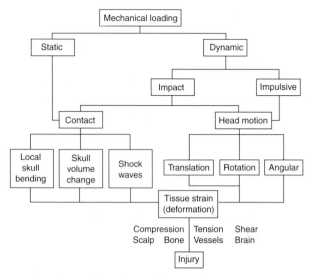

FIGURE 5.41 *Mechanical events that contribute to primary brain injury. (Reproduced from* Greenfield's Neuropathology, *7th edn, 2002 by kind permission of Arnold.)*

injuries have been known to be unaccompanied by concussion, while other apparently slight damage has often been followed by prolonged unconsciousness even ending in death. The well-known aphorism of Munro (1938) must be kept in mind that: 'Any type of head injury can give rise to any type of intracranial damage.'

The mechanism of brain damage

The brain may be injured in the following ways:

■ by direct intrusion, either by a foreign object such as a penetrating weapon, bullet or other missile – or fragments of skull in a compound fracture where the skull is disrupted. In these open wounds the mechanism of the damage to the brain is obvious, though of course it may be compounded by the second type of injury described below
■ by deformation of the brain in closed head injuries. Here the mechanism of injury is complicated and variable, with several competing theories of causation that have been put forward since the eighteenth century (Ledran 1751, Morgagni 1761). A public debate was held in 1766 in Paris, where rival theories of coup and contrecoup brain damage were hotly defended at the Academy of Surgeons.

The brain is almost incompressible and purely axial impact may give rise to little or no damage. It is extremely rare, however, for an impact not to impart some rotatory

movement and it seems agreed that this component is the main culprit in causing brain damage. What is now clear is that no actual blow or fall need be suffered by the head to cause severe and even fatal brain damage. It is the change in velocity – either acceleration or deceleration – with a rotational rather than solely axial element, that leads to damage. The surface of the head need never contact any hard object or surface, though recent research indicates that the quantum of energy delivered by impact is of a far greater order of magnitude that non-impact violence, which lessens the former conviction that shaking, as in child abuse, is a common and potent mechanism in the production of intracranial damage.

In most head injuries – notably traffic accidents and falls – there is marked deceleration of the moving head on contact with a fixed surface but, in many criminal and combat injuries, the head is accelerated by a blow. In either case the initial sudden change in velocity is applied to the scalp and skull, the latter then transmitting the change to the brain via the anatomical suspensory system within the cranium. This system is slightly flexible and consists of the falx and tentorium, which divide the cranial cavity into three major compartments; these contain the two cerebral hemispheres, the cerebellum and the brainstem. When violent relative movements take place between the brain and the dura, forming the partitions of the cranium, the cerebral tissue can become damaged against both the sharp edges and the flat surface of these membranes. In addition, vessels traversing the subdural and subarachnoid spaces can be torn by such relative movements, especially in old people where cerebral atrophy may have widened these spaces.

Among the competing theories of impact brain damage are:

■ the rotational shear force theory
■ the pressure gradient theory
■ the vibration theory
■ the transmitted wave force theory
■ the brain displacement theory
■ the skull deformation theory.

These hypotheses overlap and most are correct in some aspect. Because experiments on primates and mechanical models have been pursued vigorously in recent years, it is now widely accepted that there are marked pressure changes within the cranium on impact (Yanagida *et al.* 1989). When a head falls against the ground, pressure momentarily increases at the impact point but falls to a negative value diametrically opposite. As these suction or cavitation effects are more damaging to neural and meningeal tissue than pressure, this is good evidence for claiming that contrecoup damage is largely a result of this vacuum effect.

The actual physical disruption of cerebral tissue is caused, according to both Gurdjian and Holbourn, by one or more of the following processes:

1 compression of the constituent units, by their being forced together
2 tension of the units, which pulls them apart
3 sliding or 'shear' strains, which move adjacent strata of tissue laterally. The usual homely example is given of a pack of playing cards being displaced, so that each card slides upon its neighbour.

Transient deformation of the skull almost certainly contributes to brain damage (Rowbotham 1964). The area of the skull beneath an impact becomes momentarily depressed even if it does not fracture and therefore may impinge on the underlying brain causing compression, as in 1, above. This is responsible for the typical cone-shaped contusions on the cortex, with the base at the surface, as the impact – possibly via short-lived oscillations of decreasing amplitude – injures the cortex and passes a diminishing force down into the deeper layers.

Simultaneously, other areas of the skull must bulge outward to accommodate the deformation – the so-called 'struck-hoop' action – when it is suggested that a 'rarefaction' remote from the impact may cause tension damage, as in 2, above.

More important is 3, being laminar deformity or 'shear stress' caused by the angular rotation of the head. As the head is pivoted on the first cervical vertebra, almost any impact on jaw, face or cranium will produce an angular momentum, the acceleration being conveyed first to the skull.

Alternatively, if the head is moving and is suddenly arrested, then the skull will decelerate first and the momentum of the brain will cause it to continue in motion, again almost certainly with some rotatory component.

In either the deceleration or acceleration mode, the skull and brain cannot change their velocities simultaneously and the brain will speed up or slow down only by virtue of the restraint provided by the dural septa and the configuration of the interior of the skull. In other words, the brain is either retarded or set into motion secondarily by the skull, especially by the dural septa and the bony prominences.

This restraint will occur first – and with maximum effect – on the most superficial layers of the cortex. These in turn will drag on the next deepest layer and so on until the difference in velocity is equalized – but this will have been at the expense of laminar tearing of the cerebral tissue and its associated blood vessels. In addition to this shearing damage, the brain may be forced against the sharp edge of the tentorial opening and the lower edge of the falx, causing damage to the base of the cerebrum, the corpus callosum and the brainstem. Impact against the side wall of the skull

and against the falx may cause diffuse contusion of the cortex. The cerebellum tends to suffer less damage, as it is much smaller and lighter than the cerebrum and there is less room for relative movement in the more tightly enclosed posterior fossa. The configuration of the interior of the cranium is thought to be partly responsible for the common localization of cerebral damage at the tips and undersurface of the frontal and temporal lobes. The rough floor of the anterior fossa, the sharp edge of the wing of the sphenoid and the massive bar of the petrous temporal bone are in contrast to the smooth inner surface of the vault of the skull.

Cerebral contusion

When either linear or, more often, laminar stresses are applied to the cortex, this soft tissue may disrupt. Part of the injury is directly upon the neurocellular structure, but damage to vessels is an important component. If the cortex still retains its shape, but is bruised and swollen, this constitutes 'contusion'. A greater degree of disruption, sufficient to produce macroscopic tearing, is termed 'laceration', but the difference is only one of degree. In gross head injuries, such as crushing, missile wounds and other major penetration, the degree of laceration may lead to partial or even complete extrusion of the brain from the cranial cavity.

In the usual type of cortical contusion seen in a closed head injury, the cortex is blue or red from haemorrhage, though if survival has lasted for some time, there may be added discoloration from associated cortical infarction. The haemorrhage may be diffuse or may be punctate and is often a mottled purplish red when confined to the cortex. Extension into the underlying white matter tends to be pure red in fresh lesions. The lesion is often wedge-shaped, with the base on the surface, tapering away into the deeper layers.

Cerebral laceration

Laceration of the cortex is an extension in severity of contusion in which mechanical separation of the tissue can be seen. When widespread, but relatively superficial, the cortex appears to have a 'red velvet' appearance, which becomes progressively more tattered as the severity increases.

When it is even more severe, the cerebral surface becomes fissured, fragments of cortex may detach and deep lacerations run into the depths of the hemisphere, sometimes reaching even the deep ganglia or ventricles. There may be deep haemorrhage and – especially in the frontal and temporal lobes – the lacerations may be continuous with areas of traumatic haemorrhage. In cerebral lacerations and most contusions, the pia mater and often the arachnoid are torn, so that blood from damaged cortical vessels leaks into the subarachnoid and even subdural spaces. The corpus callosum is commonly torn, especially at its posterior end. This must be distinguished from damage caused by clumsy removal of the brain at autopsy (as must tears of the cerebral peduncles), but when genuine, may represent either a guillotine effect of the free lower edge of the falx or differential lateral movement of one hemisphere relative to the other, again because of unilateral restraint by the falx. Lacerations and contusions are most often found in those areas of the brain where the cortex is most likely to come into contact with irregularities in the internal profile of the skull. The undersurface of the temporal lobes and the orbital surface of the frontal lobes suffer most often.

Traumatic intracerebral haemorrhage

Substantial areas of haemorrhage, either infiltrating the brain tissue or forming actual haematomas, are common in severe head injuries. Some are primary, occurring at the time of impact or soon afterwards; others are secondary and caused by changes in intracranial pressure or bleeding into infarcts caused by vascular damage. These are all seen more often since artificial ventilation has been available, as victims of severe head injuries now survive longer so that there is time for secondary lesions to become apparent.

In the cerebral hemispheres, deep haemorrhage can be caused by coup or contrecoup mechanisms (see below) and may be situated anywhere within the hemispheres. They may rupture into the ventricular system or through the overlying cortex. In some severe contrecoup lesions, there may be large haematomas in one or both frontal lobes with overlying cortical contusion and laceration. These may rupture through the cortex into the meningeal spaces, forming what is sometimes called a 'burst lobe'. Such haemorrhages sometimes pose a problem for the pathologist when they occur in older subjects, especially those with hypertension and perhaps cerebral atherosclerosis. When a scalp injury is present – and perhaps even a fractured skull – it may be difficult to decide if a head injury (such as a fall) was responsible for the cerebral haemorrhage, or whether a sudden 'stroke' caused by a natural cerebral haemorrhage resulted in the fall. The problem is discussed further in the chapter on natural death, but briefly, the presence of left ventricular (cardiac) hypertrophy, a history of hypertension and the site of the (usually solitary) haemorrhage tends to point to a natural bleed. This is especially so if the large size of the lesion seems inconsistent with the degree of head injury sustained. Hypertensive lesions tend to be in the thalamus, external capsule, pons and cerebellum, and are more often occipital than frontal or temporal. Having said that, on occasions it can be impossible to differentiate the two conditions.

Primary brainstem haemorrhage

Secondary brainstem bleeding is dealt with under 'cerebral oedema' so here we are concerned with haemorrhage that occurs at the time of injury. As mentioned above, hypertensive haemorrhages not associated with trauma can occur in the midbrain, especially the pons. These tend to be large, explosive lesions that greatly swell the pons and disrupt the central part of the stem, usually with a ragged rim of white matter around the periphery. Traumatic haemorrhage in the brainstem is often a well-circumscribed lesion, sometimes rounded, which lies laterally in the tegmentum, the shape of the midbrain being undistorted (unlike a secondary bleed into an elongated stem).

The typical site is between the aqueduct and the outer end of the substantia nigra. Primary stem haemorrhages are usually associated with occipital impacts and the victim is often unconscious from the time of the injury, as opposed to the lucid interval and gradual decline of those who suffer secondary stem lesions because of a developing cerebral oedema or space-occupying meningeal haematoma.

Coup and contrecoup damage

Whatever the underlying mechanics of cerebral damage, one aspect is of considerable practical importance to the pathologist. When a mobile head is struck with an object, the site of maximum cortical contusion is most likely to be beneath or at least on the same side as the blow. This is the so-called 'coup' lesion. When a moving head is suddenly decelerated, as in a fall, though there might still be a 'coup' lesion at the site of impact, there is often cortical damage on the opposite side of the brain – the 'contrecoup' lesion.

The mechanism of the 'coup' and 'contrecoup' injuries has long been debated – at least since the time of the famous Paris meeting of 1766. The controversy has been continued, especially by Courville (1942) and by Holbourn (1943), but no satisfactory resolution has been agreed though the work on intracranial pressures by Yanagida *et al.* seems to provide proof that a 'vacuum' occurs at the contrecoup site.

The following practical points should be considered:

■ There may be no coup damage at all, only contrecoup.
■ There need be no fracture of skull, even in the presence of severe coup and contrecoup lesions.
■ The most common site for contrecoup injury is in the frontal and temporal lobes. It is often at the tips and on the undersurface of these lobes, and may be symmetrical, if a fall on the occiput has occurred.
■ In temporal or parietal impacts, the contrecoup lesions are likely to be diametrically opposite on the

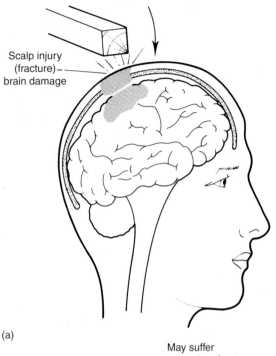

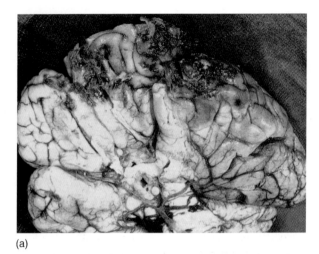

(a)

Scalp injury
(fracture) –
brain damage

(a)

May suffer
secondary fracture

Temporal and
frontal contusion

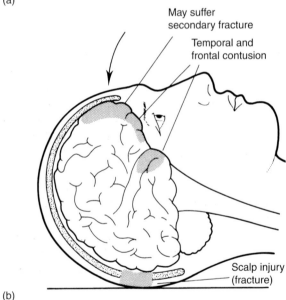

Scalp injury
(fracture)

(b)

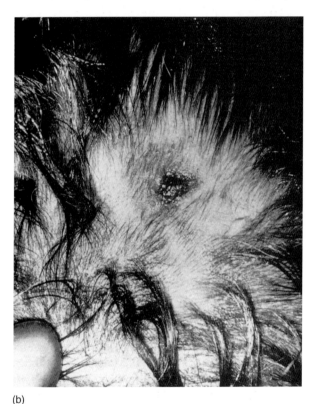

(b)

FIGURE 5.42 *(a) 'Coup' brain damage to fixed head. (b)
'Contrecoup' brain damage to moving (decelerated) head.*

FIGURE 5.43 *(a) Typical contrecoup injury to the tips of the frontal
and temporal lobes of a brain. The victim was pushed over in a
brawl and fell backwards, striking his occiput and causing a small
scalp laceration (b). There was no contusion to the posterior part of
the brain.*

contralateral surface of the brain, but exact geometrical
correspondence is not necessarily present.

■ It is virtually unknown for a fall on the frontal
region to produce occipital contrecoup. This is thought
to be due to the anatomical configuration of the
floor of the cranium, but the reasons are by no means
understood.

■ In a temporal impact, the contrecoup damage may be
not be on the contralateral hemisphere, but on the

opposite side of the ipsilateral hemisphere from impact
against the falx cerebri.

■ The degree of contrecoup damage may be severe,
sufficient to cause blood-filled cavitation in the deep
cortex and underlying white matter, especially in the
frontal lobes and tips of the temporal lobes.

- With severe frontal contrecoup from a fall on the occiput, the transmitted force may be sufficient to fracture the thin bone of the floor of the anterior fossa. Such cracks in the roofs of the orbits may allow meningeal haemorrhage to seep into the orbits and appear as 'black eyes'. In assaults where a fall has occurred, care must be taken not to attribute such periorbital bleeding to direct punches.
- Though contrecoup contusion is classically caused by deceleration of a falling head, it can also occur when a **fixed** head is struck. If the victim is already lying on the ground or against some other unyielding surface, a heavy blow on the upper side may cause typical contrecoup lesions either in the contralateral temporal or parietal cortex, or against the falx on the inner side of the ipsilateral lobe. In these circumstances, there is often coup damage as well. No external scalp injury need be visible.
- The interpretation of contrecoup lesions is most reliable in the form of cortical contusions or lacerations. Meningeal haemorrhage, either subdural or subarachnoid, may also arise in association with a contrecoup lesion, but its diagnostic value is virtually nil compared with cortical damage when interpreting a falling or fixed head injury. Where no associated cortical contusion is present, it is quite unsafe to rely upon a unilateral meningeal haemorrhage as an indicator of the type of head injury.

Concussion

Concussion is a clinical, not a pathological entity, but the pathologist must consider it, as it is related to intracranial lesions and he is often questioned about it in court proceedings. Concussion, according to Wilson (1946), is 'a disorder of cerebral function which follows immediately upon the impact of a force to the head'. A more full definition is offered by Trotter (1914): 'a transient paralytic state due to head injury which is of instantaneous onset, does not show any evidence of structural cerebral injury and is always followed by amnesia from the actual moment of the accident'.

Some neurologists would also include post-concussion symptoms within the definition of concussion, even in the absence of initial coma, following a head injury. There may also be evidence of depressed medullary function, which can affect cardiorespiratory action. Denny-Brown and Russell (1941) showed that the rate of change of velocity of the head was important in producing concussion, which rarely developed if the speed threshold was less than ~8.5 m/s (28 ft/s).

It is an extremely common, but not inevitable, sequel to any significant mechanical insult to the brain. Though in general terms its duration is loosely related to the severity of the injury, there are many exceptions. Gross skull and brain damage have occurred with little or no apparent concussion, though concussion may be so transient that the subject may not even fall to the ground. Relatively minor head injuries have given rise to prolonged unconsciousness so, once again, it is most unwise to be dogmatic about retrospective estimates of concussion.

There is considerable controversy about the cause of concussion, from the unacceptable 'traumatic neurosis' on the one hand (which cannot be true) to claims for the inevitable demonstration of physical lesions on the other.

Courville (1953) has discussed the condition in depth and there seems to be no reason to doubt that some mechanical process does temporarily disrupt the function, if not necessarily the structure, of the neuronic apparatus. Changes in the nucleus and cytoplasm of neurones, the composition of the cerebrospinal fluid and in the electro-encephalograph have all been inconstantly reported (see 'Diffuse neuronal and axonal injury' below).

True concussion may last for seconds or minutes. If prolonged unconsciousness extends into hours, days or longer, then there is likely to be some structural brain damage. Occasionally what appears to be simple concussion proves to be fatal, causing respiratory paralysis, though at autopsy no significant lesions are found.

Where a victim of 'simple' concussion dies of some incidental non-neurological condition, autopsy usually reveals no macroscopic damage, though sometimes there is slight cerebral oedema and scattered non-specific petechial haemorrhages may be found. There seems to be a connection between concussion and rotatory movements of the head, which are usually responsible for obvious structural damage because, when a head is fixed before impact, loss of consciousness may not occur. The classic example is trapping of a head against a wall or being jammed between buffers.

That shear stresses are instrumental in causing neurone damage seems confirmed by the frequency in which concussion occurs in boxing contests, where a blow on the jaw is the ultimate in producing a rotational movement of the cranium.

Concussion may be followed by a 'post-concussion state' characterized by headaches, unsteadiness and anxiety. This seems a genuine phenomenon, though it has been pointed out that it may be overlain by a 'compensation syndrome' whilst civil litigation is in progress over responsibility for the accident, which often clears up rapidly once the claim is settled.

Retrograde amnesia is almost inevitably associated with concussion, though, like concussion itself, it may be so transient as to escape notice. A protective mechanism, it seems to be caused by loss of sensory input before the latter is transferred to permanent memory storage in the brain.

Though commonly only of minutes' duration, it can extend to several days before the head injury. Though there is often a later recovery of much of this lost period, the memory of events immediately before the incident rarely returns, which may fortuitously be a protective device. Concussion has been attributed to several causes, including the undoubted vasomotor disturbances that take place after a head injury. Another theory is the impaction of the brain into the foramen magnum or tentorial opening, but the most acceptable hypothesis is 'diffuse neuronal injury'.

DIFFUSE NEURONAL AND AXONAL INJURY

According to Graham *et al.* (2002), diffuse brain damage exists in four principal forms: diffuse vascular injury, diffuse axonal injury, hypoxic brain damage and diffuse brain swelling. Diffuse vascular injury consists of multiple small haemorrhages throughout the brain and is virtually restricted to patients, who die within 24 h, whereas the latter three are encountered in patients who survive long enough to reach the hospital. Recent research and new immunohistochemical methods have shown that traumatic axonal injury is much more common than previously realized, and that axons can also be diffusely damaged by other processes than head injury. Therefore, Geddes *et al.* (2000) suggested new definitions of the terminology to get rid of the incoherent use of terms in the literature:

■ Axonal injury (AI) is a non-specific term referring to damage to axons of any aetiology.
■ Traumatic axonal injury (TAI), is a damage to axons caused by trauma, which may vary from small foci of axons to more widespread brain damage, diffuse TAI is the most severe form of traumatic axonal damage (originally termed 'DAI').
■ Diffuse axonal damage (DAI), first described as a clinicopathological syndrome of widespread axonal damage throughout the brain, including the brainstem, should not be used as a term without reference to the aetiology, because axonal injury may be caused by other pathological processes.

Experimental work has suggested that diffuse axonal injury is primarily a non-impact rotational acceleration–deceleration phenomenon, deformation by stretching probably being the most significant factor. A low level of injury causes transient changes in the permeability of the axolemma, gradually leading to ionic changes, accumulation of fluid and axonal swelling and eventually, with an increasing grade of injury, to intracellular Ca^{2+} accumulation, proteolysis and collapse of the cytoskeleton.

The disruption of axons leads to bulbous and clubbed 'retraction balls or globes' on the axons in the cerebral hemispheres, cerebellum and brainstem. Disturbance of axonal transport causes accumulation of substances in damaged fibres, that can be demonstrated immunohistochemically. At present, β-amyloid precursor protein (βAPP) is considered to be the most reliable indicator of axonal damage, revealing axonal injury within 2–3 hours of the insult, whereas it takes about 12–18 hours for axonal bulbs to become visible on routine or silver stains. However, one should keep in mind that βAPP is not specific to head injury but is an indicator of derangement of fast axonal transport, which has also been demonstrated in other pathological conditions.

It is preferable to examine the brain after proper fixation, usually after 10–14 days in 4 per cent buffered formaldehyde and, where possible, consultation with a neuropathologist with experience in forensic practice. Due to the diffuse nature of the axonal injury, extensive and systematic sampling is essential, as the diagnostic yield is directly related to the number of blocks taken. In addition to any obvious focal pathology, the minumum set of samples should include corpus callosum and parasagittal posterior frontal white matter, splenium of the corpus callosum, deep grey matter to include posterior limb of the internal capsule, cerebellar hemisphere, midbrain including the decussation of superior cerebellar peduncle, and pons including superior or middle cerebellar peduncles. In addition to these, it may also be advisable to include corpus callosum and parasagittal anterior frontal white matter and temporal lobe including hippocampus (Geddes *et al.* 2000).

Retraction globes are most numerous in the corpus callosum, the superior peduncles, the parasagittal white matter, the medial lemnisci and the corticospinal tracts, but can be seen anywhere in the white matter. The retraction globes or axonal bulbs have been shown to lose positive staining for βAPP after about a week but to persist in adjacent varicose axons up to 30 days. After some weeks in those who survive long enough, clusters of microglia, presumably part of a repair process, congregate at the site of ruptured axons. These are best seen in 20 μm thicker sections stained with cresyl violet. One problem with the microscopic evidence of both microglial clusters as well as diffuse axonal injury (as demonstrated by βAPP expression), is that neither of them is specific as a marker for trauma: retraction globes may also be seen around the periphery of natural lesions such as cerebral infarcts and haemorrhages and microglial clusters have been reported in viral/HIV encephalitis, previous global hypoxia and fat embolism. Geddes *et al.* (2000) conclude in their excellent review that 'the demonstration of traumatic axonal damage is likely to be of limited use in most forensic situations, except perhaps to confirm that there has been a head injury'.

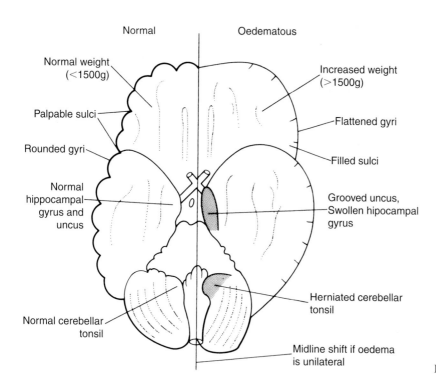

Normal   Oedematous

Normal weight
(<1500g)

Increased weight
(>1500g)

Palpable sulci

Flattened gyri

Rounded gyri

Filled sulci

Normal
hippocampal
gyrus and
uncus

Grooved uncus,
Swollen hipocampal
gyrus

Normal cerebellar
tonsil

Herniated cerebellar
tonsil

Midline shift if oedema
is unilateral

FIGURE 5.44 *Signs of cerebral oedema.*

Cerebral oedema

Swelling of the brain tissue may be a local phenomenon around almost any lesion, be it contusion, laceration, tumour or infarct, but here we are more concerned with generalized oedema. Swelling of the brain is extremely common after a substantial head injury, especially in children. Though it is an almost inevitable accompaniment of almost all intracerebral damage as either a local or general phenomenon, it can occur as the sole abnormality – and not infrequently prove fatal, particularly in young victims.

Oedema may well be related to diffuse neuronal injury and to concussion itself. It is the most common cause of raised intracranial pressure, being seen more often than localized space-occupying lesions such as haematomas and tumours, though of course these often coexist with cerebral oedema.

As with concussion, its cause is obscure and hence is the source of considerable controversy. The amount of fluid in the brain increases and the total weight may increase by at least 100 grams, mainly in the white matter. The site of the excess fluid is obscure, as the cut brain surface does not appear wet as do connective tissues elsewhere in an oedematous body. It was formerly thought that there was no true extracellular space in neural tissue and that the fluid must therefore be intracellular, but electron microscopic studies have revealed an extracellular compartment, which is much wider in the white matter (up to 80 nm) than in the grey matter (up to 20 nm), which explains the preference of oedema for the white matter.

The autopsy features of cerebral oedema are readily recognized. On removing the calvarium, the dura is stretched and tense, the brain bulging through the first incision in the membrane. The gyri are pale and flattened, and the sulci filled, giving the normally corrugated cerebral surface a smoothness that can easily be felt at autopsy. The cut surface is pale and, especially in children, the ventricles may be reduced to slits by the swelling of the adjacent white matter.

Severe cerebral oedema causes the larger volume cerebral hemispheres to press down upon the tentorium and herniate through the midbrain opening. The hippocampal gyrus may impact in the opening, lesser degrees causing grooving of the unci. Both these effects may lead to haemorrhage and necrosis at the sites of pressure, especially where the sharp edge of the tentorium cuts into the cerebral tissue. The tonsils of the cerebellum may be impacted or 'coned' into the foramen magnum, and sometimes are forced down into the upper part of the spinal canal. The pathologist must be careful not to mistake the normal anatomical grooving that often exists around the cerebellar tonsils for 'coning'. There should be other signs of brain swelling and true tonsillar herniation will show discoloration or even necrosis of the ischaemic, trapped tissue.

Cerebral oedema may be the only intracranial abnormality found at autopsy after a substantial head injury has occurred. This seems to be more commonly found in children and, in the absence of any other demonstrable lesions, the cause of death has to be attributed to this swelling of the brain, compressing the vital centres in the brainstem.

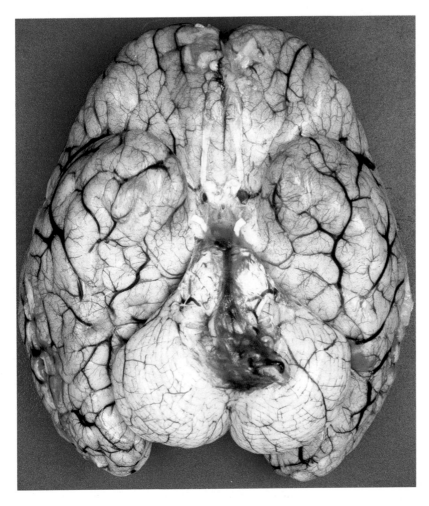

FIGURE 5.45 *Tonsillar herniation as a consequence of lumbar puncture in a patient with increased intracranial pressure. The pressure gradient has forced the cerebellar tonsils into foramen magnum and caused compression of the brainstem and patient's death. (Reproduced by kind permission of Professor H Kalimo.)*

Obviously, many other cases of cerebral oedema resolve either spontaneously or with treatment, so that fortunately no opportunity arises to prove its existence by post-mortem examination. Such oedema is, however, not infrequently found during surgical exploration for a meningeal haemorrhage, the latter sometimes being presented though often only brain swelling is demonstrated.

Cerebral oedema may be self-potentiating, in that once it begins as a result of direct brain trauma, the consequent rise in intracranial pressure then impairs the venous return from the intracranial sinuses. The pressure is insufficient to restrict the arterial inflow, so further congestion and swelling occur. This may lead to worsening cerebral hypoxia and oedema to the stage of actual cerebral infarction and brain death – again, a distressing common syndrome seen especially in child victims of head injuries, usually from road accidents.

In addition to mechanical damage, cerebral oedema can be caused or worsened by hypoxia. Many head injuries may be associated with damage to other parts of the body, such as the thorax – and because the airway may be compromised in many unconscious victims, there may be an element of

hypoxia in a considerable proportion of cases of cerebral oedema. Capillary permeability may be increased in a number of states, leading to weakening of the so-called 'blood–brain barrier' formed by the capillary endothelium and basement membrane, together with the astrocyte footplates. Cerebral oedema, either traumatic or hypoxic, can develop with surprising rapidity, especially in children. Macroscopic evidence of brain swelling can be seen at autopsy in cases where the interval between trauma or onset of hypoxia and death was less than one hour.

Several methods are available to reverse oedema, including hyperventilation, which acts by providing full oxygenation and reducing the peripheral carbon dioxide tension, thus causing constriction of arterioles and a reduction in brain volume and transudation.

HISTOLOGICAL DIAGNOSIS OF EARLY CEREBRAL HYPOXIA

Unfortunately for the pathologist, most of the hypoxic conditions seen in forensic practice cause death too quickly for any recognizable histological changes to develop. Acute deaths from strangulation, suffocation and choking occur within minutes or less, even excepting the sudden vasovagal type of cardiac arrest.

There are, however, occasions when a longer period of survival occurs after an acute hypoxic episode and in some of these there may be the opportunity to detect histological changes in the central nervous system. Probably a minimum of 2–4 hours of survival is necessary for unequivocal changes to be observed, though some neuropathologists claim to detect signs after as little as 1 hour. More cautious investigators prefer 4 hours as the minimum. A short post-mortem interval is a considerable advantage in searching for these changes, as they are subtle and can be overlaid by post-mortem autolysis, even if the latter is slight.

It may be helpful to seek the assistance of a neuropathologist in detecting or confirming the relatively minor changes seen in a brain affected by hypoxia, but with experience, a good knowledge of the normal appearances and a laboratory that is able to turn out constantly good-quality sections and uniform staining, any forensic pathologist can build up a considerable expertise in this localized aspect of neuropathology. The parts of the brain most suitable for seeking evidence of hypoxic damage are the hippocampus (especially Sommer's area), the cerebellar folia, the globus pallidus in the basal ganglia, and the boundary zones of the cerebral cortex where the grey matter is most vulnerable because it lies at the terminal reaches of the arterial supply (for example, at the occipitotemporal junction where the watershed between middle and posterior cerebral arteries lies). The third and fourth cortical layers are best for displaying the histological changes of hypoxia.

The following is a summary of the stages and changes that may be seen using different staining methods. The brain should be prefixed by suspension in formol saline for several weeks, though if this is impossible, small blocks should be wet-cut from the target areas of the brain mentioned above and immediately fixed in a large volume of formalin.

Stage 1

The earliest change is microvacuolation in the neurone cytoplasm, which may be seen in 2–4 hours. The cell outline remains smooth and its size is normal but, internally, small vacuoles appear in the cell body, and the proximal parts of the axon and dendrites. There may be a slight eosinophilia in haematoxylin and eosin stains and a violet colour in Luxol Fast Blue.

The microvacuolar change is said to begin earlier in small neurones and last for a shorter time, being present for up to 4–6 hours after insult in large cells and 2–4 hours in cerebellar Purkinje cells, though these times are arbitrary.

Stage 2

In the next stage, more prolonged hypoxia causes distortion in the shape of the neurones, the cell body becoming shrunken and staining darker with aniline dyes. The Nissl granules become fine and are dispersed more widely throughout the cell. Some vacuoles remain, the cytoplasm shows marked eosinophilia in haematoxylin and eosin, and is bright blue to mauve in Luxol Fast Blue stain. The nucleus becomes triangular and may be placed eccentrically in the cell body. The nucleolus becomes obscured and the nucleus stains a darker blue than normal with Luxol Fast Blue. This change is seen after up to 6 hours survival or later in large cells.

Stage 3

The ischaemic cell stage, described last, becomes worse during the following day or two if survival continues. The cell shrinks further, becoming narrow and tapered in many cases. Eosinophilia and blueness when stained with Luxol Fast Blue persists, but small spherical or irregular bodies begin to adhere to the exterior of the cell membrane. These incrustations persist longer than the remnants of the cytoplasm, which vanish, leaving the bare nucleus. The dark, shrunken nucleus becomes more apparent and survives for a number of days before karyolysis occurs.

Stage 4

Homogenizing cell damage is best seen in the Purkinje cells, in which the cytoplasm is uniformly eosinophilic with no Nissl granules. The nucleus stays dark and triangular until it vanishes and leaves a pale 'ghost' of the cell body with a vague perimeter.

There are parallel changes in the glial elements as well as in the neurones. From 4 to 12 hours after a hypoxic insult there may be an increase in the number of astrocytes around damaged neurones. There is a proliferation of astrocytes (which show mitoses) some 4–6 days later if the patient survives. This is most noticeable in the cerebellum and persists for 10–14 days. Fibrous astrocytes proliferate, but not the oligodendroglia. Microglia transform into rod cells, which may lie at right angles to the edge of the cortex, radially in the hippocampus and in the molecular layer of the cerebellar cortex. A later stage of cerebral hypoxic damage is the accumulation of lipid droplets and scavenging of myelin. Groups of microglia around dead neurones (neuronophages) may be obvious even at lower powers of the microscope.

SECONDARY BRAINSTEM LESIONS

When severe brain swelling (or a space-occupying lesion such as a large subdural or extradural haematoma) causes raised intracranial pressure above the tentorium, amongst the possible sequelae is compression of the midbrain against the free edge of the tentorium. This may be unilateral, causing grooving of a cerebral peduncle (called 'Kernohan's notch') associated with subpial petechial haemorrhages and often hemiplegia. When symmetrical, the oedema forces the undersurface of the cerebrum against the tentorium so that the hippocampal gyrus is squeezed into the opening. This elongates the midbrain in an anteroposterior direction as well as grooving the uncus and, in extreme cases, infarcting part of the parahippocampal gyrus. In addition, the distortion stretches, and compresses the paramedian and nigral vessels that supply the midbrain, leading to haemorrhages and infarcts in the upper pons and midbrain. Damage to cranial nerves and to the circulation of the cerebrospinal fluid may be added complications. The calcarine cortex on the medial aspect of the occipital lobe may be infarcted by the posterior cerebral artery being trapped around the edge of the tentorium by the cerebral herniation.

Secondary lesions are almost exclusively midline or paramedian haemorrhages, or haemorrhagic necrosis placed centrally in the upper pons and midbrain, though some may be obliquely placed in the substantia nigra. They may be difficult to distinguish from primary brainstem haemorrhages that arise at or soon after the original head injury – the secondary lesions tend to obscure the primary, rather than the converse. In children, the typical stem haemorrhages may not be present as in adults, but instead the medulla oblongata may be buckled or kinked due to fixation of the upper spinal cord by the denticulate ligaments (see work by Crompton).

SPINAL INJURIES

The spine and head should be thought of as part of the same system in relation to trauma. In recent years, a closer association – both skeletal and neurological – has been acknowledged between the two structures. For instance, interruption of ascending fibres in the cervical cord has been shown to be associated with neuronal chromatolysis in the brainstem and Spicer and Strich have shown that haemorrhage into spinal root ganglia may be associated with head injury. Electroencephalographic changes have been shown to occur in half the victims of cervical spine whiplash injury.

Though all segments of the spine are vulnerable to trauma, the cervical part holds the most interest for the forensic pathologist, mainly because of its close association with head injuries and vehicular accidents. The upper two cervical vertebrae provide most of the rotational movement of the head, whilst the lower neck allows flexion and extension. Violent force applied to the head tends to damage those parts of the neck corresponding with this functional

distinction. Spinal damage may be caused by compressional, hyperflexion and hyperextension stress.

Compression damage

This occurs when the victim falls from a height either onto his feet or his head, though in the latter case, head injuries may overshadow damage to the spine, as well as absorbing most of the impact.

When a person falls a long distance onto the feet, the kinetic energy of the deceleration may be absorbed by fractures of the feet, legs and pelvis, but can be transmitted up the spinal column. This can be fractured at one or more points, or the force may cause the upper cervical spine to impinge on the base of the skull and cause a 'ring fracture' around the foramen magnum as the spine is rammed into the posterior fossa.

A fall onto the head may also cause the 'burst atlas' injury, where the impact of the occipital condyles in an axial direction wedge the superior atlantal articulating facets apart and split the ring of the vertebra. The posterior arch can also be fractured in hyperextension by compression between the occiput and the posterior spine of the axis.

Compression fractures of vertebral bodies may occur, most commonly in the lower dorsal and upper lumbar zone, particularly T12 and L1. There is less chance of spinal cord injury compared with the angulation injuries described below, unless posterior extrusion of a disc or backward displacement of fragments of a disrupted vertebral body occurs.

Hyperflexion and hyperextension injury

Of the two, hyperextension is much more dangerous in causing spinal damage, possibly because flexion is protected by contraction of the strong posterior neck muscles, whereas the weak anterior longitudinal ligament is incapable of preserving the integrity of the cervical spine during hyperextension. In frontal or rearward motor vehicle crashes, which comprise 80 per cent of accidents, there is usually a hyperflexion and hyperextension component to the spines of the occupants, though head restraints and seatbelts restrict the range of movement.

Where a car undergoes violent frontal deceleration, the subject's head will swing down into hyperflexion and, unless restrained, will then strike the fascia or windscreen, and rebound into hyperextension.

When the vehicle is struck from the rear, the head will fly into hyperextension first unless a head-rest is available; such collisions often then smash the vehicle into the one in front, when a deceleration hyperflexion takes place.

Whatever the cause, a whole range of lesions can follow, both in the cervical, and to a lesser extent into the thoracic and lumbar segments. Bleeding into the surrounding muscles,

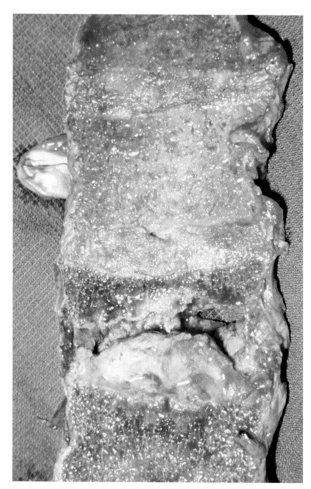

FIGURE 5.46 *Crushing of a thoracic vertebral body with disintegration of the adjacent disc following a violent hyperflexion in a car driver sustaining a deceleration injury. These lesions are best displayed at autopsy by cutting a longitudinal slice down the anterior aspect of the spinal column with an electric saw.*

rupture of the anterior longitudinal ligament, and tearing of intervertebral discs and of the annulus fibrosus may occur.

Nerve roots may be torn or compressed, and the spinal canal may be narrowed, distorted or even almost obliterated by fracture dislocations of the vertebrae. Compression, ischaemia, haemorrhage and even pulping of the spinal cord is the most serious complication. In older persons with cervical spondylosis, further narrowing of the canal by trauma may cause neurological effects that would not occur in younger subjects.

The most common part of the spine to be injured is the region of the upper two cervical vertebrae. In a series of fatal motor car accidents reported by Mant (1978), 35 per cent of passengers and 30 per cent of drivers suffered cervical spine damage. Of these the most common was a dislocation of the atlanto-occipital joint and Mant claims that one-third of all victims of fatal motor vehicle accidents

suffer this lesion, even though it is often undetected at autopsy. The mechanism of fracture of the atlas is said to be an axial impact via the head, when the occiput is held rigidly in line with the spine by contracted neck muscles. This most frequently occurs when the vertex of the lowered head violently strikes the windshield of a decelerating vehicle. Fracture or dislocation of the atlas or fracture of the odontoid of the axis can all occur from this type of impact. Hyperextension injuries tend to force the vertebral body forwards and, if there is significant displacement, the arch is intruded into the spinal canal with the consequent risk of cord damage. In addition, hyperextension – especially in the presence of cervical cord enlargement – can cause the ligamentum flavum to corrugate and intrude into the anterior part of the spinal canal to impinge upon the cord. When the injury is due to hyperflexion, dislocation of a vertebra causes it (or its fragments) to tilt backwards, again compromising the lumen of the spinal canal.

Dislocation of cervical vertebra can occur under many conditions. An anterior dislocation can be caused by a fall onto the back of the head and a unilateral dislocation is common when a head strikes a windscreen. Posterior dislocation may be caused by blows to the jaw or face that jolt the head backwards with a hyperextension element. Falling onto the face, especially from a height (such as down a staircase), is a likely cause. Fracture of the odontoid peg of the axis can occur from a variety of violent movements of the head on the neck, and is sometimes associated with fracture of the skull or mandible. Where gross injury to the spinal column is inflicted – such as a relatively high-speed motor vehicle or railway accident – the cord may be transected by a guillotine action of the two displaced fragments. This is most often seen on the upper or mid-thoracic region, from direct impact or gross 'whiplash' effects. The thoracic aorta at this level is often torn at the point where the descending arch meets the spine, even in the absence of a spinal fracture.

Damage to the cervical spine in hanging is rarely seen in the usual suicidal hangings in which sudden death is caused by carotid compression or – much less often – asphyxia. The drop in such cases is small or even absent, the subject merely slumping his weight against the neck restraint. Spinal damage can occasionally occur, however and the author has seen a fractured neck when a heavily built soldier stepped from a lavatory seat with the rope attached to the overhead cistern.

Judicial hanging with a long drop causes a severe fracture dislocation (rather than fracture) of the cervical spine, often with complete severance of the two fragments and transection of the spinal cord. Where such hanging is carried out with the knot of the suspension point beneath the chin, a violent hyperextension is produced that often fractures the axis and dislocates it from the third cervical vertebra. With a heavy person and a long drop, there may be complete decapitation.

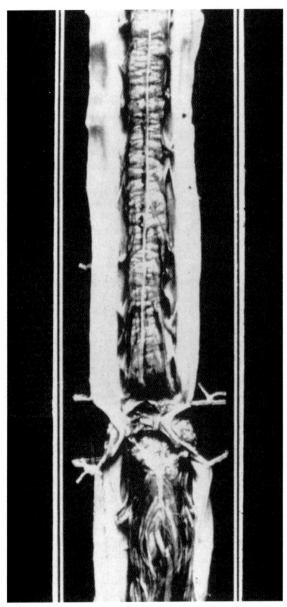

FIGURE 5.47 *Crushing and transection of the lower spinal cord following a hyperflexion fracture of the lower thoracic vertebrae. The spinal cord ends at about the lower border of the first lumbar vertebra, the cauda equina occupying the remainder of the lumbar spinal canal. This injury occurred several years before death, and the dura is constricted and adherent to the remnants of the cord. At autopsy the cord and its membranes should be pinned out and fixed for a proper examination to be made.*

Spinal cord injury

Most damage to the spinal cord arises from intrusion of some part of the spinal column into the canal, be it bony fragments or displacement, ligamentum flavum, disc annulus or extruded nucleus pulposum.

There may be bleeding into the space outside the spinal dura causing a space-occupying lesion in the canal that can compress the cord, or bleeding may occur within the dura, either from ruptured vessels or from haemorrhage in the cord itself. Damage to the cord may also occur in the absence of any apparent intrusion into the canal, in a manner similar to that seen in the brain in closed head injuries without a fracture. Haematomyelia and oedema may develop without any obvious mechanical defect at that level in the spinal column. Such injuries must be attributed to some momentary collision of the cord against the wall of the canal or a transient deformity of the profile of the canal that did not exceed the threshold for either fracture, dislocation or ligament rupture of the vertebral column.

The damage in the cord may extend for several segments above and below the point of impact. A haemorrhage within the cord tends to occupy the central grey matter more than the white columns, because of the softer and more vascular nature of the former tissue. Infarction of the cord can occur either in association with contusion, or because the local blood supply – often the anterior spinal artery – has been damaged.

An originally firm cord may undergo liquefaction ('myelomalacia') over several days or even longer, with progressive worsening of neurological symptoms.

REFERENCES AND FURTHER READING

Adams JH. 1982. Diffuse axonal injury in non-missile head injury. *Injury* **13**:444–5.

Adams H, Mitchell DE, Graham DI, *et al.* 1977. Diffuse brain damage of immediate impact type. Its relationship to 'primary brain-stem damage' in head injury. *Brain* **100**:489–502.

Adams JH, Graham DI, Murray LS, *et al.* 1982. Diffuse axonal injury due to nonmissile head injury in humans: an analysis of 45 cases. *Ann Neurol* **12**:557–63.

Adams JH, Graham DI, Gennarelli TA. 1983. Head injury in man and experimental animals: Neuropathology. *Acta Neurochir Suppl (Wien)* **32**:15–30.

Adams JH, Doyle D, Graham DI, *et al.* 1984. Diffuse axonal injury in head injuries caused by a fall. *Lancet* **2**:1420–2.

Adams JH, Doyle D, Graham DI, *et al.* 1985. Microscopic diffuse axonal injury in cases of head injury. *Med Sci Law* **25**:265–9.

Adams JH, Doyle D, Graham DI, *et al.* 1985. The contusion index: a reappraisal in human and experimental non-missile head injury. *Neuropathol Appl Neurobiol* **11**:299–308.

Adams JH, Doyle D, Graham DI, *et al.* 1986. Gliding contusions in nonmissile head injury in humans [published erratum appears in *Arch Pathol Lab Med* 1986 Nov;**110**:1075]. *Arch Pathol Lab Med* **110**:485–8.

Adams JH, Doyle D, Graham DI, *et al.* 1986. Deep intracerebral (basal ganglia) haematomas in fatal non-missile head injury in man. *J Neurol Neurosurg Psychiatry* **49**:1039–43.

Adams JH, Doyle D, Ford I, *et al.* 1989. Diffuse axonal injury in head injury: definition, diagnosis and grading. *Histopathology* **15**:49–59.

Adams JH, Doyle D, Ford I, *et al.* 1989. Brain damage in fatal non-missile head injury in relation to age and type of injury. *Scott Med J* **34**:399–401.

Adams JH, Graham DI, Gennarelli TA, *et al.* 1991. Diffuse axonal injury in non-missile head injury. *J Neurol Neurosurg Psychiatry* **54**:481–3.

Adams JH, Corsellis JA, Duchen LW. 1992. *Greenfield's neuropathology*, 5th edn. Edward Arnold, London.

Adams JH, Jennett B, McLellan DR, *et al.* 1999. The neuropathology of the vegetative state after head injury. *J Clin Pathol* **52**:804–6.

Adams JH, Graham DI, Jennett B. 2000. The neuropathology of the vegetative state after an acute brain insult. *Brain* **123**(Pt 7):1327–38.

Adams JH, Graham DI, Jennett B. 2001. The structural basis of moderate disability after traumatic brain damage. *J Neurol Neurosurg Psychiatry* **71**:521–4.

Adelson L. 1974. *The pathology of homicide*. Thomas, Springfield.

Blumbergs PC, Jones NR, North JB. 1989. Diffuse axonal injury in head trauma. *J Neurol Neurosurg Psychiatry* **52**:838–41.

Bostrom K, Helander CG, Lindgren SO. 1992. Blunt basal head trauma: rupture of posterior inferior cerebellar artery. *Forensic Sci Int* **53**:61–8.

Bromilow A, Burns J. 1985. Technique for removal of the vertebral arteries. *J Clin Pathol* **38**:1400–2.

Caffey J. 1946. Multiple fractures in the long bones of infants suffering from chronic subdural haematoma. *Am J Radiol* **56**:163–73.

Cameron JM, Mant AK. 1972. Fatal subarachnoid haemorrhage associated with cervical trauma. *Med Sci Law* **12**:66–70.

Casson IR, Siegel O, Sham R, *et al.* 1984. Brain damage in modern boxers. *JAMA* **251**:2663–7.

Coast GC, Gee DJ. 1984. Traumatic subarachnoid haemorrhage: an alternative source. *J Clin Pathol* **37**:1245–8.

Contostavlos DL. 1971. Massive subarachnoid hemorrhage due to laceration of the vertebral artery associated with fracture of the transverse process of the atlas. *J Forensic Sci* **16**:40–56.

Contostavlos DL. 1995. Isolated basilar traumatic subarachnoid hemorrhage: an observer's 25 year re-evaluation of the pathogenetic possibilities. [letter; comment] *Forensic Sci Int* **73**:61–74.

Corsellis JA, Bruton CJ, Freeman Browne D. 1973. The aftermath of boxing. *Psychol Med* **3**:270–303.

Courville CB. 1942. Coup-contre coup mechanism of craniocerebral injuries: some observations. *Arch Surg* **45**:19–43.

Courville CB. 1953. *Commotio cerebri*. San Lucas Press, Los Angeles.

Courville CB. 1964. *Forensic neuropathology*. Callaghan and Co, Mundelein.

Critchley M. 1957. Medical aspects of boxing particularly from a neurological standpoint. *Br Med J* **1**:357–62.

Crompton MR. 1971. Brain stem lesions due to closed head injury. *Lancet* **1**:669–71.

Crompton R. 1985. *Closed head injuries*. Edward Arnold, London.

Dalgaard J. 1957. Brain injuries as a cause of oesophagogastroduodenal ulceration. *J Forensic Med* **4**:110–27.

Dawson SL, Hirsch CS, Lucas FV, *et al.* 1980. The contrecoup phenomenon. Reappraisal of a classic problem. *Hum Pathol* **11**:155–66.

Deck JH, Jagadha V. 1986. Fatal subarachnoid hemorrhage due to traumatic rupture of the vertebral artery. *Arch Pathol Lab Med* **110**:489–93.

Denny-Brown D. 1945. Cerebral concussion. *Physiol Rev* **25**:296–325.

Denny-Brown D, Russell WR. 1941. Experimental cerebral concussion. *Brain* **64**:93–164.

Dowling G, Curry B. 1988. Traumatic basal subarachnoid hemorrhage. Report of six cases and review of the literature. *Am J Forensic Med Pathol* **9**:23–31.

Duhaime AC, Gennarelli TA, Thibault LE, *et al.* 1987. The shaken baby syndrome. A clinical, pathological, and biomechanical study. *J Neurosurg* **66**:409–15.

Duhaime AC, Alario AJ, Lewander WJ, *et al.* 1992. Head injury in very young children: mechanisms, injury types, and ophthalmologic findings in 100 hospitalized patients younger than 2 years of age. *Pediatrics* **90**:179–85.

Edherg S, Angrist A. 1967. Intra-cranial pressure changes following impact of human cadaver heads. *J Forensic Sci* **12**:60–8.

Editorial. 1973. Boxing brains. *Lancet* **2**:1064–5.

Farag AM, Franks A, Gee DJ. 1988. Simple laboratory experiments to replicate some of the stresses on vertebro-basilar arterial walls. An investigation of possible mechanisms of traumatic subarachnoid haemorrhage. *Forensic Sci Int* **38**:275–84.

Fell DA, Fitzgerald S, Moiel RH, *et al.* 1975. Acute subdural hematomas. Review of 144 cases. *J Neurosurg* **42**:37–42.

Flamm ES, Demopoulos HB, Seligman ML, *et al.* 1977. Ethanol potentiation of central nervous system trauma. *J Neurosurg* **46**:328–35.

Ford R. 1956. Basal subarachnoid haemorrhage and trauma. *J Forensic Sci* **1**:117–26.

Freytag E. 1963. Autopsy findings in head injuries from blunt forces: statistical evaluation of 1367 cases. *Arch Pathol* **75**:74–80.

Garfield J. 2002. Acute subdural haematoma in a boxer. *Br J Neurosurg* **16**:96–9; discussion 99–101.

Geddes JF, Whitwell HL, Graham DI. 2000. Traumatic axonal injury: practical issues for diagnosis in medicolegal cases. *Neuropathol Appl Neurobiol* **26**:105–16.

Geddes JF, Hackshaw AK, Vowles GH, *et al.* 2001. Neuropathology of inflicted head injury in children. I. Patterns of brain damage. *Brain* **124**:1290–8.

Geddes JF, Vowles GH, Hackshaw AK, *et al.* 2001. Neuropathology of inflicted head injury in children. II. Microscopic brain injury in infants. *Brain* **124**:1299–306.

Gennarelli TA. 1983. Head injury in man and experimental animals: clinical aspects. *Acta Neurochir Suppl (Wien)* **32**:1–13.

Gennarelli TA. 1993. Mechanisms of brain injury. *J Emerg Med* **11**(Suppl 1):5–11.

Gennarelli TA, Graham DI. 1998. Neuropathology of the head injuries. *Semin Clin Neuropsychiatry* **3**:160–175.

Gennarelli TA, Thibault LE. 1982. Biomechanics of acute subdural hematoma. *J Trauma* **22**:680–6.

Gennarelli TA, Thibault LE, Adams JH, *et al.* 1982. Diffuse axonal injury and traumatic coma in the primate. *Ann Neurol* **12**:564–74.

Gennarelli TA, Thibault LE, Tipperman R, *et al.* 1989. Axonal injury in the optic nerve: a model simulating diffuse axonal injury in the brain. *J Neurosurg* **71**:244–53.

Gentleman SM, McKenzie JE, Royston MC, *et al.* 1999. A comparison of manual and semi-automated methods in the assessment of axonal injury. *Neuropathol Appl Neurobiol* **25**:41–7.

Goonetilleke UK. 1980. Injuries caused by falls from heights. *Med Sci Law* **20**:262–75.

Graham DI. 2001. Paediatric head injury. *Brain* **124**:1261–2.

Graham DI, Adams JH. 1971. Ischaemic brain damage in fatal head injuries. *Lancet* **1**:265–6.

Graham DI, Adams JH. 1972. *The pathology of blunt head injuries*. In: Critchley M (ed.), *Scientific foundation of neurology*. Heinemann Medical Publications, London.

Graham DI, Lantos PL (eds). 2002. *Greenfield's neuropathology*, 7th edn. Arnold, London/ New York/New Delhi.

Graham DI, McLellan D, Adams JH, *et al.* 1983. The neuropathology of the vegetative state and severe disability after non-missile head injury. *Acta Neurochir Suppl (Wien)* **32**:65–7.

Graham DI, Lawrence AE, Adams JH, *et al.* 1988. Brain damage in fatal non-missile head injury without high intracranial pressure. *J Clin Pathol* **41**:34–7.

Graham DI, Ford I, Adams JH, *et al.* 1989. Fatal head injury in children. *J Clin Pathol* **42**:18–22.

Graham DI, Clark JC, Adams JH, *et al.* 1992. Diffuse axonal injury caused by assault. *J Clin Pathol* **45**:840–1.

Graham DI, McIntosh TK, Maxwell WL, *et al.* 2000. Recent advances in neurotrauma. *J Neuropathol Exp Neurol* **59**:641–51.

Graham DI, Raghupathi R, Saatman KE, *et al.* 2000. Tissue tears in the white matter after lateral fluid percussion brain injury in the rat: Relevance to human brain injury. *Acta Neuropathol (Berl)* **99**:117–24.

Gurdjian ES, Webster JE. 1958. *Head injuries*. Churchill, London, UK.

Gurdjian ES, Webster JE, Lissner HR. 1949. Studies on skull fracture with particular reference to engineering factors. *Am J Surg* **78**:736–42.

Gurdjian ES, Webster JE, Lissner HR. 1950. The mechanism of skull fracture. *Radiology* **54**:313–39.

Harris LS. 1991. Postmortem magnetic resonance images of the injured brain: effective evidence in the courtroom. *Forensic Sci Int* **50**:179–85.

Harwood-Nash CE, Hendrick EB, Hudson AR. 1971. The significance of skull fractures in children. A study of 1,187 patients. *Radiology* **101**:151–6.

Hijdra A, Vermeulen M, van Gijn J, *et al.* 1984. Respiratory arrest in subarachnoid hemorrhage. *Neurology* **34**:1501–3.

Holbourn AH. 1943. Mechanics of head injuries. *Lancet* **245**:438–41.

Huelke DF, O'Day J, Mendelsohn RA. 1981. Cervical injuries suffered in automobile crashes. *J Neurosurg* **54**:316–22.

Imajo T. 1996. Diffuse axonal injury: its mechanism in an assault case. *Am J Forensic Med Pathol* **17**:324–6.

Imajo T, Kazee AM. 1992. Diffuse axonal injury by simple fall. *Am J Forensic Med Pathol* **13**:169–72.

Imajo T, Roessman U. 1984. Diffuse axonal injury. *Am J Forensic Med Pathol* **5**:217–22.

Imajo T, Challener RC, Roessmann U. 1987. Diffuse axonal injury by assault. *Am J Forensic Med Pathol* **8**:217–19.

Jafari SS, Maxwell WL, Neilson M, *et al.* 1997. Axonal cytoskeletal changes after non-disruptive axonal injury. *J Neurocytol* **26**:207–21.

Jafari SS, Nielson M, Graham DI, *et al.* 1998. Axonal cytoskeletal changes after nondisruptive axonal injury. II. Intermediate sized axons. *J Neurotrauma* **15**:955–66.

Jamieson KG, Yelland JD. 1968. Extradural hematoma. Report of 167 cases. *J Neurosurg* **29**:13–23.

Johnson CP, Lawler W, Burns J. 1993. Use of histomorphometry in the assessment of fatal vertebral artery dissection. *J Clin Pathol* **46**:1000–3.

Johnson CP, How T, Scraggs M, *et al.* 1994. The poor biomechanical response of the vertebral artery applied longitudinal force. *J Pathol* **Suppl**:234.

Johnson DL, Boal D, Baule R. 1995. Role of apnea in nonaccidental head injury. *Pediatr Neurosurg* **23**:305–10.

Johnson J. 1969. Organic psychosyndromes due to boxing. *Br J Psychiatry* **115**:45–53.

Johnson P, Burns J. 1995. Extracranial vertebral artery injury – evolution of a pathological illusion? [letter; comment] *Forensic Sci Int* **73**:75–8.

Kaur B, Rutty GN, Timperley WR. 1999. The possible role of hypoxia in the formation of axonal bulbs. *J Clin Pathol* **52**:203–9.

Kerr D. 1954. *Forensic medicine*, 5th edn. A. & C. Black, Edinburgh, p. 114.

Knight B. 1979. Trauma and ruptured cerebral aneurysm. *Br Med J* **1**:1430–1.

Kubo S, Kitamura O, Orihara Y, *et al.* 1998. Immunohistochemical diagnosis and significance of forensic neuropathological changes. *J Med Invest* **44**:109–19.

Leadbeater S. 1994. Extracranial vertebral artery injury – evolution of a pathological illusion? [see comments] *Forensic Sci Int* **67**:33–40.

Leadbeater S. 1995. Letter to editor. *Forensic Sci Int* **73**:78–9.

Ledran H. 1751. *Observatis des chirurgies*. Osmont, Paris.

Leestma JE. 1988. *Forensic neuropathology*. Raven Press, New York.

Li L, Smialek JE. 1994. The investigation of fatal falls and jumps from heights in Maryland (1987–1992). *Am J Forensic Med Pathol* **15**:295–9.

Lindenberg R. 1955. Lesions of the corpus callosum following blunt mechanical trauma to the head. *Am J Pathol* **31**:297–301.

Lindenberg R, Freytag E. 1957. Morphology of cerebral contusions. *Arch Pathol* **63**:23–6.

Lindenberg R, Freytag E. 1960. The mechanism of cerebral contusions: a pathologic-anatomic study. *Arch Pathol* **69**:440–4.

Lindenberg R, Freytag E. 1970. Brainstem lesions characteristic of traumatic hyperextension of the head. *Arch Pathol* **90**:509–15.

Lindsay KW, McLatchie G, Jennett B. 1980. Serious head injury in sport. *Br Med J* **281**:789–91.

Lundberg GD. 1985. Brain injury in boxing. *Am J Forensic Med Pathol* **6**:192–8.

Madro R, Chagowski W. 1987. An attempt at objectivity of post mortem diagnostic of brain oedema. *Forensic Sci Int* **35**:125–9.

Maloney AFJ, Whatmore WJ. 1969. Clinical and pathological observations in fatal head injuries: a five year survey of 173 cases. *Br J Surg* **56**:23–30.

Mansell PW, Hunt AC. 1968. Major head injuries in fights and brawls. *Med Sci Law* **8**:181–7.

Mant AK. 1978. Injuries and death in motor vehicle accidents. In: Mason JK (ed.), *Pathology of violent injury*. Edward Arnold, London.

Mant AK. 1993. Injuries and death in motor vehicle accidents. In: Mason JK (ed.), *Pathology of violent injury*, 2nd edn. Edward Arnold, London.

Marek Z. 1981. Isolated subarachnoid hemorrhage as a medicolegal problem. *Am J Forensic Med Pathol* **2**:19–22.

Marlet JM, Barreto Fonseca JdP. 1982. Experimental determination of time of intracranial hemorrhage by spectrophotometric analysis of cerebrospinal fluid. *J Forensic Sci* **27**:880–8.

Martland MS. 1928. Punch drunk. *JAMA* **91**:1003–5.

Mawdsley C, Ferguson SR. 1963. Neurological disease in boxers. *Lancet* **2**:795–7.

McCormick WF. 1980. The relationship of closed-head trauma to rupture of saccular intracranial aneurysms. *Am J Forensic Med Pathol* **1**:223–6.

McCrory P. 2002. Boxing and the brain. Revisiting chronic traumatic encephalopathy. *Br J Sports Med* **36**:2.

McKissock H. 1960. Extradural haemorrhage; observations on 125 cases. *Lancet* **2**:167–74.

Missliwetz J. 1995. Fatal impalement injuries after falls at construction sites. *Am J Forensic Med Pathol* **16**:81–3.

Mitchell DE, Adams JH. 1973. Primary focal impact damage to the brainstem in blunt head injuries. Does it exist? *Lancet* **2**:215–18.

Miyazaki T, Kojima T, Chikasue F, *et al.* 1990. Traumatic rupture of intracranial vertebral artery due to hyperextension of the head: reports on three cases. *Forensic Sci Int* **47**:91–8.

Moar JJ. 1987. Traumatic rupture of the cervical carotid arteries: an autopsy and histopathological study of 200 cases. *Forensic Sci Int* **34**:227–44.

Morgagni J. 1761. *De sedibus et causis morborum per anatomen indagatis.* Typographia Academia, Lovanii.

Moritz AR. 1942. *Pathology of trauma.* Lea & Febiger, Philadelphia.

Munro D. 1938. *Cranio-cerebral injuries.* Oxford University Press, Oxford.

Munro D, Merritt HH. 1936. Surgical pathology of subdural haematoma. Based on a study of 105 cases. *Arch Neurol Psychiatry* **35**:64–78.

Oehmichen M. 1994. Brain death: neuropathological findings and forensic implications. *Forensic Sci Int* **69**:205–19.

Oehmichen M, Raff G. 1980. Timing of cortical contusion. Correlation between histomorphologic alterations and post-traumatic interval. *Z Rechtsmed* **84**:79–94.

Oehmichen M, Eisenmenger W, Raff G, *et al.* 1986. Brain macrophages in human cortical contusions as indicator of survival period. *Forensic Sci Int* **30**:281–301.

Oehmichen M, Meissner C, Schmidt V, *et al.* 1999. Pontine axonal injury after brain trauma and nontraumatic hypoxic-ischemic brain damage. *Int J Legal Med* **112**:261–7.

Oehmichen M, Theuerkauf I, Meissner C. 1999. Is traumatic axonal injury (AE) associated with an early microglial activation? Application of a double-labeling technique for simultaneous detection of microglia and ai. *Acta Neuropathol (Berl)* **97**:491–4.

Oehmichen M, Ochs U, Meissner C. 2000. Histochemical characterization of cytotoxic brain edema. Potassium concentrations after cerebral ischemia and during the postmortem interval. *Exp Toxicol Pathol* **52**:348–52.

Oehmichen M, Meissner C, Konig HG. 2001. Brain injury after survived gunshot to the head: reactive alterations at sites remote from the missile track. *Forensic Sci Int* **115**:189–97.

Oppenheimer DR. 1968. Microscopic lesions in the brain following head injury. *J Neurol Neurosurg Psychiatry* **31**:299–306.

Povlishock JT. 1992. Traumatically induced axonal injury: pathogenesis and pathobiological implications. *Brain Pathol* **2**:1–12.

Povlishock JT. 2000. Pathophysiology of neural injury: therapeutic opportunities and challenges. *Clin Neurosurg* **46**:113–26.

Povlishock JT, Christman CW. 1995. The pathobiology of traumatically induced axonal injury in animals and humans: a review of current thoughts. *J Neurotrauma* **12**:555–64.

Raisanen J, Ghougassian DF, Moskvitch M, *et al.* 1999. Diffuse axonal injury in a rugby player. *Am J Forensic Med Pathol* **20**:70–2.

Roberts AH. 1970. *Brain damage in boxers.* Pitman Medical, London.

Root I. 1992. Head injuries from short distance falls [see comments]. *Am J Forensic Med Pathol* **13**:85–7.

Rowbotham OF. 1964. *Acute injuries of the head*, 4th edn. Churchill Livingstone, Edinburgh.

Royal College of Physicians of London. 1969. *Report on the medical aspects of boxing.* Royal Collage of Physicians of London, London.

Schellhas KP, Latchaw RE, Wendling LR, *et al.* 1980. Vertebrobasilar injuries following cervical manipulation. *JAMA* **244**:1450–3.

Schellinger PD, Schwab S, Krieger D, *et al.* 2001. Masking of vertebral artery dissection by severe trauma to the cervical spine. *Spine* **26**:314–19.

Shapiro HA, Gordon I, Benson SD. 1988. *Forensic medicine – a guide to principles*, 3rd edn. Churchill Livingstone, Edinburgh.

Sheffield EA, Weller RO. 1980. Age changes at cerebral artery bifurcations and the pathogenesis of berry aneurysms. *J Neurol Sci* **46**:341–52.

Sherriff FE, Bridges LR, Sivaloganathan S. 1994. Early detection of axonal injury after human head trauma using immunocytochemistry for beta-amyloid precursor protein. *Acta Neuropathol (Berl)* **87**:55–62.

Simonsen J. 1967. Fatal subarachnoid haemorrhage in relation to minor head injuries. *J Forensic Med* **14**:146–55.

Simonsen J. 1976. Massive subarachnoid haemorrhage and fracture of the transverse process of the atlas. *Med Sci Law* **16**:13–6.

Simpson RH, Berson DS, Shapiro HA. 1985. The diagnosis of diffuse axonal injury in routine autopsy practice. *Forensic Sci Int* **27**:229–35.

Skold G. 1985. Injuries to pathologically changed cervical vertebrae. *Am J Forensic Med Pathol* **6**:163–6.

Smith DH, Chen XH, Xu BN, *et al.* 1997. Characterization of diffuse axonal pathology and selective hippocampal damage following inertial brain trauma in the pig. *J Neuropathol Exp Neurol* **56**:822–34.

Smith DH, Nonaka M, Miller R, *et al.* 2000. Immediate coma following inertial brain injury dependent on axonal damage in the brainstem. *J Neurosurg* **93**:315–22.

Somerville A. 1961. Subarachnoid haemorrhage due to trauma without visible external injury. *Med Sci Law* **2**:67–9.

Spicer EJ, Strich SJ. 1967. Haemorrhages in posterior-root ganglia in patients dying from head injury. *Lancet* **2**:1389–91.

Spillane JD. 1962. Five boxers. *Br Med J* **2**:1205–6.

Storey PB. 1969. The precipitation of subarachnoid haemorrhage. *J Psychosom Res* **13**:175–82.

Strassman G. 1949. Formation of haemosiderin and haematoidin after traumatic and spontaneous cerebral haemorrhages. *Arch Pathol* **47**:205–10.

Strich SJ. 1961. Shearing of nerve fibres as a cause of brain damage due to head injury: a pathological study. *Lancet* **2**:443–7.

Strich SJ. 1970. Lesions in the cerebral hemispheres after blunt head injury. *J Clin Pathol Suppl R Coll Pathol* **4**:166–71.

Strich SJ. 1976. Cerebral trauma. In: Blackwood W, Corsellis JAN (eds), *Greenfield's neuropathology*, 3rd edn. Edward Arnold, London, pp. 327–60.

Symonds CP. 1940. Concussion and contusion of the brain. In: Brock (ed.), *Injuries of the skull, brain and spinal cord*. Baillière, London.

Symonds CP. 1962. Concussion. *Lancet* **1**:1–5.

Tatsuno Y, Lindenberg R. 1974. Basal subarachnoid hematomas as sole intracranial traumatic lesions. *Arch Pathol* **97**:211–5.

Terespolsky PS. 1972. Post-traumatic epilepsy. *Forensic Sci* **1**:147–65.

Thiagaraj D, Ming T, Cyn A. 1983. Patterns of injury in deaths due to falling from heights. *Proc First Asian Pacific Congr Legal Med*, p. 399.

Tomei G, Spagnoli D, Ducati A, *et al.* 1990. Morphology and neurophysiology of focal axonal injury experimentally induced in the guinea pig optic nerve. *Acta Neuropathol (Berl)* **80**:506–13.

Tomlinson BE. 1970. Brain-stem lesions after head injury. *J Clin Pathol Suppl R Coll Pathol* **4**:154–65.

Trotter W. 1914. Concussion. *Br J Surg* **2**:271–91.

Vanezis P. 1979. Techniques used in the evaluation of vertebral artery trauma at post-mortem. *Forensic Sci Int* **13**:159–65.

Vanezis P. 1984. *Vertebral artery trauma.* Medical Faculty, University of Bristol, Bristol.

Vanezis P. 1986. Vertebral artery injuries in road traffic accidents: a post-mortem study. *J Forensic Sci Soc* **26**:281–91.

Vanezis P. 1989. *Pathology of neck injury.* Butterworths, London.

Vanezis P, Chan KK, Scholtz CL. 1987. White matter damage following acute head injury. *Forensic Sci Int* **35**:1–10.

Voigt GE. 1981. Small hemorrhages in the brain stem. A sign of injury? *Am J Forensic Med Pathol* **2**:115–20.

Wang H, Duan G, Zhang J, *et al.* 1998. Clinical studies on diffuse axonal injury in patients with severe closed head injury. *Chin Med J (Engl)* **111**:59–62.

Weber W. 1984. Experimentelle Untersuchungen zu Schädelbruchverletzungen des Säuglings. [Experimental studies of skull fractures in infants] *Z Rechtsmed* **92**:87–94.

Wilkinson AE, Bridges LR, Sivaloganathan S. 1999. Correlation of survival time with size of axonal swellings in diffuse axonal injury. *Acta Neuropathol (Berl)* **98**:197–202.

Wilson JV. 1946. *The pathology of traumatic injury.* Livingstone, Edinburgh.

Yamashima T, Friede RL. 1984. Why do bridging veins rupture into the virtual subdural space? *J Neurol Neurosurg Psychiatry* **47**:121–7.

Yanagida Y, Fujiwara S, Mizoi Y. 1989. Differences in the intracranial pressure caused by a 'blow' and/or a 'fall' – an experimental study using physical models of the head and neck. *Forensic Sci Int* **41**:135–45.

Zhang X, Niu W. 1993. A study of enzymohisto-chemistry of cerebral cortical injury. *Forensic Sci Int* **59**:19–24.

Zuo ZJ, Zhu JZ. 1991. Study on the microstructures of skull fracture. *Forensic Sci Int* **50**:1–14.

C H A P T E R 6

Chest and abdominal injuries

The major categories of wound previously described can be inflicted on any part of the body. In forensic practice certain areas are particularly vulnerable or have special medico-legal significance. Head injuries are so important that they have been discussed in a special chapter, but here consideration will be given to other regions, especially the chest and abdomen.

CHEST INJURIES

Damage can be sustained to either the chest wall or to the contents.

FORENSIC ANATOMY

The most important aspect is the relationship of the visceral contents to external landmarks. This is best described by reference to diagrams, where the relationship of pleural cavities, lungs, heart, mediastinum and diaphragm is depicted. It should be appreciated that, from the forensic aspect, the spleen and most of the liver and stomach are thoracic organs in that they lie largely beneath the costal margin, and are vulnerable to both stabbing and blunt injury to the chest.

Penetrating injuries, especially by knife to the lower lateral wall of the thorax, may enter the peritoneal cavity as well as

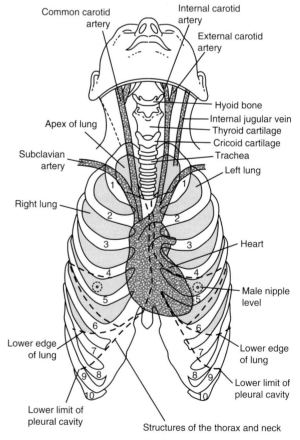

FIGURE 6.1 *Surface anatomy of heart, lungs and neck structures.*

the pleural spaces, perforating the diaphragm en route. The stomach, being largely within the rib cage, may often be penetrated. The common stab wounds of the heart may also include diaphragmatic and upper abdominal injuries. A knife can enter the front of the lower thorax, pass through either or both ventricles, and exit through the pericardial surface of the diaphragm to enter the upper surface of the liver. The orientation of the heart is often not appreciated after it is removed as an isolated organ, as the tendency is to visualize it as hanging with the apex downwards. In fact, it sits flat on the diaphragm on the lateral edge of the right ventricle, with the inferior vena cava passing immediately downwards into the abdomen.

INJURIES TO THE CHEST WALL

Respiration is dependent on the integrity of the rigid chest wall and, if the expansion is prevented or severely limited, then air entry will be correspondingly diminished. The integrity can be compromised either by severe mechanical failure of the rib cage or by penetration of the pleural cavities.

Fractures of ribs are common, but do not greatly embarrass respiration unless:

- they are so numerous that they prevent expansion of the thorax
- broken ends penetrate the pleura and lungs
- pleural and muscular pain limit respiratory effort.

Where many bilateral fractures are present, especially on the anterolateral sides of the thorax, the condition of 'flail chest' may be present, usually with multiple fractures of some ribs and sometimes with added fracture(s) of the sternum. As a result of loss of rigidity of the chest cage, attempts at expanding the thoracic volume during inspiration are impaired. The loose section is sucked inwards during inspiration, this clinical sign being known as 'paradoxical respiration'. Dyspnoea and cyanosis may develop and extreme degrees of flail chest are rapidly incompatible with life because of progressive hypoxia.

The flail chest is caused by frontal violence, most often sustained in motor vehicle accidents – where the victim is thrown against the steering wheel or fascia – or in stamping assaults, where the shod foot is violently applied to the supine body. In any substantial chest injury, broken rib ends may be displaced inwards, the jagged tips ripping the parietal and visceral pleura. This may cause a pneumothorax or a haemothorax, or both, from penetration of the lungs, with the formation of a bronchopleural fistula. In gross chest injuries there may be compound fractures of ribs that allow a pneumothorax to form from external communication with the atmosphere, but this is rare in civil practice, though common in battle casualties.

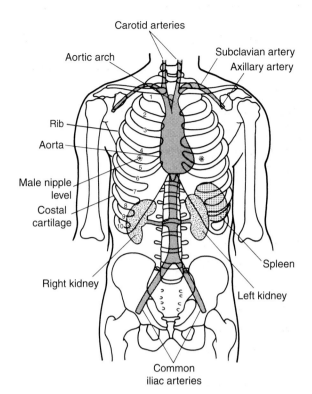

FIGURE 6.2 *Anterior view of trunk showing surface relations of heart and aorta.*

Rib fractures are most often seen in the anterior or posterior axillary lines caused by falls onto the side. The upper ribs are less often fractured, except by direct violence from kicking, heavy punching or traffic accidents. The fracture sites almost always show bleeding beneath the periosteum or the parietal pleura if the fractures occurred during life – though it must be admitted that (rarely) undoubted ante-mortem fractures may be totally bloodless, whereas some post-mortem cracks may exhibit slight oozing from the marrow cavity into the adjacent tissues. Attempts at resuscitation, especially external cardiac massage, now provide a common cause for extensive rib fractures (up to 40 per cent) and make the task of the pathologist much more difficult when trying to differentiate original trauma from the effects of enthusiastic first aid (Leadbeatter and Knight 1988). Bleeding may or may not be seen in these resuscitation fractures and, as the attempts at revival are, by definition, perimortal in timing, it is often impossible to say if they were immediately ante-mortem or post-mortem.

As the bracing action of adjacent intercostal muscles may conceal any mobility of the ribs when being examined at autopsy, it is a useful procedure to slit all the intercostal muscles with a knife when chest injury is suspected to allow any mobility to be detected more easily. In the osteoporosis of senility and some diseases, the ribs may be so fragile as to be breakable by finger pressure. Allowance must be made for this fragility in interpreting the cause of the fractures.

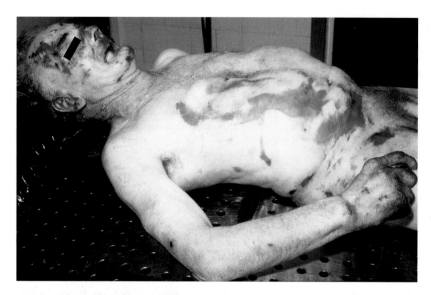

FIGURE 6.3 *Extensive abrasions and deformity of the chest in a man found by the roadside. All his ribs and sternum were fractured, resulting in a 'flail chest'. It was thought to be a road accident until bovine hairs were found on his clothing. He had been crushed by a bull and then tossed over the field wall.*

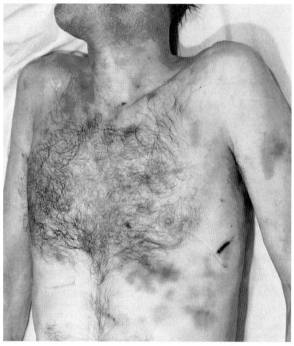

FIGURE 6.4 *Extensive bruising of the chest caused by kicking and stamping, resulting in multiple rib and sternal fractures. Over the left costal margin there is a pattern suggestive of the sole and heel of a shoe.*

In infants, especially victims of child abuse, rib fractures are common and may be an important diagnostic sign of abuse in doubtful cases. Where a small infant is squeezed from side to side, as when adult hands are clamped in each axilla or lower on the lateral sides of the chest, the hyperflexion can easily break ribs in their posterior segments, usually near their necks. The ribs are levered against the transverse processes of the vertebrae by excessive anterior flexion, which explains the tendency to fracture in the paravertebral gutter. Fresh fractures will be obvious, both on radiography and at autopsy. Within

about 2 weeks (though this is very variable), callus will form and be visible both on X-ray and by direct post-mortem inspection. It is extremely difficult to date such callus.

It is said by paediatricians and radiologists that anterior rib fractures are rare in infancy other than from child abuse; though this is probably generally correct, care must be taken to exclude bony injury from the now almost universal attempts at resuscitation (even though infant ribs are very pliable). In very young infants, the possibility of older fractures dating back to birth injury cannot be dismissed, though again these are rare.

The sternum may be fractured by stamping or other frontal impacts, but far more force is necessary than with ribs. If posterior displacement of a fragment occurs, the underlying heart or great vessels may be severely damaged.

HAEMORRHAGE AND INFECTION IN THE CHEST

Any injury to the chest wall or lung surface that breaches blood vessels and the pleural lining can lead to a haemothorax. Intercostal and, less often, mammary arteries can bleed into the pleural cavities, but most massive haemorrhage comes from large vessels in the lung or mediastinum. The lung hilum can be torn or penetrated by stabs wounds. Another obvious source of a haemothorax is the heart itself, though there must also be a defect in the pericardial sac before the blood can reach the chest cavity. Several litres of blood may accumulate in the chest, either as liquid or clot, or usually a mixture of both. Death may occur from loss of circulating blood volume, even if there is relatively little external bleeding.

Many intrathoracic haemorrhages may be fatal with virtually no external blood loss, a fact that the police often find

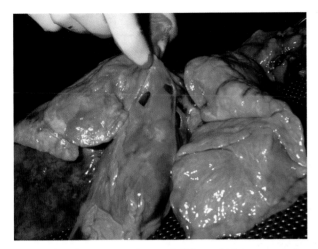

FIGURE 6.5 *Penetrating stab wound of chest, which has traversed the lung. The blade has passed through the upper lobe, crossed the interlobar fissure and re-entered the lower lobe. Death was caused by a haemothorax from severed branches of the pulmonary vessels within the lung.*

hard to credit if there is little blood at the scene of a fatal stabbing. A knife that passes obliquely into the chest through intercostal muscles may puncture a great vessel or heart chamber, allowing a fatal cardiac tamponade or haemothorax, yet the valve-like overlap of the tissues after withdrawal of the blade may seal up the external wound almost completely and prevent significant bleeding, especially as the blood inside the chest is not under any appreciable pressure.

The same may apply to a gunshot wound, where bleeding can be virtually absent if the wound is uppermost after death. Where the body lies above the wound, of whatever type, then considerable post-mortem gravitational leakage can take place.

Whatever the source of the bleeding, post-mortem haemorrhage can add very considerably to the volume found in the chest at autopsy. Due to the great variability of post-mortem coagulation – and subsequent lysis – much of the blood found at autopsy may not have been there at the moment of death. It is impossible to quantify this additional leakage in retrospect, but the ever-present possibility makes it unwise to be dogmatic about the amount of blood loss prior to death.

Infection following a chest wound is uncommon in forensic practice, as most deaths occur from haemorrhage within a relatively short time before infective sequelae have time to be established. Where survival is longer, then effective medical care usually prevents secondary infection. However, cellulitis, pleural inflammation and even empyema may supervene, especially where some dirty weapon is used, or where clothing or other foreign material has been carried into the wound. Infection may be of many types, but staphylococci, *Proteus*, coliforms and *Clostridium perfringens* are commonly found on culture.

PNEUMOTHORAX

There are three types of pneumothorax:

1 a simple type where a leakage through the pleura allows air to enter the pleural cavity, but where the communication rapidly closes. The lung partly collapses, but if death does not supervene the air is soon absorbed. If the communication remains open, then a bronchopleural fistula ensues with air in the pleural cavity but, as it is not under pressure, like type 2, it will not bubble out when the autopsy 'water test' is attempted. Radiology is then the best means of demonstrating the air in the pleural cavity.

2 when the leak in the pleura (or rarely the chest wall) has a valve-like action, air is sucked into the pleural cavity at each inspiration, but cannot escape on expiration. This pumping action leads to a 'tension pneumothorax', which causes complete collapse of the lung onto its hilum and a shift of the mediastinum to the opposite side. It is this type of pneumothorax that may be demonstrated at autopsy by penetrating an intercostal space under water, though radiology is a much better method of detection of all types of pneumothorax.

3 when an injury of the chest wall communicates with the pleural cavity, a 'sucking wound' may form with direct passage of air from the exterior. This type is most often seen in military surgery, and may be complicated by haemorrhage and infection.

A common traumatic cause of pneumothorax is a stab wound of the chest that allows direct communication with the exterior, though usually the layered skin and intercostal muscles closes the track when the weapon is withdrawn. The knife often enters the lung, however, so that air can enter the pleural cavity from the bronchi.

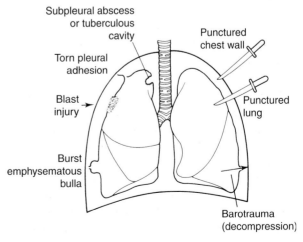

FIGURE 6.6 *Common causes of pneumothorax.*

Natural disease can also cause a pneumothorax, which can lead to sudden death. Common causes are a ruptured emphysematous bulla, a tuberculous lesion at the lung periphery, or a tear at the site of a fibrous pleural adhesion. This may initially appear suspicious, as in a case seen by the author (BK) in which a teenage boy bent down to tie a shoelace and fell dead. At autopsy the only finding was a pneumothorax that had been caused by a single pleural adhesion that had torn the visceral pleura. This illustrates the fact that sometimes a pneumothorax can cause sudden unexpected death, presumably via some vagal cardioinhibitory mechanism.

INJURIES OF THE LUNGS

Bruising of the lungs is common in both open and closed chest injuries. Any substantial impact on the chest can contuse the lung surface or deeper parts. This may be beneath the area of impact or 'contrecoup' damage on the opposite surface. Deceleration injuries are seen in falls and traffic accidents, most commonly along the posterolateral surfaces where a vertical line of subpleural bruising occurs, often in the paravertebral gutter. The outline of ribs may be imprinted in lines of contusion on the pleural surface of the lungs. Bruising may be so severe as to form subpleural blood blisters, which may rupture to release blood or air into the pleural cavities.

In all severe chest injuries the central parts of the lung may show bleeding, sometimes sufficient to form actual haematomas with breakdown of lung tissue. Osborn describes 'pincer contusions' of the lung, where the expanded lower margins of the lungs become trapped in the narrow costophrenic angles.

Laceration of the lung can occur in blunt injuries and even lobes or parts of a lobe may be detached. The hilum may tear and the pulmonary ligament below the hilum is a frequent site of haemorrhage. Vessels in the hilum (especially pulmonary veins) or those more peripherally, may be ripped, causing severe intrapleural or mediastinal haemorrhage. In children, lung injuries can occur without fracturing of the ribs, because of the greater elasticity of the latter and the ability of the chest wall to deform.

Penetrating injuries of the lungs are common, usually from stabbing by knives. The wounds may end in the lung parenchyma or in large vessels, or may be 'through-and-through' injuries that emerge to cause further damage to the heart or great vessels. They assist the pathologist by delineating the track and the direction of the stabbing, but due allowance must be made for the marked variation in topography during inspiration, compared with the collapsed state seen at autopsy.

Blast injury is dealt with elsewhere, but the lungs are the most vulnerable organs to this type of injury due to their large tissue–air interface.

INJURIES OF THE HEART

The heart is vulnerable to both penetrating and blunt injuries. A common form of homicide is a stab wound of the chest which penetrates the heart. The entry point may be anywhere over the praecordium or adjacent areas if the angulation of the track is sufficient. Sometimes the sternum is penetrated by a forceful blow that reaches the underlying heart, but most stab wounds enter via the intercostal spaces, or through a rib or costal cartilage.

Rarely, an upward stab from the abdomen reaches under the costal margin to penetrate the diaphragm. The right ventricle is often injured by a stab wound as it presents the largest frontal area, but the anterior interventricular septum and the left ventricle are also vulnerable. A shallow stab wound may enter the myocardium and not reach the lumen of the ventricle. In such a case there may be little disability unless a coronary vessel is severed, which may either cause death from myocardial insufficiency (if a major artery is transected) or cardiac tamponade.

More often – especially in the right ventricle – the knife passes into the cavity. In the thin right ventricle this usually

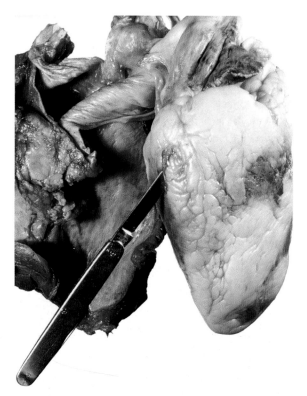

FIGURE 6.7 *Even a small penknife can inflict a fatal wound. This injury was caused by a boy to a police officer when the latter was apprehending him for some minor offence. Though the blade was only about 6 cm long, this is sufficient to enter alongside the sternum and puncture the ventricular wall.*

leads to copious bleeding into the pericardial sac even though the intraventricular pressure is relatively low because of the inability of the thin wall to close the defect by muscle overlap and contraction.

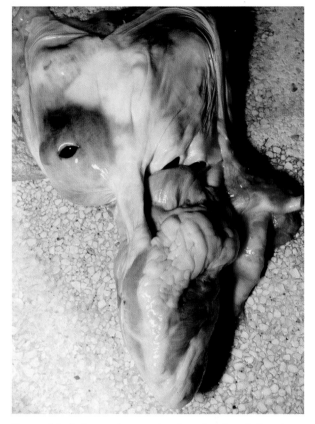

FIGURE 6.8 *Stab wound penetrating the pericardium (reflected upwards) with a wound in the corresponding point on the heart. Death was caused by cardiac tamponade from leakage of blood from the ventricular lumen.*

In the left ventricle, the contraction of the layered thick wall may partly or wholly seal the wound, and bleeding can be slight. It is, however, more common for persistent bleeding to occur and, if the drainage from the pericardial wound is less than the leakage from the ventricle, eventually a tamponade will develop. These variables make it impossible to calculate how long the victim was able to carry on with his activities, often a matter of dispute at a criminal trial. In general, wounds in the right ventricle are more dangerous than in the left because of the absence of the muscular 'self-sealing' effect.

Many stab wounds of the heart are transfixing or 'through-and-through' injuries, the knife entering one wall and emerging through another. If the left ventricle carries both wounds, the rapidity of bleeding may still not be torrential. Some of these wounds pass downwards and transfix the heart, then exit through the lower wall of the right ventricle and pass on via the diaphragm to end in the liver.

Blunt injuries of the heart are seen in civilian practice mainly in traffic accidents, falls from a height and in stamping assaults, though any heavy impact (including a punch) can cause fatal damage. There are usually multiple rib and sometimes sternal fractures, with or without a flail chest. Occasionally there can be heart damage in an intact chest cage, especially in a child with a pliable thorax. Fatal blunt damage of the heart may occur, however, without a mark on the skin of the thorax nor damage to the bony chest cage. The cardiac injuries are usually on the front of the organ, especially to the right ventricle, though posterior bruising and laceration can occur if the heart is compressed against the thoracic spine, as in stamping assaults and steering wheel impacts.

All degrees of damage can occur, from mere epicardial bruising to lacerations that open the ventricular lumen widely.

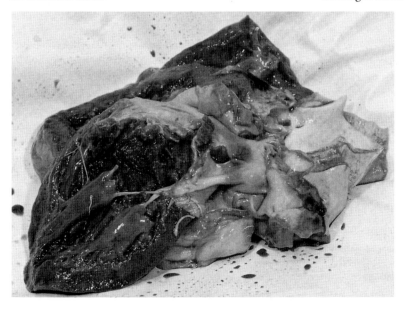

FIGURE 6.9 *Ruptured interventricular septum as a result of impact on the front of the chest. The septum can tear without damage to the outer walls of the heart.*

Internal damage to the heart may be present, without external signs of injury to either the heart or the external chest wall. The interventricular septum may be ruptured as a sole lesion, the mechanics of which seem obscure. In gross injuries, such as aircraft crashes, the whole heart may be avulsed from its root, to be found lying loose in the thorax. Histological damage, especially contraction band necrosis, can be found even when there is no macroscopic abnormality. A comprehensive review of cardiac contusions has been made by Sagall (1971).

HAEMOPERICARDIUM AND CARDIAC TAMPONADE

Bleeding into the pericardial sac may occur from the surface or the cavities of the heart, or from the intrapericardial segments of the roots of the great vessels, particularly the aorta and pulmonary artery. Most causes of haemopericardium are from natural disease, such as a ruptured myocardial infarct or a ruptured dissecting aneurysm of the aorta (Chapter 25), but it is not an uncommon sequel to injury to the chest. When the damage has been caused by a stab that has perforated the pericardial sac, bleeding can escape into the pleural cavities, mediastinum or even abdomen if the diaphragm is penetrated. Death may occur from sheer blood loss if the haemorrhage can escape from the confines of the pericardium, but another common lethal condition is 'cardiac tamponade'.

In the tamponade, blood accumulates in the pericardial sac faster than it can escape, either because the bleeding rate exceeds the drainage or because the exit hole in the pericardium becomes blocked by blood clot. In cases where the bleeding is from a contusion or laceration of the heart, there is no escape route from the sac. When sufficient blood accumulates, the pressure in the pericardial sac increases and begins to prevent the passive filling of the atria during diastole. The cardiac output falls, as does the systemic blood pressure and the venous pressure rises. If unrelieved, death will follow, though the time that this takes is variable and almost impossible to calculate retrospectively on pathological findings. It has been stated (Moritz 1942) that about 400–500 ml of blood is sufficient to cause death, though this seems a greater volume than is usually seen in tamponades. Where trauma to the heart co-exists, it is difficult to apportion the relative contribution to death of the tamponade as opposed to the other injuries.

INJURIES TO GREAT VESSELS

The most vulnerable vessel is the aorta, which most commonly suffers injury in deceleration trauma from both road

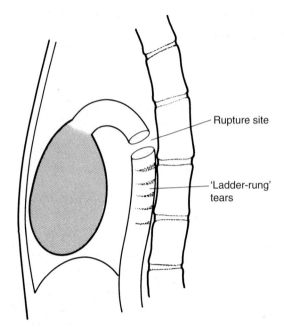

FIGURE 6.10 *The usual site of rupture of the aorta in deceleration injury.*

and air accidents, as well as from falls from a height. When the thorax is suddenly decelerated, the heart – being relatively mobile in the chest – attempts to continue in the original direction. This causes severe traction on the root of the heart, and a common sequel is complete or partial rupture of the aorta in the descending part of its arch. In falls from a height, Fiddler (1946) claims that the lesion is the result of the abdominal and thoracic viscera being forced caudalwards by the abrupt deceleration when landing on the feet or buttocks. Tannenbaum and Ferguson (1948), however, postulate that the mechanism is a sudden rise in intra-aortic pressure. Lasky (1974) has reviewed the biomechanics of impact injury of the aorta.

According to Fiddler, rupture occurs almost constantly at a point 1.5 cm distal to the attachment of the ligamentum arteriosum, the remnant of the ductus. The lower thoracic aorta is closely bound to the anterior longitudinal ligament on the front of the dorsal spine, until it reaches the termination of the arch, where it curves forwards. This appears to be the weak point and transection occurs at this level, sometimes so cleanly that it looks like a surgical incision. The tear is annular and at right angles to the axis of the aorta. Sometimes, there may be multiple parallel intimal tears near the main transection, the so-called 'ladder-rung tears'. In deceleration trauma, these incomplete tears, which affect only the intima and inner media, may be found without major transection; where death is delayed, false aneurysms and dissections may be diagnosed on aortograms.

The pulmonary artery is much less vulnerable to blunt trauma than the aorta but, in stamping assaults and steering

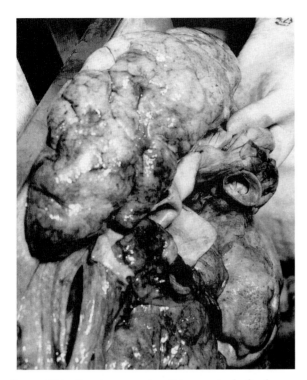

FIGURE 6.11 *Complete transection of the aorta in the distal part of the arch. The victim was a car driver who suffered a severe deceleration impact. There is also some slight pulmonary bruising; the lungs are asthmatic.*

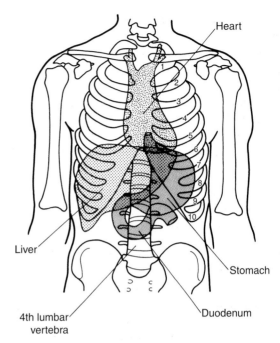

FIGURE 6.12 *Surface anatomy of liver, stomach and heart.*

wheel impacts, it may be damaged by depressed rib cage and sternal fractures. The pulmonary artery and vein branches may also be damaged in the root of the lung, where hilar tears are not uncommon. The great vessels are often involved in penetrating injuries, notably stab wounds. Stabs of the upper part of the chest may pass directly into the arch of the aorta, especially on the right side of the sternum. Here even a shallow injury may reach the aorta and the authors have seen several cases in which a short-bladed penknife has caused death in this way.

Stabs that are either too high, or are directed too laterally to puncture the chambers of the heart may penetrate the ascending aorta or the pulmonary artery. If the wound is below the reflection of the pericardium, a haemopericardium and perhaps cardiac tamponade may result. Other stab wounds may injure the heart valves or may enter the root of the lung to penetrate the large primary branches of the pulmonary artery or veins, causing gross bleeding into the corresponding pleural cavity or the mediastinum.

ABDOMINAL INJURIES

As with the thorax, the damage caused by blunt and penetrating trauma of the abdomen depends upon the location of the injury. In addition, the large area of the anterior abdomen occupied by the intestine provides a target for perforation with consequent chemical or infective peritonitis.

Open or penetrating wounds need little description, as they follow the characteristics of stab-like injuries in general. The liver, and especially the spleen, may bleed extensively, causing a haemoperitoneum. The intestine and mesentery are the other major targets, wounds often being multiple, because of the overlapping nature of the coils and their mesentery. The stomach, being partially protected by the rib margin, is less often penetrated from the abdomen, but is not uncommonly involved in chest stabbings that pass downwards through the diaphragm. The kidneys are rarely stabbed except from a thrust in the back.

Closed or blunt injury to the abdomen is common from both accidents and assault. Impact on the abdomen by a car steering wheel was more common before the widespread use of safety-belts and air-bags and still occurs in severe deceleration accidents. The liver, intestine, spleen and mesentery are most vulnerable. Crushing between two vehicles, or between a vehicle and a wall is another mechanism for abdominal trauma, and may also be seen in railway and industrial accidents where squeezing between two opposing surfaces occurs. In homicides, assaults and child abuse, kicking, stamping and heavy punching can also cause blunt injury to the abdomen.

Whatever the mechanism of infliction, the following features may be present:

■ Bruising of the abdominal wall, both of the skin and the underlying muscles, is often (but by no means

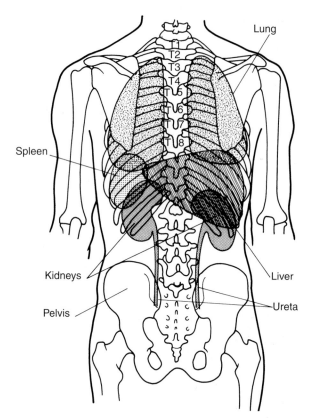

FIGURE 6.13 *Posterior view of trunk to show surface relations of organs.*

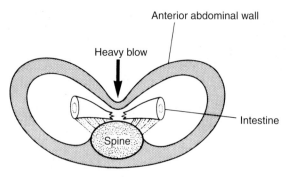

FIGURE 6.14 *Injury or rupture of intestine or mesentery in violent blow to the upper central abdomen. Because of its small size and the thin abdominal wall, the infant duodenum is especially vulnerable.*

invariably) seen in abdominal trauma. Where subcutaneous bleeding is profuse it may track from the initial area of impact to become more diffuse and may cover a large area of abdominal wall, especially in the lower segment. Blood may track down the inguinal canal and appear in the scrotum or labia.

More often there are discrete bruises on the abdominal skin, associated in some instances with surface abrasions. Kicks will usually leave scuffed abrasions if tangential, unless protected by clothing. Fingertip or knuckle bruises may be seen, especially in child abuse. In infants, bruises may be seen on the sides of the abdomen where adult fingers have forcibly gripped or lifted the child, though these are more common in the axillary line of the chest.

Severe or fatal intra-abdominal injury may be present, however, without any mark on the skin. This can occur if clothing protects or if a blunt impact is applied over, a relatively large surface. In child abuse, for example, the liver, mesentery or duodenum can be ruptured with no external sign whatsoever.

■ Extensive bleeding into the peritoneal cavity, usually from rupture of a solid viscus or bleeding from the mesentery.

■ Bruising or rupture of the stomach and diaphragm. The stomach is less vulnerable than the intestines, but

may be lacerated by a heavy blow in the upper abdomen, especially when full of food or fluid.

■ The intestine and its mesentery are frequently damaged in abdominal trauma. Extensive bruising of the gut and its vascular mesentery may occur, mainly from being crushed against the prominent lumbar vertebrae in the midline. The duodenum and jejunum are particularly vulnerable to transection from being compressed against the spine, especially in children, where a heavy blow in the central or upper abdomen can cut through the third part of the duodenum almost as cleanly as a scalpel. Laceration of the mesentery is not uncommon both in traffic accidents and assaults. The same mechanism of compression against the lumbar spine causes bruising and tearing of the central parts of the mesentery, which usually occurs towards the intestinal margin of the membrane. Multiple fenestrations may be seen, presumably because folds of mesentery overlie each other and are injured when in apposition.

Severe and intractable bleeding can occur in circumstances where surgical treatment is often not offered because the condition is unrecognized. Kicks and punches in the abdomen may be sustained by drunken persons who may be apparently unaware of the seriousness of their injuries until collapse and death supervene perhaps hours later.

In a case seen by the author (BK), a man was involved in a fight and then allegedly assaulted the police. He was forcibly restrained and may have been struck in the abdomen by a knee. He remained apparently well, though drunk, in a police cell for more than 5 hours, before collapsing and dying on his way to the lavatory, never having complained of any abdominal pain. Autopsy revealed several litres of blood in his peritoneal cavity, which had escaped from several large tears in the mesentery. Similar bleeding from mesenteric lacerations has been seen in abused infants,

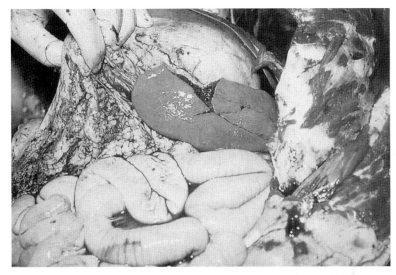

FIGURE 6.15 *Laceration of the spleen following lower chest impact during a road traffic accident.*

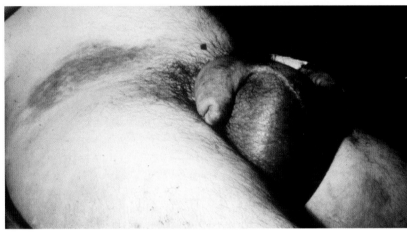

FIGURE 6.16 *Abdominal wall bruising with fatal intraperitoneal haemorrhage from a ruptured mesentery. There is also a large haematocele from a gang attack in which repeated kicking occurred.*

where the thin abdominal wall provides little protection from blows on the abdomen.

Injury to the mesentery may damage local arteries without causing severe bleeding, but may occlude or thrombose them, with infarction of the bowel as a consequence. Perforation may be delayed for a day or two and in children and old people there need not be the dramatic symptoms of the onset of peritonitis that is usually seen in clinical surgical practice.

The colon is rarely injured unless the abdominal injury is gross. One well-known lesion is rupture of the rectum or sigmoid by a high-pressure air hose being placed in or near the anus as a practical joke.

■ Rupture of the spleen is a common surgical emergency after trauma but may be first found at autopsy if undiagnosed, or if death occurs from lack of speedy surgical treatment, or if other injuries made recovery impossible. An enlarged spleen is more vulnerable and more fragile than a normal organ. Malaria, glandular fever and other infections increase the risk of rupture. The 'stiletto' dagger was specifically designed in medieval Italy for puncturing the enlarged malarious spleen by an upward blow under the left costal margin.

The spleen can be damaged either from impact on its surface or from traction on its pedicle. The rupture may be immediate or may be delayed if a large subcapsular haematoma and underlying tear are held intact for a time by the capsule. This delay can last for a number of days or even weeks.

■ Rupture of the liver is also a common lesion following serious abdominal trauma, such as fall from a height or a crush injury between two wagons. It is seen especially in traffic accidents, either from impact of the driver on the rim or centre of the steering wheel or by the unrestrained passenger being thrown against the fascia. A pedestrian can also suffer a ruptured liver either as a primary impact from a vehicle or as secondary damage from being thrown to the ground.

A more recent cause of liver injury is enthusiastic external cardiac massage. Even if death has already taken place, there may still be a significant amount of blood oozing from the liver tears into the peritoneal

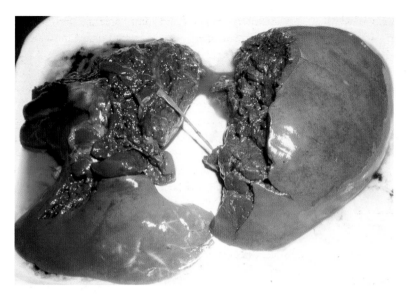

FIGURE 6.17 *Complete bisection of the liver in a high-speed deceleration during a traffic accident. The abdomen of the driver was hurled against the steering wheel as he was projected through the windscreen.*

cavity. Moritz (1942) has described six varieties of hepatic laceration, but such a differentiation is of little practical use. The liver may show one or more linear cracks, most often on the convex upper surface, which may be of any severity from superficial subcapsular tears to complete transection of the organ. Not infrequently, several roughly parallel tears are seen on the upper surface, obviously from the same type of mechanical stress. The surface lacerations may extend deeply into the liver and may even appear on the opposite surface. Occasionally, there may be internal tears that do not communicate with the surface. As in the spleen, a subcapsular haematoma can reach a large size before bursting into the peritoneal cavity, causing a delay in collapse or death.

Infants readily suffer liver damage from trauma and it is a well-known component of the child abuse syndrome. Liver tears can occur during the process of birth, particularly in breech presentation.

Injuries to the kidney. Being deeply situated at the back of the abdomen in the paravertebral gutter, the kidneys are rarely damaged by frontal trauma, but may be involved in kicks or heavy blows to the loin. Traffic impacts, mainly in pedestrians, can damage the kidney, but kicking is another cause of this rather uncommon injury. When a victim is lying on the ground, a swinging boot can conveniently enter the slightly raised arch between the rib margin and hip, where the kidney is situated.

Perirenal haemorrhage is much more common than damage to the actual organs themselves, but when they are injured, all grades of damage from comminuted pulping through transection to shallow surface lacerations may be seen. Like the mesentery and spleen, damage to vessels may lead to post-injury infarction. The suprarenal

vessels can be damaged by impact and, statistically, the right suprarenal artery is more often involved in traffic accidents in Britain because the direction of traffic tends to favour lesions on that side. It is, however, difficult to differentiate direct trauma to the suprarenal vessels from the common post-stress haemorrhages, often bilateral, of the Waterhouse–Frederichsen type. These occur quite commonly a few days after any trauma, surgical operation or infection, and are rarely diagnosed by clinicians (Knight 1980) (see Chapter 13).

FOREIGN BODIES IN THE GUT

Though not usually a feature of trauma, foreign bodies and material are not infrequently found in the alimentary system in forensic practice, both clinically and at autopsy.

Disorders of the mental state may lead to extraordinary numbers of objects being swallowed, which may be present anywhere from mouth to anus, but especially in the stomach. Betz *et al.* (1994) describe two such deaths, where, in one, 2000 cm³ of debris, including broken glass, was in the alimentary tract; the other suffered intestinal obstruction due to ingestion of a large quantity of his own hair.

Similar aberrations may lead to insertion of foreign objects into the rectum, urethra, bladder and vagina. The authors have seen large objects of various types, e.g. potatoes in the rectum, lengths of broom handle and wood in the colon (one penetrating the liver) and a banana and a beer can in the vagina. Sexual perversions, masturbation and heterosexual or homosexual activities may account for these, as well as frank mental abnormality.

In recent years, the smuggling of narcotics through ports and airports has commonly been accomplished by 'body-packing', the drugs being concealed in condoms, which are then either swallowed or, less often, inserted into the rectum or vagina. Deaths have occurred in these body-packers, usually by rupture of a package within the gut, so that a massive dose of heroin or cocaine is released with all the attendant toxic effects. Rarely, the mass of illicit material may cause intestinal obstruction, leading to a surgical emergency, which the carrier does not wish to be investigated, for obvious reasons.

INJURIES TO THE PELVIS AND PELVIC ORGANS

The bony pelvis suffers a variety of fractures and dislocations in severe trauma:

- Where great pressure is applied to the front of the abdomen or pubic area – as in running over by a vehicle wheel – the pelvis may be splayed open, the symphysis parting and one or both sacroiliac joints becoming dislocated.
- An impact from the side may shatter the superior and, less often, the inferior pubic ramus, and again dislocate the sacroiliac joint on that side.
- A fall from a height onto the feet may transmit the force up the legs either to dislocate the hips or even to drive one or both femoral heads through the acetabulum. If the hip joints remain intact, the pelvic girdle may crack and again the sacroiliac joints may be sheared apart.
- A kick or heavy fall onto the base of the spine may fracture the coccyx or sacrum.

The pelvic organs with the exception of the bladder are generally protected from all but the most severe trauma. When it is full, the bladder can be ruptured by heavy blows or kicks on the lower abdomen. The empty bladder is rarely injured by blunt trauma. The male urethra is also vulnerable to direct trauma, such as falling astride a solid object like a gate, or being kicked in the crutch, both of which compress the urethra against the undersurface of the pubis.

The external genitals may suffer injury, apart from the sexual assaults discussed in Chapter 18. The scrotum is vulnerable to severe bruising, especially from kicks: a large haematocele may develop. Scrotal and vulval injuries can occur from falling astride an object or in traffic accidents. Impact of a bicycle wheel between the legs is one such cause.

COMPLICATIONS OF ABDOMINAL INJURY

The most common fatal sequel to intra-abdominal trauma is haemorrhage from any of the contained organs. The spleen

and mesentery tend to bleed most copiously and quickly, though even here there can be a delay of many hours before serious symptoms are obvious – and, in the case of a subcapsular laceration of the spleen, the time can be far longer. The liver tends to ooze more slowly unless a major injury opens a large vessel or an extensive area of hepatic tissue.

The mesentery contains numerous blood vessels that are not covered by parenchymatous tissue as in the liver or spleen, so bleeding is usually brisk from significant tears – although, as illustrated by the case described above, even this injury can lead to delayed death.

Because all bleeding in the abdomen, unless it is from a wound of the aorta, takes time to accumulate, restriction of the victim's activity immediately after the injury need be minimal or absent unless there are other factors involved. It is never safe for a pathologist to declare that rapid immobility must have ensued, unless there are other gross injuries.

As mentioned in relation to intrathoracic bleeding, some of the blood found at autopsy within the peritoneal cavity may have accumulated there after death, adding to the true ante-mortem volume.

In spite of common surgical experience, even severe intra-abdominal injuries leading to bleeding need not necessarily be painful, especially in the commonly associated circumstance of the victim being under the influence of alcohol.

Perforation of the gastrointestinal canal is another serious complication of trauma, though often death ensues from the totality of injuries before infection can become established. As in natural perforated peptic ulcer, penetration of the stomach or duodenum will cause a chemical peritonitis that can be a cause of severe and immediate shock – perhaps a major factor in a rapid death. Rupture of the small or large intestine is less damaging but, if survival continues, will inevitably lead to generalized peritonitis unless vigorously treated. Open wounds of the abdomen, including stabbing, will introduce organisms from the outside into the peritoneal cavity. In addition to infection, trauma to the intestine may cause an intractable ileus; if the pancreas is damaged, there may be widespread fat necrosis in the mesentery and omentum.

REFERENCES AND FURTHER READING

Adams JE, Davis GG, Heidepriem RW, 3rd, *et al.* 2002. Analysis of the incidence of pelvic trauma in fatal automobile accidents. *Am J Forensic Med Pathol* **23**:132–6.

Albrektsen SB, Thomsen JL. 1989. Detection of injuries in traumatic deaths. The significance of medico-legal autopsy. *Forensic Sci Int* **42**:135–43.

Betz P, van Meyer L, Eisenmenger W. 1994. Fatalities due to intestinal obstruction following the ingestion of foreign bodies. *Forensic Sci Int* **69**:105–10.

Bowen DA. 1970. A survey of injuries to the liver and spleen in forensic autopsies. *J Forensic Med* **17**:12–19.

Canfield TM. 1969. Suicidal gunshot wounds of the abdomen. *J Forensic Sci* **14**:445–52.

Cohle SD, Hawley DA, Berg KK, *et al.* 1995. Homicidal cardiac lacerations in children. *J Forensic Sci* **40**:212–18.

Cotton JM, Cooke JC, Monaghan MJ. 2000. Forensic echocardiography: a case in point. *Echocardiography* **17**:193–4.

Darok M, Beham-Schmid C, Gatternig R, *et al.* 2001. Sudden death from myocardial contusion following an isolated blunt force trauma to the chest. *Int J Legal Med* **115**:85–9.

Davis C. 1963. Spontaneous rupture of the stomach. *Arch Surg* **32**:170–6.

Denton JS, Kalelkar MB. 2000. Homicidal commotio cordis in two children. *J Forensic Sci* **45**:734–5.

Fiddler J. 1946. *The pathology of traumatic injury.* Livingstone, Edinburgh.

Frazer M, Mirchandani H. 1984. Commotio cordis, revisited. *Am J Forensic Med Pathol* **5**:249–51.

Gunther WM, Symes SA, Berryman HE. 2000. Characteristics of child abuse by anteroposterior manual compression versus cardiopulmonary resuscitation: case reports. *Am J Forensic Med Pathol* **21**:5–10.

Hale HW. 1965. Pulmonary contusions. *J Trauma* **5**:647–52.

Knight B. 1980. Sudden unexpected death from adrenal haemorrhage. *Forensic Sci Int* **16**:227–9.

Lasky I. 1974. *Human aortic laceration due to impact.* In: Wecht C (ed.), *Legal medicine annual.* Appleton Century Crofts, New York.

Leadbeatter S, Knight B. 1988. Resuscitation artefact. *Med Sci Law* **28**:200–4.

Lloyd RG. 1982. Delayed rupture of stomach after blunt abdominal trauma. *Br Med J Clin Res Ed* **285**:176.

Loop FD, Hofmeir G, Groves LK. 1971. Traumatic disruption of the aortic valve. *Cleveland Clin Q* **38**:187–94.

Mackintosh AF, Fleming HA. 1981. Cardiac damage presenting late after road accidents. *Thorax* **36**:811–13.

Maron BJ, Poliac LC, Kaplan JA, *et al.* 1995. Blunt impact to the chest leading to sudden death from cardiac arrest during sports activities. *N Engl J Med* **333**:337–42.

McCormick GM, 2nd, Young DB. 1995. Spontaneous rupture of the spleen. A fatal complication of pregnancy. *Am J Forensic Med Pathol* **16**:132–4.

Menzies RC. 1978. Cardiac contusion: a review. *Med Sci Law* **18**:3–12.

Moritz AR. 1942. *The pathology of trauma.* Lea & Febiger, Philadelphia.

Murphy GK. 1985. A single fatal penetrating chest wound from shattered wind-blown glass. *Am J Forensic Med Pathol* **6**:332–5.

Noon GP, Boulafendis D, Beall AC, Jr. 1971. Rupture of the heart secondary to blunt trauma. *J Trauma* **11**:122–8.

Ormstad K, Rajs J, Calissendorff B, *et al.* 1984. Difference between in vivo and postmortem distances between anterior chest and heart surface. A combined autopsy and in vivo computerized tomography study. *Am J Forensic Med Pathol* **5**:31–5.

Orr CJ, Clark MA, Hawley DA, *et al.* 1995. Fatal anorectal injuries: a series of four cases. *J Forensic Sci* **40**:219–21.

Ortmann C, Pfeiffer H, Brinkmann B. 2001. Immunohistochemical alterations after intravital and post-mortem traumatic myocardial damage. *Int J Legal Med* **115**:23–8.

Osborn GR. 1943. Findings in 272 fatal accidents. *Lancet* **245**:277–84.

Puffer P, Gaebler M. 1991. [Traumatic diaphragmatic rupture in a forensic medicine autopsy sample.] *Beitr Gerichtl Med* **49**:149–52.

Sagall EL. 1971. Contusion of the heart: medical and legal considerations. In: Wecht C (ed.), *Legal medicine annual.* Appleton Century Crofts, New York.

Simonsen J. 1983. Injuries sustained from high-velocity impact with water after jumps from high bridges. A preliminary report of 10 cases. *Am J Forensic Med Pathol* **4**:139–42.

Stajduhar-Djuric Z. 1960. Penetrating wounds of the ascending aorta and heart. *J Forensic Med* **7**:147–52.

Tannebaum I, Ferguson JA. 1948. Rapid deceleration and rupture of the aorta. *Arch Pathol* **45**:503–5.

Teresinski G, Madro R. 2001. Pelvis and hip joint injuries as a reconstructive factors in car-to-pedestrian accidents. *Forensic Sci Int* **124**:68–73.

CHAPTER 7

Self-inflicted injury

Injuries that are deliberately self-inflicted are common and their examination is a frequent task for both pathologists and clinical forensic practitioners. These events consist of suicide, attempted suicide and suicidal gestures, the latter lacking the intention to kill though death may inadvertently ensue. In addition, there is non-suicidal self-inflicted trauma, as described below.

One of the most difficult decisions that can face pathologists, medical examiners and legal authorities, such as coroners, is the differentiation between homicide, suicide, accident and other self-inflicted injury. Though it is not the legal function of a pathologist to attribute motive, his experience and training are often the factors that lead the official authority to make a decision as to the classification of the manner of death or injury. One such situation is fatal auto-erotic activities, described in Chapter 15.

In addition, when a pathologist is assisting the police in the early stages of a death investigation, his opinion and decision about the manner of the death may be crucial in initiating or aborting a homicide investigation – an onerous decision which may have serious and expensive consequences if wrong. It is therefore a most important function of the forensic pathologist to decide on the evidence of a death scene and subsequent autopsy whether murder, suicide or accident is the most likely explanation.

Self-inflicted injury, when not suicidal, is often not fatal and the pathologist is usually not consulted unless he also includes clinical forensic medicine in his work. The pathologist may, however, be asked for his opinion, as he is a specialist in trauma and may be able to provide the most useful opinion available. In other cases, self-inflicted injury, which the victim did not intend to be fatal, may end in death from a variety of causes and thus the pathologist will be directly involved.

SUICIDAL INJURIES

This discussion is confined to physical trauma, self-poisoning being considered later in the book.

Suicides may injure themselves in many different ways, some bizarre in the extreme. The pathologist must always be alert to the possibility that such injuries are not true suicides, but some manifestation of peculiar practices that have taken a course unintended by the victim. A prime example is masochistic asphyxia, which is still sometimes mistaken for suicide (Chapter 15). Even more serious is the homicide that appears to be a suicide, though the reverse also occurs.

Suicides, apart from poisoning, may use one (or even more) of the following methods, though the list is by no means exclusive:

- stabbing and cutting
- firearms and explosives
- jumping from a height
- jumping into water
- burning
- suffocation, e.g. plastic bag
- hanging and strangulation
- electrocution
- road and railway injuries.

Most of these modes are discussed in the appropriate chapters.

Suicidal knife wounds

Many incised and stab wounds are self-inflicted, either from motives of self-destruction, from mental aberrations or deliberately for some form of gain. These must be differentiated from each other, and from accidental and homicidal wounding.

Sometimes the distinction may be difficult and even impossible, but the experience of the forensic pathologist is paramount in assisting investigative agencies to come to the correct conclusion. Suicide, attempted suicide and suicidal gestures commonly employ cutting weapons as the means of injury. There are certain features that are quite reliable pointers to these motives, though they are by no means infallible:

■ Suicidal knife wounds favour certain 'sites of election', which are predominantly the throat, the wrists and the front of the chest. As with most violent methods, cut throat and chest stabbing is predominantly seen in men – though cutting wrists is not uncommon in women.

■ Suicidal wounds are typically multiple, often being characterized by a number of preliminary trial cuts, called 'tentative incisions'. These are most often seen on the throat and wrists, where the person often makes a series of shallow incisions, presumably hesitating while gaining courage to make a final decisive cut. In many suicidal attempts the subject abandons this method after a few trial incisions and uses some other method of self-destruction. Although the presence of tentative incisions is strong presumptive evidence of suicide, exceptions do occur, and the pathologist must take all other aspects of the scene into account before giving an opinion to the investigators. In fact, the almost absolute statements of some older textbooks that tentative incisions must indicate suicide, is to be disregarded. The author (BK) has dealt with two recent murders in which 'typical' suicidal injuries were present on wrist or throat causing considerable doubt to the investigators until other factors clarified the situation.

■ A suicidal cut throat usually has these trial incisions; there may be only one or two, or there may be scores of trial cuts. If successful, there will be one or more deep incisions superimposed, which may destroy some of the previous shallow cuts. The classical description of the cut throat is of incisions starting high on the left side of the neck below the angle of the jaw, which pass obliquely across the front of the neck to end at a lower level on the right. This assumes that the victim is right-handed, the obliquity being reversed in a left-handed person. The cuts are said to be deeper at their origin, becoming shallower as they cross the throat, tailing off into surface cuts at the extremity.

This description, though hallowed by repetition in many textbooks, is often incorrect and many cut throats have horizontal cuts that show no variation in depth at either end. Most suicides appear to raise the chin to provide better access to the throat, so that the skin is stretched when cut. This tends to cause straight-edged incisions, rather than the jagged cut (the so-called 'dentele' toothed incision) seen when a knife is drawn over loose skin. Throwing back the head moves the carotid bundle under the protection of the sternomastoid muscles and, if the cuts are confined to the centre of the front of the neck, only the larynx or trachea may be damaged, rather than large blood vessels.

Death from a cut throat depends on the nature and extent of local damage to the neck. Severe haemorrhage

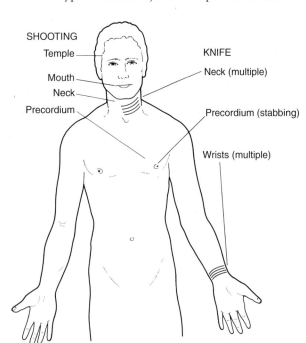

FIGURE 7.1 *Sites of election in violent suicide.*

SHOOTING
Temple
Mouth
Neck
Precordium

KNIFE
Neck (multiple)
Precordium (stabbing)
Wrists (multiple)

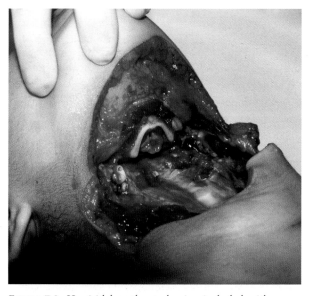

FIGURE 7.2 *Homicidal cut throat, showing single slash with no tentative cuts. Clean-cut edges with no sign of repetitive strokes, severing muscles, larynx and some large vessels.*

from the jugular veins, or less often the carotid arteries, may lead to death from exsanguination. If the larynx or trachea is opened, then even relatively minor haemorrhage from local vessels may cause blockage of the airways by blood and clot, though many slashed air-passage victims survive. A rare cause of death is air embolism, caused by aspiration into cut jugular veins while standing or sitting with the neck at a higher level than the thorax. The possibility that the victim of a cut throat may have died from some unrelated cause must always be borne in mind. Many suicides either use multiple methods of suicide to ensure success – or may abandon the pain of a cut throat for some other mode, such as poison or a fall from a height.

■ Deliberate cutting of the wrists is rarely effective as the sole method of suicide, but it is a common injury. Many suicides from other causes are seen at autopsy to have scars on the wrists from previous unsuccessful attempts or gestures. The usual site is on the flexor surface at the level of the skin flexion creases. As with the neck, there may be a number of shallow tentative incisions, but commonly several deep gashes are made without trial cuts. The left wrist is the more common target, because of right-handed dominance (86 per cent in men, 93 per cent in women).

As with the neck, there is a tendency for the victim to hyperextend the wrist before making the cut, which causes the radial artery to slip into the shelter of the lower end of the radius. The knife cuts may then miss major blood vessels and merely divide flexor tendons, though many cuts are too shallow to cause anything

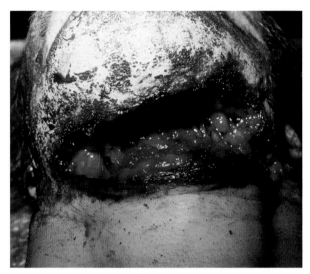

FIGURE 7.3 *Gaping laceration in front of neck of a mental patient, who on leave from a psychiatric hospital, had used a frame saw to commit suicide (see also Figure 7.4).*

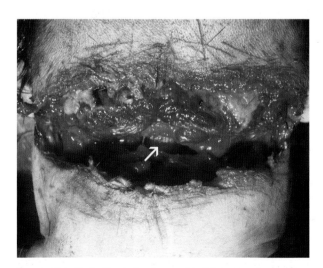

FIGURE 7.4 *Back of neck showing marks of the saw teeth around the laceration and medulla at the bottom (arrow). Mental patient who, on leave from a psychiatric hospital, had used a frame saw to commit suicide (see also Figure 7.3).*

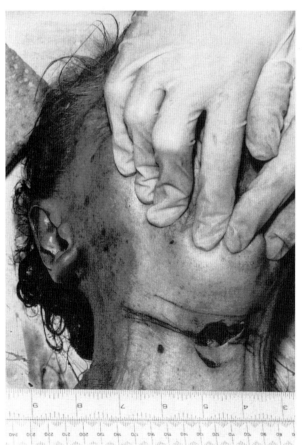

FIGURE 7.5 *Homicidal cut throat, simulating a suicide. There are several apparently 'tentative cuts', but the deep penetrating central laceration and adjacent stab wound is atypical. The face is congested and shows some petechiae from prior pressure on the neck.*

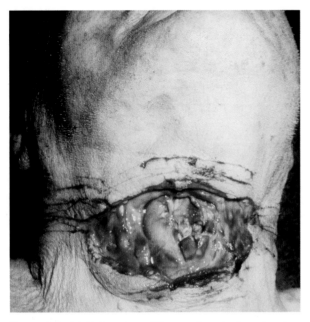

FIGURE 7.6 *Suicidal cut throat. The wounds are horizontal, rather than the more common sloping-down from left to right in a right-handed person. The numerous 'tentative cuts' are the hallmark of self-infliction, though there are rare exceptions. The larynx has been entered and death was due to aspiration of blood into the air passages. The great vessels in the neck were undamaged.*

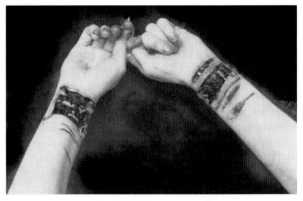

FIGURE 7.8 *Knife wounds of wrists in a suicidal attempt. Even though these are more severe than usually seen, no damage to the radial arteries was effected and death was the result of a subsequent cut throat. The victim was a woman of 31, unusual in that cut wrists and throat are much more common among men.*

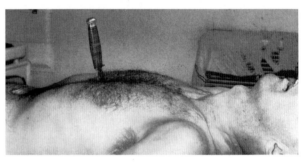

FIGURE 7.9 *Suicidal stab wound of heart. The front of the chest is one of the suicidal sites of predilection; multiple stabs do not exclude self-infliction.*

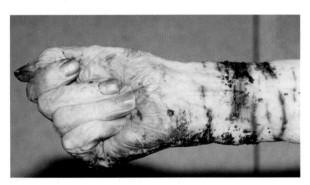

FIGURE 7.7 *Numerous self-inflicted cuts on the wrist, as part of a futile suicide attempt. Most of these attempts fail and the person turns to another method of self-destruction.*

but superficial damage. Most cut wrists are but an accompaniment to other more effective methods of self-destruction. Once again, the presence of tentative cuts, though very significant, cannot be unquestioningly accepted as an exclusion of homicide.

■ Suicidal injuries of the chest are almost always stab wounds. Sometimes linear incised cuts are made over the precordium or more widely over the front of the chest; these may be multiple, parallel and sometimes criss-cross, but rarely do any serious damage. Stab wounds are usually over the left side of the chest where common knowledge places the heart, but they may be alongside the sternum or even on the right side. The wound is often single, but multiple wounds are not uncommon. Though naturally a series of severe wounds always raises the presumption of homicide, many undoubted suicides can inflict a number of injuries upon themselves, each potentially fatal. The author (BK) has seen a suicide in a doctor, where eight severe knife wounds of the lower chest had created a large external defect and detached a portion of liver.

Suicidal knife wounds are not often made in the abdomen, though they do occur, sometimes to the extent of disembowelling. The author (PS) has seen a suicide of a person, who removed several meters of the gut through a single and relatively small incision before dying of exsanguination. There is usually frank mental abnormality present in these cases, which merge into the self-mutilation described below.

■ Stab wounds of the neck are uncommon in suicide, but are recorded (such as those described by Gee and Watson 1989, where actual transfixion of the neck was achieved).

The position of the clothing in suicidal knife wounds is equivocal. It is more common for the self-stabber to lift the garments to expose the area of chest or abdominal skin to be attacked, but exceptions are common and the point has little diagnostic significance.

Suicidal firearm wounds

The characteristics of gunshot wounds are fully discussed in Chapter 8 but, as far as suicide is concerned, the following salient features may be repeated:

- Women rarely shoot themselves. In Britain, a shot woman is a murdered woman until proved otherwise, though – as always – exceptions do occur, especially in communities where firearms are commonplace, such as farming or hunting areas.
- The weapon must always be present.
- The range must be within arm's length, depending upon the nature of the weapon and excluding some mechanical device to fire the gun. The pathologist may be asked if a dead person could have reached the trigger of a rifle or long shotgun, which may have been placed against the neck, head or chest. Having first established that the entry wound was close contact, the length of the gun from muzzle to trigger can be measured and compared with the distance from wound to tip of finger. It must be remembered, however, that the length of the limb after death, especially if rigor is present, is not necessarily the same as in life when mobile joints and muscles may have allowed a slightly longer reach than that measured after death. Allowance must also be made for lateral or other flexion of the trunk, and mobility of the shoulder girdle before declaring dogmatically that the victim could not have fired the gun and therefore did not shoot himself.
- Sites of election are the temple, the neck, the mouth and the chest. Suicides rarely shoot themselves in the eye or abdomen. The lifting of clothing to expose bare skin, usually in the chest, is very variable, and has even less significance in differentiating suicide from homicide or accident than in knife wounds.
- Shooting in anatomically inaccessible sites cannot be suicide.
- It is not true that suicides always shoot themselves in the head on the same side as their dominant hand.
- It is difficult to differentiate homicide from accident, even though the circumstances may be suggestive. The distance of discharge may be beyond arm's reach in both, the weapon may be missing in both, inaccessible sites may be shot in both and sites of suicidal election may not be used in both.

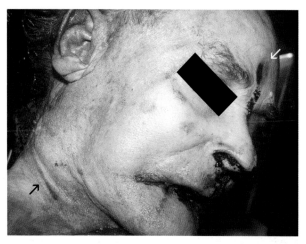

FIGURE 7.10 *A combination of two suicide methods, by firearm and hanging. The man had stood on a stool with a noose around his neck and then shot himself through the forehead. The entrance wound is seen in the forehead (white arrow) and the double ligature mark around the neck shows ecchymoses on the ridge between the two furrows (black arrow).*

Suicide by submersion

This is a common mode of self-destruction, in both men and women. It has a marked geographical variation as a favoured method of self-destruction, naturally depending on the availability of water – it is relatively infrequent in Egypt, but very common in the west of Ireland.

Either large bodies of water, such as rivers, lakes or seas may be used – or the bathtub. The pathology of immersion deaths are dealt with in Chapter 16, but the following features will assist identifying suicides:

- Other means of self-destruction may also be present, such as drug overdose: in baths, associated electrocution is not uncommon, especially in the former West Germany (Bonte 1983).
- Suicide notes may or may not be present, but those who kill themselves usually remove top clothes, hats and spectacles that may be left on the river bank; as usual, exceptions are commonplace.
- Other injuries on the body may be the result of agonal or post-mortem damage in the water.

Suicide by burning

Heat injuries are dealt with in Chapter 11, but suicide from burns has recently increased in Western countries (where it was formerly almost unknown), though in Asia it has always been relatively common. The spread to the West followed political self-martyrdom modelled on that practised by some Vietnamese protesters. There are no particular medical features to distinguish suicide from accident or homicide, this being a circumstantial matter. It is almost invariable, however, for some container of inflammable accelerant to be within reach. The myth of 'spontaneous combustion' is discussed in Chapter 11.

Suicide by 'asphyxia'

The pathology is described in Chapters 14 and 15, but the following facts are pertinent to suicide:

- The masochistic or sexual asphyxias must be carefully distinguished from homicide and suicide. Some asphyxial deaths with sexual aspects appear to be suicidal in nature – or at least, the inevitability of a fatal outcome must have been apparent to the victim (Knight 1979).
- Hanging, though not usually truly asphyxial, is a common mode of suicide, especially (though not exclusively) in men. It is also common as a sequel to homicide, especially in domestic murders, where the perpetrator often commits suicide by this means.
- Plastic bag suicide is increasing in incidence, the means being universally available.
- Suicidal ligature strangulation is not uncommon and sometimes causes difficulty in differentiation from murder. The winding of several turns of ligature and the tying of multiple knots is still consistent with suicide, even though it is hard to understand how, in some cases, death appears to have been caused by reflex cardiac arrest rather than the more florid 'asphyxial' mode of death.

    Sometimes a stick or other object is inserted under a ligature and twisted to tighten the cord against the neck. This is called a 'Spanish windlass', the stick becoming jammed against the body to prevent the tightened ligature from becoming loose once the twisting is completed. Though usually suicidal, this device is sometimes used for murder.

Jumping from a height

'Precipitation' – jumping from a height – is another mode of suicide where the circumstances rather than the autopsy findings determine the motivation. It may sometimes be possible to deduce, by measuring the distance from the jumping point to where the body strikes the ground, the fact that the victim must have actively projected himself outwards rather than fallen close to the wall or cliff face. Some experiments on this aspect have been carried out (Goonetilleke 1980). The

injuries may be variable, depending on the attitude of the body when striking the ground, contact with obstacles during the fall and the height of the drop.

Head injuries are common and are described in Chapter 5. If the fall is onto the feet, damage may occur at any point from the ankles to the skull. The legs may fracture, the hip joints may impact, the pelvis may split, the spine may be fractured (especially vertebral body compression, hyperflexion or hyperextension lesions), or the base of the skull may be imploded as a ring fracture.

It is extremely difficult, to the point of impossibility, to deduce the height of the fall from the nature and severity of the injuries, as was evident from the medical testimony in the Helen Smith inquest in Leeds in 1982.

Some persons will be killed from a fall from a standing height, whilst other may make remarkable escapes without injury from a very high fall. The rare survivals in falls from a great height – usually when some cushioning effect, such as snow, exists – may still defy mechanical explanation.

SELF-INFLICTED INJURIES OTHER THAN SUICIDE

Two main classes exist: those where some abnormality of mind leads the victim to mutilate his body – and those in which deliberate injuries are inflicted for motives of gain. Those caused by mental aberration are usually bizarre in either their multiplicity or their site.

Some mentally disordered persons may inflict hundreds of small wounds upon themselves, which may be additional to the actual cause of death, if death has taken place. Forensic physicians, such as police surgeons, may be called upon to examine living victims of this type.

The arms may be covered with scores of parallel superficial incisions from a knife, razor or broken glass. These may cross each other in groups and again are more frequent on the non-dominant side, usually the left. Small stabs may be made on the chest or temples. In a case seen by the author (BK), there were more than 200 knife-point stabs on each temple and the centre of the forehead. Another well-recognized syndrome is self-mutilation of the genitals, almost invariably by men. Paranoid schizophrenics, often with a strong religious flavour to their delusions, are known to attack themselves in this manner. The penis, scrotum and testes may be removed, and death from intractable haemorrhage can follow. In one of the cases illustrated, there was also perforation of the eyeballs and 40 stab wounds on the top of the head, as well as a complete circumferential cutting of the throat, all with the same blunt scissors that performed the castration. The forensic implications arose from

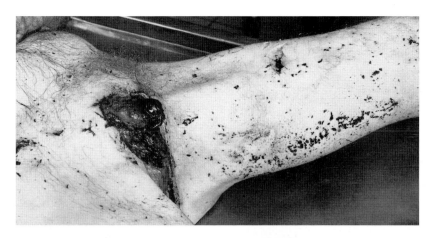

FIGURE 7.11 *Complete self-amputation of the scrotum and penis with scissors.*

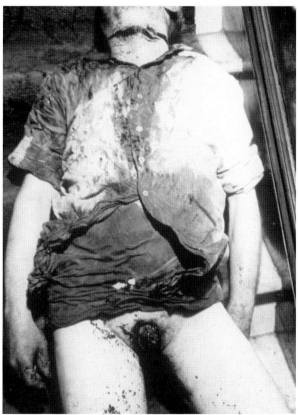

FIGURE 7.12 *Self-mutilation thought by the police to be a bizarre homicide. The genitals have been amputated, the throat cut through 360°, the eyeballs punctured and the scalp stabbed many times, all with scissors. The dead man had paranoid delusions of a religious nature.*

the initial suspicions of the police that a sadistic homicide had taken place.

Self-inflicted injuries, usually non-fatal unless some complication has arisen, may be motivated by some form of gain. The most common is fabrication of injuries to simulate an assault, either to divert attention from the person's own theft or to arouse sympathy. Fabricated accidental injuries are usually a form of malingering, as in the armed forces, or in fraudulent attempts to obtain compensation. In other cases, the 'victim' may claim that a specific person assaulted them, from motives of hate or spite. Others may injure themselves and then waste police time by insisting on a futile search for a non-existent assailant, the motive often being impossible to discover, even by a psychiatrist.

Though these matters are usually seen by the clinical forensic physician, the pathologist may be asked for an opinion where no other medico-legal doctor is available, or if death supervenes. The so-called 'Münchausen syndrome' consists of repeated simulations of illness or the infliction of repeated minor injuries, with the object of gaining admission to hospital, or obtaining medical care and attention.

The following features assist in the recognition of self-inflicted incised injuries:

- The cuts are usually superficial and rarely any danger to life, unless they become infected. Occasionally, they may penetrate the full thickness of the skin, but not in sensitive areas like the face.
- The incisions are regular, with an equal depth at origin and termination, unlike more serious wounds that tend to be deeper at the start and tail off to the surface.
- The cuts are usually multiple and often parallel. They avoid vital and sensitive areas like the eyes, lips, nose and ears, usually being drawn on the cheeks and jaws, temples and forehead, sides of the neck, chest, shoulders, arms and backs of hands and thighs. This is inconsistent with an attack by another person, as the victim is unlikely to stand still to allow these multiple delicate and uniform injuries to be carefully executed.
- In right-handed persons, most of the injuries are on the left side, especially the sides of the face and left hand.
- When the incisions are made on areas covered by clothing, the relevant garments may show either no cuts or cuts that do not match the injuries in position or direction.

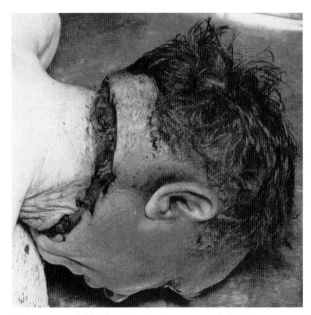

FIGURE 7.13 *Self-inflicted scissors injury around the full circumference of the neck.*

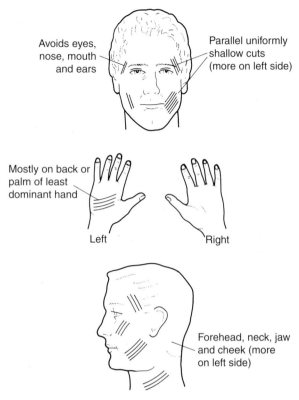

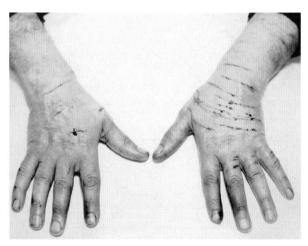

FIGURE 7.15 *Characteristics of non-fatal self-inflicted injuries.*

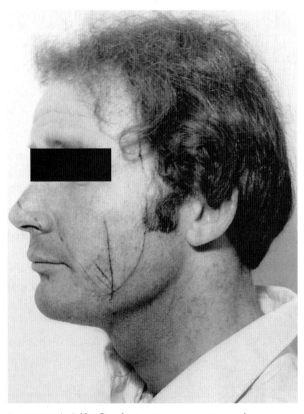

FIGURE 7.14 *Self-inflicted injury in an attempt to produce an excuse during shop-breaking. Surprised by the police, he cut himself with broken glass to claim that he had been assaulted by the robbers whilst trying to defend the premises. There were similar shallow, straight cuts on the other side of the face and on the backs of the hands.*

FIGURE 7.16 *Cuts on the backs of the hands in the man shown in Figure 7.14. He was right handed and most of the shallow incisions are on the left hand.*

In summary, the whole range of injuries and surrounding circumstances may suggest to the experienced patholo-gist that the lesions do not constitute a genuine assault. This diagnosis may be virtually immediate on first looking at the 'victim' and may be almost intuitive after some experience – though this is of little use when giving legal testimony, when every opinion has to be backed up by hard fact and reasoned opinion.

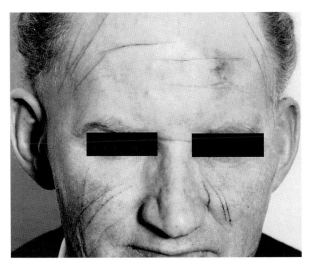

FIGURE 7.17 *Self-inflicted injury in the living. The 'victim' alleged that he had been attacked and robbed. The superficial, uniform, mostly parallel scratches avoid the eyes, nose and mouth.*

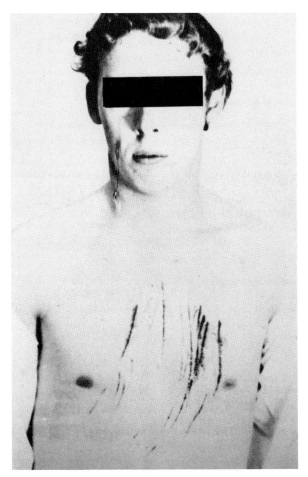

FIGURE 7.18 *Extensive self-inflicted cuts on the chest. The youth persistently claimed to the police that he had been attacked, but the cuts in his shirt were horizontal. He later confessed, explaining that he wanted to get his father's sympathy over some domestic crisis.*

The so-called 'Münchausen syndrome' and the 'Münchausen syndrome by proxy' lie within the realm of the forensic psychiatrist, but a pathologist or clinical forensic physician may be called upon to confirm – or even first detect – that the injuries are self-inflicted.

The Münchausen syndrome refers to adults who injure themselves or feign signs of illness, in order to gain medical attention and often admission to hospital. They can be a plague to casualty departments until recognized. More sinister is the Münchausen syndrome by proxy, where a parent will repetitively injure her child – occasionally fatally – to gain the same attention from doctors and medical facilities. The relationship with child abuse, of which it is a variety, must be recognized.

REFERENCES AND FURTHER READING

Anderson WR, Hudson RP. 1976. Self-inflicted bite marks in battered child syndrome. *Forensic Sci* **7**:71–4.

Asher R. 1951. Munchausen's syndrome. *Lancet* **1**:339–40.

Bonte W. 1978. [Ritual finger amputations. A contribution on the diagnosis of intentional self mutilation using an axe]. *Arch Kriminol* **162**:17–22.

Bonte W. 1983. Self-mutilation and private accident insurance. *J Forensic Sci* **28**:70–82.

Bonte W, Rudell R. 1978. [Accident or planned self mutilation? Probability of accidental injuries during chopping]. *Arch Kriminol* **161**:143–52.

Carney MW. 1978. Self-inflicted bleeding and bruising. *Lancet* **1**:924–5.

Dotzauer G, Iffland R. 1976. Self-mutilations in private-accident-insurance cases. *Z Rechtsmed* **77**:237–88.

Eckert WG. 1977. The pathology of self-mutilation and destructive acts: a forensic study and review. *J Forensic Sci* **22**:242–50.

Faller-Marquardt M, Ropohl D, Pollak S. 1995. Excoriations and contusions of the skin as artefacts in fictitious sexual offences. *J Clin Forensic Med* **2**:129–35.

Fanton L, Schoendorff P, Achache P, *et al.* 1999. False rape: a case report. *Am J Forensic Med Pathol* **20**:374–7.

Gaillard Y, Pepin G. 1998. Case report of an unusual use of lidocaine during episodes of self mutilation. *J Forensic Sci* **43**:235–8.

Gatter K, Bowen DA. 1980. A study of suicide autopsies 1957–1977. *Med Sci Law* **20**:37–42.

Gee DJ, Watson A. 1989. *Lecture notes in forensic medicine*, 5th edn. Blackwell Scientific Publications, Oxford.

Gibbon KL. 1998. Munchausen's syndrome presenting as an acute sexual assault. *Med Sci Law* **38**:202–5.

Goonetilleke UK. 1980. Injuries caused by falls from heights. *Med Sci Law* **20**:262–75.

Greenspan GS, Samuel SE. 1989. Self-cutting after rape. *Am J Psychiatry* **146**:789–90.

Guarner J, Hanzlick R. 1987. Suicide by hanging. A review of 56 cases. *Am J Forensic Med Pathol* **8**:23–6.

Halprin KM. 1966. The art of self-mutilation. I. Neurotic excoriations. *JAMA* **198**:777.

Halprin KM. 1966. The art of self-mutilation. II. Delusions of parasitosis. *JAMA* **198**:1207.

Harris CN, Rai K. 1976. The self-inflicted wrist slash. *J Trauma* **16**:743–5.

Jordan FB, Schmeckpeper K, Strope M. 1987. Jail suicides by hanging. An epidemiological review and recommendations for prevention. *Am J Forensic Med Pathol* **8**:27–31.

Karger B, DuChesne A, Ortmann C, *et al.* 1997. Unusual self-inflicted injuries simulating a criminal offence. *Int J Legal Med* **110**:267–72.

Kleiner GJ. 1984. *Suicide in pregnancy*. John Wright, Bristol.

Knight B. 1979. Fatal masochism – accident or suicide? *Med Sci Law* **19**:118–20.

Knight BH. 1968. Two cases of self-inflicted injuries in the living. *Med Sci Law* **8**:264–6.

Kohr RM. 1990. Suicide by chloroform ingestion following self-mutilation. *Am J Forensic Med Pathol* **11**:324–8.

König H. 1996. [Discrimination of sharp injuries produced in order to feign assaults and such of real cases]. In: Saternus KS, Kernbach-Wighton G (eds), *Research in Legal Medicine*. Schmidt-Römhild, Lübeck.

Koops E, Puschel K. 1990. [Self-mutilation and autophagia.] *Arch Kriminol* **186**:29–36.

Leslie J, Taff ML, Patel I, *et al.* 1984. Self-inflicted ocular injuries. A rare form of self-mutilation. *Am J Forensic Med Pathol* **5**:83–8.

Peschel O, Betz P, Eisenmenger W. 1997. Self-mutilation with needles. *Med Sci Law* **37**:175–8.

Pollak S, Saukko P. 2000. Clinical forensic medicine. Self-inflicted injury. In: Siegel JA, Saukko PJ, Knupfer GC (eds), *Encyclopedia of Forensic Sciences*. Academic Press, San Diego, San Fransisco, New York, Boston, London, Sydney, Tokyo.

Püschel K, Hildebrand E, Hitzer K, *et al.* 1998. [Self-mutilating hand and finger injuries among physicians suspected of insurance fraud]. *Versicherungsmedizin* **50**:232–40.

Riepert T, Schneider P, Urban R. 1999. [Self-injury or attempted murder – analysis of an unusual case.] *Arch Kriminol* **203**:19–26.

Rothschild MA, Raatschen HJ, Schneider V. 2001. Suicide by self-immolation in Berlin from 1990 to 2000. *Forensic Sci Int* **124**:163–6.

Shiono H, Takaesu Y. 1986. Suicide by self-inflicted stab wound of the chest. *Am J Forensic Med Pathol* **7**:72–3.

Sneddon I, Sneddon J. 1975. Self-inflicted injury: a follow-up study of 43 patients. *Br Med J* **2**:527–30.

Tsunenari S, Idaka T, Kanda M, *et al.* 1981. Self-mutilation. Plastic spherules in penile skin in Yakuza, Japan's racketeers. *Am J Forensic Med Pathol* **2**:203–7.

Zlotnick C. 1999. Antisocial personality disorder, affect dysregulation and childhood abuse among incarcerated women. *J Pers Disord* **13**:90–5.

CHAPTER 8

Gunshot and explosion deaths

Though the majority of missile wounds are caused by firearms, other devices such as crossbows, captive-bolt guns, air weapons and even catapults can launch lethal projectiles. In the bombing deaths now so commonly associated with terrorism, missile fragments cause more deaths than the blast effects, so, overall, an understanding of projectile trauma is essential.

THE MECHANICS OF MISSILE INJURY

With the exception of deceleration injuries, all mechanical trauma, whether punching, stabbing or kicking, is caused by the transfer of energy from an external moving object to the tissues and nowhere is this more obvious than in shooting. For damage to occur, some or all of the kinetic energy of the missile has to be absorbed by the target tissues, where it is dissipated as heat, noise and mechanical disruption. When a missile passes completely through soft tissues, it may retain much of its original kinetic energy and fail to transfer any appreciable amount to the tissues, which may remain relatively intact apart from the immediate bullet track. If the latter is in a limb muscle, there may be no serious effects if

major blood vessels are not involved, though the same track in brain, lung or heart may prove fatal.

To ensure transfer of energy to the tissues, some missiles are especially designed or modified to slow up or stop within the body. Soft-headed bullets will flatten on impact and some are designed to fragment. The 'dumdum' bullet, which has a scored nose, and the military missile with an air-cavity within the tip are intended to splay open on impact to increase the 'braking' or deceleration effect, and transfer more energy for disruption. Explosive-tipped bullets, such as those used in the assassination attempt on President Reagan, are not designed to cause damage by the tiny detonation, but drastically to deform the missile to cause maximum deceleration. Weapons designed to be fired in confined spaces, such as those for combating hijack attempts in an aircraft, may be of relatively low velocity and have a deceleration feature incorporated to ensure the absence of an exit wound, and thus limited travel of the missile to avoid puncture of the pressurized passenger cabin.

The trajectory of the missile also determines how much and how fast its energy is given up to the target. Shotgun pellets are spherical, so the orientation of impact is not relevant, but all conical bullets may acquire an erratic course in the tissues. They may tumble end-over-end, especially when nearing the limit of range; they may 'wag' or 'yaw' from side to side of their axial trajectory; the base may rotate around the axis, with the tip remaining on the straight path; and they may 'precess' or 'nutate' with complex spiral or circular movements about the axis.

Whatever the deviation, it offers more contact between the projectile and the tissues, allowing more transfer of energy and thus greater tissue damage. The amount of kinetic energy possessed by a projectile accords to the familiar formula of half the product of the missile mass and the square of its velocity. Modern military science takes advantage of the squaring of the velocity to develop weapons that have a missile of small mass but exceedingly high velocity to provide the maximum kinetic energy for tissue damage.

The mode of injury depends on the velocity of the missile. Relatively slow projectiles are those travelling at up to the speed of sound in air (340 metres/second or 1100 feet/second), which of course includes all non-explosively propelled missiles like crossbow bolts and air-rifle pellets, as well as most revolver bullets. These mechanically thrust aside the tissues along a track only slightly wider than the missile. The tissues are lacerated or crushed, secondary damage occurs from rupture of blood vessels and other structures, and secondary and tertiary damage is caused by displaced bone and cartilage fragments.

Above the speed of sound in air, a missile passing through tissue sends a shock wave of compression ahead of the laceration track, this wave being propagated at about the speed of sound in water (1500 metres/second or 4800 feet/second). Though this wave lasts only for a brief period, it raises the tissue pressure to extreme values, up to thousands of kilopascals. In tissues like brain, liver and muscle, this can cause severe disruption within a wide zone around the bullet track, and can be propagated down hollow fluid-containing vessels to cause distant vascular damage.

High-velocity projectiles produce yet another phenomenon, that of cavitation. The missile accelerates the molecules of the tissues adjacent to the track, so that they continue to move centrifugally outwards even after the missile has travelled onwards. This forms a cavity around the track that is far wider than the diameter of the projectile. It reaches a maximum size within milliseconds and then pulsates with decreasing amplitude so that a fusiform cavity rapidly follows in the wake of the bullet. When the bullet stops or leaves the organ, the cavity rapidly subsides, but the track of damage persists in a tubular zone much wider than the actual missile. In high-velocity bullets from military weapons – for example, 980 metres/second (3185 feet/second) this cavitation effect is the most damaging mechanism; in addition to the physical damage, the near-vacuum sucks infected dirt and clothing fibres into the depths of the wound (Owen-Smith 1981). Solid organs such as brain and liver are affected more than spongy matrices like lung. Those tissues that contain most water are most severely damaged by penetrating

missiles and high-velocity missile damage is proportional to the specific gravity of the tissue injured.

In most of the shooting cases seen by forensic pathologists, death will have occurred rapidly but, where it is delayed, secondary damage from infarction, local necrosis of muscle and organs, and infection must always be borne in mind. High-velocity weapons in particular can cause vascular damage at a distance from direct trauma, stretching and thrombosis, leading in turn to ischaemic lesions such as infarcts.

TYPES OF WEAPON

The nature of firearm wounds varies considerably with the type of weapon employed. A general knowledge of the main features of the various types of gun in common use is essential, though there is no need for the pathologist to master the unnecessary mass of detail on firearm construction offered by some forensic medicine textbooks. Indeed, much of this is solely the province of the firearms examiner, not the doctor. The inordinate amount of detail sometimes provided is perhaps symptomatic of the fascination which firearms hold for many men – but rarely women.

In the context of wounding, guns are of two main types.

The smooth-bore weapon or 'shotgun'

A shotgun consists of one or more metal barrels of relatively wide diameter, which are smooth on the inner surface. They fire a variable number of spherical lead shot (pellets), which emerge from the end (muzzle), from where they gradually diverge in the form of a long, narrow cone. Exceptionally, a shotgun may fire a few large projectiles or even a single slug, but these are rarely met with in forensic practice, the usual load of pellets totalling scores or hundreds. Special types of projectile are described later. A shotgun often has two barrels, either side by side or 'up-and-under'. One barrel may be parallel sided (the 'cylinder') and the other slightly tapered towards the muzzle (the 'choke'). The latter will produce a narrower cone of shot and this affects estimates of range derived from the size of the wound. There are several gradations of choke, such as 'improved cylinder', 'modified choke', 'half-choke' and 'full-choke'.

Some modern weapons have the facility for removing one particular type of barrel and replacing it with another degree of choke. Modern accessories can convert a cylinder barrel to a choke barrel – for example, variable choke such as Poly-Choke, Kutts Compensator and Weaver-Choke are available, especially in the USA.

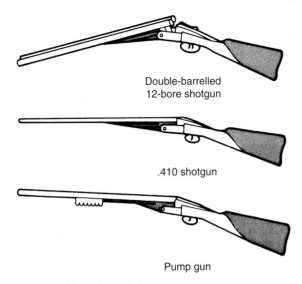

FIGURE 8.1 *Types of smooth-bore weapon.*

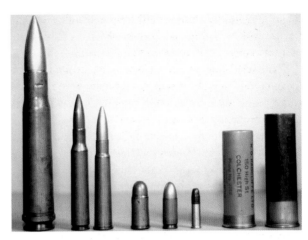

FIGURE 8.3 *Various types of ammunition. From the right, there are two twelve-bore shotgun cartridges, .22 rifle, .38 automatic pistol and .45 revolver bullets and two military rifle shells. On the left is a cannon shell, which is unlikely to be encountered in civilian forensic pathology.*

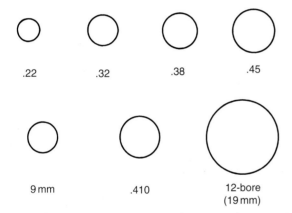

FIGURE 8.2 *Relative calibre of common weapons.*

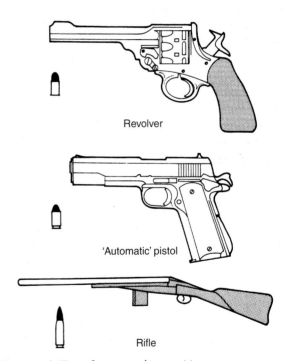

FIGURE 8.4 *Types of weapon and ammunition.*

Another typically American modification is the ability to fire a single projectile through the smooth bore. A number of devices intended for hunting are available, but they may be involved in a human fatality. One of the older types is the solid round 'pumpkin ball' or the Brenneke rifled slug, but more recent devices include the Foster rifled slug and the French Blondeau, which is a dumb-bell-shaped projectile.

Shotguns come in two main sizes, which determine the nature of the wound. The first is the 'twelve-bore', usually called 'twelve-gauge' in North America, which has a diameter of about 19 mm or 0.738 inches. The other is the smaller 'four-ten', usually single-barrelled with a diameter of 10.6 mm or 0.410 inches.

SHOTGUN AMMUNITION

The ammunition for the shotgun is a cartridge made of a cardboard or plastic cylinder fitted into a metal base. This carries a percussion detonator that is struck by the spring-loaded firing pin when the trigger is pulled. The cartridge contains a charge of propellant, above which are 'wads' or pistons of felt, and cardboard or plastic discs, or both. Above these is the charge of shot, which varies greatly in number and size, finally covered by a card or plastic disc.

This description is of the old, classical cartridge but modern ammunition has a variety of devices incorporated into the cartridge to improve efficiency and accuracy. These include the Power Piston, a proprietary name for one of a class of cartridges which holds the shot inside a polythene cup and which itself may contribute to the wound at short range. Other modern cartridges may have plastic granules as a filler between the shot; this brightly coloured material may be found inside the wounds.

Tampering with the contents of cartridges may markedly alter the spread and other characteristics of the shot and hence the resulting wound. The shot may be fused into a mass by pouring paraffin wax or even molten pitch into the cartridge. The cardboard or plastic cylinder may be partly cut through at the level of the wads, so that, on firing, the upper part of the casing is blown out to restrain the divergence of the pellets.

The propellant has also changed in recent years, so that the old black gunpowder has been largely replaced by cleaner explosives that do not produce the same volume of soot and unburnt propellant, which may be deposited in and around the close-range wound.

'Country' guns

In developing countries, in some rural and poor areas of other countries, in subversion and terrorism, and sometimes in juvenile hands, weapons and ammunition may be 'homemade'. These are common in India, where the name 'country gun' is well understood; they are also made in Sri Lanka and other Asian areas, but may be encountered anywhere.

The author (BK) had experience of such weapons in the terrorist campaign in Malaya in the 1950s, where crude weapons were made in the jungle from pieces of water-pipe attached to roughly carved wooden stocks, with a primitive firing mechanism. The guns were muzzle-loaded with black powder and the projectiles were often wood-screws, nuts and bolts and irregular fragments of metal or even stones.

In civilian practice in Britain, two similar weapons have been seen, both made by juveniles out of electrical conduit pipe, using potassium chlorate–sugar propellant. In one, the user was killed when the device exploded; the other one successfully propelled a small screwdriver across several fields to (slightly) injure a cow.

Terrorists in Northern Ireland have also manufactured some of their own weapons, but these were relatively sophisticated, being made in clandestine but well-equipped workshops.

The problem for the pathologist with such guns is that few of the criteria to be described apply to the injuries, especially where random, irregular missiles such as woodscrews are employed. Local knowledge and experience are essential for the interpretation of these wounds.

The rifled weapon

Handguns, rifles, air rifles and military weapons differ from shotguns in that they fire one projectile at a time through a thicker barrel that has spiral grooves machined on its inner surface. The elevations between the grooves are the 'lands', which grip the bullet as it passes down the barrel and give it a rotatory movement. This has a gyroscopic effect that increases the stability of the bullet's trajectory and hence the accuracy.

Handguns, which cause over 50 per cent of all homicides in the USA, comprise the revolver and the automatic pistol. The revolver has a rotating cylinder carrying a variable number of shells, which are brought into the firing position one by one, each time the trigger is pulled. The revolver has a low muzzle velocity of the order of 500 feet/second (150 metres/second). The 'automatic', more accurately called a 'self-loading' pistol, has its shells in a spring-loaded magazine, each spent round being ejected and a new one positioned by means of the gas pressure developed at each discharge. The muzzle velocity may be 1000–1200 feet/second (300–360 metres/second).

Rifles are long-barrelled guns that may be single-shot, bolt-loaded or self-loading and used for hunting, target-shooting or for military purposes. Military weapons come in a vast range of types, most of them now either 'self-loading', which means that the trigger has to be pulled for each shot – or truly 'automatic', when the weapon will continue to fire while the trigger is depressed until the magazine is empty. The muzzle velocity varies greatly, from 1500 to 5000 feet/second (450–1500 metres/second).

AMMUNITION FOR RIFLED WEAPONS

The variety of types of rifled ammunition is even greater than the range of weapons designed to fire them, but all conform to a general pattern. There is a metal cylinder, closed at one end, which is the 'shell' or cartridge, carrying a percussion detonator in the base, either centrally or peripherally. The shell is loaded with explosive propellant such as nitrocellulose and the bullet is firmly clamped into the open end. The bullet may be composed of a variety of metals, often compound. A lead core may be covered in a nickel or steel jacket, but there are many other variations. The detonator may contain elements such as barium, bismuth mercury or antimony.

Both shotgun and rifled weapon ammunition have a common purpose when detonated – to produce large volumes of hot gas under pressure that expel the bullet or shot from the barrel. One gram of black powder produces about 3000 ml and nitrocellulose produces some 13 000 ml of gas, which consists of carbon dioxide, monoxide, nitrogen, hydrogen sulphide, hydrogen, methane and many other substances, all at high temperatures.

WOUNDS

Though the construction and performance of weapons is of vital interest to the forensic firearms examiner, the relevance to the pathologist is concentrated in those aspects which affect the nature of the wound:

▨ whether the weapon is smooth-bore or rifled;
▨ if rifled, the muzzle velocity of the weapon;
▨ the nature of the projectile(s);
▨ the nature of the propellant;
▨ the degree of choke, if any;
▨ the range of discharge;
▨ the angle of discharge.

WOUNDS INFLICTED BY A SMOOTH-BORE SHOTGUN

The following constituents of the cartridge emerge on the discharge of a shotgun and all may contribute to the wound:

▨ lead pellets
▨ soot in the form of smoke and debris
▨ unburnt and burning propellant particles
▨ flame and hot gases under pressure
▨ carbon monoxide
▨ wads – either felt, cardboard or plastic
▨ detonator constituents
▨ fragments of the cartridge case.

When a shotgun is fired, a compact mass of shot emerges from the muzzle and then begins to disperse, the divergence increasing progressively as the distance lengthens. A tongue of flame and hot gas follows the shot. High pressure and temperature exists just outside the muzzle, but this rapidly expands and cools. This gas is composed of oxides of nitrogen, carbon dioxide, hot air and other compounds, but the one of interest to the pathologist is carbon monoxide. Soot from the combustion of propellant is expelled, along with some flakes or grains of propellant that may be still burning. The wads are also expelled, their nature depending upon the type of cartridge. Some modern ammunition may contain other devices that may contribute to the wound.

Chemical traces of the elements in the detonator or percussion cap cannot be seen, but may be vital laboratory evidence, where barium, antimony and other metals can be recovered on analysis or by means of the scanning electron microscope. Fragments of the cartridge case may also be ejected, especially if it has been tampered with, as described earlier.

The most important deduction that a pathologist is asked to make is the estimation of the range of discharge of the gun, as this may substantially influence the distinction between accident, suicide and homicide. The appearance of the wound is greatly modified by variation in range and it is convenient to describe them in terms of increasing range of discharge.

Shotgun contact wound

SHAPE

Where the muzzle is placed tightly against the surface of the abdomen, thorax, limb or neck, the consequent wound will

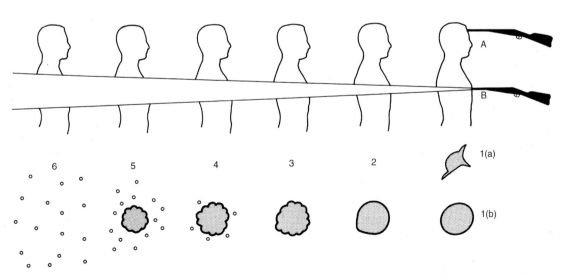

FIGURE 8.5 *Variation in appearance of a shotgun wound at increasing range of discharge: 1(a), split wound from contact over bone; 1(b), usual round contact wound; 2, close but not contact range up to about 30 cm (variable); 3, 'rat-hole' wound from 30 cm to about a metre (variable); 4, satellite pellet holes appearing over a metre; 5, spread of shot increases, central hole diminishes; 6, uniform spread with no central hole over about 10 m. All these ranges vary greatly with barrel choke, weapon and ammunition.*

be single and circular, of a size approximately equal to the bore of the weapon, though a .410 wound may be smaller because of the relatively greater effect of elastic contraction of the skin. The edges of the wound may be crenated by individual shot, but usually this feature is not noticeable.

SOILING AND BURNING

In a tight contact wound, the skin forms a seal around the muzzle, preventing much escape of hot gas and soot, so that soiling and burning are minimal or absent. The recoil, which takes the muzzle away from the skin, may, however, loosen the seal and, if the muzzle is not pressed firmly, flame, gas and soot may escape sideways and affect the skin in the immediate vicinity. Where clothing is interposed between the muzzle and skin, soot is much more likely to escape sideways and may be found in each layer of fabric, as well as on the underlying skin. The cloth may be singed at the edge of the hole and there may be a ring of burning around the skin wound.

MUZZLE IMPRESSION

There may be a muzzle impression in a tight contact wound made by firm mechanical pressure or impact of the metal rim against the skin. Many textbooks quite wrongly attribute this to 'recoil', though of course recoil takes the muzzle away from the skin, not towards it. The true explanation of a muzzle mark is either that the assailant physically kept the weapon pressed hard against the skin or – more often – that the subcutaneous expansion shortly to be described, lifts the skin forcibly up against the muzzle. A muzzle mark is a most useful indication to the pathologist of a contact wound. Actual bruising can occur around the muzzle imprint, though this is more likely to be the result of deep contusion from the effects of the blast. Rarely, a double-barrelled weapon may make a ring-like mark adjacent to the entry wound.

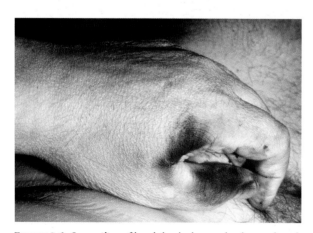

FIGURE 8.6 *Soot-soiling of hand that had grasped a shotgun barrel.*

CARBON MONOXIDE

Carbon monoxide in the gases combines with haemoglobin and myoglobin to give a pink coloration to the interior of the wound track and adjacent tissues. This diminishes in concentration along the track, but can still be present in its depths – and even at an exit wound, if there is one. The presence of carboxyhaemoglobin and myoglobin has been advocated as a test for distinguishing the exit from the entrance wound, especially where decomposition has blurred the morphological appearances. This test must be used with caution, though if quantitative measurements are made it can still be a valid exercise.

CONTACT WOUNDS OVER BONE

When the wound is made over a site with underlying bone, the wound may have a different appearance. Especially in

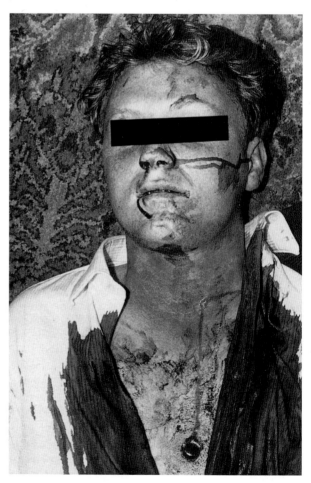

FIGURE 8.7 *Homicidal firearm wound with a twelve-bore shotgun. The wound shows a clear muzzle impression, the barrel having been pressed against the skin at discharge. There is almost no smoke soiling, the muzzle having forced a firm seal against the thin shirt and skin.*

the scalp, but also over the back of the neck, sternum, shoulder, hip and other areas where the soft tissue lies thinly over bone, the large volume of discharge gases cannot dissipate, as they can into the abdomen, chest, or mass of muscle. When the gas is forced through the skin, it is reflected back by the underlying hard layer and momentarily raises a dome of skin and subcutaneous tissue. This is rammed back against the muzzle to increase the pressure of contact further, sometimes producing a muzzle mark. When the gas volume is large, as with a twelve-bore gun, this dome may then split, causing a cruciate, stellate or ragged wound, with skin flaps. This is less likely with a .410 because the cartridge is smaller, but it can occur, as of course it can with rifled weapons.

The close discharge of a shotgun

When the muzzle is held near the skin, but not actually in contact with it, a number of helpful signs are produced. Once again the appearance is naturally modified by clothing, which must always be carefully preserved and subjected to forensic scientific examination. Where clothing is present, then it will trap most, but not necessarily all, of the soot and powder grains. It will reduce the flame effects, though if the fabric is ignited even momentarily, this can diffusely scorch the skin.

Assuming that the body surface is uncovered, a close discharge – one between actual contact and about 15 cm (6 inches) – is likely to show the following features:

■ Singeing of hairs around the wound, unless the skin is hairless. The fine downy hairs of the trunk and limbs may be burnt away, though this is unlikely with dense, long, head hair. Where the distance is greater, the keratin of the hair may melt with the flame and then

solidify on cooling, causing a 'clubbed' appearance of the hairs because of rounded bulges at the tips.
■ Burning of the skin, unless protected by head hair. There may be a wide flare or narrow rim of hyperaemia or even blistering from the flame of incandescent gas blown from the muzzle.

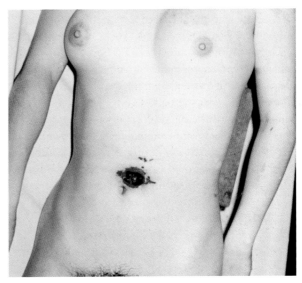

FIGURE 8.9 *Firm contact wound from a twelve-bore shotgun. The clothing has prevented any soot soiling, but there are minor peripheral abrasions from impact of a belt. As the abdomen was distensible, the gas expansion has not caused splitting of the skin at the wound edges.*

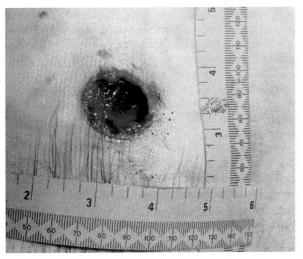

FIGURE 8.10 *Contact wound from a twelve-bore shotgun fired through clothing. There is some abrasion of the wound edges, but no irregularity from the close-packed pellets, which have not begun to disperse. The clothing has protected the skin from smoke and powder soiling. The circular wound indicates discharge at right angles to the body surface.*

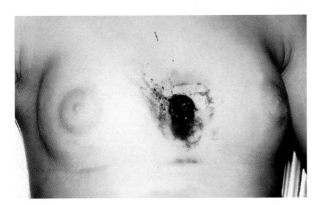

FIGURE 8.8 *Suicidal firearm wound from a twelve-bore shotgun. The wound shows a muzzle impression with soot soiling, the double-barrelled shotgun having been pressed against the skin at discharge.*

The tissues within and around the wound may be cherry-pink from absorption of carbon monoxide.

There will be 'smoke soiling' or 'soot staining' of the skin, from carbon deposition. This spreads more widely than powder tattooing, but does not carry as far as the heavier propellant grains. This effect is much less or even absent with modern 'clean' propellants.

This soot or smoke soiling is easily washed off the skin, and care must be taken at autopsy to obtain all photographs and trace samples before allowing the bloodstains to be washed from the body. Tattooing will not wash off, though adherent unburnt propellant may be physically detached from the tiny burns during any washing or swabbing process.

Burning, partly burnt and unburnt propellant flakes and grains may pepper the surrounding of the wound. As stated above, these carry further than smoke staining, but usually spread over a smaller area. The incandescent particles cause small burns on the skin, but the unburnt flakes (such as nitrocellulose) may be seen as small glistening particles on the skin, sometimes coloured.

The wound will be circular if the weapon is held at right angles to the skin and elliptical if slanted, often with undercut edges on one side. Depending partly on the size of the pellets, 'nibbling' or crenation of the edge may be seen, though this is usually imperceptible

in close discharges. The edge of the wound will be blackened and there will be soot in the exposed tissues. There may be annular bruising around the wound and distant bruising a few centimetres away as a result of tissue damage from the entry of gases. Other bruises or abrasions may be seen in the vicinity from objects such

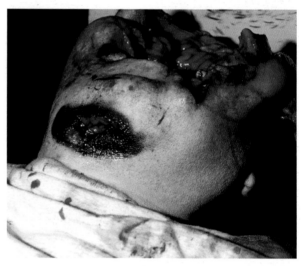

FIGURE 8.12 *Suicidal twelve-bore shotgun wound. The entrance is in one of the 'sites of election', in the neck, and the circular smoke fouling indicated a close or even contact discharge.*

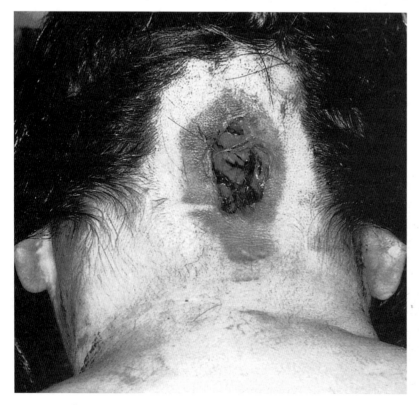

FIGURE 8.11 *Close-range twelve-bore shotgun wound of the head. This homicidal discharge was made through thick layers of fabric, which has filtered out any smoke or powder soiling. However, there is a wide zone of skin burning due to the muzzle gases. The wound is oval due to the downward angulation of the weapon.*

as buttons or buckles being hurled against the skin by the gas pressure.

■ Any felt or cardboard wads or plastic cups from the cartridge will be within the depths of the wound.

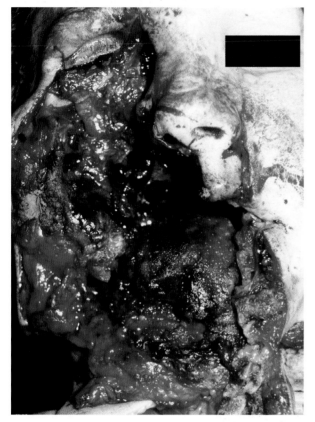

FIGURE 8.13 *Suicidal twelve-bore shotgun wound. The entrance is one of the 'sites of election', in the neck (see Figure 8.14).*

Short- to mid-range shotgun discharge

From about 15 cm (6 inches) to 2 m (6 feet), considerable variation occurs in the appearance of the wound. The shorter range will provide a similar picture to that of close discharge, but the soot soiling diminishes and over 20–40 cm it may vanish. Powder tattooing near the wound periphery may persist for somewhat further than this.

At the upper end of this range the edges of the wound will become crenated and scalloped, especially with larger shot. This is sometimes called the 'rat-hole' or 'rat-nibbling' from its resemblance to rodent teeth marks. From 2 m upwards, the number of satellite pellet holes will progressively increase around the main wound.

It must be emphasized that these are useful generalizations, but that marked variations occur between different weapons, different barrels of the same weapon and different ammunition fired from the same gun. Only test firing can give a measure of the length of the flame, the distance and pattern of soot staining and powder tattooing, the beginning of pellet spreading and the distance over which the wads are projected. As a rough rule-of-thumb, which is often incorrect, hair singeing occurs over the first 30 cm (1 foot), soot staining can be seen for the first half-metre (20 inches) and a single large hole persists for at least 1 m (3 feet).

Mid- to distant-range shotgun wounds

Here, test firing is even more vital for an estimate of range, as the variation is great. The choke as opposed to cylinder barrel on the same gun will provide different appearances at

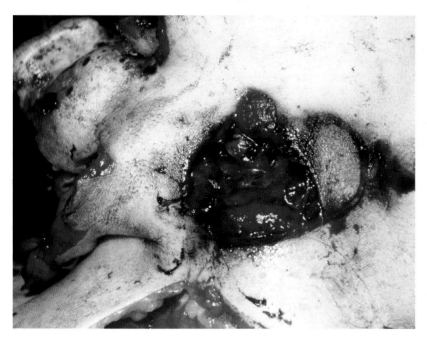

FIGURE 8.14 *Suicidal contact entrance wound in the neck. One barrel of a double-barrelled shotgun was used, the unfired barrel causing a muzzle mark (see Figure 8.13).*

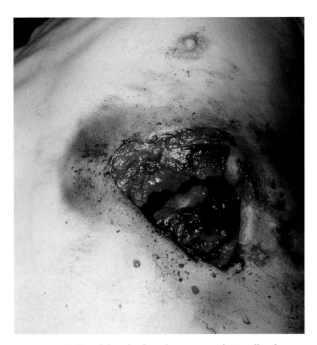

FIGURE 8.15 *Suicidal twelve-bore shotgun wound. Not all such wounds are circular – this one has torn a large defect in the chest wall because of its tangential orientation. The smoke smudging is extensive, having overshot and been deflected from the wound interior. The precordium is another site of election for suicidal shooting.*

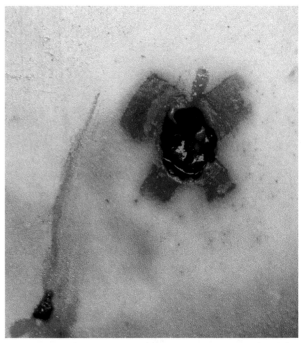

FIGURE 8.16 *Characteristic capital 'X'-shaped bruise caused by opening up of the plastic cup containing the shotgun pellets and surrounding the circular entrance wound from a homicidal short-range discharge.*

the same range. Once beyond 2 m, there will be no burning or smoke staining, rarely will there be powder tattooing and the presence of the wads will be variable. Sometimes the latter fall away within 2 m, but they can sometimes be found in a wound up to 5 m distant. Often the wad takes a lower trajectory and may strike the body below the shotgun wound. It may penetrate the skin, causing a second lacerated wound or it may only bruise the skin. Some of the plastic cup devices now used open up in flight to form a square-edged star or capital 'X' shape. This can strike the skin at or near the shotgun wound and produce a characteristic bruise or abrasion of a similar shape. The spread of pellets, which usually begins at a metre or two range, increases progressively, the central 'rat-hole' diminishing at the same rate.

There is an old (and extremely inaccurate) rule-of-thumb which states that the diameter of the spread in inches is roughly equal to the range in yards (metric: one-third of the spread in centimetres equals the range in metres). This of course applies to a circular wound or the narrow diameter of an oblique elliptical wound; it is of no use other than a quick first check to indicate if suicide can be excluded, but expert examination and test-firing are essential.

At distant ranges, beyond 6–10 m, the central hole may shrink to nothing. There will naturally be no wad injuries, no

smoke, flame or tattooing, and no way of determining range except to say that it must be within the maximum discharge distance of that particular weapon, which may be 30–50 m. At such ranges the shot will not be lethal and the pellets, if they penetrate the skin, will lie just in the subcutaneous tissues. Death may occur, however, from an unlucky shot in the eye or from natural disease precipitated by pain and shock.

The direction of a shotgun injury

It has already been stated that, where the discharge has been at right angles to the body surface, the shape of the wound will be symmetrical and circular. A shotgun blast traces out a shallow cone from the muzzle and simple geometry demands that where this cone intersects a plane (the skin), a circle will result only when the cone is at 90° to the plane. In all other positions an ellipse will be traced out, its elongation increasing as the angle between them decreases. This pattern applies not only to the pellet spread but to soot deposition and provides a ready indication of the direction. In addition to the surface features, the internal wound assists in orientating the discharge:

■ The wound edges may be shelved, the tissues being undercut below the margin distal to the origin of the

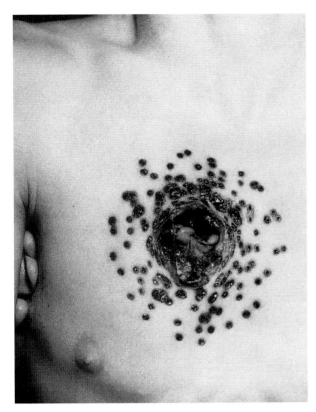

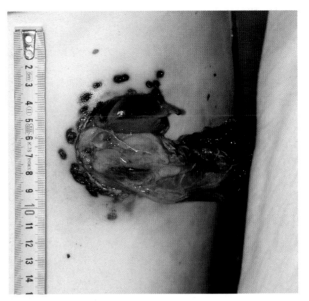

FIGURE 8.18 *Homicidal close-range shotgun wound from a twelve-bore weapon.*

FIGURE 8.17 *Shotgun wound from a twelve-bore weapon. The circular outline indicates that the discharge was perpendicular to the skin surface. The central hole was caused by the entry of a confluent mass of shot, though there were no wads in the wound. The diameter of the peripheral pellet pattern was about 12 cm, which suggests that, approximately, the range was about 4 m. Test firing must always be carried out, however, to obtain a more exact estimate. Whatever the actual range, it is clear that it could not be suicidal.*

discharge. The appearances are similar to those seen in some knife wounds, where an oblique stab leaves tissue visible at one edge and undercut on the other. In firearm wounds this is better seen in injuries from a single rifled projectile than from the more diffuse mass of shotgun pellets, but is still sometimes apparent in the latter.

■ The track of the wound in the deep tissues can be established and this line projected backwards to indicate the discharge direction relative to the body. Again, a missile from a rifled weapon usually gives a clearer picture than those from a shotgun, but a general estimate can be obtained from a knowledge of the positions of the surface wound and the mass of pellets. Examination of a radiograph may be of more assistance that the laborious search from pellets at autopsy. Whatever the type of missile(s), considerable deviation caused by deflection by bone and other tissues can

occur, so that the final resting place of the projectile may be far off the initial track. Thus the actual path through the tissues before ricochet must be established, if possible.

Other features of shotgun wounds

■ Exit wounds are uncommon in the trunk as the energy possessed by each pellet is small because of its tiny size and the relatively low muzzle velocity of the weapon. The 'four-ten' will almost never exit and even the twelve-bore rarely causes a through-and-through wound of the adult chest or abdomen. The pellets often penetrate the distal chest wall, but are held up beneath the skin of the further side of the trunk. Commonly a bruise may be seen in the deep tissues of the frustrated exit site and lead shot may be felt under the skin, which is tough enough to prevent the final exit phase.

In the head, neck and limbs, and in children and small thin adults, the twelve-bore commonly causes an exit wound which may be extremely large and ragged, with gross tissue destruction exposed. One of the most common is that seen when a twelve-bore is discharged suicidally into the mouth; this may disrupt the head, and expel most of the brain through a massive skull and scalp defect – the so-called 'burst head'.

■ The internal track is more diffuse than that caused by a rifled weapon, though where the discharge is contact or close, the compacted mass of shot travels as a unit

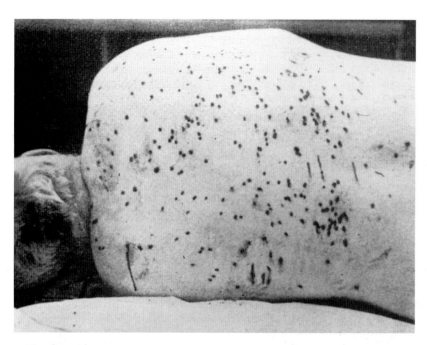

FIGURE 8.19 *Pellet injuries from a distant twelve-bore shotgun discharge. The range was about 25 m and the shot lies just under the skin. Death was caused by coronary heart disease, cardiac arrest being precipitated by the shock of injury.*

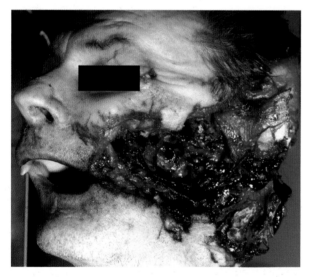

FIGURE 8.20 *Tangential shotgun wound of face. The edge of the dispersal cone of pellets and gas has ploughed through the cheek, and removed the ear. The facial bones and base of the skull were fractured.*

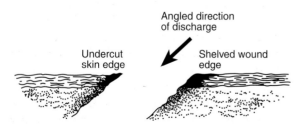

FIGURE 8.21 *Shelving and undercutting of entry wound in oblique discharge.*

for some distance into the tissues before dispersing. In general, the internal damage caused by a shotgun is diffuse and is caused by direct mechanical disruption by the gas and shot, which enter at relatively low velocity. There is no cavitation effect as is seen in high-velocity injuries, the tissue being physically smashed by the impact of a heavy load of pellets and, in the case of near discharges, by the large volume of hot propellant gases.

■ Secondary damage is caused by the mass of pellets striking bone and releasing fragments that then act as secondary missiles, damaging adjacent tissues and sometimes emerging to form exit wounds. These may sometimes cause confusion to inexperienced observers, including police officers, who may wrongly suspect multiple shots or the use of some other type of weapon.

■ Wad wounds can be caused by the non-metallic contents of a shotgun cartridge. These can vary from trivial bruises to fatal lacerations. The latter may occur when a blank cartridge is discharged at close range, the wad and accompanying gas breaching the body surface. As mentioned earlier, the new devices now often used in shotgun ammunition may cause characteristic wounds, such as the square cruciate mark from the wings of the opened plastic cup which contains the shot. Felt and plastic wads travel a variable distance from the gun muzzle, depending on many factors, such as the type of cartridge, the amount of propellant load and the nature of the wads. The wads fall away much more quickly than the lead shot because of their low weight and high air resistance. At contact and close ranges

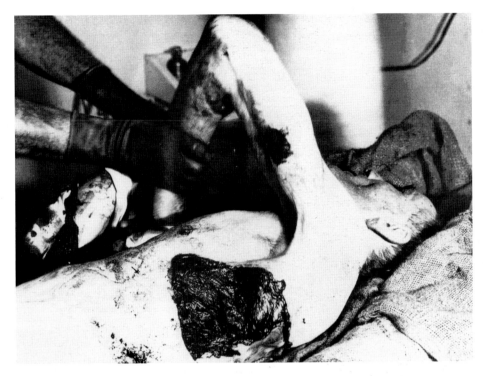

FIGURE 8.22 *A tangential shotgun wound of the side of the chest. When the victim was first found it was not appreciated that he had been shot. The discharge passed under the slightly abducted arm, injuring the upper arm as well as the thorax. Though most of the shot passed to the rear of the victim, some were found in the pleural cavity.*

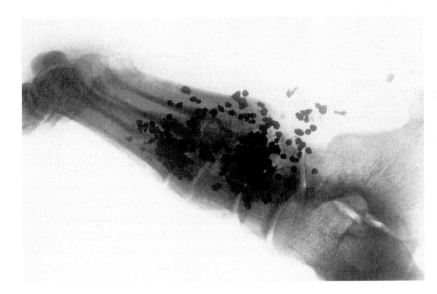

FIGURE 8.23 *Radiography should be carried out before autopsy in all deaths from firearms. The extent of dispersal of shot can be assessed – as in this film – and, in single bullet injuries, the position and possible fragmentation can be detected in order to assist in recovering the missile.*

they will almost always enter the wound and should be recovered at autopsy in order to assist in identifying the type of ammunition.

Beyond a metre or two, the wad may drop sufficiently to miss the main wound and strike the skin at a lower point. From 2 to 5 m, the wads may or may not strike the body, and further than this distance it is almost certain that the wads will fall to the ground. As with all variables associated with firearm wounds, however, it is essential for test firing to be performed wherever possible. The pathologist should not be

dogmatic or impracticably precise about distances, but offer a bracket of reasonable probability.

Tangential wounds can offer considerable difficulty in recognition to the inexperienced observer. Some pathologists, as well as clinicians and police officers, have attributed certain wounds to knives or blunt injuries, when in fact they have been gunshot wounds. The shallow cone of a shotgun discharge may pass any part of the body so that the central axis is clear of the tissues, but the periphery strikes the body surface tangentially. The most common position is probably the side of the chest, in the lower axilla. If the arm is raised it may escape damage, but sometimes an opposing injury is seen on the chest wall and inner part of the upper arm. Another area is the side of the face, where a glancing gun blast may gouge the face and perhaps carry away an ear.

The appearance of the wound depends, of course, on the range and the depth to which the cone of shot and gas penetrates. On the side of the chest, a large elliptical area may be ripped from the surface to expose underlying muscle and ribs. If a close discharge, then the nature of the injury will be clear from the usual burning and soiling of the muzzle gases, but a more distant shot may cause a clean wound that can give rise to doubt about causation. Radiography will usually reveal lead shot in the tissues, unless the contact is extremely superficial.

In the chest – even if shot penetration is minimal – severe damage to the pleura and lungs may occur from the impact, and death may occur from a haemothorax with or without lung laceration or contusion. When the side of the head is hit, shattering of skull or facial bones can occur and intracranial damage is common, even though no metallic projectiles enter the cranium. Rifled weapons can also cause tangential wounds and some features of skidding across the surface and re-entry wounds have been mentioned earlier. There is not usually the wide gouging of tissue seen in smooth-bore injuries, but the glancing passage of a high-velocity missile can open up a severe longitudinal laceration. The lateral transfer of energy can cause severe internal damage in both chest and skull, even though the missile does not enter the cavities. The skull may be extensively fractured, with widespread underlying damage, and in the absence of any projectile and a deficient knowledge of the circumstances, some such injuries have erroneously been ascribed to blunt trauma.

WOUNDS FROM RIFLED WEAPONS

Injuries from rifled weapons vary greatly according to the velocity of the projectile, as discussed at the beginning of this chapter, but there are some characteristics common to all types. Unlike shotguns there is only one missile in each discharge, though an automatic weapon may well cause multiple wounds in close succession which impact upon the same area of the body. Occasionally, because of some defect in the weapon, two bullets may be fired at once, or a fragment of metal may detach from cartridge, barrel or bullet, so that two missiles may strike simultaneously; this is described later.

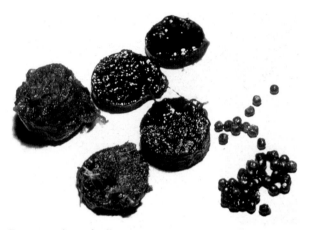

FIGURE 8.24 *Lead pellets and felt cartridge wads from a twelve-bore shotgun wound. It is important to recover at least a sample of pellets and the wads so that the type of cartridge can be identified.*

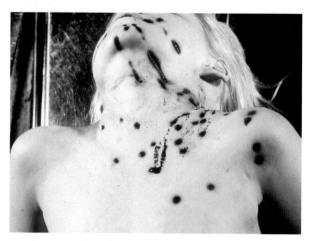

FIGURE 8.25 *Pellet injuries from a distant twelve-bore shotgun discharge (see also Figure 8.26). The child had been walking behind a hunter carrying a shotgun on his shoulder, the barrel pointing down. When the hunter was ducking to avoid branches of a tree the shotgun was triggered by a branch.*

Contact wounds

When a weapon is fired in contact with the skin, the appearances can vary according to whether the muzzle was firmly pressed against the surface so as to form a tight seal – or whether it was merely held in loose contact, so that the backward jerk of recoil can permit a small gap to appear. Yet another permutation is when clothing is interposed between the muzzle and the skin.

When a rifled weapon is held firmly against the body surface during discharge, the resulting wound is in many respects similar to that from a shotgun. A twelve-bore wound

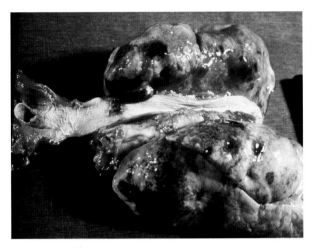

FIGURE 8.26 *Pellet injuries puncturing the oesophagus and both lungs (see also Figure 8.25).*

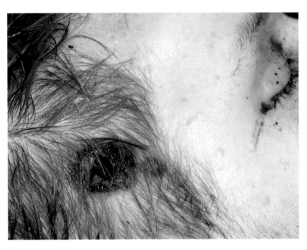

FIGURE 8.28 *Suicidal contact wound with muzzle mark from a 9 mm pistol (see also Figure 8.29 for corresponding exit wound).*

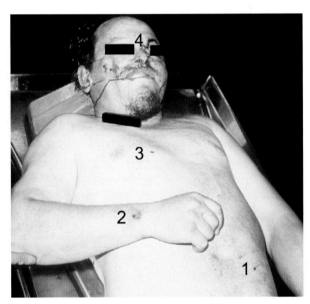

FIGURE 8.27 *Hunting accident in which the man was hit by four pellets from a distant twelve-bore shotgun discharge. Pellet no. 1 punctured the abdominal skin and was found in the subcutaneous fat; pellet no. 2 bruised the right wrist; pellet no. 3 penetrated the chest wall and was found in the pericardial fat tissue without any injury to the heart; pellet no. 4 hit the corner of the left eye and travelled through the left cerebral hemisphere, causing death.*

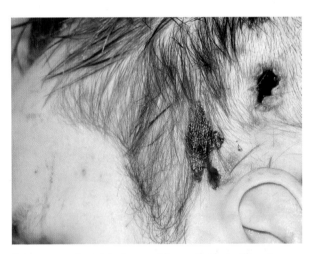

FIGURE 8.29 *Suicidal exit wound from a 9 mm pistol (see also Figure 8.28 for corresponding entrance wound).*

is usually much larger, but a .410 can closely resemble a large-calibre rifled weapon injury. Over deep soft tissues, such as the limbs, abdomen, neck and usually chest, the wound will be small and circular. There will be burning and blackening of the immediate wound edges, but if the seal between muzzle and skin is tight, there will be little or no sideways escape of flame and soiling unless clothing is interposed.

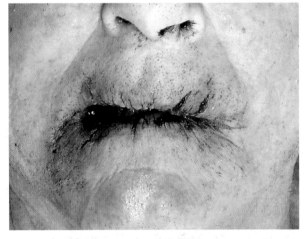

FIGURE 8.30 *Numerous tears in the lips due to expansion of muzzle gases from a 9 mm pistol fired in the mouth.*

Within the wound, there will be some flecking with soot in the tissues, the amount varying with the 'cleanliness' or otherwise of the particular ammunition. Most rifled weapon ammunition is 'clean', compared with many shotgun cartridges, so that soot may be absent altogether. There is usually an areola of hyperaemia that extends beyond the diameter of the muzzle and carbon monoxide will be absorbed by the haemoglobin and myoglobin in the vicinity of the skin wound and in the deeper track. There may be bruising, sometimes extensive, though this is rarely symmetrical and is often absent. The expansion of the tissues by gas entry tends to force the skin even harder against the end of the barrel and a 'muzzle imprint' may be formed. In rifled weapons, especially handguns, there are more features at the end of the barrel than in shotguns, so complex imprints may be made of foresights and mechanisms for self-loading in 'automatics'.

If the contact wound is over a bony support, especially the skull, then the same phenomenon occurs as in shotgun wounds. The muzzle gases entering the subcutaneous tissues cannot expand by displacing adjacent soft structures and are reflected from the bone to raise a dome of gas that often splits the entry hole. This results in a linear, cruciate or stellate tear that may well destroy the original puncture. As the volume of gas produced is usually less than that formed by the large mass of propellant in a twelve-bore shotgun cartridge, the tear is smaller – though the charge in some older rifles and sporting guns may be comparable.

When the contact is loose, burning and soiling in the immediate vicinity of the muzzle may occur – again modified as in the case of shotguns, by the interposition of clothing between muzzle and skin. The fabric allows a lateral passageway for diffusion of soiling, as the muzzle cannot make such a good seal as against skin.

If the skin of the gun hand remains in firm contact with the weapon steel for a longer period of time, rust stains may develop as seen in Figure 8.34. In experiments carried out by Ulrich and Zollinger (2001) in the living as well as corpses, the formation of rust stains depends on the firmness of the contact, humidity of the skin and the environment, contact time and the state of the weapon surface. The shortest period of time necessary for the formation of rust under the most favourable circumstances, as reported by Ulrich and Zollinger, was 135 minutes for a corpse and 27 minutes for a living person.

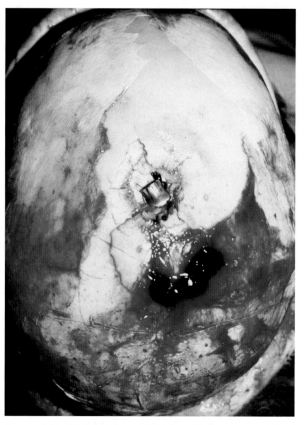

FIGURE 8.31 *Slightly deformed full-jacketed bullet in the middle of the cone-shaped exit wound on top of the skull. Homicidal entrance wound under the chin.*

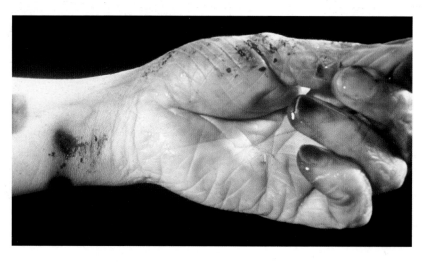

FIGURE 8.32 *Wrist of a homicide victim, who had raised her left hand to ward off the attack, showing a 'clean' exit wound of a full-jacketed bullet in the middle and soot-soiled entrance wound beneath it.*

Blow back into the barrel – 'back spatter'

Contact wounds – and also close-range discharges – may cause blood and tissue fragments to enter the muzzle, sometimes penetrating for several centimetres, this being

called 'back spatter'. There appears to be a momentary suction effect after the pressure of the gas blast subsides, possibly as a result of rapid relative cooling in the barrel. This seems to aspirate material into the muzzle and pieces of skin, hair and adipose tissue have been found inside the weapon. Sometimes blood and tissue may soil the hand or arm of the person firing the gun, a matter of considerable significance in forensic science.

Close-range wounds

When there is a short distance between the muzzle and body surface, the appearances of the wound will vary accordingly to the type of ammunition used. The wound

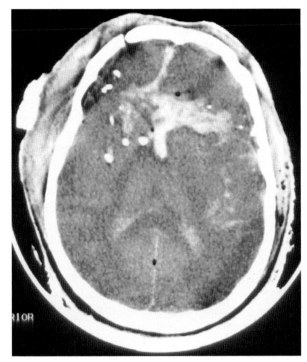

FIGURE 8.33 *Intravital CT scan of a 23-year-old male who in the course of a 'Russian roulette' shot himself in the right temple with a .357 calibre Magnum revolver. Extensive injury of the cranium and brain with several X-ray positive particles probably due to the disintegration of the bullet. (From the files of the Department of Radiology of Turku University Hospital reproduced by kind permission of Professor M Kormano.)*

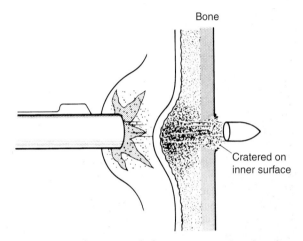

FIGURE 8.35 *A firm contact discharge against tissue overlying bone (such as the skull) causes gas to rebound from the rigid base. This raises a dome under the skin that can split to give a ragged entrance wound. This effect is by no means invariable.*

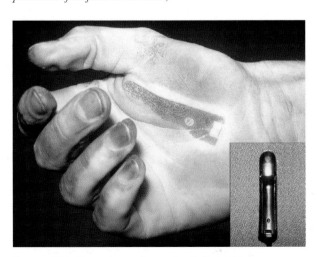

FIGURE 8.34 *Rust stains on the gun-hand of a suicide corresponding to the shape of the grip.*

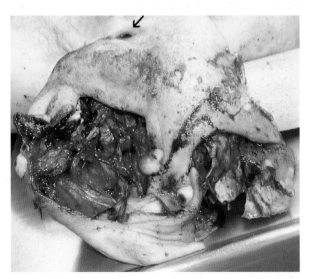

FIGURE 8.36 *Suicidal contact wound in the neck (arrow) from a 7.62 calibre rifle with destruction of the head.*

will almost invariably be circular as the tearing due to gas intrusion is unlikely to occur. The wound edges may be inverted, but at close range the rebounding gases may level up or even evert the margins. As will be described in medium-range wounds, there will be an abrasion collar.

Burning

Modern propellant produces less flame than the black powder of older shotgun cartridges, but within a few centimetres of bare skin there is likely to be burning of the skin with singeing of hairs. Even where hairs are not destroyed, they may be 'clubbed', that is, the keratin melts at the tip and resolidifies as a tiny blob. Hyperaemia around the wound is usual and some bruising can occur, which may be more evident as the post-mortem interval increases.

It is sometimes claimed that the flame effects extend from the muzzle a distance equal to the length of the barrel, but the truth of this rule-of-thumb is doubtful, though it may be a very rough approximation.

Soot or smoke soiling and powder tattooing

Though most propellant is now 'clean', some soot may be seen around the wound. In addition, there will be tiny burns from specks of incandescent propellant, the so-called 'powder tattooing'. These may pepper the vicinity of the entry hole in a roughly symmetrical pattern, which may assist in

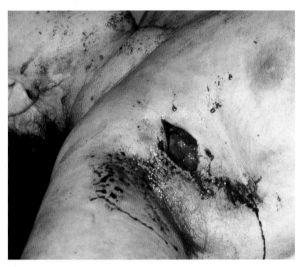

FIGURE 8.37 *A typical slit-like exit wound of a homicidal firearm wound from a hunting rifle with entrance wound in the back.*

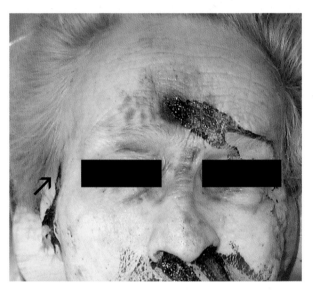

FIGURE 8.39 *Entrance wounds from a 7.65 calibre automatic pistol in the forehead and right side of the face (arrow) of a homicide victim, with soot soiling.*

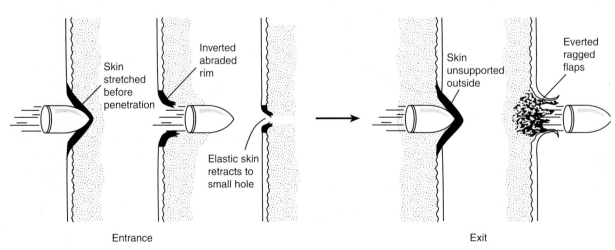

Entrance

Exit

FIGURE 8.38 *Entrance and exit wounds.*

determining the angle of impact. Particles of propellant carry further than smoke, so tattooing around the entrance wound in the absence of soot indicates a greater distance. The soot rarely carries more than 15 cm (6 inches) from a pistol, whereas powder grains will travel 30–45 cm (12–18 inches).

These distances are approximate and can be doubled for a rifle compared with a handgun. The length of the barrel is another variable and a rule-of-thumb for pistols in this respect states that the distance from which powder residues can reach the skin is about twice the length of the barrel. It must be emphasized once again that test firing is essential for any hope of accuracy.

'Fouling' refers to tiny lesions around the entry wound caused by fragments of metal expelled by the discharge. These come either from the surface of the missile or from the interior of the barrel. Friction between the bullet and the rifling may gouge off pieces of lead, jacket, or barrel steel and hurl them at the skin, where they become embedded. These particles, like powder burns, will not wipe off at autopsy, whereas soot soiling can easily be removed with a damp sponge. Even fragments of the shell case may become detached and blown out of the barrel.

Minute flakes of unburnt explosive or inert filler may land on the same area of skin; these tend to glisten and may be orange or blue, depending on the manufacturer. It is important that a forensic scientist or police scene of crime officer has the opportunity to retrieve these before the wound is washed. If no such person is available, the pathologist should swab the area with a water-damped plain swab, or preferably cut out the skin around the wound and preserve it unfixed (refrigerated if necessary). These specimens should be sent for expert forensic examination, as they may indicate the nature of the ammunition and may be matched to that in the possession of a suspect. As with contact wounds, carboxy-haemoglobin and myoglobin will be present in the wound track in diminishing concentrations as the range increases.

The estimation of range is dealt with later, but here it is again emphasized that until test firing is carried out with a similar weapon and ammunition, only an approximate estimate can be offered from the appearances of the wound.

Medium-distance wounds

Unlike the shotgun, once the discharge of a rifled weapon is greater than a metre, there is nothing to indicate increasing range, until perhaps the erratic trajectory of extreme distance suggests maximum range. From perhaps less than half a metre to up to several kilometres the entry wound of a high-velocity rifled weapon appears the same. The typical appearance of the entry wound has been likened to that caused by 'driving a dirty pencil through the skin'. The central aperture is circular

and may be inverted – that is, the margins are driven inwards by the passage of the missile – though this feature is often absent.

The size of the hole is rarely equal to the diameter of the missile and therefore the calibre of the weapon cannot instantly be determined by inspection of the wound – in spite of the apparent ease with which television drama doctors and detectives can instantly spot 'a thirty-two' or a 'thirty-eight'. When the bullet strikes the skin, the latter is stretched for a minute fraction of a second until penetration occurs, so that the missile perforates expanded skin. Immediately after entry, the skin undergoes elastic recoil and the resulting hole is usually smaller than the diameter of the bullet unless the range is so close that gas entry – or gas rebound – contributes to the size of the defect.

The abrasion collar

The skin immediately around the central hole is discoloured, the so-called 'abrasion collar'. This may be only a narrow rim or may be equal in width to the central defect. The collar is due to the inversion of the skin during penetration by the missile so that the sides of the bullet are 'wiped' by a tiny tube of skin, the epidermis of which is abraded by heat and friction.

The width of the abrasion collar is determined by the degree of inversion and hence the length of the skin tube. The collar is caused by friction and heat as the missile chafes the skin.

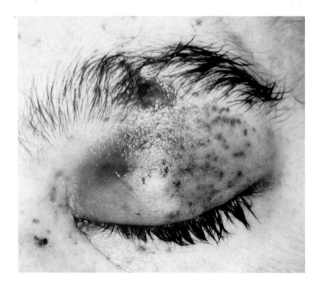

FIGURE 8.40 *Close-range pistol entrance wound. The eyelid and lower forehead show tiny burns from propellant flakes landing on the skin. The eyes are blackened by fractures of the floor of the anterior fossa.*

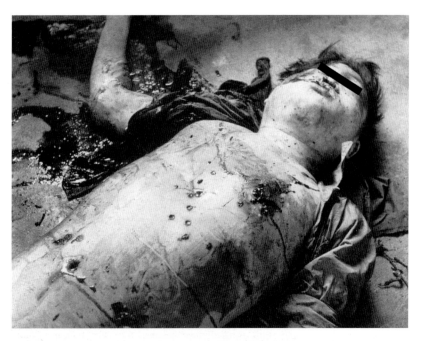

FIGURE 8.41 *Multiple entry wounds from a military self-loading weapon. The wounds are in line and approximately evenly spaced. Each is a typical entry, with an inverted appearance and an abrasion collar. There were massive exit wounds on the back, caused by .303 bullets from a Bren gun used by a Malayan patrol.*

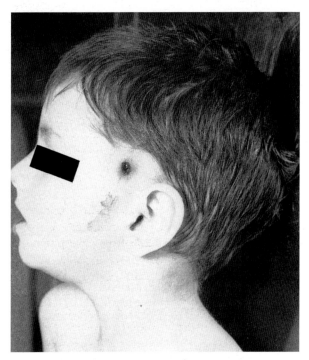

FIGURE 8.42 *Entrance of a .22 rifle bullet at a few inches range. There is slight smoke soiling around the wound, which has a well-marked abrasion collar. In fact, two shots were fired in quick succession through the same hole, which is slightly ovoid because of the non-congruence of the two shots (see Figure 8.49).*

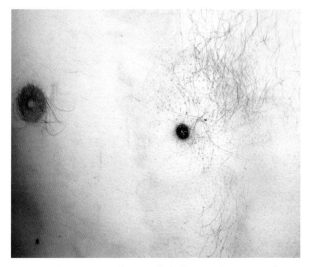

FIGURE 8.43 *Entrance of a .22 rifle bullet in a shooting accident.*

separation of the outer layer, due to the impact of the bullet knocking the deeper layers down away from the keratinized surface.

The grease ring

The inner edge of the abrasion collar may be black, as a result of heating effects and to the rubbing-off of dirt, lubricating oil, or grease and metal particles from the bullet. This is often called the 'grease ring' or 'ring of dirt', and may be absent if the missile was clean.

There may also be bruising around the wound from mechanical damage to adjacent subcutaneous blood vessels,

In addition to the true abrasion collar, there is often a slightly wider circle of peeled keratin, where the stratum corneum of the skin is raised to form a slightly frayed edge around the entry wound. This appears due to mechanical

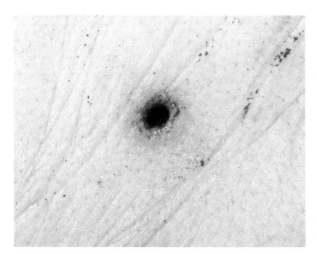

FIGURE 8.44 *Entrance wound in the back of a rifle bullet fired from across a room. There is thus no burning or soiling, and only minimal bruising at the margins of an almost circular inverted entry.*

but no other features, apart from the keratin ring, are present in the surrounding skin. No burns, soot or powder can be found beyond a variable distance that will not exceed a metre in the case of a rifle, and half that distance with a handgun.

Extreme trajectory wounds

Over most of their flight path, rifled weapon missiles maintain a fairly constant attitude. Soon after emergence from the muzzle, the bullet may 'precess', with the tip on the axis of travel and the base rotating in a diminishing circle about the axis. This soon settles down and causes no observable difference in the contact wound. For most of the distance of travel, the bullet remains steady, with only minor variations from axial stability. When the extreme range is approached, however, the reduced velocity allows instability of the flight path. The bullet begins to wobble and yaw, and may even tumble, that is, turn end-over-end. If the missile strikes the body in this phase, the impact may be sideways or even backwards, as well as being in an irregular lateral motion. A bullet striking sideways may leave an almost rectangular entry wound. The wound will then be similarly irregular, and there may be difficulty in recognizing it as a firearm wound or in differentiating it from a laceration caused by other means.

The direction of discharge

As with smooth-bore weapons, a close range discharge may provide information about the angle of the shot because of the geometry of any smoke soiling, powder tattooing, or

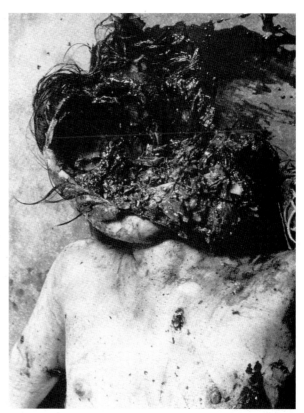

FIGURE 8.45 *Disintegration of the head of a young female terrorist in the Malayan emergency from a single bullet entering the external auditory meatus. The weapon was a F-N rifle with a high muzzle velocity; the impact of the missile on the base of the skull instantly converted the kinetic energy into a virtual explosion.*

burns on the skin. An impact at right angles will produce a circular zone of discoloration on the skin, while an oblique angle will result in an elliptical mark, the length of which increases as the angle decreases. As rifled weapons produce relatively little soiling except at close range, this clue is of less assistance than with shotguns.

Again as with smooth-bore guns, the edges of the wound may be shelved or 'undercut' when the discharge enters at an oblique angle. Tissue may be seen in the floor of the wound at one side, which indicates the direction from which the bullet came. Muscular contractions may distort this picture, however and it is not always present, though minute inspection (using a lens if necessary) may reveal shelving in the deeper layers of the skin rather than in the tissues below. More useful is the shape of the abrasion collar, which will be asymmetrical if the bullet enters at an angle, even through the central hole often remains circular. The other means of determining direction, which is not usually available with shotguns, is the trajectory between entrance and exit wounds. These can be joined and projected in direction of approach to indicate the site of discharge. Two important conditions attach to this interpretation, however:

- If the bullet strikes a solid object, either bone or even a firm organ, it may be diverted within the body to exit well off the original trajectory.
- The posture of the victim's body at the instant of impact must be taken into account. It is too often assumed, especially by lawyers, that all persons are injured – in whatever fashion – whilst standing passively in the 'anatomical position'. Nothing is further from the truth, as people, especially in conditions of fight, fright or flight, may be moving or dodging in a variety of postures, which change by the second. For example, in one of the author's (BK) cases, a woman accidentally shot by a police officer had the anterior entrance wound much higher than the exit in her back. This did not mean that she was shot from above, but that she was leaning forward when the bullet hit her. Much more bizarre examples occur from time to time, such as another case seen by the author (BK) in which a puzzling high-angle wound in the chest was later proved to have been fired from an upstairs window as the victim was knocking on the front door below.

Bullet wounds in bone

Where a bullet passes through bone, especially the thin bone of the skull, the well-known pattern of 'cratering' can usually be seen, though there are exceptions. Using the cranium as the best example, the initial contact of the missile punches a clean hole through the outer table of the skull. Where the bullet emerges internally, the inner table is then unsupported and a cone-shaped plug is detached, forming a crater that is appreciably larger than the external hole. If the bullet traverses the cranium and penetrates the opposite side, the same pattern occurs, this time with the small hole on the inner table and the crater on the outside. In addition to these penetrating defects, there are often fissured, sometimes comminuted, fractures running away from the central holes.

However, though this is the classical picture, a number of exceptions have been reported in the literature, where the cratering has been reversed or is otherwise atypical (Bhoopat 1995).

A shotgun usually destroys a large area of the skull, but similar shelving may be seen on the edges of bone fragments if a bolus of shot strikes the bone. Individual pellets rarely penetrate, but the massive cranial damage from close range of contact shotgun discharges is largely the result of the rapid and violent increase in intracranial pressure caused by the entry of a large volume of gas, as well as the bolus of shot and wads.

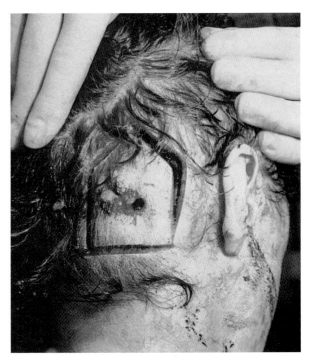

FIGURE 8.46 *Bullet entrance wound, showing the removal of a wide area of skin for forensic examination, the hair having already been removed and preserved before photography. The autopsy incision around the wound is wide, to include any discharge residue and burned skin. The shape of the incision is obviously asymmetrical, to indicate the orientation of the sample after removal from the body.*

Where several bullets have struck the cranium, the sequence of shots can usually be determined using Puppe's rule, which is applicable to any multiple blunt force causing skull fractures. Madea and Staak (1988) have developed this rule in relation to bullet injuries: the test depends on the observations of the fracture lines either when they intersect each other or when they intersect a cratered lesion, so that one can determine which crack or defect must have been formed first.

Where bones other than skull are hit by a bullet or shot, comminuted fractures are frequent and may be the cause of extensive secondary injury. Part of the kinetic energy of the missile is transferred to the bone and fragments may be violently displaced into the adjacent tissues. They may be extruded from the body altogether, leaving secondary exit wounds in the skin. These may give rise to difficulty in interpretation, as both lay persons and doctors may mistake them for lacerated or even stab wounds, unrelated to the firearm incident. Fractures of bone from gunshot impact may be of any variety, and radiography is necessary to detect and orientate fragments of bone and differentiate them from missiles and missile fragments.

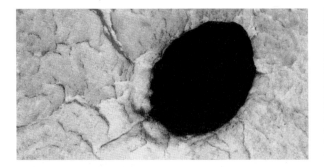

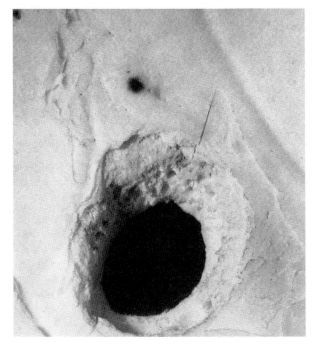

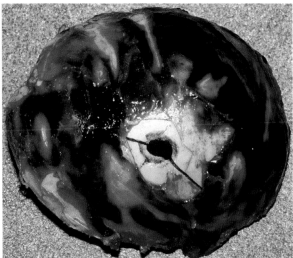

FIGURE 8.48 *Cone-shaped exit wound of the calvarium, with radial fractures in left parietal bone.*

FIGURE 8.47 *The entrance wound of a bullet into a skull. Externally the defect is clean-cut and slightly ovoid because of the oblique impact of the missile. Internally, the inner table of the cranium is cratered, the bevel being caused by lack of support from the diploë. The exit hole on the opposite side of the skull showed a reversal of this pattern, with the cratering on the exterior surface.*

EXIT WOUNDS

When a gunshot wound completely traverses the part of the body struck, an exit wound will result.

Shotgun exit wounds

When smooth-bore weapons are involved, the residual energy of the individual pellets (which have a small mass and a relatively low initial velocity) is usually insufficient for them to emerge through the wider parts of the body, such as the chest and abdomen. Wounds of the limbs, neck and head may well be 'through-and-through' with a twelve-bore shotgun and occasionally, though rarely, with the small 'four-ten'. The range has an effect on the possibility of a shotgun exit wound, as contact or close-range discharge will allow the compacted mass of shot to act like a single bolus – in addition to which, the large volume of intruded gas assists in disrupting the tissues and clearing a path for the missiles, especially in the head. A shotgun blast into the mouth may well remove much of the back of the head as an exit wound, but this is in part caused by the explosion of the cranium by the gas, the so-called 'burst head', which can occur in any gunshot wound of the head, whether into the mouth or elsewhere.

The appearance of a shotgun exit wound is totally random, depending on the anatomical part injured and the addition of any bone or tissue fragments blown out in the discharge. Typically, it is a jagged, irregular laceration with everted edges that exposes deep tissues and comminuted bone fragments beneath. A shotgun injury of the chest or abdomen often just fails to exit on the opposite side, because the toughest obstruction, other than bone, is the skin. It is not uncommon to be able to palpate lead shot under the skin in the contralateral position after it has traversed the body and been trapped by the skin.

As a contact shotgun discharge may produce a large, ragged, entrance wound, this may resemble the exit wound, if present. Differentiation is usually simple, however, because of the burning and soiling present around the entrance. It has been said that the presence of carbon monoxide in the tissues marks the entrance wound, even in decomposed bodies, but carbon monoxide can in fact be detected right through a close shotgun discharge, though the concentration should be greater near the entrance.

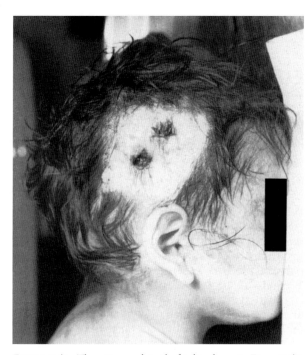

FIGURE 8.49 *The exit wounds in the fatality shown in Figure 8.42. The two bullets have diverged inside the head from their common entrance wound and emerged separately. The exit wounds are typically stellate, everted and clean. With small-calibre missiles, such as a .22, there is often no exit wound, but here the small head and thin skull provide less resistance to complete traversing.*

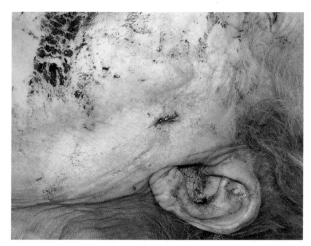

FIGURE 8.50 *Atypical slit-like exit wound of a 7.65 cal. bullet (see also Figure 8.39).*

Exit wounds from rifled weapons

As stated above, many wounds from rifled guns are 'through-and-through', especially from high-velocity military weapons. The muzzle velocity is important in determining whether a single bullet will completely traverse the body. A high-velocity missile (of the order of 800 metres/second or 3000 feet/second) is likely to pass right through the body unless it strikes a large bony structure like the spine, large limb bone or base of the skull. As discussed at the beginning of the chapter, this may be inefficient in terms of wounding capability, as much of the kinetic energy fails to be transferred to the tissues to cause damage, although the cavitating effects of a high-speed missile in vital tissues may be extremely damaging. Much modern military ammunition consists of a small bullet with a large propellant charge to provide maximum muzzle velocity. This, by the familiar physics equation, provides substantial kinetic energy. The bullet is designed to fragment on impact, so that all the energy is transferred and an exit wound may not occur. In some shootings of this nature the pathologist may have difficulty in retrieving any metallic missile material, even after identifying it radiographically, as the fragmentation may reduce the bullet to granules and dust. If the missile does not strike bone or cartilage, it is

likely to emerge on the other side of the body, even through the thickness of the chest or abdomen. Of course, in many cases where bone is penetrated (especially the skull or ribs), the bullet will still emerge, but this is considered below.

If a fairly intact bullet emerges, not having been seriously deformed or fragmented, the exit wound is likely to be a small everted defect, either circular or with torn edges. The classical description is of a stellate wound, with triangular skin flaps at the margin, where the bullet has pushed out against unsupported skin. Many wounds may be cruciate or linear slits, however, and others are as circular as the entrance wound, which can give rise to some difficulty in interpretation.

It is naturally important to confirm the direction of the shot, but where a bullet has come from any distance between half a metre and near the extreme range of the weapon, then both entrance and exit wounds can look remarkably similar. There will be no burning or soiling to indicate the entry and identification will depend upon the close examination of the margins of the wounds. Where the entry was covered by clothing, fibres of fabric may have been driven into the wound, which can never occur at the exit.

Though the exit is usually everted, this may not occur if the skin is supported at the moment of penetration. A firm brassière band or an elasticated trouser waistband can press on the skin and prevent eversion, as can a plaster or fibreboard wall, if the victim was leaning against it. In these instances, there may even be a spurious 'abrasion collar', which is really caused by the emerging bullet slamming the wound periphery against the resisting surface. In difficult cases the pathologist or a deputy should examine clothing and the scene, to see if there are any such factors that will help in arriving at a definite answer as to direction.

Usually, the abrasion collar and frayed keratin ring of the entrance wound will be of diagnostic significance, as it is

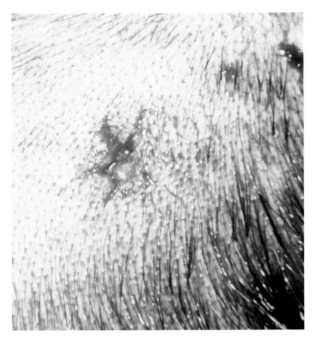

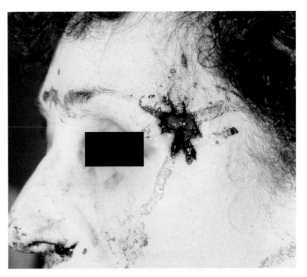

FIGURE 8.53 *Exit wound of the bullet responsible for the wound seen in Figure 8.46, showing the classical everted, split edges, with no soiling of the surrounding skin.*

FIGURE 8.51 *Typical exit wound from a 9 mm bullet. The wound in the scalp is everted, stellate and quite clean, the missile having been wiped by its passage through the tissues.*

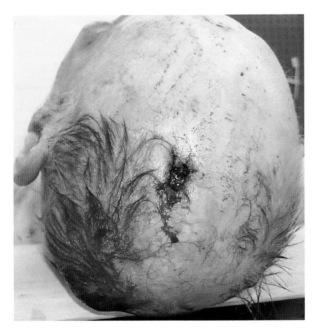

FIGURE 8.52 *Exit wound of a 9 mm pistol fired into the mouth.*

absent in the exit wound, except as detailed above. Occasionally, however, the abrasion collar of the entrance wound is merely a narrow rim that needs close inspection to detect. Where the bullet has struck bone or fragmented, the exit wound may be of any size or shape, and may be multiple. If bone is shattered, pieces can be driven out through the skin, causing wounds that may be mistaken for lacerations from blunt or even incised weapon violence. Where the bullet has hit bone within the body, the bullet may emerge sideways causing a longer or otherwise distorted exit wound.

Of the many bizarre findings in gunshot wounds, re-entry can pose some problems. One case seen by the author had two entrance and one exit wounds, with a single bullet in the body. The victim had been standing against a wall when shot from the front: the bullet emerged through his back, ricocheted from the wall and re-entered his body.

Penetration of two parts of the body is quite common, a single missile causing several wounds. The most usual is a through-and-through wound of the arm or leg, the bullet then re-entering the abdomen or chest. Placing the limb in the appropriate position immediately clarifies the situation and can considerably aid an estimation of direction.

Glancing or tangential rifled weapon wounds

Though the large gaping wounds caused by a glancing blast from a shotgun are rarely seen with rifled weapons, some strange wounds can occur. A bullet may strike the body surface at a shallow angle, enter and then re-emerge some distance away, having travelled superficially under the skin. Within the skull, a missile may enter, follow the internal curve of the calvarium and exit some distance away. Cases are on record of such wounds causing relatively little damage, having traversed the meninges, rather than the brain substance.

When the body surface is irregular, such as the breast, buttocks or groin, several re-entries and exits can take place.

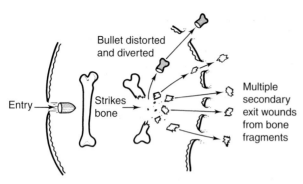

FIGURE 8.54 *Diversion of trajectory of bullet on striking bone. The secondary effects can be more damaging than those from the missile.*

In these instances, extensive bruising may mislead examiners into assuming that some blunt injury has occurred, if the firearm nature of the wound is overlooked.

A bullet striking at a small angle with the surface may follow the curvature of the skull or a rib and emerge some distance away after having made a track in the subcutaneous tissues. Alternatively, a bullet can pass tangentially across the surface, causing a linear graze or even a laceration, which may lead to great difficulties in interpretation if the circumstances are unknown. Gunshot wounds in the axilla or across the side of the thorax may gape widely, looking quite unlike a firearm injury to an unsuspecting medical examiner.

FIREARM DAMAGE TO INTERNAL ORGANS

This may be of any nature, but broadly falls into two categories:

- Contusion and laceration from low-velocity impact. Where a mass of shotgun pellets and gas strike tissues or an organ the damage is simple mechanical disruption, with widespread haemorrhage from local vessels. Similar, though less extensive, damage is likely from a low-velocity rifled bullet or slug, which pushes the tissues apart as it ploughs through an organ or muscle. Secondary damage can occur from fragmentation of bone or bullet, which produces further traumatizing missiles within the tissues. The danger to life that ensues naturally depends upon the target tissues – a clean wound through the thigh may cause only temporary disability, whereas the same wound through heart or brain may well be rapidly fatal.
- High-velocity missiles produce disproportionate damage relative to their diameter because of cavitation effects, described at the beginning of the chapter. This

is particularly damaging in solid organs, such as the brain and liver. The track may be many times wider than the diameter of the bullet, and may consist of pulped and haemorrhagic tissue left behind by the pulsating cavitation effect caused by the lateral transfer of energy as the missile passes through.

ESTIMATING THE RANGE OF DISCHARGE

This is one of the most important aspects of the interpretation of firearm wounds. Though guidelines can be offered, it cannot be emphasized too strongly that every weapon and batch of ammunition will vary, so that medical opinion must always defer to the results of test firing with the same gun and similar shells. Allowance must also be made for the effect of interposed clothing.

Rifled weapons

TIGHT CONTACT OVER SOFT TISSUES

- Possible muzzle impression.
- Circular hole with abrasion collar.
- Bruising.
- Local reddening from heat and monoxide.
- Little or no surface burning.
- Little or no propellant soiling or powder tattooing.

TIGHT CONTACT OVER UNDERLYING BONE

- Split or cruciate wound.
- Local reddening and monoxide.
- Bruising.
- Little or no surface burning or propellant soiling.
- Abrasion collar partly lost on skin tags.

DISCHARGE FROM LESS THAN 15 CM (6 INCHES)

- Circular hole with abrasion collar.
- Flame burn on surrounding skin.
- Burnt hairs.
- Soot and smoke soiling (depending on ammunition).
- Small punctate burns from propellant tattooing.
- Unburnt propellant flakes.
- Little or no monoxide in tissues.

DISCHARGE FROM 15 TO 30 CM (6 TO 12 INCHES)

- No soot, but perhaps powder tattooing, depending on barrel length.

- No monoxide.
- Rarely, flame burns.

DISCHARGE FROM MORE THAN 40–60 CM (16–24 INCHES)

- Circular hole with abrasion collar.
- No burning, soiling, burnt hairs or monoxide.

FAR DISTANT DISCHARGE AT LIMIT OF RANGE

- Larger, irregular hole with irregular abrasion rim caused by tumbling bullet.
- No other features.

Smooth-bore shotguns

TIGHT CONTACT DISCHARGE OVER SOFT TISSUES

- Single circular wound about diameter of muzzle.
- Smooth margin.
- Often muzzle imprint.
- Blackened edge.
- No surrounding smoke soiling unless clothing allows leakage.
- Deep bruising.
- Pink tissues.
- Wads in wound.

TIGHT CONTACT DISCHARGE OVER SKULL OR BONY AREA

As last type, but wound may be ragged and split from gas rebound.

DISCHARGE WITHIN A FEW CENTIMETRES

- Circular wound, unless oblique discharge.
- Smooth or slightly crenated margin.
- No satellite pellet holes.
- Surrounding soot soiling.
- Punctate powder burns.
- May be unburnt powder flakes.
- Burning of surrounding skin.
- Burnt hairs.
- Pink monoxide in tissues.
- Wads in wound.

DISCHARGE FROM 30 CM (12 INCHES)

- Circular 'rat-hole' wound with nibbled margins.
- No satellite pellet holes.

- Soot soiling may persist.
- Powder tattooing present.
- Little or no monoxide.
- Still burning of skin and hairs.
- Wads in wound.

DISCHARGE FROM 1 TO 5 M (39 TO 195 INCHES)

- Central 'rat-hole' wound.
- Satellite pellet holes around periphery.
- No burning.
- No soot.
- Maybe slight tattooing at 1 m.
- No monoxide.
- Wads not in wound at upper part of this range.

DISCHARGE OVER 5 M (195 INCHES)

- Diffuse pellet pattern.
- Probably no central hole.
- No burning, soot, tattooing, monoxide, no wads.

All the foregoing data are very variable, being dependent upon the individual weapon and ammunition. Test firing must be used to validate the pathological interpretation.

AIRGUN INJURIES

Air rifles and pistols produce wounds that have some of the characteristics of both shotguns and explosive rifled weapons. The missile is single and fired through a rifled barrel, but is small and resembles a shaped (waisted) shotgun pellet.

The muzzle velocity is relatively low, but some more sophisticated rifles, such as the German Weirauch, can produce more than 12 foot-pounds of energy and the pellet can easily penetrate a wooden door – and the human skull.

Two calibres are common, the .177 and the .22 inch, the latter naturally being the more dangerous. The .177 can, however, penetrate the thin temporal bone of a child. Wounds from an air weapon are rarely fatal except when the head is struck – and children are the usual victims. The pellet can enter the skull and traverse the whole width of the brain, but never produce an exit wound, being usually found in the contralateral meninges. The track may be surprisingly wide for such a low-velocity missile.

Apart from fatal head wounds, a number of eye injuries occur from airguns, the pellet lodging within the globe, the orbit or the adjacent air-sinuses. Radiology is obviously of prime importance in locating the missile, prior to surgical removal.

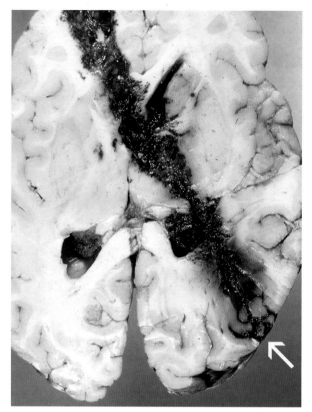

FIGURE 8.55 *Track through a child's brain made by a .177 inch air-rifle pellet (arrowed). Although a relatively low-velocity missile, the track is much wider than the pellet from lateral transfer of kinetic energy.*

There are no particular features of an air weapon wound, as, of course, there are none of the heat, powder or soot effects of an explosive gun. The entry wound is small, but may show an abrasion ring. There is never an exit wound, unless the tissue traversed is extremely narrow.

HUMANE (VETERINARY) KILLERS AND INDUSTRIAL 'STUD-GUNS'

Explosive weapons of a specialized type are used in abattoirs and by veterinary surgeons to dispatch large animals.

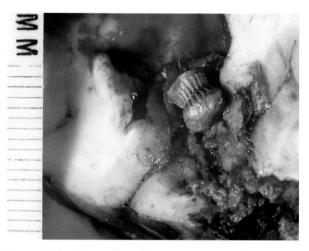

FIGURE 8.56 *Airgun pellet in brain tissue.*

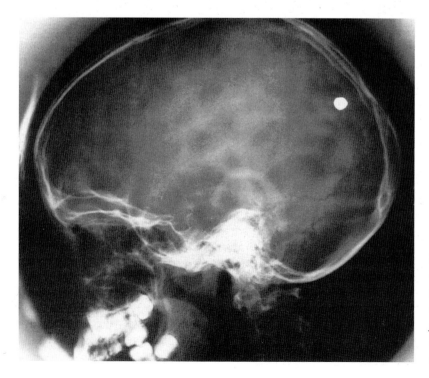

FIGURE 8.57 *Radiography can assist in locating a missile before autopsy, so that random searching does not cause instrument damage to the delicate striation pattern used for weapon identification. Here there is a lead pellet in the occipital lobe, with a bone defect in the extreme front of the skull.*

They may be of the 'captive-bolt' type, which consists of a metal rod, the distal end of which is propelled for a few centimetres from the muzzle of the weapon by a blank cartridge inserted in a chamber behind the proximal end. The captive bolt inflicts a clean, penetrating injury, about 5 cm deep, which can be mistaken for a stab-like injury.

Another variety consists of a metal barrel on the distal end of which is a heavy flange, which is placed against the head of the animal. A cartridge carrying a 0.31 inch (8 mm) bullet is inserted into the proximal end of the barrel and a firing pin struck with a mallet. The injuries from this resemble a contact wound from a conventional weapon, though the base of the flange may have embossed concentric circles to prevent slipping, which may produce an unusual patterned imprint on the skin surrounding the wound.

Another type is the Webley veterinary pistol, which is of .32 calibre and is virtually identical with a conventional gun. Humane killers may cause injuries on humans either accidentally or suicidally, homicide being rare. The nature of the weapon will almost always be apparent from the circumstances, including the presence of the weapon. Death may be delayed due to complications, as in one case seen by the author (BK) where a farmer died of tetanus after accidentally shooting himself in the knee with a humane killer.

Devices used in industry and especially the building trade, are similar to humane killers. These are the 'stud-guns' used

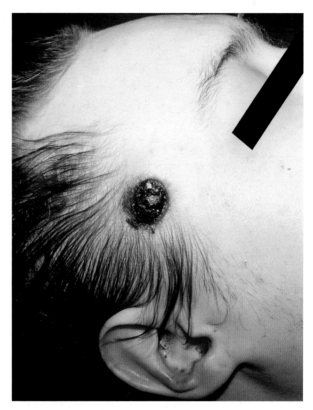

FIGURE 8.59 *Suicidal contact wound from a humane veterinary killer (see also Figure 8.60).*

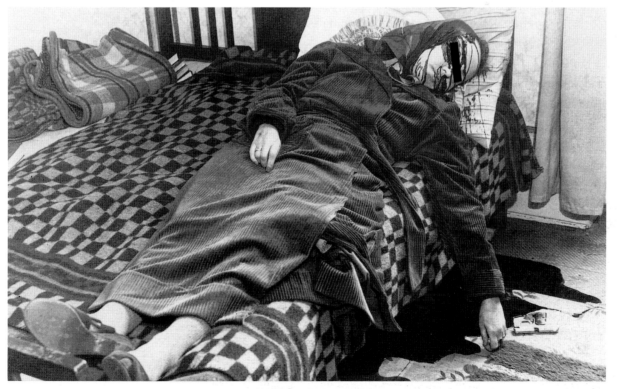

FIGURE 8.58 *A relatively unusual photograph in Britain, in that the suicide is of a woman and an automatic pistol is used. Note the massive haemorrhage on the floor, which illustrates the possible extent of post-mortem bleeding.*

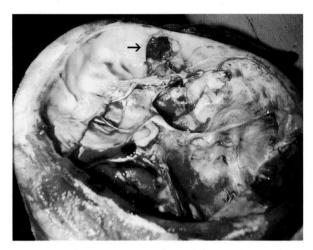

FIGURE 8.60 *Defect of the right frontal bone (arrow) from a humane veterinary killer (see also Figure 8.59).*

for driving a hardened metal pin or threaded stud into masonry, or other wood or metal structures as a rapid and convenient means of attachment. An explosive cartridge, often of .22 calibre, is used to drive a piston that acts as a hammer on the pin or stud. Many accidents and the occasional suicide have occurred from these tools, which resemble a long pistol, with a flat faceplate attached to the muzzle for pressing against the structure. Some accidents occur because the guns are used on relatively flimsy partitions, and the stud traverses the structure and flies on to injure or kill someone on the other side.

RUBBER AND PLASTIC BULLETS

A relatively recent innovation in firearms is the use by police and security forces of projectiles for riot control. Originally rubber bullets were used, being compressed into smooth-bore weapons. These have been abandoned in Britain in favour of 'baton rounds', more commonly known as 'plastic bullets'. They have been used in large quantities in Northern Ireland, some 43 000 having fired up to 1985. These projectiles have not yet been used in the mainland of Britain, though many police forces hold stocks. Elsewhere in the world, they are used extensively for riot control.

The baton round is a solid cylinder of polyvinylchloride 38 mm in diameter and 10 cm long, weighing 135 g. When fired from a smooth-bore weapon it has a muzzle velocity of about 250 km/hour and an effective range of 50–70 m. It should not be fired at a person under about 20 m range. It is used to disperse riots and discourage stone-throwers by striking them sufficiently hard to cause pain and bruising, but no serious injury. The bullet is about the same weight as a

cricket ball, but travels twice as fast as the best bowler could deliver it. In Britain, the bullets were made by Pains-Wessex-Schermuly, but later by Brocks Fireworks and also by the Ministry of Defence. Many injuries and some deaths have been reported from their use. Fractures of the face and skull, eye damage including blinding, broken ribs and limbs, and contusions of liver, lung and spleen have occurred.

Police are instructed to fire at the lower half of the body, to avoid the more serious injuries arising from hitting the head or chest. The death rate is said to be 1/18 000 rounds fired, compared with rubber bullets which had a mortality rate of 1/4000 rounds.

DEATHS FROM EXPLOSION

Deaths from the effects of explosive substances or devices occur in both civil and 'military' circumstances, though the latter now include a considerable proportion of terrorist activities rather than conventional wars. Civil tragedies are usually industrial, as in individual incidents in mines and quarries, or on a larger scale, such as the detonation of chemical stores, ships or factories.

The nature of explosive trauma

Several different factors cause injury following an explosion, and the relative importance of each varies considerably with the type of detonation. For example, pure blast effects are far more important with high-explosive projectiles designed for purely military use than with the home-made terrorist bombs, the lethality of which may be primarily caused by flying fragments. Death and injury from explosives is caused by:

- blast effects
- impact of projectiles derived from the explosive device
- impact from surrounding objects and debris impelled by the explosion
- burns from hot gas and incandescent objects
- secondary injuries from falling masonry, beams and furnishings dislodged by the explosion.

A blast consists of a wave of compression passing rapidly through the air – or water in the case of a submarine explosion, such as a mine. The velocity of the shock wave depends on the distance from the epicentre, being many times the speed of sound at the start, but rapidly decreasing as it spreads out. The compression wave is followed by a transient zone of low pressure (below atmospheric), so that a rapid double change in pressure is suffered by the body. The magnitude of the blast varies with the energy released and also with the distance from the epicentre, the intensity obeying the inverse square law. With all but powerful military high explosives, the blast effects of most terrorist devices fall off so rapidly with distance that only those in the immediate vicinity will suffer severe damage from blast. Not uncommonly, this type of victim is the bomb-setter himself, when a premature detonation occurs.

A blast causes the most damage at an interface between tissues in contact with the atmosphere, which is why the lung usually suffers the most. About 100 lb/inch^2 (690 kPa) is the minimum threshold for serious damage to humans. The shock wave can pass through solid, homogeneous tissues such as liver and muscle, causing little or no damage, but in the lung there is marked variation in density between the alveolar walls and the contained air so that damping of the shock wave occurs and energy is absorbed, with disruptive effects.

There is controversy about whether pulmonary damage occurs from direct transmission of the shock wave through the thoracic wall, or through the oronasal orifices and air passages. In any event, the autopsy signs are of subpleural patchy haemorrhages, often in the line of the ribs, intrapulmonary haemorrhage and bullae at the lung margins. The air passages may be filled with bloody froth causing airway obstruction and hypoxia in addition to the primary damage.

Microscopically the alveolar walls can be shredded by the acceleration and consequent tearing of the air-sac wall when the shock waves traverses the lung. Desquamated alveolar and bronchial epithelium is seen lying free. Large areas of haemorrhage are seen, with either the alveolar pattern still visible or the architecture completely disorganized. Pulmonary haemorrhage in explosive incidents is often not caused solely by the blast, but may be from direct impact on the chest from flying objects, aspiration of blood from nasopharyngeal injuries and from bleeding following aspiration of stomach contents.

The ear may suffer severe damage from a blast, but this is not easily discernible at autopsy. Clinical examination and testing (obviously in the living) reveals many lesions, but these are of little relevance to the pathologist.

The gastrointestinal system suffers from the effects of a blast because, like the lung, it contains air and gases, and is thus not a uniform medium for transit of the shock wave. Once again haemorrhage is the most common lesion, usually small foci of the order of a centimetre in size. They may form circumferential bands around the intestine or may be confined to the serous coat as focal haemorrhages. The caecum and colon are more often injured than the ileum, jejunum and stomach, probably because they are larger and often contain more gas. Occasionally ruptures of the gut occur if the blast is violent and the victim in near proximity.

Victims of explosions in water suffer a reverse order of gastrointestinal to lung damage. The former is more

common and may be manifested as haemorrhages under the serous coats and mucosa. Perforations may occur and, in survivors, peritonitis is not uncommon. The perforations are often multiple and in any part of the intestine. Lung damage is less common in water and some instances may be caused by impact transmitted up through the diaphragm.

Missile injuries in explosions

It is again emphasized that unless a sophisticated high-explosive military device is involved, or if the victim is virtually adjacent to a lower energy terrorist bomb, blast effects will rarely be the sole cause of death. The body will, however, be vulnerable to impact from solid fragments originating from the bomb casing or a container or conveyance, such as a car in which the bomb was concealed. Fragments of metals, from tiny splinters to large chunks or sheets, will be projected at high speed. The smaller ones will not travel more than a few metres, but larger, heavier pieces can fly over considerable distances and can cause serious or fatal injuries in just the same way as projectiles from a firearm. In the open, debris is scoured away, including dust and dirt, which can impinge on the body to injure and discolour it. At autopsy the body may appear pigmented from this dust blasting, the clothing causing a shadow effect similar to bathing suit protection from sunburn. A more common appearance is a 'peppering' as a result of the numerous small missiles causing bruises, lacerations and abrasions. The lacerations are often puncture wounds, of varying size and depth. Burns may also discolour the body, especially those areas unprotected by clothing. Flash burns from the bomb itself only affect those nearby unless the device is massive, though singeing of hair and eyebrows is not uncommon. Other burns may be caused by ignition of clothing, or by the building or vehicle catching alight from the bomb effects –or from gas or petrol ignition.

A massive bomb, or one where the victim is virtually on top of the device, may totally disrupt the body and fling unidentifiable pieces over a wide area. Alternatively, part of the body may be totally destroyed, sometimes the remainder of the victim being remarkably intact. The legs may be blown off or the abdomen disrupted, or the hands and arms torn away. In terrorist attacks these effects may be seen in the person who was planting the bomb or carrying it to the place chosen for detonation. A premature explosion, sometimes during the act of setting the timer, may cause these localized injuries.

The pathologist may be able to assist in reconstructing the events, as localized severe trauma obviously indicates the relative position of the bomb and the victim at the time of detonation. If the lower legs are destroyed, then the person was standing near the device that lay on the ground. Punctured wounds and bruises on the front of the thighs and trunk will indicate that he was facing the bomb. If the thighs, pelvic region and abdomen are damaged, the bomb may have been carried on the lap – and if the hands, chest and face are the most affected areas, the deceased may have been bending over the device.

The autopsy in explosion deaths

The salient features have already been described and much of the autopsy is directed at listing the injuries, as in any

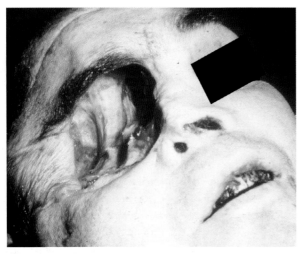

FIGURE 8.61 *Localized injury by an explosive device. The soldier picked up an apparently 'dud' smoke shell, which then detonated. He lived for some weeks, the injury having partly healed, though part of the face and skull were destroyed.*

other trauma death. The interpretation outlined above, however, may be most important for the investigators.

There are some more specific matters in an explosion death which the pathologist must bear in mind. Firstly, trace evidence may be vital to the forensic scientists and bomb experts, who are trying to trace the maker of a terrorist device. X-rays should be taken of all bodies before autopsy to identify any radio-opaque objects. Not only will this assist in detecting lethal missiles not visible from the surface, but it may reveal small metal objects that form part of the bomb mechanism, such as small springs or contacts from the timer or detonator. These may be invaluable in allowing the experts to recognize the handiwork of a particular bomb-maker or terrorist group. Such radiography may also reveal the unexpected, which in the past has included a bullet, the victim having been blown up after death from shooting. Even prior to radiography, there may be much that the pathologist has to do. Though many explosion victims are relatively intact, where extensive disruption has occurred, the fragments have to be collected and sorted out in the mortuary.

A major initial problem is to discover how many bodies are represented and to try to allot the correct fragments to the right individuals. Where there are a number of victims and a large pile of small fragments, this task may be difficult or impossible, but it is naturally of paramount importance to determine how many victims are involved and to determine the sex of each. This is largely an anatomical exercise, akin to the sorting of multiple skeletal remains. Careful identification of all recognizable structures, such as prostate, uterus, breasts, scalp, eyes, for example, is needed in addition to more gross sorting of limb and trunk fragments. Radiology may again assist in matching contained skeletal structures, but much of

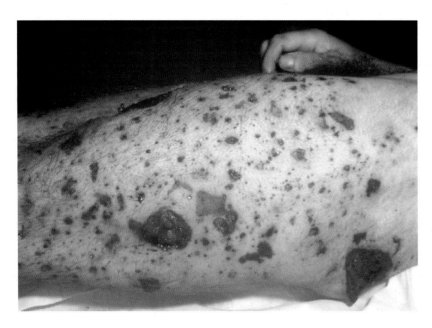

FIGURE 8.62 *Numerous wounds and peppering by debris projected in a terrorist bomb blast. Blast injuries occur only in close proximity to the device – most injury is caused by flying projectiles. (Reproduced by kind permission of Professor TK Marshall.)*

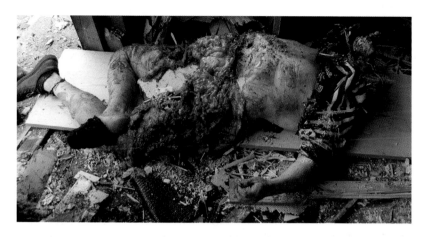

FIGURE 8.63 *Anterior aspect of a man who had constructed an explosive device using dynamite. The device probably detonated prematurely, the blast disrupting the head and abdominal region.*

the debris accumulated after a large explosion consists mainly of skin and attached tissues.

In spite of the most thorough police search of the scene, considerable proportions of some bodies are never recovered, having been disrupted into tiny fragments and mixed with the masonry and other debris of the bomb site. The collected fragments have to be washed clean from the inevitable dirt that coats them and sorted into groups by anatomical similarity. Non-human tissue is discarded, as animal material is not uncommonly admixed. The completed piles of tissue are then resorted by any apparent similarity, such as racial pigmentation, hair colour and sex. Limbs and large joints are then sorted, allotting them to left and right from anatomical considerations.

The difficulties of such a task was emphasized by Professor TK Marshall, whose experiences in Northern Ireland make his writings on the subject the definitive guide to such tragedies. In one of his incidents, eight victims were accounted for, when a single penile fragment forced the inevitable conclusion that there were in fact nine victims, not eight, though no other recognizable part of this ninth man was ever discovered. He had presumably been the bomb-carrier and had been completely disintegrated.

REFERENCES AND FURTHER READING

Adelson L. 1984. Bullet embolism with radiologic documentation. A case report. *Am J Forensic Med Pathol* **5**:253–6.

Aguilar JC. 1983. Shored gunshot wound of exit. A phenomenon with identity crisis. *Am J Forensic Med Pathol* **4**:199–204.

al Alousi LM. 1990. Automatic rifle injuries: suicide by eight bullets. Report of an unusual case and a literature review. *Am J Forensic Med Pathol* **11**:275–81.

Amatuzio JC, Coe JI. 1981. Homicide by exploder ammunition. *Am J Forensic Med Pathol* **2**:111–13.

Anonymous. 1968. Nail-gun injuries. *Br Med J* **1**:462.

Betz P, Pankratz H, Penning R, *et al.* 1993. Homicide with a captive bolt pistol. *Am J Forensic Med Pathol* **14**:54–7.

Bhoopat T. 1995. A case of internal beveling with an exit gunshot wound to the skull. *Forensic Sci Int* **71**:97–101.

Black AM, Burns BD, Zuckerman S. 1942. Wounding mechanism of high velocity missiles. In: Pugh WS (ed.), *War medicine*. F. Hubner & Co, New York.

Breitenecker R. 1969. Shotgun wound patterns. *Am J Clin Pathol* **52**:257–62.

Brissie RM, Collum ES. 1980. Shotgun wounds: multiple probes and shielding effects as adjuncts to determining position of the decreased at time of injury. *J Forensic Sci* **25**:528–32.

Callender GR. 1943. Wound ballistics; mechanism of production of wounds by small bullets and shell fragments. *War Med* **3**:337–45.

Clark MA, Micik W. 1984. Confusing wounds of entrance and exit with an unusual weapon. *Am J Forensic Med Pathol* **5**:75–8.

Clark MA, Smith TD, Fisher RS. 1981. Russian roulette with an exploding bullet. A case report. *Am J Forensic Med Pathol* **2**:167–9.

Coe JI. 1982. External beveling of entrance wounds by handguns. *Am J Forensic Med Pathol* **3**:215–19.

Coe JI, Austin N. 1992. The effects of various intermediate targets on dispersion of shotgun patterns. *Am J Forensic Med Pathol* **13**:281–3.

Conradi SE. 1982. New aluminum-jacketed ammunition: The case of the 'invisible' jacket. *Am J Forensic Med Pathol* **3**:153–5.

Copeland AR. 1985. Concepts in survival from lethal handgun wounds. *Am J Forensic Med Pathol* **6**:175–9.

Cragg J. 1967. Nail-gun fatality. *Br Med J* **4**:784–5.

Dada MA, Loftus IA, Rutheerford GS. 1993. Shotgun pellet embolism to the brain. *Am J Forensic Med Pathol* **14**:58–60.

de la Grandmaison GL, Brion F, Durigon M. 2001. Frequency of bone lesions: an inadequate criterion for gunshot wound diagnosis in skeletal remains. *J Forensic Sci* **46**:593–5.

DiMaio VJ. 1981. Penetration and perforation of skin by bullets and missiles. A review of the literature. *Am J Forensic Med Pathol* **2**:107–10.

DiMaio VJ, Copeland AR, Besant Matthews PE, *et al.* 1982. Minimal velocities necessary for perforation of skin by air gun pellets and bullets. *J Forensic Sci* **27**:894–8.

Dixon DS. 1984. Pattern of intersecting fractures and direction of fire. *J Forensic Sci* **29**:651–4.

Eckert WG. 1981. Exploding bullets. A hazard to the victim, physician, and investigator [editorial]. *Am J Forensic Med Pathol* **2**:103–4.

Eisele JW, Reay DT, Cook A. 1981. Sites of suicidal gunshot wounds. *J Forensic Sci* **26**:480–5.

Elsayed NM. 1997. Toxicology of blast overpressure. *Toxicology* **121**:1–15.

Freytag E. 1963. Autopsy findings in head injuries from blunt forces: statistical evaluation of 1367 cases. *Arch Pathol* **75**:74–80.

Geurin PF. 1960. Shot-gun wounds. *J Forensic Sci* **5**:294–9.

Glattstein B, Zeichner A, Vinokurov A, *et al.* 2000. Improved method for shooting distance estimation. Part III. Bullet holes in cadavers. *J Forensic Sci* **45**:1243–9.

Goonetilleke UK. 1976. A stud (cartridge) gun suicide (a case report). *Med Sci Law* **16**:181–4.

Green GS, Good R. 1982. Homicide by use of a pellet gun. *Am J Forensic Med Pathol* **3**:361–5.

Guileyardo JM, Cooper RE, Porter BE, *et al.* 1992. Renal artery bullet embolism. *Am J Forensic Med Pathol* **13**:288–9.

Gulmann C, Hougen HP. 1999. Entrance, exit, and reentrance of one shot with a shotgun. *Am J Forensic Med Pathol* **20**:13–16.

Hawley DA, Pless JE, Palmer H. 1987. Tumbling abrasions. Injuries from ricocheting bullets. *Am J Forensic Med Pathol* **8**:229–32.

Hudson P. 1981. Multishot firearm suicide. Examination of 58 cases. *Am J Forensic Med Pathol* **2**:239–42.

Hunt AC, KonVanda M. 1962. The patterns of injury from humane killers. *Med Sci Law* **2**:197–202.

Jacob B, Huckenbeck W, Daldrup T, *et al.* 1990. Suicides by starter's pistols and air guns. *Am J Forensic Med Pathol* **11**:285–90.

James WR. 1962. Fatal air rifle pellet wound of the brain. *Med Sci Law* **2**:153–4.

Janssen W, Kulle KJ, Gehl A, *et al.* 2001. [Unintentional gunshot during police intervention.] *Arch Kriminol* **207**:1–11.

Janssen W, Miyaishi S, Koops E, *et al.* 1996. [Gunshot fatalities in connection with hunting and hunting rifles – causes, prevention and expert evaluation.] *Arch Kriminol* **197**:1–15.

Johnson GC. 1985. Unusual shotgun injury. Gas blowout of anterior head region. *Am J Forensic Med Pathol* **6**:244–7.

Jones AM, Graham NJ, Looney JR. 1983. Arterial embolism of a high-velocity rifle bullet after a hunting accident. Case report and literature review. *Am J Forensic Med Pathol* **4**:259–64.

Kage S, Kudo K, Kaizoji A, *et al.* 2001. A simple method for detection of gunshot residue particles from hands, hair, face, and clothing using scanning electron microscopy/wavelength dispersive X-ray (SEM/WDX). *J Forensic Sci* **46**:830–4.

Karger B, Stehmann B, Hohoff C, *et al.* 2001. Trajectory reconstruction from trace evidence on spent bullets. II. Are tissue deposits eliminated by subsequent impacts? *Int J Legal Med* **114**:343–5.

Kleiber M, Stiller D, Wiegand P. 2001. Assessment of shooting distance on the basis of bloodstain analysis and histological examinations. *Forensic Sci Int* **119**:260–2.

Knight B. 1982. Explosive bullets: a new hazard for doctors [editorial]. *Br Med J Clin Res Ed* **284**:768–9.

Lee KA, Opeskin K. 1995. Gunshot suicide with nasal entry. *Forensic Sci Int* **71**:25–31.

Madea B, Staak M. 1988. Determination of the sequence of gunshot wounds of the skull. *J Forensic Sci Soc* **28**:321–8.

Marshall T. 1988. A pathologist's view of terrorist violence. *Forensic Sci Int* **36**:57–67.

Marshall TK. 1976. Deaths from explosive devices. *Med Sci Law* **16**:235–9.

Marshall TK. 1978. Violence and civil disturbance. In: Mason JK (ed.), *The pathology of violent injury.* Edward Arnold, London.

Marshall TK. 1978. The investigation of bombings. In: Wecht C (ed.), *Legal medicine annual 1979*. Appleton Century Crofts, New York.

McCorkell SJ, Harley JD, Cummings D. 1986. Nail-gun injuries. Accident, homicide, or suicide? *Am J Forensic Med Pathol* **7**:192–5.

Menzies RC, Scroggie RJ, Labowitz DI. 1981. Characteristics of silenced firearms and their wounding effects. *J Forensic Sci* **26**:239–62.

Millar R, Rutherford WH, Johnson S, *et al.* 1975. Injuries caused by rubber bullets: a report on 90 patients. *Br J Surg* **62**:480–6.

Milroy CM, Clark JC, Carter N, *et al.* 1998. Air weapon fatalities. *J Clin Pathol* **51**:525–9.

Murphy GK. 1980. The study of gunshot wounds in surgical pathology. *Am J Forensic Med Pathol* **1**:123–30.

Oehmichen M, Meissner C, Konig HG. 2000. Brain injury after gunshot wounding: morphometric analysis of cell destruction caused by temporary cavitation. *J Neurotrauma* **17**:155–62.

Opeskin K, Cordner S. 1990. Nail-gun suicide [see comments]. *Am J Forensic Med Pathol* **11**:282–4.

Ornehult L, Eriksson A. 1987. Accidental firearm fatalities during hunting. *Am J Forensic Med Pathol* **8**:112–19.

Owen-Smith MS. 1981. *High velocity missile wounds*. Edward Arnold, London.

Petty CS. 1966. Firearms and the forensic pathologists. American Society of Clinical Pathologists. *Council on Forensic Pathology Meeting*. Commission on Continuing Medical Education, Washington.

Petty CS. 1969. Firearms injury research: the role of the practicing pathologist. *Am J Clin Pathol* **52**:227–81.

Petty CS, Hauser JE. 1968. Rifled shotgun slugs, wounding and forensic ballistics. *J Forensic Sci* **13**:114–23.

Pollak S, Ropohl D, Bohnert M. 1999. Pellet embolization to the right atrium following double shotgun injury. *Forensic Sci Int* **99**:61–9.

Quatrehomme G, Iscan MY. 1997. Bevelling in exit gunshot wounds in bones. *Forensic Sci Int* **89**:93–101.

Quatrehomme G, Iscan MY. 1998. Analysis of beveling in gunshot entrance wounds. *Forensic Sci Int* **93**:45–60.

Quatrehomme G, Iscan MY. 1998. Gunshot wounds to the skull: comparison of entries and exits. *Forensic Sci Int* **94**:141–6.

Rao VJ, May CL, DiMaio VJ. 1984. The behavior of the expanding point 25 ACP ammunition in the human body. *Am J Forensic Med Pathol* **5**:37–9.

Ratanaproeksa O, Hood I, Mirchandani H. 1988. Single gunshots with multiple entrances. *Am J Forensic Med Pathol* **9**:212–14.

Rocke L. 1983. Injuries caused by plastic bullets compared with those caused by rubber bullets. *Lancet* **1**:919–20.

Rosenhead J. 1985. Plastic bullets – a reasonable force? *New Scient* **17**:26–7.

Rothschild MA, Liesenfeld O. 1996. Is the exploding powder gas of the propellant from blank cartridges sterile? *Forensic Sci Int* **83**:1–13.

Shaw J. 1972. Pulmonary contusion in children caused by rubber bullets. *Br Med J* **4**:764–5.

Smith OC, Berryman HE, Lahren CH. 1987. Cranial fracture patterns and estimate of direction from low velocity gunshot wounds. *J Forensic Sci* **32**:1416–21.

Spitz WU, Wilhelm RM. 1970. Stud gun injuries. *J Forensic Med* **17**:5–11.

Stahling S, Karlsson T. 2000. A method for collection of gunshot residues from skin and other surfaces. *J Forensic Sci* **45**:1299–302.

Steindler R. 1983. The case of the mysterious dum-dum bullet. *Am J Forensic Med Pathol* **4**:205–6.

Steindler RA. 1982. An expanding .25 ACP bullet. *Am J Forensic Med Pathol* **3**:119–21.

Stephens BG. 1983. Back spatter of blood from gunshot wound observations and experimental simulation. *J Forensic Sci* **28**:437–9.

Stone IC. 1992. Characteristics of firearms and gunshot wounds as markers of suicide. *Am J Forensic Med Pathol* **13**:275–80.

Subke J, Haase S, Wehner HD, *et al.* 2002. Computer aided shot reconstructions by means of individualized animated three-dimensional victim models. *Forensic Sci Int* **125**:245–9.

Thali MJ, Kneubuehl BP, Dirnhofer R, *et al.* 2001. Body models in forensic ballistics: reconstruction of a gunshot injury to the chest by bullet fragmentation after shooting through a finger. *Forensic Sci Int* **123**:54–7.

Thali MJ, Kneubuehl BP, Zollinger U, *et al.* 2002. The 'skin-skull-brain model': a new instrument for the study of gunshot effects. *Forensic Sci Int* **125**:178–89.

Thali MJ, Kneubuehl BP, Zollinger U, *et al.* 2002. A study of the morphology of gunshot entrance wounds, in connection with their dynamic creation, utilizing the 'skin-skull-brain model'. *Forensic Sci Int* **125**:190–4.

Torre C, Varetto L, Ricchiardi P. 1986. New observations on cutaneous firearm wounds. *Am J Forensic Med Pathol* 7:186–91.

Ulrich U, Zollinger U. 2001. [Development of rust stains on the skin due to contact with a gun.] *Arch Kriminol* **208**:32–41.

Warren MW, Falsetti AB, Kravchenko II, *et al.* 2002. Elemental analysis of bone: proton-induced x-ray emission testing in forensic cases. *Forensic Sci Int* **125**:37–41.

Zuckerman S. 1940. Experimental study of blast injuries to the lung. *Lancet* **2**:219–24.

Transportation injuries

Injuries and fatalities occur in all forms of transportation but numerically road traffic accidents account for the great majority worldwide. In developed countries, they are the most common cause of death below the age of 50 years, and in young men this trend is even more marked. The pattern of injury, fatal and otherwise, varies considerably depending upon whether the victim is a vehicle occupant, a motorcyclist, a pedal cyclist or a pedestrian.

THE DYNAMICS OF VEHICULAR INJURY

A number of elementary physical facts help to explain the complex pattern of traffic injuries, especially those sustained by the occupants of a vehicle.

- Tissue injury is caused by a change of rate of movement. A constant speed, however rapid, has no effect whatsoever as is evident from space travel or the rotation of the earth. It is the change of rate that is traumatic – that is, acceleration or deceleration.
- Change of rate is conveniently measured in 'gravities' or 'G forces'. The amount that a human body can tolerate depends greatly on the direction in which the force acts. Deceleration of the order of 300 G can be sustained without injury and even 2000 G can be survived for a short time, if it acts at right angles to the long axis of the body. The frontal bone may resist 800 G without fracture and the mandible 400 G, as can the thoracic cage.

- During acceleration or deceleration the tissue damage produced will depend upon the force applied per unit area, just as a sharp knife penetrates more easily than a blunt one used with the same force. If a car driver is brought to rest from 80 km/hour by striking 10 cm² of his head on the windscreen frame, the damage will be vastly more severe than if the same decelerative force was spread over 500 cm² of a safety belt.
- Between 60 and 80 per cent of vehicular crashes (either into a fixed structure or into another vehicle) are frontal, causing violent deceleration. Another 6 per cent are rear impacts, which accelerate the vehicle and its occupants. Of the remainder, about half are sideswipes and the rest 'roll-overs'.
- In the common frontal impact, there is never instant arrest of the vehicle, even when it runs into a massive, immovable structure. The vehicle itself deforms from the front so that there is always a deceleration distance and time, albeit small. In fact, much of the manufacturers' design research now goes into making deliberate provision for the crumpling or 'concertinaing' of the front and rear of the car, leaving a central rigid cell that comprises the passenger compartment. The object is to extend the stopping distance and time, so that the G value acting on the occupants is reduced.
- The value of the G forces can be calculated from the formula: $G = C(V^2)/D$, where V is velocity in km/hour, D is the stopping distance in metres after impact, and C is a constant 0.0039. (If V is in mph and D is in feet, C becomes 0.034.) For example, if a car

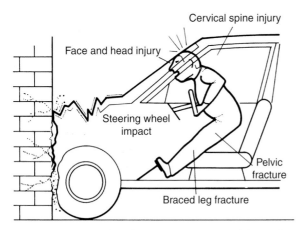

FIGURE 9.1 *Major points of injury to an unrestrained driver of a vehicle in deceleration impact.*

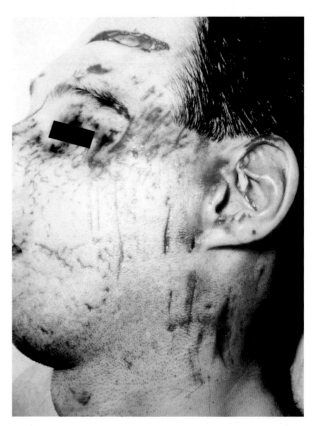

FIGURE 9.2 *Facial lacerations from a shattered windscreen in an unrestrained driver. The toughened glass breaks into small fragments, which produce the characteristic 'sparrow-foot' marks. The laceration on the forehead was made by the windscreen rim.*

travelling at 80 km/hour runs into a stone wall that it penetrates for 25 cm, plus 50 cm crumpling of the front of the car, the deceleration would amount to about 33 G. If an occupant was rigidly belted into his seat (a practical impossibility), he would also suffer the same deceleration, which would be survivable. If, however, he was unrestrained, he would continue forwards momentarily at 80 km/hour and suffer massive G forces, the magnitude of which would depend on his deformation stopping distance (a few centimetres of tissue compression) when he struck the internal car structures in front of him.

PATTERN OF INJURY OF VEHICLE OCCUPANTS

The type of vehicle (other than motorcycles) in theory makes little difference to the mechanism of injury, but most statistical surveys divide them into cars and light vans under 1.5 tonnes, on the one hand and heavier vehicles, such as trucks and buses, on the other, though the latter have different features more akin to passenger aircraft.

Heavy goods vehicles naturally suffer less than cars and light vans in crashes because of their far greater mass and strength, and also due to their height above the ground. Structural damage from impact with other smaller vehicles is less and often sustained below the level of the driver. Given smaller deceleration forces, however, the cab occupants are vulnerable to the same injury patterns.

Light vans are virtually identical to cars with respect to the front-seat occupants. In fact they may be more at risk, as modern vans tend to be flat-fronted and thus have little or no 'crumple' potential to increase the stopping time. Concentrating on cars, the most common vehicular casualty,

the pattern of injury varies according to the position of the occupant.

The driver

Numerous investigations have been made by road research organizations and car manufacturers using dummies and actual corpses, together with sophisticated recording equipment and high-speed cinematography. These have established a detailed picture of the sequence of events in automobile crashes. When the most common event – frontal impact – occurs, the unrestrained driver first slides forwards so that his legs strike the fascia/parcel-shelf area, and his abdomen or lower chest contacts the lower edge of the steering wheel. The body then flexes across the steering wheel and begins to rise. The heavy head goes forwards, and there is flexion of the cervical and thoracic spines. The upward and forward component causes the head to strike the windscreen, the upper windscreen rim or the side pillar. The windscreen is often perforated by the head or face, and the whole body may be ejected through the broken glass, to land on the bonnet or even on the roadway ahead.

Another factor causing injury is the intrusion of structural parts into the passenger compartment. Though modern cars are designed to maintain a rigid central passenger compartment, if the impact is gross, the engine or front-wheel assembly may be forced back into the seating area, intruding upon the driver. Similarly, the roof or front corner pillar (the so-called 'A'-frame) may cave in on top of the driver.

One effect of column, engine, or gearbox intrusion may be to force the floor up and backwards against the driver's feet and legs. The control pedals also take part in intrusion, and, in the usual desperate braking and declutching, the reflex pressure of feet on rising pedals and floor may cause transmitted force up the legs and into the pelvic girdle. The steering column was formerly a more dangerous item for intrusion, being forced back to 'stab' or crush the driver's chest or abdomen. Modern design has reduced this danger

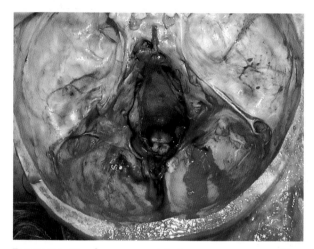

FIGURE 9.3 *Ring fracture around the foramen magnum caused by an impact on the crown of the head in a car driver, who lost the control of his vehicle and crashed into a tree.*

by making the column telescopic, hinged or otherwise collapsible, but injuries still occur – sometimes from the wheel itself breaking and penetrating the chest. Additionally, the door may burst open and the driver, if unrestrained, ejected sideways onto the road, especially in a crash that has a roll-over component.

In a rear impact, the driver is violently accelerated and, if no rigid head restraint is fitted to the seat, severe hyper-extension of the neck occurs, often followed by the sequence of deceleration events when the car is cannoned into the vehicle or other obstruction in front, causing the popular, if inaccurate name of 'whiplash'.

In side impacts, the injuries depend upon the amount of intrusion of the driver's door and side panels. Restraint devices can offer no protection, though modern vehicles usually have strengthened side-impact bars built within the doors.

This range of traumatic events can produce the following lesions in drivers not wearing seatbelts or protected by airbags:

- Impact against the fascia can cause abrasions, lacerations and fractures of the legs around knee or upper shin level.
- Pressure of feet on the floor, especially when it is intruded by the engine, can cause fractures anywhere from foot to femur. The leg can also be injured by violent contact with the fascia or dashboard and the hip joint may be dislocated posteriorly. Not uncommonly the pelvis is fractured, often at one or both sacroiliac joints. In Mant's (1978) series of 100 driver fatalities there were 22 pelvic injuries and 31 of the lower limb.
- Impact of the abdomen and chest against the steering wheel may cause severe internal injuries, usually rupture of the liver (50 per cent) and, less often, spleen (36 per cent). There may be bruising of the skin surface, but this is often absent even in the presence of

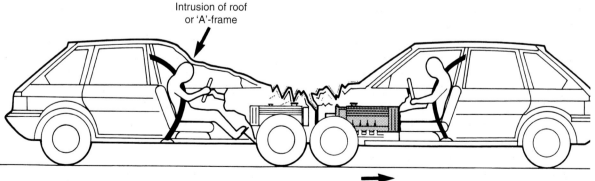

Intrusion of roof or 'A'-frame

Intrusion of engine and front suspension

FIGURE 9.4 *When vehicle structures impinge on the occupants even belt restraints offer little protection. The engine, front suspension, roof and 'A' frame are frequent intruders.*

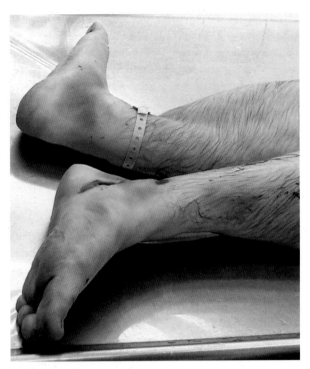

FIGURE 9.5 *Bruising, laceration and bilateral leg fractures of a car driver in a frontal impact.*

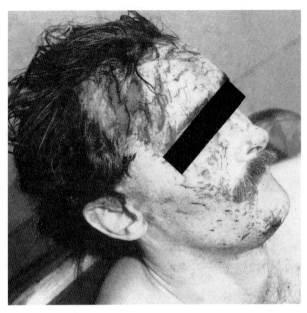

FIGURE 9.6 *Facial injuries in a car driver unrestrained by a seatbelt. Following a deceleration impact his face struck the windscreen, causing the typical small cuts from broken safety glass and lacerations of the temple from striking the windscreen rim or 'A' frame.*

severe internal injuries. Laceration of the skin is rare unless the steering wheel snaps and penetrates the trunk. Other steering-wheel lesions include bruising of the lungs, fractured ribs and sternum, cardiac contusion and haemothorax or pneumothorax or both. Almost 70 per cent of Mant's series had broken ribs.

- Upper limb injuries are less common but may occur from transmitted force through gripping the steering wheel or from impact against the windscreen, pillars, intrusive roof, bonnet or ground when held up in a reflex protective position. Only 19 per cent of Mant's series had arm injuries.
- The most obvious injuries are often those to the face and head as a result of projection against and ejection through, the windscreen. The unrestrained driver rises and flexes forwards so that his forehead and skull are likely to contact the upper rim of the windscreen, leading to lacerations. The face frequently suffers multiple cuts from contact with the shattered safety glass. In most European vehicles the glass is of the toughened, not laminated, variety and, when broken, it shatters into small cubes with relatively blunt edges. These still cause superficial lacerations, often in short 'V-shaped' or 'sparrow-foot' patterns. In themselves they are not a danger to life, but indicate an impact sufficient to hurl the driver on or through the glass. Damage to the eyes is common.

- The impact against the windscreen rim or corner pillar – or after ejection – can cause any type or degree of head injury, including scalp laceration, fractured skull, intracranial haemorrhage or brain damage. In Mant's series there were 42 skull fractures in 100 drivers. This was less than in the front-seat passengers, a figure at variance with Eckert's (1959) series of 300 in the USA, where drivers suffered twice as many head injuries as the passenger, though it is not stated how many accidents were to vehicles occupied only by the driver.
- Hyperflexion of the cervical spine when the head swings can cause fractures or dislocation. There is often a double component in that the hyperflexion of deceleration is followed by a rebound hyperextension when the head strikes an obstruction in front. Rear impacts also cause the double 'whiplash' effect, as already mentioned.

One injury that is frequently overlooked at autopsy is the atlanto-occipital dislocation, which Mant found in a third of his series. Other fractures can occur anywhere in the cervical spine, often at about C5–6. Seatbelt restraint cannot prevent cervical spine damage, though a rigid head restraint can reduce injuries resulting from hyperextension. The thoracic spine is less often damaged, but in unrestrained drivers the same 'whiplash' effect can fracture or dislocate the upper dorsal spine, often around T5–6–7.

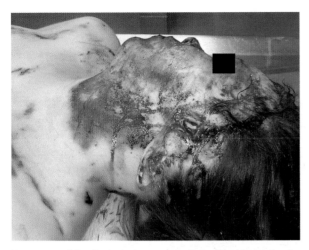

FIGURE 9.7 *Mixed injuries in a restrained car driver from a head-on collision. Death was caused by ruptured aorta.*

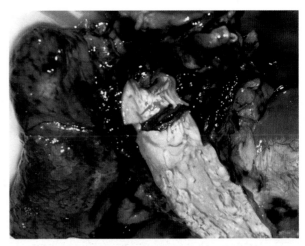

FIGURE 9.8 *Ruptured aorta in which car occupant, unrestrained by seatbelt, suffered severe deceleration. Aorta has torn in the usual place, the distal arch where the curve of the vessel meets the thoracic spine.*

A more common thoracic injury associated with deceleration is the ruptured aorta. It may be associated with a severe whiplash effect on the thoracic spine, as the aorta is tethered to the anterior surface of the vertebrae where the distal arch joins the straight descending segment. Probably the most common reason for aortic rupture, however, is the 'pendulum' effect of the heart within the relatively pliable thoracic contents. When the thorax is violently decelerated, the heavy cardiac mass attempts to keep moving ahead and may literally pull itself off its basal mountings, the most rigid part of which is the aorta. Separation takes place at the point where the aorta is attached to the spine at the termination of the arch.

The appearance of the aortic rupture is often of a clean-cut circular break, almost as sharp as if it had been transected with a scalpel. Sometimes there are additional transverse intimal tears adjacent to the main rupture, the so-called 'ladder tears', as they can resemble the rungs of a ladder. These may be present when no actual rupture has occurred and may be found as an incidental finding at autopsy. Sometimes they are deep enough to allow a local dissection of blood to seep into the intima, when death has not been virtually instantaneous. Rarely, a major dissection may lead to delayed death some hours or even days later. Ruptured aorta is a common lesion in traffic accidents – in a two-car crash, the author (BK) has seen three transected aortas among the four fatalities.

The frequency of such tears is common enough for a warning always to be offered to the autopsy prosector not to use undue force on the neck and thoracic structures when removing the organ pluck from the body. Rough handling during this stage can produce artefactual ladder tears in the aorta.

■ Other chest injuries can be caused by impact with the steering wheel, ejection through the windscreen or impact with the road. There may be bruising or laceration on the chest from the steering wheel, though padding, collapsible columns, less fragile wheels, airbags and seatbelts have reduced the incidence of this formerly common lesion. Beneath the skin, sternal and rib fractures are common, though fatal visceral injuries can occur without rib fractures in young people because their ribs are more pliable.

■ The heart may be damaged even in the absence of external marks or thoracic cage fractures. Bruising of the epicardium and underlying myocardium is not uncommon and the posterior surface may be damaged from impact against the spine. In high-speed impacts, the heart may be completely avulsed from its base and be found lying loose in the chest. Less severe degrees of damage may lacerate the ventricles or atria, and cause gross haemorrhage. Coronary artery thrombosis has been described following contusion over a coronary artery. Penetrating injuries from sternum, ribs or external objects may lacerate the heart directly. Subendocardial haemorrhages on the left side of the interventricular septum and opposing papillary muscles are not a sign of impact, but an index of catastrophic hypotension. They are also seen in head injuries; they can occur within the space of a few beats, as the author (BK) has seen these prominent lesions in an avulsed heart after a military aircraft crash.

■ The lungs are frequently injured, either from stabbing by fractured ribs penetrating the pleura or from blunt impact. The latter often leads to a line of bruising down the posterior part of the lung where it lies in the paravertebral gutter. There may be air bullae or blood blisters under the pleura overlying the bruised areas and a pneumothorax or haemothorax may result. The interior of the lung may be pulped even in the presence of an intact visceral pleura, from transmitted force or massive variations in intrathoracic pressure during the impact. The lung often shows areas of bleeding under the pleura, which may be from direct contusion, from aspiration of blood from other damaged areas of lung or from blood sucked down the air passages from injuries in the nose or mouth.

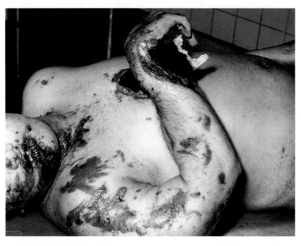

FIGURE 9.9 *Penetration of the wrist and chest by a wooden component of a bus seat. The victim drove his car at speed into a bus and part of the resulting debris penetrated his left ventricle.*

■ The major abdominal injury is a ruptured liver, which may be damaged in any part. A common lesion is central tearing of the upper surface, which may extend deeply and even transect the organ. Less serious damage is often seen in the form of shallow, sometimes multiple, parallel tears on the upper surface of the right lobe. Subcapsular tears can occur with the formation of a subcapsular haematoma, which can rupture later. The spleen also shows shallow tears in some accidents, often around the hilum; in rare cases, it may be avulsed from the pedicle. The mesentery and omentum often show bruising and, rarely, there is laceration and fenestration sufficient to cause a lethal haemorrhage.

■ Ejection injuries are common, and lethal in both driver and passengers. This is particularly likely to happen in roll-over accidents. Much research has been pursued by manufacturers to develop anti-burst door locks, which have improved safety. Where there has been considerable distortion of the vehicle frame, however, nothing can prevent the doors from opening or even being torn off. It has been shown by Moore and Tourin's study (1954) at Cornell that ejection injuries followed steering-column lesions as the second most frequent type of trauma and, if a victim was ejected, there was a fivefold greater chance of dying than if he was retained in the vehicle. Moore and Tourin found that when doors burst open a third of the car occupants were ejected.

Almost any kind of injury, usually multiple, may be sustained after ejection, either from contact with the road surface or (in a significant proportion) from being struck by other vehicles, especially on motorways.

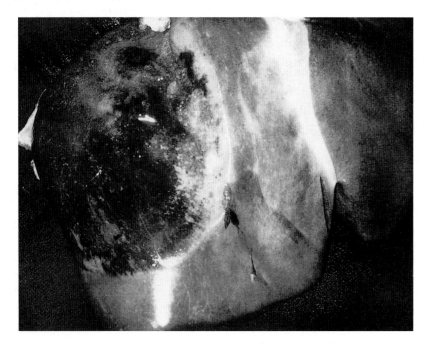

FIGURE 9.10 *Large subcapsular haemorrhage of the liver in a driver who struck the rim of the steering wheel during severe deceleration. Such subcapsular lesions can remain intact for hours or even days, then rupture into the abdominal cavity.*

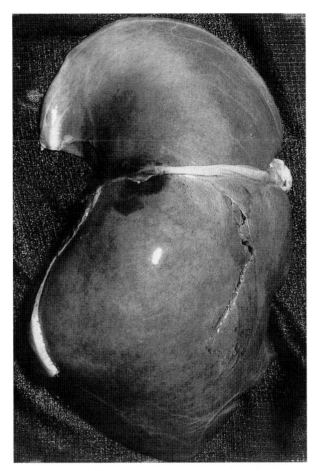

FIGURE 9.11 *Anterior tear through the full thickness of the liver; there is also a haemorrhage around the suspensory ligament. The victim was a car driver who was impacted against the steering wheel in a frontal crash.*

The front-seat passenger

In Western countries, far more drivers than passengers are killed or injured, but this reflects the fact that a high proportion of cars contain only a driver – a third in Mant's series. In countries with a lower ratio of vehicles to population the converse is true and indeed many accidents are due to gross overcrowding of passenger vehicles. The pattern of injuries is similar to that of the driver, but this position in the car is even more dangerous, as indicated by the title of a safety film made by the French Michelin Tyre Company – *La place du mort*.

Though there is no steering wheel to impact into the chest, its absence also denies the slight protection offered to the driver in reducing the collision with the windscreen, perhaps by giving him something to brace against. Another factor may be that the driver gives his attention constantly to the road and so has momentary warning of an impending crash, compared with the passenger who may be oblivious of imminent disaster and fail to 'brace up' ready for the

impact. This may explain the greater number of skull fractures and brain damage in unrestrained passengers in Mant's series, the percentages being 55 per cent and 42 per cent, compared with 64 per cent and 53 per cent, respectively. However, these figures were compiled before seatbelts and airbags became commonplace or even mandatory.

Rear-seat occupants

Before the more widespread use of front seatbelts – now mandatory in many countries – it was thought that the rear-seat position was fairly safe, as indeed it is compared with the front seats.

When the widespread use of seatbelts dramatically reduced the deaths and serious injuries amongst front-seat occupants, the dangers of the back seats became much more obvious. One series showed that 49 per cent of rear-seat passengers in car crashes sustained serious or moderately serious injuries. Campaigns and legislation similar to the previous crusade were waged on behalf of the rear-seat occupants, and the use of these has now become mandatory in Britain and some other countries.

During violent deceleration, unrestrained occupants in the rear are projected forwards and strike the back of the front seats, including head-rests where fitted. They may be thrown over the seats, striking and adding further injuries to the front-seat occupants and may even be ejected through the windscreen, which is broken by them or by the people in front.

In roll-over accidents, they share in the general trauma of being churned inside the passenger compartment, when multiple injuries can occur from contact with fitments, such as mirrors, door handles and window winders. Design changes have reduced these hazards by making handles smoother or countersunk and mirrors that easily snap off their mountings. Ejection is another common cause of death and serious injury in rear-seat occupants, a wide range of head, chest and limb injuries being seen.

THE EFFECT OF SEATBELTS

As stated, many countries now have legislation making the wearing of front and rear seatbelts mandatory. Where no laws exist, persuasion seems to have little effect, in spite of the fact that it is uncontested that their use reduces deaths and serious injury by a factor of 20–25 per cent, as seen in the Australian experience in Victoria and New South Wales. A similar reduction was attained in Britain after the introduction of mandatory laws. Not only did the death rate drop substantially, but facial injuries and especially eye damage was dramatically reduced.

Seatbelts are now almost all of the lap-strap and shoulder diagonal type, the so-called 'three-point attachment belt'. The simple lap-strap is now fitted only in aircraft, where it is really only of token effectiveness. Most car belts are now of the 'inertia-reel' type, which allow slow movement but jam at a sudden tug. The advantage, apart from the comfort, is that they automatically tighten up around the body, as a slack belt is not only less effective but can actually constitute a danger. More complex restraints, such as double shoulder harness and crotch strap, are fitted only in light aircraft, gliders and racing cars. Though far more effective, their use would be socially unacceptable in ordinary road vehicles, as would head-band restraints, which are almost the only way of preventing hyperflexion damage to the cervical spine.

The various forms of strap restraints act by:

▪ Holding the occupant back against the seat, so that forward projection against the steering wheel, windscreen and corner 'A' frame is prevented. The head, though still subject to hyperflexion, is prevented from smashing through the glass and the body cannot be projected through the screen onto the bonnet or roadway. The belt cannot cope with backward intrusion of the engine, floor, roof or corner pillar if those structures reach the occupant sitting in the original seat position. The effectiveness of the belt is also dependent on the secure fixation of the seat to the vehicle floor.

▪ The belt restrains the occupants within the vehicle in the event of a door bursting, as ejection greatly increases the risk of death or serious injury. A belt is relatively ineffective in a side impact, except in that it reduces injuries from ejection. It has been reported, however, that head injuries were fewer in restrained victims of side-swipes, though the reason is not clear.

It has been claimed (mainly in insurance disputes) that seatbelts can worsen this sort of injury by holding the occupant in more dangerous proximity to the intruding impact. There would seem few occasions, however, in which even the unrestrained occupant could voluntarily escape from any significant degree of sudden lateral intrusion from a speeding vehicle.

▪ Extending the deceleration time and distance by substantial stretching of the belt fabric, which may lengthen by many centimetres during a violent arrest. To be effective the belt must be held tightly against the body to get the maximum restraint, either by adjusting the buckle or using an inertia reel. The belt should never be used again, as it cannot stretch further and may break on the next application of tension.

▪ Spreading the area of application of deceleration forces. As stated earlier, the body has to absorb whatever G forces are applied to it, as calculated by the $G = C(V^2)/D$ equation. If these are absorbed by a focal impact covering a few square centimetres over the skull, fatal injury may well ensue. The same deceleration diffused against the thorax and abdomen by 500 cm² of belt may leave no injury or merely surface bruising.

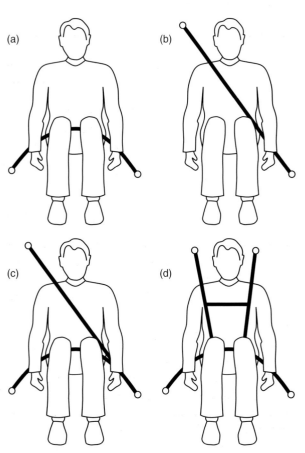

FIGURE 9.12 *Types of seatbelt restraint: (a) simple lap-strap (dangerous to aorta), (b) diagonal only (can slip underneath), (c) diagonal plus lap-strap (usual car type), and (d) shoulder harness (used in aircraft and racing cars).*

Seatbelt injuries

There is no doubt that seatbelts can themselves cause injury, occasionally of considerable severity. This was one of the arguments of the vociferous anti-seatbelt lobby that opposed legislation in several countries, but it is largely illogical, because an impact that causes seatbelt injuries would almost invariably have caused even worse injuries or death if no seatbelt had been worn.

Another invalid criticism of restraints was that they impede escape from a burning vehicle. Fires involving passenger car crashes are, however, quite rare. A report by Bako *et al.* (1970) from Canada showed that, of 1297 vehicle fatalities, only 24 were from burns, a mere three in passenger cars.

Incorrectly adjusted or positioned straps such as a twisted belt, which reduces the area of contact, can increase the danger of injury. Loose straps allow the body to move relative to the belt before sudden restraint occurs, decreasing the distance between the passenger and facing structures.

Where the person is too small for the harness, such as a child or a small woman, the body may slide from under the strap – the so-called 'submarining' – or it may act as a garrotte around the neck. Some women find that the diagonal strap compresses the breast even in normal use, so that the greatly increased tension during deceleration is likely to injure the gland.

Pregnant women also have problems with belts but, although uterine and fetal injuries have been recorded in accidents, the incidence is relatively low and without the belt the consequences would have been as bad or probably worse.

Injuries from seatbelts can vary from the trivial to the fatal. Bruising is the most common and may be seen either under the diagonal or the transverse component of the three-point belt. It is more common with the single aircraft-type lap-strap because of the smaller area of pressure. Bruising may occur in the abdominal or chest wall, but the dangerous lesions are visceral. The abdominal contents suffer most, especially from single lap-straps. Rupture of the mesentery, or the small or large intestine, usually occurs from acute flexion over a lap-strap. The full bladder can be ruptured as can the caecum. The abdominal aorta can be crushed and the lumbar spine suffer a compression fracture or be dislocated through a disc in the midlumbar region. The posterior arch, pedicles or transverse processes may also be damaged.

The diagonal strap usually prevents serious abdominal injury as it prevents hyperflexion, but it may contribute to thoracic injury. Bruising of the skin and underlying muscles and fractures may accompany a broken clavicle or sternum where the belt crosses them. Several authors (listed at the end of this section) have made detailed studies of seatbelt injuries.

Airbags

In recent years, the use of airbags has spread from only the most expensive vehicles to many standard production cars. The device consists of a large fabric bag, which is normally folded into the steering-wheel hub in the case of the driver position and into the fascia in front of the front-seat passenger.

A sensitive deceleration device triggers the ignition of sodium azide, a solid and highly toxic explosive propellant, which is converted in milliseconds to nitrogen gas. The deploying airbag can reach speeds up to over 300 km/h (>200 mph). Deflation is also rapid, so that residual car control and escape from the vehicle is not impeded.

The inflated bag is designed to interpose itself between the occupant and the frontal structures of the passenger cabin, to cushion the impact and prevent forceful contact and hyperflexion.

In addition to the life-saving capabilities, airbags can also cause serious and even fatal injuries either by the airbag itself or the module cover overlying it in the steering wheel or in the fascia on the passenger side. Injuries can be inflicted at any stage of the deployment process, depending on the posture and possible objects between the occupant and the deploying airbag or the module cover. They vary from facial bruising, partial or complete amputation of fingers to dislocated and fractured arms or cervical spine and fatal head injuries. Eye injuries are common and range from mild corneal abrasions and chemical burns from contact with unburned sodium azide or the alkaline byproducts of combustion, which are released into the passenger compartment, to globe rupture from blunt trauma or perforation by interposed objects.

THE VULNERABILITY OF CHILDREN IN VEHICLES

This is a particular problem with several aspects. Many countries have brought in laws to protect children in cars because of their special vulnerability.

First, it is an understandable, but highly dangerous, indulgence for adults to allow small children to travel unrestrained in the front seat of a car. Some parents even allow them to stand gripping the fascia edge immediately below the windscreen, an invitation to facial and eye damage even in minor accidents. The seating of a child on the mother's lap is hazardous, as on violent deceleration either mother and child pitch against the windscreen – or the child flies out of the arms of a belt-restrained mother. The close proximity to the fascia and windscreen causes many deaths and facial injuries, especially to the eyes.

Adult-secured seatbelts will not properly accommodate a child (or even a small adult), because the fixation point on the door pillar is too high even if the straps can be shortened sufficiently to be made tight. The diagonal may pass across the throat and, unless special drop-plates are fitted to the door pillars, the restraint is often worse than useless.

Though some European countries already forbid children under 14 years to travel in front seats, the medical profession in Britain campaigned for similar legislation, as they had done for motorcyclists to wear helmets many years before.

As discussed above, a similar campaign has been successfully waged for rear-seat restraints for children and adults. Banished from the front, children were thought to be safe in the back of the car, but many have died and far more have been injured from being projected against the seat backs, front passengers and internal fitments. Special seats secured on top of the regular seating are required and, for a baby, the cot must be lashed down with equally robust restraints. In 1988, legislation was introduced into the British Parliament to make compulsory the restraint of children in rear seats: from 1991, this law also became applicable to adults.

INJURIES TO MOTORCYCLISTS

Though there are fewer motorcycles than four-wheeled vehicles, especially in developed countries, the rate of injury and death amongst motorcyclists is far higher than among car drivers. For example, in England and Wales in 1989 there were more deaths amongst male motorcyclists between the ages of 16 and 24 than with comparable car drivers (343 compared with 323) even though the ratio of motorcycles to cars is very small in Britain. In the 25–44 age group, 192 motorcyclists died compared with 381 car drivers.

The two extremities of the body suffer most in motorcycle accidents, though Larsen and Hardt-Madsen's analysis in Denmark in 1988 also showed high injury rates for chest and abdomen.

■ Because the rider inevitably falls to the ground, head injuries are common and often severe, causing 80 per cent of deaths according to Bothwell (1962). Though crash helmets are mandatory in most countries, the severity of the impact often defeats the protective effect of the helmet.

Impact with the road surface or another vehicle at speed causes skull fractures at any part of the head, but often temporoparietal. A common complication is a basal skull fracture, especially a 'hinge' fracture. This transverse crack across the floor of the skull, crossing the petrous base or behind the greater wing of the sphenoid bones through the pituitary fossa to the opposite side, has also been called 'the motorcyclist's fracture'.

Another type is the ring fracture around the foramen magnum in the posterior fossa caused by an impact on the crown of the head. The neck suffers quite often and Mant found cervical spine fractures in over a quarter of his series. Brain damage may be severe, even with a helmet in place. Cortical contusion and laceration, sometimes contrecoup, may be gross enough to cause brain tissue to extrude through compound fractures of the skull. In Mant's series of motorcyclists, 60 per cent had skull fractures and almost 80 per cent had brain damage.

■ The legs are often injured, either by primary impact with another vehicle or fixed road structures, or by

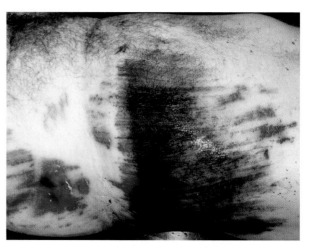

FIGURE 9.13 *Severe brush abrasions or 'friction burns' in a motorcyclist, who came off his machine and skidded across the road surface.*

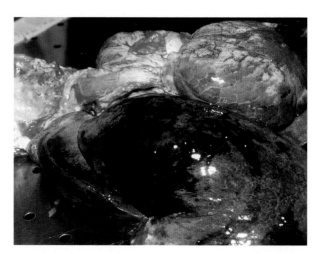

FIGURE 9.14 *Pulmonary contusions in a motorcyclist, who collided with a truck and was hurled into a signpost. Death was caused by a cranial fracture and multiple injuries of the internal organs.*

becoming trapped by part of the motorcycle frame. Lacerations, friction burns and fractures – often compound – are common. Mant recorded leg or pelvic fractures in 55 per cent of his cases.

■ Any part of the body may suffer injury, but less often than the extremities. Falling from the machine, especially at speed, can cause rib fractures and visceral damage, especially rupture of the liver and spleen.

■ An injury common with motorcycles is the 'tail-gating' accident, where a rider drives into the back of a truck so that the machine passes underneath, but the head of the motorcyclist impacts upon the tail-board. Decapitation may occur in the most extreme cases, but severe head and neck injuries are almost inevitable.

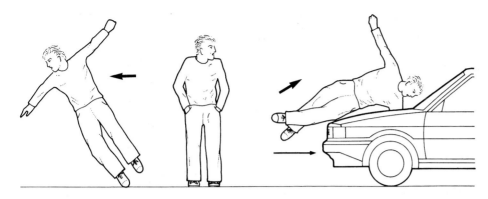

FIGURE 9.15 *A pedestrian struck by the front of a car may be projected forwards or lifted onto the vehicle.*

Trucks in many countries must now have strong bars fitted at the rear to prevent this 'tail-gating', which may also happen to motor cars, the rear of the truck smashing into the windscreen and driver.

Safety helmets act both by providing a rigid barrier against impact, which depends partly on the shock absorbing padding within the helmet and by providing a smooth surface, which is designed to skid across the road surface, thus lengthening the stopping distance and time to reduce the G force of deceleration. Their strength is designed to be finite to control the rate of deceleration but in massive impacts seen at high speeds the helmet may be penetrated or the head and brain damaged by the transmission of blunt force. Crash-bars are another safety measure on motorcycles, being fitted in front of the engine to project on each side and protect the legs if the machine falls over. Unless extremely strong, however, such bars can themselves trap the legs if they bend backwards on impact.

INJURIES TO PEDAL CYCLISTS

These form a less severe counterpart of motorcycle lesions, as the pedal cycle has the same instability but far lower speeds. Once again, head injuries figure largely in accidents, as the height above the ground is considerable and the rider suffers from the passive fall, added to by any forward motion or projection from impact by a motor vehicle. Helmets are now worn by many cyclists and naturally afford considerable protection.

Other injuries are from the primary impact from a striking vehicle, which may hit the rider around thigh, hip or chest level. Secondary damage to the shoulder, chest and arm may occur from striking the ground, when friction grazes are common. (A unique injury, though not fatal, was entrapment of the leg between wheel spokes with compression of the soft tissues of the calf, when the leg penetrated the wheel.)

INJURIES TO PEDESTRIANS

Worldwide these are easily the most common road fatalities, probably accounting for more than 50 per cent of the third of a million road deaths each year. In the densely populated areas of the globe where vehicles are greatly outnumbered by people, such as Southern Asia, parts of Africa, and the Middle East and Central America, pedestrian casualties form a significant part of the total mortality.

Most pedestrians are struck by motor cars or trucks, and the type of vehicle makes a difference to the dynamics of the impact, which – unlike injuries to vehicle occupants – is an **acceleration** not a **deceleration** process.

Primary injuries are caused by the first impact of the vehicle on the victim, while secondary injuries are caused by subsequent contact with the ground. Some writers also use the term 'tertiary injuries' to describe the impact with the ground, reserving 'secondary' for additional contact with the vehicle, as when the pedestrian is hurled up against the windscreen. The usual sequence of events is as follows:

■ The height of the car bumper bar ('fender') is well below the centre of gravity of the adult pedestrian, which lies in the abdominal region. Thus the first impact tends to knock the legs from under the victim and rotate them towards the oncoming vehicle. Depending on the profile of the front of the car, the struck pedestrian is either thrown forwards in the direction of travel if the bonnet-front is high and blunt – or scooped up onto the bonnet top, as with many slope-fronted modern vehicles.

■ If thrown forward, secondary injuries will be suffered as a result of striking the ground, as well as the primary impact on legs and often the hips. If the car speed is appreciable (anything over 20 km/hour is sufficient), the body can be thrown into the air or knocked down flat with a severe impact. The secondary injuries may fracture the skull, ribs, pelvis, arm or thigh.

A further hazard is being run over by the vehicle if the victim is projected directly in front. Sometimes he may be dragged by the under-belly of the car, and seriously soiled and injured, perhaps appearing at the rear if the vehicle does not stop quickly. Many impacts are on the front corner of the car and the pedestrian may then be knocked diagonally out of the path of the car. If thrown into the centre of the roadway, the person can be run down by a different vehicle overtaking in another lane or by one coming in the opposite direction on a single carriageway.

■ If scooped up, the victim will land on either the bonnet or against the windscreen or corner-supporting pillar (the 'A' frame). The flat bonnet usually does relatively little damage, though linear abrasions, brush grazes, or friction burns may be seen. Violent contact with the windscreen, especially the rim or side pillars, is the most frequent cause of severe head injury from primary impact.

Scooping-up can occur at speeds as low as 23 km/hour (about 15 mph; below 19 km/hour the body will usually be projected forwards). If the speed is high, the victim can be thrown up onto the car roof, sometimes somersaulting so that the head strikes the roof. He can then slide or be flung right over the back of the car, landing behind it in the roadway. This is more likely to happen if the car does not brake, but literally drives from under the body.

■ In most cases, the scooped pedestrian falls or is flung off on one side of the car or the other, again to suffer secondary injuries in the road and perhaps be run over by another vehicle. The usual pattern of events is that, at the instant of contact – or even slightly before – the driver will apply the brakes violently. The scooped-up victim will acquire the speed of the car by the time he lands on the bonnet, but then the vehicle decelerates. As the adhesion to the shiny surface is small, the newly acquired velocity of the body will cause it to slide off the front of the car as the latter brakes. The victim then hits the ground in front of the car, sustaining secondary injury – and may even be run over during the residual motion of the vehicle before it finally stops.

■ In a high-speed impact, which may be anything over 50 km/hour (31 mph), the body can be flung high in the air and for a considerable distance, either to the side or in the path of the car – or even backwards over the roof. In general, the severity of the injuries – both primary and secondary – will be the more severe the higher the speed.

It is impossible to estimate the speed of impact from the nature of the injuries. These can be fatal even at slow speeds of the order of 10 km/hour (6 mph), yet

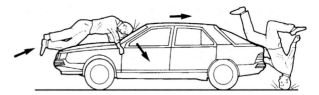

FIGURE 9.16 *At speeds of over 23 km/hour (15 mph) a pedestrian can be 'scooped up' onto a car, suffering head injuries against the windscreen. He may then fall off sideways or – at higher speeds – be thrown over the roof.*

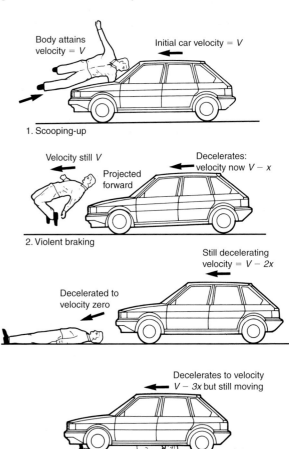

1. Scooping-up

2. Violent braking

4. Running over

FIGURE 9.17 *Sequence of events when a carried pedestrian is projected forwards during braking.*

occasionally high-speed impacts can produce only minor damage. In Ashton's (1975, 1978) series half the deaths occurred at speeds less than 48 km/hour (30 mph).

In child victims, although the general pattern of injuries is similar, their shorter height and smaller weight affects the mechanics of impact. The primary contact is higher up their body, so they tend to be hit forwards rather than rotated upwards, though many do become scooped up onto the bonnet. Children tend to be projected further by impact and may be hurled in

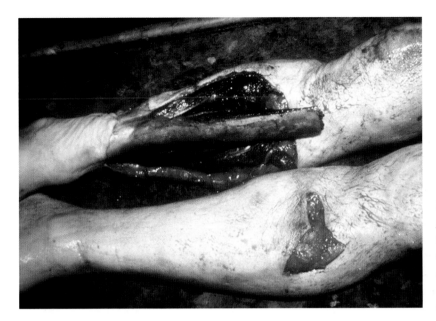

FIGURE 9.18 *Primary injury to a pedestrian struck by a car. There is damage to both legs at about the same level, with a compound fracture of the right leg. These are sometimes called 'bumper fractures'. The height of the injuries above heel level should always be measured at autopsy.*

the air at lower speeds than with adults. They are also more prone to be run over by reversing vehicles, especially trucks, as they often play between parked vehicles and – being small – are less visible to the driver. Recent safety measures on trucks include audible reversing warnings that are automatically linked to the gear-shift lever.

▦ When a pedestrian is struck by a larger vehicle, such as a van, truck or bus, the initial point of impact is higher and may cause primary damage to pelvis, abdomen, shoulder-girdle, arm or head. Because of the profile of these vehicles, there is no scooping-up effect, and the victim is usually projected forwards to suffer secondary damage from road contact and sometimes to be run over.

▦ The nature of pedestrian injuries reflects these dynamic effects.

The most common trauma is to the legs, some 85 per cent of pedestrian casualties having lower limb injuries. Abrasions and lacerations to the upper shin and knee area are typical of car bumper contact, and fractures of the tibia and fibula, often compound, are so common that they are present in a quarter of fatalities, according to Eckert. The femur is fractured less often, but is no rarity. The midshaft may be broken or the head may be driven into the acetabulum, together with a fractured pelvis. In children, because of their small stature, the femur may be fractured by the low bumper bar. At autopsy, the skin of the lower legs should be incised to seek deep bruising, as the clothing often protects the surface from obvious marking.

When a bumper (fender) strikes a leg, the tibia is often fractured in a wedge-shaped manner; the base of the wedge indicates the direction of the impact (often from behind), the front of the wedge pointing away from the side of contact.

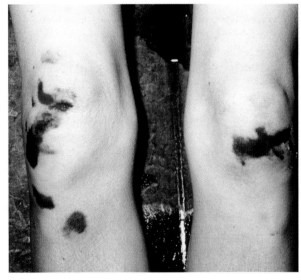

FIGURE 9.19 *Abrasions and laceration at knee level in a pedestrian struck by a car bumper. Their anterior position indicates that the victim was facing the vehicle at the moment of contact, but this may be a last-instant turn during final awareness of the car's proximity.*

If the leg is weight-bearing at the time of the impact, the tibial fracture tends to be oblique, whereas if not stressed, as when being lifted during walking, the fracture line is often transverse. When both shins are damaged, the level may be different on each side; this indicates that the person was moving at the time, with one leg raised in walking or running. Sometimes the level of injury appears too low for the normal bumper height of most cars, but this may indicate that the vehicle was braking violently at the moment of impact, going down on its suspension as the front wheels decelerated or locked, unless dip compensators were fitted.

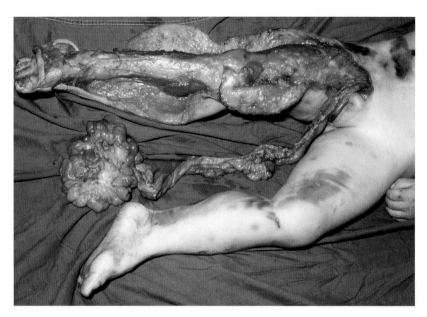

FIGURE 9.20 *Injuries caused by being run over by a bus. The large rotating wheel has 'flayed' the right leg, stripping the skin and subcutaneous tissues from the muscles. The passage of the adjacent double wheel over the abdomen has extruded the intestines through the perineum.*

Because of impact with the windscreen, pillars and roof, together with secondary contact with the ground, the head is the next most frequently damaged region – and the one which leads to most causes of death. Any type of injury may be sustained, as described in Chapter 5. Traffic accidents are the most frequent cause of skull fracture, especially of the base. Fractures of chest, arm and pelvis and injuries to the abdomen follow in frequency. Often the injuries are concentrated on one side, usually on the opposite side to the point of primary impact, because the body was thrown down onto the road. Because of rotation and the variable posture from being thrown off the car structure, however, the injuries are often widespread and may show no particular pattern.

Soft tissue injuries are common and, apart from abrasions, bruises and lacerations, muscle laceration and crushing can occur. A characteristic lesion from running-over, as opposed to knocking-down, is the 'flaying' injury, where a rotating motor wheel tears the skin and muscle from a limb or head. The rotatory effect against a fixed limb may strip off almost all tissue down to the bone. When a wheel passes over the abdomen or pelvis, multiple parallel striae or shallow lacerations may occur near the contact area because of ripping tension in the skin.

When a wheel passes over the pelvis, abdomen or head, there may be great internal damage with little surface injury. The weight of a large vehicle can virtually flatten a head, crushing the cranial vault. Often the brain is extruded through scalp lacerations, as may be the intestine through an abdominal wound. The pelvis may flatten out when run over, the symphysis or superior rami breaking, and one or both sacroiliac joints becoming detached. Any type of intra-abdominal injury may occur from ruptured liver and spleen to perforated intestine, lacerated mesentery and fractured

lumbar spine. In the chest, ribs, sternum and thoracic spine may fracture, and heart and lung damage occur from crushing or laceration from jagged ribs. A 'flail chest' is sometimes produced when a heavy wheel runs across the supine body, breaking all the ribs on each side in the anterior axillary line.

Patterned injuries may be important, in that they can assist the police in identifying a vehicle in a 'hit-and-run' accident. The most common is a tyre pattern outlined in intradermal bruising and these should be measured carefully and photographed. These marks are usually caused by the skin being forced into the grooves of the tyre tread, the edge of the raised rubber tracing out the pattern. The elevated parts do not leave bruises, but may imprint dirt on the skin.

Paint fragments and glass shards are also trace evidence that must be carefully retained, as the forensic laboratory may be able to identify the make and model of vehicle involved, and match the fragments when a suspect car is examined.

Parts of the vehicle may leave patterned imprints on the skin, such as headlamps, mirrors or other components. Safety regulations for manufacturers have now almost eliminated the dangerous devices such as bonnet mascots, projecting door handles and non-flexible mirrors that used to adorn older cars. Metallic and plastic objects may still be found in the tissues from time to time, however; the author (BK) has recovered a door handle from the interior of the liver and a chromium bonnet insignia from a cerebral hemisphere. Any such artefacts must be preserved for the police in cases in which the identity of the vehicle is not known.

In Britain, where traffic drives on the left side of the road, it is more common for pedestrians to be struck on the right side as they walk off the pavement. Many, however, are struck facing the vehicle, from turning during last-minute awareness, and some are hit from behind.

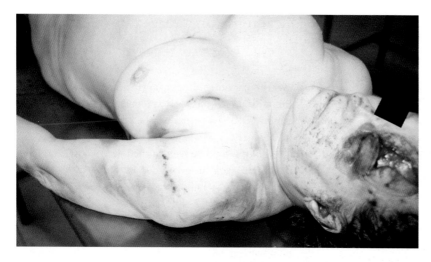

FIGURE 9.21 *A patterned injury in a pedestrian struck by a truck. The circular bruise and abrasion over the front of the shoulder are from a headlamp rim. There is also a well-demarcated imprint around the left eye from some other projection on the vehicle.*

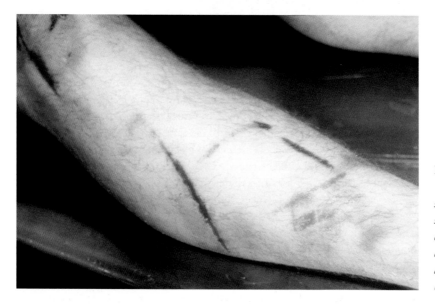

FIGURE 9.22 *Primary pedestrian injury. The pattern is caused by the bumper bar striking the leg. The height from the heel should always be measured for the police to compare with the vehicle – though during extreme braking, many vehicles will dip down at the front, thus lowering their bumper height.*

These factors will all affect the distribution of injuries, but it is too hazardous to try to reconstruct unwitnessed events in any detail from a study of the injuries. Suprarenal haemorrhage is more common in the right gland than the left after a traffic injury in Britain (Johnson, unpublished communication), but this observation must be modified by the fact that many such haemorrhages occur several days after the trauma and are usually the result of general systemic effects, rather than direct impact.

CAUSE OF DEATH IN TRAFFIC ACCIDENTS

In gross injuries this is often obvious, as in the crushed head with extrusion of brain or rupture of the aorta. Often multiple injuries make it difficult to decide which was the most serious and mortal lesion, but in such cases it is quite acceptable to use the term 'multiple injuries', preferably listing several of the most lethal.

When death occurs on the road or soon afterwards, there is usually macroscopic evidence of gross musculoskeletal or organ damage, severe haemorrhage, blockage of air passages from blood, or traumatic asphyxia from fixation of the chest caused by crushing some part of a vehicle.

Delayed death can be caused by continuing bleeding, secondary haemorrhage, renal failure from hypotension and/ or extensive muscle damage, fat embolism, local infection, chest or other systemic infections, myocardial or cerebral infarction and other sequelae discussed in Chapter 13.

The presence of natural disease is always an important consideration in all transportation deaths, as a possible cause or contribution to the accident. In pedestrians, a sudden collapse

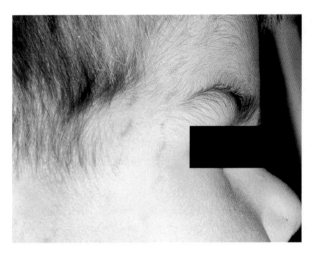

FIGURE 9.23 *Intradermal bruising on the forehead of a live boy who was found wandering in the street with amnesia for recent events. He had been struck by a 'hit-and-run' car, which left identifiable tyre marks on the skin. An astute casualty officer had a photograph taken as the marks faded in a few hours.*

in the roadway may lead to fatal injuries when a vehicle comes along – or even a dead body being run over by the next car.

Similarly, defects in sight or hearing may have contributed to the accident, though this is almost never detectable at autopsy, unless there are gross corneal or lens abnormalities. Of course, the possibility of drug or alcohol intoxication in the pedestrian victim must always be considered.

Where drivers or pilots are concerned – or even shipmasters – the presence of disease or intoxication may be a vital element, with both civil and criminal connotations possible.

Generally speaking, sudden natural disease does not often cause road vehicles to go out of control, as there seems to be a sufficient warning in most instances of cardiac or cerebral disablement, to allow the driver to pull over and stop.

Even the regular medical checks on older drivers legally enforced by some countries are no warranty that sudden collapse will not occur the very next day. The same applies to air pilots, as the VC-10 crash at London Airport proved some years ago, when the hypertensive pilot with coronary artery disease collapsed on take-off after an altercation with his co-pilot.

Schmidt *et al.* (1990) analysed 39 deaths at the wheel in Germany and found that 97 per cent had cardiovascular disease and 90 per cent had coronary heart disease. This was confirmed in a more recent retrospective study covering a 15-year time period in Munich, Germany, ranging from 1982 until 1996. Ischaemic heart disease was the underlying cause of death in 113 (84%) of the 147 natural deaths at the wheel. Morild (1994) found that 14 of 133 traffic deaths in Norway had died of natural disease, again predominantly coronary atherosclerosis.

The autopsy on a road traffic death

The autopsy is in general identical to the usual procedure, but with special attention to the following points:

■ As criminal proceedings against a driver may follow, legal matters such as identity of the body and continuity of evidence must be assured, as discussed in Chapter 1.

■ The body should be seen clothed, if brought dead to the mortuary or hospital, so that injuries can be matched against soiling and damage to the garments. Often this is not possible, especially if temporary survival allowed admission to a hospital or accident department, but where practicable the clothing should be preserved and examined by the pathologist. In any event, the clothes should be retained by the police for submission to the forensic science laboratory, usually when criminal proceedings are likely.

■ Blood samples must be retained for blood grouping and now perhaps even 'DNA fingerprinting' in case a 'hit-and-run' vehicle is found with blood or tissue traces upon it. Sometimes hair samples may be required for the same purpose. Where death occurs within 12 or even 24 hours of the time of the accident, blood analysis for alcohol is essential, whether in the driver or pedestrian (see Chapter 28). Where possible, screening for drugs of dependence and common medicinal substances that might have caused drowsiness should be carried out. In combination with alcohol, even low levels of sedative, hypnotic and antihistamine drugs may be relevant in the causation of an accident. In certain cases, where leakage of carbon monoxide is suspected, the circumstances will suggest analysis of the blood for carboxyhaemoglobin concentration.

■ The external examination, as in all trauma deaths, is vital and should be detailed, accurate and fully recorded. The height of major or patterned injuries above heel level must be noted, in order to compare these against dimensions of a vehicle. Patterned injuries must be photographed with a scale in view. Any foreign bodies or particles, either in the clothing, hair, on the skin or in the wounds, must be carefully retained for forensic science examination, especially in a 'hit-and-run' accident, where the identity of the vehicle may be vital.

All types of trace evidence may be found by a pathologist, from paint flakes and glass debris (which may be traced to a certain make, age, type and even individual vehicle) to parts of the vehicle structure. In past years, the author (BK) has retrieved a Renault door handle from inside a liver and an Austin bonnet insignia from within a brain.

A full autopsy must be carried out, not merely a catalogue of injuries. The presence of any natural disease is relevant, especially if it might have contributed to the accident, either by causing a driver to lose control or ability to drive, or a pedestrian to exercise proper caution or behaviour in the roadway. Old and recent cardiac and cerebral lesions are particularly important, as is any evidence of a fit, such as a bitten tongue, or old meningeal adhesions over cortical damage. It is almost impossible to assess visual acuity at autopsy, but obvious lesions such as lens opacities must be noted. Similarly, it is virtually impossible to give any opinion on acuity of hearing from autopsy findings unless there is a gross neurological abnormality in the auditory tract.

SUICIDE AND HOMICIDE BY MOTOR VEHICLE

There is little that the pathologist can contribute to the elucidation of motivation in traffic accidents, as it is circumstantial and sometimes forensic-laboratory evidence that is more likely to reveal a non-accidental cause. Homicidal traffic deaths are rare, though the author (BK) has been involved in one incident where racial hatred led to the running-down of youths of one ethnic group – and another where a man repeatedly crashed the near-side of his own car in an effort to kill his passenger (his wife). There are no specific pathological features that can assist, except that the incident is likely to occur at relatively high speed, without braking effects. The victims of homicide by other means – or persons rendered unconscious first – may be deliberately placed in motor vehicles which are then crashed, preferably with a subsequent fire. The author (BK) dealt with one such case where a husband placed the body of his strangled wife in his car and secretly pushed it over the edge of a mountain road. Unfortunately (for him), he left the ignition key in the 'off' position. This faking of a vehicular 'accident' to conceal homicide is by no means unknown, the author (BK) being involved in another case where a police officer disposed of the body of his wife who died in suspicious circumstances, by crashing her car and smashing the windscreen with a hammer to add to the effect.

In such circumstances, the pathologist's role is to match the injuries with a traffic accident, to detect any which are atypical. For instance, focal depressed fractures of the skull of the type caused by a weapon are unusual in a car occupant unless there was a localized intrusion of the vehicle roof. The ante-mortem nature of the injuries should be demonstrated, though this is not always possible. When there is a fire, some evidence of ante-mortem burns, soot inhalation or carbon monoxide absorption should be sought, though – as mentioned in Chapter 11 – some flash petrol fires may kill before any monoxide is absorbed. Where the victim was unconscious though not dead, no such differentiation is possible. Full analysis for alcohol and stupefying drugs must be made if there is any suspicion.

Attempts at deliberate self-destruction by the use of a motor vehicle are said to be not uncommon (Selzer and Payne 1962), though this is difficult to prove in most cases. Once again, the evidence is more likely to be based on circumstantial rather than medical evidence – a matter for the investigating authorities rather than the pathologist. Driving at speed into the path of an oncoming truck or into a solid obstruction at the roadside are the methods employed, though it is hard to prove in the absence of definite evidence. It has been said that the imprint of the accelerator pedal on the undersurface of the shoe may be an indication, though this can never be the only indication. A witnessed lack of other causative factors may offer some corroboration, but this is police business, not pathology.

RAILWAY INJURIES

These are not uncommon, especially in countries with many 'level crossings' (called 'grade crossings' in the USA), where a public road crosses a railway track with either no barrier at all or with only a flimsy lifting pole. Many vehicles are struck each year by passing locomotives.

Few rail passengers are killed or injured in moving trains compared with accidents to railway staff and to other types of accident on railway property. Track workers may be run down and some die from electrocution from overhead cables. The pathology of all these is no different from accidents elsewhere, the interest lying in the occupational epidemiology and preventive aspects.

One worrying development in recent years is the malicious damage caused to trains, either by placing objects on the tracks, which may cause a derailment, or the dropping of objects from bridges. The author (BK) has conducted an autopsy on a driver killed by a concrete block dropped from a bridge, which smashed through the windshield of his cab.

The other fairly common railway fatality is the suicide who lays himself in front of an approaching train. Decapitation is the most common injury and the obvious features are the local tissue destruction, usually with grease, rust or other dirt soiling of the damaged area.

The usual search for alcohol and other drugs must be made, as suicides often employ multiple methods to ensure self-destruction. As well as lying down before a locomotive,

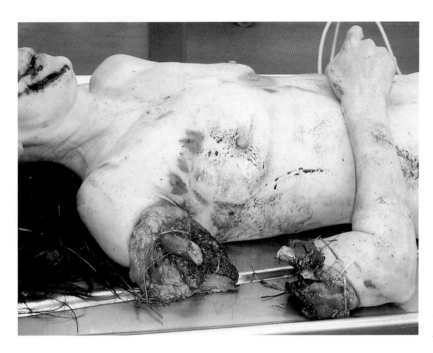

FIGURE 9.24 *Amputation of the right arm and bruising of the face and chest in a pedestrian struck by a passing locomotive.*

another common method of suicide in large cities is to jump from the subway platform of an underground 'tube' or 'metro' system. Here injuries are sometimes complicated by high-voltage electrical lesions, as the typical traction voltage of an electric railway is in excess of 600 volts.

REFERENCES AND FURTHER READING

Ahmed M. 1978. Motorcycle spoke injury. *Br Med J* **2**:401.

AMA Committee on Medical Aspects of Automotive Safety. 1963. Automobile safety belts during pregnancy. *JAMA* **221**:20–1.

Anonymous. 1977. Safety of children in cars [leading article]. *Br Med J* **1**:2.

Anonymous. 1979. Motorcycle and bicycle accidents [special correspondent]. *Br Med J* **1**:39–41.

Anonymous. 1979. Pedestrian accidents [special correspondent]. *Br Med J* **1**:101–4.

Ashton SJ. 1975. The cause and nature of head injuries sustained by pedestrians. *2nd Conference of Biomechemical Serious Trauma*, Lyon, France.

Ashton SJ, Mackay GM. 1978. Pedestrian injuries and death. In: Mason JK (ed.), *The pathology of violent injury.* Edward Arnold, London.

Baik S, Uku JM, Joo KG. 1988. Seat-belt injuries to the left common carotid artery and left internal carotid artery. *Am J Forensic Med Pathol* **9**:38–9.

Baker SO. 1979. Motor vehicle occupant death in young children. *Pediatrics* **64**:860–5.

Baker SP, Spitz WU. 1970. Age effects and autopsy evidence of disease in fatally injured drivers. *JAMA* **214**:1079–88.

Baker SP, Spitz WU. 1970. An evaluation of the hazard created by natural death at the wheel. *N Engl J Med* **283**:405–9.

Bako G, Mackenzie WC, Smith ES. 1970. What is the risk of being burned in a motor vehicle crash? A survey of crash fatalities in alberta. *J Traffic Med* **4**:20–4.

Bothwell PW. 1962. The problem of motor cycle accidents. *Practitioner* **188**:475–6.

Burke DC. 1973. Spinal cord injuries and seatbelts. *Med J Aust* **2**:801–6.

Buttner A, Heimpel M, Eisenmenger W. 1999. Sudden natural death 'at the wheel': a retrospective study over a 15-year time period. 1982–1996. *Forensic Sci Int* **103**:101–12.

Byard RW, Green H, James RA, *et al.* 2000. Pathologic features of childhood pedestrian fatalities. *Am J Forensic Med Pathol* **21**:101–6.

Christian MS. 1975. Non-fatal injuries sustained by back seatbelt passengers. *Br Med J* **1**:320–2.

Christian MS. 1976. Non-fatal injuries sustained by seatbelt wearers: a comparative study. *Br Med J* **2**:1310–12.

Clarke J, Milroy C. 1993. Pedestrian injuries and death. In: Mason JK (ed.), *Pathology of trauma*, 2nd edn. Edward Arnold, London.

Copeland AR. 1991. Pedestrian fatalities. The metropolitan dade county experience, 1984–1988. *Am J Forensic Med Pathol* **12**:40–4.

Cunningham K, Brown TD, Gradwell E, *et al.* 2000. Airbag associated fatal head injury: case report and review of the literature on airbag injuries. *J Accid Emerg Med* **17**:139–42.

Davis GG, Alexander CB, Brissie RM. 1997. A 15-year review of railway-related deaths in Jefferson County, Alabama. *Am J Forensic Med Pathol* **18**:363–8.

Denaner RM, Fitchett VH. 1975. Motorcycle trauma. *J Trauma* **15**:678–81.

DiMaio DJ. 1971. A survey of sudden unexpected deaths in automobile drivers. *Proc 3rd Int Assoc Accident Traffic Med*, pp 75–80.

Eckert W. 1959. Traumatic pathology of traffic accidents; review of 302 cases. *J Forensic Sci* **4**:3–20.

Eckert WB. 1977. *Transportation injuries.* In: Tedeschi L, Eckert WB (eds), *Forensic medicine.* Saunders, Philadelphia.

Edland SF. 1971. The suicide crash. *Proc 3rd Int Assoc Accident Traffic Med*, pp 81–3.

Fisher P. 1965. Injury produced by seatbelts: report of two cases. *J Occup Med* **7**:211–16.

Foster GR, Dunbar JA, Whittet D, *et al.* 1988. Contribution of alcohol to deaths in road traffic accidents in Tayside 1982–6. *Br Med J Clin Res Ed* **296**:1430–2.

Gadd CC. 1966. The use of a weighted impulse criterion to estimating injury hazard. *Proc Tenth Stapp Car Crash Conference.* Society of Automotive Engineers, New York, p. 164.

Gissane W, Bull JP. 1964. Motorway fatalities. *Br Med J* **1**:75–6.

Gissane W, Bull JP, Roberts B. 1970. Sequelae of road injuries. *Injury* **1**:195–200.

Goldberg BA, Mootha RK, Lindsey RW. 1998. Train accidents involving pedestrians, motor vehicles, and motorcycles. *Am J Orthop* **27**:315–20.

Guichon DM, Myles ST. 1975. Bicycle injuries: one-year sample in Calgary. *J Trauma* **15**:504–6.

Hall RR, Fisher AJ. 1972. The influence of car frontal design on pedestrian trauma. *Accid Anal Prev* **4**:47–51.

Hamilton JB. 1968. Seat belt injuries. *Br Med J* **2**:485–6.

Harruff RC, Avery A, Alter-Pandya AS. 1998. Analysis of circumstances and injuries in 217 pedestrian traffic fatalities. *Accid Anal Prev* **30**:11–20.

Hawley DA, Clark MA, Pless JE. 1995. Fatalities involving bicycles: a non-random population. *J Forensic Sci* **40**:205–7.

Hendrickx I, Mancini LL, Guizzardi M, *et al.* 2002. Burn injury secondary to air bag deployment. *J Am Acad Dermatol* **46**:S25–6.

Hotz GA, Cohn SM, Popkin C, *et al.* 2002. The impact of a repealed motorcycle helmet law in Miami-Dade county. *J Trauma* **52**:469–74.

Huelke DF, Chewin WA. 1968. *The energy-absorbing steering column.* Highway Safety Research Institute, Ann Arbor, Michigan.

Huelke DF, Davis RA. 1969. *A study of pedestrian fatalities in Wayne County, Michigan.* University of Michigan, Ann Arbor, Michigan.

Huelke DF, Gikas PW. 1967. Ejection – the leading cause of death in automobile accidents. *Conf Proc Soc Automative Eng*, New York.

Huelke DF, Gikas PW. 1968. Causes of death in automobile accidents. *JAMA* **203**:1100–3.

Huelke DF, Kaufer H. 1975. Vertebral column injuries and seat belts. *J Trauma* **15**:304–18.

Huelke DF, Sherman HW. 1971. Automobile occupant ejection through the side door glass. *Conf Proc Soc Automative Eng*, Detroit.

Huff GF, Bagwell SP, Bachman D. 1998. Airbag injuries in infants and children: a case report and review of the literature. *Pediatrics* **102**:e2.

Jamieson KG, Kelly D. 1973. Crash helmets reduce head injuries. *Med J Aust* **2**:806–9.

Jenkins J, Sainsbury P. 1980. Single-car road deaths – disguised suicides? *Br Med J* **281**:1041.

Jones AM, Bean SP, Sweeney ES. 1978. Injuries to cadavers resulting from experimental rear impact. *J Forensic Sci* **23**:730–4.

Kamdar BA, Arden GR. 1974. Road traffic accidents fatalities – a review of 142 post-mortem reports. *Postgrad Med J* **50**:131–6.

Karger B, Teige K, Buhren W, *et al.* 2000. Relationship between impact velocity and injuries in fatal pedestrian-car collisions. *Int J Legal Med* **113**:84–8.

Kelsch G, Helber MU, Ulrich C. 1996. [Craniocerebral trauma in fall from bicycles – what is the effect of a protective helmet?] *Unfallchirurg* **99**:202–6.

Knight B. 1976. An unnecessary risk to children. *Br Med J* **1**:180.

Larsen CF, Hardt Madsen M. 1988. Fatal motorcycle accidents in the county of Funen (Denmark). *Forensic Sci Int* **38**:93–9.

Lee WB, O'Halloran HS, Pearson PA, *et al.* 2001. Airbags and bilateral eye injury: five case reports and a review of the literature. *J Emerg Med* **20**:129–34.

Lifschultz BD, Donoghue ER. 1994. Deaths due to forklift truck accidents. *Forensic Sci Int* **65**:121–34.

Mackay GM. 1969. Some features of traffic accidents. *Br Med J* **4**:799–801.

Mackay GM. 1975. One engineer's view of human injury. *Injury Br J Accident Surg* **9**:179–83.

Mant AK. 1978. Injuries and death in motor vehicle accidents. In: Mason JK (ed.), *The pathology of violent injury* (and 2nd edition, 1993). Edward Arnold, London.

Mason MA. 1988. Restraining infants in cars. *Br Med J* **296**:1345–6.

McCarrol JR. 1962. Fatal pedestrian automotive accidents. *JAMA* **180**:127–30.

McCarthy M, Gilbert K. 1996. Cyclist road deaths in London 1985–1992: drivers, vehicles, manoeuvres and injuries. *Accid Anal Prev* **28**:275–9.

McDonald QH. 1979. Children's car seat restraints: when top-tether straps are ignored, are these restraints safe? *Pediatrics* **64**:848–55.

Moore J, Tourin B. 1954. *Study of automotive doors opening under crash conditions.* Cornell University, New York.

Morild I. 1994. Traffic deaths in western Norway. A study from the county of Hordaland 1986–1990. *Forensic Sci Int* **64**:9–20.

Morton J. 1968. The suicide driver. *Traffic Saf* **68**:37–40.

Mouzakes J, Koltai PJ, Kuhar S, *et al.* 2001. The impact of airbags and seat belts on the incidence and severity of maxillofacial injuries in automobile accidents in New York state. *Arch Otolaryngol Head Neck Surg* **127**:1189–93.

Murphy GK. 1976. Death on the railway. *J Forensic Sci* **21**:218–26.

Ostrom M, Eriksson A. 2001. Pedestrian fatalities and alcohol. *Accid Anal Prev* **33**:173–80.

Pearlman JA, Eong KG, Kuhn F, *et al.* 2001. Airbags and eye injuries: epidemiology, spectrum of injury, and analysis of risk factors. *Surv Ophthalmol* **46**:234–42.

Petersen PJ, Petty CS. 1962. Sudden natural death among automobile drivers. *J Forensic Sci* **7**:274–7.

Rowe BH, Rowe AM, Bota GW. 1995. Bicyclist and environmental factors associated with fatal bicycle-related trauma in Ontario. *Can Med Assoc J* **152**:45–53.

Schmidt P, Haarhoff K, Bonte W. 1990. Sudden natural death at the wheel – a particular problem of the elderly? *Forensic Sci Int* **48**:155–62.

Selzer ML, Payne CE. 1962. Automobile accidents, suicides and unconscious motivation. *Am J Psychiatry* **119**:237–44.

Sevitt S. 1968. Death after road traffic accidents. *Med Sci Law* **8**:271–87.

Sevitt S. 1968. Fatal road accidents: injuries, complications and cause of death. *Br J Surg* **55**:481–4.

Sevitt S. 1973. Fatal road accidents in Birmingham: times to death and their causes. *Injury* **4**:281–93.

Shennan J. 1973. Seat belt syndrome [letter]. *Br Med J* **4**:786.

Simpson K. 1960. The interpretation of the surface pattern of vehicular injuries. *Med Sci Law* **1**:420–8.

Smith WS, Kaufer H. 1969. Patterns and mechanisms of lumbar injuries associated with lap seat belts. *J Bone Joint Surg Am* **51**:239–54.

Solheim K. 1964. Pedestrian deaths in Oslo traffic accidents. *Br Med J* **1**:81–3.

Transport and Road Research Laboratory. 1974. *Pedestrian injuries.* Department of the Environment, London.

Van der Linden WJ. 2002. Dislocated fracture of the mandibular condylar process after airbag deployment: report of a case. *J Oral Maxillofac Surg* **60**:113–15.

Whent P. 2000. Rail accident investigation. In: Siegel JA, Saukko PJ, Knupfer GC (eds), *Encyclopedia of forensic sciences.* Academic Press, San Diego, San Francisco, New York, Boston, London, Sydney, Tokyo, vol 1, pp. 42–47.

Wilks PM. 1967. Safety in car design. *Proc R Soc Med* **60**:955–8.

Wolf RA. 1962. The discovery and control of ejection in automobile accidents. *JAMA* **180**:220–2.

Wyatt JP, Martin A, Beard D, *et al.* 2001. Pedestrian deaths following collisions with heavy goods vehicles. *Med Sci Law* **41**:21–5.

CHAPTER 10

Abuse of human rights: deaths in custody

Regrettably, abuse of human rights is so widespread on a global scale that some reference must now be made in forensic pathology texts to the physical manifestations of torture. It is stated by Amnesty International (2001) that in a third of the member states of the United Nations torture of one kind or another is practised, in spite of them being signatories to United Nations resolutions banning these atrocities. According to Amnesty International's worldwide report on torture based on a 3-year investigation (2000), currently more than 150 countries routinely torture people compared with 98 countries in their previous report in 1984.

Although most torture does not result in death, there are sufficient cases of physical abuse of human rights that progress to fatality that a number of organizations offer expertise when any alleged case needs to be investigated, usually calling upon forensic pathologists to assist them in such circumstances. These include Amnesty International (based in London), Physicians for Human Rights (PHR), the Medical Foundation for the Treatment of Victims of Torture (London) and many others.

EVIDENCE OF FATAL PHYSICAL ABUSE

In many instances the autopsy appearances of fatal abuse are no different from those by any other homicide, and the confirmation of lethal torture must depend upon circumstantial and other corroborative evidence, which is no concern of this book. For example, if a political detainee is kicked to death, the physical findings may be identical to those of a murder by kicking in a street crime. Similarly, head injuries,

shooting and suffocation may show no variation from the same modes of death outside a political context.

Certain features may arouse suspicion or provide definite evidence that the death had political overtones. The word 'political' is used in a wide sense as many abuses of human rights are not directed or even condoned by higher levels of government, though often there is an indifference to being informed about such activities. Many instances of illegal death and injury are perpetrated by the military or the security forces – and even here, the level of command that directs or condones the abuse varies greatly. In general, the civil police and the regular prisons are usually not the perpetrators of gross abuse, though there are many exceptions. It tends to be the armed forces, clandestine security police, and special detention camps that are most often guilty of torture and illegal executions.

One of the features that characterizes torture and abuse is that the victim is usually either in detention or some form of custody, or is temporarily in the power of the authorities, even if that means that soldiers have just burst into a private house. All deaths in custody – discussed later in the chapter – should be examined with care, as much to ensure that the guardians are cleared of any suspicion of ill-treatment as to discover any ill-treatment itself. The fatal event may be quite different from the non-fatal abuse, as a victim who is beaten may be disposed of by shooting. As in all forensic work, the pathological investigations can only be part of the overall enquiry, another example of cooperation and teamwork between all disciplines.

One of the major differences – and great problems – in the investigation of torture and abuse of civil rights is that the authorities in the state where it occurred may be totally uncooperative and, indeed, wholly hostile to impartial enquiry. It is through respected international agencies, such as the Red Cross, Amnesty International and Physicians for Human Rights, that pathologists have the best chance of being allowed access to the relevant material, and the organizations mentioned above are willing to undertake or assist legitimate investigations anywhere in the world.

One particular problem associated with human rights abuse is the frequent long delay before being able to examine the victim. In the living, they may have been detained for months or years after the ill-treatment, or may have been exiled or in hiding before they have the opportunity to be seen by an impartial medical observer, by which time acute injuries will have healed, bruises absorbed and wounds and burns scarred over. In the dead, long-term post-mortem changes are common: the body may have been buried and exhumed before examination.

Even skeletal material is all that is sometimes available, as in the 'lost children' of Argentina or in the killing fields of Uganda. Problems of identification are often difficult. Contemporary photographs of injuries are often of poor quality and the facilities for autopsy are primitive in some of the less developed countries. When the suspicion, lack of cooperation and often open hostility of the local authorities is added, the task for the visiting pathologist is formidable indeed.

The following types of injury may confirm or arouse suspicion of torture, though, as stated, virtually any type of injury can be inflicted deliberately to extract information, punish or degrade the victims or to exterminate them. Repetition of a particular injury, such as 'tramline' bruises from beating, is suspicious, because in ordinary assaults and homicides such excessive and perhaps regularly placed repetitive lesions would be unusual.

■ Beating is one of the most common forms of torture and can take many forms, varying both with the weapon used and the part of the body injured. Blows both to the head and to other parts of the body were present in all the cases reported by Hougen (1988). Unless severe and repeated, beating is not often the sole cause of death, though this can occur from haemorrhage, sepsis, injured internal organs, or from sheer exhaustion and pain in an already debilitated victim. The blows may be inflicted by fist or foot, but are more often applied with a weapon. The use of a whip or lath-like instrument is common, but metal or wooden bars, clubs, batons, rifle butts or belts may be used. More recently, lengths of plastic hosepipe or tubing have come into favour in some parts of the world.

Many of these produce a characteristic skin lesion, namely a single- or double-edged linear bruise. The bruise may be a line of confluent petechial haemorrhages or a continuous mark of red skin. The 'tramline' bruise is a double line of parallel marks with a pale unbruised zone between them, caused by the impact of a rectangular or circular-sectioned object. This is described in more detail in Chapter 4.

The bruising may be intradermal, when it reproduces the pattern of the weapon well. If a leather whip with, for example, plaited thongs, is struck against the skin, the pattern may be imprinted clearly on the skin.

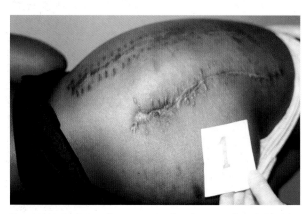

FIGURE 10.1 *A scar about one year after the original injury. The female victim was shot while escaping from an East African concentration camp. The wound was opened surgically and healed imperfectly with keloid formation. The other surgical incision is of more recent origin. Such scars will remain unaltered for life, apart from possible increase in the keloid formation.*

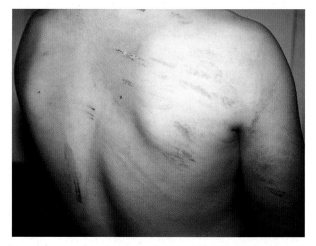

FIGURE 10.2 *Recent bruising inflicted within the previous 2 days, from blows by lengths of plastic tubing about 15 mm wide. The injuries show parallel 'tramlining' typical of impact from a cylindrical weapon. The assailants were vigilantes administering a punishment beating to an alleged collaborator in a Middle Eastern country.*

Buckles on belts and other recognizable artefacts may occasionally be useful in identifying the weapon. Where the bruising is deeper, no such pattern is likely. The skin may be broken, causing abrasions or lacerations and, if the full thickness is breached, healing will cause scars, which may even be recognizable as 'tramlines'.

Repeated beating leaves multiple marks, which though overlapping and often criss-crossing, may have a generally similar orientation that indicates that the attacker stood in a relatively fixed position to the victim. For example, lashing across the back may leave marks running from top right to bottom left, suggesting that a right-handed perpetrator stood to the left of the victim.

The use of a multi-thonged whip, such as a 'cat-o'nine-tails' will leave a series of marks, again generally in the same orientation. The thongs tend to be narrow and may cause linear marks with tramlining. There may be metal tags or knots on the end of each thong, which can cause focal damage. The back is the most frequent target, but whipping and beating may be applied to the buttocks, thighs, front of chest, breasts and abdomen, lower legs, soles of the feet, and even perineum and genitals.

Beating of the soles of the feet with canes or rods is a torture rooted in antiquity and this so-called 'falanga' may leave relatively little to see, even though it is extremely painful and debilitating. The tough tissue and thick fascial planes of the foot do not readily reveal bruising, though it may be found on deep dissection in victims who have been killed by some other means.

If injuries were inflicted months before examination, little or nothing may be found unless the skin was broken, when scarring will have taken place. Sometimes, however, faint red lines may be seen in pale-skinned people and in those with appreciable racial melanin pigment there is often hyperpigmentation along the lines of injury. Where severe damage has been caused and sometimes where there is scar tissue, depigmentation may be seen.

- Burns are unfortunately common and may be either the actual cause of death or visible as recent or scarred evidence of previous torture. All kinds of burns may be suffered. The author (BK) has seen extensive burns from molten rubber dripped onto victims from motor tyres suspended overhead, hot irons applied to skin, ignited kerosene-soaked rags wrapped around limbs and numerous burns from cigarettes pressed into the skin. Knowledge of local practices, such as the burning motor tyre 'necklace', can help identify burns in typical sites. Where molten liquids have been dripped from above onto a bound-up victim, there may be shadow areas that indicate the direction of contact, which makes any innocent explanation highly unlikely. In survivors, scarring occurs in all but the most superficial burns, and may lead to large, unsightly cicatrized areas. In victims of African origin, large keloids may form, and further complicate the damage and attempts at surgical treatment.

- Cutting and stabbing may be inflicted with a variety of weapons, but wounds from knives and bayonets are most common in the context of torture and extrajudicial execution. The features are identical to

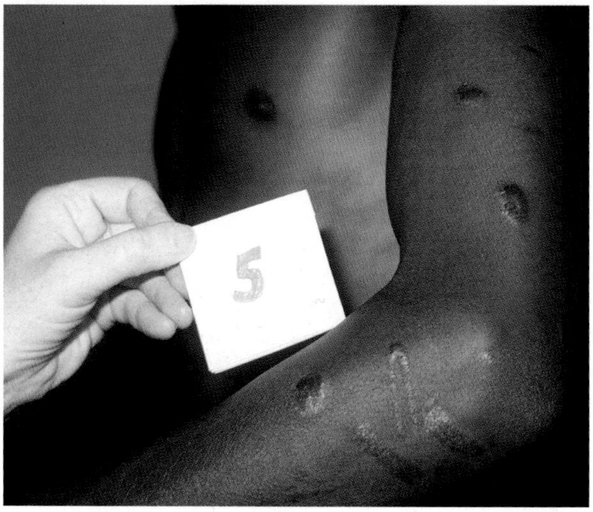

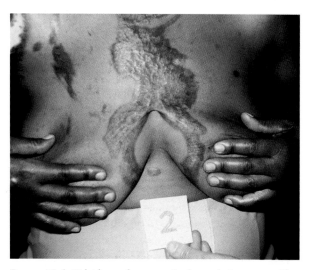

FIGURE 10.3 *Scars from beating with a thin metal rod in an East African torture camp. Though more than a year old, the 'tramline' nature of one of the scars is outlined in keloid.*

FIGURE 10.4 *Keloid scars from extensive burns during torture. The elderly lady was tied to a chair and a burning motor tyre suspended over her. The shadowed area between the breasts indicates the downward trickle of molten burning rubber. Her face was also extensively scarred.*

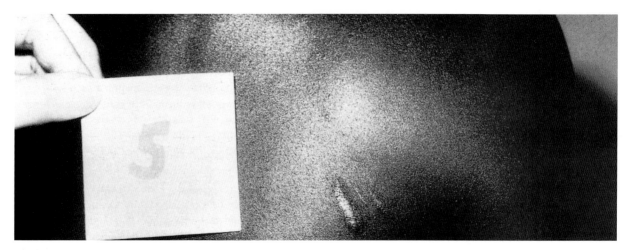

FIGURE 10.5 *The scar of a bayonet stab wound inflicted many months earlier in a Ugandan torture camp. Though scars are usually of little help in interpreting the cause of the injury, here the elliptical shape of the original stab wound can still be seen as a keloid scar and even the sharp upper end of the blade edge, as opposed to blunter lower end.*

those described in Chapter 4. The site on the body may be anywhere, but the chest and upper arms seem to be favourite targets. The scars of old stab wounds, such as those from a bayonet, may still be recognizably elliptical many months or years after infliction.

- Clubbing and blunt injury is extremely common, either to cause death or as a form of abuse. It is sometimes dispensed almost casually, as when guards lay about themselves with rifle butts against the inmates of detention camps. Again the features are non-specific and are described in the chapter on wounding. The head is the most common target, but the legs and knees are also often struck. Blows on the back or side of the neck can be particularly lethal from vertebrobasilar artery damage (Chapter 5).

- Deaths from suffocation and drowning are not common, though non-fatal practices of this kind are well-known methods of abuse. Repeated dipping of the victim's head under water or even foul liquid such as sewage is called 'submarining', and may cause drowning, air-passage occlusion or a later pneumonia. Enveloping the head in an opaque plastic bag is more a means of disorientation than physical torture, but partial suffocation by similar means may eventually prove fatal.

- Electrical torture is common and well documented. Either mains voltage of 110 or 240 V is used – which carries the risk of fatal cardiac arrhythmia as well as local burning – or a magneto delivering high voltage, which is painful but not lethal. The latter will not leave any significant skin marks, as the amperage is so low.

  The later demonstration of electrical injury is difficult, as healed lesions have few characteristic features. The acute injuries which may cause burns and

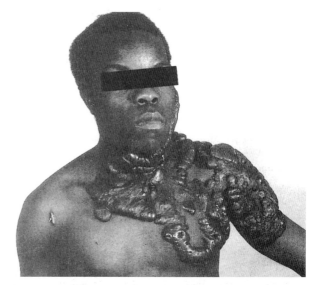

FIGURE 10.6 *Extensive keloid scars following deliberate burning of a 16-year-old student in an East African concentration camp. An electric hot plate was pressed against his neck and kerosene-soaked rags were ignited on his arm.*

death are described in Chapter 12. Karlsmark and his co-authors have made a special study of the pathology of electrical torture. The current may be applied anywhere, but the genitals are sites favoured by torturers, especially the penis and scrotum. The female nipples are also targets.

- Injuries to the ears can rarely be demonstrated at autopsy, but a favourite torture is the 'telefono', consisting of repeated slapping of the sides of the head by the open palms of the assailant. This may rupture the tympanic membranes and injure the inner ear.

- Suspension is a common torture, though again not often fatal in itself. If the victim is seen relatively soon after the ordeal then abrasions, bruises and chafing marks may be found at ligature sites, usually on legs, arms and sometimes genitals.
- Shooting is not a method of torture in the accepted sense, but is a common means of execution or of non-fatal punishment, such as the 'knee-capping' perpetrated in Northern Ireland, where opponents and suspected traitors are shot either through the knee joint or the lower thigh.
- Sexual abuse is also common and in women, rape – sometimes multiple – may leave physical signs as described in Chapter 18.

Medical examiners of alleged victims of torture must be careful not to misinterpret non-torture lesions as evidence of abuse, as such lapses will be seized upon by opponents wishing to discredit the medical opinion, either for political or immigration reasons. Forrest's guide (Forrest *et al.* 1995) lists most of these, which include innocent occupational, sporting or other accidents, tribal marks, skin infections, variations in pigmentation, traditional scarification, healing marks, stretch marks, etc.

EXTRAJUDICIAL EXECUTION

Many hundreds of thousands – indeed probably millions – of victims have been assassinated in recent years by governmental agencies acting quite outside the legal system. Because of ethnic origin, tribal feuds or political views, whole sections of populations have 'disappeared' on a scale sometimes amounting to genocide as in Rwanda, Cambodia, Bosnia and Kosovo. It is common knowledge that these disappearances are usually explained by murder, either on a mass scale or by continuous individual or group extermination by 'extermination squads'. Specific instances are not the concern of a textbook, but as recent years have shown, severe excesses have taken place in most continents leading to several forensic exercises directed towards identification of victims and proving methods of torture.

When vanished people have been presumed to have been killed by troops or security agencies, the evidence is usually very late in coming to light, so that forensically, much of the work consists of skeletal identification and investigations into causes of death. Where the bodies have decomposed or skeletalized, shooting or head injuries may be the only mode of death to leave any telltale evidence on exhumation. Autopsy examination may resemble mass-disaster procedures where there are large numbers of victims. The talents of odontologists and anthropologists, and the techniques of

archaeology may be needed in such cases, as described by Clyde Snow in relation to the 'lost children' of Argentina or more recently in Bosnia and Herzegovina, Croatia and Kosovo. The vast numbers of skeletal remains in the Lowero triangle of Uganda have so far had no such attention.

DEATH IN CUSTODY

The occurrence of death while a person is either in the custody of the police, or the inmate of a prison, raises public interest and emotions that require careful handling and investigation. There is often an immediate complaint or rumour of ill-treatment by the relatives or the media. A meticulous autopsy is a necessary part of the investigation needed to dispel – or sometimes confirm – allegations that an act of commission or omission on the part of the custodians has led to, or contributed to, the death. This applies in all countries and has no relationship to the preceding section, when political issues may be suspected as a cause of the death. The two aspects are not always totally separate, however, as countries with excellent human rights records have sometimes been suspected of occasional lapses of standards where custodial deaths are concerned.

Most of the cases dealt with by a forensic pathologist will concern civil police forces and the regular prison service. Many countries, including Britain, have strict legislative rules that make all deaths in custody, whether police or prison, reportable for medico-legal investigation by the appropriate law officer (the coroner in England and Wales), in addition to a searching internal enquiry by officers from a different police force (e.g. in Finland the National Bureau of Investigation).

An autopsy will inevitably be held, regulations in UK making this a case for an accredited forensic pathologist. It is sometimes helpful if the pathologist visits the scene of the death, especially if it was caused by hanging or some form of mechanical trauma.

There are several situations in which death may occur in custody. The deceased may die during or soon after arrest by police officers, as there is often a struggle in which the offender is resisting arrest, sometimes violently. It may be a physical struggle, especially when police officers are attempting to control or overpower a resisting offender. In these situations, the use of so-called personal defence sprays has increased, as they have been shown to be very effective in incapacitating an aggressor. They cause acute ocular irritation, lachrymation, conjunctivitis, blepharospasm and extreme discomfort. Most of these sprays contain *o*-chlorobenzylidene malononitrile (CS), 2-chloroacetophenone (CN), oleoresin capsicum (OC), or a combination of these ingredients as the active agent. Capsacain (8-methyl-*N*-vanillyl-6-nonenamide) is a neurotoxin component of cayenne pepper. It stimulates excitatory afferent sensory neurones, causes hypothermia, neurogenic inflammation and pain, followed by subsequent desensitization. Although these sprays have been considered to be relatively safe, unexpected deaths have been reported after the exposure to oleoresin capsicum (OC) spray devices. Pepper spray has been suspected to induce bronchoconstriction. Chan and co-workers (2002) tested the effect of (OC) spray inhalation on respiratory function in 35 healthy subjects by itself and combined with restraint but could not find evidence of hypoxaemia or hypercapnia in either group. OC exposure did not result in abnormal spirometry, hypoxaemia, or hypoventilation when compared to placebo in either sitting or prone maximal restraint position. In another study on clinical toxicity of OC, in Kansas, Watson *et al.* (1996) reported on 81 emergency department patients who had been investigated after exposure to OC. Ocular burning and redness were the most common presenting symptoms. None of the patients required hospitalization due to OC toxicity. Corneal abrasions and respiratory symptoms occurred in seven and six patients, respectively. In case of death after OC exposure, a thorough autopsy, with ancillary investigations, including complete histology and toxicological analysis with assessment of the circumstances and symptomatology, is necessary to assess whether the exposure to OC spray has been causative, contributory, or unrelated to death.

On other occasions, the offender may threaten police officers with a knife, gun or blunt weapon, and the police have to subdue him either by sheer physical force – truncheons or riot sticks – or by the use of firearms. The most common event is the arrest of a drunken offender and this poses extra problems, discussed below. Other drugs, such as cocaine, cannabis, amphetamine and hallucinogens, rather than opiates such as morphine, heroin and barbiturates, may also be involved.

The physical overpowering of a suspected offender poses definite risks to health and life, and has been the subject of numerous controversial enquiries and litigation in many countries. The police usually outnumber the offender, sometimes by a considerable margin, but even a one-to-one struggle can be dangerous for either party. The following risks exist, though the list is by no means comprehensive.

■ Traumatic asphyxia may occur where several policemen fall upon a resisting subject to overpower him. The author (BK) has dealt with several deaths where a number of large police officers piled on top of a prisoner fighting maniacally, to apply handcuffs. When they got up, the man was not breathing and died in hospital shortly afterwards. Death was caused by traumatic asphyxia, the weight of the men on top of him causing

chest compression and prevention of respiratory movements. The appearances are described in Chapter 14.

■ Arm-locks or neck-holds applied by police officers to resisting persons are other causes of deaths during arrest. These have been particularly notorious in the USA, where police officers have been trained to apply neck-holds as a form of restraint, but similar deaths have been seen elsewhere. The arm-lock is applied either from behind or with the head of the offender tucked under the police officer's arm against his waist. The dangers are compression of the front or sides of the neck, and death can occur either from reflex cardiac arrest or cerebral ischaemia during carotid compression, or asphyxia from airway obstruction, though the latter is unlikely as the sole mechanism. According to American writers such as Reay and Eisele (1982, 1986), there are two types of neck-hold – the 'bar arm control' and the 'carotid sleeper'. The former is alleged to be more dangerous; the officer's forearm is pulled across the front of the larynx to occlude the airway. The carotid sleeper uses the two sides of the 'V' formed by the flexed upper and lower arm to compress the carotids and produce transient cerebral ischaemia. Both varieties are dangerous, however, as there is the ever-present hazard of reflex cardiac arrest from vagal stimulation from the carotid sinus and sheath, as well as the potential danger of neck traction and hyperextension causing subarachnoid haemorrhage from vertebrobasilar artery damage.

■ Postural (positional) asphyxia has been reported to have caused sudden deaths in persons after the use of the 'hogtie', 'hobble' or prone maximal restraint and even in situations where a person has been placed in a prone position in the rear compartment of a police car. In an experiment with healthy subjects, the restraint position resulted in a restrictive pulmonary function pattern but did not cause clinically relevant changes in oxygenation or ventilation. It has been postulated that the hogtie restraint position by itself does not cause respiratory compromise to the point of asphyxiation but other factors, e.g. acute intoxication by alcohol or drugs, are responsible for the sudden deaths of individuals placed in this position.

■ Blunt injury may occur from the use of fist, arm or leg – or the use of a weapon such as a truncheon, riot stick or pistol butt. During a struggle, usually with one or more police officers who are attempting to subdue a fighting offender, injuries may be received by either side. All types of blunt injury may be sustained, some potentially fatal and these are discussed in Chapter 4. Head injuries may occur during a scuffle from falls either against the ground, or against a wall or other obstruction. A heavy punch in the face may cause nasopharyngeal bleeding that can block the air passages, especially in a person affected by alcohol. A blow on the side of the neck can cause reflex cardiac arrest or a subarachnoid haemorrhage from vertebrobasilar vascular damage.

A backward blow from the point of an elbow can be damaging, if it strikes the face, neck or abdomen. Kicking and stamping are unusual, but not unknown, in custodial deaths. A blow in the abdomen can also be serious if delivered with sufficient force. Though in an adult a fist blow is not very likely to cause serious harm, it can in a slighter young person. The use of the elbow, knee or a head butt can deliver extreme force, especially from a fit, muscular police officer, as well as from an offender.

The author (BK) has seen fatal intraperitoneal bleeding amounting to three litres in a drunken man arrested after a scuffle with two police officers, in which there were allegations that one struck or fell on the man with his knee. Several hours later the prisoner collapsed and at autopsy there were several large tears in the mesentery.

Alcohol is a frequent cause of death in custody. Not only is it the major factor in provoking aggression and violent resistance, with the consequences mentioned above, but it can have other effects which lead to death while in the care of the police. Acute alcoholic poisoning, described more fully in Chapter 28, may lead to death while the victim is thought to be 'sleeping it off' in a police cell. When blood alcohol levels rise to above 350 mg/100 ml there is an increasing risk of coma and central respiratory depression. Although most responsible police forces have standing orders about placing drunken prisoners in the semiprone position and observing them at frequent intervals, a quiet drunk may still slip into irreversible coma and respiratory arrest.

At lower blood alcohol levels there is still the risk of aspiration of vomit and choking on gastric contents. Though drunken prisoners are placed in the safest posture for drainage, they can still vomit and choke when unobserved, between visits by the often busy police station officers. At autopsy, caution must be observed before ascribing death to aspiration of vomit, as this is a common agonal phenomenon in deaths from other causes. Where an otherwise healthy person dies with a high blood alcohol concentration in these circumstances, however, gross blocking of the trachea and bronchi with vomit forms one of the most convincing arguments for acceptance of aspiration as the cause of death if no other factors can be identified.

Alcohol also contributes to accidents during custody, especially head injuries, which come about because of falls to the ground, falls down steps and stairs, and being run over by traffic, as a result of the ataxia and incoordination of the drunken state. Falls onto a hard surface are often on the occiput and the frequent finding of frontal and temporal contrecoup brain damage at autopsy is good evidence of a deceleration injury rather than an assault with a weapon.

Some falls may occur during custody or in transit from the site of arrest to the police station – others have happened before arrest, but the ill-effects and death may become manifest during the stay in the police cell, when the police are often blamed either for allowing or causing the injury – or for not summoning or providing urgent medical attention. Drugs, especially those causing excitement, such as amphetamine, cocaine or hallucinogens, may also lead to physical damage, but alcohol remains by far the most common.

Drugs are commonly available within prisons and overdose or hypersensitivity deaths are occasionally seen amongst prisoners, as they are in the outside world.

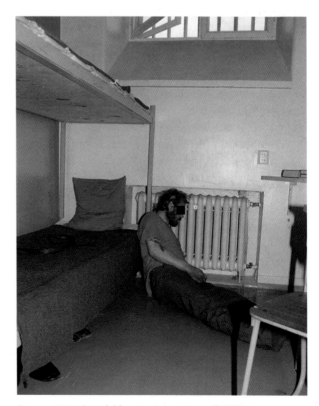

FIGURE 10.7 *Suicidal hanging in a prison cell. This is an infrequent but regular tragedy, which, in spite of strenuous efforts by prison officers and designers of cells, occurs because of the determination of the prisoner to defeat the safeguards. The belt used as ligature has been removed and lies on the bed.*

■ Suicide in custody is not uncommon, and often leads to accusations and recriminations from the relatives over lack of supervision. There has recently been a spate of such deaths in Britain, especially amongst young offenders on remand awaiting trial. It is such a well-recognized hazard of custody that most police forces deprive the prisoner of any objects, such as belts, braces (suspenders), cord or even bootlaces, that could be used to hang himself in his cell. In addition, the police cell may be specifically designed to avoid any convenient suspension points, such as hooks, bars or even internal door handles. In spite of these precautions, prisoners regularly manage to find some means of killing themselves. Strips of bedding material, sleeves of clothing and handkerchiefs have all been used for self-suspension. As described in Chapter 14, hanging can be successfully accomplished by traction on the neck at low levels and need not occur from high suspension points, so prisoners have killed themselves by attaching ligatures to bed-heads, chairs and other unlikely objects in the cell.

Accusations that apparent suicidal hangings were in reality homicides by the custodians can usually be resolved by the autopsy showing no signs of bruising, abrasions or a struggle. It would seem impossible to hang a conscious person against his will without leaving some signs of restraint. The proposition that the hanging was a ligature strangulation is usually disproved by the rising angle of the ligature mark, which most commonly sets under the angles of the jaw and has a defect in the skin mark where the suspension point pulls the ligature away from the surface. A homicidal strangulation usually encircles the neck and a cross-over point is often seen. The level is lower, nearer the horizontal (Chapter 14).

Where a true hanging mark is caused by a ligature with a slip-knot, there may also be a full circle of skin abrasion and compression. If the suspension point is low, as might happen in a cell using a doorknob or a bed-frame, then the direction of pull can be oblique. If the body also leans over against the direction of pull, the resultant mark can be virtually horizontal and, unless the situation is fully assessed – preferably by a visit to the scene with the body *in situ* – confusion can occur, as with the controversy over the death of Rudolph Hess in 1988, whilst an inmate in Berlin's Spandau prison.

■ Death may be from purely natural causes, usually cardiovascular in origin, which happened to have occurred during detention. It must be admitted, though it is almost impossible to provide objective proof, that the emotional and sometimes physical upset of being arrested and confined may have affected the blood

pressure and heart rate sufficiently, by an adrenaline response, to have precipitated an acute cardiac crisis in the presence of severe pre-existing disease.

The presence of diabetes, epilepsy, asthma or other diseases that can potentially cause sudden or unexpected death should be sought by medical history and autopsy appearances (Chapter 25).

REFERENCES AND FURTHER READING

Amnesty International. 2001. *Amnesty international report 2001*. Amnesty International, London.

Billmire DF, Vinocur C, Ginda M, *et al.* 1996. Pepper-spray-induced respiratory failure treated with extracorporeal membrane oxygenation. *Pediatrics* **98**:961–3.

Blaauw E, Vermunt R, Kerkhof A. 1997. Deaths and medical attention in police custody. *Med Law* **16**:593–606.

Bloom AI, Zamir G, Muggia M, *et al.* 1995. Torture rhabdomyorhexis – a pseudo-crush syndrome. *J Trauma* **38**:252–4.

Bork K, Nagel C. 1997. Long-standing pigmented keloid of the ears induced by electrical torture. *J Am Acad Dermatol* **36**:490–1.

Brkic H, Strinovic D, Kubat M, *et al.* 2000. Odontological identification of human remains from mass graves in croatia. *Int J Legal Med* **114**:19–22.

Bro Rasmussen F, Henriksen OB, Rasmussen OV, *et al.* 1982. [Aseptic necrosis of bone following phalanga torture.] *Ugeskr Laeger* **144**:1165–6.

Brown L, Takeuchi D, Challoner K. 2000. Corneal abrasions associated with pepper spray exposure. *Am J Emerg Med* **18**:271–2.

Busker RW, van Helden HP. 1998. Toxicologic evaluation of pepper spray as a possible weapon for the Dutch police force: risk assessment and efficacy. *Am J Forensic Med Pathol* **19**:309–16.

Chan TC, Vilke GM, Neuman T. 1998. Reexamination of custody restraint position and positional asphyxia. *Am J Forensic Med Pathol* **19**:201–5.

Chan TC, Vilke GM, Clausen J, *et al.* 2002. The effect of oleoresin capsicum 'pepper' spray inhalation on respiratory function. *J Forensic Sci* **47**:299–304.

Copeland AR. 1984. Deaths in custody revisited. *Am J Forensic Med Pathol* **5**:121–4.

Corovic N, Durakovic Z, Zavalic M, *et al.* 2000. Electrocardiographic changes in ex-prisoners of war released from detention camps. *Int J Legal Med* **113**:197–200.

Dalton V. 1999. Death and dying in prison in Australia: national overview, 1980–1998. *J Law Med Ethics* **27**:210, 269–74.

Epstein RJ, Majmudar PA. 2001. Pepper spray in the eye. *Ophthalmology* **108**:1712–13.

Fernandez M, Pissiota A, Frans O, *et al.* 2001. Brain function in a patient with torture related post-traumatic stress disorder before and after fluoxetine treatment: a positron emission tomography provocation study. *Neurosci Lett* **297**:101–4.

Fitzpatrick JJ. 1984. Role of radiology in human rights abuse. *Am J Forensic Med Pathol* **5**:321–5.

Forrest D. 1995. The physical after-effects of torture. *Forensic Sci Int* **76**:77–84.

Forrest D, Knight B, Hinshelwood G, *et al.* 1995. A guide to writing medical reports on survivors of torture. *Forensic Sci Int* **76**:69–75.

Frost R, Hanzlick R. 1988. Deaths in custody. Atlanta city jail and Fulton county jail, 1974–1985. *Am J Forensic Med Pathol* **9**:207–11.

Fruehwald S, Frottier P, Eher R, *et al.* 2000. Prison suicides in Austria, 1975–1997. *Suicide Life Threat Behav* **30**:360–9.

Giles HG, Sandrin S. 1992. Alcohol and deaths in police custody. *Alcohol Clin Exp Res* **16**:670–2.

Gniadecka M, Danielsen L. 1995. High-frequency ultrasound for torture-inflicted skin lesions. *Acta Derm Venereol* **75**:375–6.

Goldfeld AE, Mollica RF, Pesavento BH, *et al.* 1988. The physical and psychological sequelae of torture. Symptomatology and diagnosis [published erratum appears in *JAMA* 1988 Jul 22–29;**260**(4):478]. *JAMA* **259**:2725–9.

Goldney RD. 1993. Deaths in custody. *Med J Aust* **159**:572–3.

Gordon E, Knight B. 1985. *Uganda: evidence of torture.* Amnesty International, London.

Granzow B, Puschel K. 1998. [Fatalities during imprisonment in Hamburg 1962–1995.] *Arch Kriminol* **201**:1–10.

Hiss J, Kahana T. 1996. Medicolegal investigation of death in custody: a postmortem procedure for detection of blunt force injuries. *Am J Forensic Med Pathol* **17**:312–14.

Hougen HP. 1988. Physical and psychological sequelae to torture. A controlled clinical study of exiled asylum applicants. *Forensic Sci Int* **39**:5–11.

Jandoo R. 1987. Human rights abuses and the medical profession. *Forensic Sci Int* **35**:237–47.

Johnson HR. 1982. Deaths in police custody in England and Wales. *Forensic Sci Int* **19**:231–6.

Karch SB, Stephens BG. 1999. Drug abusers who die during arrest or in custody. *J R Soc Med* **92**:110–13.

Karlsmark T, Thomsen HK, Danielsen L, *et al.* 1984. Tracing the use of electrical torture. *Am J Forensic Med Pathol* **5**:333–7.

Kirschner RH. 1984. The use of drugs in torture and human rights abuses. *Am J Forensic Med Pathol* **5**:313–15.

Lacroix JS, Buvelot JM, Polla BS, *et al.* 1991. Improvement of symptoms of non-allergic chronic rhinitis by local treatment with capsaicin. *Clin Exp Allergy* **21**:595–600.

Lanphear BP. 1987. Deaths in custody in Shelby county, Tennessee, January 1970–July 1985. *Am J Forensic Med Pathol* **8**:299–301.

Lee RJ, Yolton RL, Yolton DP, *et al.* 1996. Personal defense sprays: effects and management of exposure. *J Am Optom Assoc* **67**:548–60.

Levine LJ. 1984. The role of the forensic odontologist in human rights investigations. *Am J Forensic Med Pathol* **5**:317–20.

Levine M. 1998. Deaths in police custody. *Med Leg J* **66**:97–108.

Lifschultz BD, Donoghue ER. 1991. Deaths in custody. *Leg Med* 45–71.

Lok V, Tunca M, Kumanlioglu K, *et al.* 1991. Bone scintigraphy as clue to previous torture [letter] [see comments]. *Lancet* **337**:846–7.

Luke JL, Reay DT. 1992. The perils of investigating and certifying deaths in police custody. *Am J Forensic Med Pathol* **13**:98–100.

Macdonald HA. 1998. Possible idiosyncratic reaction to OC spray. *N Z Med J* **111**:327.

Mercy JA, Heath CW, Jr., Rosenberg ML. 1990. Mortality associated with the use of upper-body control holds by police. *Violence Vict* **5**:215–22.

Mirzaei S, Knoll P, Lipp RW, *et al.* 1998. Bone scintigraphy in screening of torture survivors. *Lancet* **352**:949–51.

Mirzaei S, Knoll P, Keck A, *et al*. 2001. Regional cerebral blood flow in patients suffering from post-traumatic stress disorder. *Neuropsychobiology* **43**:260–4.

Missliwetz J, Denk W. 1991. [Maltreatment by police officers?] *Arch Kriminol* **187**:1–12.

Morrison S. 1996. Custodial suicide in Australia: a comparative study of different populations. *Med Sci Law* **36**:167–77.

Norfolk G, Cartwright J. 1996. Deaths in police custody are being analysed retrospectively. *Br Med J* **312**:911.

Patel F. 2000. Custody restraint asphyxia. *Am J Forensic Med Pathol* **21**:196–7.

Patel V. 1996. Deaths in police custody. *Br Med J* **312**:56.

Petersen HD, Rasmussen OV. 1992. Medical appraisal of allegations of torture and the involvement of doctors in torture. *Forensic Sci Int* **53**:97–116.

Pollanen MS, Chiasson DA, Cairns JT, *et al*. 1998. Unexpected death related to restraint for excited delirium: a retrospective study of deaths in police custody and in the community. *Can Med Assoc J* **158**:1603–7.

Primorac D, Andelinovic S, Definis-Gojanovic M, *et al*. 1996. Identification of war victims from mass graves in croatia, bosnia, and herzegovina by use of standard forensic methods and DNA typing. *J Forensic Sci* **41**:891–4.

Rainio J, Hedman M, Karkola K, *et al*. 2001. Forensic osteological investigations in Kosovo. *Forensic Sci Int* **121**:166–73.

Rainio J, Lalu K, Penttila A. 2001. Independent forensic autopsies in an armed conflict: investigation of the victims from Racak, Kosovo. *Forensic Sci Int* **116**:171–85.

Rasmussen OV. 1990. Medical aspects of torture. *Dan Med Bull* **37**(Suppl 1):1–88.

Rasmussen OV, Lunde I. 1980. Evaluation of investigation of 200 torture victims. *Dan Med Bull* **27**:241–3.

Rasmussen OV, Skylv G. 1992. Signs of falanga torture [letter]. *Lancet* **340**:725.

Reay DT. 1998. Death in custody. *Clin Lab Med* **18**:1–22.

Reay DT, Eisele JE. 1982. Death from law enforcement neck holds. *Am J Forensic Med Pathol* **3**:253–8.

Reay DT, Eisele JE. 1986. Law enforcement neck holds. *Am J Forensic Med Pathol* **7**:177–87.

Reay DT, Hazelwood RR. 1970. Death in military police custody and confinement. *Milit Med* **135**:765–71.

Reilly CA, Crouc DJ, Yost GS, *et al*. 2001. Determination of capsaicin, dihydrocapsaicin, and nonivamide in self-defense weapons by liquid chromatography-mass spectrometry and liquid chromatography-tandem mass spectrometry. *J Chromatogr A* **912**:259–67.

Reilly CA, Crouch DJ, Yost GS. 2001. Quantitative analysis of capsaicinoids in fresh peppers, oleoresin capsicum and pepper spray products. *J Forensic Sci* **46**:502–9.

Richmond PW, Fligelstone LJ, Lewis E. 1988. Injuries caused by handcuffs [see comments]. *Br Med J* **297**:111–12.

Ross DL. 1998. Factors associated with excited delirium deaths in police custody. *Mod Pathol* **11**:1127–37.

Ruttenber AJ, Lawler-Heavner J, Yin M, *et al*. 1997. Fatal excited delirium following cocaine use: epidemiologic findings provide new evidence for mechanisms of cocaine toxicity. *J Forensic Sci* **42**:25–31.

Savnik A, Amris K, Rogind H, *et al*. 2000. MRI of the plantar structures of the foot after falanga torture. *Eur Radiol* **10**:1655–9.

Skinner M. 1987. Planning the archaeological recovery of evidence from recent mass graves. *Forensic Sci Int* **34**:267–87.

Skylv G. 1992. The physical sequelae of torture. In: Basoglu M (ed.), *Torture and its consequences: current treatment approaches*. Cambridge University Press, Cambridge.

Smith CG, Stopford W. 1999. Health hazards of pepper spray. *N C Med J* **60**:268–74.

Snow CC, Levine L, Lukash L, *et al*. 1984. The investigation of the human remains of the 'disappeared' in Argentina. *Am J Forensic Med Pathol* **5**:297–9.

Steffee CH, Lantz PE, Flannagan LM, *et al*. 1995. Oleoresin capsicum (pepper) spray and 'in-custody deaths'. *Am J Forensic Med Pathol* **16**:185–92.

Stover E, Nightingale EO. 1985. The medical profession and the prevention of torture. *N Engl J Med* **313**:1102–4.

Tedeschi LG. 1984. Human rights and the forensic scientist. *Am J Forensic Med Pathol* **5**:295–6.

Tedeschi LG. 1984. Methodology in the forensic sciences. Documentation of human rights abuses. *Am J Forensic Med Pathol* **5**:301–3.

Thomsen AB, Eriksen J, Smidt-Nielsen K. 1997. [Neurogenic pain following Palestinian hanging.] *Ugeskr Laeger* **159**:4129–30.

Thomsen AB, Eriksen J, Smidt-Nielsen K. 2000. Chronic pain in torture survivors. *Forensic Sci Int* **108**:155–63.

Thomsen JL. 2000. The role of the pathologist in human rights abuses. *J Clin Pathol* **53**:569–72.

Thomsen JL, Helweg Larsen K, Rasmussen OV. 1984. Amnesty International and the forensic sciences. *Am J Forensic Med Pathol* **5**:305–11.

Tunca M, Lok V. 1998. Bone scintigraphy in screening of torture survivors. *Lancet* **352**:1859.

Vesaluoma M, Muller L, Gallar J, *et al.* 2000. Effects of oleoresin capsicum pepper spray on human corneal morphology and sensitivity. *Invest Ophthalmol Vis Sci* **41**:2138–47.

Watson WA, Stremel KR, Westdorp EJ. 1996. Oleoresin capsicum (cap-stun) toxicity from aerosol exposure. *Ann Pharmacother* **30**:733–5.

Zollman TM, Bragg RM, Harrison DA. 2000. Clinical effects of oleoresin capsicum (pepper spray) on the human cornea and conjunctiva. *Ophthalmology* **107**:2186–9.

CHAPTER 11

Burns and scalds

Damage to the tissues arising from the application of heat is commonly encountered in forensic pathology and sometimes provides a challenging problem in the distinction between ante-mortem and post-mortem burning, which may have serious criminal aspects.

HEAT INJURY

This may arise following a defect in body temperature control or, more commonly, from the external application of heat. Mammalian tissues can survive only within a relatively narrow range of temperatures, approximately 20–44°C.

When external heat is applied, the extent of damage depends upon:

- the applied temperature
- the ability of the body surface to conduct away the excess heat
- the time for which the heat is applied.

The temperature/time relationship is important, for it is sometimes forgotten that relatively low temperatures, even as little as 44°C, can cause damage if sustained long enough. This is attested by many negligence lawsuits concerning unconscious patients burned by forgotten hot-water bottles.

The degrees of thermal damage were investigated by Moritz and Henriques (1947), who found that the lowest temperature that would cause damage was 44°C, though it required no fewer than 5 hours before a burn appeared. Only 3 seconds was needed, however, if the object was at 60°C.

Radiant heat can also cause severe damage, as is obvious from overexposure to sunlight or artificial sunlamps. The long-term effects also include malignant changes, now more important because pollution-induced changes in the stratosphere are allowing more ultraviolet radiation to reach the earth's surface. In forensic practice it is more often seen when an old or disabled person falls unconscious within close range of a gas, electric or coal fire, those areas of skin unprotected by clothing becoming burned, often to a blistered state. It can be difficult or impossible to tell how much of such a condition is ante-mortem or post-mortem, as the presence of reddening and blistering cannot always be depended on as criteria of vital infliction. Mottled pigmentation and reddening of the fronts of the legs (erythema ab igne) is a familiar sign in those addicted to sitting before an open fire.

CLASSIFICATION OF THE SEVERITY OF BURNS

An arbitrary, but useful, classification is used (mainly for surgical purposes) to denote the severity of both burns and scalds. The older six-stage classification of Dupuytren has given way to Wilson's three-stage nomenclature:

- **First degree:** erythema and blistering without loss of dermis. There is capillary dilatation and transudation of fluid into the tissues, causing swelling. A split may occur in the epidermis to form a blister with an upper cap of pale skin enclosing fluid, surrounded by a zone of hyperaemia. If small (< 1 cm) this blister may resorb, otherwise it will burst, leaving a reddened base. A first-degree burn will heal without scarring.

■ **Second degree:** destruction of the full thickness of skin. The epidermis is coagulated or charred, and a central zone of necrotic tissue is surrounded by first-degree burns or a zone of hyperaemia, or both. The central necrosis sloughs in due course and the epidermis grows in from the margins. The injury cannot heal without scarring, which usually contracts during the healing process, causing puckering and distortion of the surface.

■ **Third degree:** destruction of deeper tissues below the skin. This can be of any severity, from damage to subcutaneous fat to loss of muscle, bone and even a whole limb.

The area involved is traditionally estimated by the surgical 'Rule of Nines', which is sufficient for prognostic purposes, though for the pathologist a more precise anatomical description of the areas burned is essential for his autopsy report.

If the burns are widespread, then large areas of skin may be damaged and functionless. A large area involved may be more dangerous to life than a deeper, more localized burn. It is generally considered that 30–50 per cent involvement of the total body surface is incompatible with survival. Old people can die at considerably lower percentages than this, while children appear more resistant.

MOIST THERMAL DAMAGE – SCALDS

A 'scald' refers to tissue damage from hot liquids, usually water. Other hot fluids include oils, molten rubber, other liquid chemicals and steam. Molten metals are usually at such a high temperature that the results are similar to dry burns. The water scald is a common domestic accident, especially to children and old people, that group at the extremes of life who are vulnerable to so many types of accident.

A scald, unless from some superheated oil, does not cause charring, carbonization or singeing of surface hairs, as does dry heat. It resembles a first-degree dry burn (see later) in

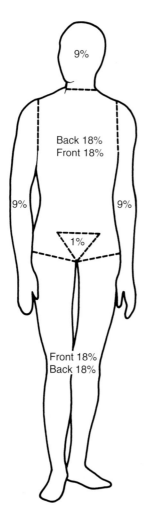

FIGURE 11.1 *The 'Rule of Nines' for calculating the area burned. It does not apply to infants whose body proportions are different from adults. About 60 per cent surface burns can be survived by children and young people up to 20 years of age but this rapidly decreases with advancing age.*

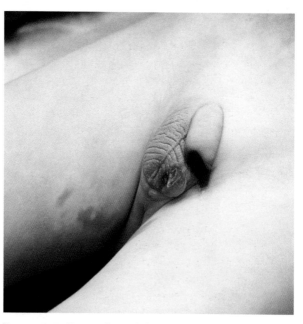

FIGURE 11.2 *First- and second-degree burns on the right thigh and scrotum of a 5-year-old diabetic child, who had been treated by a quack, who had promised the parents to cure the child by hot baths. Death was caused by the untreated diabetes.*

that there is reddening, desquamation and blistering, but the shape of the scald tends to be different. There is usually a sharply demarcated edge, corresponding to the limits of contact of the fluid. If due to immersion in hot water, such as a bath, there will be a horizontal fluid level, though this may be made irregular by splashing. When tipped or splashed, the hot liquid runs under gravity so that trickle patterns may be seen, which may enable the medical examiner to determine the posture of the victim when scalded.

The intensely red base of a severe scald may at first be covered by wrinkled, macerated epidermis. The scalded skin may swell and exude serum. Infection may supervene but where the burns are extensive, death usually results from the systemic effects of shock, fluid and electrolyte disturbance, and secondary chest infections. The severity of a scald depends on the duration of contact with the skin, as well as the temperature. When hot water is splashed, tipped or thrown, it has only a momentary contact, falling away under gravity. The large surface area allows rapid cooling, so damage must occur in a short time, which necessitates the temperature being high if severe damage is to be caused. Often the water is boiling, especially in the kitchen accidents that, sadly, occur to children with such regularity. The interposition of clothing may have two opposite effects; it may protect the underlying skin from the hot liquid, especially if poorly permeable, but it may also hold the hot liquid in contact with the skin for a longer time, especially if the fabric is absorbent.

The appearance of scalds may resemble dry burns except for the distribution and the fact that, if due to immersion, the severity of the skin damage is usually uniform over the whole of the burnt area up to the sharply demarcated margin. When hot or boiling water has been poured or splashed onto the body, the worst scalds will be at the area of initial contact where the fluid was hottest, but decrease in severity as the cooling liquid runs away. In children who pull containers of hot liquid down on themselves, the scalds tend to be on the face, neck, chest and arms, with 'shadow areas' of undamaged skin in the axillae and on the back.

BURNS FROM DRY HEAT

More common than scalds, burns due to dry heat may be caused by high temperature applied to the body surface by conduction or radiation. Convection is merely a variant of conduction in this respect; as hot gas impinges on the surface, the molecules transfer their high energy in a similar fashion to the direct contact of a hot solid.

Radiation causes damage through the conversion of infrared frequencies into thermal heat on absorption at the

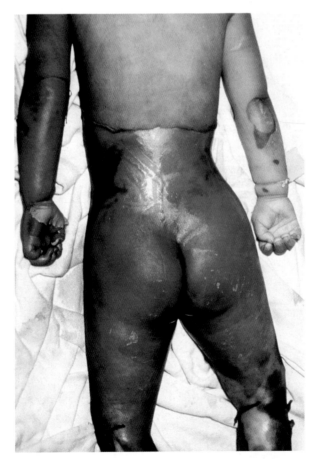

FIGURE 11.3 *Scalds or wet burns in a child accidentally left in a hot bath while her mother went to answer the telephone. This illustrates that time, as well as temperature, is a factor in causing heat damage to skin. The child died some days later from an intercurrent chest infection.*

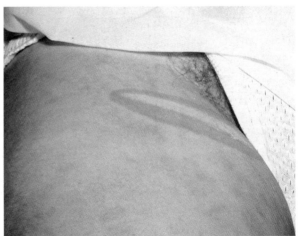

FIGURE 11.4 *A burn on the inner sides of each upper thigh in a young woman. These are suggestive of the application of a hot-water bottle in an attempt at resuscitation after a criminal abortion. The victim died of air embolism following the use of a Higginson syringe.*

skin interface. As with scalds, the tissue damage is a function of temperature and time. A warm water-pipe will cause a burn if left long enough in contact with the same area of skin, but the vast majority of dry burns are due to high temperatures acting for a shorter time.

Where the time is extended beyond that needed for initial burning, the tissues may be charred, carbonized or completely destroyed, as in cremation.

The severity of dry burns

The Wilson classification of severity of burns is given above, with three degrees according to the depth of tissue damage:

■ Erythema leads to redness and swelling of the skin. Blisters may form either within the thickness of the epidermis or at the epidermal–dermal junction.

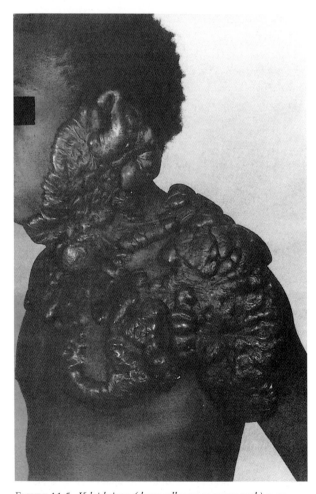

FIGURE 11.5 *Keloid tissue (dense collagenous overgrowth) more often follows burns than other injuries. It is especially prevalent and profuse in negroid persons. This East African youth was tortured in a political camp with hot metal and burning kerosene, resulting months later in exuberant keloid.*

■ Destruction of the full thickness of the skin, which may be total or incomplete. If epidermal structures survive, such as the deeper parts of hair follicles, then epithelialization may occur from islands within the burned area. If not, slow coverage with more probability of extensive scarring will occur from invasion of epidermis at the periphery.
■ Destruction of subcutaneous tissues, such as fat, muscle and even bone, is the most serious grade of burning, though, as mentioned elsewhere, it may be less dangerous to life than larger areas of more superficial burns.

GROSS APPEARANCES AT AUTOPSY

The body may present a wide range of damage from mere reddening over wide areas to almost total cremation, in which a search may have to be made at the scene of the fire to collect or even discover the remnants.

Usually, where leathery coagulation or charring has not occurred, ante-mortem burns will be reddened and often blistered. The latter have a marginal red zone of variable width, usually 5–20 mm across. Blisters may be present either in the main burn or as islands beyond the periphery. Most ante-mortem blisters will have a bright red base when burst and an erythematous areola. The whole of the burned area may form one large blister or be a coalescence of blisters. These are usually collapsed at autopsy, so that sheets and shreds of white epidermis lie across an angry red base.

Where the burns are more severe, the skin may be stiffened, yellow–brown and leathery, a half-way stage to actual carbonization. Drying after death of areas that were weeping serum leads to a stiff, parchment-like surface. Post-mortem heating and deposition of smoke may mimic or overlie the ante-mortem appearances, the surface often being blackened by soot deposition.

Hair is singed or completely burnt away in severe burns. In lesser degrees it may survive and the ends of the hairs may be 'clubbed'. Here the keratin melts at the distal end nearest the heat, then resolidifies on cooling, forming a terminal blob on the shaft like an unlit match. Eyelashes, eyebrows, pubic, axillary and general body hair may all suffer this scorching. Where skin has actually ignited, the subcutaneous fat acting as a fuel, black brittle masses will occupy the tissues merging into cooked, dry muscle beneath, which in turn grades into more moist and normal-looking soft tissue at greater depths. Beneath burns of any degree, the deeper tissues may be affected, especially muscle, which becomes pale, brownish and obviously 'part-cooked'. This is often a post-mortem phenomenon caused by the dead body remaining in a heated environment and such cooked muscle may

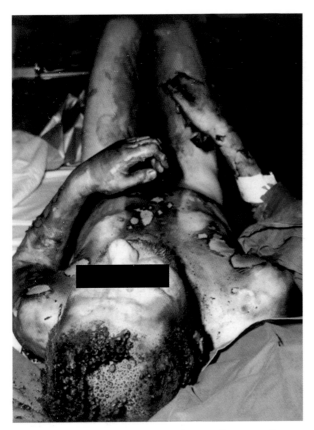

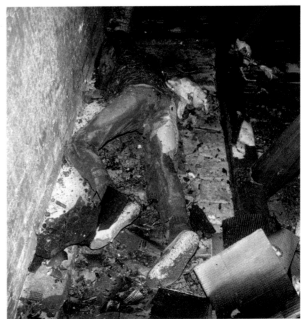

FIGURE 11.7 *Dead bodies in fires pose a problem for pathologists and investigators. Death was shown to have occurred after the fire began from soot in the lungs and carboxyhaemoglobin in the blood. There were no ante-mortem burns and there was a high blood-alcohol concentration.*

FIGURE 11.6 *Second and third degree burns and singeing of hair on a suicide who doused himself with petrol and set himself to fire.*

extensively underlie normal skin, which shows no evidence of ante-mortem burning, especially if protected by clothing. It is the general high temperature of the environment over a relatively long period which produces this 'parboiled' appearance, similar to the cooking effect of a slow oven.

Where heat has been intense and continuous, all soft tissue down to bone may be consumed and the bone itself may be blackened. The most extreme stage is conversion of the bone to brittle greyish-white splinters, sometimes with loss of skeletal structures, leading to absent feet, hands or limbs. It is rare for the whole body to be completely consumed, even in deliberate cremations, but only a fraction of the original body mass may remain, often almost inseparable from the burned surroundings. Where much smoke has been generated, as in most house fires, the skin will be discoloured where exposed. Sharply demarcated areas of soot deposition may coincide with burning from hot gas. Even the thinnest layer of clothing may protect completely from both these effects.

Muscle contractures are common where substantial heat has reached the body. This is almost always a post-mortem occurrence, as deep-heating effects sufficient to cook muscle are incompatible with life. The muscle becomes shortened by dehydration and protein denaturation. The flexors, being

bulkier than the extensors, contract more and force the limbs into a position of general flexion, the so-called 'boxer's' or 'pugilistic' attitude. Contraction of the paraspinal musculature often causes a marked opisthotonos. Froth, often pink-stained, may appear at the mouth and nostrils as a result of pulmonary oedema caused by heat irritation of the air passages and lungs. The tongue frequently protrudes and may be scorched.

SPURIOUS 'WOUNDS' IN BURNS

Heated skin contracts markedly and splits often appear. This may lead inexperienced observers (such as police) to suspect that ante-mortem wounds have been inflicted, the fire being used to cover up a criminal offence. These splits may be anywhere, but are especially seen over extensor surfaces and joints, as well on the head. Some, especially those at elbows and knees when the limbs are flexed across brittle skin, are caused by firemen handling the body during recovery.

The possibility of true wounds being present must always be kept in mind, as many homicides have been concealed in fires. The false split will show no bleeding in the deeper tissues and its position is usually suggestive. The differentiation may be difficult or even impossible, however, especially when severe heat damage in the area makes examination of the underlying tissue impracticable.

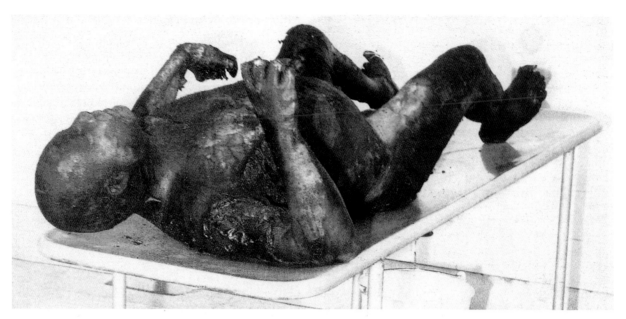

FIGURE 11.8 *Heat flexures of the limbs, part way towards the 'pugilistic attitude' formed when the arms are raised higher. The elbows, knees and wrists are strongly flexed because muscle contraction is stronger in the flexor groups. The victim was the captain of a Russian ship who set fire to his cabin during a bout of heavy drinking.*

The other major false lesion is the 'heat haematoma' in the extradural space. When severe heat is applied to the cranium, a mass of blood resembling a true extradural haematoma may form between the skull and the dura. This may arise either from venous sinuses or be virtually 'boiled' out of the diploic space in the skull through emissary venous channels. The blood is spongy from gas bubbles and tawny or chocolate brown. The exterior of the skull overlying the haematoma is usually charred and the scalp burnt away. If it is a purely post-mortem phenomenon, the heat haematoma will have a similar level of carboxyhaemoglobin to the blood, whereas if it was an ante-mortem lesion sustained before the fire began, it will be free from monoxide, as discussed in more detail below. Where the heat is intense the spurious haematoma may be outside a grossly shrunken dura, which compresses the brain into a cooked mass. The dura may split under the tension and allow brain tissue to ooze out into the large space within the cranium, where it may form a mass of frothy paste (Kondo and Ohshima 1994). These changes may be present without a haematoma, but the latter is often present. In the absence of a skull fracture, other than one due to heat, this haematoma should not be ascribed to trauma.

ANTE-MORTEM VERSUS POST-MORTEM BURNS

In severe conflagrations, either in buildings or vehicles, the terminal state of the body often does not reflect the condition at the time of death. Indeed, many deaths will have occurred before any heat reaches the body, death being caused by the inhalation of smoke. It may be difficult or impossible for the pathologist to determine the extent of ante-mortem damage if the ensuing fire later reaches the body and causes post-mortem burning. The exposed skin surface may be reddened in both ante-mortem and post-mortem burns, the classical distinction of a 'red flare' or 'vital reaction' being unsafe as an index of infliction before death. The author (BK) has seen several cases of undoubted post-mortem burns, one at least 30 minutes after fatal strangulation, where an extensive 'red flare' was caused during attempts at disposal of the body by fire.

Blisters can form post-mortem, but are pale yellow unless on scorched skin. There is rarely a red base or erythematous areola, though this sign cannot be depended upon absolutely. The contained fluid is thin and clear. Traditionally most authors claim that differentiation can be made between an ante-mortem and a post-mortem blister by an analysis for protein and chloride in the fluid. The blister formed in life is said to contain more protein and chlorides, but no absolute figures are offered and the authors have yet to meet a pathologist who does this as a routine. One suspects that the test is another of the apocryphal procedures that have been handed down from textbook to textbook without verification.

Most useful of all in fatalities is the presence of carbon monoxide in the circulating blood and carbon particles in the air passages and lungs, and this is dealt with in the section on inhalation of fumes. They do not necessarily prove that any burns were ante-mortem, but that the victim was still alive when the fire was in progress, which is not the same conclusion. The extradural heat haematoma may be investigated in a different way to determine its time of origin. If it is a true traumatic lesion produced before the fire began, it should contain no carboxyhaemoglobin. A spurious heat haematoma is formed from blood that will contain carboxyhaemoglobin if the victim has absorbed this gas during the fire. It must be appreciated, however, as

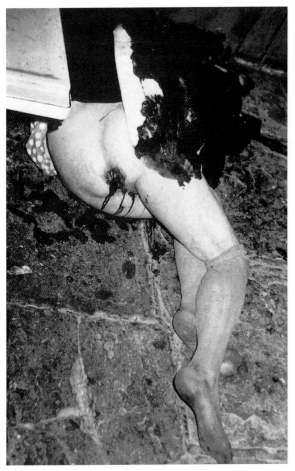

FIGURE 11.9 *Substantial destruction of the body by fire. The upper half of the victim has virtually vanished, including skeletal structures, leaving the lower part intact. The gas stove was ignited with a match after a delay while gas was escaping, causing a near-explosion that consumed the upper part of the body, the fat burning with clothing acting as a 'wick'. Such events have given rise to the myth of 'spontaneous combustion'.*

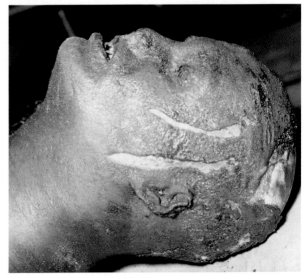

FIGURE 11.10 *Post-mortem injuries caused by heat simulating head injuries. The fire service were concerned about an apparent preconflagration assault, but such skin splits are commonly seen as a result of heat contracture of the tissues. The scalp on the top of the head has been burned through and the skull is charred. Beneath this is a spurious 'heat haematoma', sometimes confused with a traumatic extradural haemorrhage.*

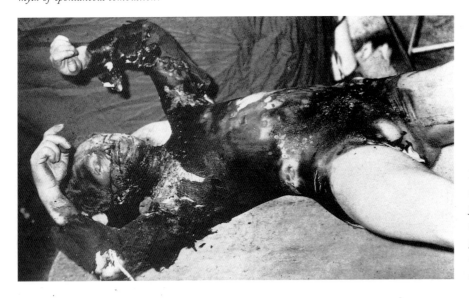

FIGURE 11.11 *Post-mortem burns in a victim recovered from a house fire. Note the raised arms caused by heat contractures and the complete protection against burning afforded by clothing on the legs. There is extensive skin splitting on the chest.*

discussed below, that not all persons alive during a fire accumulate carboxyhaemoglobin in their blood.

If there is carboxyhaemoglobin absorption, then the heat haematoma will also yield it on analysis. The use of this test, again related in most classical texts, is, however, extremely limited.

FUMES AND FIRES

The majority of fatal dry burns in civilian practice occur in conflagrations in buildings, rather than in vehicles or aircraft. In many of these tragedies death is not caused by burns, but to inhalation of fumes produced by the combustion of the building structure and contents. Indeed, most burns seen by forensic pathologists are post-mortem, either because the victim was already dead from smoke inhalation or because severe post-mortem burning obliterates the lesser degrees of burns present up to the moment of death.

Death from inhaling fumes may be caused in several ways:

■ Thermal damage to the air passages and lungs from the direct effect of hot gases. At autopsy the tongue, pharynx and especially glottis may be scorched, lesser degrees causing a greyish-yellow blanching of the mucosa. The interior of the larynx, trachea and main bronchi may be thickened and blanched, or reddened and inflamed, if the temperature is too low actually to burn the lining.

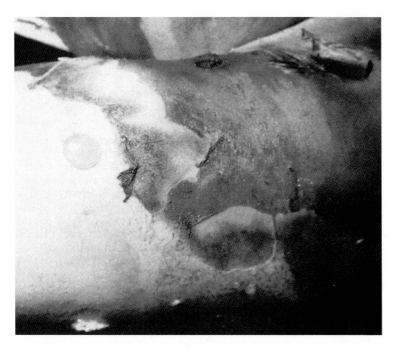

FIGURE 11.12 *It can be difficult or impossible to differentiate between ante-mortem and post-mortem burns when they are sustained near to the time of death. Here the blister with no erythema at the base could either be post-mortem or ante-mortem, as reddening of the margins and adjacent skin can occur for at least an hour after death. It is preferable to call doubtful lesions 'peri-mortal'.*

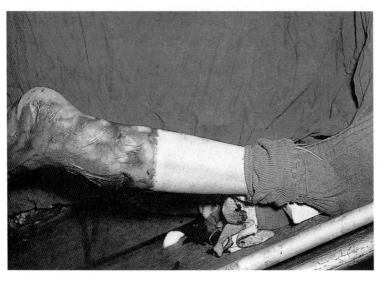

FIGURE 11.13 *Post-mortem smoke soiling and superficial burns on the leg of a house-fire victim who died of smoke inhalation. Note the complete protection of the skin, which had been covered only by a sock.*

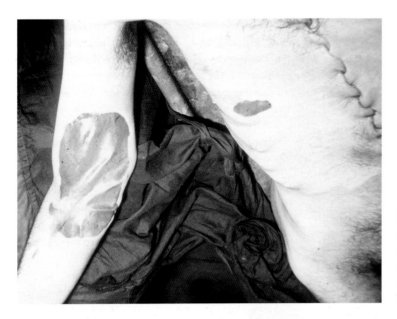

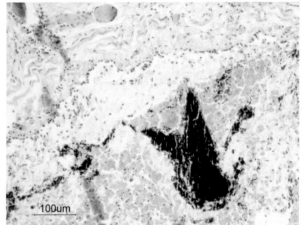

FIGURE 11.14 *Post-mortem burn on the arm and chest caused by a hot-water bottle being left over the heart in an attempt at resuscitation. The lesion is sharp-edged, there is no erythematous margin, and the surface is brown and leathery from post-mortem drying.*

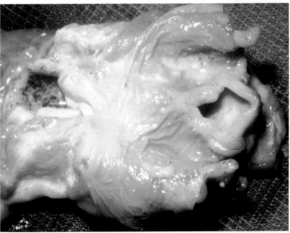

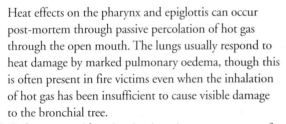

FIGURE 11.15 *Larynx of a house-fire victim showing heat blanching of the epiglottis and glottal entrance from breathing hot gas. The lower cut end of the trachea shows copious soot-containing mucus, also indicating respiration during the fire.*

FIGURE 11.16 *A small bronchus from a fire victim, showing histological evidence of soot deposition, together with desquamation of the epithelium and plugging with cellular debris. (Van Gieson; original magnification ×10.)*

Heat effects on the pharynx and epiglottis can occur post-mortem through passive percolation of hot gas through the open mouth. The lungs usually respond to heat damage by marked pulmonary oedema, though this is often present in fire victims even when the inhalation of hot gas has been insufficient to cause visible damage to the bronchial tree.

■ Carbon monoxide poisoning is an important aspect of most fires – indeed it is the major or even sole cause of death in many victims of conflagrations, especially in house fires. When any combustible material burns in air, most of the carbon in organic material, such as timber, fabric and furnishings, is converted to carbon dioxide. Carbon monoxide is also produced, however, and, where the access of oxygen is limited or exhausted by the ongoing combustion, larger volumes of the monoxide are produced. Slow, smouldering fires with little flame are likely to produce more monoxide, as with burning bedclothes and mattresses. At the other extreme, rapid flash fires with flames fanned by moving draughts and those involving volatile fuels, such as petrol or kerosene, produce relatively little monoxide – though much depends upon the free access of air.

In many house fires, where the seat of the fire is originally remote from the victim, death may occur from carbon monoxide poisoning long before the flames reach the body.

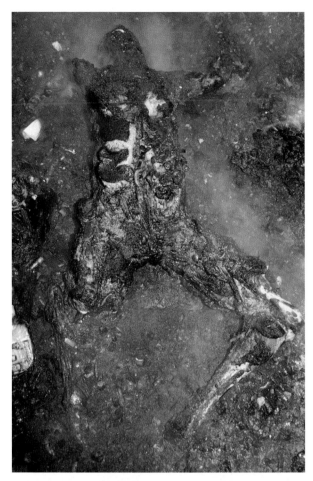

FIGURE 11.17 *Charred body at the scene of fire showing the 'pugilistic attitude' and post-mortem skin splits on the chest.*

A person may be asleep in an apartment or house, and die without ever waking if large volumes of monoxide creep through the rooms. Burns are often post-mortem in such cases and, where extensive charring occurs, the differentiation between ante-mortem and post-mortem damage may be impossible.

It is often a comfort for bereaved relatives to be told that their loved ones were either already dead or unconscious before the agony of burning reached them, and the pathologist may be able to emphasize this at any inquest or inquiry. Unfortunately, where the bodies are found in positions obviously indicating escape or concealment, such an explanation loses its conviction – though even then it may well be that coma from monoxide poisoning overtook them before burning began.

The pathology of carbon monoxide is dealt with in another section of this book, but it may be repeated here that the autopsy signs are primarily that of a cherry-pink coloration of the skin, blood and tissues. Where smoke staining or extensive charring has occurred, there may be little skin to examine, though there is usually some in a protected position under the body. The blood and tissues usually have the characteristic colour but, when the person is anaemic or exsanguinated, this may be hard to detect. A high saturation with monoxide is usually unmistakable at autopsy, though sometimes certain types of artificial light in the autopsy room, such as some fluorescent tubes, make the cherry-pink colour difficult to confirm. The colour may be better seen if blood is diluted with water against a white background, such as a porcelain autopsy table or sink. Nothing replaces laboratory analysis of a sample, however, and this must be done in

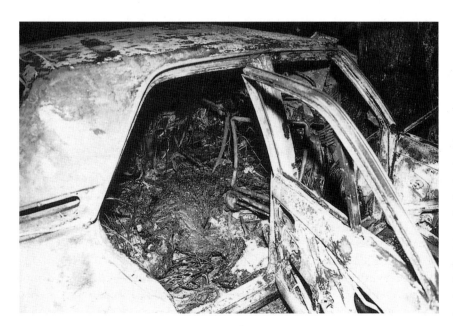

FIGURE 11.18 *The finding of a body in a burnt-out car is always suspicious, but is usually accidental or suicidal. Radiography should always be carried out to exclude firearm injuries. Carboxyhaemoglobin levels are often low or even absent in a rapid flash gasoline fire; this makes the diagnosis of being alive during the fire difficult, especially when there may also be little soot to foul the air passages.*

every case of death from fire, irrespective of the subjective appearance of the skin, blood and tissues.

The saturation of haemoglobin with carbon monoxide varies greatly from one fatal case to another. Many variable factors exist such as the concentration in the atmosphere, the time of exposure and local changes in oxygen content. When carbon monoxide is the sole cause of death, a blood saturation of at least 40 per cent is required, except in old and debilitated persons where deaths have been reported at 25 per cent. Many fatalities will display 50–60 per cent saturation, though levels in general are less than in pure carbon monoxide poisoning, such as car exhaust suicides or industrial exposure, where concentrations of up to 80 per cent may occur. In fires, additional factors such as other toxic fumes and reduction of the atmospheric oxygen may operate, resulting in death at lower carboxyhaemoglobin concentrations.

Yoshida *et al.* (1991) published data from 120 house-fire victims in Japan, in which only nine people had carboxyhaemoglobin (HBCO) concentrations below 10 per cent, the range being from 1 to 95 per cent saturation. Of 31 victims in whom cyanide analyses were made, two had high cyanide and low HBCO.

The variability of monoxide poisoning may be illustrated by the fact that two bodies lying side by side in a burned house may have widely differing blood saturations – indeed, sometimes one victim may have a zero blood monoxide saturation. Children often have much lower levels than adults in the same situation, but even two adults may differ in their carboxyhaemoglobin concentrations, the explanation being unclear. Local variations in draughts, levels above the floor and respiration rates may account for these anomalies.

Carbon monoxide in the blood is a valuable indicator that the victim was alive after the fire began. Where a dead body is disposed of by arson no absorption can take place, as the gas can gain entry only through the pulmonary interface. Thus the presence of more than a smoker's level of 5 per cent saturation of the blood with carboxyhaemoglobin means that breathing occurred after the fire began. It is vital, however, to appreciate that the converse is not true. **The fact that a body in a fire does NOT have carboxyhaemoglobin in the blood does NOT mean that they must have been dead before the fire began.** The records of all forensic departments have examples of this occurrence and therefore it is illogical – and sometimes legally dangerous – to draw the unwarranted inference that such a victim must have been already dead before the fire began, however common the generalization may be. In rapid flash fires, especially where gasoline or kerosene are involved, the monoxide level is more likely to be low or even negative, than in the slower conflagration with restricted access of oxygen that occurs in a burning building.

Toxic substances in fumes

In recent years it has been appreciated that a number of toxic substances other than carbon monoxide may be present in the fumes from fires. Cyanides are predominant and the blood of fire victims may often be shown to have high levels of this toxic compound. Nitric oxide, phosgene and other more complex substances may be liberated, especially when modern plastic polymers are burned. Furnishings, upholstery, paints, lacquers, varnishes and actual structural components are increasingly made from polystyrene, polyurethane, polyvinyl and other plastic materials. These are particularly liable to generate toxic gases when ignited (Anderson *et al.* 1981, 1982).

Caution must be employed when interpreting the analysis of cadaver blood for cyanide, as this substance can be produced in significant concentration by post-mortem decomposition. Particular care must be taken in preservation of samples, which should have fluoride added, and in ensuring there is no delay before analysis so that further decomposition is kept to a minimum. Where cyanides, oxides of nitrogen and other toxic substances are inhaled during a fire, carbon monoxide is inevitably absorbed as well. It then becomes difficult to apportion the relative blame for the death among these different toxic agents – and where there are also ante-mortem burns, the differentiation may be impossible. If the pathologist considers that he cannot identify any ante-mortem burns, then the most logical cause of death is 'inhalation of smoke'. If vital burns are present then, according to the circumstances, these can be given as the cause of death, with or without the addition of 'carbon monoxide or smoke inhalation'.

INHALATION OF SOOT

As well as the inhalation of carbon monoxide, victims in a fire usually breathe in carbon particles present in the sooty smoke. Once again this is more pronounced in a building fire than a vehicle blaze, though there are many exceptions. The combustion of timber floors, roofs, furniture, and the fabric of furnishings and carpets produces large volumes of dense black smoke. Every pathologist attending the scene of a house fire is aware of the thick layer of soot than clings to every surface and may hang in fronds from the ceilings. It is little wonder that such material suspended in the air finds its way into the respiratory passages of the victims.

As a marker of ante-mortem inhalation, it is almost as useful as carbon monoxide. Soot particles may enter the open mouth of a corpse, stain the tongue and pharynx, and may even passively reach the glottis. No significant amount can pass the vocal cords and enter the trachea after death, however, so carbon in the lower respiratory tract is a certain

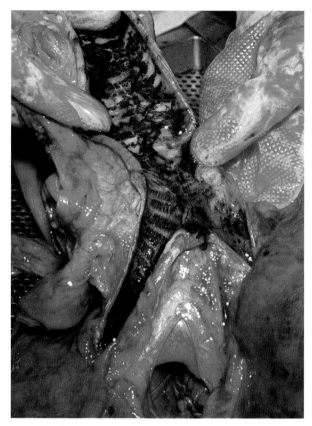

FIGURE 11.19 *Soot in the tracheal mucus, a sign of breathing while the fire was in progress. Though soot can passively reach the glottis after death if the mouth is open, it cannot reach the lower air passages in any significant quantity. Histology of the smaller bronchi offers complete proof of active respiration.*

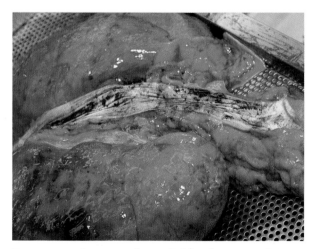

FIGURE 11.20 *Soot in oesophagus of a house-fire victim indicating respiration during the fire.*

indicator of breathing during the fire. Histological demonstration of soot in the more peripheral bronchi, out as far as the terminal bronchioles, is absolute proof of such respiratory function. The carbon is usually mixed with mucus

adherent to the tracheal and bronchial walls because of heat irritation of the mucosa. Often there is swallowed soot and mucus in the stomach, and again this is evidence of life during the smoky phase of the fire.

ATYPICAL LOCALIZED BURNING AND 'SPONTANEOUS COMBUSTION'

Some very strange instances of fatal burning occur and most experienced forensic pathologists have recollections of apparently inexplicable cases.

A human body may sometimes burn away almost completely, yet the surrounding fire damage is minimal. These almost invariably occur near a hearth or open fire-grate or chimney. The burning may be confined to the body, its clothing, and a narrow zone of floor or carpet. The author (BK) has seen a circumscribed hole burned through a hearthrug and the floorboards beneath, with an ashed body lying in the space under the floor. He also remembers a pair of undamaged house slippers, with feet still within, the legs burned off at ankle level and no remaining body above, apart from ashed material lying on the adjacent floor. Both these deaths occurred in front of a fireplace with an open chimney.

It seems extraordinary that virtually a whole adult body can be consumed, including the skeleton, with minimal surrounding fire damage, but many such cases are on record and have helped to substantiate the myth of 'spontaneous human combustion'.

Experiments carried out many years ago by Professor David Gee (personal communication) indicated that body fat can burn slowly, using the clothing as a 'wick', similar to a candle flame.

Most cases have in common the fact that there was a source of ignition in an open fire and a chimney which can provide a constant updraught – and often the victims are alcoholics. Though it is not suggested that alcohol plays any part in the burning process, the confusion, instability and lack of judgement which goes with inebriation may well precipitate the ignition process.

As indicated above, the myth of 'spontaneous combustion' is one which refuses to go away, as endless unsubstantiated reports, and newspaper, magazine and television features have continued to fascinate a credulous public ever since Charles Dickens included a description of a case in his novel *Bleak House*.

Numerous allegations have been made of people bursting into flames as they walk down the street, but as yet, no photographs or film has been produced; in fact, the majority of the retrospective claims for this phenomenon have been of bodies next to some source of ignition and where alcohol was involved – as indeed was Dickens' original example.

REFERENCES AND FURTHER READING

Anderson RA, Harland WA. 1982. Fire deaths in the Glasgow area: III. The role of hydrogen cyanide. *Med Sci Law* **22**:35–40.

Anderson RA, Watson AA, Harland WA. 1981. Fire deaths in the Glasgow area: I. General considerations and pathology. *Med Sci Law* **21**:175–83.

Anderson RA, Watson AA, Harland WA. 1981. Fire deaths in the Glasgow area: II. The role of carbon monoxide. *Med Sci Law* **21**:288–94.

Ballantyne B. 1977. In vitro production of cyanide in normal human blood and the influence of thiocyanate and storage temperature. *Clin Toxicol* **11**:173–93.

Bohnert M, Rost T, Faller-Marquardt M, et al. 1997. Fractures of the base of the skull in charred bodies – post-mortem heat injuries or signs of mechanical traumatisation? *Forensic Sci Int* **87**:55–62.

Bohnert M, Schmidt U, Perdekamp MG, et al. 2002. Diagnosis of a captive-bolt injury in a skull extremely destroyed by fire. *Forensic Sci Int* **127**:192–7.

Brown RF. 1978. Injuries by burning. In: Mason JK (ed.), *The pathology of violent injury.* Edward Arnold, London.

Bull JP. 1963. Burns. *Postgrad Med J* **39**:717–25.

Bull JP. 1971. Revised analysis of mortality due to burns. *Lancet* **2**:1133.

Cattaneo C, DiMartino S, Scali S, et al. 1999. Determining the human origin of fragments of burnt bone: a comparative study of histological, immunological and DNA techniques. *Forensic Sci Int* **102**:181–91.

Curry AS, Price DE, Rutter ER. 1967. The production of cyanide in post mortem material. *Acta Pharmacol Toxicol Copenh* **25**:339–44.

Dyer RF, Esch VH. 1976. Polyvinyl chloride toxicity in fires. Hydrogen chloride toxicity in fire fighters. *JAMA* **235**:393–7.

Eckert WG, James S, Katchis S. 1988. Investigation of cremations and severely burned bodies. *Am J Forensic Med Pathol* **9**:188–200.

Gerling I, Meissner C, Reiter A, et al. 2001. Death from thermal effects and burns. *Forensic Sci Int* **115**:33–41.

Gormsen H, Jeppesen N, Lund A. 1984. The causes of death in fire victims. *Forensic Sci Int* **24**:107–11.

Hill IR. 1986. The immediate problems of aircraft fires. *Am J Forensic Med Pathol* **7**:271–7.

Karlsmark T, Aalund O, Danielsen L, et al. 1988. The occurrence of calcium salt deposition on dermal collagen fibres following electrical injury to porcine skin. *Forensic Sci Int* **39**:245–55.

Katcher ML. 1981. Scald burns from hot tap water. *JAMA* **246**:1219–22.

Kojima T, Nishiyama Y, Yashiki M, et al. 1982. Postmortem formation of carbon monoxide. *Forensic Sci Int* **19**:243–8.

Kondo T, Ohshima T. 1994. Epidural herniation of the cerebral tissue in a burned body: a case report. *Forensic Sci Int* **66**:197–202.

Levine B, D'Nicuola J, Kunsman G, et al. 1996. Methodologic considerations in the interpretation of postmortem carboxyhemoglobin concentrations. *Toxicology* **115**:129–34.

Lokan RJ, James RA, Dymock RB. 1987. Apparent post-mortem production of high levels of cyanide in blood. *J Forensic Sci Soc* **27**:253–9.

Matsubara K, Akane A, Maseda C, et al. 1990. 'First pass phenomenon' of inhaled gas in the fire victims. *Forensic Sci Int* **46**:203–8.

Moritz AR, Henriques FC. 1947. Studies of thermal injury: the relative importance of time and surface temperature in the causation of cutaneous burns. *Am J Pathol* **23**:695–704.

Noguchi TT, Eng JJ, Klatt EC. 1988. Significance of cyanide in medicolegal investigations involving fires. *Am J Forensic Med Pathol* **9**:304–9.

Quatrehomme G, Bolla M, Muller M, et al. 1998. Experimental single controlled study of burned bones: contribution of scanning electron microscopy. *J Forensic Sci* **43**:417–22.

Richards NF. 1977. Fire investigation – destruction of corpses. *Med Sci Law* **17**:79–82.

Rothschild MA, Raatschen HJ, Schneider V. 2001. Suicide by self-immolation in Berlin from 1990 to 2000. *Forensic Sci Int* **124**:163–6.

Sajantila A, Strom M, Budowle B, et al. 1991. The polymerase chain reaction and post-mortem forensic identity testing: application of amplified D1S80 and HLA-DQ alpha loci to the identification of fire victims. *Forensic Sci Int* **51**:23–34.

Schmidt P, Musshoff F, Dettmeyer R, et al. 2001. [Unusual carbon monoxide poisoning.] *Arch Kriminol* **208**:10–23.

Schuberth J. 1997. Gas residues of engine starting fluid in postmortem sample from an arsonist. *J Forensic Sci* **42**:144–7.

Schwerd W, Schulz E. 1978. Carboxyhaemoglobin and methaemoglobin findings in burnt bodies. *Forensic Sci Int* **12**:233–5.

Sigrist T. 1999. ['Crow's feet wrinkles' as a sign of preserved consciousness.] *Arch Kriminol* **203**:103–7.

Soares-Vieira JA, Billerbeck AE, Iwamura ES, *et al.* 2000. Post-mortem forensic identity testing: application of PCR to the identification of fire victim. *Sao Paulo Med J* **118**:75–7.

Strom CM, Rechitsky S. 1998. Use of nested PCR to identify charred human remains and minute amounts of blood. *J Forensic Sci* **43**:696–700.

Sweet DJ, Sweet CH. 1995. DNA analysis of dental pulp to link incinerated remains of homicide victim to crime scene. *J Forensic Sci* **40**:310–14.

Teige B, Lundevall J, Fleischer E. 1977. Carboxyhaemoglobin concentrations in fire victims and in cases of fatal carbon monoxide poisoning. *Z Rechtsmed* **80**:17–21.

Yoshida M, Adachi J, Watabiki T, *et al.* 1991. A study on house fire victims: age, carboxyhaemoglobin, hydrogen cyanide and hemolysis. *Forensic Sci Int* **52**:13–20.

Zhu BL, Ishida K, Quan L, *et al.* 2001. Post-mortem urinary myoglobin levels with reference to the causes of death. *Forensic Sci Int* **115**:183–8.

CHAPTER 12

Electrical fatalities

The passage of a substantial electrical current through the tissues can cause skin lesions, organ damage and death. This injury is commonly called 'electrocution', though some would use this term only if death occurs. Fatalities are usually accidental, in both a domestic and industrial environment. Suicides from electricity have increased in recent years, especially in Germany. Homicide is rare but is recorded and, in the USA, electricity has again become a means of judicial execution.

PHYSICAL FACTORS

The severity of tissue damage 'including death' is directly related to a number of physical factors, which include current, voltage, resistance and time. For biological damage to occur, the body must be incorporated into an electrical circuit, so that there is a passage of electrons through the tissues. A mere accumulation of electrons in the form of a static charge can do no harm; scientists in the ball of a Van de Graaf static generator may be at a potential of more than a million volts (V), but experience nothing other than their hair standing on end. Similarly, a person outdoors in a thunderstorm may accumulate a high charge from the capacitance effect of an overhead cloud but, unless the insulation of the air breaks down to allow a lightning strike at or near the person, no ill-effects will occur.

In electrocution there must be a pathway for electrons across part of the body which, in fatal cases, contains vital structures. The current enters at one point (most often a hand being used to hold, touch or manipulate some electrical device) and then leaves the body at an exit point, usually to the earth or the neutral conductor of the electricity supply. The pathway of the current will depend mainly on the relative resistance of various potential exit points. It tends to take the shortest route between entry and best exit, irrespective of the varying conductivity of different internal tissues. If a person places a finger on a 240 V conductor while standing with damp shoes on a wet concrete floor, then an appreciable current will pass from hand to feet, with possibly fatal results. If, however, the person is standing on a carpeted upstairs wooden floor, the poor earth return will allow only a small current to flow and all that may be suffered is a painful muscular spasm.

In another variant of the upstairs scene, should the neutral wire of the supply be touching the skin of the same finger a few centimetres away from the live conductor, a severe local burn may occur but no danger to life, because the high resistance through the feet to earth will prevent any significant current flow passing through the thorax.

Should the person upstairs happen to be turning a bath tap with the other hand, the contact with the opposite finger would allow a current to pass to earth via the tap and metal water-pipes from hand to hand across the thorax – an extremely dangerous position.

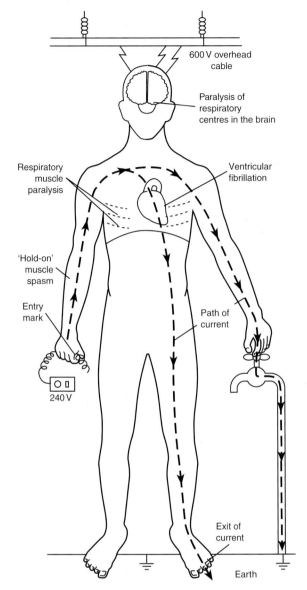

600 V overhead cable

Paralysis of respiratory centres in the brain

Respiratory muscle paralysis

Ventricular fibrillation

'Hold-on' muscle spasm

Entry mark

240 V

Path of current

Exit of current

Earth

FIGURE 12.1 *Pathways of current in electrocution.*

The pathologist is concerned with fatal electrocution and three major events may occur, which are a threat to life:

■ The most common is the passage of a current across the heart, usually when a hand is brought into contact with a live conductor, and the body is earthed either through the feet or the opposite hand. It has been claimed that the most dangerous is contact with the right hand and exit through the feet, as this causes the current to pass obliquely along the axis of the heart. Compared with the other variables of voltage, skin resistance and time, this hypothesis seems immaterial, though this route increases the current across the heart by a factor of 1.5–2.5 compared with left-hand entry.

The fatal process is a cardiac dysrhythmia, usually a ventricular fibrillation ending in asystole.

■ Less often, the passage of a current across the chest and abdomen may lead to respiratory paralysis from spasm of the intercostal muscles and diaphragm.

■ Rarely, the current passes through the head and neck, usually in circumstances when the head of a worker on overhead power lines comes into contact with the conductor. In such instances, there may be a direct effect on the brainstem so that cardiac or respiratory centres are paralysed.

It is commonly said that tolerance can be gained to electric shock and that professional electricians often work on live 240 V conductors with impunity. It seems more likely that expectation of a shock decreases sensitivity, but only for brief contacts, less than would be required for physiological or structural damage.

ELECTRICAL CONSIDERATIONS

Electrons are moved around a circuit by the 'potential difference' between two points, which may be looked upon as the 'pressure' of the electricity, measured in volts (V). The number of electrons flowing constitutes the 'current', analagous to the volume of electricity and is measured in amperes, though in the present discussion, milliamperes (mA) are more relevant to biological effects. The tissues also have 'resistance' to the electrical flow. There is a mathematical relationship between potential difference, current and resistance – the well-known Ohm's law – in which the current varies directly with the voltage and inversely with the resistance. This law has considerable relevance to biological electrical damage.

Alternating and direct current

In spite of the folklore of electricians there is no doubt that direct current (d.c.) is less dangerous than alternating current (a.c.); a current of 50–80 mA a.c. can be fatal in seconds, whereas 250 mA d.c. for the same time is often survived. Alternating current is four to six times as likely to cause death, partly because of the 'hold-on' effect described below, which is the result of tetanoid muscle spasm and prevents the victim from releasing the live conductor.

Alternating current is also much more likely than direct current to cause cardiac arrhythmias. The passage of a.c. at 100 mA for only one-fifth of a second is likely to cause ventricular fibrillation and arrest. High amperage d.c. (above 4 A) may even cause an arrhythmic heart to revert to sinus rhythm, as in medical defibrillation.

The usual frequency of a.c. is 50 cycles/second (cps), though some American and European systems run at 60 cps. Alternating current between 40 and 150 cps is most dangerous in terms of ventricular fibrillation, and regrettably the usual mains supply lies in the centre of this range. Above 150 cps, fibrillation is progressively less likely as the frequency increases: at 1720 cps the heart is 20 times less likely to fibrillate than at 150 cps.

Current

The degree of damage to the tissues is proportional to the actual quantity of electricity flowing through them. This quantity is expressed by the number of electrons per unit time and strictly speaking should be measured in 'coulombs', which is the product of amperes and seconds, though amperes are usually accepted as an index of the current flow. According to Ohm's law, current depends on the applied voltage, the resistance of the tissue and, for tissue damage, the time for which the current is flowing.

In forensic pathology, we are concerned with fatal electrocution and, as most deaths are the result of cardiac dysrhythmias, the most important measure of current is that which leads to acute heart failure. Estimates vary among authors, but it is generally considered that the passage of 50–80 mA across the heart for more than a few seconds is likely to cause death. The most that can be tolerated voluntarily by most people is 30 mA applied to the hand, which results in painful muscle contractions. Consciousness is likely to be lost at about 40 mA and, as stated, currents sustained for some seconds at over 50–80 mA carry a substantial risk of death.

Voltage

To produce a potentially fatal current across the chest, a certain minimum voltage must be applied to the skin surface. As the latter has a relatively high resistance (see below), Ohm's law dictates that an appreciable voltage is required to produce the 50 mA or so needed for ventricular fibrillation. Most fatalities occur with the domestic voltage of 240, though the common alternative in parts of the USA and Europe of 110 V is still lethal in many instances.

It is uncommon to encounter deaths at less than 100 V, mainly because there are few sources of supply between 110 V and the 12 V or 24 V used in vehicle electrical systems. These are almost always innocuous, though Polson (1963) has reported a fatality at 24 V in a man pinned beneath an electrical vehicle for several hours. That case emphasizes the importance of the time element in electrical injury. Extremely high voltages, such as those encountered in power transmission systems and in electronic equipment, may paradoxically be safer on some occasions, as the shock may physically fling the subject off the conductor, thus reducing the contact time below the threshold for cardiac damage.

Resistance

The major barrier to an electrical current is the skin, which has a far higher resistance than internal tissues. That is why skin electric burns occur, as the resistivity causes energy transfer from the electron flow to the skin. Once inside the dermis, the semi-fluid cytoplasm, and especially the vascular system filled with electrolyte-rich fluid, passes the current through the body quite easily. The resistance of skin varies greatly according to the thickness of the keratin-covered epidermis; that on the soles and finger-pads is greater than the thin skin elsewhere. The average resistance is between 500 and 10 000 ohms for areas other than the horny hand and foot pads, which may offer 1 million ohms resistance when dry.

A more potent factor is the dryness or dampness of the skin, which greatly affects its resistance. While dry palm skin may have a resistance of the order of 1 million ohms, when wetted this may fall to only 1200 ohms. Jellinek (1932) found the horny skin of a workman to have a dry resistance of from 1 to 2 million ohms; Jaffe (1928) stated that sweating could reduce skin resistance from 30 000 to 2500 ohms. When the current begins to pass, there is a further marked drop in resistance, as a result of electrolytic changes in the skin, which may fall to only 380 ohms. Thus for a fixed voltage, such as the mains supply of 240 V, the resultant current will be far greater if the skin is wet from sweating or external moisture. This emphasizes the dangers of bathrooms and using electrical equipment in damp surroundings. Where alternating current is concerned (as in most forensic cases), resistance is replaced by 'impedance', but this is not relevant to the pathological aspects.

EFFECTS UPON MUSCLE

One effect of electricity that has practical implications is the spasm that occurs in skeletal muscle if the current reaches between 10 and 40 mA at 50 cps. When, as most often happens, the entry point is in the hand, the stronger flexor muscles of the arm go into spasm and cause a 'hold-on' effect. This means that any object being held in the hand is involuntarily clenched and, as it is likely to be the faulty electrical appliance or a wire, the object cannot be released and the current thus continues to flow. This adds to the time element and progressively worsens the risk of both cutaneous burns and the risk of cardiac or respiratory arrest. Tingling may be felt in the skin with a current of only 1 mA and 'hold-on' can begin at a current as low as 9–10 mA.

MODE OF DEATH

As already stated, most deaths from electricity are from cardiac arrhythmias, usually ventricular fibrillation ending in arrest. This is caused by the passage of current through the myocardium, especially in the superficial epicardial layers and possibly across the endocardium. The current has a profound effect directly upon the myocardial syncytium, the possible dislocation of the pacemaking nodes and conducting systems being ill-understood. When death occurs from cardiac arrest, the body remains either pale or only slightly congested, the autopsy appearances being unhelpful apart from the presence of any external electrical marks.

The second (and far less common) mode of death is respiratory arrest, in which the passage of current through the thorax causes the intercostal muscles and diaphragm to go into spasm, or become paralysed. In either case, respiratory movements are inhibited and a congestive–hypoxic death occurs. The brainstem is affected rarely, when the current enters through the head. Either cardiac arrest or respiratory paralysis can then supervene.

Many electrical deaths are not observed, the person being found dead later, so that the mode of death is unknown. Sometimes the witnessed mode of death is hard to explain on physiological grounds, in that there appears to be a delay (often some minutes in duration) between the shock and the death. In the interval, the victim may be conscious and even apparently recovering. It is difficult to know why a sudden cardiac arrest should take place after the current is switched off, but presumably some fundamental damage has been caused on an intracellular level to cardiac or neural tissue.

Finally, when discussing the mode of death, it must always be remembered that non-electrical trauma is quite common. In a series reported by Bissig (1960), some 15 per cent of cases had injury from falls and other associated trauma. In industrial accidents and when working on power lines, victims of shock may be thrown from a height, or suffer violent muscular spasms that may lead to fractures and other serious injury.

THE CUTANEOUS ELECTRIC MARK

The point of contact on the body surface may leave skin lesions, which are either called 'electrical burns' or 'electrical marks', though the term 'Joule burn' is gaining in popularity. These are the sites of entry of the current, but another mark or marks may also appear where the body was earthed or

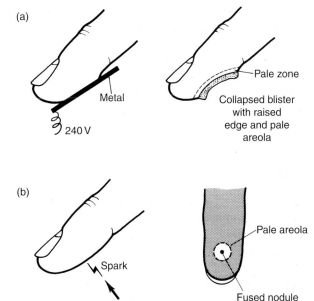

FIGURE 12.2 *(a) Firm contact electric mark, and (b) spark burn across air gap.*

'grounded'. It must be emphasized here that fatal electrocution may occur with no skin mark whatsoever, making the diagnosis entirely dependent upon the circumstances of the death. An extreme example is electrocution in the bath, when the large surface area for entry plus the low skin resistance caused by the water abolishes the possibility of a focal burn.

An electrical mark may not be externally obvious, as the current can be applied to the genitals, anus or abdomen in sexual perversions or through the mouth, especially in children. Infants may place a live plug between their lips and sustain electrical burns on the tongue or buccal mucosa, which may not be readily apparent on external examination at autopsy.

When a current passes, there may or may not be a visible lesion, depending upon:

- the density of the current passage in terms of skin area and
- the conductivity, usually varying with the moisture content.

The skin lesion is a thermal burn from heating of the epidermis and dermis as the current passes. Theoretically, the heat generated can be determined from the formula $GC = C2R/4.187$, where GC is the heat in gram calories per second, C is the current in amperes and R the resistance in ohms. If the electron flood passes through a relatively wide area, then the resistance per unit area is small (especially if the skin is damp) and thus the heating effect is proportionately diminished. For example, a person resting the palm of the hand on a flat metal plate which is electrified will pass a far

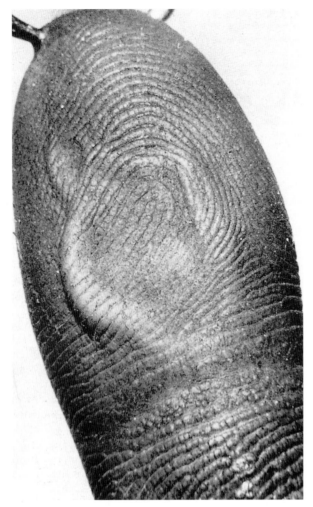

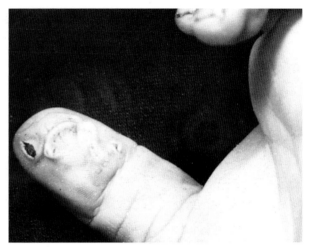

FIGURE 12.4 *Firm contact blister and adjacent spark burn from 240 V mains supply. The victim was holding a faulty electric drill. There were no other marks on the body.*

FIGURE 12.3 *Firm contact electric marks on a fingertip. Two blisters have been formed by the heat of local skin resistance; they have collapsed on cooling.*

smaller current per square centimetre of skin than another touching the plate with the tip of a finger. The first is likely to have no demonstrable lesions, while the second will have a blistered burn or a keratinized nodule, depending on the firmness of the contact.

The temperature in the tissues directly under the contact point can easily reach 95°C. Tissue damage can occur within 25 seconds when the temperature reaches a mere 50°C. The focal electric mark is largely a thermal burn and even some of the histological features to be described later, which were once thought to be peculiar to the electrical current, are now generally ascribed to thermal effects. There are some features, however, which are characteristic of an electrical cause.

▪ When the skin has been in firm contact with an electrical conductor, the passage of the current through the high skin resistance heats up the tissue fluids and produces steam. This may split the layers of the epidermis or the epidermal–dermal junction and produce a raised blister. This may rupture if the current continues or if the area is relatively large.

When the current ceases, the blister cools and collapses, giving the familiar appearance seen at autopsy. The collapsed blister is often annular, producing a raised grey or white ring with an umbilicated centre. The mark sometimes reproduces the shape of the conductor, especially where this is a linear wire or a shaped metal object. Where the tip of a wire or rod is at right angles to the skin, a focal pit is created, sometimes penetrating quite deeply into the skin.

▪ Where the contact is less firm, so that an air gap (albeit narrow) exists between skin and conductor, the current jumps the gap as a spark. In dry air 1000 V will jump several millimetres and 100 kV about 35 cm. This is at extremely high temperatures (about 4000°C), as in the sparking plug of a petrol engine, and causes the outer skin keratin to melt over a small area. On cooling, the keratin fuses into a hard brownish nodule, usually raised above the surrounding surface, the so-called 'spark lesion'.

▪ In many electrical burns these two types are combined, as a result of movement of the hand or body against the conductor and sometimes because of irregularity of the shape of the conductor. Where the time has been prolonged, the voltage is high, or the conductor is large, the burn may be correspondingly severe with large areas of peeled blistered skin, charred keratin, and a mixture of hyperaemia, deep scorching and shed epidermis.

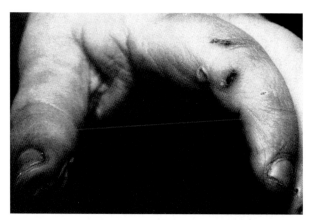

FIGURE 12.5 *Collapsed blisters and a spark burn from holding a faulty power tool.*

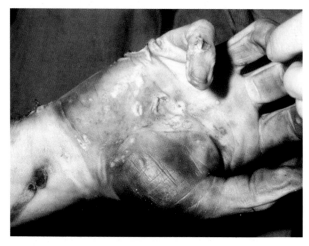

FIGURE 12.6 *Multiple electrical burns on a hand, with blisters showing the typical pale raised margins and areas of peeling epidermis. There is a blackening from metallization as the current was passing for several hours; the victim was an electrician who fell into an air-conditioning plant.*

■ A characteristic feature of the electric mark, which is the most useful indicator of the nature of the lesion, is the common occurrence of an areola of blanched skin at the periphery. Presumably because of arteriolar spasm from the direct effects of the current on vessel-wall musculature, the pallor survives death and is virtually pathognomonic of electrical damage. Often there is a hyperaemic border outside the blanching, though reddening may also be seen inside the pale zone, as the outermost rim of the heated burn area. Occasionally, an alternating spectrum of blister-reddening-pallor-reddening can be observed centrifugally from the centre of the lesion. When the burn is linear, such as that from a bare wire pressed against the skin, the 'areola' takes the form of a pale zone parallel to the central burn.

■ When the marks are minimal, all that may be seen are tiny white discs representing minute flat blisters where the epidermis has split, but no reddening or areola has formed – or at least, has not persisted until the time of autopsy. These can be hard to find and, as they are likely to be present on the palmar surface of the hands (the usual site from grasping an electrical appliance), the strong flexion of rigor mortis may bring the fingers down to the palms, so obscuring any lesions. It is essential in all autopsies to examine the flexor surface of the fingers by forcible breaking of the rigor – and, where electrocution is a possibility, minute inspection of the hands must be carried out, even if the flexor tendons at the wrist have to be cut to release the rigor clenching of the fingers.

■ In high-voltage burns, such as those sustained from high-tension grid transmission cables, where the voltage is in the multi-kilovolt range, sparking may occur over many centimetres. This can cause multiple spark lesions giving rise to a 'crocodile-skin' effect. Both linesmen and copper thieves working on high pylons may suffer non-electrical injuries from being thrown to the ground, or they may sustain gross charring burns or even limb fractures from both direct electrical energy and the muscle spasm caused by a massive bolt of electricity.

■ Earthing or 'grounding' lesions are not often seen, but should be looked for on the contralateral hand and on the feet. The lesions may be similar, though less severe. In a case seen by the author (BK), in which a workman pushed a metal wheelbarrow over a live cable lying in a pool of water, the entry burns were on the hands, but on the soles of both feet the electrical burns matched the metal studs in his boots where the current earthed through damp socks and leather.

In another case, a homicide in a bath, there were no entry burns but the current went to earth by contact of the breasts with the metal taps.

■ When the current has flowed for an appreciable time, even at a domestic voltage of 240, the effects may be severe. Charring and more extensive peeling and blistering of skin may occur, with deep muscle damage and cooking of the tissues. This is partly because of the fact that the initial damage lowers skin resistance so that progressively more current flows and therefore more burning and necrosis follows.

Much of this damage seen at autopsy may have occurred post-mortem, if death from cardiac arrest occurs early in the event and, where the victim is alone, there is no one to remove his body from the source of the current. It has been

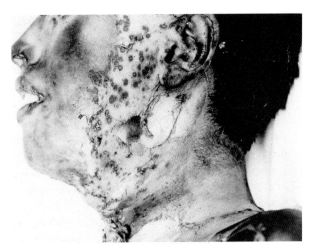

FIGURE 12.7 *Multiple burns from high-voltage (multi-kilovolt) supply lines of the grid system. The appearance is sometimes called 'crocodile skin' and is caused by arcing of the current over a considerable distance. The victim was a boy who went bird-nesting amongst the switch gear of a power station.*

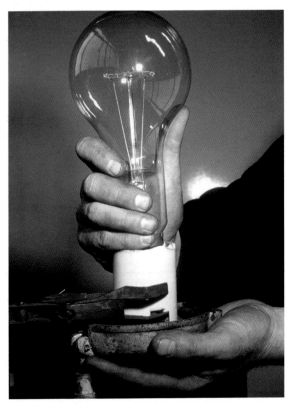

FIGURE 12.8 *Reconstruction of a fatal electrocution. While replacing a bulb a workman dropped dead, even though the light was not illuminated. The circuit had been improperly 'wired through' – that is, the switch had been placed in the neutral wire, instead of the live. The porcelain holder was broken so that his little finger touched the brass base of the bulb, thus completing the circuit across the chest to the other hand, which held an earthed base-plate. The only electrical mark was on the little finger.*

conclusively shown by Polson and others that post-mortem burns can be inflicted on a dead body, the appearances being similar in terms of blistering and burning, though the red flare of 'vital reaction' will be absent if death has occurred some time before.

PATTERNED ELECTRIC MARKS

As with many other injuries, a pattern of the shape of the causative object may sometimes be identified. When the electrical conductor is a wire, a linear burn may occur. The shape and spacing of electrical plugs or contacts may be seen, and faulty electrical equipment may impress its shape into the skin. These marks may be useful when the pathologist tries to reconstruct the events – and indeed, may indicate for the first time that the death was caused by electricity, when the unwitnessed events are particularly obscure.

As electric shock and burns are commonly seen in torture victims in abuse of human rights, a pattern may be useful in determining what object was used and give evidence of deliberate repetition. The deliberate use of a male-pin plug connected to the mains supply, then pressed against the skin, may give a series of regularly spaced marks, consisting of hyperaemia, blistering, areola formation or even charring.

METALLIC TRACES IN ELECTRICAL MARKS

When a current passes from a metal conductor into the body, a form of electrolysis occurs so that metallic ions are embedded in the skin and even in the subcutaneous tissues. This occurs with both d.c. and a.c. because of the combination of metallic ions with tissue anions to form metallic salts. These may be invisible to the eye, but detectable by chemical, histochemical and spectrographic techniques. They persist for some weeks during life and resist a moderate amount of post-mortem change. Where gross they may be observed directly on the skin, and where copper or brass conductors are involved a bright green imprint may be obvious. Where an electric arc forms, vaporized metal may be deposited on the skin, often extensive enough to be visible to the naked eye. In high-voltage contacts, the skin of a wide area may be brown or greyish, partly from heat effects, but partly from metallization.

Recently, using the scanning electron microscope, it has become possible to see tiny globules of molten metal on the skin at and near an electrical mark, deposited there by the almost inevitable 'mini-arcing' that accompanies any electrical contact. Chemical tests for metallic deposits include that devised by Adjutantis and Skalos (1962), which is a simple touch-test using elution on strips of filter paper. Copper, iron, aluminium, zinc or nickel are dissolved in nitric or hydrochloric acid, and the solution tested with a variety of simple but specific reagents.

INTERNAL APPEARANCES

In fatal electrocution, gross findings in the internal organs may be absent and even histological changes are a matter of controversy. Because the internal tissues are largely aqueous and contain conductive electrolytes, the current pathway is usually too diffuse to cause thermal damage. The absence of visceral damage is made up for by physiological and functional abnormalities, mainly in muscle and nervous tissue.

The usual mode of death is cardiac arrhythmia leading to ventricular fibrillation and arrest. In these deaths there is little to find at autopsy apart from the skin lesions. It is claimed that epicardial petechiae may occur, but these are too non-specific to be of any use. The body is either pale or only slightly congested, in contrast to the **few** deaths that occur from respiratory paralysis.

In the latter group the intercostal muscles and diaphragm go into spasm or are paralysed, which leads to marked congestion and cyanosis of the face, with similar changes in the lungs. There may be some petechiae on the pleura, though this again is such a non-specific finding as to be unhelpful as a diagnostic sign. At autopsy, the usual signs of a congestive death are found, with dark blue–red post-mortem hypostasis.

A number of other signs of electrocution have been claimed, but they are rarely confirmed by personal experience. These include intracerebral petechiae, which are probably part of the general congestive state in respiratory paralysis.

HISTOLOGICAL APPEARANCES

These are rather controversial, as some changes formerly claimed to be specific for electrical lesions have been shown to be thermal.

The skin mark consists of vacuolation in the epidermis and sometimes dermis, caused by the gas spaces from the heated tissue fluids splitting the cells apart. The affected tissues become more eosinophilic. The cap of epidermis may be detached and raised into a blister, with a large space beneath. The cells of the epidermis are often elongated, with the nuclei of the lower layers orientated and horizontally stretched; this was once claimed to be an electromagnetic

effect, but the same appearance can be seen in purely thermal burns and in hypothermic lesions.

Changes in the brain have been described, even when the cause of death was cardiac. Focal petechial haemorrhages, spaces around small blood vessels and tears in white matter have been described. Electron microscopy reveals a variety of changes, especially in the nuclei of skin cells, which are deformed with clumped chromatin. Janssen (1984) has compiled a review of electrical histological lesions in his book on forensic histology, but it seems evident that there is little that is absolutely pathognomonic of electrical as opposed to purely thermal burns.

Histochemical reactions for metallization can also be carried out, though, again, metals can be transferred into the skin by purely thermal means if hot metallic objects are pressed against the skin.

Scanning electron microscopy appears to be the best way of distinguishing between electrical and thermal damage, as the punctate nature of the deposition and the possibility of chemical analysis by electron microprobes offer a sophisticated means of identifying the metallic deposit. Internal organs reveal no true diagnostic lesions of electricity. The wavy appearance of the myocardial fibres and their fragmentation may be suggestive, but by no means diagnostic. Contraction bands within the fibres, especially of a 'bark-like' appearance, have been described but, again, are non-specific, though they are often seen in the subepicardial myocardium after resuscitation that includes electrical defibrillation. However, they are identical to catecholamine effects on the myocardium and so may not be electrical in origin.

ELECTROCUTION IN THE BATHROOM

The bathroom is a common site for electrical tragedies. Accidents, suicides and even homicides occur there because of its vulnerability to electrical shock. The bathroom is electrically the most dangerous place in a house as there is a moist atmosphere, ample water, good earthing through metal taps and pipes, and a wet, unclothed body – all of which are conducive to low electrical resistance and hence high tissue currents. Accidents are common, usually as a result of the careless use of electrical appliances, such as hairdryers and room heaters. Most European countries have strict regulations about electrical installations in bathrooms because of the danger. In Britain, no wall switch is permitted for the light, a ceiling switch operated by an insulating cord being mandatory. No power sockets are allowed except for a shaver socket which incorporates a step-down transformer

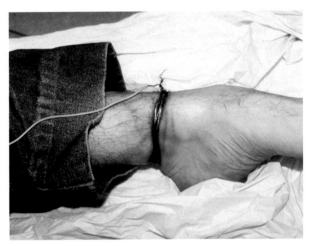

FIGURE 12.10 *Suicide by electricity. Both wrists were wired in this fashion to a 240 V supply socket, the circuit being completed from arm to arm across the chest.*

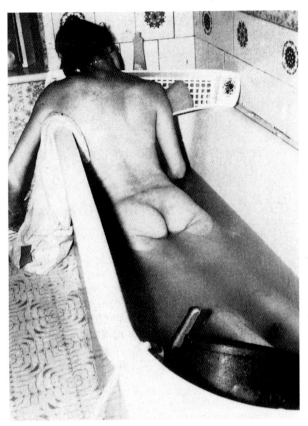

FIGURE 12.9 *Homicidal electrocution in the bath. An electric heater was dropped into the water with the wire to the earth terminal deliberately disconnected. The 240 V supply entered the body diffusely through the water and completed the circuit by earthing through contact with the breasts against the metal taps, leaving electrical marks on the skin.*

with a low maximum current output. In spite of this, people unwisely use extension leads or plug into light sockets to operate a variety of appliances.

SUICIDE BY ELECTRICITY

There has been a remarkable increase in the number of suicidal electrocutions in recent years, especially in the bath. Bonte *et al.* (1986) have described an increasing number of cases in the former West Germany, drawing attention to the unusual demarcation of post-mortem hypostasis in such deaths, where the water level during electrocution appears to limit the subsequent appearance of the hypostasis. Various circuit arrangements are made by suicides in baths: these range from the pulling of an electrical appliance into the water to complex connections to metal soap dishes and wiring up contacts on the body. There may even be arrangements to break the circuit when the bathroom door is opened to safeguard those who find the body. The

circumstances are rarely in doubt except that some less sophisticated cases may be difficult to differentiate from the many other accidents that occur in bathrooms. Rarely, other more bizarre deaths associated with electricity occur, as seen in Figure 12.11.

HOMICIDE BY ELECTRICITY

Homicide is occasionally committed by electricity, the author (BK) having dealt with two such incidents and his co-author (PS) with one. The first took place in the bath and provided good illustrations of the electrical aspects of fatal shock. A young woman was found dead in her bath, slumped forwards in a kneeling position with one breast resting against a chrome tap. The left arm was trailing over the edge of the bath, in which was the usual level of water plus an electric fan-heater immersed near the feet. The heater was connected by a long cable to a 240 V 13 A socket in an adjacent bedroom. Significantly, the third 'earth' wire had been deliberately disconnected from the earth pin inside the plug. Subsequent forensic tests showed that the enamel lining of the metal bath was an excellent insulator so that earthing of the current through the bath water could only occur via the chrome waste pipe. The circuit was completed, however, with fatal results, by the woman falling (or being pushed) against the tap, so that she sustained an electrical burn on the breast. She also had another typical burn on the inside of her left arm near the axilla, where the insulating enamel of the bath ceased at the turned-over edge. Forensic tests showed that there was a progressive gradient of voltage down the bath from over 200 V near the heater to virtually zero near the earthed waste pipe. The current had preferentially taken a course

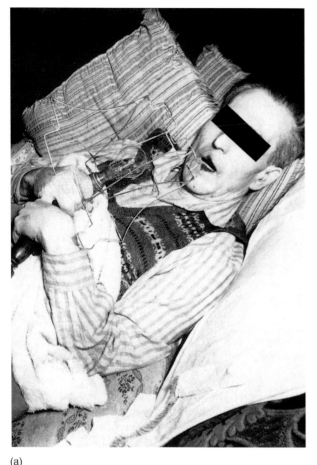
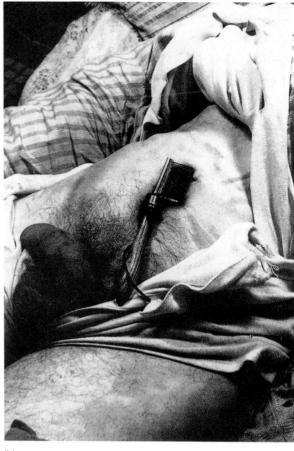

(a) (b)

FIGURE 12.11 *(a) The deceased man had electrical marks on his fingers and lips, which were stained green from metallization from the brass fittings of the table lamp. (b) In addition, he had a metal comb resting over a large electric burn on his abdomen, also wired up to the lamp socket. No circumstantial evidence of suicidal intent could be discovered and some masochistic exercise was suspected.*

through the victim's body from feet to exit through breast and arm, rather than through the higher resistance of the fresh water.

It was also shown that, when the earth safety wire was reconnected, the voltage at the top of the bath fell to negligible levels, even though the fuse did not blow. The woman's husband, after several denials, eventually confessed to dropping the heater into the bath – and also to borrowing a book from the public library the previous day entitled *The do-it-yourself home electrician!*

The other homicide, which could not be proved for lack of evidence or a confession, concerned the wrapping of bare electric wires around a woman's neck. The wire was thick 30 A cooker cable with 40 cm of insulation stripped except for the extreme tips. The woman's husband, a professional electrician, provided the unlikely explanation that he was using this to test his electric shaver!

The third homicide went first undetected as the perpetrator, the husband of the victim, had staged it as an accident.

The wife was supposed to have been ironing in the kitchen early one morning and been electrocuted by a faulty cord of the iron, the water-pipe of the sink providing the contact to the earth. In addition to the SOCs, an electrician, but not the pathologist, was called to the scene to investigate the faulty device, but nothing suspicious was detected. Ironically, in spite of the clumsy way in breaking the insulation of the cord and leaving only a couple of millimetres of the naked wire visible, a picture of the faulty cord and iron landed in a textbook for electricians, pointing out the dangers of faulty household appliances. At autopsy the only finding was an electrical burn on the chest. Eight years later, when the husband was in detention in the course of an investigation due to a stolen money transport, he wrote a very detailed confession of the murder of his wife. He had attached two copper electrodes to an extension cord and, while the wife was asleep, pressed them to her chest. In court, in spite of the withdrawal of his confession, he was sentenced to a long imprisonment. Several details, which came out in the course

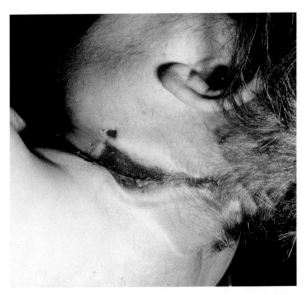

FIGURE 12.12 *Electrical burn around the neck from a mains wire being held against the skin. The typical pale areola and peeled skin blistering can be seen. There was suspicion of homicide, but it could not be proved.*

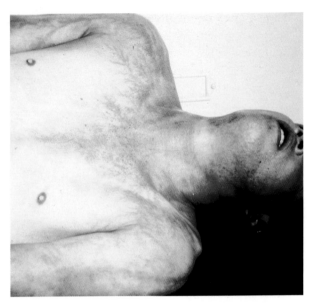

FIGURE 12.13 *The fern-like, arboresque pattern seen over the shoulders and chest in a victim of lightning stroke. Although this is always mentioned in descriptions of lightning deaths, it is seen only in a small minority of cases.*

of the criminal investigation, implied, although it was never proven, that the man had first attempted to kill his wife by feeding her diazepam tablets without her knowledge, and when this had failed, electrocuted her. It is hindsight and fruitless to contemplate what might have happened if the pathologist had been to the scene. The lesson of the case is, however, that if electrocution is suspected, it certainly is worthwhile to take a look at the scene of death.

In tropical and subtropical countries deaths from lightning are not uncommon and, even in higher latitudes, occasional tragedies occur where numbers of people are killed or injured in single episodes. An example was at the Ascot race meeting in 1955. The physics of a lightning strike are complex and not fully understood. Gigantic voltages and amperages are involved when a highly charged thundercloud discharges via a huge arc to the ground.

Lightning deaths cannot be other than accidental and provide no real problems for the forensic pathologist. Occasionally the nature of the death may be uncertain if a dead body is discovered in the open with no marks upon it, but usually there will be reports of a lightning strike nearby and artefacts, such as torn and scorched clothing and magnetized metallic objects in the pockets, may assist in explaining the event.

It is well known that injury from lightning is capricious and unpredictable. Two people can stand side by side during a flash and one may be mutilated and killed while the other is unharmed. The physical damage in fatal cases can vary from virtually nil to gross burning, fractures and tissue destruction. Cutaneous marks may be present, the well-known 'fern-like' or 'arboresque' pattern, also referred to as 'Lichtenberg' figures (because of their similarity to the pattern described by a German physicist, Georg Christoph Lichtenberg, in 1777) being much less common than the standard texts suggest. Irregular red marks, often linear first-degree burns, may follow skin creases, especially if damp from sweating. These marks may be many inches long and generally follow the long axis of the body towards the ground. Frank blistered or charred burns are also present in some cases.

An excellent picture of the Lichtenberg figures was taken by Domart and Garet, published in the *New England Journal of Medicine* in 2000, showing a 54-year-old man struck by lightning. With the exception of numbness and paraesthesia of the left shoulder, flank and leg, he felt well on the arrival at the emergency department. The serum creatine kinase and myoglobin concentrations were slightly elevated. After a 24-hour observation period, the patient was sent home and two days later, on a follow-up visit, the fern-leaf pattern of marks had disappeared.

The clothing may be torn off and this can sometimes raise the suspicion of foul play if the lightning aspect is obscure. The clothing is typically ripped open as if by an internal explosion, and belts and boots may be similarly ruptured. Metal objects in the pockets may be fused or magnetized, as may be metal buttons and tooth fillings. Burns on the skin may be adjacent to metal objects in or on the clothing.

There is often a smell of singeing or burning about the body and its clothing. The hair may be scorched and there is often a head injury, caused either by the lightning strike itself or by falling to the ground.

REFERENCES AND FURTHER READING

Adjutantis G, Skalos S. 1962. The identification of the electrical burn in cases of electrocution by the acro-reaction test. *J Forensic Med* **9**:101–4.

Anders S, Matschke J, Tsokos M. 2001. Internal current mark in a case of suicide by electrocution. *Am J Forensic Med Pathol* **22**:370–3.

Arden GB, Harrison S, Lister J. 1956. Lightning accident at ascot. *Br Med J* **2**:1450–3.

Arnold R, Giebe W, Winnefeld K, *et al.* 2002. [An initially unexplained death during prison sentence. Diagnostic verification by atomic absorption spectrometry.] *Arch Kriminol* **209**:14–19.

Bailey B, Forget S, Gaudreault P. 2001. Prevalence of potential risk factors in victims of electrocution. *Forensic Sci Int* **123**:58–62.

Bissig H. 1960. Über Niederspannungsunfälle. *Elektromedizin* **5**:154–60.

Bonte W, Sprung R, Huckenbeck W. 1986. [Problems in the evaluation of electrocution fatalities in the bathtub.] *Z Rechtsmed* **97**:7–19.

Bornstein FP. 1962. Homicide by electrocution. *J Forensic Sci* **7**:516–17.

Critchley M. 1934. Neurological effect of lightning and electricity. *Lancet* **1**:68–70.

Domart Y, Garet E. 2000. Images in clinical medicine. Lichtenberg figures due to a lightning strike. *N Engl J Med* **343**:1536.

Dutra FR. 1981. Electrical burns of the skin. Medicolegal investigation. *Am J Forensic Med Pathol* **2**:309–12.

Eriksson A, Ornehult L. 1988. Death by lightning. *Am J Forensic Med Pathol* **9**:295–300.

Harrison SH, Arden GP. 1957. Electrical burns. *Br J Clin Pract* **10**:117–20.

Holder JC. 1960. An unusual method of attempted suicide. *Med Leg J* **28**:41–3.

Jacobsen H. 1997. Electrically induced deposition of metal on the human skin. *Forensic Sci Int* **90**:85–92.

Jaffe RH. 1928. Electrical injury. *Arch Pathol* **5**:837–70.

Janssen W. 1984. Injuries caused by electricity. In: *Forensic histopathology*. Springer, Berlin.

Jellinek S. 1932. *Elektrische verletzungen*. Barth, Leipzig.

Klintschar M, Grabuschnigg P, Beham A. 1998. Death from electrocution during autoerotic practice: case report and review of the literature. *Am J Forensic Med Pathol* **19**:190–3.

Lee WR, Zoledziowski S. 1964. Effects of electric shock on respiration in the rabbit. *Br J Ind Med* **21**:135–48.

Marcinkowski T, Pankowski M. 1980. Significance of skin metallization in the diagnosis of electrocution. *Forensic Sci Int* **16**:1–6.

Mellen PF, Weedn VW, Kao G. 1992. Electrocution: a review of 155 cases with emphasis on human factors. *J Forensic Sci* **37**:1016–22.

Moncrief JA, Pruitt BA, Jr. 1971. Hidden damage from electrical injury. *Geriatrics* **26**:84–5.

Morgan EW. 1958. Atrial fibrillation and subdural haematoma associated with lightning strike. *N Engl J Med* **259**:956–9.

Pasetti M, Viterho B. 1965. Ultrastructural modifications in the skeletal muscles of electrocuted mice. *Med Sci Law* **5**:29–36.

Perper J. 1977. *Electrical injuries*. In: Wecht C (ed.), *Legal medicine annual 1976*. Appleton Century Crofts, New York.

Pierucci G, Danesino P. 1980. The macroscopic detection of metallization in the latent current mark. *Z Rechtsmed* **85**:97–105.

Polson CJ. 1963. *Essentials of forensic medicine*. Pergamon Press, Oxford.

Polson CJ, Gee DJ, Knight B. 1985. *Essentials of forensic medicine*, 4th edn. Pergamon Press, Oxford.

Puschel K, Brinkmann B, Lieske K. 1985. Ultrastructural alterations of skeletal muscles after electric shock. *Am J Forensic Med Pathol* **6**:296–300.

Puschel K, Lockemann U, Bartel J. 1995. Postmortem investigation of serum myoglobin levels with special reference to electrical fatalities. *Forensic Sci Int* **72**:171–7.

Robinson DW, Nasters F, Forrest WJ. 1965. Electrical burns an analysis and review of 33 cases. *Surgery* **57**:385–90.

Shaw D, York-Moore ME. 1957. Neuropsychiatric sequelae of lightning strike. *Br Med J* **2**:1152–4.

Somogyi E, Rozsa G, Toro I, *et al.* 1967. Electron microscopic observations on the epidermis of the electrocuted skin of rats. *Med Sci Law* **7**:152–5.

Thomsen HK, Danielsen L, Nielsen O, *et al.* 1981. Early epidermal changes in heat- and electrically injured pig skin. I. A light microscopic study. *Forensic Sci Int* **17**:133–43.

Thomsen HK, Danielsen L, Nielsen O, *et al.* 1981. Early epidermal changes in heat- and electrically injured pig skin. II. An electron microscopic study. *Forensic Sci Int* **17**:145–52.

Torre C, Varetto L. 1986. Dermal surface in electric and thermal injuries. Observations by scanning electron microscopy. *Am J Forensic Med Pathol* **7**:151–8.

Werne AH. 1923. Death by electricity. *NY State Med J* **118**:498–502.

Wright RK, Davis JH. 1980. The investigation of electrical deaths: a report of 220 fatalities. *J Forensic Sci* **25**:514–21.

Zhang P, Cai S. 1995. Study on electrocution death by low-voltage. *Forensic Sci Int* **76**:115–19.

CHAPTER 13

Complications of injury

Serious bodily injury, from whatever cause, may either lead to virtually instantaneous death from destruction of vital organs and structures, or may cause delayed death from complications of the original injury. This delay may be short, as in torrential haemorrhage or acute respiratory failure, or it may be progressively longer, stretching into hours, days, weeks or even years. For example, the author (BK) dealt with a death in which a glider crash 15 years previously had to be implicated as the sole reason for the death, as the victim suffered a fractured spine, a paraplegia, paralysed bladder and recurring ascending urinary infection leading to death in renal failure from bilateral pyelonephritis.

Many even more delayed deaths can be found in the records of most experienced forensic pathologists. As long as a direct chain of events can be traced from the injury to the death, then the former must be considered to be the basic cause, a fact which may have profound legal implications both for civil compensation and criminal responsibility. Some of the most difficult problems in forensic pathology – and some of the most arduous testimony and cross-examination in court – concern deaths from which post-traumatic complications are disputed as being causative factors.

HAEMORRHAGE

Bleeding may occur externally through lacerations and incised wounds or via natural passages, such as the bronchi and trachea, oronasal passages, ears, vagina, urethra or rectum. Internal bleeding comprises contusions, which are leakages of blood into tissue spaces from rupture of vessels and free bleeding into body cavities, notably the pericardium, peritoneum, pleura and cranium.

The volume varies greatly, from the tiny petechiae of ruptured venules to the massive amounts seen in a ruptured aorta. As a primary cause of death it is not only the total volume that is lethal, but the rapidity and the site of the bleeding. When the leakage is slow the body can compensate for the loss of a far greater volume, both by adjustment of the vascular bed and by restoration of the blood volume by transfer from other aqueous compartments.

As to site, it is obvious that a small quantity of bleeding into the brainstem is likely to be lethal, whereas the same volume exuded into the pleural cavity would be of little consequence. Bleeding usually begins at the time of injury, though there is often a momentary delay at the instant of infliction. When a sharp blade cuts the skin, it is a matter of common observation that the blood may hesitate for a second or so before welling out. This is caused by transient spasm of local vessels from the stimulus of the injuring object. Bleeding then continues until normal haemostasis plugs the vessels.

In some injuries involving arteries, the musculoelastic vessel may retract and its wall invaginate, so that an almost immediate seal prevents copious haemorrhage. Occasionally even gross injuries, such as the amputation of a limb by a railway wheel, may be almost devoid of significant bleeding, because the crushing effect may combine with arterial wall retraction to seal the cut vessel effectively. It can sometimes be more dangerous partly to transect an artery than to divide it completely, as retraction cannot then take place. Failure of haemostasis is a haematological matter, but may have medico-legal connotations if an injury (which includes a surgical procedure) is performed on someone who has a haemorrhagic diathesis either from natural disease, or from therapeutic anticoagulant treatment, such as heparin or warfarin.

Delayed bleeding may be seen in a number of conditions. In trauma, especially traffic accidents, organs, such as the liver, spleen or (sometimes) lung, may be injured within their capsules or covering membranes, which initially remain intact. A good example is a subcapsular haematoma of the liver, which may be large and grow even larger as continued bleeding strips more capsule from the parenchymal surface. Eventually, the blister may rupture and the now unrestrained bleeding area can pour into the peritoneal cavity. Trauma can also weaken the wall of an artery or vein, leading to a false aneurysm, which can later rupture. An arteriovenous fistula can also form and later burst.

Infections can also develop in trauma sites and involve vessels in the vicinity, so that an abscess or cellulitis can secondarily lead to severe haemorrhage when the vessel wall is eroded. This is rare except among poorly treated accident or battle casualties, as are mycotic aneurysms that result from infected emboli impacting in a branch of an artery and causing local septic necrosis.

It is sometimes difficult to know how much of a haemorrhage found at autopsy may be accounted for by post-mortem bleeding. There is little doubt that the volume may increase after death, but, except in serous cavities, such as the pleura and peritoneum, or externally from the body surface, in most cases this is a small proportion of that which leaked under arterial pressure during life, due to the tissue pressures opposing passive bleeding.

However, a haemothorax from a ruptured aorta may amount to several litres and much of this may be in the

form of a large shaped clot. A clot can form post-mortem, so its presence cannot be taken as an index of *in vivo* formation, but the source of the bleeding will usually be obvious and any post-mortem addition will not affect the interpretation. Copious external bleeding can continue after death, especially from the scalp, particularly if the head is dependent after death.

INFECTION

Infection used to be so common after open wounds that it was the norm rather than the exception. Prior to the introduction of sulphonamides and antibiotics, many criminally inflicted wounds, which in themselves were not a danger to life, became fatally infected so that an assault became a homicide. This illustrates the fallacy of comparing murder rates in the last century with today, as the survival rate because of rapidly available ambulance and resuscitation services, blood transfusion, emergency operations and antibiotics is vastly greater now than in former times, when even a trivial injury was often fatal.

The types of post-traumatic infection are legion and vary greatly from country to country. Purulent wound infection from Gram-positive cocci, Gram-negative bacilli, anaerobes, such as *Clostridium perfringens*, and other more common organisms, is the most frequent, but in some countries tetanus and anthrax are common dangers. The whole matter is one of clinical microbiology, and the main forensic relevance is to prove a chain of causation between the original injury and a death from intercurrent infection. There may be medico-legal issues involved, such as failure to give or delay in giving antibiotic cover, which can have both civil and criminal legal consequences. A criminal assault that ends in death because of a neglected infection does not exonerate the perpetrator from all responsibility, even though there has been a *novus actus interveniens* in the form of defective medical treatment.

PULMONARY EMBOLISM

This is a most important topic in forensic pathology, as the medico-legal implications of a fatal pulmonary embolus are common and profound. Pulmonary embolism is the most underdiagnosed cause of death where no autopsy is performed; it has been estimated that, in the USA – and probably elsewhere – less than half of fatal pulmonary emboli are recognized clinically.

As with infection, an originally non-lethal injury may end in death because of venous thrombosis and pulmonary embolism, making what might be a simple accident or a

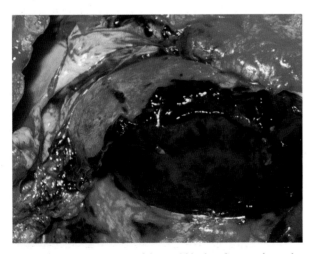

FIGURE 13.1 *Massive intra-abdominal bleeding from a subcapsular haematoma of the liver due to blunt abdominal trauma.*

common assault into a grave legal issue. The victims of many forms of trauma are at risk from pulmonary embolism because:

- Tissue trauma increases the coagulability of the blood for several weeks, the peak being between one and two weeks.
- Injury to the tissues, especially the legs or pelvic region, may cause local venous thrombosis in the contused muscles or around fractured bones.
- The injury may confine the victim to bed, either because of general shock and debility (especially in old people) or because the trauma itself necessitates recumbency, as in head injuries, severe generalized trauma or injury affecting the legs. In either case, recumbency leads to pressure on the calves and immobility causes reduced venous return and stasis because of lessened muscular massage of the leg veins. The common result is thrombosis of the deep veins of the legs, which can extend proximally into the popliteal and femoral vessels, forming a dangerous source of venous thromboemboli. Small emboli may break off and impact in more peripheral branches of the pulmonary arteries, sometimes causing pulmonary infarcts that may be precursors of a massive embolus that impacts in the major lung vessels and causes rapid death.

At autopsy, such large emboli are readily visible and can usually be easily distinguished from post-mortem clot. The latter is dark red, soft and jelly-like, with a shiny, glistening surface. It is often separated into 'chicken-fat' plasma clot and dark red-cell clot by sedimentation after death. When pulled out of the vessels it forms a cast of the branches, albeit shrunken by clot retraction. It is less evident in peripheral branches and, when the lung is sliced post-mortem, clot does not pour out of cut small vessels.

Conversely, ante-mortem embolus (especially if a number of days old) is firm, though brittle and has a dull, matt, striated surface from fibrin lamination. Older thrombus tends to be greyish-red and varies in colour from place to place. Although it may appear to be a cast of the large vessel in which it is impacted, it may often be unravelled to form a long length that obviously originated in a leg vein. Side branches, or the stumps thereof, may be seen that do not correspond to the branches of the pulmonary artery in which they lie.

Post-mortem clot may be adherent to the ante-mortem embolus and sometimes forms a sheath around it, so that the true nature is obscured unless a careful examination is made. On cutting the lung with a knife, ante-mortem emboli may be seen in the more peripheral vessels, often standing up slightly 'proud' above the surface, like toothpaste coming from a tube.

The importance of the differentiation between ante-mortem emboli and post-mortem clot is emphasized, as the legal issues hanging upon the unequivocal diagnosis may be very important. Histological confirmation of an ante-mortem origin must be made if there is any doubt. Pulmonary infarction does not occur from fatal massive pulmonary embolism, as death is too rapid. There may be infarcts present in the lungs but these must be caused by previous smaller emboli, at least a day earlier and probably much longer.

Medico-legal aspects of pulmonary embolism

Pulmonary embolism is the most underdiagnosed condition in British death certification, frequently being unsuspected as the cause of death by clinicians. Several investigations into the medico-legal aspects have been made (Knight 1966; Knight and Zaini 1980; Zaini 1981) and the peak incidence at about 2 weeks after trauma confirmed. In Knight's survey, more than three-quarters of the victims had predisposing factors such as injury, surgical operation or immobility in bed, but the remaining 20 per cent were ambulant and apparently healthy. This has important medico-legal implications because, if fatal pulmonary embolism can strike an appreciable proportion of the population who have not suffered one of the recognized predisposing factors, then the cause–effect relationship after trauma is weakened. If the standard of proof in criminal trials must be 'beyond reasonable doubt', then the fact that up to 20 per cent of pulmonary embolism deaths have not followed trauma or immobility must surely remove the cause–effect relationship from near-certainty to mere probability, which is sufficient for a civil decision, but not for a criminal conviction. This is a legal matter for the judge, however, who may or may not let the matter go to the jury – and if it does, for the jury to decide. There is marked variation in these decisions from case to case.

After the lung appearances have been examined and pulmonary embolism confirmed, the source of the embolus must be sought. In almost all cases this will be found in the vessels draining into the femoral veins, though rarely pelvic vessels are involved (usually in relation to pregnancy or abortion). Here pelvic veins may be thrombosed, with extensions into the iliac system and exceptionally into the inferior vena cava. An even more rare source is from jugular thrombosis, sometimes seen as extensions of intracranial venous sinus thrombosis. Axillary and subclavian vein thrombosis is equally unusual, the legs accounting for the vast majority of emboli.

In the usual leg vein thrombosis, various autopsy techniques are available to seek the site of obstruction. Extensive dissection is favoured by some, in which the femoral vein is exposed through a skin incision, this being continued distally as far as necessary to find the residual thrombosis. Of course, after a massive pulmonary embolus, by definition a large part of the source thrombus has been detached and therefore the pathologist has to search further distally to find the remnants. This makes dissection an extensive and disfiguring process, so alternative techniques can be used.

Zaini found that many thrombi begin far distally, even in the dorsum of the foot. He used a flexible wire with a blunt terminal knob (a Bowden cable from a bicycle brake) inserted down the femoral vein until it was arrested, then cut down from the skin at that point to examine the peripheral veins. Alternatively, transverse or longitudinal incisions can be made into the calf of the leg to examine the deep veins. The soleus and gastrocnemius muscles are transected to view their contained veins, but often the thrombus is found in the interosseous veins between tibia and fibula. If ageing of the thrombus is attempted histologically, then it should not be expressed from the vein, but the vein should be taken out with adjacent muscle, as it is the junction between thrombus and vein wall that offers the most information about the maturity of the thrombus.

Dating of pulmonary emboli and deep vein thrombi

As discussed above, it can be a matter of considerable medico-legal importance to know if a pulmonary embolus arose prior to, or subsequent to, some traumatic event. A major difficulty is that the embolus may be the most recent addition to an extending venous thrombosis that is considerably older.

It is also difficult to use histological criteria to date the free embolus from the lungs, as it is the thromboendothelial junction that provides the most information. The best method, therefore, is to examine the residual thrombus, almost always in the leg veins, to see if the oldest part could have formed as far back in time as the suspected traumatic event. For this, the vein wall with the contained thrombus is required. A segment of thrombosed vein, if necessary with adjacent muscle, should be dissected out of the leg. The presence of thrombus will have been confirmed prior to removal by transverse cuts across the calf or thigh muscles containing the veins. Sometimes the original site of thrombosis may be as far distal as the dorsum of the foot.

The thrombus-containing vein is processed in the usual way and subjected to various histological stains. Though accuracy about dating is impossible, the following is a useful scheme to provide at least an approximate idea of the duration of thrombosis in the section of vein under study – remembering always that other segments or other veins may have thrombi of different dates.

▪ Platelet and red-cell appearances give no useful information. Red cells begin to haemolyse between 24 and 48 hours to form amorphous masses, but many intact red cells survive for weeks.

▪ Using phosphotungstic acid-haematoxylin stain (PTAH), fibrin can be seen as purplish strands on the first day, but they aggregate into small masses with a meshwork of thicker strands and sheets by 4 days. After 2 weeks, the fibrin becomes more deeply purple stained, but begins to be absorbed by about the twenty-fifth day. Using Martius Scarlet Blue stain (MSB), the early pink fibrin strands become fringed by scarlet in about a week.

▪ Endothelial proliferation is most useful in the first week, as buds begin to arise from the vessel wall about the second day and proliferate during the first week. Clefts lined by endothelium are seen around the periphery of the thrombus against the vein wall. Artefactual contraction caused by fixation shrinkage must be excluded by seeking endothelial nuclei. These endothelial buds anchor the thrombus to the vein wall, and represent the first stage of healing and recanalization. They are usually noticeable by about the fourth day when they begin growing into the fibrin mass and breaking it up into compartments.

▪ Collagen fibres do not appear for about 5–10 days, often much later. Fibroblasts may be seen as early as 2 or 3 days, but tend to appear towards the end of the first week and reach a maximum at 2 or 3 weeks, reaching a maximum at about 4 weeks. Elastic fibres appear late, not before 28 days and often much later. They reach their maximum density in about 2 months, mainly in the walls of recanalizing vessels.

▪ Haemosiderin, blue granules demonstrated by Perl's reaction, may be seen by the end of the first week and reach a maximum in 3 weeks. It does not seem to be present as early in thrombi as in extravascular haemorrhages, such as bruising or meningeal bleeding, where it can be seen in 2 or 3 days.

▪ Capillaries begin to appear on the second day as endothelial buds, but do not contain red cells until about 2 weeks. Over the next 3 months, substantial canalization occurs by widening and merging of these channels. The full lumen may be restored within 6–12 months, but endothelial thickening and haemosiderin deposits in the vein wall may form permanent evidence of a former thrombus.

▪ Leucocytes, both polymorph and mononuclear, are inconsistent markers; sometimes they do not appear at all. Polymorphs may be seen within the first day – sometimes in profusion – but they vanish rapidly, often by the next day when mononuclears take their place.

Covering of the thrombus surface by endothelium is rapid and may begin on the first day and be complete within a few days. Various authors have given 24–72 hours as the time required. Naturally, the size of the thrombus surface is a variable factor. Also, only sections taken where the thrombus does not fully fill the vein lumen will provide an opportunity for observing the endothelial covering.

FAT AND BONE MARROW EMBOLISM

Another important sequel to trauma – fat embolism – is the subject of considerable controversy about the source of the lipoid; this does not, however, detract from the autopsy significance of its detection.

A great deal has been written about the pathophysiology of fat embolism and it is now evident that it is not just a simple extrusion of marrow or adipose tissue material by mechanical trauma. The work of Sevitt (1962), Bergentz (1961), Edland (1971), Ellis and Watson (1968), Buchanan and Mason (1982), and many others must be studied for detailed accounts of the suggested pathogenesis.

Wherever the fat comes from, embolism is most often seen after injury to bone or fatty tissue. In simplistic terms, where skeletal structures containing fatty marrow are damaged or where subcutaneous fat is compressed or lacerated, fat globules commonly appear in the pulmonary capillaries – and where they are numerous they somehow leak through the lungs into the systemic circulation where they can cause severe disability or death from impaction in vital organs, such as brain, kidney or myocardium. Not only fat, but cellular haematopoietic tissue from bone marrow, can be liberated into the venous system and reach the lungs.

The clinical manifestations of fat embolism depend on the volume of fat reaching the lungs. If substantial, ventilatory problems can ensue because of vascular obstruction and pulmonary oedema. The most dramatic symptoms occur, however, with systemic fat embolism when globules reach the brain and cause a range of neurological abnormalities, usually coma and death from brainstem involvement.

There is usually a delay between trauma and cerebral fat embolism while fat builds up in the lungs, so that a 'lucid interval' occurs, which may be confused clinically with the development of an extradural or subdural haemorrhage. Sevitt stated that of patients with multiple bone fractures, no fewer than 45 per cent had pulmonary fat emboli and 14 per cent had cerebral embolism.

Fat embolism is also associated with burns, barotrauma, soft tissue injury, osteomyelitis, diabetes, surgical operations on fatty tissues (especially mastectomy), septicaemia, steroid therapy, acute pancreatitis and the fatty liver of alcoholism, though fractures remain the most potent cause of the condition. In burns, there is some doubt whether pulmonary fat embolism is a true ante-mortem process, or whether fat can be melted out of tissues and organs in the perimortal period. Mason's (1968) experience in rapid air-crash fires was that fat embolism was not present, but Sevitt's hospital series revealed embolism in 47 per cent of deaths from burns.

Pulmonary fat embolism

After trauma, fat commonly appears in the lungs and can be demonstrated there histologically in the majority of cases of fractures and injury to fatty parts of the body such as the buttocks. Indeed, Lehman and Moore (1927) showed that half of a series of non-trauma deaths had histological evidence of fat in the lungs. Mason found fat in the lungs of 20 per cent of his series of non-trauma deaths, but emphasized that quantitatively the amount was small in contrast to that found in cases of fatal trauma. He used a simple scale for assessing the histological severity of embolism as seen in Oil Red-O frozen sections of lung:

- Grade 0: no emboli seen
- Grade 1: emboli found after some searching
- Grade 2: emboli easily seen
- Grade 3: emboli present in large numbers
- Grade 4: emboli present in potentially fatal numbers.

In systemic fat embolism, no such grading is possible; they are either absent or scanty, or they are abundant.

In most instances, pulmonary fat embolism is merely a phenomenon and not a clinical syndrome and the difference between the two seems closely related to the amount of fat impacted in the lung vessels. When clinically manifest it appears as acute respiratory insufficiency, the incidence being up to 2 per cent in long bone fractures and as much as 10 per cent in multiple fractures, especially with pelvic injuries. In small to moderate amounts, fat in the lungs gives rise to no disability, but large amounts, easily seen by a cursory glance at any field of a fat-stained histological section, give rise to acute respiratory distress. Marked pulmonary oedema is the pathological marker for this syndrome, but caution must be employed, as cerebral fat embolism can also cause pulmonary oedema by its effect upon the brain.

Systemic fat embolism

Here the fat penetrates the lung capillaries and appears in the major circulation, so that it can be carried to any organ or structure, including the skin, where it can cause petechial-like

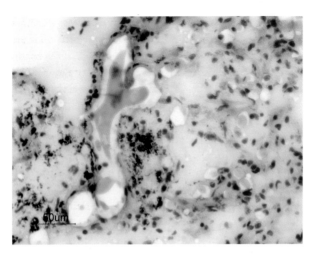

FIGURE 13.2 *Pulmonary fat embolism (Oil Red-O frozen section of lung; original magnification ×20).*

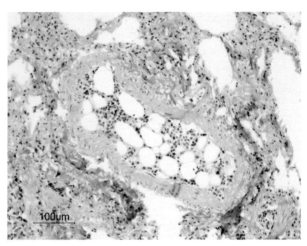

FIGURE 13.3 *Pulmonary bone marrow embolism (van Gieson staining, original magnification ×10).*

lesions. Systemic fat embolism is the fatal manifestation, except where pulmonary loading is so great that it causes respiratory distress. The brain, kidneys and myocardium are the most vulnerable target organs, the brainstem being the one that is most likely to lead to death from impaction of fat globules in its capillaries.

Autopsy findings in fat embolism

When fat is released through the lungs into the systemic circulation, a number of target organs and tissues exhibit abnormalities demonstrable at autopsy, either by gross or histological examination.

Petechial haemorrhages are the typical lesion, caused by the impaction of fat droplets in small venules. These may be seen in the skin of any part of the body, but especially over the front of the chest and on the face and eyelids. Internally they can be widespread but are classically seen in the white matter of the brain, both cerebral and cerebellar hemispheres, as well as the brainstem. Microscopically, when frozen sections are stained by Oil Red-O or other fat stain, the cerebral petechiae will show a central fat globule or globules, and others will be visible without haemorrhage.

In the myocardium, fat may be seen in the interfibre capillaries and in the kidney glomeruli may be stuffed with stained fat. There can be fat in the retina and in the optic nerve, which, in survivors, can cause visual impairment.

Fat embolism is markedly underdiagnosed, both clinically and at autopsy. The more often and the more thoroughly it is sought, the more often it is found. Mild to moderate degrees of pulmonary fat embolism, without systemic overspill, however, must not be given as a cause of death unless there are corroborative clinical features.

Bone marrow embolism

Bone marrow embolism is almost wholly a pulmonary phenomenon, as only in quite exceptional circumstances can cellular material penetrate the lung capillaries. It is quite common in association with fractures of long bones or in multiple bone injuries, though again the frequency with which it is seen is directly related to both awareness and the thoroughness of the search. Where marrow is found, the degree of fat embolism is usually substantial. The common concurrence of fat and cellular embolism is strong evidence of a marrow source for embolic fat, as pointed out by Mason, who found marrow cells in 81 per cent of his cases that had a grade 2 or more lung loading with fat, on a scale of 0–4. According to both Sevitt and Mason, the finding of both substantial fat and marrow emboli in the lungs is definite evidence of ante-mortem infliction of any discovered trauma. For these elements to reach the lungs there must be a competent circulation, albeit for a short time after the trauma.

With the possible exception of burns, any injury inflicted after cessation of effective cardiac function cannot transmit fat or marrow to the pulmonary capillary bed. This is therefore a useful forensic marker on some occasions, such as differentiating between ante-mortem and post-mortem fractures in a body recovered from water. Systemic embolism is not seen in rapid deaths following trauma: there is an interval averaging 24 hours before lung percolation takes place.

Foreign body embolism

A number of other objects may be found as emboli during forensic autopsies and histology. The lung granulomata of

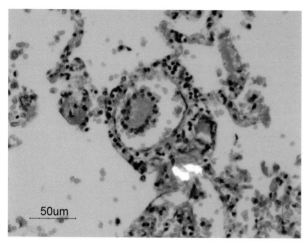

FIGURE 13.4 *Small foreign body granuloma with giant cells and birefringent particles as seen in polarized light in the lung of a drug addict (HE, original magnification ×20).*

talc, etc., seen in the lungs of intravenous drug users, are emboli from contaminants introduced into the venous system by syringe and needle. Shotgun pellets and bullets may enter the circulation via tissue damage and embolize to various sites including coronary arteries. In fat and bone marrow embolism, even fragments of bone and cartilage have been found as emboli in the lungs.

Amniotic fluid embolism is discussed elsewhere.

ADULT RESPIRATORY DISTRESS SYNDROME

Following severe lung injury, such as gross impact upon the thorax or blast injury from explosion, or from aspiration of gastric contents, infections, toxins, systemic shock, irritant gases, near-drowning and many other causes, the lung epithelium may suffer 'diffuse alveolar damage'. Clinically the victim may suffer marked dyspnoea and progressive respiratory failure, becoming hypoxaemic. Pathologically the lungs show a stiff oedema that progresses to a rigid, infiltrated lung if survival is long enough. At autopsy the lungs are hard and retain their shape after removal, having a 'dry-oedema' appearance, being almost double in weight in some instances.

Histologically the initial changes are shedding of type I pneumocytes with intra-alveolar exudates, the formation of hyaline membrane and patchy alveolar haemorrhage. This destructive phase is then replaced after a few days with a proliferative stage, when type II pneumocytes begin to fill the alveoli and a mononuclear response infiltrates the interstitial areas. The alveolar proliferation organizes, if survival continues, and eventual pulmonary fibrosis may seriously

incapacitate the half who survive. A typical progression is seen in paraquat poisoning, though here there are virtually no long-term survivors.

A condition that is similar to the appearances of adult respiratory distress syndrome is the so-called 'respirator lung', which develops when a patient dies after an appreciable period of mechanical ventilation. It may appear within a few days, but usually supervenes after many days or weeks on a ventilator. The gross appearances are of a stiff, rigid lung, which, though heavy, does not usually appear obviously oedematous. Microscopically, proteinaceous fluid and a mixture of proliferative cells may be seen in the alveoli.

RENAL FAILURE FOLLOWING TRAUMA

Known for many years, this is a common sequel to extensive muscle damage or to burns that affect considerable areas of skin, as well as from certain poisons. It was formerly ascribed most often to 'acute tubular necrosis', but recent experimental work has thrown some doubt upon this as an accurate clinicopathological entity. When muscle is crushed, severely torn or otherwise rendered ischaemic, where extensive burns are suffered, or where poisons, such as mercuric salts or carbon tetrachloride are given, destruction of the renal tubular epithelium may be seen.

Unfortunately for histological diagnosis, a similar change occurs during post-mortem autolysis. In burns and muscle damage, the tubules may also be blocked with brown casts of myoglobin and these two changes of distal tubular necrosis and casts were thought to cause the profound oliguria or anuria often associated with trauma and burns. In biopsy as opposed to autopsy material, however, the tubular damage has been found to be minimal and the casts may be a sequel to reduced filtration rather than to tubular damage, so the validity of 'acute tubular necrosis' as an explanation of renal failure following trauma has been questioned. The true mechanism is still obscure, but may well involve the juxtaglomerular apparatus and the renin–angiotensin system, as well as disseminated intravascular coagulation effects on the glomeruli.

DISSEMINATED INTRAVASCULAR COAGULATION

The importance and frequency of this condition has been increasingly recognized in recent years, as it may follow a whole range of traumatic, infective and other acute events. Widely known as 'DIC', it has a number of other names indicating that it is a consumption coagulopathy associated with the blood clotting mechanism.

In DIC there is an abnormal activation of the coagulation process within the blood vessels caused by a wide variety of factors related to the blood itself, the vessel walls and to blood flow. Damaged tissue from trauma and burns can trigger thromboplastin-initiated coagulation: entry of tissue cell elements, especially from erythrocytes, brain and placenta are particularly potent. Particulate matter such as micro-organisms or microemboli of all types (including fat and air emboli, especially those from decompression) can precipitate coagulation via factor XII. Vascular endothelial damage and stasis of blood flow can have a similar effect.

Whatever the causes – and they are extremely complex – fibrinogen is consumed and fibrin precipitated in vessels, leading to both vascular obstructive effects and to a haemorrhagic diathesis from depletion of the coagulation system. Platelets are also consumed, adhering to the fibrin thrombi. Fibrinolysis is activated and there is a dynamic contest between intravascular coagulation and its removal.

After death there can be post-mortem fibrinolysis (Mole 1948), which lessens the ease with which fibrin deposits can be detected: staining techniques are also an imperfect method of visualizing the fibrin, so that a careful search must be made in autopsy histology for fibrin remnants. Lungs, kidney, liver and adrenals are the most likely organs to yield positive results.

Microvascular obstruction, leading sometimes to frank infarction as well as reduced function, together with bleeding, form the major dangers of DIC in a forensic context.

AIR EMBOLISM

Most examples of air embolism have a medico-legal significance as the entry of air into the circulation usually comes about as a result of trauma, sometimes surgical or therapeutic, from barotrauma or from criminal intervention.

Air embolism consists of an interruption of the circulatory system by bubbles of air (or other gas) that gain access to the circulation, usually through the venous side. It is an 'airlock', familiar to plumbers and owners of diesel engines, where the normal flow of liquid through tubes is wholly or partially blocked by air.

In the animal body the major disability is in the heart, as air is compressible and the contractions of the heart fail to move on the bolus of gas, being designed to pump an incompressible liquid. The air must enter on the venous side to be sucked towards the heart, causing pulmonary air embolism. The air usually remains in the right side of the heart, pulmonary trunk and arteries, and in the pulmonary vessels, rarely emerging on the pulmonary vein side. Death is usually immediate, but can be delayed by up to about 2 hours.

In the surgical context, aspiration of air into neck veins may occur while operating on the head or neck (especially thyroid and neurosurgical operations) with the patient in a sitting position. When the atria are below any breach in a vein, there is a suction effect that can draw in air; this can also happen in suicidal or homicidal cut throat. Refilling of a therapeutic pneumothorax has also led to fatal air embolism, either because the lung is punctured or an adhesion has torn the visceral pleura. In either case air under pressure may enter an exposed vein.

Some accidents have arisen during transfusion or infusion, and may form the basis for a medical negligence action. Now that flexible, collapsible fluid or blood containers are widely used the danger is less, but where rigid bottles are still used, the need for a vent tube may allow air to enter the connecting tubing when a bottle is allowed to empty completely. This in itself is innocuous, but if a fresh bottle is then connected, the new flow will drive all the air in the tubing into the vein.

Even more dangerous is the practice of connecting pressurized air or oxygen to the vent in order to hasten the transfusion speed: if the bottle is allowed to empty, gas under pressure enters the vein.

Arterial air embolism is rare, but can occur in lacerations of the lungs, refilling of an artificial pneumothorax or in some forms of barotrauma where the lung is ruptured in a diver who ascends too rapidly from a great depth. The 'bends' are also a type of gas embolism, in which dissolved nitrogen appears in gaseous form in the blood. This is caused by a sudden release of pressure on the return of a diver to atmospheric conditions after being supplied with air at high pressure. Death can be the result of air locks in the cerebral vessels or of ventricular fibrillation from coronary air embolism (Moore and Braselton 1940).

Criminal abortion accounted for many deaths from air embolism in former years (and still does in some parts of the world), from the insufflation of the uterus by a Higginson syringe (Chapter 19). Though therapeutic abortion by suction aspiration of the uterine contents is an extremely safe procedure, several somewhat inexplicable deaths have occurred from air embolism. The mechanism is obscure but may have been caused by muscular rebound of the uterus sucking air into the cervix. Some homicides, including 'mercy killings' committed by doctors, have been caused by deliberate injection of air into peripheral veins. The volume of air needed to cause fatal embolism has been hotly debated for years, but no real consensus has emerged, estimates varying from 10 to 480 ml (Polson 1963). If the volume of the right side of the heart is accepted as the minimum space that has to be filled, about 100 ml would appear to be a reasonable volume. In the rare event of air gaining access to the arterial system, presumably much less would be required to be effective; it would have to be introduced into a carotid artery to be of much danger, as this is the only way it could gain access to the cerebral circulation. To reach the coronary vessels – always mentioned in books, but virtually never seen – the blood would have to enter the pulmonary veins to reach the root of the aorta via the left side of the heart. Virtually all of the few cases of arterial air embolism have arisen in relation to dysbarism, where bubbles have either been generated within the vessels by decompression, or have entered the arterial system in the lungs from tears in the lung tissue.

Certainly air injected into a limb artery would do no harm at all, especially as most of the gas is likely to be absorbed very rapidly by the tissues. Thus the ingenious plot in Dorothy L Sayer's novel, *Unnatural Death*, where 'a hypodermic of air was injected into an artery' would have failed on two counts: site and volume!

The autopsy in suspected air embolism

When the circumstances indicate the possibility of fatal air embolism, special precautions must be taken over the autopsy. A pre-autopsy chest radiograph must be taken, as this is by far the best way of demonstrating air in sufficient quantities to be fatal. A chest radiograph is also essential in any kind of barotrauma as it may also indicate a pneumothorax, a lesion so often the cause of air embolism.

Almost the only mechanism of death is 'pump failure' of the right side of the heart. Air fills the great veins, right atrium and right ventricle, causing a froth that cannot be pumped on by the heart in systole because air is compressible. It is unlikely that air will penetrate the pulmonary capillaries in any quantity, unless some vascular shunts are present, so froth is unlikely to be seen in the left side of the heart, except in dysbarism.

Following radiography – in place of it, as second-best – the body must be carefully inspected for any tissue swelling, especially in the upper thorax and neck region, where crepitant gas bubbles may form surgical emphysema from leakage from lung damage or pneumothorax, or both, in dysbarism.

The head should be dissected first, not to detect air bubbles in the cortical veins, as almost every textbook erroneously states, but to look for air in the cerebral arteries. Descriptions and photographs of air segments in the cerebral veins are part of the mythology of forensic pathology, handed on uncritically from one book and one author to another. There is no way in which air bubbles can reach the pial veins on the brain surface. They cannot get there

via the venous system, as there is no way in which they could struggle against the flow in the jugular veins, pass through the complex arrangement of intracranial venous sinuses retrograde to the circulation and dispose themselves over the cortical surface. Neither can they reach the same veins by penetrating the capillary bed of the brain, in the rare instances of arterial air embolism. As was demonstrated almost 30 years ago, these bubbles are artefacts and can be seen in many routine autopsies where there can be no question of air embolism.

The basal arteries should be inspected for air, however, which can reach them during episodes of dysbarism where air gains access to the arterial system in the lungs during decompression. The calvarium is removed gently and the dura opened. The brain is carefully lifted and small artery forceps clamped on the intracranial part of both internal carotid arteries and vertebral arteries. The vessels are then cut below these before the brain is removed from the skull in the usual manner. The whole pluck can then be submerged in water and the ends of the vessels watched for escaping bubbles when the clamps are removed.

The thorax is opened in the fashion appropriate for the detection of a pneumothorax, with puncture of an intercostal muscle beneath a pool of water supported by the reflected skin flap. This is done on each side, remembering that a positive result can only be expected in a **tension** pneumothorax.

The abdomen should next be examined, especially where air may have gained access through the uterus. The intestines should be gently displaced and the mesenteric veins examined for air bubbles. The inferior vena cava, the common iliac veins and the various pelvic veins should be scrutinized, and, if necessary, opened under water by pouring water into the opened abdominal cavity.

The sternum and costal cartilages are then removed carefully, preferably keeping the manubrium and upper ribs intact at this stage to avoid damage to the great vessels in the thoracic inlet. The superior vena cava should be inspected for bubbles. The pericardium is opened and the right and left ventricles punctured under water.

Bajanowski *et al.* (1998, 1999) consider that an aspirometer has to be used for the detection, measurement and storage of gas originating from the heart ventricles. It should be filled completely with distilled water containing two drops of Tween 80 to reduce the surface tension of the water to prevent adherence of small air bubbles to the wall of the aspirometer. Subsequently the gas should be analysed by gas chromatography and the results assessed according to the criteria defined by Pierucci and Gherson (1968, 1969) before the diagnosis 'air embolism' is justified.

If air embolism substantial enough to have caused death is present, frothy blood will be quite evident oozing from

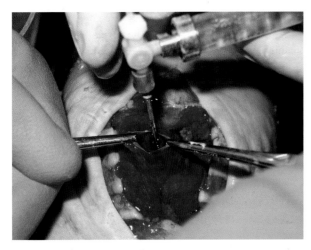

FIGURE 13.5 *An aspirometer should be used to recover air from the heart ventricles for subsequent analysis by gas chromatography.*

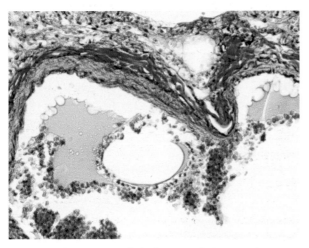

FIGURE 13.6 *Leucocyte and platelet accumulation around an empty space, 'air bubble' in blood, considered by some authors as evidence of venous air embolism. (Reproduced by kind permission of Professor E Lignitz.)*

the ventricular lumen, almost invariably the right. If this is apparent, however, it will almost certainly already have been seen on the pre-autopsy radiograph.

If there has been a considerable delay between death and autopsy, the air can dissipate, presumably dissolving into the tissues. Any degree of decomposition of the body negates a diagnosis of air embolism, because of the production of gases of putrefaction.

SUBENDOCARDIAL HAEMORRHAGE

A striking feature of many forensic autopsies, especially on victims of severe trauma, is the presence of well-marked haemorrhage under the endocardium of the left ventricle. This is often so striking as to provide an indication of some catastrophic event shortly before death.

Though the haemorrhages have been described since the last century, they were specifically studied in the 1930s by Sheehan in cases of abortion and acute haemorrhage associated with pregnancy; they were formerly known as 'Sheehan's haemorrhages'.

The lesions are seen in the left ventricle, on the interventricular septum, and on the opposing papillary muscles and adjacent columnae carneae of the free wall of the ventricle. The haemorrhages are flame-shaped and confluent, not petechial, and tend to occur in one continuous sheet rather than patches. The bleeding is in a thin subendocardial layer, but when severe may actually raise the endocardium into a flat blister that can be palpable on the smooth septum. The mechanism of production is obscure, but they are commonly seen in the following circumstances:

- After sudden, profound hypotension, either from severe blood loss or from 'shock' in the widest sense.
- After intracranial damage, from head injuries, cerebral oedema, surgical craniotomy or large intracranial tumours. Sudden intracranial decompression also seems to be associated with subendocardial bleeding.
- Obstetric catastrophes seem particularly prone to produce these haemorrhages, as found by Sheehan. Death from ante-partum or post-partum haemorrhage, ruptured ectopic gestation, abortions of various types and ruptured uterus often reveal these lesions.
- Various forms of poisoning, especially acute heavy-metal toxicity, particularly arsenic. The most profound subendocardial haemorrhages ever seen by the author (BK) were in a massive suicidal poisoning with arsenious oxide: the endocardium was raised into a large blood blister on the interventricular septum.

The haemorrhages can appear extremely rapidly, within a few heart beats. The author (BK) has seen well-marked lesions in a heart that was avulsed from its base during the crash of a military aircraft, obviously causing virtually instantaneous death. The common factor seems to be sudden hypotension and it has been suggested that, if the intraventricular pressure drops precipitously, the existing blood pressure in the coronary system is then unsupported across the endocardium by an equal pressure within the ventricular lumen, so that rupture of the superficial vessels occurs. There are flaws in this theory, one being the common incidence in intracranial lesions. Experimental work in goats has shown that prior vagotomy prevents the occurrence of subendocardial haemorrhages, suggesting that the phenomenon is mediated by the autonomic nervous system. To support this hypothesis, they are known to be part of Virchow's triad of 'pulmonary oedema, gastric erosions and subendocardial haemorrhage' seen in head injuries and cases of raised intracranial pressure.

SUDDEN DEATH FROM SUPRARENAL HAEMORRHAGE

Though not common, haemorrhage into the adrenal glands is a well-recognized terminal event, usually after some trauma to the body not related to direct injury to the suprarenal vessels themselves.

Originally these haemorrhages were thought to be confined to meningococcal septicaemia in children, the lesion being called the 'Waterhouse–Friderichsen syndrome'. It is now recognized that adrenal haemorrhage is part of a general response to stress, of which meningococcal infection is only one of a wide range.

In a recent 5-year period, the author (BK) found 16 cases of 'adrenal apoplexy' (to give it its old name) in the autopsy records of a forensic pathology service that performed 4890 autopsies in that period, giving an incidence of about 0.3 per cent.

Of these 16 cases, more than half (9) were bilateral. There were more male than female subjects, probably because of the greater amount of trauma in men. Three were infants, all with meningococcal infections.

None of the adult cases was diagnosed or even suspected clinically. Most were traffic accidents, the remainder being post-operative, other trauma or poisoning, together with several cases of hypertension and chronic renal failure. The most frequent common denominator was trauma, whether that trauma was direct injury or surgical trauma. The sudden collapse and rapid death usually occurred a few days after the trauma, varying from 2 to 21 days.

At autopsy one or both of the adrenal glands are found to be swollen, sometimes to the size of a large walnut (3–5 cm) the cortex being tightly stretched around a large haematoma occupying the medulla. The haemorrhage is usually dark red and fairly fresh, though occasionally an area of brown bleeding indicates a previous episode.

The late Professor Hugh Johnson, of St Thomas' Hospital, London, collected between 150 and 200 autopsy cases of suprarenal haemorrhage (unpublished) and considered that they fell into six main groups:

- Trauma of all types. Johnson was of the opinion that the predominance of right-sided gland haemorrhages was a result of the frequency of right-sided impacts on pedestrians in Britain because of the side of traffic flow.
- Perinatal, newborn or stillborn infants, especially when they were breech births or had fetal anoxia.
- Infancy and childhood, especially meningococcal and disseminated intravascular coagulation.
- Infective and post-operative septicaemia, often with Gram-negative organisms. Sometimes there was direct surgical trauma to the gland, as in gastric surgery.
- Tumour: haemorrhage into a secondary deposit or invasion of adrenal vasculature.
- Thrombosis of central vein with adrenal infarction.

REFERENCES AND FURTHER READING

Adams V, Guidi C. 2001. Venous air embolism in homicidal blunt impact head trauma. Case reports. *Am J Forensic Med Pathol* **22**:322–6.

Adkins RB, Foster JH, O'Saile D. 1962. Experimental study of the genesis of fat embolism. *Ann Surg* **156**:515–27.

Allardyce DB. 1971. The postmortem interval as a factor in fat embolism. *Arch Pathol* **92**:248–53.

Bajanowski T, West A, Brinkmann B. 1998. Proof of fatal air embolism. *Int J Legal Med* **111**:208–11.

Bajanowski T, Kohler H, DuChesne A, *et al.* 1999. Proof of air embolism after exhumation. *Int J Legal Med* **112**:2–7.

Bergentz SE. 1961. Studies on the genesis of post-traumatic fat embolism. *Acta Chir Scand* **282**:1–72.

Beyer A. 1979. Shock lung. *Br J Hosp Med* **21**:248–52.

Bonnell H, French SW. 1982. Fatal air embolus associated with pneumatosis cystoides intestinalis. *Am J Forensic Med Pathol* **3**:69–72.

Bowen DA, McKim Sycamore E. 1976. Traumatic air embolism. *Med Sci Law* **16**:56–8.

Buchanan D, Mason JK. 1982. Occurrence of pulmonary fat and bone marrow embolism. *Am J Forensic Med Pathol* **3**:73–8.

Bunai Y, Yoshimi N, Komoriya H, *et al.* 1988. An application of a quantitative analytical system for the grading of pulmonary fat embolisms. *Forensic Sci Int* **39**:263–9.

Butler BD, Hills BA. 1985. Transpulmonary passage of venous air emboli. *J Appl Physiol* **59**:543–7.

Cebelin MS, Hirsch CS. 1980. Human stress cardiomyopathy. Myocardial lesions in victims of homicidal assaults without internal injuries. *Hum Pathol* **11**:123–32.

Chau KY, Yuen ST, Wong MP. 1995. Seasonal variation in the necropsy incidence of pulmonary thromboembolism in Hong Kong. *J Clin Pathol* **48**:578–9.

Chau KY, Yuen ST, Wong MP. 1997. Clinicopathological pattern of pulmonary thromboembolism in chinese autopsy patients: comparison with caucasian series. *Pathology* **29**:263–6.

Dada MA, Loftus IA, Rutherfoord GS. 1993. Shotgun pellet embolism to the brain. *Am J Forensic Med Pathol* **14**:58–60.

Edland J. 1971. Post-traumatic fat embolism. In: Wecht C (ed.), *Legal medicine annual*. Appleton Century Crofts, New York.

Ellis HA, Watson AJ. 1968. Studies on the genesis of traumatic fat embolism in man. *Am J Pathol* **53**:245–51.

Erhen J, Nadvornik F. 1963. The quantitative demonstration of air embolism. *J Forensic Med* **10**:45–8.

Fineschi V, Centini F, Mazzeo E, *et al.* 1999. Adam (MDMA) and eve (MDEA) misuse: an immunohistochemical study on three fatal cases. *Forensic Sci Int* **104**:65–74.

Flute PT. 1970. Coagulation and fibrinolysis after injury. *J Clin Pathol Suppl R Coll Pathol* **4**:102–9.

Freiman DG. 1965. Frequency of pulmonary thrombo-embolism in man. *N Engl J Med* **24**:1278–82.

Gottlieb JD, Ericsson JA, Sweet RB. 1965. Venous air embolism: a review. *Anesth Analg* **44**:773–9.

Gresham GA, Kuzynski A, Rosborough D. 1971. Fatal fat embolism following replacement arthroplasty for transcenvical fractures of the femur. *Br Med J* **2**:617–18.

Guileyardo JM, Cooper RE, Porter BE, *et al.* 1992. Renal artery bullet embolism. *Am J Forensic Med Pathol* **13**:288–9.

Hamilton PJ, Stalker AL, Douglas AS. 1978. Disseminated intravascular coagulation: a review. *J Clin Pathol* **31**:609–19.

Hartveit F, Lystad H, Minken A. 1968. The pathology of venous air embolism. *Br J Exp Pathol* **49**:81–6.

Havig O. 1977. Deep vein thrombosis and pulmonary embolism. An autopsy study with multiple regression analysis of possible risk factors. *Acta Chir Scand Suppl* **478**:1–120.

Irniger W. 1962–3. Histological determination of the age of thromboses and embolisms. *Virchows Arch A Pathol Anat Histopathol* **236**:220–37.

Jackson CD, Gerendyke RM. 1965. Pulmonary and cerebral fat embolism after closed-chest cardiac massage. *Surg Gynecol Obstet* **120**:25–8.

Janssen W. 1967. [On the pathogenesis and forensic evaluation of brain hemorrhages following cerebral air embolism.] *Dtsch Z Gesamte Gerichtl Med* **61**:62–80.

Johnson HR. 1973. Delayed air embolism. *Forensic Sci* **2**:375–7.

Jörgensen L. 1964. Experimental platelet and coagulation thrombi. *Acta Pathol Microbiol Scand Sect A Pathol* **62**:189–223.

Kerner T, Fritz G, Unterberg A, *et al.* 2003. Pulmonary air embolism in severe head injury. *Resuscitation* **56**:111–15.

King P. 1970. Fat embolism syndrome. *Med J Aust* **2**:1190–1.

Knight B. 1966. Fatal pulmonary embolism: factors of forensic interest in 400 cases. *Med Sci Law* **6**:150–4.

Knight B. 1980. Sudden unexpected death from adrenal haemorrhage. *Forensic Sci Int* **16**:227–9.

Knight B, Zaini MR. 1980. Pulmonary embolism and venous thrombosis. A pattern of incidence and predisposing factors over 70 years. *Am J Forensic Med Pathol* **1**:227–32.

Knight L, Velentine EH. 1962. Spontaneous bilateral adrenal haemorrhage. *JAMA* **14**:1312.

Lau G. 1995. Pulmonary cartilage embolism: fact or artefact? *Am J Forensic Med Pathol* **16**:51–3.

Lehman EP, Moore RM. 1927. Fat embolism including experimental production without trauma. *Arch Surg* **14**:621–6.

Lequire VS. 1959. A study on the pathogenesis of fat embolism based on human necropsy material and animal experiments. *Am J Pathol* **35**:999–1003.

Levy V, Rao VJ. 1988. Survival time in gunshot and stab wound victims. *Am J Forensic Med Pathol* **9**:215–7.

Lignitz E, Lignitz G, Puschel K. 1995. [Lung embolism as the cause of death in legal medicine.] *Versicherungsmedizin* **47**:203–7.

Loehry CA. 1966. Pulmonary emboli in young adults. *Br Med J* **1**:1327–8.

Mackay DG. 1965. *Disseminated intravascular coagulation: an intermediary mechanism of disease.* Hoeber, New York.

Malhotra MS, Wright HC. 1960. Air embolism during decompression under water. *J Physiol* **151**:32–5.

Mason JK. 1968. Pulmonary fat and bone marrow embolism as an indication of ante-mortem violence. *Med Sci Law* **8**:200–6.

Melinek J, Livingston E, Cortina G, *et al.* 2002. Autopsy findings following gastric bypass surgery for morbid obesity. *Arch Pathol Lab Med* **126**:1091–5.

Mole RH. 1948. Fibrinolysin and the fluidity of the blood postmortem. *J Pathol Bacteriol* **60**:413–17.

Moore RM, Braselton CW. 1940. Injections of air and of carbon dioxide into a pulmonary vein. *Ann Surg* **112**:212–18.

Morell MT, Dunhill MS. 1968. The postmortem incidence of pulmonary embolism in a hospital population. *Br J Surg* **55**:5–10.

Nordstrom M, Lindblad B. 1998. Autopsy-verified venous thromboembolism within a defined urban population – the city of Malmo, Sweden. *APMIS* **106**:378–84.

Pierucci G. 1985. [Post-mortem diagnosis of gas embolism.] *Pathologica* **77**:145–55.

Pierucci G, Gherson G. 1968. [Experimental study on gas embolism with special reference to the differentiation between embolic gas and putrefaction gas.] *Zacchia* **4**:347–73.

Pierucci G, Gherson G. 1969. [Further contribution to the chemical diagnosis of gas embolism. The demonstration of hydrogen as an expression of 'putrefactive component'.] *Zacchia* **5**:595–603.

Polson CJ. 1963. *Essentials of forensic medicine*. Pergamon Press, Oxford.

Rappaport H, Raum M, Horrell JB. 1951. Bone marrow embolism. *Am J Pathol* **27**:407–43.

Robertson H. 1938. A clinical study of pulmonary embolism. *Am J Surg* **16**:3–21.

Rouse DA, Hargrove R. 1992. An unusual case of gas embolism. *Am J Forensic Med Pathol* **13**:268–70.

Sandritter W, Staeudinger M, Drexler H. 1980. Autopsy and clinical diagnosis. *Pathol Res Pract* **168**:107–14.

Sanz P, Reig R, Borras L, *et al.* 1988. Disseminated intravascular coagulation and mesenteric venous thrombosis in fatal amanita poisoning. *Hum Toxicol* **7**:199–201.

Sevitt S. 1962. *Fat embolism*. Butterworth, London.

Sevitt S. 1970. Thrombosis and embolism after injury. *J Clin Pathol* **23**:86–90.

Sevitt S. 1973. Coronary thrombosis following injury and burns. *Med Sci Law* **13**:185–91.

Sevitt S, Gallagher N. 1961. Venous thrombosis and pulmonary embolism: a clinico-pathological study in injured and burned patients. *Br J Surg* **48**:475–81.

Shapiro HA. 1965. Death from delayed air embolism. *J Forensic Med* **12**:3–7.

Shapiro HA, Robertson JK. 1962. The significance of blood in the pleural cavity observed after death. *J Forensic Med* **9**:5–8.

Simpson JG, Stalker AC. 1973. Disseminated intravascular coagulation. In: Douglas (ed.), *Clinics in haematology*, vol. 2. W. B. Saunders, Philadelphia.

Simpson K. 1959. Fat embolism. *J Forensic Med* **6**:19–22.

Slater DN. 1988. Bone marrow emboli [letter]. *Am J Forensic Med Pathol* **9**:357–8.

Stalker AC. 1978. Issue: disseminated intravascular coagulation. In: Mason JK (ed.), *Pathology of violent injury*. Edward Arnold, London.

Stamatakis JD, Kakkar VV, Lawrence D, *et al.* 1978. The origin of thrombi in the deep veins of the lower limb: a venographic study. *Br J Surg* **65**:449–51.

Start RD, Cross SS. 1999. Acp. Best practice no 155. Pathological investigation of deaths following surgery, anaesthesia, and medical procedures. *J Clin Pathol* **52**:640–52.

Stein PD, Henry JW. 1995. Prevalence of acute pulmonary embolism among patients in a general hospital and at autopsy. *Chest* **108**:978–81.

Suzuki T, Ikeda N, Umetsu K, *et al.* 1984. Pulmonary fat embolism as an ante-mortem reaction in traumatic immediate death. *Med Sci Law* **24**:175–8.

Suzuki T, Ikeda N, Umetsu K. 1987. Pulmonary bone marrow embolic phenomena. Antemortem reactions in traumatic immediate death. *Am J Forensic Med Pathol* **8**:283–6.

Thali MJ, Yen K, Plattner T, *et al.* 2002. Charred body: virtual autopsy with multi-slice computed tomography and magnetic resonance imaging. *J Forensic Sci* **47**:1326–31.

Timperley WR. 1978. Disseminated intravascular coagulation in forensic pathology. *Med Sci Law* **18**:108–16.

van Ieperen L. 1985. Gas embolism as a cause of death. *Am J Forensic Med Pathol* **6**:240–3.

Voigt J. 1966. Adrenal lesions in medico-legal autopsies. *J Forensic Med* **13**:3–15.

Williams G. 1956. Experimental studies in arterial ligation. *J Pathol Bacteriol* **72**:569–74.

Wilson D, Cooke EA, McNally MA, *et al.* 2001. Changes in coagulability as measured by thrombelastography following surgery for proximal femoral fracture. *Injury* **32**:765–70.

Zaini MRS. 1981. *Medicolegal aspects of pulmonary embolism*. Medical Faculty, University of Wales, Cardiff.

Zaitoun AM, Fernandez C. 1998. The value of histological examination in the audit of hospital autopsies: a quantitative approach. *Pathology* **30**:100–4.

CHAPTER 14

Suffocation and 'asphyxia'

Though traditionally every textbook of forensic medicine has a chapter entitled 'Asphyxia', it is a partial misnomer, as many of the conditions described under this heading are not truly asphyxial in nature. It is difficult to find a succinct alternative, however, unless each subcondition is described individually – and some deaths have a mixed aetiology. The conventional title is therefore retained in this book, though it is emphasized that 'asphyxia' is both inappropriate and inaccurate when applied to many of the mechanisms of death formerly ascribed to this cause.

THE NATURE OF 'ASPHYXIA'

Common usage has led to the term 'asphyxia' being equated with 'lack of oxygen', though etymologically the word means 'absence of pulsation'. Interestingly – if fortuitously – this original sense is sometimes more accurate in certain deaths associated with pressure on the neck, where cardiac arrest – certainly a prime reason for absence of pulsation – is the fatal mechanism, rather than hypoxia.

Reverting to the usual meaning of asphyxia, a whole series of disturbances can lead to lack of oxygen. The basic purpose of respiration is to convey atmospheric oxygen to the peripheral tissue cells. Anything that interferes with oxygen transfer can be called 'asphyxia', though other terms such as 'hypoxia' or 'anoxia' are more accurate, and should be preferred. The following conditions may legitimately be considered to be defects in the chain of respiration and hence are examples of asphyxia:

- Absence or reduction of oxygen tension in the external atmosphere, such as reduced barometric pressure or replacement of oxygen by an inert gas, such as nitrogen or carbon dioxide.

- Obstruction of the external respiratory orifices, as in smothering or gagging.

- Blockage of the internal respiratory passages, at either pharyngeal, laryngeal, tracheal or bronchial level.

- Restriction of the respiratory movements of the thorax, preventing the inspiration of air through patent respiratory passages, as in the so-called 'traumatic asphyxia' or in paralysis from brainstem or cord damage, or the use of curare-like drugs.

- Disease of the lungs that prevents or reduces gaseous interchange. Extensive pneumonia, pulmonary oedema, adult respiratory distress syndrome, diffuse fibrosis and many other conditions may lead to hypoxia, but these are rarely of forensic concern.

- Reduction in cardiac function leading to impairment of the circulation of oxygenated blood may be considered as a type of 'asphyxia', sometimes called 'stagnant anoxia'. Again, the condition is rarely relevant to forensic problems.

- A reduced ability of the blood to transport oxygen can also be thought to be asphyxial in nature, such as severe anaemias and the replacement of the oxygen-combining power of haemoglobin by carbon monoxide.

- Finally, an inability of the peripheral tissue cells to utilize the oxygen delivered to them by the bloodstream is seen in conditions such as cyanide poisoning, where the cytochrome-oxidase enzyme systems are inactivated.

Several schemes of classification of asphyxia have been devised, such as those of McIntyre (1969) and Shapiro (1988).

MECHANICAL 'ASPHYXIA'

The usual relevance of asphyxia in a forensic context is in mechanical asphyxia, rather than some of the internal conditions mentioned above, which are more likely to arise as a result of natural disease or toxic conditions.

The normal oxygen content of blood varies according to the age and health of the subject. Young to middle-aged adults have almost complete saturation of their arterial blood with oxygen, at a level of 90–100 mmHg (12–13.5 kPa), whilst persons over 60 may drop to between 60 and 85 mmHg (8–10 kPa). These normal values in the younger group may be contrasted with those sufferers from mild hypoxia of about 60 mmHg (8 kPa), and those in severe to fatal hypoxia when oxygen tension falls to between 40 and 20 mmHg (5–3 kPa).

Unfortunately for pathologists, post-mortem analysis of oxygen levels in the blood is of no value in the retrospective diagnosis of hypoxia, as changes soon after death rapidly distort the distribution of gases and make the results meaningless.

Definition of terms

A number of different names have been used to describe the various types of mechanical 'asphyxia', some of which are confusing or inexact:

- **Suffocation** is a general term used to indicate death from deprivation of oxygen, either from lack of the gas in the breathable environment or from obstruction of the external air passages.
- **Smothering** is more specific, in that it indicates blockage of the external air passages, usually by a hand or soft fabric. A variety of suffocation may be called **gagging** where fabric or adhesive tape occludes the mouth to prevent speaking or shouting. While the nasal passages remain patent, air can enter, but later blockage by mucus or oedema may lead to death.
- **Choking** refers to blockage of the upper airways by some foreign body, but is also used for manual strangulation.
- **Throttling** refers to strangulation, usually by hand, the word rarely being applied to ligature strangulation.
- **Strangulation** is the most specific term, indicating the use either of the hands or a ligature as a means of applying external pressure to the neck. **Garrotting** has been used for ligature strangulation, but more accurately refers only to a Spanish method of judicial execution. Other methods exist in various parts of the world, such as the Indian technique of pressing a flexible stick or 'lathi' across the front of the neck.

- **Mugging** originally meant the application of pressure to the neck by means of an arm crooked around from the rear, but more recent American usage has widened the term to mean any kind of robbery with violence. More recently still the **arm-lock** has been used as means of restraint by law enforcement officers, sometimes with fatal results.

As an aside, in some deaths during arrest, usually where a violent struggle occurs between several police officers and a drunken or drugged offender, the death of the latter occurs where no neck or chest pressure can be implicated. Though the mechanism is obscure and impossible to demonstrate objectively at autopsy, it has been provisionally ascribed to a catecholamine-induced cardiac arrhythmia from an exaggerated adrenal response.

As most of these victims are given energetic cardiopulmonary resuscitation, any markers of this catecholamine effect, such as contraction-band necrosis in the myocardium, cannot be differentiated from resuscitative artefacts.

THE CLASSIC SIGNS OF 'ASPHYXIA'

For many years the autopsy diagnosis of an asphyxial death was made by reference to a set of findings that have come to be known as the 'classic signs of asphyxia'. Unfortunately, it is now quite clear that most of these signs are so non-specific that little reliance can be placed on them in the absence of other confirmatory evidence. They are scathingly referred to by Lester Adelson (1974) as the 'obsolete diagnostic quintet'.

In many cases of undoubted fatal hypoxia these signs are absent and, conversely, they are often present in some degree in conditions that can be shown to be non-hypoxic in origin. The major difficulty for the pathologist is that 'asphyxia' cannot reliably be equated with 'hypoxia'. There are no truly distinctive autopsy signs of pure hypoxia and most of the alleged criteria are caused by factors other than a lack of oxygen.

To confuse the issue further, some apparently hypoxic states lead to sudden or rapid death before there is time for oxygen lack to take effect, such as often happens when a victim enters a space devoid of oxygen, has the trachea suddenly blocked by food or has a plastic bag pulled over the head.

Each of the 'classic features' must be looked at in depth.

Petechial haemorrhages

These are small pin-point collections of blood lying in the skin, the sclera or conjunctivae and under thoracic serous membranes such as the pleura or pericardium. They vary in size from a tenth of a millimetre to about two millimetres. If larger than this, they are more accurately called 'ecchymoses'.

Petechiae are often known as 'Tardieu's spots', but this eponym should be restricted to those lying in the visceral pleura, where they were described by the Parisian Professor Ambroise Tardieu in 1866, in the bodies of infants who he claimed had been 'overlain'. A further common error is to attribute the petechiae to the rupture of **capillaries**, whereas they actually emanate from small venules – capillary bleeding would be invisible to the naked eye.

Petechiae are caused by an acute rise in venous pressure that in turn causes overdistension and rupture of thin-walled peripheral venules, especially in lax tissues, such as the eyelid, and in unsupported serous membranes, such as the pleura and epicardium. It is traditionally claimed that hypoxia of the vein wall is an added factor, but there is no experimental proof of this conjecture, which seems unlikely considering the rapid formation of these lesions when venous pressures rise; for example, petechiae can appear almost instantly after violent sneezing or coughing before any hypoxia is possible.

Petechiae are seen most often in the face and eyes of victims of compression of the neck or fixation of the chest. In the former, where strangulation by either hand or ligature has occurred, occlusion of the jugular veins prevents venous drainage from the head, whilst almost always allowing the arterial supply to continue via the more deeply placed and much less compressible carotid and vertebral arteries. There is a rapid rise in venous pressure in the head, leading to engorgement of the veins. The consequences are swelling of the tissues, both from an increase in intravascular volume and from rapid transudation of fluid into the tissues, followed by showers of petechial haemorrhages in unsupported areas, such as the skin of the upper eyelids, the forehead, the skin behind the ears, the circumoral skin, and the conjunctivae and sclera of the eye. The same venous engorgement often leads to frank bleeding from the nasal mucosa and the external auditory meatus.

In the internal tissues and organs, petechiae are most often seen on serous membranes in the thorax, where the presence of a body cavity leads to lack of support for the superficial venules and hence predisposes to rupture when venous pressure rises. They are almost never seen in the peritoneal serosa and it has been postulated that, in the chest, attempts at breathing against a closed airway may lead to a sudden extreme decrease in intrapleural pressure causing petechiae in the same way as suction on the skin can cause a shower of pin-point haemorrhages. As described by Tardieu, petechiae in the thorax are often seen on the visceral pleura, especially in the interlobar fissures and around the hilum.

Petechiae are also common on the surface of the heart, especially on the epicardium around the atrioventricular groove, particularly on the posterior surface, though these have been shown to appear or worsen as a post-mortem phenomenon. In infants and children, the thymus or thymic remnants may show numerous petechiae. It is claimed that in the sudden infant death syndrome these are confined to the cortex, whereas in other 'asphyxial' conditions they are scattered throughout the gland; this is doubtful.

Petechiae are rarely seen in the parietal pleura or the peritoneum except in haemorrhagic diatheses. In the brain, petechiae occur in the white matter and there may be larger patches of bleeding in the subarachnoid space where superficial vessels have ruptured because of acute venous engorgement. The same mechanism often produces profuse petechiae and ecchymoses under the scalp. In regard to the scalp, caution must be observed as numerous haemorrhages can be caused as a common autopsy artefact during the reflection of the scalp flaps.

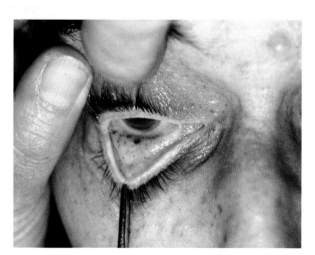

FIGURE 14.1 *Petechial haemorrhages in the eye in manual strangulation. There are also some petechiae on the facial skin.*

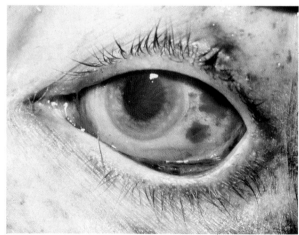

FIGURE 14.2 *Scleral haemorrhages in manual strangulation. These are larger than the usual petechiae, but the latter are present inside the lower lid.*

Petechiae may also disappear with lengthening post-mortem interval. Betz *et al.* (1994) have shown that in putrefaction and freshwater immersion, conjunctival petechiae may vanish.

THE SIGNIFICANCE OF PETECHIAE

A number of factors cause difficulty in the interpretation of petechial haemorrhages. First, there is no doubt that both cutaneous and visceral petechiae, especially the latter, can both appear and enlarge as a post-mortem phenomenon. Gordon and Mansfield (1955) have shown that the presence and number of petechiae is a function of the post-mortem interval, in common with other haemorrhagic artefacts such as those found behind the larynx by Prinsloo and Gordon (1951).

Posture also has an effect on the appearance of haemorrhages. They are commonly seen, along with larger ecchymoses, on the front or back of corpses who have died from a variety of causes in which mechanical asphyxia is absent. They are often present in normal post-mortem hypostasis, especially where the mode of death was congestive as in

many types of natural heart disease. Their appearance in the hypostatic areas is also time-related, the longer the post-mortem interval, the more likely – and more prominently – they are to occur.

Where some abnormal posture is present – such as the deceased being slumped out of bed or otherwise found with the head lower than the body – marked congestion, cyanosis and petechial haemorrhages are common.

Occasionally the abnormal posture may have occurred during life, such as in overdose victims, drunks and senile persons, who have fallen into a position with the upper part of the body lowermost. This may embarrass respiration and contribute to death and the ante-mortem component may be difficult or impossible to distinguish from post-mortem accentuation of the congestive-petechial appearances.

Another problem in the autopsy interpretation of petechiae is that not all punctate lesions in the pleura are petechiae. Zaini and Knight (1982) showed that many such apparent petechiae were either intravascular venous pools, subpleural microbullae or pigment foci.

In summary, petechial haemorrhages are highly unreliable indicators of an asphyxial process, taking this to mean a hypoxic state. They are the result of venous engorgement, usually from mechanical obstruction of venous return to the heart – or in the thorax, from attempts to inspire against a blocked airway. Petechiae and ecchymoses are common non-specific autopsy findings and many are post-mortem in origin, especially in dependent positions. They

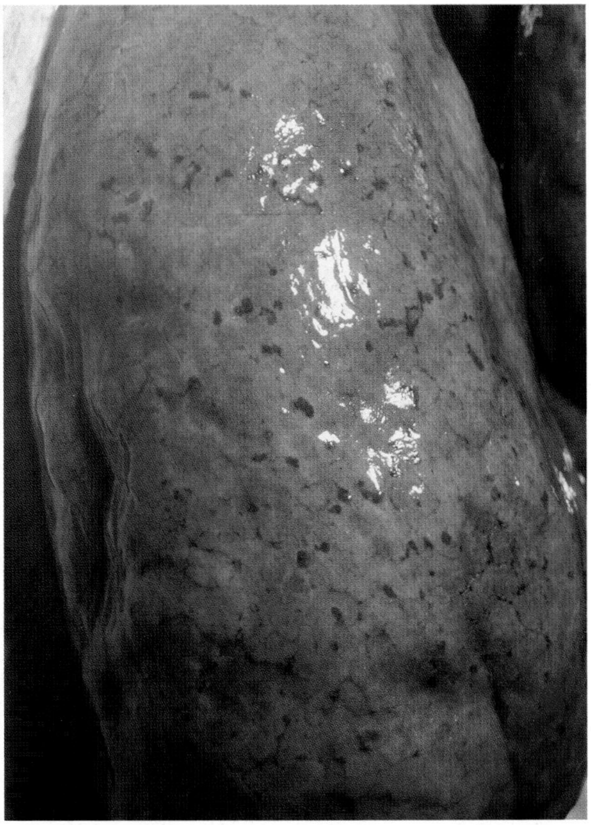

FIGURE 14.3 *Subpleural petechial haemorrhage – the true 'Tardieu spots' – in manual strangulation. These are no longer considered to be specific for 'asphyxia' and a few petechiae can frequently be found in many autopsies unassociated with asphyxia.*

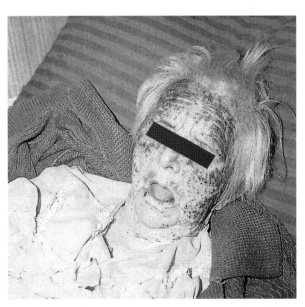

FIGURE 14.4 *Dense confluent skin haemorrhages in the face of an old lady who had slipped from her bed and was found with her head on the floor and her legs on the bed. The signs of this 'postural asphyxia' may well have been accentuated by post-mortem worsening of the hypostatic haemorrhages.*

may occur in many non-asphyxial states and, in the lungs, some petechiae can be found in the interlobar fissures and around the hilum in most routine autopsies.

Conversely, in some types of death where oxygen deprivation is to be expected (such as drowning, plastic-bag suffocation and entering an atmosphere devoid of oxygen), petechiae are seldom demonstrable.

The most significance must be placed on facial and ocular petechiae, because showers of pin-point haemorrhages in the eyelids, conjunctivae, sclera and facial skin require urgent explanation unless the body was face down or head down.

Congestion and oedema

The next 'classic' sign of asphyxia is congestion. This is even more non-specific than petechiae and once again is the result of obstructed venous return. When the neck is compressed, the face, lips and tongue become swollen and reddened. The true colour change of congestion is usually darkened by the onset of cyanosis. Internal organs also become congested and in strangulation this is most notable in the tongue, pharynx and larynx above the level of venous obstruction. In pressure on the chest, failure of respiratory movements cause an intense rise in venous pressure, accompanied by cyanosis.

Congestion is often associated with tissue swelling if the venous obstruction continues. The oedema is the result of rapid transudation through capillary and venule walls, again mainly a function of back pressure in the venous system. Hypoxia of the vascular endothelium is alleged to allow increased permeability, but generalized hypoxia from other causes does not produce the tissue swelling seen in strangulation.

Tissue fluid also escapes rapidly into the brain in strangulation that continues for even a few minutes, though here the well-known effect of hypoxia might be an added factor. Pulmonary oedema, causing excess fluid to enter the alveoli, is often found in hypoxic deaths. Here the mechanism is more obscure, but is probably a combination of hypoxia and raised pulmonary vessel pressure. In strangulation, froth may sometimes be so profuse as to emerge from the mouth and nostrils – yet in other throttlings, it may be absent. Pulmonary oedema is such a common and non-specific phenomenon in a whole range of fatal conditions that it has little diagnostic significance.

Cyanosis

The colour of blood depends upon the absolute quantity of oxyhaemoglobin and reduced haemoglobin present in the erythrocytes. The normal pink colour of well-oxygenated skin may change to purple or blue when oxygen is lacking – indeed, the word 'cyanosis' is derived from the Greek, meaning 'dark blue'. Cutaneous cyanosis, however, depends on the absolute amount of reduced haemoglobin, rather than the proportion of reduced haemoglobin to oxyhaemoglobin. It is not apparent in marked anaemia, even if the ratio of oxyhaemoglobin to reduced haemoglobin is low. There must be at least 5 g of reduced haemoglobin per 100 ml blood before cyanosis becomes evident, irrespective of the total amount of haemoglobin.

In the common forensic event of constriction of the neck, cyanosis almost invariably follows congestion of the face, as venous blood containing much reduced haemoglobin after perfusing the head and neck is dammed back and becomes more blue as the blood accumulates. If and when the airway becomes blocked, then impaired oxygenation in the lungs leads to a diminution in the oxygen content of arterial blood. This will lead to a darkening of all organs and tissues, and will accentuate the cyanosis of the face. This does not happen in the first phases of strangulation, however, and depends on complete or substantial occlusion of the airway, or restriction of the respiratory excursions of the chest.

Cyanosis produced during life may be partly or wholly overshadowed by hypostasis, which may be a deep purple or blue, and may be mistaken for true cyanosis – indeed, some pathologists refuse to use 'cyanosis' in respect of the dead, claiming that it cannot reflect the ante-mortem situation.

'Engorgement of the right heart and fluidity of the blood'

Descriptions of an abnormal fluidity of the blood seen at autopsy in asphyxial deaths are part of forensic mythology and can be dismissed with little discussion. Post-mortem clotting in the heart and venous system is a most erratic process, as is the eventual dissolution of those clots by the action of fibrinolytic enzymes (Mole 1948). It is irrelevant in the diagnosis of asphyxia.

Engorgement of the chambers of the right side of heart and the great veins is also a non-specific autopsy observation, useless as a marker of an asphyxial process. Any type of congestive death, including primary heart failure from many diseases, leads to terminal engorgement of the right ventricle and atrium as part of the generalized rise in venous and intracardiac pressure.

The autopsy diagnosis of 'asphyxia'

Thus there are no specific autopsy findings for 'asphyxia', taking this in its hypoxic sense. As stated earlier, the so-called 'classic signs' have been well described by Adelson (1974) as the 'obsolete diagnostic quintet'. He goes on to observe that 'the co-existence of these findings, in themselves, does not prove that death resulted from mechanical asphyxia. All these phenomena are non-specific and are in no way peculiar to this mode of death. Inasmuch as they are observed frequently in deaths arising from unquestioned natural disease, they are of no value in proving that death resulted from mechanical asphyxia'.

Other salutary cautions on the significance of 'asphyxial signs' may be found in the important publications of Gordon and Turner (1951), Camps and Hunt (1959), Shapiro (1953) and Swann and Brucer (1949).

It is impossible to make a post-mortem diagnosis of acute hypoxia by measuring the blood gases, as rapid changes after death – and indeed agonal changes – make analysis worthless. Only by a careful assessment of the history and circumstances of the death, exclusion of other causes and a cautious evaluation of the signs described above can any conclusion be reached. Most important of all is the finding of a cause for airway obstruction or other local trauma, such as prolonged pressure on the neck or chest, obstruction of the airways, postural causes or occlusion of the external respiratory orifices.

It cannot be emphasized too strongly that the mere finding of any of the non-specific features, such as congestion and petechiae, without firm circumstantial or preferably physical evidence of mechanical obstruction of respiration, is quite insufficient to warrant a speculative diagnosis of asphyxia. If such collateral evidence is not forthcoming, then the cause of death must be left undetermined.

Histological and biomechanical diagnosis of anoxia/'asphyxia'

Many attempts have been made to find markers of hypoxia, anoxia and 'asphyxia' by means of laboratory techniques, including histology, histochemistry and various biochemical methods. Although many claims have been made for their usefulness, the fact that such tests are virtually never put forward in criminal or civil litigation makes it self-evident that they are not reliable.

This is hardly surprising, given the vague and contentious nature of the 'asphyxial' condition, where the mechanisms are diverse and even the nomenclature is unstandardized. If the target for research is narrowed down to severe hypoxia at a tissue or cellular level, then perhaps more success might be expected, by being able to demonstrate cellular damage by one or more of the great battery of techniques now available. However, even this limited objective is not yet attained with the degree of reliability required for legal purposes. The

extensive strangling, drowning and gassing of legions of small animals may have produced many theses and papers, but has had no practical impact upon a long-standing problem in forensic pathology. Cell death, especially in neurones or myocytes, due to ischaemic/hypoxic damage is the most common focus for research, but the problem in a forensic context is that a considerable period of hypoxia – usually a minimum of many minutes or even hours – is needed before changes can be detected, even in experimental circumstances. In human autopsy material, the ever-present post-mortem and agonal changes interfere with the subtle early signs of hypoxic damage.

Histological changes in the lung and also chemical markers in blood or vitreous, such as hypoxanthine, have been claimed to indicate generalized hypoxia, but the application of such techniques in routine practice has not been fruitful.

SUFFOCATION

Although not a specific term, suffocation usually refers to a death caused by reduction of the oxygen concentration in the respired atmosphere, formerly called a 'vitiated atmosphere'. It is less often used to include smothering or choking. Reduction of atmospheric oxygen may occur in a wide variety of situations. Decompression, such as cabin failure of aircraft at high altitudes, causes a dramatic fall in the partial pressure of oxygen and hence reduced penetration of the gas through the alveolar wall. Other factors, however, such as the direct effects of a partial vacuum and often mechanical trauma from the near-explosive situation may overshadow the hypoxic aspects.

More common is the reduction of oxygen in the atmosphere by physical replacement by other gases, or chemical changes such as combustion. In fires, the loss of respirable air may be a potent factor in causing death, though other complications, such as the presence of toxic gases such as carbon monoxide, cyanide and many other poisonous substances liberated by the burning of plastics, may cause death more quickly than pure hypoxia. Carbon dioxide, which though not itself poisonous, is irrespirable and may accumulate in fires, and in wells and shafts in limestone. In former years, vagrants sleeping for warmth near limekilns were sometimes suffocated by this heavy gas creeping over them.

Carbon dioxide is also the cause of deaths in a more modern agricultural setting – the grain silo. Here, many tons of grain are stored in gas-tight towers; the seed produces carbon dioxide that settles to the bottom of the tower. When a blockage occurs in the gravity discharge, farm workers may enter the tower to clear the obstruction. Although safety precautions demand venting before the men enter, some workers still suffer a sudden death on encountering an atmosphere rich in carbon dioxide.

A similar hazard exists in ships' tanks or other industrial metal chambers, in which oxygen is replaced by nitrogen. This happens because the damp steel walls become rusty and use up much of the contained oxygen in forming ferric oxides. In all these deaths associated with replacement of oxygen with an inert gas, rapid death is common before hypoxia can have had any physiological effect. For example, the author (BK) has dealt with two deaths in which seafarers entered closed ships' tanks and virtually fell dead off the entry ladder. The presumed mechanism, which was far too quick to be hypoxic, was considered to be some overstimulation of the chemoreceptor system, leading to a parasympathetic 'vasovagal' cardiac arrest.

Even where death was not witnessed as sudden, the 'classic signs' of asphyxia are almost always absent. In domestic circumstances, death may be seen where a heating apparatus has removed oxygen from the atmosphere in the absence of ventilation. Though oxides of carbon are usually formed, a kerosene or natural gas appliance may kill from pure hypoxia, especially where left burning all night in a small room where the occupants lie sleeping. The effect may be accentuated by the victims having blocked up cracks in the doors and windows to keep out draughts. An open wood or coal fire does not present the same hazard, as it requires a flue or chimney in order to burn. In all such deaths, carbon monoxide poisoning must first be excluded by blood analysis, as it is a common accompaniment to lack of oxygen, especially as the reduction in oxygen availability tends to make the heat source produce progressively more monoxide than dioxide during combustion.

In a different variety of hypoxic death, persons – especially children – may asphyxiate by being confined in a small airtight space. Examples include boxes and discarded refrigerators; the danger of the latter is so well known that in Britain it is illegal to dump a refrigerator in a place with public access, unless the self-locking handle is rendered inoperative.

In all such 'hypoxic' deaths (though some are patently due to vasovagal cardio-inhibitory mechanisms) it is very rare to find any petechial haemorrhages, as these are mainly the result of venous obstruction, which is absent in these circumstances. In the true hypoxic deaths, there may be congestion and cyanosis, though even these are often absent and the autopsy findings are essentially negative.

SMOTHERING

This term refers to death from mechanical occlusion of the mouth and nose, though sometimes 'suffocation' is used to include this class of death. The smothering agent is usually fabric, an impervious sheet or a hand, though occasionally (especially in industrial accidents) a mobile solid, such as sand, mud, grain or flour may be responsible for blocking the air passages. In the 1966 Aberfan disaster in South Wales, more than 140 victims – almost all children – were smothered when semi-liquid coal slurry from a collapsing mine tip swept over their school.

In smothering, death may occur either by the occluding substance pressing down upon the facial orifices, or by the passive weight of the head pressing the nose and mouth into the occlusion. Deliberate homicide is seen usually in the old, the debilitated and in infants. It is extremely difficult to prove homicide from objective findings.

In relation to infants, the matter will be further discussed in the chapter on sudden infant death syndrome, but it is essential to appreciate that the smothering of babies, whether intentional or accidental, is both rare and difficult to prove. The so-called 'classic signs' of asphyxia, for what they are worth, are rarely present in proven suffocation – and as intrathoracic petechiae are common in undoubted 'cot deaths', these signs cannot therefore be accepted in isolation as evidence of suffocation.

Pressure marks on the face can rarely be distinguished from post-mortem postural changes, where circumoral and circumnasal pallor is caused merely by passive pressure of the dependent head after death, preventing the gravitational hypostasis from entering these areas.

Even where the head is found supine, variation in colour is still common on the face, with contrasting white and pink patches, which usually change as the post-mortem interval lengthens. Unless there are bruises or abrasion on the cheeks, around the mouth, lips or lesions within the lips or mouth, it is dangerous to overinterpret mere colour variations from

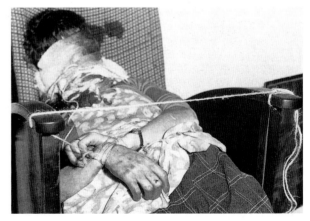

FIGURE 14.5 *Smothering from a towel being tied over the face. Death was contributed to by head injuries, also inflicted by the aged husband, who died within a few hours of natural causes from hypertensive heart disease.*

alterations in the amount of blood in the facial capillary bed, which is almost always a post-mortem phenomenon.

Even a confession from the mother is not always reliable – cases are on record where a mother has falsely confessed to smothering her child to rationalize the inexplicable events of a true sudden infant death syndrome fatality.

A similar situation exists with the elderly, who may be victims of a 'mercy killing', often a euphemism for the exhaustion of patience of long-suffering caring relatives. A pillow placed over the face of a sleeping octogenarian leaves no signs, **unless a struggle develops**, when protracted attempts at respiration against obstruction may lead to congestion, cyanosis and sometimes facial and conjunctival petechiae.

'Overlaying' of infants

This alleged condition has an ancient pedigree, being mentioned in the Old Testament. In Chapter III of the First Book of Kings, Solomon has to adjudicate between two women who both claim the same child, as the other infant was 'overlain'. This event, some 3000 years ago, has been mentioned at intervals through history, as in Wales in AD 1188, when Giraldus Cambrensis records that the Lord punished a woman for preventing her husband joining the Third Crusade, by causing her infant son 'to be overlain in the night'.

When an infant was found dead in the morning in the maternal bed (as separate cots or cribs are a relatively modern invention), it was assumed that the mother had turned over onto the baby in her sleep and suffocated it. When infants began to be placed in cots, the deaths continued unabated and it seems obvious that most of these were victims of the sudden infant death syndrome (SIDS). Whether or not overlaying really exists is doubtful and seems incapable of proof, given that any infant found dead in bed with no physical signs at autopsy could, by definition, be a SIDS.

The recent marked decline in numbers of SIDS in Britain has coincided with a campaign to discourage mothers from putting their infants to sleep face down – but, as yet, no definite cause-and-effect relationship has been proved, so any consequent strengthening of the 'overlaying' hypothesis cannot be substantiated.

Plastic bag suffocation

Although an increasingly common form of suicide in Britain, plastic bag suffocation may also be homicidal or accidental. In all these types, the essential mechanism is that a hood of impervious substance, usually polythene or other plastic, is placed over the head down to neck level.

The plastic is usually in the form of an open-ended bag, either transparent or a 'supermarket' shopping bag.

Although many suicides tie the open end of the bag around their neck with cord or a tie, this is not necessary for a fatal result. Indeed, even flat sheets of polythene have killed infants when placed on the face. The mechanism is not understood, as it was formerly but erroneously thought to be the result of the clinging effect of static electricity.

Plastic bag suffocation can be rapid and leave no signs whatsoever. In the author's (BK) series of accidental, suicidal and three homicidal deaths from plastic bags, not one had any petechial haemorrhages or, indeed, any signs of 'asphyxia' at all, the faces being pale and uncongested. In another case, a person was convicted of murder by plastic bag, yet was only arrested after a spontaneous confession 6 weeks after an autopsy that had revealed no signs whatsoever of an asphyxial cause of death. As with hypoxic atmospheres, it seems that the mechanism of death in plastic-bag facial occlusion is some rapid cardio-inhibitory mode, rather than a purely hypoxic process. This conclusion is strengthened by the causes mentioned above, where flat sheets of plastic, not bags, have killed infants by clinging to the face, which of necessity must have been rapid deaths.

At autopsy, unless the bag is still present, these cases can present great difficulty. In fact, as in the homicide mentioned above, unless a confession or other corroborative evidence is forthcoming, the pathologist may never even know that he has dealt with an occult suffocation. Where the bag

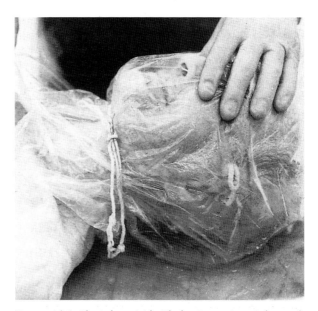

FIGURE 14.6 *Plastic bag suicide. The bag is sometimes tied around the neck, as in this case, but this is not necessary for a fatal outcome. The deaths are not asphyxial in the hypoxic sense; facial congestion and petechiae are almost always absent.*

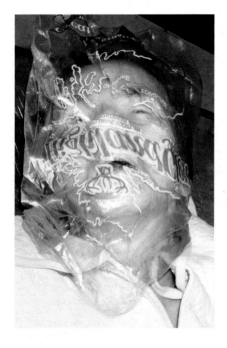
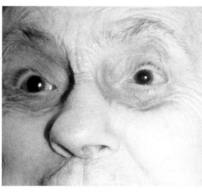

FIGURE 14.7 *Plastic bag suicide, with an open bag placed loosely over the head. As usual there are no congestive petechial signs in the face.*

is still in place, a search must be made for other indications of suicide, such as drug analysis and futile injuries, such as slashed wrists. Masochistic activities, described later in this chapter, are sometimes, though not often, associated with plastic bag suffocation.

It is sometimes said that moisture seen inside the bag indicates that it was put on during life, the water being from respiration. It is rare for this to be an important issue, as placing a bag on a corpse's head would seem excessively unusual; in any event, the test is invalid, as evaporation from the skin, nose and mouth can produce beads of moisture inside, whether the victim is dead or alive.

Autopsy signs of suffocation

Where smothering is suspected, local signs must be sought to try to substantiate pressure on the face. Such signs include bruising around the mouth, chin and nose, though these are rarely seen except in the more violent incidents. Pressure of the lips on the teeth or dentures may cause the buccal surfaces to be bruised or abraded, though lacerations are rare unless a blow has been administered. It must be remembered that as small infants and many old people have no teeth, these injuries are less likely. The dangers of accepting areas of facial pallor as 'pressure marks' when the face shows post-mortem hypostasis has already been mentioned. In the early stages of post-mortem discoloration of the skin, variable colouring may not be truly 'hypostatic' as mottling and patchy variation is common due to uneven vasodilatation after death. It takes some time for gravity to pull cutaneous blood down to lower levels.

Smothering may occur accidentally where a person who is incapacitated from one of a variety of causes lies face down on a surface that is impervious to air. Drunkenness, epilepsy, drug overdose, coma or stupor from natural disease, may lead to this. Though it has long been proved in connection with 'cot death' that woven fabrics of most types can still admit enough air to support quiet respiration when placed over the mouth and nose, fabric that becomes saturated with saliva, nasal mucus or vomit may form an impervious seal that ceases to allow the passage of air. The weight of the inert head also distorts the nose and presses the nostrils and mouth so hard against a mattress or pillow that this adds to the airway stenosis.

In these instances, congestion and cyanosis are common, but when the body is examined after death, some of these findings may be postural and hypostatic in nature. As always, however, it must be recognized that skin haemorrhages often appear post-mortem in dependent hypostasis.

Gagging

Smothering may also occur where a pad or gag is fixed over the face, as sometimes happens in robbery with violence. A householder, caretaker or night-watchman may be tied up and silenced by having a scarf, tie or other fabric tied around his face. At first this admits air, but when it becomes progressively soaked with saliva or mucus it may become impervious and lead to an asphyxial death, again usually without any petechiae in the face or eyes.

A similar situation arises when a gag is thrust into the mouth to silence a watchman or security officer. Another variant is adhesive tape applied over the mouth. Though the nasal airway may originally be quite patent, any later obstruction from oedema and mucus, or movement of the gag backwards into the nasopharynx, may cause an unforeseen death and turn a robbery charge into a homicide.

CHOKING

This term refers to blockage of the internal airways, usually between the pharynx and the bifurcation of the trachea. Death can be the result of pure hypoxia from occlusion of the airway, when all the attendant signs of congestion, cyanosis and perhaps petechiae may be present, usually where the victim struggles to breathe for an appreciable period. As described below, however, a large proportion of deaths occur suddenly before any possible hypoxic manifestations have time to take effect; these fatalities must be caused by neurogenic cardiac arrest, either purely neurogenic or accelerated by excess catecholamine release from the adrenaline response.

Causes of choking include the following.

Foreign bodies

Objects such as gags, dummies, small toys, table-tennis balls and a multiplicity of objects may be placed in the mouth and inhaled, usually by children and the mentally retarded. Occasionally adults will do the same, accidentally or by design; an example of the latter was a suicide seen by the author (BK), who died (without any asphyxial signs whatsoever) by pushing a closed pill-bottle into his pharynx.

Dentures and haemorrhage

False teeth (especially partial plates), extracted large teeth, blood clots, and frank haemorrhage following dental or ear, nose and throat operations such as tonsillectomy.

Acute obstructive lesions

Lesions of the glottis or larynx, such as the oedema of acute hypersensitivity (including insect stings), irritant vapours, inhalation of hot gas and acute infective conditions. The most dangerous of the latter is diphtheria or *Haemophilus influenzae* epiglottitis in children, which is a medical emergency sometimes requiring an immediate tracheostomy to relieve the airway obstruction. At autopsy, great thickening of the epiglottis and aryepiglottic folds by jelly-like oedema and inflammatory tissue will be found occluding the entrance to the larynx.

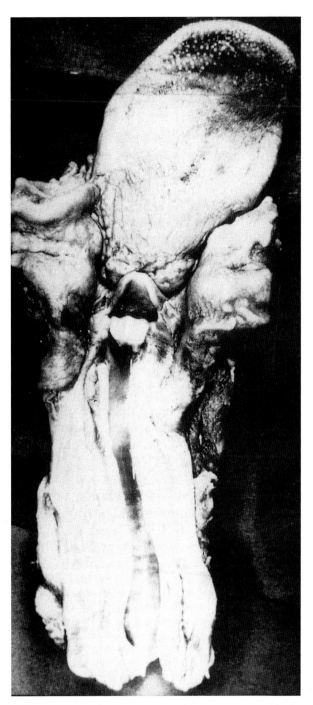

FIGURE 14.8 *Impaction of an extracted molar tooth in the larynx. Though now uncommon with modern dental and anaesthetic practices, it can still happen in less satisfactory circumstances. Blood clot from dental extraction, tonsillectomy, and other ear, nose and throat surgery can also block the airway.*

Food material

This is an important topic, as the cause of death 'aspiration of vomit' is used too often without real justification. Food

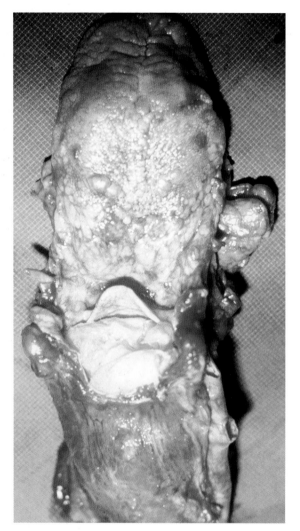

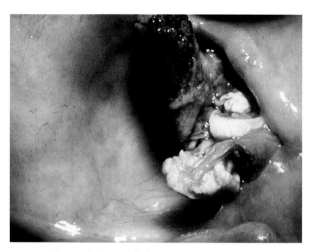

FIGURE 14.10 *Blockage of the larynx by meat. The victim was an old person with senile dementia who gulped food and who eventually died suddenly without asphyxial signs from reflex cardiac arrest.*

FIGURE 14.9 *Blockage of the larynx by a complete small orange in a mentally disturbed patient. The fruit had just been swallowed and was not regurgitated from the stomach. The face was pale and death was rapid, unaccompanied by symptoms of choking.*

may be drawn into the larynx either as it is being taken down from the mouth in the act of swallowing, or it may be regurgitated from the stomach.

▨ The first instance is rarely misinterpreted, as whole undigested food may be found in the air passages and there is usually a history of death taking place while eating. Though most commonly encountered in old persons and the mentally disturbed, it can occur in any age group. A notable example was the so-called 'café coronary' syndrome, which received considerable publicity in the USA some years ago. The most frequent victims were well-nourished businessmen, who died suddenly and unexpectedly during a meal with no signs

of respiratory distress or any of the 'classic signs of asphyxia'. Initially thought to be coronary heart disease, autopsy revealed a bolus of food, often steak, lodged in the pharynx or larynx. In any choking on food, the bolus can be quite large, such as a whole pancake, a whole tangerine or masses of meat, fruit or vegetable. Senile persons in retirement homes and mentally retarded children in institutions are also vulnerable. In such fatalities, the history and mode of death gives no hint of a hypoxic mechanism. Many cases have been observed where the victim merely sits back in their chair, dead – the mode clearly being cardiac arrest, presumably from overactivity of the parasympathetic nervous system from stimulation of the laryngeal or pharyngeal mucosa – the so-called 'vasovagal reflex' or 'reflex cardiac inhibition'.

▨ The finding of gastric contents in the air passages is by no means as significant as the presence of freshly swallowed food. First, difficulties can arise in distinguishing gastric contents from fresh food material if digestion of the former has not proceeded far – which is not always a function of the time since the last meal, as any physical or psychological disturbance can retard or completely halt digestion. The history, if available, is a better guide, unless the material is obviously partly or wholly digested. In cases of doubt, the smell and acid reaction to pH indicators may be useful.

Gastric contents are commonly found in the larynx, trachea and bronchi at autopsy when no other evidence of aspiration exists, and when there is a clear and unconnected cause of death. Knight (1976) found that no less than a quarter of a series of 100 consecutive autopsies on both adults and children contained some gastric contents in the air passages, and Pullar (1984) observed that this was a low figure compared with his series. These findings were obviously caused in the great majority of cases by agonal or post-mortem spillage.

Gardner (1958) described experiments in which barium was placed in the stomachs of recently dead patients while still in bed in the hospital wards. When X-rays were taken after they were first moved to the mortuary and thence into the autopsy room, most had barium in their tracheobronchial tree, confirming that overspill was common as a post-mortem phenomenon. Even histological evidence of leucocyte clustering around foci of gastric contents deep in the bronchi was shown by Gardner to be an early post-mortem event, not a 'vital reaction'. Leucocyte migration in the skin up to 16 hours post-mortem was demonstrated by Ali (1986).

Almost the only definite evidence of aspiration of gastric contents is either reliable witnessed observation during life or the histological finding of an advanced 'vital reaction' with infection, necrosis and a definite inflammatory reaction. This is a relatively late change and cannot be seen where death occurred within a few hours of aspiration. Finding a few foci of leucocytes around a bronchiole is of no evidential use. There is therefore no reliable method of distinguishing agonal or even early post-mortem overspill from true vital aspiration, unless clinical or other witnessed evidence is available. In most instances, it is not justifiable for a pathologist to claim that death was caused by inhalation of stomach contents without such confirmatory evidence. Unfortunately, where other lesions are absent or unconvincing at autopsy, especially in the sudden infant death syndrome, many pathologists use the presence of gastric contents in the air-passages as the primary and often the only cause of death. This unwarranted assumption may have distressing consequences, both in the field of medical negligence, deaths in custody and especially in the sudden infant death syndrome, where mothers may be misled into thinking that some negligence on their part in failing to observe vomiting, may have caused the death.

The only circumstance where a firmer opinion may be held is in acute alcoholism, though even here certainty is usually elusive. Where an undoubtedly drunken person (usually with a blood alcohol of at least 150 mg/100 ml) is found dead with massive blockage of his air passages by copious gastric contents and where other causes of death can be excluded by autopsy, then it might be reasonable to assume that regurgitation may have killed him, especially if there is other evidence of external vomit on the clothing or immediate surroundings. However, it is not an autopsy diagnosis to be made lightly.

TRAUMATIC 'ASPHYXIA'

This condition is unfortunately misnamed, as the word 'traumatic' could equally be applied to hanging or strangulation. It is well recognized now, however, as meaning mechanical fixation of the chest, and is important both because of its frequency in accidents and because it provides the most extreme demonstration of the 'classic signs' of asphyxia.

Whereas other types of mechanical asphyxia may cause obstruction of air entry into the lungs, 'traumatic asphyxia' acts by restricting respiratory movements and thus prevents inspiration. It was termed 'traumatic' because gross mechanical forces are usually the reason for the fixation of the thoracic cage. Traumatic asphyxia occurs in two main conditions:

- The chest and usually the abdomen are compressed by an unyielding substance or object, so that chest expansion and diaphragmatic lowering are prevented. Burial in earth following the collapse of an excavation is a common cause and may kill workmen even if their heads remain above the fallen soil. Similarly, burial in grain, sand, coal or minerals, may have the same effect, and is usually encountered in industrial, marine or agricultural accidents. An avalanche in a silo, hopper, or other large-scale storage container may bury the worker up to neck level and, unless rescue is rapid, asphyxia will prove fatal. Similar restriction of chest movement may be caused by the victim being pinned under an overturned vehicle, or by falling timber or masonry. Many fatalities have occurred on farms, especially in hill country, by the toppling of a tractor, pinning the driver underneath. Protection in the form of a 'roll-bar' over the driving position or the provision of a rigid cab on a tractor was specifically designed to avoid such accidents.
- Crushing in crowds also leads to traumatic asphyxia, and this has caused some mass disasters, the largest probably being in Mecca. Most of the football-ground tragedies such as Bolton, Ibrox Park (1971), Lima (1964), Hillsborough (1989) and the Heisl Stadium in Belgium (1986) have been the result of crushing in crowds out of control. A similar mechanism led to 173 deaths in wartime London, when a panic on the stairs of Bethnal Green underground station, used as an air-raid shelter, caused the crowd to fall on those beneath.

Other forms of chest crushing arise from trapping between a vehicle and a wall, or between the buffers of two railway trucks.

Individual cases of traumatic asphyxia can occur when one person allows the whole weight of his body to fall upon another for a protracted period. This may happen in sexual intercourse, especially when one or both parties are incapacitated by drink or drugs.

Features of traumatic asphyxia

The appearances just mentioned are the hallmark of traumatic asphyxia and in no other condition, apart from postural dependency, is the degree of congestion and cyanosis so marked. When the chest is fixed, the face, neck and shoulders down to the thoracic inlet are grossly discoloured. Sometimes this colour is more red than purple. It can extend lower than the clavicles, Polson *et al.* (1985) being of the opinion that it often reaches down to the level of the third rib.

The conjunctivae are grossly congested and haemorrhagic. Rather than the petechiae seen in pressure on the neck, the conjunctivae and sclera may be so engorged with blood that the haemorrhagic tissue actually bulges out through the lids, completely obliterating the whites of the eyes. The face, lips and scalp may be swollen and congested, being dotted with petechiae and ecchymoses. There may be copious bleeding from the ears and nostrils. The whole picture is commonly an exaggeration of the appearances seen in slow death from manual strangulation, but local injury is absent and the signs extend down to or beyond the root of the neck. Where the compression has been caused by pinning under a solid object – as opposed to soil, sand or squeezing in a crowd – there may be local bruises and abrasions from the weight of a vehicle or heavy beam, but these are unrelated to the margin of the congestive–haemorrhagic zone.

Internally, the congestion is less marked than on the surface, but the lungs are usually dark and heavy and may well have subpleural petechial haermorrhages, the true 'Tardieu spots'. The right heart and all the veins above the atria are markedly distended. There may be injuries to the chest wall from the trauma of the fixating object.

It is not clear why there should be such gross venous congestion, but it is usually explained rather unconvincingly by the failure of the pulmonary circulation consequent upon the cessation of the normal expansion and collapse of the pulmonary vasculature. Shapiro suggested that the pressure on the chest forces blood back into the great veins and, as the venous valves in the subclavian vessels prevent displacement into the arms, the extra volume is forced up the valveless jugular system to congest the head and neck.

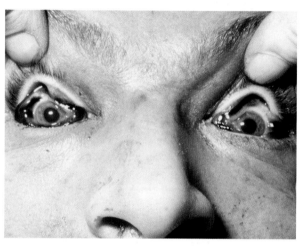

FIGURE 14.12 *Gross conjunctival haemorrhages in traumatic asphyxia. The victim was a workman who was buried up to his chest in an avalanche of ash.*

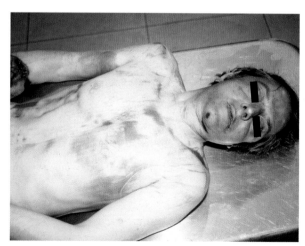

FIGURE 14.11 *Traumatic asphyxia showing gross congestion of confluent petechial haemorrhages of the face and parts of the shoulders. The victim had been buried up to the axillae in an avalanche of iron ore in a factory bunker.*

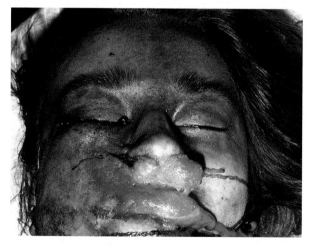

FIGURE 14.13 *Traumatic asphyxia showing gross congestion of the face and red blood-tinged froth exuding from the nostrils and mouth. The victim had lost the control of the tractor he was driving, fell out of the cab and was compressed under the overturned vehicle.*

POSTURAL ASPHYXIA

Closely allied to traumatic asphyxia is the so-called 'postural asphyxia', whose description as a separate entity is quite recent. When a person remains in a certain position for an extended time, either due to being trapped, or being in a drunken or drugged state, there may be a mechanical impediment to adequate respiratory movements. In addition, the normal venous return to the heart may be impaired.

Such positions usually entail inversion, either of the whole body or of the upper half; the syndrome and the pathophysiology are described well by Madea (1993), though most forensic pathologists will have had experience of such situations from time to time.

Persons who have been trapped upside down or even only in a 'jack-knife' position, with the upper half of their body bent acutely downwards from the waist, may have such impairment of their respiratory movements that they become hypoxic and suffer marked disturbance of their circulatory system, especially the venous return to the heart.

The author (BK) has seen two cases in which a victim has become stuck whilst trying to climb through the upper part of a window, one as a thief, the other in trying to get into a house without his key. Others have been seen where, in a state of drunkenness or other disability, they have slipped out of bed, so that their head and shoulders are on the floor, with the legs and pelvis still at a higher level on the bed. These may also suffer the same disturbance of respiratory movements, which when prolonged may lead to death.

Inversion may occur during torture: crucifixion has an element of postural asphyxia. In the case of inverted crucifixion, as in the death of St Peter, it would be the major factor, as inspiration would be impeded by the weight of abdominal viscera upon the diaphragm.

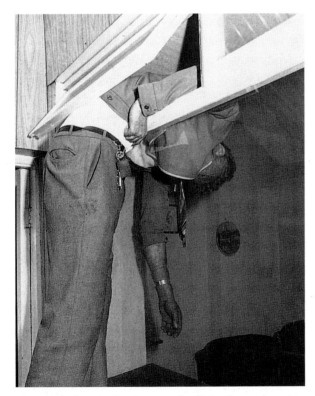

FIGURE 14.14 *Postural asphyxia in an inebriated man attempting to climb through a fanlight window. His feet slipped from the sill and he was unable to make sufficient respiratory movements against the weight of his body. Note the marked difference in congestion and cyanotic lividity between his two hands, the face and lower hand being discoloured at least partly from post-mortem hypostasis.*

REFERENCES AND FURTHER READING

Adelman HC. 1988. Asphyxial deaths as a result of aspiration of dental appliances: a report of three cases. *J Forensic Sci* **33**:389–95.

Adelson L. 1974. *The pathology of homicide: a vade mecum for pathologist, prosecutor and defense counsel.* W. B. Saunders, Philadelphia.

Ali TT. 1986. *Post-mortem autolytic changes in skin and the role of white blood cells.* Medical Faculty, University of Leeds, Leeds.

Bell MD, Rao VJ, Wetli CV, *et al.* 1992. Positional asphyxiation in adults. A series of 30 cases from the Dade and Broward County Florida medical examiner offices from 1982 to 1990. *Am J Forensic Med Pathol* **13**:101–7.

Betz P, Penning R, Keil W. 1994. The detection of petechial haemorrhages of the conjunctivae in dependency on the postmortem interval. *Forensic Sci Int* **64**:61–7.

Brinkmann B, Püschel K. 1981. [Histomorphological alterations of lung after strangulation. A comparative experimental study (author's transl).] *Z Rechtsmed* **86**:175–94.

Brinkmann B, Püschel K, Bause HW, *et al.* 1981. [Death by obstructive asphyxia: the pathophysiology of respiration and hemodynamics (author's transl).] *Z Rechtsmed* **87**:103–16.

Brinkmann B, Fechner G, Püschel K. 1984. Identification of mechanical asphyxiation in cases of attempted masking of the homicide. *Forensic Sci Int* **26**:235–45.

Bullock MJ, Diniz D. 2000. Suffocation using plastic bags: a retrospective study of suicides in ontario, canada. *J Forensic Sci* **45**:608–13.

Bywaters EG, Beal D. 1941. Traumatic asphyxia. *Br Med J* **1**:427–8.

Camps FE, Hunt AC. 1959. Pressure on the neck. *J Forensic Med* **6**:116–36.

Collins KA. 2001. Death by overlaying and wedging: a 15-year retrospective study. *Am J Forensic Med Pathol* **22**:155–9.

Ely SF, Hirsch CS. 2000. Asphyxial deaths and petechiae: a review. *J Forensic Sci* **45**:1274–7.

Flobecker P, Ottosson J, Johansson L, *et al.* 1993. Accidental deaths from asphyxia. A 10-year retrospective study from Sweden. *Am J Forensic Med Pathol* **14**:74–9.

Fred HL, Chandler FW. 1960. Traumatic asphyxia. *Am J Med* **29**:508–11.

Gardiner EE, Newberry RC, Keng JY. 1990. Avian vitreous humor concentrations of inosine, hypoxanthine, xanthine, uric acid, uracil and uridine as influenced by age and sex: their relevance as indicators of ante-mortem hypoxia. *Forensic Sci Int* **47**:123–7.

Gardner AN. 1958. Aspiration of food and vomit. *Q J Med* **27**:227–42.

Gordon I. 1976. Medicolegal aspects of rapid deaths initiated by hypoxia and anoxia. In: Wecht C (ed.), *Legal medicine annual 1975*. Appleton Century Crofts, New York.

Gordon I, Mansfield RA. 1955. Subpleural, subpericardial and subendocardial haemorrhages: a study of their incidence at autopsy and of the spontaneous development after death of subepicardial petechiae. *J Forensic Med* **2**:31–50.

Gordon I, Turner R. 1951. Deaths from rapid anoxia. *Am Med Assoc Arch Pathol* **2**:316.

Haddix TL, Harruff RC, Reay DT, *et al.* 1996. Asphyxial suicides using plastic bags. *Am J Forensic Med Pathol* **17**:308–11.

Haugen RK. 1963. The café coronary. *JAMA* **186**:142–4.

Hood I, Ryan D, Spitz WU. 1988. Resuscitation and petechiae. *Am J Forensic Med Pathol* **9**:35–7.

Hunt AC, Camps FE. 1962. Plastic bag deaths. *Br Med J* **1**:378–9.

Keil W, Kondo T, Beer GM. 1998. Haemorrhages in the posterior cricoarytenoid muscles – an unspecific autopsy finding. *Forensic Sci Int* **95**:225–30.

Knight B. 1976. The significance of gastric contents in the air passages. *Forensic Sci Int* **14**:398–402.

Luke J. 1971. The pathology, diagnosis and certain medical-legal aspects of death by homicidal smothering in adults. In: Wecht C (ed.), *Legal medicine annual 1971*. Appleton Century Crofts, New York.

Madea B. 1993. Death in a head-down position. *Forensic Sci Int* **61**:119–32.

McIntyre J. 1969. The classification of asphyxia. *Br J Hosp Med* **2**:1113–15.

Mole RH. 1948. Fibrinolysin and the fluidity of the blood postmortem. *J Pathol Bacteriol* **60**:413–17.

Morita M, Tabata N. 1988. Studies on asphyxia: on the changes of the alveolar walls of rats in the hypoxic state. II. The hypoxic state produced by carbon dioxide and methane gases. *Forensic Sci Int* **39**:257–62.

Ogden RD, Wooten RH. 2002. Asphyxial suicide with helium and a plastic bag. *Am J Forensic Med Pathol* **23**:234–7.

O'Halloran RL, Lewman LV. 1993. Restraint asphyxiation in excited delirium [see comments]. *Am J Forensic Med Pathol* **14**:289–95.

Plum F, Posner JB, Hain RF. 1962. Delayed neurological deterioration after anoxia. *Arch Intern Med* **110**:18–25.

Pollanen MS. 2001. Subtle fatal manual neck compression. *Med Sci Law* **41**:135–40.

Polson CJ, Gee DJ. 1972. Plastic bag suffocation. *Z Rechtsmed* **70**:184–90.

Polson JK, Gee D, Knight B. 1985. *Essentials of forensic medicine*, 4th edn. Pergamon Press, London.

Ponka JL, Lam CR. 1948. Effect of asphyxia on blood coagulation in dogs. *Proc Soc Exp Biol Med* **68**:334–6.

Prinsloo I, Gordon I. 1951. Postmortem dissection artefacts of the neck and their differentiation from ante-mortem bruises. *S Afr Med J* **25**:358–61.

Pullar P. 1984. Mechanical asphyxia. In: Mant AK (ed.), *Taylor's medical jurisprudence*, 13th edn. Churchill, London.

Purdue B. 1992. An unusual accidental death from reverse suspension [see comments]. *Am J Forensic Med Pathol* **13**:108–11.

Rao VJ, Wetli CV. 1988. The forensic significance of conjunctival petechiae. *Am J Forensic Med Pathol* **9**:32–4.

Reay DT, Howard JD, Fligner CL, *et al.* 1988. Effects of positional restraint on oxygen saturation and heart rate following exercise. *Am J Forensic Med Pathol* **9**:16–18.

Reay DT, Fligner CL, Stilwell AD, *et al.* 1992. Positional asphyxia during law enforcement transport [see comments]. *Am J Forensic Med Pathol* **13**:90–7.

Schleyer F. 1963. On adventitial haemorrhages of the thoracic blood vessels. *J Forensic Med* **10**:3–5.

Schmunk GA, Kaplan JA. 2002. Asphyxial deaths caused by automobile exhaust inhalation not attributable to carbon monoxide toxicity: Study of 2 cases. *Am J Forensic Med Pathol* **23**:123–6.

Shapiro H. 1975. Asphyxia. In: Gordon I, Shapiro H (eds), *Forensic medicine: a guide to principles*. Churchill Livingstone, London.

Shapiro H. 1988. Asphyxia. In: Gordon I, Shapiro H, Berson S (eds), *Forensic medicine: a guide to principles*, 3rd edn. Churchill, Edinburgh.

Shapiro HA. 1953. Is asphyxia a pathological entity recognizable at post-mortem? *J Forensic Med* **1**:65–8.

Shapiro HA. 1955. Tardieu spots in asphyxia. *J Forensic Med* **2**:1–4.

Simpson CK. 1943. Traumatic asphyxia. *Lancet* **2**:309–10.

Sturner WQ, Sullivan A, Suzuki K. 1983. Lactic acid concentrations in vitreous humor: their use in asphyxial deaths in children. *J Forensic Sci* **28**:222–30.

Swann HE. 1960. Occurrence of pulmonary oedema in sudden asphyxial deaths. *Am Med Assoc Arch Pathol* **69**:89–93.

Swann HE. 1964. The development of pulmonary oedema during the agonal period in sudden asphyxial deaths. *J Forensic Sci* **9**:360–4.

Swann HE, Brucer M. 1949. Cardiorespiratory and biochemical events during rapid anoxic death: fulminating anoxia. *Tex Rep Biol Med* **7**:511–16.

Swann HE, Brucer M. 1949. Cardiorespiratory and biochemical events during rapid anoxic death: obstructive anoxia. *Tex Rep Biol Med* **7**:593–9.

Tamaki K, Sato K, Katsumata Y. 1987. Enzyme-linked immunosorbent assay for determination of plasma thyroglobulin and its application to post-mortem diagnosis of mechanical asphyxia. *Forensic Sci Int* **33**:259–65.

Tardieu A. 1855. Memoire sur la mort par suffocation. *Ann Hyg Pub Med Leg (Series 11)* **6**:371–82.

Zaini MR, Knight B. 1982. Sub-pleural petechiae and pseudo petechiae. *J Forensic Sci Soc* **22**:141–5.

CHAPTER 15

Fatal pressure on the neck

This provides one of the most complex and controversial areas of 'asphyxial' deaths, as the mechanism is uncertain and the frequency of such deaths makes them a common problem for both forensic pathologist and jurist.

Pressure on the neck may arise from manual strangulation, ligature strangulation, hanging, direct blows, arm-locks and a variety of accidental lesions, such as entanglement with cords or falling onto the neck.

Strangulation was formerly thought to be a pure asphyxia as a result of 'cutting off the air' by occlusion of the airway during the constriction of the neck. Since the end of the nineteenth century, however, it has been recognized that the rapidity of death in many cases made it impossible for hypoxia to be the sole or even major cause. Many victims died almost immediately and exhibited none of the so-called 'classic' signs of asphyxia.

Others, though showing these signs, still died too quickly for it to be reasonably argued that lack of oxygen had proceeded to a fatal stage. It was common knowledge that most people could hold their breath for over a minute and that some pearl divers could be physically active and yet not breathe for at least 3 minutes, so the much more rapid onset of death seen in many cases required further explanation.

MECHANISM OF DEATH IN PRESSURE ON THE NECK

A number of anatomical and physiological factors must be considered in analysing the effects of pressure on the neck.

Airway occlusion

This may occur either from direct compression of the larynx or trachea, or from a lifting of the larynx so that the pharynx is closed by the root of the tongue being pressed against the soft palate and roof of the mouth. The latter explanation is far more likely, as the strong cartilages of the larynx will resist all but the most extreme compression. Various experiments have been attempted to quantify the force needed to close the airway and blood vessels, but it is difficult to translate the often conflicting results to the degree of violence actually used in fatal events. For example, Brouardel (1897) calculated that the force needed to close the trachea was of the order 15 kg, far more than that required to occlude the blood vessels.

Occlusion of the neck veins

This factor is almost solely responsible for the appearance of the 'classic' signs of congestion, cyanosis, oedema and petechiae above the line of constriction. The external jugular system is most vulnerable, but any significant pressure encircling the neck will also obliterate the lumen of the internal jugular system, causing a rapid rise in venous pressure in the head, especially if the carotid arteries are still patent, which is usually the case. Brouardel's experiments suggest that a ligature with a tension of 2 kg blocks the jugular return; Reuter (1933) found an even lower figure.

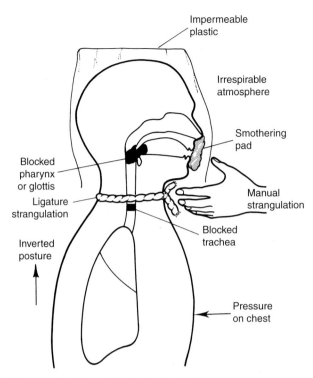

FIGURE 15.1 *Causes of mechanical asphyxia.*

Compression of the carotid arteries

This is much less common than venous occlusion, as the higher internal pressure of the carotid arteries resists occlusion and they are situated much more deeply. The carotids are largely obscured by the sternomastoid muscles. If bilateral occlusion of the carotids is achieved, almost immediate unconsciousness will ensue, as the supply of arterial blood to the brain by the vertebral circulation is insufficient to maintain cortical function, which depends mainly upon the anterior and middle cerebral arteries that arise from the carotid supply. Occlusion of the vertebral arteries by neck compression seems virtually impossible despite some claims to the contrary.

If the carotid circulation is totally occluded for an unremitting period of 4 or more minutes, then irreversible cerebral damage may occur. The time for this to happen is variable and the minimum has been disputed for many years, but the consensus of opinion is that permanent brain damage is very unlikely if the supply has been cut off continuously for less than 4–5 minutes. Total recovery has often been recorded after total ischaemia of considerably longer than this, even in normothermic conditions, with 9–14 minutes being quoted. Where the body has been subjected to low temperature, far longer times have been recorded, including an anecdotal case of a boy falling into the cold water of a Scandinavian harbour and being totally submerged for 40 minutes, with total recovery of cardiac and cerebral function.

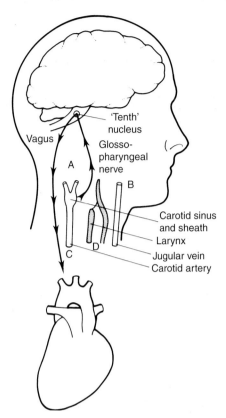

FIGURE 15.2 *Possible effects of pressure on the neck: (A) carotid sinus reflex leading to cardiac arrest; (B) jugular venous compression leading to cyanosis and petechiae; (C) carotid artery compression leading to unconsciousness; and (D) airway obstruction leading to hypoxia.*

Nerve effects

Pressure on the baroreceptors situated in the carotid sinuses, the carotid sheaths and the carotid body, can result in bradycardia (slowing of the heart), or in total cardiac arrest. This is an example of the physiological mechanism that monitors and adjusts blood pressure and heart rate.

This mechanism acts through a reflex arc in which the afferent (sensory) nerve impulses arise in the carotid complex of nerve endings, but not – as is sometimes alleged – in the vagus nerve trunk itself.

These impulses pass up to the brain via the glossopharyngeal nerves to the tenth nucleus in the brainstem, then return via the vagus (efferent) supply to the heart and other organs. This reflex arc acts through the parasympathetic side of the autonomic nervous system and is independent of the main motor and sensory nerve pathways. It is often claimed, admittedly without much concrete evidence, that fear, apprehension, struggling and possibly the effect of drugs such as alcohol, may heighten the sensitivity of this vagal mechanism. The release of catecholamines during such adrenal responses may well sensitize the myocardium to such neurogenic stimulation.

The vagal reflex has profound implications in relation to pressure or blows on the neck. Sometimes called 'vagal inhibition', 'vasovagal shock' or 'reflex cardiac arrest', the rapid onset of heart stoppage may antedate any evidence of congestive or 'asphyxial' signs, causing death immediately or within seconds, or at any time thereafter.

It is a matter of some dispute as to whether this reflex can cause immediate cardiac arrest or whether there has to be a period of marked slowing of the heart with negligible cardiac output – or whether an arrhythmia such as ventricular fibrillation precedes such an arrest. Probably any combination can occur, but it is an indisputable fact that collapse and apparent death can occur immediately on the application of pressure to the neck. Overstimulation of nerve endings in the carotid sinus or adjacent arterial sheath may be brought about by direct pressure from fingers, or from a ligature during strangulation or hanging – or from a blow directed at the side of the neck. Severe pain, such as a blow on the larynx or genitals, may also trigger a 'vagal response'.

THE FREQUENCY OF VAGAL CARDIAC ARREST

Though different authors vary in the proportion of such deaths that they attribute to reflex cardiac arrest, they all admit to the existence of such a mechanism. In the author's (BK) own series of fatal pressure on the neck from a variety of causes, the 'classical signs', denoting vascular and perhaps sometimes airway obstruction, were present in slightly less than half the cases. The remaining deaths presented with an absence of congestion, cyanosis and petechiae, the pale faces indicating that cardiac arrest had taken place before the congestive signs had time to appear.

One aspect which is uncertain – and virtually incapable of experimental proof in humans – is whether vagus-mediated cardiac arrest can be spontaneously reversible. Where an arrhythmia leads to arrest, resuscitation by cardiac massage or direct current electrostimulation has an excellent chance of revival – though in most forensic situations, such assistance is often lacking or too late.

However, it is not known whether cardiac arrest caused by the vasovagal reflex, can spontaneously revert to normal rhythm some minutes later – or whether it inevitably leads to death if no timely resuscitation is offered. This may have forensic relevance, as the author (BK) has been involved in several cases where pressure on the neck has lead to a comatose, but heart-beating victim, who later dies on artificial ventilation from irreversible brain damage. In the absence of medical data, the problem then arises as to whether the brain damage was caused by prolonged carotid artery occlusion from neck pressure – or was the result of a momentary neck

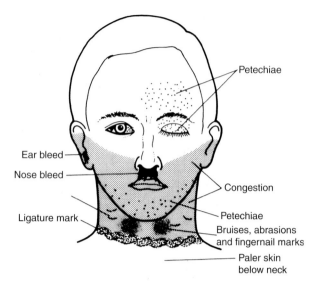

FIGURE 15.3 *Classical features of strangulation when cardiac arrest is delayed.*

pressure which caused reflex cardiac arrest, with spontaneous reversion to normal rhythm more than five minutes later, by which time irreversible cerebral damage had occurred.

Medico-legal aspects

This phenomenon has considerable legal as well as medical significance, as sudden death from 'vagal inhibition' can occur with total unexpectedness even with relatively slight pressure to the neck. Keith Simpson and Polson recorded cases many years ago in which a soldier at a dance playfully 'tweaked' his partner's neck and was mortified to see her drop lifeless to the floor. Many such cases are on record and every forensic pathologist of any experience has examples in his own records. Where it can be shown that the death occurred rapidly and without prolonged manual gripping of the neck, the defence may be raised that neither death nor serious injury was contemplated by the accused. It would be much harder to establish this lack of intent if the grip was maintained long enough to lead to florid congestion and petechiae in the face.

A combined mechanism of injury and the duration of neck compression

It is important to remember that the cardiac arrest mode of death may be mixed with the congestive–petechial mode in that, though the first stages of pressure may continue for long enough for congestive–asphyxial signs to appear (perhaps a minimum of 15–30 seconds), a change in grip may then allow the fingers to impinge on the carotid structures and lead to reflex cardiac arrest. Thus the progression of the pure 'asphyxial' process may be abruptly terminated at any point along its pathway to death by the superimposition of 'vagal inhibition', so that the intensity of the congestive changes may be of any degree in any given death.

The duration for which pressure must be maintained is often a contentious issue in criminal trials, as the 'inadvertent squeeze' which causes rapid vasovagal cardiac arrest is likely to be viewed as less culpable than a prolonged, unremitting gripping of the throat.

It is virtually impossible to measure the average minimum time of gripping that will produce congestion, cyanosis and petechiae from venous occlusion. As so often is the case in forensic medicine, animal experiments are useless for this purpose and obviously few cases of strangulation homicide are ever reliably witnessed, especially by some dispassionate observer with a stopwatch! Even in non-fatal cases – which incidentally, can produce far more florid examples of facial and eye haemorrhages than deaths – there is almost never any independent, accurate measurement of the time for which the neck was compressed.

It has been arbitrarily suggested that 15–30 seconds is probably the minimum period which will give rise to petechiae in the eyelids, conjunctivae and facial skin, but this really is 'picking a figure from the air', with little scientific justification.

Some years ago, the British Home Office and the Royal College of Pathologists set up a small working party to study this problem, composed of several experienced forensic pathologists and a respiratory physiologist – but the project was soon abandoned because of a total lack of reliable data.

Though it is easy to demonstrate that facial congestion develops within a few seconds of total jugular occlusion, petechiae – the only lasting sign after the venous return is re-opened – do not appear as quickly from neck pressure. However, they can occur from sudden, transient rises in venous pressure, such as sneezing or coughing – whooping-cough is a well-known example – and during the Valsalva experiment of forcibly trying to expire against a closed glottis. Eye petechiae and retinal haemorrhages can also occur during the chest compression of energetic cardiac massage during resuscitation.

CAUSES OF REFLEX CARDIAC ARREST

Vagal inhibition of the heart from stimulation of the carotid neural complex may occur in any form of pressure on the neck, but is much more common in manual strangulation than with a ligature, hanging excepted. Fingers seem more prone to dig deeply and find the structures under the anterior edge of the sternomastoid muscle. Perhaps the movements of the fingers, especially during the shifting postures of a struggle, more readily impinge upon the carotid bifurcation than the more static position of a ligature.

The majority of hangings, however, present with a pale face, free from congestive–haemorrhagic signs.

This seems to be caused by the more precipitate impact of the noose on the carotid structures when the victim's weight abruptly bears down, though Polson favoured actual carotid occlusion and hence cerebral ischaemia as the common cause of death in hanging. The scarcity of carotid intimal damage in suicidal hangings does not favour this view.

Blows to the throat

Another cause for sudden cardiac arrest is a blow to the neck or throat. This is the basis of the so-called 'commando punch' and some of the oriental martial arts also contain this in their repertoire – often forbidden because of its potential lethality. The edge of the hand is brought forcibly across the side of the neck or the front of the larynx.

Direct violence to the carotid region naturally causes gross stimulation of the afferent nerve endings. Blows directly to the larynx indirectly stimulate the sinus region or the laryngeal sensory nerve endings may themselves trigger the cardio-inhibitory reflex.

It is well known that the hypopharynx and larynx are particularly sensitive to stimulation, which accounts for the sudden deaths from impaction of food in the larynx, or from the flooding with cold water that causes some sudden immersion deaths. The testicles and uterine cervix also have a similar reputation for leading to sudden cardiac death, if unexpectedly overstimulated, especially when the myocardium is pre-sensitized by catecholamines released by fear or emotion.

MANUAL STRANGULATION

A common method of homicide, manual strangulation is most often encountered when the physical size and strength of the assailant exceeds that of the victim. It is most commonly seen in domestic homicides when a husband kills his wife, in sex-related murders when the victim is again a woman, and in child killings, when the killer is an adult. Manual strangulation is rarely committed by a woman except on a child and a man rarely kills another man of equal physique.

Autopsy appearances in manual strangulation

The autopsy findings fall into two groups, namely, the local signs of violence, and the signs of the mechanism of death, where discernible.

■ Bruising on the neck is the result of the assailant's attack, whereas abrasions may be from either victim or

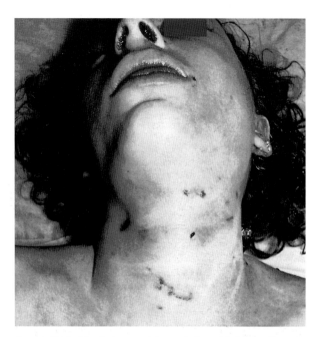

FIGURE 15.4 *Classical manual strangulation with fingernail marks and abrasions on the neck, congestion of the face, slight protrusion of the tongue and bleeding from the nose.*

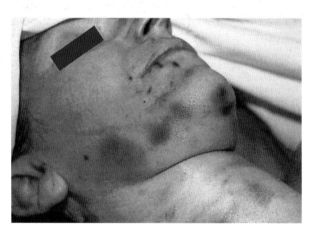

FIGURE 15.5 *Bruising on the neck and jaw margin in manual strangulation. Separate bruises along the jaw are due to high finger pressure – where a larger area of abrasion or bruising is present in this region, consideration must be given to pressure from an arm-lock.*

assailant. The bruises are mainly discoid, but may run together into larger areas of confluent bruising. The discoid marks are from finger-pads and are about 1–2 cm in size, though where the fingers skid across the skin surface, longer, irregular marks may occur, especially along the jaw margins. The bruises tend to cluster at the sides of the neck, often high up under the angles of the jaw. Some may overlap the jaw line and trespass on the chin, but others can be lower on the neck spreading down to the inner ends of the clavicles.

As a result of the shifting grip, often caused by the struggles of the victim, bruising can be anywhere, even at the posterolateral sides of the neck, and on the upper chest over the sternum and collar bones. Some may be seen in the grooves on either side of the larynx, over the anterior edge of the sternomastoid. They are also common over the prominence of the larynx and at the level of the cricoid.

As in most of the cases seen by a pathologist, death will have taken place at or about the time of the attack, most bruises will be fresh, being dark red or purple. Some may be so severe as to form actual superficial haematomas raised slightly above the skin surface. Bruises may often be seen in an asymmetrical pattern, with just one or two on one side of the neck, and a larger group on the opposite side. This may well suggest that a thumb was applied on one side and a group of fingers on the other; this may well be correct, but is not necessarily so and may be fortuitous if a shifting grip caused several reapplications of fingers.

It is sometimes tempting to use such asymmetrical grouping to decide 'handedness', that is to suggest that one bruise on the right side of the victim's neck and a group on the left means that a right-handed assailant gripped from the front. The grouping may not be genuine, however, and because it can be fortuitous, it cannot be definitely determined that it was the right hand nor that it was not placed around the neck from the back. Overinterpretation must be avoided, as in all fields of forensic medicine and 'Sherlock Holmesian' opinions as to the handedness, size of hand, and orientation of attacker and victim in strangulation must be suitably restrained if both justice and the credibility of pathologist are to be preserved.

■ Abrasions on the neck: scratches may be caused by the assailant or the victim, usually from fingernails. As with bruising, rough finger-pads (especially from a male hand on the delicate skin of a female neck) may abrade the epidermis and underlying bruises may be overlain by diffuse abrasions, again often seen along the margin of the jaw line.

Linear scratches are the hallmark of fingernails and, when a woman strangles a child, the often longer nails of the woman may leave obvious marks. Whether male or female, the scratches are of two types: when the pressure is static, straight or curved marks up to a centimetre in length are made; when the nails skid down the skin, linear lines may result, sometimes several centimetres in length.

A static nail mark is often semi-lunar in shape, but caution must be used in interpreting the posture of the hand from this shape. Though it would seem obvious that the concavity of the mark should face the finger-pad, experiments by Shapiro *et al.* in 1962 showed that the converse may be true. This is caused by fixation of the skin at the centre where the nail digs in, with escape at the margins, so that when the traction relaxes, the mark appears inverted, with the convexity facing the finger-pad. However, experiments by others, including the author (BK), show that this phenomenon is by no means invariable and often the marks are the result of the nails being applied in the expected direction.

Scratches are the result of the victim's attempts at pulling away the strangling hand. As most victims are women, the nails may be long and the scratches more severe than those from the assailant, which are often absent altogether. These defence scratches may run in parallel lines from grouped fingers and run in a vertical direction in the long axis of the neck, though they are often random.

In the autopsy on a strangled victim it is good practice to take fingernail scrapings or clippings for full forensic science investigation. These should be preserved and labelled so that each clipping or scraping is individually identified – or failing that, at least the left- and right-hand material should be kept separate. Skin fragments or blood under these nails may provide blood typing or DNA characteristics that can be matched to an alleged assailant – and other valuable trace evidence, such as hairs and fibres might be trapped in a torn fingernail – though admittedly, the number of occasions when such evidence has been gained is extremely small.

The alleged assailant should always be examined medically to correlate any injuries that may have been inflicted on him by the fingernails of the victim, such as facial or hand scratches. If he is examined soon after the offence, his own fingernail scrapings should be taken, especially if the victim has neck abrasions, so that comparison studies can be made between any debris found and the tissue types of the victim.

Internal appearances in manual strangulation

Internally, the bruises described above may be visible to a greater or lesser extent in the tissues of the neck. Often they are quite superficial and are confined to the dermis, but some may be visible to an appreciable depth in the muscles and other structures in the neck.

The platysma muscle may be bruised, but the sternomastoid and the deeper strap muscles that run vertically along the larynx may show patchy bleeding, not always corresponding exactly to the position of surface bruises.

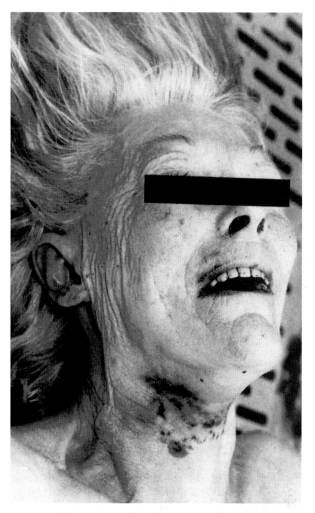

FIGURE 15.6 *Manual strangulation with bruising from the assailant and fingernail abrasions from the victim. The face is pale as a result of rapid vasovagal cardiac arrest before congestive signs could develop.*

They may contain infiltrated blood or even frank haematomata, especially the sternomastoid.

At autopsy, it is essential to release the blood in the venous system before dissecting the neck to avoid or reduce artefactual haemorrhages that can occur in the region. It may be easiest to reflect the scalp and remove the brain before dealing with the neck, to release venous engorgement. Alternatively, after the skin of the neck has been carefully flayed off in a wide 'V' incision, the internal jugular vessels can be incised before any further manipulation to release the venous pressure, but removal of the skull is preferable.

Radiography of the neck may be carried out before any dissection to determine the state of the cervical spine and the laryngeal cartilages, though the author (BK) has never found this to be particularly helpful, preferring to X-ray the isolated larynx before dissection.

When examination of the deep neck structures begins, careful removal of the overlying tissues layer by layer is required, seeking genuine haemorrhage as each set of muscles is exposed. There may be bruising into the thyroid capsule and into any of the strap muscles. The vascular bundles must be handled carefully and the large veins opened with scissors. The carotids can be opened *in situ*, or after the laryngo-oesophageal pluck has been removed.

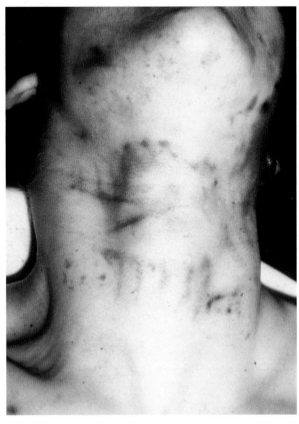

FIGURE 15.7 *Manual strangulation, showing scattered bruises from the fingers of the assailant, but also a pattern of abrasions under the chin and below the larynx, caused by the nails of the victim whilst attempting to pull off the strangling fingers.*

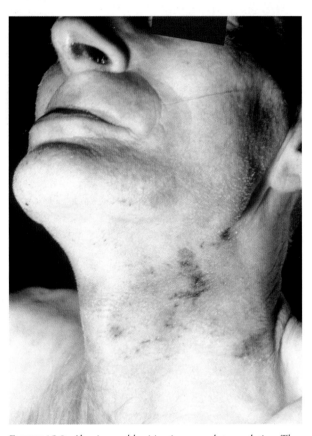

FIGURE 15.9 *Abrasion and bruising in manual strangulation. The face is pale, indicating a rapid sudden death; much of the skin damaged is directly over the position of the underlying carotid sinus.*

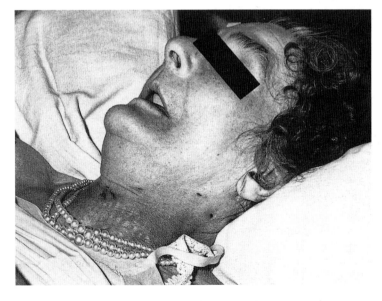

FIGURE 15.8 *Illustration of the need for all doctors to be observant and vigilant. This lady was seen in bed by a family doctor and pronounced a 'heart attack' victim. Later examination revealed facial congestion, fingernail marks on the neck and the impression of her necklace on the skin by strangling hands.*

Spurious bleeding behind the larynx

Bleeding over the front and sides of the larynx is usually genuine, if the venous pressure has been released beforehand, but great caution must be employed in interpreting bleeding behind the larynx and pharynx.

In any autopsy, substantial haemorrhage may be seen over the posterior surface of the oesophagus and on the anterior longitudinal ligament of the cervical spine. This is a common post-mortem artefact, described fully by Prinsloo and Gordon (1951) and sometimes known by their name. In the absence of any other neck lesions, especially bleeding in the lateral and anterior parts of the neck, no reliance can be placed on this haemorrhage. It tends to develop more as the post-mortem interval lengthens and even releasing the venous pressure in the neck by removal of the brain, or opening the jugulars early, does not ensure its absence. To avoid the Prinsloo and Gordon artefact, a special technique of dissecting the neck is recommended by Shapiro (1988). Another artefact in the neck, much easier to recognize as false, is 'banding' of the oesophagus, especially when the tissues are congested. These bands are pale areas in the mucosa caused by post-mortem hypostasis being prevented from settling by the external pressure of adjacent anatomical structures, including parts of the larynx, trachea and aortic arch. Banding is common in routine non-trauma autopsies, but has been misinterpreted by inexperienced pathologists as evidence of strangulation.

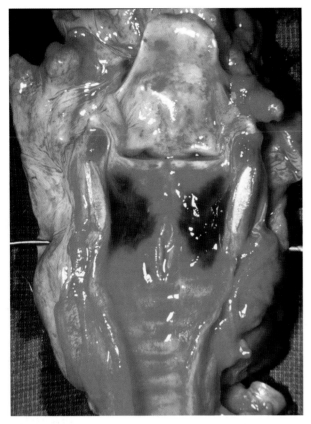

FIGURE 15.10 *Mucosal haemorrhages in the interior of the larynx immediately below the vocal cords, in manual strangulation. This is a common finding and the mechanism is uncertain. It can occur as here – in the absence of generalized congestive–petechial changes – and appears to be caused by local trauma.*

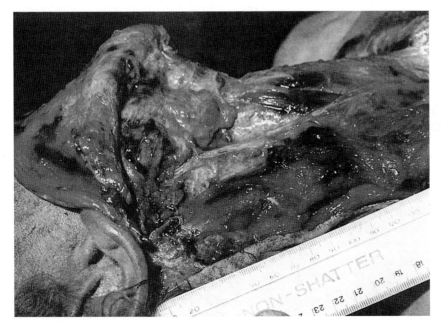

FIGURE 15.11 *Dissection of the neck in a victim of manual strangulation. There are extensive areas of bleeding in the strap muscles, the lower part of the larynx and on the submandibular gland and jaw margin. Removal of the brain before dissection of the neck reduces the risk of artefactural haemorrhages in this region.*

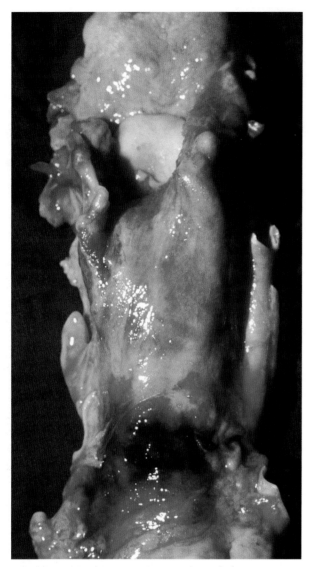

FIGURE 15.12 *Artefactual post-mortem haemorrhage on the posterior surface of the oesophagus in a natural death. This was fully described by Prinsloo and Gordon, and is a reason for draining the blood from the venous system of the head and neck before beginning to dissect.*

Forensic anatomy of the larynx

The larynx consists of a large 'V'-shaped thyroid cartilage, which has a prow-like prominence anteriorly and is open at the back. Below this is the smaller cricoid cartilage, which is narrow at the front, but expands posteriorly to occupy the lower part of the space left by the open thyroid cartilage.

At the upper margin of the posterior wing of the thyroid on each side, are the superior horns or 'cornuae', which are connected by the thyrohyoid membrane to the greater horns of the hyoid bone which lies immediately above.

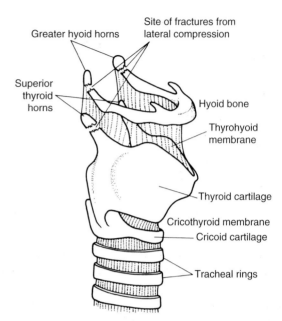

FIGURE 15.13 *The forensic anatomy of the larynx. The hyoid and thyroid bones fracture either from direct lateral compression, or from traction from the thyrohyoid membrane when it is compressed.*

The hyoid bone lies at the root of the tongue, and consists of a central horizontal 'body', to which are attached two long 'greater horns', which sweep backwards and slightly upwards above the upper margin of the thyroid cartilage and superior horns. The hyoid often has natural joints, sometimes even with synovium, which lie at the junction of the body with the greater horns.

There are two lesser horns on the upper surface of the body that have no forensic anatomical significance. The hyoid calcifies at variable times: the body is usually calcified, but the horns may calcify irregularly, both in space and time. In teenagers and young adults they are usually cartilaginous and the joints mobile. In middle and later life, the hyoid and thyroid horns calcify and become more brittle. The cricoid cartilage is a modified upper tracheal ring but can also become partly calcified as age increases; no meaningful ages can be placed on any calcification, but traumatic fractures can occur at any time except in children and most teenagers, in whom fractures are rare.

Injury to the larynx

During manual strangulation the larynx may become damaged in various ways. The pressure is mainly bilateral, so that the sides of the larynx are squeezed. Particularly vulnerable structures are the four 'cornuae' or horns, which protect backwards to maintain the patency of the airway around the glottis. Lateral pressure of the fingers can displace any of the

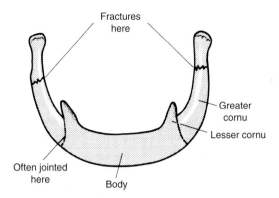

FIGURE 15.14 *The hyoid bone.*

four horns inwards, either by direct pressure or by pressure on the thyrohyoid membrane, which then drags the horns medially. In young persons, the horns are so pliable that they return to their normal position on release of the pressure but, variably beyond the third decade, they may be sufficiently calcified to fracture.

The appearance of a fractured horn is of a loose or even flapping termination. The horn usually displaces medially, but is held by the thyrohyoid ligament. At autopsy it is advisable to cut down this ligament carefully between thyroid cartilage and hyoid to destroy the 'splinting' effect that may support a broken horn. As will be discussed later, however, there will be a haemorrhage at the fracture site that will make the lesion obvious. In the case of the hyoid, care must be taken not to misinterpret a natural joint as a fracture. These are more medial than the usual site of fracture, which is likely to be within a centimetre of the tip. The jagged edge of the fracture line may be exposed, especially in an older person with a brittle horn. Radiography before dissection is an excellent way of confirming a fracture, identifying natural joints and detecting any other fractures in the thyroid or cricoid cartilage.

Though the hyoid bone has received most attention in publications as being the marker of violence to the larynx, in fact the thyroid horns are far more vulnerable. Simpson (1985) found that, in 25 successive deaths from manual strangulation, there were 22 fractures of thyroid horns but only one fractured hyoid. Though this ratio is not typical of the experience of most pathologists, there is no doubt that the superior horn of the thyroid is much more fragile and more vulnerable than the greater horn of the hyoid bone. Although fractures of the horns are more common with advancing age, they can on rare occasions be found even in teenagers. Care must be taken, however, not to confuse mobility at natural joints with a fracture (Evans and Knight 1982).

Conversely, undoubted severe violence to the neck in older persons does not necessarily cause horn fractures. The frequent persistence of joints at the base of the greater horns of the hyoid may allow movement and so avoid fractures when compressed. The cricoid and the main ala of the thyroid cartilage may be cracked, but this is an index of much greater pressure from strangling fingers. The plates may break in a spiral or oblique fashion and the cricoid may crack anteriorly through the narrow bridge rather than at the wider posterior plate. Fractures of these larger areas are also found in direct blunt violence such as punching, kicking or arm-locks, often as part of general severe damage and disruption of the entire larynx.

Significance of laryngeal fractures

Laryngeal cornual fractures are, of course, merely indicators of pressure applied to the neck and are not themselves relevant in terms of a threat to life. This is sometimes misunderstood by laymen, especially police and lawyers, who have been misled by the importance that pathologists attach to the finding of a fractured horn into thinking that the injury itself is a significant contribution to the death.

Such fractures, if proved to be genuine, are certainly significant in proving the application of violence to the neck, but certain precautions must be observed in their interpretation. The sole finding of a fractured horn, where there is no other injury to the skin, subcutaneous tissues, muscles or rest of the larynx is of little value unless there is firm circumstantial evidence of violence to the throat.

When a fracture of a laryngeal horn is found, it must first be proved to be ante-mortem in origin. Post-mortem fractures undoubtedly occur, either from mishandling the body during transit or from incorrect autopsy techniques – though the frequency of the latter has been overestimated.

It is certainly possible to damage the larynx post-mortem by allowing the neck to fall against a hard surface or sharp edge during removal from the place of death, or during handling in the mortuary. Such damage, however, is more likely to occur to the laryngeal plate of the thyroid cartilage or to the cricoid, rather than to the laterally placed horns, though these can be broken. Damage at autopsy is usually caused by an inexperienced pathologist or autopsy-room technician, especially when forensic expertise is lacking. Clumsy removal of the tongue and neck structures can break the thyroid or hyoid cornuae, especially in old persons where they are calcified and brittle and when any natural joints are ankylosed.

This may be one justification for radiography before autopsy, but probably the danger of artefactual breakage has been overestimated, especially where a gentle removal technique is employed.

Proof of ante-mortem laryngeal fracture

This must be obtained by demonstrating haemorrhage at the fracture site. It is usually obvious to the naked eye and can be confirmed histologically. Sometimes the bleeding is prominent, with a blood bleb under the periosteum or perichondrium at the fracture line, and the broken end of a calcified horn may be palpable and even slightly crepitant. Where no macroscopic evidence of bleeding is found, careful histology of the fracture site will almost always reveal some red-cell extravasation, but this evidence is of less value because microscopic – and even slight macroscopic – oozing can occur from a post-mortem fracture of a horn. Bleeding is therefore a 'one-way' criterion: if there is no haemorrhage, the fracture must be post-mortem, but if there is a small bleed, then the lesion can be either ante-mortem or post-mortem. Naturally the findings must be taken in conjunction with other evidence of neck injury and, if there are surface bruises, scratches, muscle bleeding, intralaryngeal and tongue haemorrhage, then a minimal bleed at a fractured horn can be accepted as probably ante-mortem.

Conversely, it must again be emphasized that the solitary finding of a fractured laryngeal horn, even with slight associated bleeding, is not in itself sufficient evidence of ante-mortem trauma to the neck.

Other causes of fractured laryngeal horns

The hyoid and thyroid horns can be broken other than by manual strangulation. Ligature strangulation and hanging can certainly cause these lesions, though not as often as manual throttling. Direct violence can also break the cornuae, but usually only as part of more diffuse laryngeal damage. A punch or kick in the throat can disrupt the larynx and break the horns as part of general damage. Even wide, blunt pressure can fracture the horns, however, such as an arm-lock from behind squeezing the larynx against the cervical spine. It has been said that such direct violence from the front tends to splay the fractured horns laterally, whereas in manual strangulation the horn tends to fall inwards – but this is too tenuous a claim to be of much practical value.

In accidents, the larynx can be damaged. In falls, the larynx is usually protected by the prominences of the chin and chest, but if the fall is onto a ridged object, such as gate or chair-back, then a focal impact can injure the throat. The author (BK) has seen a death in a housebreaker, who slipped when trying to climb through a sash window. He fell with his throat across the top of the window-frame and died – presumably of a vagal cardiac arrest – being found suspended by his neck next morning with fractures of the laryngeal cartilages.

Other laryngeal injuries in strangulation

Other injuries to the larynx include splitting of the ala of the thyroid cartilage, often either in the midline or obliquely across the left or right plate. This may be part of a violent strangulation, seen by Green (1973) in 12 per cent of his series – but is more often seen in blows to the front of the neck, either by fist or the edge of the hand, or a kick or any other kind of substantial trauma directed at the front of the neck.

The cricoid cartilage, a circle shaped like a signet ring that lies below and partly within the thyroid cartilage, may also be fractured by manual throttling when pressure is applied rather lower than usual. Again, this cartilage tends to break either across the front midline or obliquely. Though an uncommon injury, a severe displacement of a broken cricoid – especially if accompanied by mucosal tearing and bleeding – may project backwards into the airway and cause a partial obstruction.

The interior of the larynx may also show indications of pressure on the neck. This usually takes the form of haemorrhage into the mucosal lining and is most often seen immediately below the vocal cords. Bleeding may be intense here, but its cause is obscure. It can occur with no other damage to the cartilages of the larynx and it is then hard to equate it with direct physical pressure as it lies on the protected inner surface.

Similar, but less intense, haemorrhage is sometimes seen on the surface of the epiglottis, which more often shows a shower of petechial haemorrhages if the death was not sudden.

Such haemorrhage inside the larynx is often a bright, fiery red, unlike the dark cyanotic discoloration that is seen in the pharynx, root of tongue and larynx in congestive–asphyxial deaths, and is caused by obstructed venous return rather than direct trauma. At autopsy the base of the tongue should always be sliced, as deep haemorrhages may be present, usually at the sides of the tongue, deep congestion being more central or across the whole posterior part of the tongue.

Damage to the carotid arteries

Though the sudden 'vagal inhibition' type of death caused by pressure on the baroreceptors of the carotid sinus and sheath is quite common, it is unusual to find anatomical confirmation of injury to these structures.

There may be deep haemorrhage in the neck tissues surrounding or adjacent to the bifurcation of the common carotid artery, but this is often absent in these cases of cardiac arrest – and conversely, such bleeding may be found in the slow 'asphyxial' deaths, as part of the generalized diffuse bleeding into the tissues.

Rarely, careful dissection of the carotid arteries may reveal an intimal tear or bleeding into the walls of the vessels at or near the carotid sinus. A delicate technique is required and artefactual damage must be carefully excluded, especially that from the point of scissors used to slit open the artery. Such tears are more often found when a forcible impact or a more focal pressure has been applied, such as from a thin ligature that can cut deeply and abruptly into the neck, especially in hanging. Generally, little or no morphological confirmation is to be expected in the cardiac arrest type of death, following pressure on the neck. The diagnosis is one of exclusion, based on the absence of any congestive–cyanotic–petechial appearances, together with some circumstantial history of sudden death whilst pressure is being applied to the neck.

As already mentioned, one problem is that pressure may be maintained for long enough – perhaps a minimum of 15–30 seconds – to produce these signs, yet not cause death, but death then supervenes abruptly because a vagus-mediated cardiac arrest is superimposed on the early asphyxial mode. In the absence of any structural damage to the carotid apparatus, autopsy cannot differentiate between the two mechanisms and only the history (which is rarely available for obvious reasons) can assist in interpreting the sequence of events.

STRANGULATION BY LIGATURE

Pressure on the neck may be effected by constricting all or part of the circumference of the neck by a ligature. This is sometimes called 'garrotting', though strictly this refers to the tightening of a noose around the neck by twisting a rod within the ligature, a form of judicial execution once employed in Spain, from which also comes the description of the twisting device as a 'Spanish windlass'. This method had a refinement in which the back of the neck was forced against a sharp spike which penetrated the spinal cord.

In forensic practice, if hanging is excepted as a separate entity, most ligature strangulations are homicidal. Some are suicidal and a few accidental, usually in children.

The nature of the ligature

The ligature may consist of a wide variety of objects, some not obviously suitable for the purpose, yet effective in causing death. Cords, wires, ropes and some belts are strong and relatively thin, so that they tend to cut deeply into the neck if the tension is great. Softer fabrics, however, in the form of scarves, ties, towels, stockings, tights and even strips of bed-linen may be used and may cause some problems in interpretation if they are removed from the scene before the

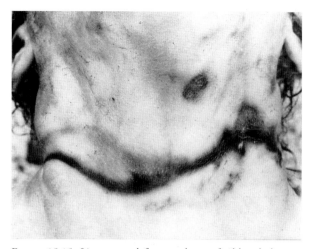

FIGURE 15.15 *Ligature mark from a nylon scarf. Although the fabric was broad, the tension bands from the tightly stretched material have produced a definite line that could be mistaken for a cord or wire.*

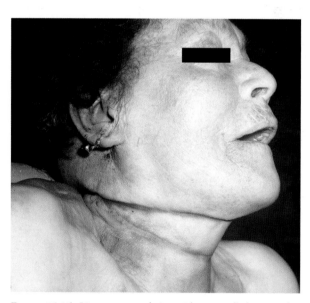

FIGURE 15.16 *Ligature strangulation with a generally horizontal course for the two strands of cord that diverge from the skin at the back of the neck.*

investigation begins. The ligature may be applied as one turn around the neck – or even less, as homicides have been perpetrated by the assailant pulling a U-shaped ligature against the front and sides of the neck, while standing at the back. Even a flexible rod, such as bamboo cane or – in India – a flat 'lathi', can act as a ligature if the two ends are forcibly pulled back from behind against the front of the throat.

In the majority of cases, however, the ligature is crossed over itself after passing a full circle around the neck – and several turns may be wound around, secured with one or more knots. These multiple turns are not uncommon in

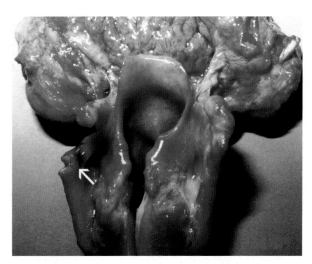

FIGURE 15.17 *Fracture of the left laryngeal horn (arrow) with haemorrhage. The body was recovered from a lake based on the confession of the perpetrator. Further findings were haemorrhage in the fractured cricoid cartilage, bruising on the neck and petechiae in the conjunctivae and larynx.*

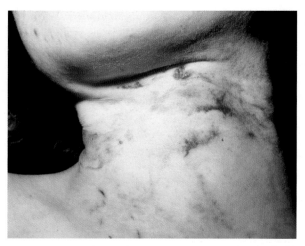

FIGURE 15.19 *In the case shown in Figure 15.18. When the scarf was removed, typical bruises and abrasions of manual strangulation were seen in addition to the ligature mark.*

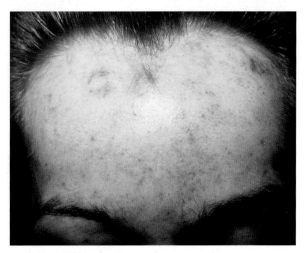

FIGURE 15.18 *Typical appearance of congested, cyanosed forehead, with multiple petechiae in the skin, in a woman strangled manually and by ligature. Circular bruising probably due to knuckle blows. The scarf tied around the neck initially suggested only ligature strangulation.*

suicide, where two, three, or even more circles are wound around, often with complex knots. The presence of these more complicated ligatures by no means confirms homicide – in fact they are more common in suicide, where the determined victim is eager to succeed. The ligature may be tightened even further by means of the 'Spanish windlass' mentioned above, which consists of some rod-like object, which may be a ruler, stick or screwdriver inserted between the ligature and the skin, and twisted around several times. The rod may be held in position by being wedged under the

chin or against the shoulder or chest. This device may be seen in either homicides or suicides.

The ligature mark

The appearance at autopsy naturally depends on the nature and texture of the ligature. When there is a pronounced pattern, such as the weave of a cord or the plaiting of a thong, the same pattern may be imprinted into the skin. In homicide, where the ligature has been removed by the killer, such a pattern may be of great value in tracing its origin. When a fabric has been used, such as a scarf or towel, the marks on the neck are more difficult to interpret. A broad, flat band may leave no mark whatsoever, but it usually leaves one or more linear marks on the skin of the neck, often discontinuous. These may fade if the body is not seen soon after death and if the surface has not been abraded.

A fabric ligature may leave a sharply defined mark, which may be misinterpreted as being caused by a narrow cord or wire. The reason for this is that when a broad piece of cloth is tightly stretched, one or more bands appear that are under greater tension than the rest. It is these that mark the skin, and no sign may be left that a wider area was lying on either side of the most tensed band. These marks are usually less well demarcated at the edges than a cord or rope, but can cause confusion.

When the ligature is still in position when the body is examined, it may appear to be deeply embedded in the skin, sometimes almost out of sight, and on removal a deep groove may be seen in the skin. This embedding may be accentuated by oedema of the tissues, especially above the ligature, which initially may not have been applied so tightly. The swelling can continue to develop to some

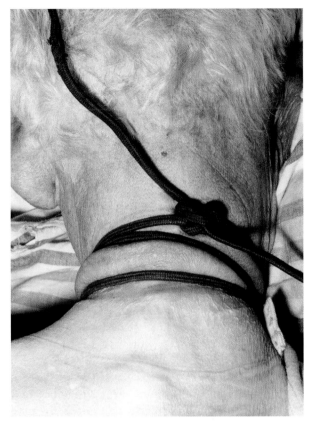

FIGURE 15.20 *Self-strangulation by ligature, with three turns around the neck and a complex knot. There was no doubt from the circumstances that the deceased man had deliberately killed himself with this telephone cord, but the mechanism of apparent vasovagal death before any congestive changes could appear remains obscure.*

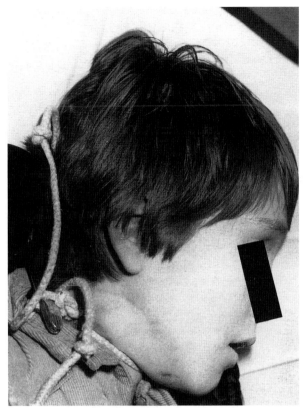

FIGURE 15.21 *Ligature strangulation by means of a 'Spanish windlass'. A penknife has been thrust through the knot to twist the ligature tight.*

extent even after death, accentuating the depth of the groove. Presumably some passive transudation of tissue fluid continues even after the circulation has stopped. In suicides, multiple turns and knots may have been applied and obviously, the degree of tightness as seen later at autopsy could not have been present during the application of the ligature, otherwise incapacity would have been so rapid that the process could not have been completed. In such cases, it is remarkable how often the mode of death still seems to be of the non-asphyxial cardiac arrest type. It might be expected that vagal stimulation could not have occurred once the expected static position was attained with the completion of ligation – but experience indicates otherwise, the mechanism remaining obscure.

The skin mark may remain red, especially if the ligature was of softer material such as cloth, but cords, ropes and wires tend to abrade the surface, which later becomes yellow or brown and parchment-like. This is seen particularly in hanging, when the friction and chafing may be greater.

The stiff, brownish-yellow appearance occurs post-mortem and tends to become more pronounced as the interval lengthens after death. The mark may be slightly wider, narrower or the same width as the actual ligature, depending partly upon how deeply it cut into the skin. There is often a narrow zone of reddened hyperaemia at either margin of the mark. This used to be taken to indicate that the ligature must have been applied during life – though by analogy with the spurious 'vital reaction' sometimes seen as a post-mortem development at the margin of burns (see Chapter 11), this sign is of doubtful reliability. Experiments by Pollak (personal communication) confirm this by the production of similar marginal reddening by applying ligatures soon after death – it seems to be due to lateral displacement of blood from the squeezed area immediately below the ligature.

THE POSITION OF THE LIGATURE MARK

The geometry of the mark is important in interpreting the fatal events. In strangulation, unlike hanging, the mark tends to encircle the neck horizontally and at a lower level. Typically it crosses immediately above or below the prominence of the

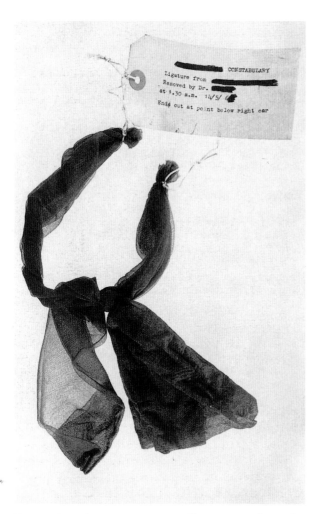

FIGURE 15.22 *At autopsy on a victim of ligature strangulation, the ligature should be cut well away from the knot, if one is present. The knot should never be untied, but preserved for forensic examination. If the ligature is in danger of unravelling, it should be tied at two places and divided between these points. (Reproduced with permission from Robert Hale Publishers.)*

Other signs of local injury in ligature strangulation

There may be scratches on the neck, but these are usually caused by the attempts of the victim to pull away the ligature. Fingernail marks, sometimes linear and vertical, may be present as in manual strangulation, but not focal abrasions or bruises. Internally there may be superficial haemorrhage under the ligature mark, though this is often minimal. Depending on the force with which the ligature was applied, there may be deep damage in the muscles of the neck, but this tends to be less than in manual strangulation. Similarly, there may be laryngeal injury, but less severe than from pressure from the hands. The hyoid bone and thyroid horns may be fractured, especially where the ligature rides at the level of the thyrohyoid ligament, but damage to the laryngeal cartilages is much less common than in manual strangulation. Gonzales found in 24 fatal manual strangulations, four hyoid fractures but nine thyroid and cricoid fractures. In 25 deaths from manual strangulation, Simpson found only one hyoid fracture but 22 with thyroid horn fractures. It is rare for the main thyroid plate or the cricoid to be fractured unless gross violence was applied with excessive pressure by a strong ligature. Uncommonly, a narrow wire may be used, the so-called 'cheese-cutter' method. Here, strong pressure over a small area – such as that delivered by a piano wire – may actually lacerate the skin, and even cut into the deeper tissues and cartilages.

Where much bruising and abrasion is seen, especially if scattered and away from the actual ligature mark, then the possibility of a combination of manual and ligature strangulation must be considered. This is not uncommon, the handling of the throat either preceding or accompanying the application of the ligature. Fractures of the laryngeal structures may be caused by this element, rather than the associated ligature. A deeply sunken narrow ligature applied with force may damage the carotid arteries and focal injury to the intima may rarely be found on careful dissection.

The mode of death in ligature strangulation

The mode of death is more often the 'classic asphyxia' picture than in manual strangulation, where sudden cardiac death is common before congestive–petechial changes have time to occur. The contrast in the appearance of the skin immediately above and below the ligature mark is often striking, with pale skin below, and a puffy, oedematous, congested, cyanotic and haemorrhagic surface above. Petechiae may abound in the eyelids, conjunctivae and facial skin, and there

larynx and passes back to the nape of the neck. In homicide, where a single turn is used, there is often a cross-over point where the two ends of the ligature mark overlap. This may be at the front, side or back of the neck, depending on the relative positions of assailant and victim.

When a knot is tied, it may leave a mark on the skin and, of course, if multiple loops are present, some or all of these will be represented on the skin. Unless the killer is pulling upwards, the mark will not be seen to rise nor will there be a gap in the mark at the highest point, as seen in most hangings.

In the later section on hanging, the point will be made that sometimes a hanging mark may resemble a ligature mark, but the converse is almost unknown.

may be bleeding from the ear and nose. This is by no means invariable, and many ligature strangulations die rapidly from vagal reflex cardiac arrest before any congestive signs have had time to appear.

This can occur in both homicide and suicide and, as mentioned earlier, the mechanism is obscure, especially where the victim – bent on self-destruction – has been able to complete multiple loops around his neck and tie several knots before dying.

Accidental ligature strangulation – which may be actual hanging if the body weight is thrown wholly or partially upon the ligature – is seen in the tragedies than occur to young children, who may become entangled in blind or curtain cords, usually when their cot or playpen is left too near a window.

ARM-LOCKS AND 'MUGGING'

The original meaning of 'mugging' has now been confused by its application, especially in North America, to any form of robbery with violence. The term strictly means throttling by pressure from an arm held around the throat. The attack is usually made from behind, the neck being trapped in the crook of the elbow. Pressure is then exerted either on the front of the larynx, or at one or both sides by the forearm and upper arm. The mechanism is further discussed in Chapter 10, as an arm-lock (or 'choke-hold') is a method of restraint used by police officers for law enforcement, but it is rapidly losing favour because of the number of inadvertent fatalities due either to 'asphyxia' or to reflex cardiac arrest. Following several fatalities during police arrests in the early 1990s, the Association of Chief Police Officers in Britain have issued recommendations that arm-locks be avoided during the restraint of violent prisoners.

The autopsy features are those of ligature strangulation with a broad object, in that signs may be minimal. Some diffuse abrasion may be seen, especially along the margin of the jaw or lower face, sometimes over a considerable area, caused by the friction of the forearm. Internally there may be diffuse bruising, but this again may be slight or even absent. The larynx may also escape damage, though if it is pressed backwards against the spinal column the thyroid horns and even the hyoid may fracture (see also Chapter 10).

HANGING

Hanging is a form of ligature strangulation in which the force applied to the neck is derived from the gravitational drag of the weight of the body or part of the body.

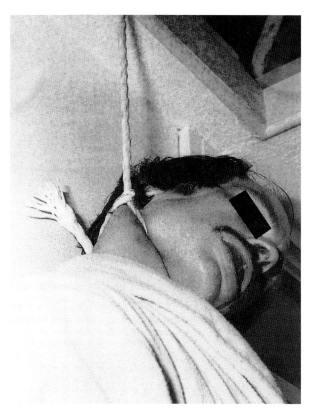

FIGURE 15.23 *Typical posture in hanging with the suspension point rising to the ear, tilting the head to the opposite side. The tongue is projecting because of upward pressure on the larynx and root of the tongue. There are no congestive appearances. As a slip-noose was used, the rope is in contact with the skin throughout the full circumference of the neck.*

Judicial hanging

The modern form of judicial execution is unrelated to the usual suicidal hangings seen in routine forensic practice, as it depends upon severe mechanical disruption of the neck structures. Until the nineteenth century judicial hanging in Britain was carried out even more barbarically by 'ordinary' hanging, where the victim was strangled at the end of a rope by his own weight. At the infamous Tyburn execution site near the present Marble Arch in London, tens of thousands were dispatched, the usual method being the placing of a rope noose around the neck of the condemned person, who stood on a cart or ladder. This support was then removed leaving the victim suspended. Some contemporary accounts suggest that many died with little further movement, but this was not the case for a considerable number and it was not unusual for the victims' relatives to pull on the victims legs to shorten the agony. It appears to have been a desire to increase the rapidity with which death occurred that 'improvements' were made, principally the use of a drop effected suddenly by means of a trapdoor. The use of a drop required the placing of the 'knot' – really a brass eyelet and rubber washer – under the left ear where it was less likely to be pulled over the head than at the occiput, a traditional site. The aim was that, when the rapidly falling body was suddenly arrested, the cervical spine would be dislocated resulting in traction on the spinal cord with consequent spinal cord or brainstem disruption. Exhumation of persons executed by this method shows that fracture was not usual but post-mortem accounts of findings indicate that cervical spine dislocation – occurring at various levels – was common with resulting cord or brainstem damage. However, the effects do seem to be variable with decapitation occurring at drop heights, which, in others, judging by contemporary descriptions of the execution, appear not even to have caused rapid unconsciousness. Though cerebral function presumably ceased immediately on cord or brainstem damage, the heart usually continued to beat, sometimes for up to 20 minutes until hypoxia caused arrest.

Suicidal and accidental hanging

Apart from the now rare 'lynching', hanging is almost always suicidal or accidental, the former being by far the most common. Hanging has many features in common with ligature strangulation. Death is, however, more often caused by reflex cardiac arrest from pressure on the carotid structures. Many more victims of hanging are found to have pale faces, rather than the congested, haemorrhagic appearance of the slower asphyxial type of death. James and Silcocks (1992), in a 15-year survey of hangings in Cardiff, found congestive–petechial features in 27 per cent, being related to the completeness of suspension.

Polson suggested that the usual pale face in hanging is caused by cerebral ischaemia from bilateral occlusion of the carotid arteries rather than a vasovagal effect, though this seems incapable of proof. In either event, the death can be taken to be rapid if no asphyxial signs are present.

Methods of hanging

Most hangings are self-suspension. This may be carried out by a wide variety of methods, but a typical method of self-suspension is to attach a thin rope to a high point such as a ceiling beam or staircase. The lower end is formed into either a fixed loop or a slipknot, which is placed around the neck while the intending suicide stands on a chair or other support. On jumping off or kicking away the support, the victim is then suspended with all or most of his weight upon the rope.

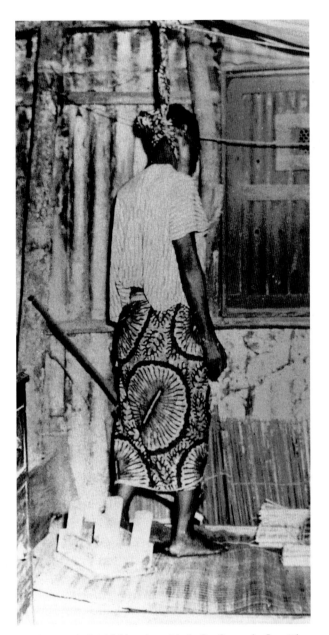

FIGURE 15.24 *Suicidal hanging with the feet flat on the floor. The deceased man stepped off the low stool, but the stretching of the cloth ligature prevented total suspension. Many suicidal hangings are successful at much lower levels, such as doorknobs and bed headboards.*

The many variations of this involve either the ligature or the height of suspension. Wires, string, pyjama cords, belts, braces (suspenders), scarves, neckties, stockings and numerous other devices may be used, depending on availability. In prison or police custody considerable ingenuity may be employed to defeat the efforts of the custodians to remove anything that could be used for self-destruction: shoelaces, stockings and torn bed-sheets have been used in prison cells.

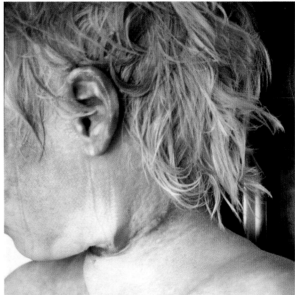

FIGURE 15.26 *Hanging deaths in children are very rare. This 7-year-old boy took his leave from his playmates and hanged himself from a bedpost under their very eyes.*

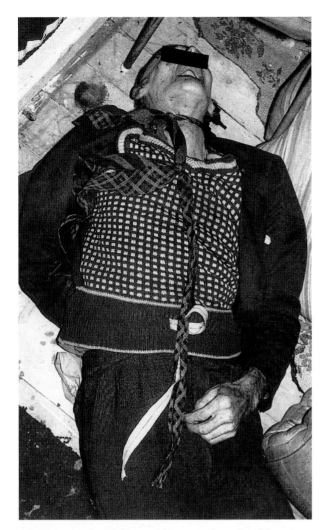

FIGURE 15.25 *Suicidal hanging by means of a necktie. The deceased man had suspended his neck from a hook on the back of a door by tying two neckties together. The hook had pulled out and he was found on the floor. Note the pale, uncongested face, indicating rapid cardiac arrest.*

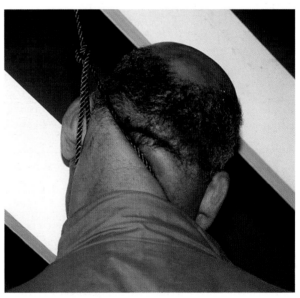

FIGURE 15.27 *Hanging with a fixed knot in the cord, so that there is a segment of skin free from the mark where the cord rises towards the knot. This was part of the common murder–suicide pattern in a domestic homicide.*

Suspension is often not high enough to keep the victim's feet clear of the floor. Commonly, when the person steps from his support, the stretch in the ligature rope is sufficient to allow the feet to reach the ground, but this by no means prevents a fatal outcome. The weight of the upper part of the body leaning into the noose is often more than enough to cause death. Successful hanging can occur from low suspension points, where the person is merely slumped with part of his weight into the ligature. Hanging can take place from doorknobs, bedposts and any other convenient low securing point. The body may be merely slumped against the door or bed or chair, with the legs and buttocks supported on the floor, so that only the weight of the chest and arms is contributing to the fatal pressure within the noose. One 'hanging' seen by the author (BK) was successfully achieved by

merely leaning the neck into the shallow curve of a low clothesline stretched between two posts in a garden.

It is unusual for a suicidal hanging to be sufficiently violent for damage to the cervical spine to occur as the length of drop is usually too short. Only occasionally will a person jump from a roof or other high place with a rope around his neck – here severe injury can occur, even decapitation if the

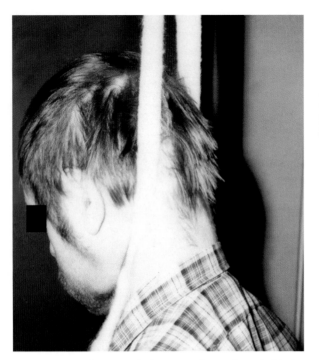

FIGURE 15.28 *This inmate had torn up a sheet and attached both ends to a water tap (not shown) and is leaning into the loop in sitting position with sparing of the back of the neck.*

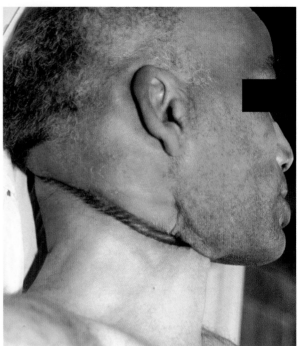

FIGURE 15.29 *A deep hanging mark showing the high position under the chin rising to the back of the neck. The spiral weave of the rope is clearly imprinted in the skin. The dark tint of the face is racial, not congestive.*

rope is strong enough. More often the jump will be from an attic trapdoor or a tree, sufficient to damage the vertebrae or atlanto-occipital joint. The author (BK) once saw a fractured cervical spine when a heavily built soldier jumped off a lavatory seat after securing a rope to the overhead cistern, but this is unusual.

The hanging mark

The mark on the neck in hanging can almost always be distinguished from ligature strangulation. The circumstances will usually indicate the fact of hanging, but sometimes the rope will break or become detached, and the deceased will be found lying with a ligature around his neck. There may then be doubt as to whether he was hanged or strangled. Obviously a search of the locus for a suspension point and signs of rope attachment will be the task of the investigators.

The hanging mark almost never completely encircles the neck unless a slipknot was used, which may cause the noose to tighten and squeeze the skin through the full circumference of the neck. In most instances the point of suspension is indicated by a gap in the skin mark, where the vertical pull of the rope leaves the tilted head to ascend to the knot and thence to the suspension point. This gap is usually seen at one or other side of the neck or at the centre of the back of the neck. Much less often it is under the chin. The knot itself

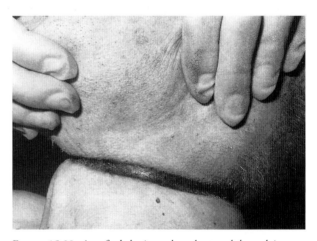

FIGURE 15.30 *A perfectly horizontal mark around the neck in a man who hanged himself from a staircase. A slipknot was used, which tightened so that the usual rising line of a hanging mark did not occur, illustrating the dangers of assuming that the usual is invariable.*

may be impressed into the skin, especially if at the side of the head, above the gap where the anterior mark begins.

The hanging mark, the features of which resemble those described earlier in strangulation, is usually deepest at the side diametrically opposite the suspension point where the maximum load-bearing occurs. Like ligature strangulation,

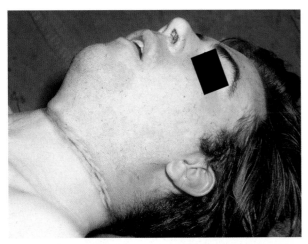

FIGURE 15.31 *A hanging mark showing the plaited imprint of a six-strand cable. There is a central line of abrasion, within a zone of pallor caused by vascular compression, outside which is a narrow band of hyperaemia. The mark is horizontal due to leaning forwards.*

the mark may be abraded, brown and dried to a parchment-like consistency after death. There may be a narrow red zone either above or below (or both sides) the ligature mark. This is not an indicator of vital reaction, as explained in relation to ligature strangulation, but is due to displacement of blood laterally from under the zone of maximum pressure.

THE POSITION OF THE HANGING MARK

The hanging mark is situated higher on the neck than in strangulation, usually being directly under the chin anteriorly, passing round beneath the jawbones and rising up at the sides or back of the neck to the usual gap under the knot.

An exception may be seen where the suspension point is low and part of the body is supported. For example, the victim may sit or slump on a chair, bed or floor with the rope attached to a point only slightly above neck level. Then the pull on the rope is almost at right angles to the axis of the body when the latter slumps away, so that the resulting mark may be almost horizontal and set at a lower level than usual on the neck. In such cases, if the body is cut down before investigators arrive, it may be much more difficult to distinguish hanging from strangulation, a fact which has been argued in more than one criminal trial or controversial death, such as that of Rudolf Hess in Spandau Prison, Berlin in 1987.

On rare occasions, hanging will take place with the suspension point at or above the point of the chin with the rope cutting into the back of the neck. Where the rope passes

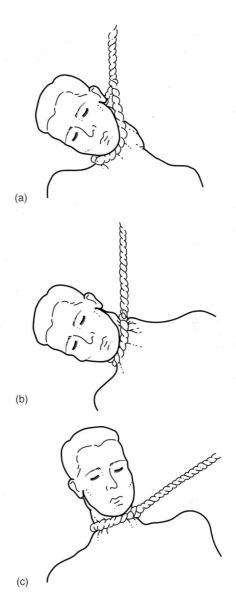

FIGURE 15.32 *The position of the hanging mark on the neck. (a) Usual position with fixed noose and high suspension point. The mark rises high to a gap. (b) If a slipknot is used, the tightness of the deeply impressed loop tends to find the smallest circumference on the neck, and may be lower and more horizontal. (c) If the suspension point is low and the subject leans away, the mark can be horizontal.*

across the jaw margins to a knot in front of the face, the mechanism of death is somewhat obscure as the laryngeal region suffers little or no compression. Fatalities, however, certainly do occur, presumably as there is still opportunity for pressure on the carotids.

Autopsy appearances in hanging

Apart from the appearances of the hanging mark, there are some other features to note. First, post-mortem hypostasis

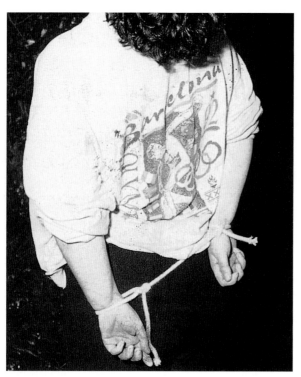

FIGURE 15.33 *The back of the victim in Figure 15.31, showing tying of the wrists. This does not indicate a homicide, unless the ligature could not have been self-applied. Some persons bent on self-destruction will try to ensure that they do not attempt to rescue themselves. A suicide note was left in this case.*

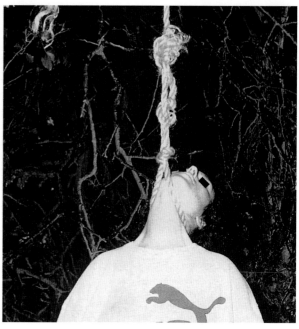

FIGURE 15.34 *Suicidal hanging with the rope in a frontal position. Even though the larynx cannot be compressed, death is due to pressure on the carotid arteries and sinuses. The face is pale, with no so-called 'asphyxial' signs.*

will occur in the legs and hands if the body has been in the vertical position for at least a few hours. When the body is cut down and laid horizontal for a considerable time, some or all of this appearance may flow back into the usual pattern.

Petechial haemorrhages are the exception rather than the rule, most series reporting them in approximately 25 per cent of cases. Such petechiae appear to occur more frequently in incomplete suspension but are frequently present in the absence of significant congestion. Congestion itself is far less usual than a pale face.

In the neck tissues there may be surprisingly little to find with an absence of laryngeal fracture or strap muscle haemorrhage being a common finding, especially if a soft ligature has been used. However, the literature suggests that an average figure for the incidence of soft tissue haemorrhage would be about 20–30 per cent of cases and for laryngeal fractures approximately 35–45 per cent of cases. Fractures of both the hyoid and thyroid may be seen.

Damage to the intima of the carotid arteries, often in the region of the sinuses, may sometimes be found on careful dissection. In hangings with an unusually long drop, severe disruption of the larynx can be found.

Mechanism of hanging

There are a number of mechanisms by which hanging may cause death, which may act independently or in concert. These include: stretching of the carotid sinus causing reflex cardiac arrest; occlusion of the carotid (and possibly vertebral) arteries; venous occlusion; airway obstruction resulting from pushing the base of the tongue against the roof of the pharynx or from crushing of the larynx or trachea; and finally spinal cord–brainstem disruption.

Whilst hanging shares some features with manual strangulation, the majority of victims of hanging are seen with pale faces rather than the congested, haemorrhagic appearance associated with the slower death resulting from pressure on the neck. This probably reflects a different mechanism, with reflex cardiac arrest and carotid occlusion more prevalent in hanging than in strangulation. Such mechanisms cause death rapidly, with unconsciousness resulting from bilateral carotid occlusion 3–11 seconds after the application of circumferential pressure.

However, the precise interplay of different mechanisms, which themselves appear only partially dependent on the completeness of suspension and the location of the noose, is impossible to determine from the pathological findings alone.

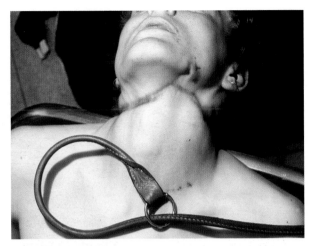

FIGURE 15.35 *Hanging by frontal suspension. A leather noose has been used so that compression has occurred round the whole periphery of the neck. The imprint of the metal ring on the jaw is well seen.*

THE SEXUAL ASPHYXIAS: AUTOEROTIC OR MASOCHISTIC PRACTICES

Though not all of this group are hangings or strangulations, this well-recognized phenomenon is conveniently considered here. The sexual asphyxias occur almost exclusively in men and only a few reports exist of women indulging in this dangerous habit, though Byard *et al.* (1990) have been able to contrast the death scenes in the two sexes, indicating that males tend to use more apparatus, whilst females are usually found naked with only a ligature in evidence.

The age of the male victims can vary widely, but is most often seen in young to middle-aged adults. The deaths that occur are obviously a small proportion of the total incidence of this strange practice. A fatal outcome is usually because of some failure of the equipment and this emphasizes the accidental nature of most of these deaths.

Accidental and homicidal hanging

Though most hangings are suicidal, accidental hangings occur from two main causes. The first is entanglement in ropes or cords; this is relatively uncommon, and is usually seen in infants and children. The straps of a baby harness, used to support or restrain an infant, have led to death on a number of occasions, the child becoming entangled in leather or plastic reins when no adult was present. Any other cords may present a similar hazard, as in several cases seen by the author (BK), where infants standing in a cot near the bedroom window became entangled in a noose formed by the control cords hanging from a nearby blind or curtain.

On rare occasions, similar tragedies have befallen adults in factories, farms or ships, where a trip or fall has precipitated the victim head-first into machinery or structures, where ropes or cords have caused hanging or strangulation.

More commonly, a totally different situation causes fatal hanging or strangulation, almost exclusively in men and most often in young men, which is described in the next section.

Homicidal hanging is very rare, outside abuse of human rights and 'lynching'. For one individual to hang another, there must be either a disparity in their size and strength – or the victim must be drugged, drunk or otherwise incapacitated by fear, illness or senility. For a conscious, presumably unwilling, victim to be hanged by another, there will inevitably be signs of resistance, such as grip bruises on the arms due to restraint, or signs of binding the arms, wrists or legs.

Features of the sexual asphyxias

The basic mechanism of the sexual asphyxias is the production of cerebral hypoxia, which in some men appears to produce hallucinations of an erotic nature.

This hypoxia is most often achieved by constriction of the neck by a ligature, which can be voluntarily tightened to produce vascular obstruction and perhaps airway stenosis. It would seem reasonable to think that vascular obstruction, either by blocking venous return – or even carotid flow – to the brain was the most likely explanation, as this would occur early. The production of cerebral hypoxia by anoxaemic anoxia through airway narrowing would surely be painful, distressing and slow in onset – hardly features which persons intent on self-gratification would welcome.

Some autoerotic procedures use other means of hypoxia, such as anaesthetic agents and a variety of volatile substances, tapering into 'solvent abuse', discussed elsewhere (Chapter 34). Whatever the mechanism, when cerebral hypoxia occurs with its attendant erotic sensations, progressive loss of voluntary control as consciousness fades allows the constrictive device to slacken, so that the subject recovers. As some fatal cases show clear evidence of repeated previous escapades, it is obvious that the mechanism usually functions quite successfully and that death was the result of some unforeseen complication.

A common practice is to place a fixed noose around the neck, so that compression will cease as soon as muscular tension on the free end is relaxed. This free end may be passed down the front or back to be fastened to the ankles, so that by extending the legs, the noose around the neck is

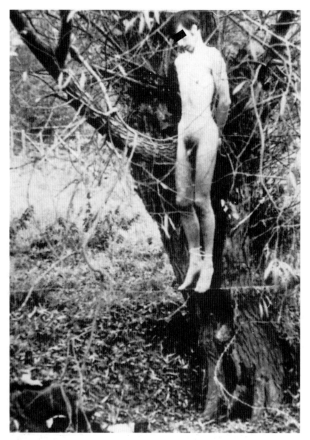

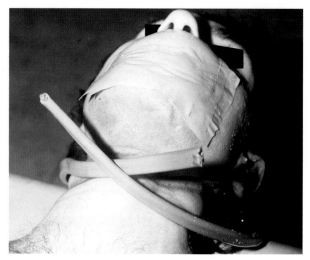

FIGURE 15.37 *A hanging in which it was not clear if there was a true sexual–masochistic element. The victim was suspended by electric cable from an attic trapdoor with his face plastered with surgical tape and the wrists tied together. Homicide could be excluded. In some deaths with an undoubted sexual element, the means used would inevitably lead to a fatal outcome, so there seems to be an overlap between masochism and suicide.*

FIGURE 15.36 *Hanging in circumstances which suggest a sexual–masochistic motive. The young man showed no signs of previous depression or suicidal tendency. He was found naked, with arms and legs tied together with wire. Though homicide was suspected at first, the bonds were loose and easily self-applied. No satisfactory explanation was forthcoming.*

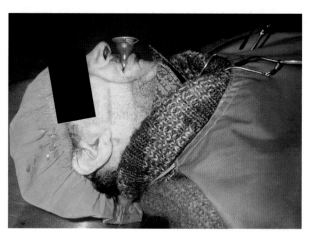

FIGURE 15.38 *Fatal sexual asphyxia in an engineer with a rubber fetish. He was found dead connected to a dental anaesthetic machine, with a rubber face mask strapped on over a rubber teat in the mouth. Bizarre pornographic material devoted to dentistry was in the vicinity. (Figure reproduced by kind permission of Dr S Leadbeatter.)*

tightened. Compression may also be attained by passing the rope over a support and hanging a weight on the end to produce tension.

Other men may secure the end to an overhead support and achieve constriction by slumping against the pull of the rope. In these and similar cases, it is difficult to understand how death can be avoided once consciousness is lost, but evidence of repetition on previous occasions indicates that enough voluntary control must be retained to allow the person to retrieve the situation after obtaining his erotic satisfaction.

Similar hypoxia may be produced by placing the head in a plastic bag, by pushing the head into a confined space, by postural contortions (often associated with bondage) that constrict the airway, or a host of other ingenious methods. One case seen by the author (BK) deliberately constructed a large sack made from impervious material, into which he crawled to attain his hypoxia. Certain features of these

deaths make them fairly easy to differentiate from suicides, a distinction which is important, though some cases are impossible to separate from deliberate attempts at self-destruction (Knight 1979).

Bondage is common, with sometimes elaborate and bizarre methods of restriction. The wrists and ankles may be tied together with cord, wire, chains, padlocks or handcuffs, for example, and it is vital for the investigators to ensure

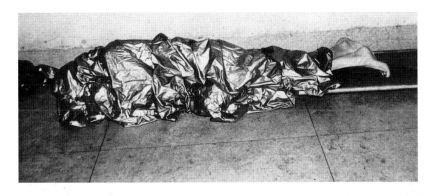

FIGURE 15.39 *A presumed instance of sexual asphyxia. The deceased was naked and had enveloped himself in a large impervious bag, which he had made himself. It seemed impossible for him to save himself once unconsciousness had occurred, but there appeared to be no suicidal tendencies in the history.*

that such bondage could have been secured by the deceased himself to exclude the possibility of homicide, usually by a heterosexual or homosexual partner involved in the ritual.

The bonds may be sexually orientated, with straps around the crutch or constricting the genital organs. In cases seen by the author (BK), one had made a metal sheath for the penis that was padlocked in place and another clamped the penis within a metal shackle.

Masks and gags may be in place, again a manifestation of restraint. The mouth may be sealed by adhesive plaster and the eyes blindfolded. Rubber or leather often features in the masks, which may have eye-slits or completely envelope the face. Transvestism is common, female attire being worn either overtly or under male clothing. False breasts and nipples may be fabricated or brassières padded with cloth. This is a common phenomenon, however, without sexual asphyxia, as any coroner's autopsy service will reveal some men (often elderly) as hidden transvestites, wearing female underclothing beneath their suits. Fetishism is often seen, especially rubber or shiny plastic or leather. Female wigs and make-up are sometimes encountered, though the syndrome does not seem to be overtly associated with homosexual activity.

Pornographic literature is often within view and may be spread around the body at the scene of death. The act is sometimes performed before a mirror and masturbation is common. The mere emission of semen found at autopsy does not confirm sexual activity in itself, however, as postmortem discharge of semen from the meatus is common in any type of death, not only in asphyxia (as used to be commonly alleged by standard textbooks). Occasionally, lewd writings are left near the body and even upon the body surface. The author (BK) has seen one where obscene graffiti were written with a ball-pen on the abdomen and around the glans penis.

Perhaps more importantly, overt suicide notes are never present, helping to distinguish the cases from definite self-destruction. Another important piece of evidence against suicide is the fact that, in some neck ligatures, the rope may be padded by fabric to avoid leaving a telltale mark on the neck – an act incompatible with an intention of suicide.

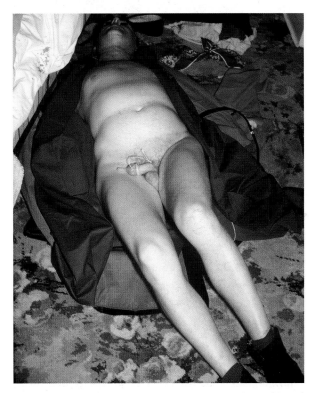

FIGURE 15.40 *A classical sexual asphyxia where the deceased has used a dog collar round the neck (removed before photography), the chain passing down to the ankles, which provide temporary traction. The common features of rubber fetishism and penile bondage were present.*

Rarely, autoerotic gratification may be achieved by the application of electric current, usually low voltage applied to the genitals. Electrical faults, such as in a transformer, may lead to a fatal outcome.

Medico-legal aspects of the sexual asphyxias

Though all these features make the true nature of the death clear to the medical examiner, it can sometimes be difficult

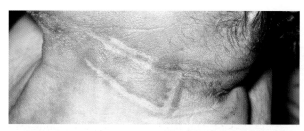

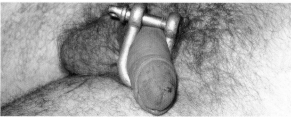

FIGURE 15.41 *A sexual asphyxia from a buckled belt applied tightly to the neck and a metal shackle on the penis. Obscene phrases were written on the glans and abdomen.*

to convince the police, the coroner or judge – and especially the relatives – that death was accidental. The stigma still attached to suicide and the revulsion felt at the perverted sexual element may cause the relatives to prefer homicide as the cause. The judicial authorities often lean towards suicide, especially when they are unaware of the existence of this strange syndrome of the masochistic or sexual asphyxias. The doctor is often the only person able to explain the relatively common occurrence of this phenomenon and assist in reaching the correct conclusion. It has to be admitted, however, that in a small minority of these deaths, it seems inevitable that the victim must have been aware of the fatal outcome, as the mechanics of the asphyxia are such that no escape could have been foreseen. In these instances the circumstances are such that a mixed motivation must have existed. For example, hanging by the neck in free suspension from a tree or from the trapdoor of an attic is a situation from which escape is impossible, even though sexual attributes such as nudity, bondage and masking were present (Knight 1979).

Where the victim is young, motivation is again less clear. Youths of 12 or 14 years are sometimes found hanged, usually without the secondary sexual or bizarre attributes listed above. There is usually nothing in the history to suggest suicide, and quite often the coroner or other legal authority will decide that death was due to 'experimenting with ropes', sometimes alleging that it followed watching lynching in cowboy films on television. It is probable that most of the obscure deaths are also associated with aberrant sexual activity, even if more positive evidence is lacking. Recognition of the true nature of most of these deaths is vital for the medical examiner, as spurious homicide investigations may be initiated if they are misinterpreted. More commonly

a false suicide verdict may result, which can have financial implications in respect of life insurance. A mistaken belief in suicide may be preferred by some families, however, rather than the shame of a publicised sexual aberration.

REFERENCES AND FURTHER READING

Adelson L. 1962. Possible neurological mechanisms for sudden death with minimum anatomical findings. *J Forensic Med* **9**:10–16.

Anscombe AM, Knight BH. 1996. Case report. Delayed death after pressure on the neck: possible causal mechanisms and implications for mode of death in manual strangulation discussed. *Forensic Sci Int* **78**:193–7.

Bockholdt B, Maxeiner H. 2002. Hemorrhages of the tongue in the postmortem diagnostics of strangulation. *Forensic Sci Int* **126**:214–20.

Bohnert M, Faller-Marquardt M, Lutz S, *et al.* 2001. Transfer of biological traces in cases of hanging and ligature strangulation. *Forensic Sci Int* **116**: 107–15.

Bowden KM. 1962. The larynx. *J Forensic Med* **9**:10–16.

Brinkmann B, Koops E, Wischhusen F, *et al.* 1981. [Compression of the neck and arterial obstruction (author's transl).] *Z Rechtsmed* **87**:59–73.

Brouardel P. 1897. *La pendaison, la strangulation, la suffocation, la submersion.* Baillière, Paris.

Byard RW, Bramwell NH. 1988. Autoerotic death in females. An underdiagnosed syndrome? *Am J Forensic Med Pathol* **9**:252–4.

Byard RW, Hucker SJ, Hazelwood RR. 1990. A comparison of typical death scene features in cases of fatal male and autoerotic asphyxia with a review of the literature. *Forensic Sci Int* **48**:113–21.

Byard RW, Hucker SJ, Hazelwood RR. 1993. Fatal and near-fatal autoerotic asphyxial episodes in women. Characteristic features based on a review of nine cases. *Am J Forensic Med Pathol* **14**:70–3.

Camps FE, Hunt AC. 1959. Pressure on the neck. *J Forensic Med* **6**:116–36.

Cooke CT, Cadden GA, Hilton JM. 1988. Unusual hanging deaths. *Am J Forensic Med Pathol* **9**:277–82.

Danto BL. 1980. A case of female autoerotic death. *Am J Forensic Med Pathol* **1**:117–21.

DiMaio VJ. 2000. Homicidal asphyxia. *Am J Forensic Med Pathol* **21**:1–4.

Ditto EWD. 1981. Electrocution during sexual activity. *Am J Forensic Med Pathol* **2**:271–2.

Duflou JA, Lamont DL, Knobel GJ. 1988. Homicide in Cape Town, South Africa. *Am J Forensic Med Pathol* **9**:290–4.

Emson HE. 1983. Accidental hanging in autoeroticism. An unusual case occurring outdoors. *Am J Forensic Med Pathol* **4**:337–40.

Evans KT, Knight B. 1982. *Forensic radiology*. Blackwell Scientific Publications, Oxford.

Ford R. 1957. Death by hanging of adolescents and young adult males. *J Forensic Sci* **2**:171–4.

Gonzalez TA. 1933. Fractures of the larynx. *Arch Pathol* **15**:55–62.

Gordon I, Shapiro HA, Taljaard JJ, *et al.* 1976. Aspects of the hyoid-larynx complex in forensic pathology. *Forensic Sci* **7**:161–70.

Green MA. 1973. Morbid anatomical findings in strangulation. *Forensic Sci* **2**:317–23.

Grellner W, Benecke M. 1997. The quantitative alteration of the DNA content in strangulation marks is an artefact. *Forensic Sci Int* **89**:15–20.

Harm T, Rajs J. 1981. Types of injuries and interrelated conditions of victims and assailants in attempted and homicidal strangulation. *Forensic Sci Int* **18**:101–23.

James R, Nasmyth-Jones R. 1992. The occurrence of cervical fractures in victims of judicial hanging. *Forensic Sci Int* **54**:81–91.

James R, Silcocks P. 1992. Suicidal hanging in Cardiff – a 15-year retrospective study. *Forensic Sci Int* **56**:167–75.

Kennedy NM, Whittington RM, White AC. 1995. Suicide by self-strangulation whilst under observation. *Med Sci Law* **35**:174–7.

Khokhlov VD. 2001. Calculation of tension exerted on a ligature in incomplete hanging. *Forensic Sci Int* **123**:172–7.

Knight B. 1979. Fatal masochism – accident or suicide? *Med Sci Law* **19**:118–20.

Koops VE, Puschel K. 1983. Obstruction of the carotid arteries and upper airway by manual strangulation. In: Holczabek W (ed.), *Beiträge zur gerichtlichen medizin*. Verlag Franz Deuticke, Vienna, vol. XLI.

Kornblum RN. 1986. Medical analysis of police choke holds and general neck trauma. *Trauma* **27**(Part I):760; **28**(Part II):13–64.

Kunnen K, Thomas F, Van der Velde E. 1966. Semimicroradiography of the larynx. *Med Sci Law* **6**:218–19.

Leth P, Vesterby A. 1997. Homicidal hanging masquerading as suicide. *Forensic Sci Int* **85**:65–71.

Lew EO. 1988. Homicidal hanging in a dyadic death. *Am J Forensic Med Pathol* **9**:283–6.

Litman RE, Swearingen C. 1972. Bondage and suicide. *Arch Gen Psychiatry* **27**:80–5.

Luke JL, Reay DT, Eisele JW, *et al.* 1985. Correlation of circumstances with pathological findings in asphyxial deaths by hanging: a prospective study of 61 cases from Seattle, WA. *J Forensic Sci* **30**:1140–7.

Mallach HJ, Pollak S. 1998. [Simulated suicide by hanging after homicidal strangulation.] *Arch Kriminol* **202**:17–28.

Maxeiner H. 1998. 'Hidden' laryngeal injuries in homicidal strangulation: how to detect and interpret these findings. *J Forensic Sci* **43**:784–91.

Michalodimitrakis M, Frangoulis M, Koutselinis A. 1986. Accidental sexual strangulation. *Am J Forensic Med Pathol* **7**:74–5.

Minyard F. 1985. Wrapped to death. Unusual autoerotic death. *Am J Forensic Med Pathol* **6**:151–2.

Muller E, Franke WG, Koch R. 1997. Thyreoglobulin and violent asphyxia. *Forensic Sci Int* **90**:165–70.

Perper JA, Sobel MN. 1981. Identification of fingernail markings in manual strangulation. *Am J Forensic Med Pathol* **2**:45–8.

Pollanen MS. 2001. Subtle fatal manual neck compression. *Med Sci Law* **41**:135–40.

Prinsloo I, Gordon I. 1951. Postmortem dissection artefacts of the neck and their differentiation from ante-mortem bruises. *S Afr Med J* **25**:358–61.

Rajs J, Thiblin I. 2000. Histologic appearance of fractured thyroid cartilage and surrounding tissues. *Forensic Sci Int* **114**:155–66.

Reay DT, Eisele JW. 1982. Death from law enforcement neck holds. *Am J Forensic Med Pathol* **3**:253–8.

Reay DT, Holloway GA, Jr. 1982. Changes in carotid blood flow produced by neck compression. *Am J Forensic Med Pathol* **3**:199–202.

Resnick H. 1972. Eroticised repetitive hangings: a form of selfdestructive behaviour. *Am J Psychother* **26**:4–8.

Reuter F. 1933. *Lehrbuch der gerichtlichen Medizin*. Urban and Schwarzenberg, Berlin.

Rogde S, Hougen HP, Poulsen K. 2001. Asphyxial homicide in two Scandinavian capitals. *Am J Forensic Med Pathol* **22**:128–33.

Rothschild M, Maxeiner H. 1992. [How extensive can injury of the larynx in self-choking be?] *Arch Kriminol* **189**:129–39.

Seabourne A, Seabourne G. 2001. Suicide or accident – self-killing in medieval England: series of 198 cases from the eyre records. *Br J Psychiatry* **178**:42–7.

Shapiro H. 1988. *Strangulation*. In: Gordon F, Shapiro H, Berson S (eds), *Forensic medicine: a guide to principles*, 3rd edn. Churchill, Edinburgh.

Shapiro HA, Gluckman J, Gordon I. 1962. The significance of the nail abrasion of the skin. *J Forensic Med* **9**:17–19.

Simonsen J. 1988. Patho-anatomic findings in neck structures in asphyxiation due to hanging: a survey of 80 cases. *Forensic Sci Int* **38**:83–91.

Simpson CK. 1985. *Forensic medicine*, 9th edn. Arnold, London.

Sivaloganathan S. 1985. Catheteroticum. Fatal late complication following autoerotic practice. *Am J Forensic Med Pathol* **6**:340–2.

Spence MW, Shkrum MJ, Ariss A, *et al.* 1999. Craniocervical injuries in judicial hangings: an anthropologic analysis of six cases. *Am J Forensic Med Pathol* **20**:309–22.

Thomas JE. 1969. Hyperactive carotid sinus reflex and carotid sinus syncope. *Mayo Clin Proc* **44**:127–39.

Walter PF, Crawley IS, Dorney ER. 1978. Carotid sinus hypersensitivity and syncope. *Am J Cardiol* **42**:396–403.

Wesselius CL, Bally R. 1983. A male with autoerotic asphyxia syndrome. *Am J Forensic Med Pathol* **4**:341–4.

Wright RK, Davis J. 1976. Homicidal hanging masquerading as sexual asphyxia. *J Forensic Sci* **21**:387–9.

Yada S, Tsugawa N, Uchida H. 1972. Demonstration of thyroglobulin in the heart blood in fatal cases of strangulation. *Acta Crim Jpn* **38**:60–8.

Immersion deaths

Many corpses are recovered from water, but not all have drowned. Of those that have drowned, pathological proof is often difficult or even impossible to obtain. The autopsy diagnosis of drowning presents one of the major problems in forensic medicine, especially when there is delay in recovering the victim.

Bodies retrieved from water may have:

- died from natural disease before falling into the water
- died from natural disease while already in the water
- died from injury before being thrown into the water
- died from injury while in the water
- died from effects of immersion other than drowning
- died from drowning.

All the above may show signs of immersion on examination, but this is rarely helpful, other than confirming that they had indeed been in water. It does not assist in differentiating the mode of death.

SIGNS OF IMMERSION

- Maceration of the skin begins within minutes in warm water, such as death in a bathtub, but in cold water is visible after a variable time, the minimum probably being 4 or 5 hours depending upon temperature. Polson's (1962) experience suggests a much longer time, from 12 to 48 hours, but sodden skin on the hands can undoubtedly occur much earlier than this.

The first signs tend to be on areas with an appreciable keratin layer (such as the fingertips, palms, backs of the hands and later the soles) where the surface becomes wrinkled, pale and sodden – the so-called 'washer-woman's skin', for obvious reasons. Areas protected by clothing develop these changes later than exposed parts so that the hands usually reveal more marked maceration than the feet during the first few days.

After prolonged immersion, wide areas of skin assume the same appearance, especially where the stratum corneum is thick or naturally creased, such as the extensor surface of knees and elbows. After some days in warmer water and up to several weeks in cold, the thick keratin of hands and feet becomes detached and eventually peels off in 'glove and stocking' fashion. The nails and hair become loosened at about the same time. Problems of obtaining fingerprints in such circumstances are dealt with later.

- Cutis anserina – or 'goose-flesh' – is a common finding in immersed bodies, but is related to cold rather than warm water. The erector pilae muscles attached to each hair follicle can contract in any type of death and cause a generalized pimpling of the skin. It is often stated that rigor mortis can produce this goose-flesh appearance, but this is doubtful, as rigor does not shorten muscles appreciably. From whatever cause, however, agonal contraction of the erector pilae is common and in immersed bodies has no diagnostic significance.

■ The distribution of post-mortem hypostasis is also of no value in immersed bodies. According to Bonte *et al.* (1986), electrocution in the bath seems cause the margin of hypostasis to correspond with the horizontal line of the water level (see Chapter 12). It is usual for most corpses to float or hang in the water with buttocks uppermost, and the head and limbs hanging down, but water movements often roll the body constantly unless in a placid lake or wide river. Other corpses may float upon the back, and gravitational staining of the skin may therefore be in any pattern if the body is subject to frequent changes or posture. The hypostasis of bodies from cold water is frequently pink, but this has no diagnostic value. The reddish colour is caused by the presence of unreduced oxyhaemoglobin in the superficial blood vessels and is the result of cold, whether ante-mortem or post-mortem. It may be seen in any body taken from a mortuary refrigerator or found in a cold environment, irrespective of immersion. In immersion, however, it does not have the typical distribution over extensor surfaces and large joints, nor the rather dusky tinge that is seen in true ante-mortem hypothermia.

■ Mud, coal-slurry, oil, silt or sand may be present on or in the body, as well as other artefacts such as seaweed, water weed, algae and small aquatic animal life of many types. Mud may be adherent to the whole body surface and clothing, or may be retained in the hair, mouth, nostrils, ears and other more protected sites. In appropriate circumstances, such deposits should be retained for scientific examination, if they might help establish where the body has travelled from in marine or riverine waters. Sand may be found deep in the respiratory passages and stomach, especially if the body has been rolled by the waves on a beach. Such deep penetration is not evidence of live aspiration. Where a body is decomposed and partly skeletalized, molluscs may colonize the bones. The author (BK) has had several cases recovered from the sea where mussels and barnacles filled the eye sockets and other crevices of the skull.

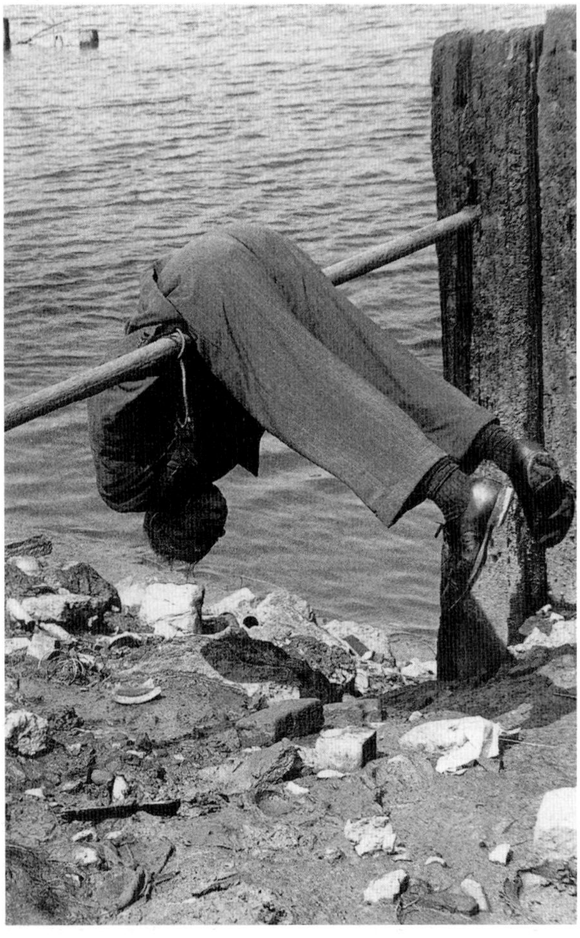

ESTIMATION OF DURATION OF IMMERSION

This is another difficult problem and one that is often too dogmatically answered by doctors with insufficient experience to appreciate the potential errors. The over-riding variable factor is water temperature, which has the most effect upon decomposition. Water pollution has little to do with speed of putrefaction, as most of the decomposing organisms come from the gut of the body itself.

FIGURE 16.1 *The diagnostic problems associated with bodies recovered from the water. In a death such as this, where a body is left by the falling tide, it may be difficult or even impossible to prove drowning, especially if the post-mortem period is long.*

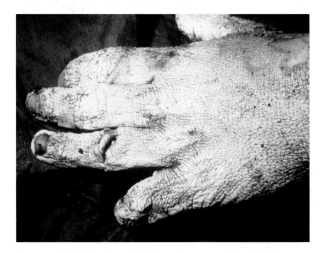

FIGURE 16.2 *Waterlogged skin ('washer-woman's hands') after 2 weeks' immersion in a temperate climate. Fingerprints can still be obtained from hands like these, with appropriate techniques.*

When a body falls into water in average temperate climates, the following is an approximate guide to timing, in conjunction with the other usual signs, such as rigor:

▪ if no wrinkling of the finger-pads is present, less than a few hours
▪ wrinkled fingers, palms and feet, progressively from half a day to 3 days
▪ early decomposition, often first in the dependent head and neck, abdomen and thighs: 4–10 days

▪ bloating of face and abdomen with marbling of veins and peeling of epidermis on hands and feet, and slippage of scalp: 2–4 weeks
▪ gross skin shedding, muscle loss with skeletal exposure, partial liquefaction: 1–2 months.

These times may be reduced or exceeded by wide margins according to animal predation, climatic changes and bodily build.

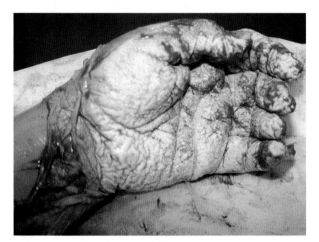

FIGURE 16.3 *Waterlogged skin after one week's immersion in a cold climate.*

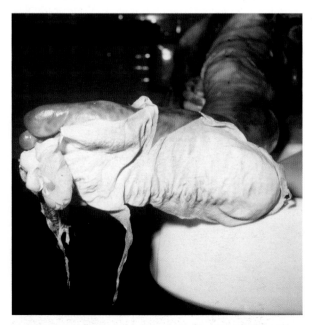

FIGURE 16.4 *Peeling of the epidermis in a 'stocking' fashion after a few weeks' immersion. The rate at which such changes occur is so variable, because of environmental factors, that no timetable can be offered to attempt to date death. In a temperate-zone summer, this stage would require at least 2 weeks and probably much longer.*

DEATH FROM NATURAL CAUSES BEFORE ENTERING THE WATER

This is relatively uncommon, but does occur. The victim may suffer one of the many causes of sudden natural death, most commonly a cardiovascular catastrophe, in circumstances where he involuntarily falls into the water. The last such instance dealt with by the author (BK) was a man returning to his yacht in a rubber dinghy, alone and in the dark. The dinghy was found empty and a search recovered the body, autopsy revealing a well-established myocardial infarct with no evidence of drowning, though the latter is never conclusive. Other instances have involved persons collapsing from natural disease while on boats, a canal tow-path or a river bank.

Of course, in the absence of witnesses it is difficult to separate such cases from those who first fall into the water and then suffer a natural death. The autopsy must be directed towards identifying the pathological lesions and to excluding, as far as is possible, any evidence of drowning.

NATURAL DEATH WHILST IN THE WATER

As discussed above, it may well be impossible to determine whether a person recovered from the water, with a potentially fatal natural disease, suffered this before or after immersion. Because of the problems (to be described later) of positively diagnosing drowning, it is difficult to exclude this as either the primary or contributory cause in someone with a lethal disease.

Cardiovascular disease is the most common reason for death in the water. A pre-existing condition may be exacerbated either by the physical exertion of swimming or struggling, or by the effects of cold. The common belief that swimming after a heavy meal is dangerous probably has some basis in fact, because of circulatory changes such as the 'splanchnic shunt'. When an acute cardiac episode occurs, such as sudden myocardial insufficiency or an arrhythmia, death may follow either from the cardiac lesion itself, or from drowning because of sudden physical incapacity.

INJURIES SUSTAINED BEFORE ENTERING THE WATER

The disposal of a murdered corpse in water is by no means uncommon, as it provides a convenient means of concealing the body, of transporting it from the scene of the crime by means of currents in river or sea, and – if discovery is delayed – of preventing identity by post-mortem decay and damage. Occasionally, accidental or suicidal injuries may be inflicted on a person before he or she enters the water. In marine, air or (rarely) road transport accidents, the victims may be injured or killed before entering the water. Persons falling from docks, bridges or ships may strike masonry or solid obstructions before hitting the water. Suicides may suffer in the same way or in exceptional circumstances, may stab themselves or cut their throats in a position where they fall into water immediately afterwards.

Whatever the means, the difficulties for the pathologist are the same, in that he must try to differentiate them from injuries sustained in the water before death occurs – and from post-mortem injuries. Often this is an impossible task, as such injuries are sustained perimortally, so that the time span involved is far too short for any of the usual criteria of ante-mortem infliction to be applied.

When the nature of the injuries is such that they could not have occurred in water, the issue is clear. Burns, missile wounds, the effect of explosions (other than compression injury) and patterned injuries may be incompatible with

infliction in water, and must therefore be related to the effects of a previous assault or some accident on board ship or aircraft.

INJURIES SUSTAINED IN THE WATER

As stated, this category is often impossible to differentiate from injuries inflicted before entering the water. Trauma in the water is common, as both an ante-mortem and a post-mortem phenomenon. Before drowning or another mode of death can supervene, the victim may be washed by waves or current against any kind of obstruction, from bridge pier to wharf, from rocks to weirs. Contact with the rough bottom of a river or a stony beach is another common cause of trauma. Damage from boats, ship's propellers, and marine or animal predators is frequent.

The issue usually becomes one of attempting to distinguish injuries sustained during life from those after death. Water complicates the problem by washing away surface bleeding from open injuries. A laceration inflicted during life will, however, usually show some bleeding into the tissues under the margins of the wound, at least until post-mortem decomposition blurs the appearances. Many decomposed bodies from water reveal green or black areas under the skin, especially in the scalp. It can be difficult or impossible to decide whether these are areas of altered blood, or merely autolytic changes. Even histological examination is often unhelpful in this respect. A similar problem exists with bruises in a decomposed body, which are often mimicked by discoloured areas of putrefaction. Post-mortem damage from animal predators is common in water and is discussed in the chapter on post-mortem changes.

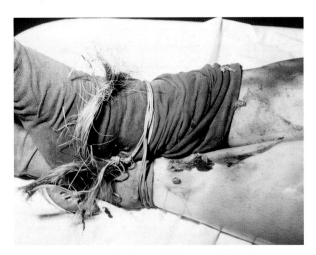

FIGURE 16.5 *Tying of the legs in a body removed from the water is suspicious, but not absolute proof of foul play. Some suicides who are good swimmers deliberately tie their legs to prevent instinctive self-preservation. In this illustration, however, the bonds were used to secure a heavy weight after homicide.*

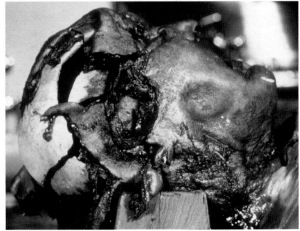

FIGURE 16.6 *Decomposed head and fractured skull of a person, who disappeared in the autumn before the river was covered with ice. The injuries have possibly been caused post-mortem by the ice packs when the body surfaced in the spring.*

In cold climates, if a body enters the cold water in late autumn, the gas formation due to putrefaction may be so slow that the sea, lake, or river will be covered with ice before the body surfaces and this takes place first in the spring when the ice is melting. In rivers, additional injuries may occur if the body gets pinned down between moving ice blocks.

Internally, there is no particular problem distinct from the examination of injured bodies in general, until post-mortem decomposition begins to obscure the appearances. This is more common in immersed bodies because of the frequent prolonged delays before the body is discovered. Bodies that have been suspended in shallow water may bear post-mortem damage from being dragged against the

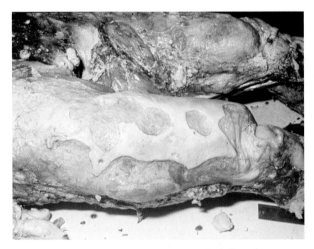

FIGURE 16.7 *Marine predator injuries on a body from the sea. The circular defects in the skin are probably made by crustaceans such as crabs.*

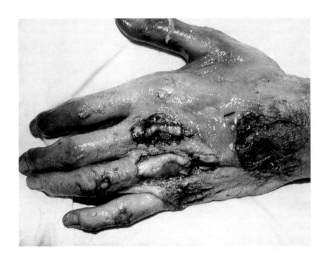

FIGURE 16.8 *Post-mortem injury to the back of the hand in a drowned person. Bodies usually hang suspended in the water with the back upwards and the knees, head and arms hanging down. In shallow water these areas may be dragged against the bottom, causing injuries similar to those shown here.*

bottom. A common posture is with the head, hands and knees hanging downwards, so that these areas (especially the backs of the hands) may suffer extensive abrasions against a rough stone or gravel bottom.

Damage from the propellers of ships and smaller boats is common in commercial waterways and where pleasure craft abound. The screw of a large vessel may inflict serious damage – even dismemberment – on a body, but more characteristic is that caused by a small, high-speed propeller, such as an outboard motor or the out-drive of a motor cruiser. These injuries are becoming more common with the increase in water-skiing, and the number of other small pleasure boats on rivers, lakes and off beaches. The characteristic lesions are parallel wounds set a few centimetres apart, often of a sliced, undercut incised nature, usually on the head or back.

DEATHS FROM IMMERSION OTHER THAN DROWNING

Irrespective of natural disease or injury, some persons who die after falling into water do not drown, in the accepted physiological sense. The great problem for the pathologist is that, even in true drowning, there may be no autopsy signs, especially if any appreciable delay has occurred before recovery or autopsy, or both. Therefore it may be difficult or impossible for him to say whether a death is a true drowning or one from the non-drowning mechanisms. All that can then be offered is that death was due to 'immersion' – and even then such a diagnosis is usually one reached by exclusion of natural disease, trauma or toxic conditions, using hearsay circumstantial evidence to arrive at a pathological diagnosis. This is why drowning and immersion deaths present one of the most difficult problems for the forensic practitioner.

In certain circumstances, death may be extremely rapid after falling into water, there being insufficient time for drowning to occur. The typical occasion is familiar to any forensic pathologist with a harbour or dockside within his area. A seaman (often the worse for drink) returns to his ship at night, misses the gangway and falls into the water. The night-watchman immediately raises the alarm and the victim is pulled from the water within a minute or two, but is dead. At autopsy, none of the typical signs of drowning are present.

Other witnessed accidents of a similar nature are relatively common, in which rapid, almost instantaneous death must be presumed, in circumstances where true drowning can be excluded by history and lack of autopsy findings. The mechanism must be attributed to a reflex cardiac arrest, of a type similar to 'vasovagal inhibition', which is discussed elsewhere. Powerful stimulation of sensitive nerve endings can induce sudden overactivity of the parasympathetic system, inducing

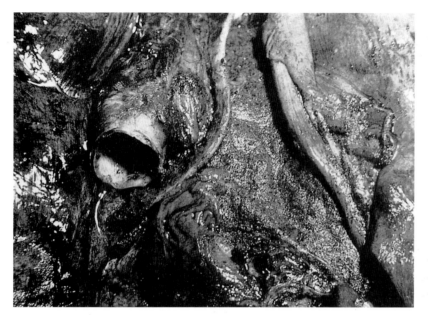

FIGURE 16.9 *The bifurcation of the trachea and main bronchi at autopsy on a body recovered from a beach. The air passages are full of sand, but this is not proof of vital aspiration of water, as foreign material can enter the bronchi by passive percolation after death.*

bradycardia and triggering cardiac arrest via the tenth cranial nerve nucleus and its vagal outflow. The afferent arc of this reflex varies from case to case, but is probably either:

- sudden immersion in cold water, causing intense stimulation of cutaneous nerve endings. Alcohol is known to potentiate such effects, perhaps by the general vasodilation of skin vessels – which would make the contrast with cold water all the more severe – and possibly by some central effects on the vasomotor centre
- sudden entry of cold water into the pharynx and larynx, and perhaps nasal passages can produce powerful stimulation of nerve endings in the mucosa. A bolus of water entering the trachea can also cause reflex cardiac arrest before there is time for airway insufficiency to have any effect.

As with any reflex cardiac arrest, there will be nothing to find at autopsy, a situation that forces this diagnosis to be speculative and based on the circumstances and exclusion of other conditions. Another mechanism that is often postulated as a cause of non-drowning immersion death is 'laryngeal spasm', leading to a hypoxic death from closure of the airway. The evidence for such a condition is tenuous, as such closure would have to operate for many minutes for hypoxia to kill, all the time keeping the larynx closed to prevent entry of water. Cyanosis is an uncommon feature of immersion deaths and in its absence it is difficult to see how laryngeal spasm could be differentiated from 'dry-lung drowning' or vasovagal cardiac arrest, the latter being a more reasonable diagnosis in those found dead after rapid recovery from the water.

Deaths in the bathtub

Fatalities in the bathroom are common, from a variety of causes, some unconnected with immersion. For example, Schmidt and Madea (1995) reported no fewer than 215 deaths in bathtubs from their Cologne Forensic Institute in 13 years, including 11 homicides.

Many suicides take place in the bathroom, from slashing of the throat or wrists, in or out of the bath. The bathroom cabinet or cupboard commonly holds razors for cutting and medicinal poisons for overdose. Electricity is more likely to be fatal in wet surroundings and a number of self-killings from electricity occur in the bathroom. Accidents include falls on slippery, wet floors or bath lining, with hard ceramic surfaces to cause head injuries.

Where gas appliances are used to heat water, the risk of carbon monoxide toxicity from faulty equipment is greater, as is also the case with electrical appliances such as hair-dryers, heaters and other devices. Although most countries have strict regulations about the electrical supply in bathrooms, people often defeat these safety measures by various means. Natural deaths from many causes may occur in the bathroom, but epileptics having unsupervised baths may have a fit and fall or drown.

Even homicide may be committed in bathrooms, by almost any means, but also from electricity and forcible immersion. The notorious multiple murders of 'The Brides in the Bath' perpetrated by George Joseph Smith early this century were probably accomplished by sudden pulling of the feet of the three women, so that their heads slid under the water. There is now a considerable literature about death in the bathtub, and all deaths in these circumstances must be investigated with particular care.

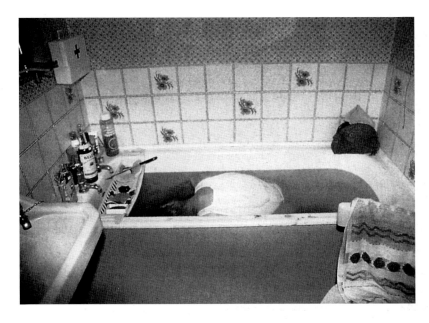

FIGURE 16.10 *Death in the bath is not uncommon and always requires careful investigation. In this case, the water is blood-stained, due to a suicidal cut throat after committing murder.*

DEATH FROM DROWNING

During the past five decades, views on the mechanism of drowning have undergone a radical change and perhaps the pendulum of opinion has swung a little too far. Until the researches stimulated by the Second World War, when large numbers of seamen and airmen were exposed to the risks of cold water, the classic view of drowning was that the victim was plunged into an airless medium and died of lack of oxygen. Following the experiments of Swann and many others (see below and references and further reading), it was recognized that, in animals, fluid and electrolyte disturbances had a major role in causing acute myocardial failure. The hypoxic element was relegated to such a secondary role that some commentators on drowning seemed to ignore the fact that the victims may have suffered 10 or more minutes without drawing a single breath of air. This criticism by no means disputes the undoubted role of fluid and electrolyte changes in drowning, but the effects of hypoxia must be considered in parallel when discussing the pathophysiology of drowning. The biochemical findings in the experimental animals did not seem to be matched by constant changes in human subjects and, in delayed and near-drowning victims, the electrolyte changes in aspiration have been shown to differ considerably from those in experimental animals.

A number of investigators long before Swann showed that blood and plasma were radically affected by drowning. In 1902, Carrara used specific gravity and other methods to demonstrate marked dilution of left heart blood in freshwater drowning and its absence in seawater, work repeated by Planck the following year with similar density techniques. Freimuth in 1955, however, used such specific

gravity methods and found similar differences in non-drowning deaths.

The classical work of Swann and his colleagues (Swann *et al.* 1947; Swann and Spafford 1951) and others was conducted on conscious dogs imprisoned in cages and immersed totally under water – which, as pointed out by Crosfill (1956), does not accurately reflect human drowning, in which submersion is intermittent at first, prolonging the process and altering the physiological effects. In summary, the findings of Swann were that in freshwater drowning there was a massive absorption of water through the alveolar membranes, which could amount to 70 per cent of the original blood volume within 3 minutes. This haemodilution caused a relative anaemia and myocardial hypoxia, as well as rapid overloading of the cardiac capacity by hypervolaemia. It was also suggested that haemolysis of red cells released potassium, a powerful myocardial toxin – yet in dogs, unlike man, sodium is the main electrolyte in the erythrocyte. In fact, because of the hypoxia and haemodilution, there was a fall in plasma potassium and sodium, which led to early ventricular fibrillation in dogs that did not occur in seawater. Such fibrillation is said to be rare in man (Rivers *et al.* 1970).

In seawater the hypertonic medium caused a withdrawal of water from the plasma into the lungs and a rise in plasma sodium concentration. This was less deleterious to heart function and helped to explain the longer survival time in seawater immersion.

Pulmonary oedema developed in both types of aqueous medium but was slight and inconstant and, where abnormal, rapidly returned to normal. Death in freshwater typically took some 4–5 minutes, whilst seawater drowning was delayed for 8–12 minutes. Occasional instances have been reported of remarkably long periods of total submersion in the sea, always in cold water where oxygen uptake is reduced: these periods may exceed 20 minutes, and at least one authenticated survival exceeded 40 minutes.

Modern commentators on the researches of Swann, such as Giamonna and Modell (1967), have pointed out the inconsistencies between animal and human responses, and emphasized the role of hypoxaemia as a result of interference with the blood–air interface in the alveoli. This once again indicates the dangers of transposing the results of animal experiments to man and poses the question of how many dogs died in vain.

THE AUTOPSY SIGNS OF DROWNING

At autopsy much depends on the delay, both in recovering the body from the water and in starting the post-mortem examination. Where a considerable period has elapsed between death and retrieval of the body, the positive signs of drowning progressively fade. Depending on temperature, a period of several days in the water is likely to minimize most changes and, once significant putrefaction has occurred, then (apart from the controversial diatom tests) there is little hope of finding positive signs of drowning.

Even when a fresh body is recovered, delay in performing the autopsy reduces the amount of evidence. The author (BK) has seen several drowned bodies soon after retrieval in which a large plume of froth has been present at the mouth, yet when commencing the autopsy several hours later, such froth had vanished and was present only in the deeper air-passages.

Froth in the air passages

The positive signs of drowning, as opposed to mere immersion, are scanty and not absolutely specific. The most useful, has just been mentioned – the presence of frothy fluid in the air passages – which in fresh bodies, often exudes though the mouth and nostrils, sometimes in the form of a plume. The froth is oedema fluid from the lungs, and consists of a proteinaceous exudate and surfactant mixed with the water of the drowning medium. It is usually white, but may be pink or red-tinged, because of slight admixture with blood from intrapulmonary bleeding. It is similar in appearance to the oedema of left ventricular failure that is commonly seen in deaths from cardiac disease such as hypertension, though some drownings exhibit a column of

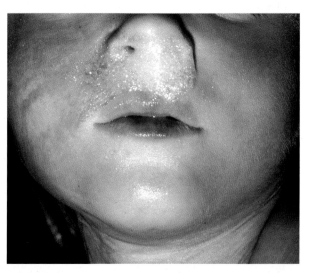

FIGURE 16.12 *Red-tinged froth exuding from the nostrils of a drowned person.*

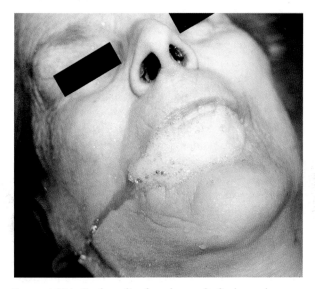

FIGURE 16.11 *Froth exuding from the mouth of a drowned person. Froth disappears with increasing post-mortem interval, though it persists in the internal air-passages for a much longer time.*

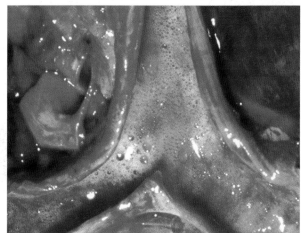

FIGURE 16.13 *Frothy fluid in the trachea and main bronchi of a person who was first strangled and subsequently fell or was thrown into sea and drowned.*

froth that is rarely, if ever, seen in natural pulmonary oedema. The froth extends into the trachea, main bronchi and smaller air passages. The lungs themselves in such cases will inevitably be waterlogged, and frothy fluid will exude from the bronchi when the lung is squeezed and from the cut surfaces when they are sectioned with a knife.

Unfortunately, although such oedema can be taken as diagnostic when combined with the appropriate circumstances and lack of other lethal pathology, the absence of waterlogging by no means excludes true drowning. The so-called 'dry-lung drowning' is not uncommon, in which the lungs appear normal in all respects, presumably because all the aspirated water has been absorbed through the alveolar walls into the plasma.

It has been suggested that this is more likely to occur if cardiac arrest takes place after removal from the water or if laryngeal spasm supervenes to prevent further water entry, so that continued circulatory function is able to clear away intra-alveolar fluid into the plasma. This theory, however, often fails to conform to the available facts of the drowning episode.

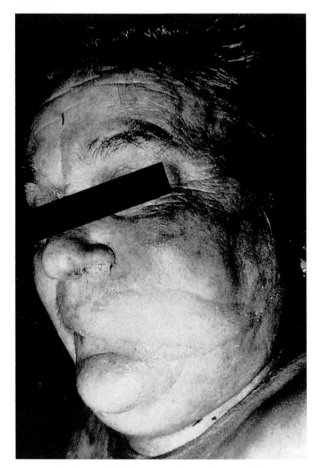

FIGURE 16.14 *Not all froth around the mouth is from drowning. This lady died in bed from hypertensive heart disease with profuse pulmonary oedema.*

Copeland (1985) measured lung weight in non-drowning deaths and deaths from salt-water and freshwater drowning. There was no significant difference in the weights of the last two, though 10–20 per cent of undoubted drownings were 'dry-lung' cases with no excess weight. Generally, the weights of a lung in drowning were around 600–700 g, whilst the non-drowned were in the 370–540 g range – though there was a considerable overlap in the two groups. The lung weights were also studied by Kringsholm *et al.* (1991) who claimed that the duration of submersion is related to lung weight. They found that 7 per cent of cases were 'dry-lung drownings' with a combined lung weight of less than a kilogram. In the remainder, the average weight of both lungs was 1411 g, compared to 994 g in controls. This was where the body was in the water less than 24 hours. After this, lung weight decreased, but pleural transudate increased. By combining the weight of lungs and transudate, more than 75 per cent of the cases lay between 1000 and 2200 g, up to 30 days.

Overinflation of the lungs

Apart from generalized waterlogging, the lungs may be markedly overinflated, filling the thoracic cavity when the sternum is removed. The normally bare area over the heart may be covered and the lungs may bulge upwards, meeting in the midline to obliterate the anterior mediastinum. The texture is rather pale and crepitant, superficially resembling that shown in asthma – for the same reasons. The older name for this condition is 'emphysema aquosum'. True pre-existing emphysema may partially mimic the distension of drowning, but in the latter, bullae are never present. The oedema fluid in the bronchi blocks the passive collapse that normally occurs at death, holding the lungs in the inspiratory position. In addition, there is often an element of over-distension caused by the valvular action of the bronchial obstruction – again similar to asthma. In drowning this may be sufficient to mark the lateral surfaces of the lungs with the impression of the ribs, leaving visible and palpable grooves after removal of the organs from the thorax. This may be one of the most valuable positive signs of drowning to be gained at autopsy.

There may be some areas of intrapulmonary haemorrhage, which give the red tinge to the oedema fluid. These areas are seldom large or intense, and the general oedema and distension tend to minimize their prominence. Some may lie near the pleural surface and can be seen as rather blurred blotches on the exterior of the lung, the blurring being partly the result of spreading haemolysis. There are almost never subpleural petechial haemorrhages in drowning, apart from the few non-specific spots that can be found in the fissures and around the hilum in virtually every autopsy, no matter what the cause of death.

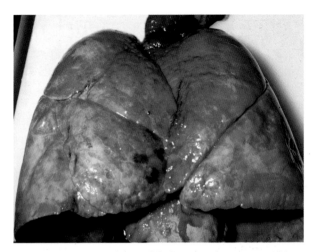

FIGURE 16.15 *Overinflation of the lungs (emphysema aquosum) in drowning with overlapping of the anterior margins and haemorrhages in the right middle lobe.*

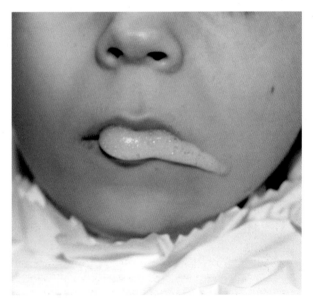

FIGURE 16.16 *A typical plume of froth from the mouth of a recently drowned boy. This will vanish as the post-mortem interval extends.*

Other organs in drowning

There are no other reliable autopsy changes in drowning. The heart and great veins have often been said to be 'dilated and engorged with fluid blood, especially the right side', but this is such a subjective and non-specific finding as to be useless, meriting no further consideration.

Many pathologists have for centuries claimed that the blood remains more fluid in drowning, and the physiological researchers of this century have confirmed the haemodilution in freshwater drowning. As a gross sign at autopsy, however, it is totally subjective and unreliable.

The stomach may contain watery fluid or even foreign material from the water, such as silt, weed or sand, but this cannot be accepted as a positive aid to the diagnosis. Many undoubted drownings show no water in the stomach, yet other cases in which a dead body was immersed reveal copious water in the stomach. The limiting factor is the tone in the oesophagus and cardiac sphincter, not the drowning process. The same applies to foreign materials in the trachea. Haemorrhage into the middle ears has been postulated as a positive sign of drowning, but in the author's (BK) own experience, it is totally unreliable. It can occur in any type of death where drowning can be definitely excluded, yet in classic instances of drowning, such bleeding may be absent. It has been said to be related to the depth to which the body sinks because of the hydrostatic pressure within the ear, but even this does not accord with the experience of most pathologists (Niles 1963).

CHEMICAL CHANGES IN THE BLOOD IN DROWNING

Because of the marked haemodilution that occurs in freshwater drowning and the electrolyte shifts in salt-water drowning, it is reasonable to expect that chemical analyses of the plasma should provide reliable evidence of drowning. Unfortunately, these theoretical hopes have not been realized in practice, mainly because of the biochemical chaos that occurs soon after death from any cause, in which the ability of live cell membranes to partition fluid and electrolytes is rapidly lost. Gettler (1921) published results of analyses of chloride content from the left and right sides of the heart, suggesting that the haemodilution from freshwater drowning would differentially reduce the plasma concentration on the left side, a difference of 25 mg/100 ml being significant. Salt-water drowning was said to produce the opposite effect. Gettler's claims have often been refuted and they are now no longer accepted. It has been shown that post-mortem changes in blood chloride concentrations occur irrespective of drowning and that the rate of change may be different on each side of the heart. Even the differentiation between freshwater and seawater drowning was discredited by the work of Durlacher *et al.* (1953), who found no reliable changes in sodium, potassium and chloride concentration. Similar results were found by Fuller (1963).

Electrolyte measurements in surviving victims of near-drowning showed no regular pattern, according to Rivers *et al.* (1970). Moritz (1944) attempted to use magnesium

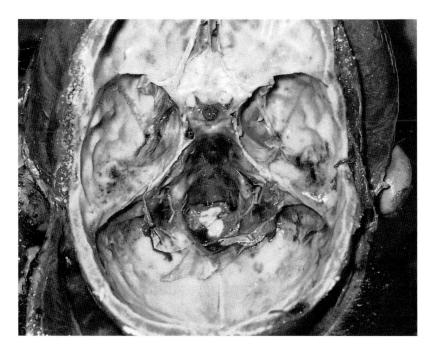

FIGURE 16.17 *Bilateral haemorrhages within the petrous temporal bones in drowning. Though claims have been made for the usefulness of this observation, its occurrence seems random, sometimes being present in non-drowning and absent in proven drowning.*

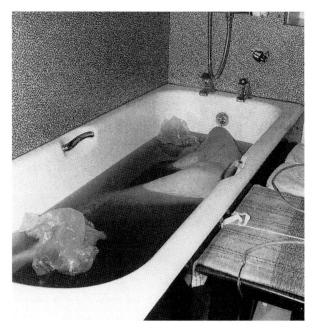

FIGURE 16.18 *Suicide in the bath. The head was enveloped in a plastic bag and an (unused) electrocution device was also present, illustrating the frequent presence of alternative methods in suicide.*

as a similar marker in drowning, but the unreliability of such analyses has prevented their being used as a routine procedure. Once again, the hazards of extrapolating the results of animal experiments to humans is highlighted by these results, as even other mammals like dogs have quite different responses to the same environmental changes.

Other chemical substances have been used as markers of drowning, such as strontium. Azparren *et al.* (1994) claim that differences in the strontium concentration of blood from left and right heart are always greater than 75 µg/l in seawater drowning.

HISTOLOGICAL CHANGES IN DROWNING

Much has been written about both light and electron microscopy of the lungs in immersion deaths, especially in continental Europe. The accounts are confusing, however, and sometimes contradictory, the consensus of opinion being that such changes are inconstant and unreliable.

Much of the work has tried to confirm histologically the genuineness of 'emphysema aquosum' in both fresh and decayed bodies, but the dilatation and rupture of the terminal air spaces can occur not only as a result of drowning, but of passive immersion in water deeper than 4 m. Dilatation of the alveoli, thinning of the walls and compression of the capillaries are easy to observe, but the significance is always ambiguous. Reh (1976) classified such lungs on the basis of reticulin fibres, but Heinen and Dotzauer (1973) showed similar changes in undrowned material. Janssen (1984) has reviewed the subject and concludes that though histological evidence may be helpful and indicative, it is never probative.

The number of macrophages in the alveoli, adjusted to the size of the alveoli where distended, was studied by Betz *et al.* (1993), who claimed a diagnostic usefulness of the method as long as no autolytic changes were present.

The weight of the spleen has been used by Haffner *et al.* (1994) as a diagnostic marker in drowning. Compared with other modes of 'asphyxia', about an 18 per cent reduction in weights and spleen–liver ratios was recorded, with a suggestion that stress, hypoxia, alcohol and cooling were responsible.

The skin changes in maceration are also well recorded, and some have been claimed to have use in dating the period of immersion (Okros 1938; Dierkes 1938). Schleyer (1951) is pessimistic on the reliability of such histological criteria.

The early formation of adipocere can be detected microscopically after 3–4 weeks; this is dealt with in the chapter on post-mortem changes.

DIATOMS AND THE DIAGNOSIS OF DROWNING

Few topics in forensic pathology have given rise to so much argument as the use of diatoms in the diagnosis of drowning.

Revenstorf in 1904 was the first to attempt to use diatoms as a test for drowning, though he stated that Hofmann in 1896 was the first to discover them in lung fluid. An excellent review of the diatom controversy was published by Peabody in 1980.

The basic premise is that when a live person is drowned in water containing diatoms (microscopic algae with a silicaceous exoskeleton), many diatoms will penetrate the alveolar walls and be carried to distant target organs such as brain, kidney, liver, and bone marrow. After autopsy, samples of these organs can be digested with strong acid to dissolve the soft tissue, thus leaving the highly resistant diatom skeletons to be identified under the microscope. Alternatively, blood can be used to seek the organisms.

When a dead body is deposited in water or when death in the water is not due to drowning, then, although diatoms may reach the lungs by passive percolation, the absence of a beating heart prevents circulation of diatoms to distant organs.

The great advantage of the diatom test, if it was reliable, would be that a positive diagnosis of drowning could be

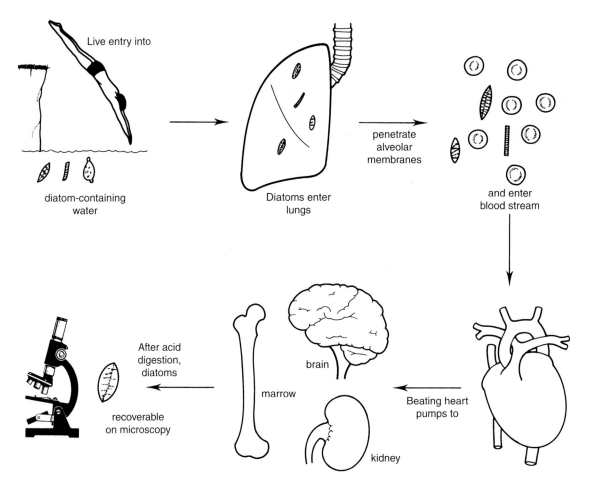

Live entry into

diatom-containing water

Diatoms enter lungs

penetrate alveolar membranes

and enter blood stream

Beating heart pumps to

brain

kidney

marrow

After acid digestion, diatoms

recoverable on microscopy

FIGURE 16.19 *The principle of the diatom test for drowning. When a dead body enters the water, diatoms cannot progress further than the lungs.*

made even in the frequently putrefied bodies that are recovered, where no hope of anatomical recognition of drowning is possible. In addition, evidence of the site of the drowning might be obtained from the ecological typing of the diatoms, especially in relation to salt-water or freshwater locations.

Meticulous attention to technique must be employed at autopsy to recover suitable samples of tissue, which must not be contaminated by the body surface or instruments, before digestion is commenced. (Technical details are given in Appendix 1.)

Diatoms belong to the class of plants known as *Diatomaceae* and consist of a box or 'frustule' composed of two valves that fit together to enclose the cytoplasmic contents. They have either radial symmetry ('centric' diatoms) or are elongated ('pennate' diatoms). The valves are highly complex in shape and are extremely resistant to decay, fossil diatoms from Jurassic times being abundant. The floor of the oceans have an area of 11 million square miles of thick diatomaceous ooze and upraised beds on land may be hundreds of feet thick, which emphasizes the vast amount of potential contaminant available.

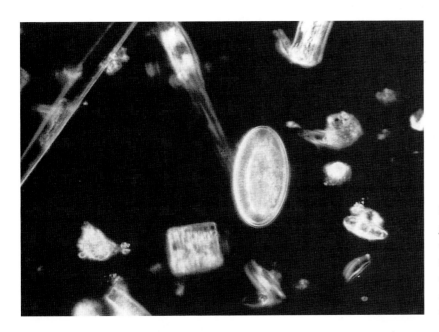

FIGURE 16.20 *Diatoms seen under dark-ground illumination (original magnification ×350). These are from fresh water. There are at least 10 000 different types and, where identification of locus of likely origin is required, the help of a biologist with expert knowledge is essential.*

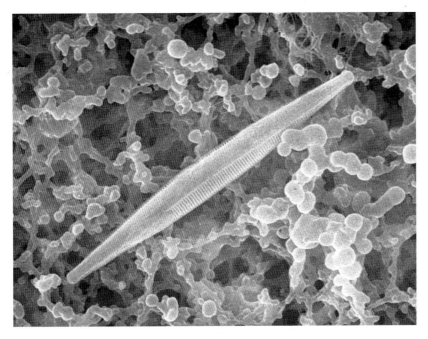

FIGURE 16.21 *Scanning electron micrograph of a diatom (original magnification ×4000, 20 kV).*

There are at least 10 000 species, and the identification of the various types is a matter for an experienced botanist or biologist, but the following general classification is useful: 'oligohalophilic' diatoms live in freshwater with a salinity less than 0.05 per cent, and 'mesohalophilic' and 'polyhalophilic' diatoms live in brackish water and seawater with a salinity higher than 0.05 per cent.

The critics of the diatom test point to certain problems:

■ Diatoms are ubiquitous, being present in soil, water supplies and in the air. Many commonly used minerals, such as kieselguhr, are largely fossil diatoms. Manufactured substances like board-chalk and abrasives – even toothpaste – contain diatomaceous raw materials. Mant, however, examined the filters of the air-conditioning system of Guy's Hospital in London and found no diatoms taken from the city atmosphere.

■ Though entry into the body is thought to be mainly through the lungs, there seems no reason why they cannot penetrate the intestinal lining, and gain access to the bloodstream and hence any body tissues.

■ Certain foods, notably shellfish, contain vast quantities of diatoms that may enter the circulation and reach the tissues.

■ Examination of the tissues of both animals and man reveal the presence of diatoms when the cause of death is other than drowning. Schellmann and Sperl (1979) found them in the tissues of 15 out of 16 non-drowned bodies, but other workers found no diatoms in 33 out of 34 bodies, including two drownings.

Foged (1983) made a detailed investigation into drowned and non-drowned bodies in Denmark, and concluded that the diatom test was quite invalid. He quoted many references both for and against the reliability of the technique, and no doubt the controversy will continue. It seems probable that there may be a quantitative difference between the numbers of diatoms recovered from the tissues in drowning and non-drowning deaths, and a careful analysis of the species identification in relation to the locus and circumstances of the death may be useful. At the present time the diatom test should be used only as an indicative aid and not as legal proof of drowning. Recently, other water organisms have been advocated as tests for drowning, including soft-bodied protozoa and crustaceans.

Japanese workers have used other methods to digest autopsy tissues to seek diatoms because it has been shown that strong acid digestion markedly reduces the yield. The new methods introduced for diatoms, such as enzymatic and detergent digestion, allowed soft-bodied microscopic organisms to be recovered and claims for better specificity for drowning have been made (Matsumoto and Fukui 1993; Funayama *et al.* 1987, 2001). Chinese workers have claimed that the spectrofluorophotometric detection in the lungs of chlorophyll derived from plankton is diagnostic, but it is not clear how this can be differentiated from plankton passively entering the lungs after death (Qu and Wang 1992).

REFERENCES AND FURTHER READING

Auer A, Mottonen M. 1988. Diatoms and drowning. *Z Rechtsmed* **101**:87–98.

Azparren J, de la Rosa I, Sancho M. 1994. Biventricular measurement of blood strontium in real cases of drowning. *Forensic Sci Int* **69**:139–48.

Betz P, Nerlich A, Penning R, *et al.* 1993. Alveolar macrophages and the diagnosis of drowning. *Forensic Sci Int* **62**:217–24.

Bhaskar GR. 1965. Diatoms in cases of drowning. *J Indian Acad Forensic Sci* **4**:2–6.

Bonilla-Santiago J, Fill WL. 1978. Sand aspiration in drowning and near drowning. *Radiology* **128**:301–2.

Bonte W, Sprung R, Huckenbeck W. 1986. [Problems in the evaluation of electrocution fatalities in the bathtub.] Probleme bei der Beurteilungen von Stromtodesfällen in der Badewanne. *Z Rechtsmed* **97**:7–9.

Bray M. 1985. Chemical estimation of fresh water immersion intervals. *Am J Forensic Med Pathol* **6**:133–9.

Budnick LD. 1984. Bathtub-related electrocutions in the United States, 1979 to 1982. *JAMA* **252**:918–20.

Budnick LD, Ross DA. 1985. Bathtub-related drownings in the United States, 1979–81. *Am J Public Health* **75**:630–3.

Byard RW, Lipsett J. 1999. Drowning deaths in toddlers and preambulatory children in South Australia. *Am J Forensic Med Pathol* **20**:328–32.

Carrara M. 1902. Electrolytes and osmotic pressure in drowning. *Vrtlschr Gericht Med* **24**:236–40.

Chiaraviglio E, del Carmen, Wolf AV. 1963. Diagnosis of drowning. *Arch Pathol* **75**:337.

Copeland AR. 1985. An assessment of lung weights in drowning cases. The metro Dade County experience from 1978 to 1982. *Am J Forensic Med Pathol* **6**:301–4.

Copeland AR. 1986. Homicidal drowning. *Forensic Sci Int* **31**:247–52.

Copeland AR. 1987. Suicide by drowning. *Am J Forensic Med Pathol* **8**:18–22.

Coutselinis A, Boukis D. 1976. The estimation of Mg^{2+} concentration in cerebrospinal fluid (C.S.F.) as a method of drowning diagnosis in sea water. *Forensic Sci* **7**:109–11.

Crosfill JW. 1956. Mechanism of drowning. *Proc R Soc Med* **49**:1051–4.

Davis JH. 1961. Fatal underwater breath holding in trained swimmers. *J Forensic Sci* **6**:391–6.

Davis JH. 1986. Bodies found in the water. An investigative approach. *Am J Forensic Med Pathol* **7**:291–7.

Devos C, Timperman J, Piette M. 1985. Deaths in the bath. *Med Sci Law* **25**:189–200.

Dierkes K. 1938. Über die Histologie der Waschhaut. *Dtsch Z Gesamte Gerichtl Med* **30**:262.

Durlacher S, Freimuth H, Swan H. 1953. Blood changes in man following drowning. *Arch Pathol* **56**:454–60.

Durwald W. 1964. Elektrotodesfälle in der Badewanne. *Arch Kriminol* **134**:164–71.

Foged N. 1983. Diatoms and drowning – once more. *Forensic Sci Int* **21**:153–9.

Fornes P, Pepin G, Heudes D, *et al.* 1998. Diagnosis of drowning by combined computer-assisted histomorphometry of lungs with blood strontium determination. *J Forensic Sci* **43**:772–6.

Foroughi E. 1971. Serum changes in drowning. *J Forensic Sci* **16**:269–82.

Fukui Y, Hata M, Takahashi S, *et al.* 1980. A new method for detecting diatoms in human organs. *Forensic Sci Int* **16**:67–74.

Fuller RH. 1963. The clinical pathology of human near-drowning. *Proc R Soc Med* **56**:33–8.

Funayama M, Aoki Y, Sebetan IM, *et al.* 1987. Detection of diatoms in blood by a combination of membrane filtering and chemical digestion. *Forensic Sci Int* **34**:175–82.

Funayama M, Mimasaka S, Nata M, *et al.* 2001. Diatom numbers around the continental shelf break. *Am J Forensic Med Pathol* **22**:236–8.

Gardner E. 1944. Death in the bathroom. *Med Leg Criminol Rev* **12**:180–95.

Geertinger P, Voigt J. 1970. Death in the bath. A survey of bathtub deaths in Copenhagen, Denmark, and Gothenburg, Sweden, from 1961 to 1969. *J Forensic Med* **17**:136–47.

Gettler AO. 1921. A method for the determination of death by drowning. *JAMA* **77**:1650–2.

Giammona ST, Modell JH. 1967. Drowning by total immersion. Effects on pulmonary surfactant of distilled water, isotonic saline, and sea water. *Am J Dis Child* **114**:612–16.

Goldhahn RT. 1977. *Scuba diving deaths; a review and approach for the pathologist.* In: Wecht C (ed.), *Legal medicine annual 1976.* Appleton Century Crofts, New York.

Gooden BA. 1972. Drowning and the diving reflex in man. *Med J Aust* **59**:583–7.

Gordon I. 1972. The anatomical signs in drowning. A critical evaluation. *Forensic Sci* **1**:389–95.

Gruspier KL, Pollanen MS. 2000. Limbs found in water: investigation using anthropological analysis and the diatom test. *Forensic Sci Int* **112**:1–9.

Haffner HT, Graw M, Erdelkamp J. 1994. Spleen findings in drowning. *Forensic Sci Int* **66**:95–104.

Heinen M, Dotzauer G. 1973. [The lung of a drowned person.] *Beitr Gerichtl Med* **30**:133–41.

Hendey NI. 1973. The diagnostic value of diatoms in cases of drowning. *Med Sci Law* **13**:23–34.

Holden HS, Crosfill JW. 1955. The significance of foreign bodies in the alveoli of the apparently drowned. *J Forensic Med* **2**:141–50.

Hurlimann J, Feer P, Elber F, *et al.* 2000. Diatom detection in the diagnosis of death by drowning. *Int J Legal Med* **114**:6–14.

Jääskeläinen A. 1967. Diatomenbefunde in Wasserleichen. *Dtsch Z Gesamte Gerichtl Med* **61**:41–7.

Janssen W. 1984. *Forensic histopathology.* Springer, Heidelberg, Germany.

Karkola K, Neittaanmaki H. 1981. Diagnosis of drowning by investigation of left heart blood. *Forensic Sci Int* **18**:149–53.

Knight B. 1981. Immersion or drowning? *Br Med J* **282**:1340–1.

Kobayashi M, Yamada Y, Zhang WD, *et al.* 1993. Novel detection of plankton from lung tissue by enzymatic digestion method. *Forensic Sci Int* **60**:81–90.

Koseki T. 1969. Investigations on the bone marrow as a material in the diatom method diagnosing of death from drowning. *Acta Med Biol* **16**:88–90.

Kringsholm B, Filskov A, Kock K. 1991. Autopsied cases of drowning in Denmark 1987–1989. *Forensic Sci Int* **52**:85–92.

Kvittingen TD, Naess A. 1963. Recovery from drowning in fresh water. *Br Med J* **1**:1315–16.

Lucas J, Goldfeder LB, Gill JR. 2002. Bodies found in the waterways of New York City. *J Forensic Sci* **47**:137–41.

Ludes B, Coste M, North N, *et al.* 1999. Diatom analysis in victim's tissues as an indicator of the site of drowning. *Int J Legal Med* **112**:163–6.

Matsumoto H, Fukui Y. 1993. A simple method for diatom detection in drowning. *Forensic Sci Int* **60**:91–5.

Mikami Y. 1959. Experimental study and practice on the detection of vegetable planktons in the bone marrow of the drowned dead body. *Acta Med Okayama* **13**:259–67.

Modell JH. 1968. The pathophysiology and treatment of drowning. *Acta Anaesthesiol Scand Suppl* **29**:263–79.

Modell JH. 1971. *Drowning and near-drowning.* Thomas, Springfield, USA.

Modell JH. 1978. Biology of drowning. *Annu Rev Med* **29**:1–8.

Modell JH, Davis JH. 1969. Electrolyte changes in human drowning victims. *Anesthesiology* **30**:414–20.

Monantay NK, Rao RD. 1964. The diagnosis of death from drowning with particular reference to 'diatom method'. *J Indian Acad Forensic Sci* **3**:21–7.

Moritz AR. 1944. Chemical methods for the determination of death by drowning. *Physiol Rev* **24**:70–88.

Mueller WF. 1969. Pathology of temporal bone hemorrhage in drowning. *J Forensic Sci* **14**:327–36.

Niles NR. 1963. Haemorrhage in the middle ear and mastoid in drowning. *Am J Clin Pathol* **40**:281–4.

Ohlsson K, Beckman N. 1964. Drowning – reflections based on two cases. *Acta Chir Scand* **128**:327–31.

Okros S. 1938. Annähernde Bestimmung der Todeszeit aus dem Hautzustand. *Dtsch Z Gesamte Gerichtl Med* **29**:497.

Pachar JV, Cameron JM. 1993. The diagnosis of drowning by quantitative and qualitative diatom analysis. *Med Sci Law* **33**:291–9.

Peabody AJ. 1980. Diatoms and drowning – a review. *Med Sci Law* **20**:254–61.

Peabody AJ. 1986. *Drowning cases: a protocol for their submission.* CRE, Aldermaston.

Pearn J. 1985. Pathophysiology of drowning. *Med J Aust* **142**:586–8.

Pearn J, Nixon J. 1977. Bathtub immersion accidents involving children. *Med J Aust* **64**:211–13.

Pearn JH, Brown JD, Wong R, *et al.* 1979. Bathtub drownings: report of seven cases. *Pediatrics* **64**:68–70.

Pollanen MS. 1998. Diatoms and homicide. *Forensic Sci Int* **91**:29–34.

Polson CJ. 1962. *Essentials of forensic medicine.* Pergamon Press, Oxford.

Qu J, Wang E. 1992. A study on the diagnosis of drowning by examination of lung chlorophyll(a) of planktons with a spectrofluorophotometer. *Forensic Sci Int* **53**:149–55.

Reh H. 1976. [About the problem of 'lungs in drowning' (author's transl).] *Z Rechtsmed* **77**:219–21.

Rivers J, Orr G, Lee H. 1970. Electrolytes in near-drowning. *Br Med J* **2**:157–60.

Rushton DG. 1961. Drowning – a review. *Med Leg J* **29**:90–8.

Schellmann B, Sperl W. 1979. [Detection of diatoms in bone marrow (femur) of nondrowned (author's transl).] *Z Rechtsmed* **83**:319–24.

Schleyer F. 1951. Zur Histologie der Waschhaut. *Dtsch Z Gesamte Gerichtl Med* **40**:680.

Schmidt P, Madea B. 1995. Homicide in the bathtub. *Forensic Sci Int* **72**:135–46.

Schmidt P, Madea B. 1995. Death in the bathtub involving children. *Forensic Sci Int* **72**:147–55.

Schneider V. 1985. [Electrocution in the bathtub.] *Arch Kriminol* **176**:89–95.

Schwar TG. 1972. Drowning: its chemical diagnosis. A review. *Forensic Sci* **1**:411–17.

Schwerd W, Lautenbach L. 1960. Mord mit elektrischem Strom in der Badewanne. *Arch Kriminol* **54**:126–49.

Sidari L, Di Nunno N, Costantinides F, *et al.* 1999. Diatom test with soluene-350 to diagnose drowning in sea water. *Forensic Sci Int* **103**:61–5.

Spitz W, Schneider V. 1964. The significance of diatoms in the diagnosis of death by drowning. *J Forensic Sci* **9**:11–18.

Sturner WQ, Balko A, Sullivan J. 1976. Magnesium and other electrolytes in bovine eyeballs immersed in sea water and other fluids. *Forensic Sci* **8**:139–50.

Swann HG. 1956. Mechanism of circulatory failure in fresh water and sea water drowning. *Circ Res* **4**:241–2.

Swann HG, Spafford NR. 1951. Body salt and water changes during fresh and sea water drowning. *Tex Rep Biol Med* **9**:356–62.

Swann HG, Brucer M, Moore C, *et al.* 1947. Fresh water and sea water drowning: a study of terminal cardiac and biochemical events. *Tex Rep Biol Med* **5**:423–37.

Terazawa K, Takatori T. 1980. Isolation of intact plankton from drowning lung tissue by centrifugation in a colloidal silica gradient. *Forensic Sci Int* **16**:63–6.

Thomas F, Van Hecke W, Timperman J. 1961. The detection of diatoms in the bone marrow. *J Forensic Med* **8**:142–4.

Thomas F, Van Hecke W, Timperman J. 1962. [Medicolegal diagnosis of death by submersion by demonstration of diatoms in the marrow of the long bones.] *Ann Med Leg (Paris)* **42**:369–73.

Timperman J. 1962. The detection of diatoms in the marrow of the sternum. *J Forensic Med* **9**:134–6.

Timperman J. 1969. Medico-legal problems in death by drowning. Its diagnosis by the diatom method. A study based on investigations carried out in Ghent over a period of 10 years. *J Forensic Med* **16**:45–75.

Timperman J. 1972. The diagnosis of drowning. A review. *Forensic Sci* **1**:397–409.

Trubner K, Püschel K. 1991. [Fatalities in the bathtub.] Todesfälle in der Badewanne. *Arch Kriminol* **188**:35–46.

CHAPTER 17

Neglect, starvation and hypothermia

Though, tragically, starvation is one of the most widespread scourges of our planet, we are here concerned with individual neglect with which starvation is often associated, either as a potentially criminal act or as a manifestation of self-neglect. As with so many conditions, the extremes of life are most affected, rather than the middle years. Infants and children are at the mercy of their parents or guardians for the provision of care and sustenance. The old are prey to senile dementias and other disorders of the mind, as well as often being devoid of spouse or caring relatives – or sometimes even the financial means to stay warm and adequately fed.

Many countries have legislation designed to protect children, on the basis that they are totally dependent upon adults for the necessities of life. In Britain, the Children Act places a responsibility upon parents, guardians or the community to care for children. The minimum requirements laid down by law are the provision of food, clothing, shelter and education. Unfortunately, these requirements are evaded in spite of official supervision and, from time to time, scandals explode in the public eye when a child has died, not from physical abuse, but from sheer neglect.

Voluntary organizations, such as the National Society for the Prevention of Cruelty to Children (NSPCC) were founded in the nineteenth century to combat the widespread neglect of children consequent upon the population explosion of the Victorian industrial revolution. Their present-day role, however, has changed radically so that now most of their efforts are directed against physical, sexual and mental abuse, rather than starvation and neglect. Notwithstanding this change of emphasis, deaths still occur from deliberate or negligent lack of provision of proper care

and nutrition of children. In general – though there are many exceptions – nutritional neglect and physical battering tend to be mutually exclusive. The abused child is usually well nourished and the emaciated child is usually uninjured.

Neglect and starvation are not synonymous, but are so often closely associated that the two conditions are usually considered together. When fatal, they may come to the attention of the pathologist either as a potentially criminal death or, when self-inflicted, in the usual course of coroners' or similar enquiries. Rarely, victims will starve from being isolated in some catastrophe, such as a mining incarceration or shipwreck, but these days a more common occurrence is a hunger strike or voluntary fast for some political or similar motive.

GENERAL FEATURES OF NEGLECT AND STARVATION

The obvious and outstanding appearance is of emaciation caused by an inadequate intake of food. A minimum of about 1500–1900 calories is needed to maintain body weight in active adults. Life is threatened when more than 40 per cent of the original body weight has been lost, though the speed of loss is relevant. Total deprivation of food will obviously kill faster than a severe reduction. Total lack of food is likely to cause death in about 50–60 days as long as adequate water is available, but this depends on weather and temperature as well as the original fitness – and fatness – of the individual. Deprivation of water will kill in about 10 days – or less in higher ambient temperatures.

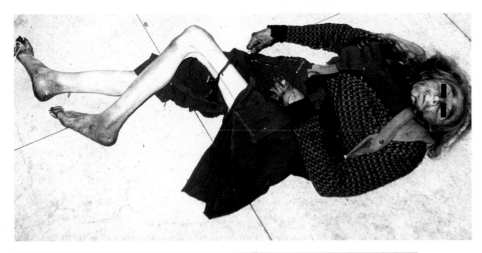

FIGURE 17.1 *Death from neglect and hypothermia in an old woman. The discoloration of the feet and hands was cyanotic.*

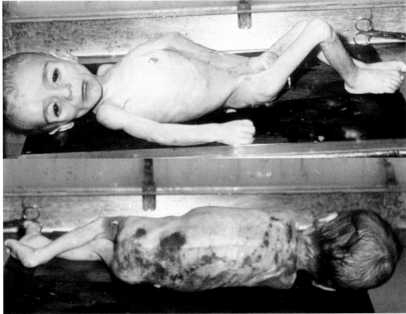

FIGURE 17.2 *Fatal neglect and starvation in an infant. The limbs are emaciated, the abdomen scaphoid and the head appears relatively large. The back shows extensive pressure ulceration. The sunken eyes and cheeks from malnutrition and dehydration constitute the 'Hippocratic facies'.*

In the numerous cases of fatal and non-fatal starvation seen at the end of the 1939–45 war in Nazi concentration camps, two main types were seen. These were the 'dry' type, in which there was emaciation, but only leg oedema, with a body weight up to half the normal. Alive, these showed marked hypotension, feeble pulse and cyanosis. The other 'wet' group had marked oedema of face, trunk and limbs, with ascites and pleural effusions. The oedema of hypoproteinaemia is caused by protein being diverted to produce energy when carbohydrate and fat are grossly deficient in the diet. In some victims, the skeleton accounted for 50 per cent of the total body weight, instead of the usual 15 per cent.

Other features are secondary to this nutritional deficiency, such as intercurrent infections, avitaminoses, skin disorders and nutritional oedema. Dehydration, hypothermia and actual necrosis of the extremities are the most severe manifestations that contribute to death.

Most fatally neglected infants are under one year of age. At autopsy great care must be taken to measure, not estimate, the full indices of size and weight. Crown–heel, crown–rump, head diameter, foot length and exact weight must be measured accurately, so that comparison may be made with standard paediatric percentile growth charts, consonant with age, birth weight, sex and race.

The diameter of limbs at major landmarks such as wrists and ankle should be measured with a flexible tape. Photographs should be taken in all major views, using colour to record skin tints and lesions, as well as the general aspect of the emaciated body. The words 'cachexia', 'emaciation' and 'marasmus' are all synonymous as used today, though 'marasmus' is confined to the description of infant victims. The so-called 'Hippocratic facies' is not confined to the emaciation of neglect, as cachexia from any cause – such as an obstructive carcinoma of the oesophagus – can give rise to the same appearance. The skin of the face is stretched tightly across the cheekbones, the cheeks are sunken and the lines of the jaw are obtrusive. The eyes are deeply sunken from loss of orbital fat, though dehydration may contribute to this manifestation.

On the trunk the ribs are prominent, with concavities in the intercostal spaces and sunken supraclavicular fossae. The abdomen is of the classical 'scaphoid' shape, being concave from costal margin to iliac crests, the latter sticking up like wings. The limbs are almost skeletal from loss of fat and muscle, and the head may appear deceptively large by contrast with the narrowed neck.

The skin surface may present differing appearances according to the length of time that nutritional loss has been suffered and the qualitative defect in the diet, especially of certain vitamins. The skin may be pale, lustrous and semi-translucent, with an almost blue tinge in infants, partly as a result of the loss of subcutaneous fat. It may also be coarse and rough, however, with flaking hyperkeratosis, though this is more often seen in aged persons, partly as a result of senile changes. Pigmentation, either diffuse or of a punctate nature, is sometimes seen.

Dehydration is a common feature, especially in infants and may be the major contribution to death. The skin is dry and wrinkled and, when pinched between the fingers, remains ridged because of loss of subcutaneous fat and fluid. The fontanelles may be depressed from loss of pressure of cerebrospinal fluid. In chronic starvation, hypoproteinaemia can lead to oedema, though this is rarely seen in forensic practice. In famines it may be widespread, associated with other nutritional disorders such as kwashiorkor.

Skin infections are common, partly as a result of nutritional loss of resistance to infections and partly because of neglect in care and hygiene, especially in infants. Pressure sores on buttocks, heels and spine may occur in both infants and old people who are lying inert because of weakness, and, in infants, urine dermatitis and lack of any skin care after defecation worsens these. Sores may be seen on any pressure or friction points, such as the elbows, knees, shoulders and occiput. Apart from pressure areas, any part of the skin surface may develop infected lesions, which often crust over after partial healing. Sores on the lips, blepharitis and conjunctivitis may also occur. The hair is dry and brittle, sometimes becoming depigmented and even gingery with chronic malnutrition.

Internally, the same loss of adipose tissue will be evident both subcutaneously and in the internal fat stores, such as the omentum, mesentery and perirenal area. The organs will be small (except the brain) and it is therefore important to weigh the major viscera to compare them with standard tables for sex and age. Organ atrophy will be more apparent in old people, but the problem then exists of distinguishing weight loss caused by nutritional defects from the usual senile atrophy. The differentiation is one of degree, as chronic starvation can reduce organs to unusually low weights. More specific internal signs will include an empty gut, which may be gas-filled and translucent from stomach to colon. Any faeces in the rectum are likely to be inspissated, especially if there has been fluid restriction and dehydration. Faecoliths may ulcerate the intestinal lining. In infant starvation, however, the stools may be fluid and offensive unless dehydration was severe. The gall bladder is distended in starvation if there has been no recent meal to stimulate emptying. The tongue may be thickly coated, but this is such a non-specific finding that it is of no practical use.

MEDICO-LEGAL PROBLEMS

In infants there may sometimes, if rarely, be physical abuse associated with neglect, so radiography prior to autopsy is essential – in fact the whole procedure must be conducted on the lines indicated for the 'battered child' (Chapter 22). In both children and adults, a major problem is cause and effect, especially where some pathological disease process is found. Did a cancer lead to cachexia or is it an incidental finding? Did pulmonary tuberculosis cause the emaciation or was the infection secondary to the nutritional deficiency? The relevance of diseases such as diabetes, Addison's disease, chronic infections and neoplasms must be evaluated. Particularly important in children are familial metabolic diseases that may be associated with failure to thrive and frank emaciation.

Where death from a wasting condition is alleged to be the result of malnutrition, either from wilful withholding of food or from indifference about its provision, a defence may be raised against criminal prosecution that the condition was caused by a natural disease. Indeed, such a claim may be true on occasions. Both the prosecution and defence medical advisers must undertake a thorough investigation using all anatomical, histological and biochemical means at their disposal to discover any such metabolic or pathological cause for fatal wasting, before attributing the death to sheer malnutrition.

INJURY CAUSED BY COLD: HYPOTHERMIA

Until about 40 years ago, injury and death from the effects of low temperature was thought to occur almost exclusively among those subjected to extremes of climate out of doors. Mountaineers, polar explorers and those exposed in some disaster on sea or land were considered to be the prime candidates for frostbite and 'freezing to death'. Only after some noteworthy medical publications, such as those by

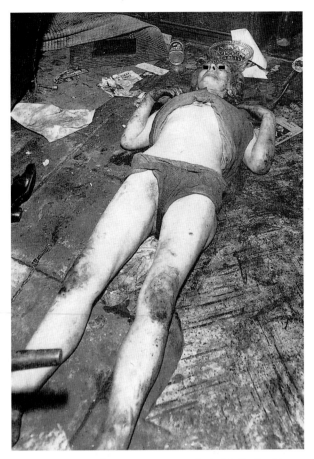

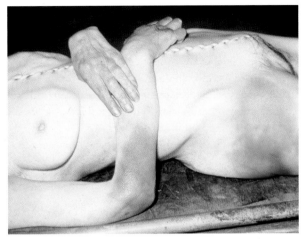

FIGURE 17.4 *A death from hypothermia showing brownish-pink discoloration over the hip and elbow.*

FIGURE 17.3 *Hypothermia in a woman of only 56. She lived in extreme squalor, with no heating and broken windows, even though she had been a state registered nurse. The knees, hands and feet showed hypothermic discoloration as well as dirt.*

Emslie-Smith (1958), Duguid *et al.* (1961) and others, was it generally appreciated that hypothermia was a common and widespread danger in temperate climates and indoors. Recognition was rapid and Special Committees of both the Royal College of Physicians and the British Medical Association produced reports on hypothermia in the 1960s.

As in so many other conditions, the aged and the infants are most vulnerable, especially as the condition is insidious and may not be suspected in time by those more active persons who are the potential guardians of those at the two extremes of life.

Factors involved in hypothermia

LOW ENVIRONMENTAL TEMPERATURE

No precise figures can be given in degrees Celsius for temperatures potentially dangerous to life, as other factors and the personal vulnerability of different individuals vary considerably. Certainly the air temperature need be nothing

like as low as was thought in former years, when profound frost was considered essential for the production of lesions. Air temperatures below 10°C are probably low enough to cause hypothermia in vulnerable persons, but air movements such as external wind or internal draughts will make things worse by markedly increasing the rate of body cooling. Damp conditions, especially of clothing, will also aid cooling from the latent heat of evaporation.

AGE AND PHYSIQUE

As stated, the elderly and the young are at greatest risk. The old person may have poor musculature and a lack of mobility, thus depressing heat production from muscular activity. Often thin, there may be a lack of insulating subcutaneous fat. Poor thyroid function is common, especially in old women, and is discussed below. Cerebral dysfunction – often from degenerative arterial disease – may lead to poor central heat regulation, a disinclination to move around, and apathy concerning personal nutrition, heating and general well-being. Depression and mental illness are not uncommon, as in the early cases reported by Emslie-Smith and by Duguid *et al.*

In infants, the body mass is small and the surface area:mass ratio large, so that heat is lost more easily. In small infants, there is naturally complete dependence on others in regard to clothing and environment.

HYPOTHYROIDISM

Myxoedema, either occult or obvious, is an important factor in hypothermia. Many elderly women have a thyroid deficiency and this is a potent factor in vulnerability to cold. The majority of victims are women over 70 and the environmental conditions in which thyroid dysfunction is a factor may be little below optimum. Cases were first reported in the 1950s by Marquand, soon followed by the paper of Angel and Sash (1960). In hypothyroid subjects, certain drugs may have a deleterious effect by precipitating hypothermia, even when the environment is relatively normal. Imipramine, chlorpromazine and diazepam are particularly hazardous. Barbiturates, phenothiazines and alcohol are also dangerous in this respect.

LACK OF FOOD, ADEQUATE CLOTHING AND INDOOR HEATING

These are factors that may be social or financial, but are often related to the depressed, apathetic state of many old people, especially those with cerebral atherosclerosis. Cause and effect are often hard to separate, as the effects of cold may bring on or worsen mental sluggishness and confusion.

The manifestations of hypothermia

The clinical manifestations are not the concern of the forensic pathologist, though when unsuspected before autopsy the history may give a clue to the fatal process.

It is sometimes claimed that hypothermia in the elderly never occurs unless there is some predisposing disability, such as cerebrovascular disease, hypothyroidism, alcoholism or diabetes, for instance. This seems too restrictive an attitude, though in general is probably true. The rectal temperature is used as the measure of severity in hypothermia. Between 37°C and 32°C there are no ill-effects beyond the normal subjective feeling of being cold, with shivering and constriction of blood vessels.

When the core temperature falls further below 32°C to 24°C, there is dulling of consciousness, a fall in respiration and heart rate, and a lowering of blood pressure. If maintained without relief, death will ensue and recovery is rare if the rectal temperature falls below about 26°C, though one remarkable case reported by Laufman (1951) recovered after falling to 18°C, albeit with severe mutilating frostbite.

Autopsy findings in hypothermia

There may be no signs whatsoever at autopsy in a death from hypothermia and thus the history may be all-important. The usual difficulties then arise as to how much the pathologist is entitled to rely upon hearsay evidence – as opposed to the objective findings of his own examination – when deciding on a cause of death. This is more fully discussed in the first chapter of this book.

Hypothermia, like some cases of epilepsy, asthma and drowning, provides some of the more difficult pathological dilemmas when there are slight, non-specific or absent autopsy findings. When a victim of hypothermia has been admitted to hospital and 'warmed-up', death may supervene at any time up to a few days later. In such circumstances the autopsy may reveal no positive findings. The skin changes will almost certainly be absent, but intra-abdominal signs may persist.

In a classical death from hypothermia the body will usually be that of an old person – almost half the Royal College of Physicians' series was over 65 years of age; most will be women. The exterior of the body may present suggestive

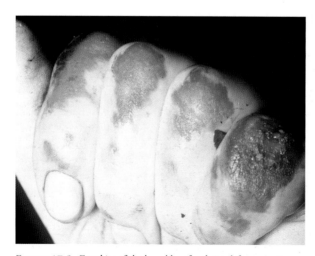

FIGURE 17.5 *Frostbite of the knuckles after being left unconscious during winter in Wales. It does not require Arctic temperatures to cause tissue damage or death.*

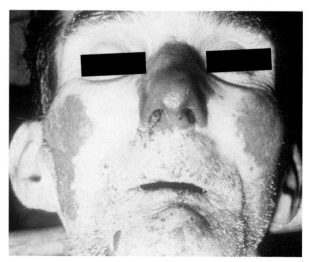

FIGURE 17.6 *Bright red discoloration of the cheeks and nose from hypothermia. The victim suffered from mitral stenosis (where malar flush is one of the clinical signs) and was in bed in an unheated room during a Welsh winter. The tissues of the nose were virtually necrotic, amounting to actual frostbite.*

signs of hypothermia, in that patches of pink to brownish-pink discoloration may be seen in certain areas. They are most often present over extensor surfaces and large joints, such as the outer sides of the hips, the elbows and the knees, and less often on the flanks and face.

The colour is similar to that seen in bodies exposed in cold water or in severe outdoor cold – and to the post-mortem pinkness that often develops in mortuary refrigerators. In hypothermia, however, the distribution over the large joints is distinctive, in addition to the pinkness of hypostasis. There may be pink patches on the cheeks, chin and nose, especially in victims who already had impaired cardiac function, such as the 'malar' flush of mitral stenosis. The slight brownish tinge often seen in the pinkness and the rather indefinite blurred edges of the patches suggest that some haemolysis may have occurred, perhaps in the early post-mortem period as well as during the terminal stages of life. The colour is presumably due to persistent oxyhaemoglobin in the skin capillaries, which, because of the low metabolic activity of the cold tissues, fail to take up the delivered oxygen. Pooling of blood in surface vessels from the breakdown of normal vasomotor control allows this unreduced haemoglobin to show through the skin. Why a normally coloured body placed after death in a mortuary refrigerator should also become pink has never been satisfactorily explained.

In addition to pink areas of skin, the extremities may be cyanosed or they may be white. Sometimes the feet are blue to the ankles, above which is pale. The hands may show blueness of the fingers or nail beds. Oedema may be seen, most often in the feet and lower legs, but many of the victims of hypothermia already have pre-existing congestive cardiac failure. Rarely there may be blistering of the skin, usually in dependent parts such as the buttocks, backs of thighs and

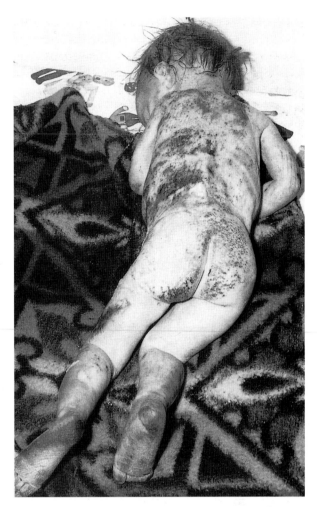

FIGURE 17.7 *Fatal child neglect. The infant has extensive skin ulceration and was underweight. Death was the result of an intercurrent chest infection.*

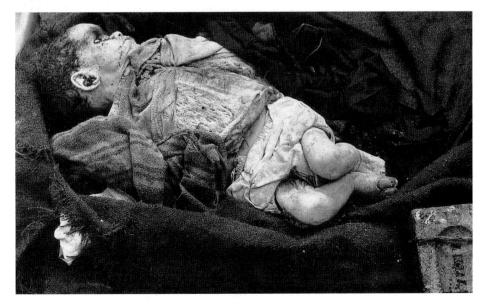

FIGURE 17.8 *This infant died of neglect, hypothermia and frostbite, having been left in an unheated farmhouse bedroom, the cardboard box that acted as a cot having crystals of frozen urine in the bedclothes. After death the child was dropped down the farm well in this sack with a brick as a weight.*

upper arms. This may or may not be in pink areas and seems to be caused by skin oedema which then breaks down.

The face, especially of an elderly woman, may show appearances suggestive of myxoedema or hypothyroidism, with coarsening of the features, puffy eyelids and loss of eyebrow hair. Internally there may be nothing specific to note, even if the external skin changes are obvious. Signs of pre-existing disease are common, especially if one subscribes to the view that hypothermia in the elderly never occurs in the absence of systemic disease. Degenerative arterial disease, senile myocardial degeneration, hypertension, chronic renal lesions and obstructive airways disease are common. More specific lesions are considered below.

ACUTE GASTRIC EROSIONS

In the authors' view, these are found much more often than pancreatitis. The stomach mucosa is frequently studded with numerous shallow ulcers, the floor of each containing a dark brown plug of altered blood. Frank haematemesis is rare, but the stomach contents sometimes contain dark acid-affected blood.

ACUTE PANCREATITIS

This is the lesion most often quoted in textbooks, but is present in less than half the deaths from proven hypothermia. It may have been diagnosed before death from an increase in serum amylase activity. The most obvious feature may be areas of stiff, yellow, fat necrosis when the pancreas is sectioned at autopsy. There may be adjacent areas of fat necrosis in the omentum and mesentery. Haemorrhage into the gland may occur, but caution has to be employed here, as post-mortem autolysis of this organ commonly gives a haemorrhagic appearance in many other modes of

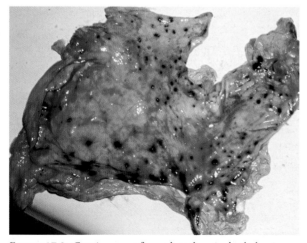

FIGURE 17.9 *Gastric mucosa from a hypothermia death showing numerous acute erosions.*

death seen at autopsy. Histologically, necrosis, leucocyte infiltration and fat necrosis may be confirmed in some instances, but in others the pancreas, even if haemorrhagic, yields little information on microscopy.

PULMONARY OEDEMA

This is common, but as it is such a common finding in any death from cardiac failure, its diagnostic value in hypothermia is almost nil.

PERIVASCULAR HAEMORRHAGES

These have been described in the brain, especially in the walls of the third ventricle, but again they are not particularly specific, especially in an autopsy population that has a high incidence of cerebrovascular disease. Sludging of blood in peripheral vessels may occur, partly from cold agglutinins. This contributes to skin oedema and necrosis, though peripheral vasoconstriction is the main cause of the infarction of frostbite. Microinfarcts are common in many organs in hypothermia, presumably from cold agglutinins blocking small vessels. Deep vein thrombosis in the legs and pulmonary embolism are occasionally found, but again cause and effect is hard to establish.

It is said that the good preservation of tissues when examined histologically is characteristic of hypothermia, as autolysis is retarded by the low temperature. In the experience of the authors, this claim is not justified.

THE 'HIDE-AND-DIE' SYNDROME

There is a peculiar aspect to some cases of hypothermic death in that it is associated with the victim undressing and hiding away from sight. The subject is usually an old person, man or woman. When found dead (usually, but not always at home), the body may be partly or even totally naked, even though the environment is cold. In addition, the victim may have burrowed his or her way into some corner or cupboard, or alternatively pulled down furniture and household articles into a heap on top of the body. In fact, the house may be in such a state of disorder that when the police break in and find a corpse amongst such chaos they may naturally suspect a homicide and robbery.

The author (BK) has seen old people who have crawled into small cupboards, the bottom of wardrobes, under low shelves, and into corners of pantries and outhouses. They have been found under piles of books pulled from a bookcase, or hidden under a mound of old clothes, newspapers and other debris.

The signs of hypothermia are usually present and the problem then arises as to whether the victim became hypothermic first, which led to mental confusion that caused the strange behaviour, or whether – as a result of some mental aberration, perhaps related to senility or other cerebral episode – they began behaving abnormally, including shedding their clothes and so became fatally hypothermic.

Though some geriatricians claim that hypothermia is almost always precipitated by some natural illness, including cerebral vascular episodes, the experience of most pathologists is that it is not common to find definite lesions of such predisposing factors at autopsy.

Biochemical markers of hypothermia have been investigated, and catecholamines appear in the blood and then urine in the early stages, but then decline, as the adrenals become exhausted (Hirvonen and Huttunen 1995). There is a variation in the adrenaline:noradrenaline ratio, all these changes being manifestations of stress induced by low temperature.

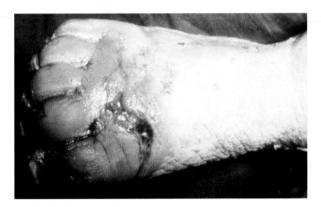

FIGURE 17.10 *Frostbite of the foot from the infant shown in Figure 17.8. The distal part of the foot is infarcted and a line of separation has appeared between the distal slough and the rest of the limb.*

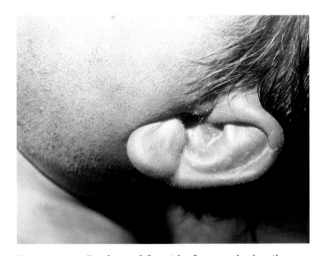

FIGURE 17.11 *Frostbite on left auricle of a man who, heavily intoxicated by alcohol, left for home at night in the Arctic winter, but lost his way at −40°C and was found dead the following day.*

DEATHS FROM EXPOSURE

Fatal hypothermia can occur in healthy adults, as well as infants and old people. This is caused by purely environmental conditions, which need not be extreme. One common group, especially in more northern countries, is the inebriated person who becomes exposed to even moderate cold. The typical circumstances are a person who gets drunk and either falls asleep outdoors in his drunken state or sustains some accident – such as a fall or even mild head injury – which incapacitates him for long enough for him to become hypothermic. Alcohol seems to have a secondary effect, apart from causing incapacity and immobility. Its vasodilating effect on skin allows heat loss to be more rapid and in higher concentrations it may have a direct action on the heat-regulating centres. Apart from drunken victims, many other classes of person may fall prey to hypothermia. Hill-walkers, climbers, yachtsmen and dinghy-sailors, swimmers, and other classes of sportsmen and women can become cold and exhausted. Every year sees deaths and rescue escapades in the hill country of Britain, even when the weather is far from Arctic in severity. Naturally the risks in colder countries and at high altitudes almost anywhere in the world are much greater. For the pathologist, the features are similar to domestic hypothermia, but there may be the added lesions of frostbite.

LOCAL INJURY DUE TO COLD: FROSTBITE

There are a number of different clinical lesions caused by the effect of prolonged cold on the extremities. 'Immersion foot' and 'trench foot' refer to damp cold damage, whereas 'frostbite' is caused by dry conditions below zero. In the context of forensic pathology, they may be found in victims of fatal hypothermia, but rarely kill in themselves unless tissue necrosis becomes infected. Severe damage with sloughing and separation of toes, or part of the foot is likely to be seen only in survivors or victims of some catastrophe on sea or mountainside, but the author (BK) has seen one case where a neglected infant was left in a urine-soaked cot at temperatures below zero for many days. When it died of a mixture of hypothermia and chest infection, the parents placed it in a sack with a brick and dropped it down a well. On recovery of the body, separation of the necrotic distal part of a foot was seen, with a red zone of inflammatory tissue on the proximal margin. Frostbite may affect only the skin or may extend deeply into the underlying tissues. Lesser degrees are reversible, but infarction and necrosis may ensue if the blood supply is cut off by vasoconstriction, sludging and thrombosis, for a sufficient time.

REFERENCES AND FURTHER READING

Angel J, Sash Z. 1960. Hypothyroidism and exposure to cold. *Br Med J* **1**:1855–9.

Benecke M, Lessig R. 2001. Child neglect and forensic entomology. *Forensic Sci Int* **120**:155–9.

Bray M. 1984. The eye as a chemical indicator of environmental temperature at the time of death. *J Forensic Sci* **29**:396–403.

Davis JH, Rao VJ, Valdes-Dapena M. 1984. A forensic science approach to a starved child. *J Forensic Sci* **29**:663–9.

Denmark LN. 1993. The investigation of beta-hydroxybutyrate as a marker for sudden death due to hypoglycemia in alcoholics. *Forensic Sci Int* **62**:225–32.

Duguid H, Simpson R, Strowers J. 1961. Exposure to cold. *Lancet* **2**:1213–19.

Elias AN, Gwinup G. 1982. Glucose-resistant hypoglycemia in inanition. *Arch Intern Med* **142**:743–6.

Emslie-Smith D. 1958. Hypothermia. *Lancet* **2**:492.

Fieguth A, Gunther D, Kleemann WJ, *et al.* 2002. Lethal child neglect. *Forensic Sci Int* **130**:8–12.

Fitzgerald FT. 1980. Hypoglycemia and accidental hypothermia in an alcoholic population. *West J Med* **133**:105–7.

Hirvonen J. 1976. Necropsy findings in fatal hypothermia cases. *Forensic Sci* **8**:155–64.

Hirvonen J. 2000. Some aspects on death in the cold and concomitant frostbites. *Int J Circumpolar Health* **59**:131–6.

Hirvonen J, Huttunen P. 1982. Increased urinary concentration of catecholamines in hypothermia deaths. *J Forensic Sci* **27**:264–71.

Hirvonen J, Huttunen P. 1995. Hypothermia markers: serum, urine and adrenal gland catecholamines in hypothermic rats given ethanol [see comments]. *Forensic Sci Int* **72**:125–33.

Hirvonen J, Lapinlampi T. 1989. Plasma and urine catecholamines and cerebrospinal fluid amine metabolites as hypothermia markers in guinea-pigs. *Med Sci Law* **29**:130–5.

Kelsey RM, Alpert BS, Patterson SM, *et al.* 2000. Racial differences in hemodynamic responses to environmental thermal stress among adolescents. *Circulation* **101**:2284–9.

Knight B. 1976. Forensic problems in practice. XI. Injury from physical agents. *Practitioner* **217**:813–18.

Kortelainen ML, Huttunen P, Lapinlampi T. 1990. Urinary catecholamines in hyperthermia-related deaths. *Forensic Sci Int* **48**:103–10.

Kreyburg L. 1946. Tissue damage due to cold. *Lancet* **1**:338–40.

Laufman H. 1951. Hypothermia. *JAMA* **147**:1201–12.

Mant AK. 1964. Some port-mortem observations in accidental hypothermia. *Med Sci Law* **4**:44–7.

Mimasaka S, Funayama M, Adachi N, *et al.* 2000. A fatal case of infantile scurvy. *Int J Legal Med* **114**:122–4.

Molnar G. 1946. Survival of hypothermia by men immersed in the ocean. *JAMA* **131**:1045–50.

Ortmann C, Fechner G, Bajanowski T, *et al.* 2001. Fatal neglect of the elderly. *Int J Legal Med* **114**:191–3.

Paton BC. 1983. Accidental hypothermia. *Pharmacol Ther* **22**:331–77.

Sadler DW, Pounder DJ. 1995. Urinary catecholamines as markers of hypothermia. *Forensic Sci Int* **76**:227–30.

Steinhauer JR, Volk A, Hardy R, *et al.* 2002. Detection of ketosis in vitreous at autopsy after embalming. *J Forensic Sci* **47**:221–3.

Tanaka M, Tokudome S. 1991. Accidental hypothermia and death from cold in urban areas. *Int J Biometeorol* **34**:242–6.

Teresinski G, Buszewicz G, Madro R. 2002. The influence of ethanol on the level of ketone bodies in hypothermia. *Forensic Sci Int* **127**:88–96.

Wedin B, Vanggaard L, Hirvonen J. 1979. 'Paradoxical undressing' in fatal hypothermia. *J Forensic Sci* **24**:543–53.

Wolf DA, Aronson JF, Rajaraman S, *et al.* 1999. Wischnewski ulcers and acute pancreatitis in two hospitalized patients with cirrhosis, portal vein thrombosis, and hypothermia. *J Forensic Sci* **44**:1082–5.

Young AJ, Castellani JW. 2001. Exertion-induced fatigue and thermoregulation in the cold. *Comp Biochem Physiol A Mol Integr Physiol* **128**:769–76.

Zhu BL, Oritani S, Ishida K, *et al.* 2000. Child and elderly victims in forensic autopsy during a recent 5 year period in the southern half of Osaka city and surrounding areas. *Forensic Sci Int* **113**:215–18.

CHAPTER 18

Deaths associated with sexual offences

The examination of living victims of sexual assaults is the province of the forensic physician or 'police surgeon', in places where such doctors exist. In many countries, any physician may be asked by the police to examine the victim of an alleged sexual offence, but this difficult and onerous task in the living victim is outside the experience of many pathologists – though in some jurisdictions, this function is combined with that of the forensic pathologist.

In this book, attention will be confined to those cases in which a sexual assault leads to death, almost always rape and homicide. Regrettably, a significant proportion of non-domestic homicides are associated with sexual offences, death occurring either because the woman rejects the sexual approaches or because a sadosexual motive colours an intended murder. The most common mode of killing is either pressure on the neck, head injuries, or, less often, stabbing. In some instances death may be the result of violence associated with the sexual activities themselves, especially in child victims when pelvic trauma may be the immediate cause of death. In this chapter, only the sexual aspects are discussed, as other modes of violent death are covered elsewhere.

EXTERNAL FINDINGS IN FATAL SEXUAL ASSAULTS

As with most forensic autopsies, a meticulous external examination is as important – and usually more important – than the internal dissection. The study of the body surface in sexual assaults is similar in both the living and dead and

may be divided into general appearances and those of the perineum. The whole body surface should be searched for sexually orientated injuries.

Mouth and lips

Bruises may be found on the lips and especially inside on the buccal surfaces, from rough kissing. The lips may have been forced back on to the edges of the teeth, causing abrasions, bruises and even laceration of the buccal surface. Swabs should be taken from the mouth in every case before substantial manipulation for examination, to seek evidence of seminal fluid from oral penetration. Though such swabs rarely yield a positive result as to the presence of spermatozoa, modern analytical methods may be able to detect other components of the seminal fluid or the presence of male epithelial cells.

Bites

Other bruises may be found on the neck, shoulders, breasts and buttocks from oral suction or biting. These are somewhat euphemistically termed 'love bites' and may range from minor lesions inflicted from enthusiastic passion to mutilating bites of a sadistic nature.

Suction lesions may comprise a circular or oval area of bruising, in which the damaged zone consists of many small intradermal petechial haemorrhages caused by sucking the skin into the mouth, the reduced air pressure rupturing the small vessels. There may be semilunar marks at the periphery from the lips, and there may be associated teeth indentations or abrasions. Such suction marks are often seen at the sides of the neck, below the ears, on the upper shoulder, and on the upper part of the breasts and around the nipples.

Actual bites may accompany suction marks or may be independent. The characteristics are described in Chapter 26, but the main features are abrasions or bruises matching the dental arches, often with discrete marks from each tooth. These may be linear if the teeth are scraped down the skin in closing the jaws. They may be superficial or deep enough to penetrate the skin as lacerations. The latter are especially common at the nipples in sexual assaults, and the nipple and part of the areola may even be partly or wholly amputated.

In sexual homicides, it is essential to obtain expert forensic odontological advice, if at all possible. In any event, photographs and measurements must be taken of these injuries and, if practicable, a cast of any teeth indentations for later comparison. Before any handling of the lesions, swabs should be taken of the surface in an effort to recover saliva, which – if the assailant was a 'secretor' – may be tested for blood-group-specific substances.

General bruising and abrasion

Apart from bruises that may be associated with the fatal assault, such as throat or head injuries, some bruises are indicative of the sexual motivation. The breasts are often manually squeezed and manipulated, causing discoid bruises of 1–2 cm on any part, especially around the nipples. Linear abrasions, usually from fingernails, may also be present. Bruises may also be seen on the thighs and buttocks, from struggles to achieve intercourse. Both the outer and inner sides of the thighs may be bruised and scratched: a typical area is the inner aspect of the upper thigh, where the legs are manually forced apart. There may be bruising around the anus from fingers opening the buttock cleft to achieve either anal or posterior vulval penetration.

Where the assault takes place on a hard or uneven surface, bruises and abrasions may be seen on the back, especially the shoulders and buttocks. If outdoors, there may be marks from stones or sticks and remnants of vegetation, such as leaves, and grass and green staining may be adherent to the skin, together with earth or dirt. Examination of the clothing is usually a function of the forensic scientist ('criminalist'), but when the pathologist examines the body *in situ*, he will naturally note damage, disarray and foreign material on the garments.

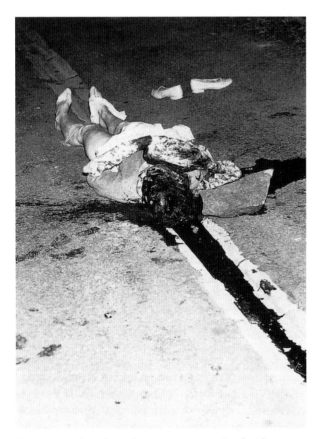

FIGURE 18.1 *Sexual assaults are sometimes associated with extreme violence, often of a sadistic nature. Here, rape has been followed by severe head injury from the large rock seen near the central gutter of this back lane.*

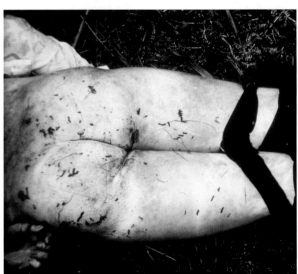

FIGURE 18.2 *In fatal rape the pathologist must note at the scene, or at the mortuary, the position and condition of clothing and presence of foreign material on the skin. Full cooperation with scene of crime officers or forensic scientists is vital in collecting trace evidence.*

Other general injuries

The hands should be carefully examined, as in all assaults. The fingernails, especially the often longer and manicured nails of younger women, may be broken from a struggle. Occasionally, there are hairs or fibres trapped in nail splits, which may have come from the assailant or his clothing. At autopsy, the nails should be cut closely to the junction with the fingers and all parings carefully collected for forensic laboratory examination. It is rarely necessary to collect those from each finger in individual packets, but each hand should be identified separately. Some pathologists or scientific officers prefer to scrape out the space under each nail with a pointed orange-stick or toothpick, carefully retaining any debris. The reason for this interest, especially in sexual assault victims, is that they may have scratched their assailants and have blood, or even skin parings, under the nails that can be identified as to blood group or individually specific DNA characteristics.

Signs of head injury and throttling are dealt with elsewhere, but some fatal trauma may be sexually orientated, especially knife injuries. Sadistic cutting or stabbing may be inflicted on sexually significant areas, especially the breasts, buttocks, perineum and lower abdomen. The vulva itself may be mutilated. These may be slashes or deeply penetrating stabs, often multiple and indeed numerous. They may be arranged in a pattern or may be mutilating, as when whole breasts are amputated. Decapitation is sometimes performed and ritual acts may be performed, with objects placed in definite sites near the body. The notorious 'Jack the Ripper' murders in London in 1888 exhibited the arrangements of disembowelled organs and this type of mutilation is another feature of some sadistic sexual homicides. Intestine or uterus may be removed, either through abdominal wounds or manually through the vagina. General injuries may be continuous with genital trauma, as in knife or broken bottle wounds of the abdomen and perineum.

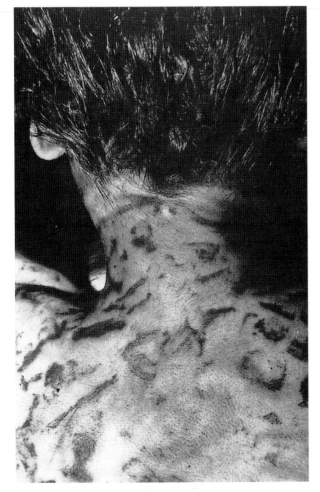

FIGURE 18.3 *Multiple superficial abrasions from undergrowth and ground debris on the back of the victim of rape. This is an indication of pressure of the unclothed body on the ground. There is a ligature mark around the neck with a cross-over point visible.*

Genital injuries

Once the pathologist has examined all the external general injuries, attention should be turned to the perineum. As with the clinical examination of sexual offences, a set routine should be used, as the incorrect order may lose valuable forensic evidence.

The vulva and anus should be inspected externally and laceration, swelling, bruising, bleeding and discharge noted. Any blood or suspected semen stains anywhere on the body or clothing should be sampled either by the pathologist or by the forensic scientist or scene of crime police officer. The pubic hair should be examined for foreign material, hairs, vegetation and dried seminal stains, and samples of hair and combings taken. The hair may be combed using a fine comb with the base of the teeth packed with cotton-wool to trap any loose fibres. Dried stains on hair may be cut away and placed in clean folded paper in an envelope, or plastic bag for transit to the laboratory. The vulval labia may show clear signs of trauma, especially in children. In forcible rapes, especially in young persons, there may be external signs of perineal tears, with laceration of the margin of the vaginal introitus or anus, sometimes causing a complete rip between the two orifices.

Caution must be used in interpreting the degree of dilatation of the anus in a dead body, as the sphincter can become patulous and wide open as a normal post-mortem change. Unless the dilatation is very marked, the sole finding of an open anus in the absence of abrasion, bruising, or semen is difficult to sustain as proof of anal penetration. This applies

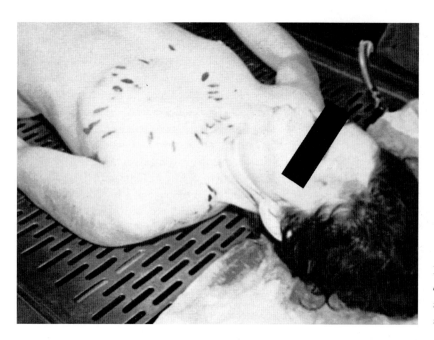

FIGURE 18.4 *Some homicides have obvious sexual connotations even if there is no genital interference. This circle of stab wounds is centred on a breast.*

to children as well as adults; in fact, post-mortem dilatation of the anus is particularly noticeable in children.

Once external examination and assessment has been made, samples should be taken for forensic biological testing, for the presence of semen and venereal infection, as well as samples for DNA profiling, which may be able to distinguish between any semen present and the vaginal secretions. If any fluid is running from the vulva or anus, it should be picked up with clean pipettes and preserved in the smallest available tube, to prevent drying from evaporation. Then cotton-wool swabs on sticks (ensuring that those used for semen detection are plain swabs, not those containing albumin or other media) should be used to take the following samples by touching gently on to the mucosal surfaces:

- the interior of the vulval labia and around the vaginal orifice
- the margins and interior of the anus
- the mid-vagina, using a speculum or broad handle of a dissecting forceps to part the lower vaginal walls gently to allow the swab to reach the area without contamination from the lower vagina
- the upper vagina, cervix and posterior fornix, again using a spatulate instrument to open the canal to give access to the swab. If more fluid contents are seen higher in the vagina, either now or during the later dissection, they should be recovered by pipette.

After samples are taken, the interior of the anus, vulva and vagina, as far as can be seen from the exterior, should be examined. Lacerations, abrasions, bruises and bleeding may be evaluated, though they can be seen in more detail at dissection. The presence and condition of a hymen is noted,

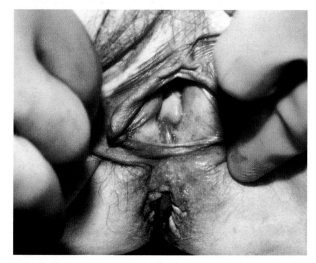

FIGURE 18.5 *Fresh bleeding and mucosal abrasion on the lower wall of the vagina in a sexual assault associated with fatal head injuries in an old lady.*

with any evidence of recent tearing. Where injuries are gross, especially in children, fistulae between the vagina and the rectum or even peritoneal cavity may be seen. There may be extrusion of intestine.

INTERNAL EXAMINATION

The order of the autopsy may be determined by the nature of the death. The fatal injuries, such as strangulation or head

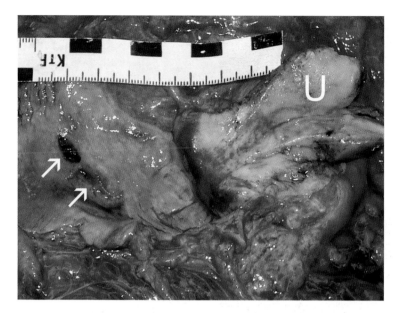

FIGURE 18.6 *Stab wounds (arrows) in the vaginal wall of a homicide victim (U, uterus).*

injuries, may be dealt with first or the pelvic region may command prime attention. The autopsy incision should be similar to that described for the examination of deaths associated with pregnancy, with an incision circumscribing the perineum, removal of the anterior part of the pelvic bones and the extraction of all the pelvic organs in continuity from ovaries to vulva and anus. This block of tissue is then dissected separately. Before this is done, the bladder should first be emptied of urine (either by catheter or through a small incision in the fundus) and the fluid retained for toxicological analysis, especially for alcohol.

The vagina should be opened with large scissors, the track of the cut depending on the assessment of any injuries seen on external examination. If there are tears or bruises in the vulva or vagina, the cut should be orientated to avoid them wherever possible; the anus is later dealt with in a similar way. The vagina is laid open to the posterior fornix and all injuries carefully examined and photographed. The cervix and uterus are examined in the same way.

Injuries may be of all types, from mere reddening or swelling to complete disruption of the vaginal canal. This may occur in small children from sheer brutality of penetration, especially if there is gross disproportion between the adult penis and infantile canal. It may also occur from instrumental injury, as it is by no means uncommon for deliberate incised wounds to be made. The author (BK) has seen abdominal knife wounds carried over the pubis into the vagina in a murdered prostitute; another murder–rape was found to have a broken milk bottle high in the vagina, to the potential hazard of the examining fingers. Vaginal injuries, especially by instrument, may continue up into the abdominal cavity, either via the posterior fornix or lateral vaginal walls. This will have been examined

through the abdominal autopsy incision before removal of the pelvic organs.

INTERPRETATION OF MINIMAL FINDINGS

As in clinical forensic practice, there is little difficulty in interpreting gross sexual interference, but problems arise when only minimal evidence is present in a death (traumatic or otherwise) where the circumstances suggest some sexual offence or activity. In such cases, the following questions need to be answered, in the light of all the available findings at the end of the autopsy and ancillary investigations:

■ Is there any evidence of sexual intercourse at any time – that is, absence of virginity as determined by an intact hymen? This does not exclude sexual activity short of penetration and technically rape can occur from even the minimal passage of a glans between the labia, which does not affect the hymen. Old intercourse may be assumed from healed hymenal tears with epithelialized 'carunculae myrtiformes' at the margins, though the prolonged use of tampons and manual manipulation can also tear a hymen. Evidence of previous pregnancy, such as abdominal striae, old damage to the cervix and breast changes are almost incontrovertible evidence of previous sexual intercourse.

■ Is there evidence of recent sexual intercourse? A recently ruptured hymen, with swelling, a raw unepithelialized edge and bleeding may be found, though admittedly it is relatively uncommon except in children and previously virginal young persons. The labia may be red and

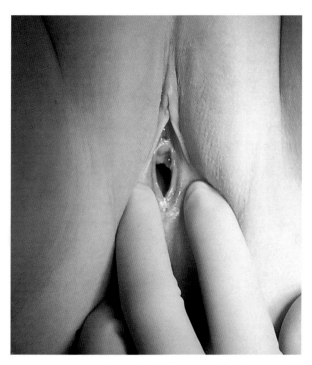

FIGURE 18.7 *External genitals of a live 8-year-old girl, a victim of repeated sexual abuse by an adult living in the neighbourhood. The lack of intact hymen, reddened and larger than normal orifice of the vagina as well as thickened skin and ulcers perianally (not shown) are in keeping with abuse.*

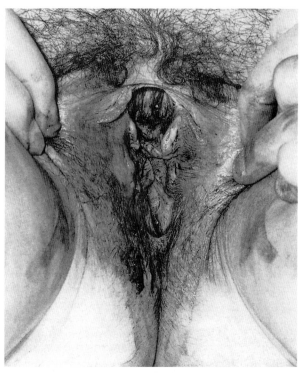

FIGURE 18.8 *Extensive bleeding from inner lacerations of the vaginal walls in a fatal rape. Blood is pooling in the posterior part of the vaginal canal. A full autopsy dissection is required, keeping the perineum en bloc with the genital tract to display any injuries and to exclude natural disease as a contribution to the bleeding.*

inflamed with slight oedema of the vaginal introitus if it is the first episode, or if there is disproportion between an adult man and a young person, even in voluntary sexual connection. The presence of semen on swabs is the best evidence, though with the use of condoms it may be absent. After vasectomy, though no sperms will be present, chemical and enzyme tests for semen remain positive. The presence of venereal disease, especially gonorrhoea, is presumptive evidence of intercourse, though it can be contracted other than by sufficient penile penetration to constitute rape.

■ If recent intercourse has taken place, was it by force? This may be all too obvious in the presence of gross injury, especially in small children. Where vaginal or rectal tearing has occurred, or where there is obvious abrasion, bruising or laceration of the vulva, anal margins or perineum, then this can hardly be compatible with voluntary intercourse. The possibility of sexually motivated injury without actual penile penetration must be considered when no semen can be recovered, as equally severe damage can be caused by digital or instrumental trauma. All kinds of foreign objects can be forcibly introduced into the vagina and rectum, and are not infrequently employed by sadistic

and perverted killers. The author (BK) has seen candles, bottles, a banana, broken glass and knives introduced into the vagina, and broom-handles and potatoes lying in the rectum.

Where injury is relatively slight and confined to hyperaemia and oedema of the vaginal or anal entrances – and where abrasion and bruising of the vulva is slight (even including fingernail scratches), although the presumption is that intercourse was by force, the possibility still exists that it was voluntary though overenthusiastic, unless, of course, the victim was a small child.

TESTS FOR SEMEN

In countries with sophisticated forensic science or police laboratories, the pathologist will not be called upon to carry out the actual techniques for the detection of seminal fluid. His role is to be a careful collector of the original samples at autopsy and, to some extent, to be able to interpret the results for the benefit of the police and the courts. He should be conversant with the general principles of the tests and aware of any potential shortcomings. In places where forensic science facilities are deficient or their availability may be delayed, the pathologist may have to conduct the more simple tests himself and the technical details are given in Appendix 1. The detection of semen depends upon the following methods:

■ Naked-eye and lens recognition is a screening method which may identify suspicious stains on clothing, skin

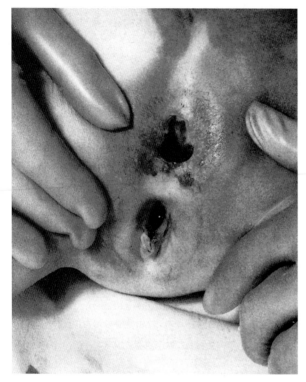

FIGURE 18.9 *Rape and buggery of a small girl who was then strangled. The vulva has a slight posterior tear and there is a large vaginal tear internally, the canal being filled with blood. The anus is widely ripped, especially posteriorly. Swabs were positive for semen in both orifices.*

and pubic hair. Liquid semen leaking from the vagina or anus may be obvious, though leucorrhoeic vaginal discharge may be mistaken for seminal fluid. Dried seminal stains are stiff and rather silvery, depending upon the nature and colour of any fabric they may be upon. On the skin they flake off readily and can easily be lost if not carefully lifted with a blade or needle into a container. Dried stains on hair should be retrieved by cutting away the clump on which they lie. Suspect smears on skin may be collected by gentle rubbing with a plain cotton-wool swab that has been moistened with water or saline. All material should be examined as soon as possible after collection.

■ Examination under ultraviolet light causes seminal stains to fluoresce a bluish-silver, but many other biological fluids and vegetable juices give false-positive

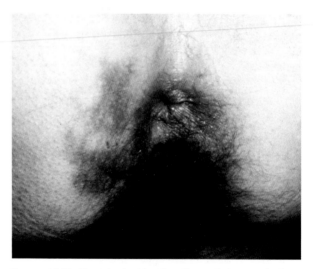

FIGURE 18.11 *Extensive bruising from fingers during a multiple anal and vaginal rape. Though penetrated by several men in a short space of time, the anus shows no injury.*

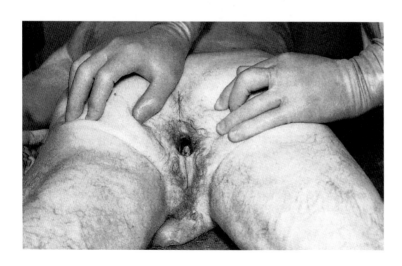

FIGURE 18.10 *A chronically dilated anus in an habitual passive homosexual. After death any anus can appear open and patulous, but this example is too large to be accepted as within normal limits. It also has keratinized, chronically abraded margins.*

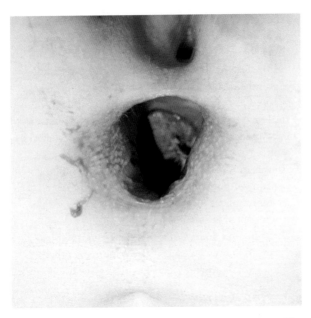

FIGURE 18.12 *The anus of a girl who has suffered penetration. The sphincter is overdilated, there is slight tearing of the anal margin, and some epidermal tags have been abraded from the surface. However, this degree of dilatation in a dead subject should not be used as the sole indication of buggery, as the post-mortem anus can be patulous in quite innocent circumstances.*

results. Many detergents, such as washing powders, also produce a confusing background fluorescence. The method is a useful screening process but cannot be used as definitive evidence of the presence of semen. Areas that fluoresce, especially on fabric, should be outlined to identify them for more specific testing.

■ Enzyme reactions are valuable, and though not absolute proof, are strong presumptive evidence of the presence of semen. They depend on detecting high concentrations of acid phosphatase originating in prostatic secretion. Acid phosphatase activity in semen is 500–1000 times greater than in any other normal bodily fluid. Also, vaginal fluid contains endogenous acid phosphatase showing considerable variation in activity depending on various factors, which complicates the interpretation of the findings. There are several methods of detecting phosphatase, including a rapid commercial 'spot' test, which should not be used as hard evidential proof.

■ Immunological methods, where animal antihuman semen sera are set up against extracts of the stain. These techniques can only be used by trained laboratory staff.

Prostate-specific antigen (PSA, p30) is a glycoprotein produced by the prostatic gland and is found in seminal plasma, male urine and blood, but not in any tissues or fluid of the female body. A positive PSA finding is a reliable indicator of semen regardless of the presence of spermatozoa or elevated acid phosphatase level. Simple and sensitive methods have been developed for analysis of the presence of PSA.

Other serological techniques may be able to determine the blood group of the semen if the ejaculator was one of the 80 per cent of the population who are 'secretors' – those who pass blood-group antigens into their saliva, sweat and semen. A problem for the forensic serologist is the admixture of semen with biological fluids from the victim, in the form of vaginal secretion and blood, but this is a complex technical matter that is usually outside the remit of the forensic pathologist, though he needs to be aware of the potential difficulties.

Recent developments have now added the DNA technique to the armamentarium of the forensic biologist; this is a remarkable advance, especially in sexual offences, as the previous problems of blood group and enzyme typing caused by the admixture of semen and vaginal secretion can now be solved in many instances. The sensitivity of detection and identification has also been enormously enhanced by amplification techniques, such as PCR (polymerase chain reaction). Y-chromosome short tandem repeat (STR) markers have been succesfully used to analyse mixed stains with a male component.

■ Until recent years, the only absolute proof accepted by the courts was the demonstration of spermatozoa in stain extracts and it remains the best evidence, though some of the sophisticated laboratory techniques such as serological and DNA identification are now equally reliable. One modern problem in using spermatozoa retrieval is the widespread and increasing incidence of vasectomy as a method of male contraception, so the seminal fluid contains no sperm; this also occurs naturally in azoospermic men. The phosphatase and some serology tests are unaffected by vasectomy. Fluorescent *in situ* hybridization (FISH) has been suggested as a sensitive and specific test for the detection of male epithelial cells in the post-coital vagina up to one week. Y-chromosome-positive epithelial cells have been identified in vaginal swabs even in cases with no ejaculation.

HOMOSEXUAL OFFENCES

As with heterosexual offences, the cause of death in fatal cases is almost always some form of general trauma, such as strangulation or head injuries. Homosexual activity, however, may be a parallel event; it is a fact that some of the most violent homicides seen by pathologists are among male homosexuals. In addition, quite a number of fatal altercations arise because a heterosexual man becomes violent when importuned by a homosexual.

The pathologist's attention will almost always be directed to the anal region of the passive participant, as the other partner or assailant is rarely dead, and any examination will be carried out by a police surgeon or clinical doctor. The examination of the victim follows closely on that for a female subject of rape, in that general injuries are sought first – including the one that caused death – together with any sexually orientated marks such as scratches anywhere on the body, but especially down the back, on the buttocks or on the thighs. Bruising around the anus and in the cleft of the buttocks is significant, especially if discoid finger bruises are seen. The anus should be inspected and the warning given earlier about the degree of dilatation in corpses should be heeded. Though most marked in children, a patulous anus can be seen in any adult post-mortem. Unless it is grossly dilated, an open anus cannot be used in isolation as an index of homosexual penetration. In recent or forcible anal intercourse, especially by a large penis upon a 'virgin' or young person, the margins of the anus may be reddened, sometimes abraded, and occasionally torn, especially in a child. There might be some eversion of the lower rectal mucosa through the sphincter. In gross anal 'rapes', especially on a young person, there may even be severe perineal tearing. At autopsy, swabs must be taken from the anal margin, and deeper in the anus and rectum. Mouth swabs should also always be taken. The presence of blood or lubricant should also be sought.

The classic description of the chronic passive homosexual has been passed down from textbook to textbook over the years, but is a rarity. The so-called 'funnel anus' is usually an anatomical variant. Some men and women have a deeply set anus as an anatomical variant, sometimes with a bridge of skin dorsally across the cleft of buttocks. This causes the anus to appear as if it was at the bottom of a funnel, but has no significance. The other classic feature was said to be silvery thickening of the skin outside and at the margins of the anus – but this is often due to chronic scratching from pruritis, rather than from prolonged friction during homosexual activities. In life, a lax anus, prolapsed mucosal rim and thickened anal margin may well be genuine signs to the experienced clinical eye, but at autopsy only acute damage and the presence of semen or lubricant is of much evidential value.

FURTHER READING

Allard JE. 1997. The collection of data from findings in cases of sexual assault and the significance of spermatozoa on vaginal, anal and oral swabs. *Sci Justice* **37**:99–108.

Allen M, Saldeen T, Gyllensten U. 1995. Allele-specific HLA-DRB1 amplification of forensic evidence samples with mixed genotypes. *Biotechniques* **19**:454–63.

Berg SP. 1955. A new method for testing for seminal stains. *Crim Pol Rev* **11**:53–7.

Carracedo A, Beckmann A, Bengs A, *et al.* 2001. Results of a collaborative study of the ednap group regarding the reproducibility and robustness of the Y-chromosome STRs DYS19, DYS389 I and II, DYS390 and DYS393 in a PCR pentaplex format. *Forensic Sci Int* **119**:28–41.

Clery JM. 2001. Stability of prostate specific antigen (PSA), and subsequent Y-STR typing, of *Lucilia (Phaenicia) sericata (Meigen)* (Diptera: Calliphoridae) maggots reared from a simulated postmortem sexual assault. *Forensic Sci Int* **120**:72–6.

Collins KA, Bennett AT. 2001. Persistence of spermatozoa and prostatic acid phosphatase in specimens from deceased individuals during varied postmortem intervals. *Am J Forensic Med Pathol* **22**:228–32.

Concheiro L, Carracedo A, Guitian F. 1982. The use of scanning electron microscopy in the examination of seminal stains. *Forensic Sci Int* **19**:185–8.

Costa MJ, Tadros T, Tackett E, *et al.* 1991. Vaginocervical cytology in victims of sexual assault. *Diagn Cytopathol* **7**:337–40.

Crouse CA, Ban JD, D'Alessio JK. 1993. Extraction of DNA from forensic-type sexual assault specimens using simple, rapid sonication procedures. *Biotechniques* **15**:641–4, 646, 648.

Dahlke MB, Cooke C, Cunnane M, *et al.* 1977. Identification of semen in 500 patients seen because of rape. *Am J Clin Pathol* **68**:740–6.

Davies A. 1978. Evaluation of results from tests performed on vaginal, anal and oral swabs received in casework. *J Forensic Sci Soc* **17**:127–33.

Davies A, Wilson E. 1974. The persistence of seminal constituents in the human vagina. *Forensic Sci* **3**:45–55.

Department of Health. 1988. *Diagnosis of child sexual abuse.* HMSO, London.

Dziegelewski M, Simich JP, Rittenhouse-Olson K. 2002. Use of a Y chromosome probe as an aid in the forensic proof of sexual assault. *J Forensic Sci* **47**:601–4.

Enos WF, Beyer JC. 1978. Spermatozoa in the anal canal and rectum and in the oral cavity of female rape victims. *J Forensic Sci* **23**:231–3.

Enos WF, Beyer JC. 1980. Prostatic acid phosphatase, aspermia, and alcoholism in rape cases. *J Forensic Sci* **25**:353–6.

Enos WF, Beyer JC. 1981. The importance of examining skin and hair for semen in sexual assault cases. *J Forensic Sci* **26**:605–7.

Gabby T, Winkleby MA, Boyce WT, *et al.* 1992. Sexual abuse of children. The detection of semen on skin. *Am J Dis Child* **146**:700–3.

Gill P, Jeffreys AJ, Werrett DJ. 1985. Forensic application of DNA 'fingerprints'. *Nature* **318**:577–9.

Hochmeister MN, Budowle B, Rudin O, *et al.* 1999. Evaluation of prostate-specific antigen (PSA) membrane test assays for the forensic identification of seminal fluid. *J Forensic Sci* **44**:1057–60.

Hooft P, van de Voorde H. 1988. In vitro changes in human spermatozoa exposed to gastric juice: laboratory findings as a support for forensic practice. *Z Rechtsmed* **101**:41–4.

Hooft P, van de Voorde H. 1992. Evaluation of the modified zinc test and the acid phosphatase test as preliminary screening methods in sexual assault case material. *Forensic Sci Int* **53**:135–41.

Hooft PJ, van de Voorde HP. 1997. Bayesian evaluation of the modified zinc test and the acid phosphatase spot test for forensic semen investigation. *Am J Forensic Med Pathol* **18**:45–9.

Jimenez-Verdejo A, Osuna E, Garcia-Olivares E, *et al.* 1994. Study of the enzymatic activity of GGT, LDH, PAP and PSA in semen stains: application to age calculation. *Forensic Sci Int* **68**:7–15.

Keil W, Bachus J, Troger HD. 1996. Evaluation of MHS-5 in detecting seminal fluid in vaginal swabs. *Int J Legal Med* **108**:186–90.

Kind SS. 1964. The acid phosphatase test. In: Curry AS (ed.), *Methods of forensic science*. Interscience, London, Vol. 3, pp. 267–87.

Maher J, Vintiner S, Elliot D, *et al.* 2002. Evaluation of the biosign PSA membrane test for the identification of semen stains in forensic casework. *N Z Med J* **115**:48–9.

Nicholson R. 1965. Vitality of spermatozoa in the endocervical canal. *Fertil Steril* **16**:758–64.

Paparo GP, Siegel H. 1979. Histologic diagnosis of sodomy. *J Forensic Sci* **24**:772–4.

Poyntz FM, Martin PD. 1984. Comparison of p30 and acid phosphatase levels in post-coital vaginal swabs from donor and casework studies. *Forensic Sci Int* **24**:17–25.

Reade DJ. 1985. Early investigations of sexual assault. *Police Surg* **April**:424.

Roberts REI. 1984. Sexual offences. In: McClay W (ed.), *Rape. The new police surgeon*. Association of Police Surgeons of Great Britain, Northampton, pp. 65–81.

Rupp JC. 1969. Sperm survival and prostatic acid phosphatase activity in victims of sexual assault. *J Forensic Sci* **14**:177–83.

Sato I, Sagi M, Ishiwari A, *et al.* 2002. Use of the 'SMITEST' PSA card to identify the presence of prostate-specific antigen in semen and male urine. *Forensic Sci Int* **127**:71–4.

Schiff AF. 1969. Modification of the Berg acid phosphatase test. *J Forensic Sci* **14**:538–44.

Schiff AF. 1975. Sperm identification – acid phosphatase test. *Med Trial Tech Q* **21**:467–74.

Sibille I, Duverneuil C, Lorin de la Grandmaison G, *et al.* 2002. Y-STR DNA amplification as biological evidence in sexually assaulted female victims with no cytological detection of spermatozoa. *Forensic Sci Int* **125**:212–16.

Simich JP, Morris SL, Klick RL, *et al.* 1999. Validation of the use of a commercially available kit for the identification of prostate specific antigen (PSA) in semen stains. *J Forensic Sci* **44**:1229–31.

Soukos NS, Crowley K, Bamberg MP, *et al.* 2000. A rapid method to detect dried saliva stains swabbed from human skin using fluorescence spectroscopy. *Forensic Sci Int* **114**:133–8.

Steinman G. 1995. Rapid spot tests for identifying suspected semen specimens. *Forensic Sci Int* **72**:191–7.

Takatori T, Sasaki T. 1980. Isolation of spermatozoa in vaginal contents by centrifugation in a colloidal silica gradient. *Forensic Sci Int* **15**:61–5.

Toates P. 1979. The forensic identification of semen by isoelectric focusing of seminal acid phosphatase. *Forensic Sci Int* **14**:191–214.

Vihko P, Mattila K, Ehnholm C. 1981. Radioimmunoassay of human prostate-specific acid phosphatase. A sensitive and specific assay for semen detection in forensic medicine. *Am J Clin Pathol* **75**:219–20.

Willott GM, Allard JE. 1982. Spermatozoa – their persistence after sexual intercourse. *Forensic Sci Int* **19**:133–54.

Willott GM, Crosse MA. 1986. The detection of spermatozoa in the mouth. *J Forensic Sci Soc* **26**:125–8.

Zarrabeitia M, Amigo T, Sanudo C, *et al.* 2002. A new pentaplex system to study short tandem repeat markers of forensic interest on X chromosome. *Forensic Sci Int* **129**:85–9.

CHAPTER 19

Deaths associated with pregnancy

Though not usually a forensic problem, deaths associated with pregnancy (other than criminal abortions) are intensively investigated in a number of countries. In Britain, the Department of Health has had an ongoing 'Confidential Enquiry into Maternal Deaths' running for many years, which publishes valuable reports at 3-yearly intervals that have helped to clarify both the clinical and pathological aspects of the problem.

The pathologist has an important role in furthering the understanding of the causes of death in pregnancy and after childbirth. A good autopsy is essential, with full histological examination and other ancillary investigations where necessary. Only in this way can the full range of causes of death be recognized, especially amniotic fluid embolism, which is a histological diagnosis.

To give an example of the range of fatal conditions that occur in association with pregnancy, the following causes are taken from the 'Confidential Enquiry' from Britain published in 1998, the figures referring to death during pregnancy and within 6 weeks of parturition in the years 1994–1996. Altogether 376 deaths were reported to or identified by the enquiry in the UK during that period. Of the 376, there were 134 (36 per cent) direct and 134 (36 per cent) indirect maternal deaths. The number of underlying causes of death of the direct maternal deaths is shown in Table 19.1.

According to a recent estimation, about 26 million legal and 20 million illegal abortions are carried out yearly throughout the world. Forensic pathological interest in pregnancy revolves almost exclusively around deaths associated with abortion, either criminal or legally induced. The term 'therapeutic abortion' is used in many countries, including

TABLE 19.1 *Number of direct maternal deaths by cause, United Kingdom 1994–1996*

Cause of death	n	Percentage
Thrombosis and thromboembolism	48	35.8
Hypertensive disease of pregnancy	20	14.9
Amniotic fluid embolism	17	12.7
Early pregnancy deaths*	15	11.2
Sepsis	14	10.4
Haemorrhage	12	9.0
Genital tract trauma	7	5.2
Anaesthesia	1	0.7
Total	134	100.0

*Ectopic pregnancy, spontaneous abortion, or termination of pregnancy, before 24 weeks' gestation.

Britain, where there is no abortion on demand, as in some countries. The description 'legal termination of pregnancy' is a wider definition for all but illegal (that is, criminal) abortions. The autopsy investigation of deaths from legal abortions has much in common with that into fatalities associated with surgical and anaesthetic procedures.

DEATHS ASSOCIATED WITH ABORTION

Though in many countries medical termination of pregnancy ('therapeutic abortion') is legal, a large area of the world still prohibits any form of abortion, either totally or except for the preservation of life of the pregnant woman. Even in those states where legal termination is possible, criminal abortions are still carried out, albeit on a small scale.

The reasons for this survival are varied, but are either because of restrictive grounds for legally available termination or to some sections of society that do not wish to avail themselves of the legal provisions. Whatever the cause, criminal abortion is associated with a considerable risk of both morbidity and mortality, especially in countries with a lower level of medical and social care.

Legal termination of pregnancy

When carried out with proper facilities, legal abortion has an extremely low mortality rate, being less than the mean death rate associated with pregnancy. The usual methods are vacuum aspiration, dilatation and curettage, or hysterotomy in later pregnancy. A few deaths are reported from time to time, the causes including:

- pulmonary embolism from leg vein thrombosis
- mishaps associated with anaesthesia
- disseminated intravascular coagulation and cerebral damage (including 'butterfly' haemorrhagic infarction in the basal ganglia) when abortion was induced by intrachorionic injection of hypertonic saline or glucose after the twelfth week (Cameron and Dayan 1960)
- air embolism following vacuum aspiration – only two cases have been reported and the mechanism is obscure, one theory being that 'elastic rebound' of the aspirated uterus sucked air into the cavity
- bleeding or infection, which failed to respond to treatment.

Death from illegal abortion

This has a much wider range of causes. The risks vary according to the skill, experience and facilities of the abortionist. When this is carried out by a doctor with aseptic and antiseptic methods, together with antibiotic cover if needed, the risk may be small compared with the crude methods of a lay person using makeshift instruments. The most common methods together with the associated dangers to health and life are as follows.

INSTRUMENTAL INTERFERENCE

The intention is to disturb the pregnancy sac so that, once damaged, it will be expelled by uterine contractions. This usually consists of dilatation of the cervical canal, which in itself also tends to dislodge the pregnancy. All manner of instruments have been used, from surgical dilators to bicycle spokes. A favourite in the hands of paramedical abortionists is the bougie or stiff catheter. When used by doctors or nurses with anatomical knowledge and sterile instruments, the risk is small, but lay persons often have no idea of the relationship of uterus to vagina. The instrument is then often pushed into the posterior fornix in the misguided belief that the cervix lies axially with the vagina. The vault of the vagina can be perforated and the instrument may even be passed through coils of intestine as far as the liver. Penetration of the lower or mid-vagina can also occur. If the cervix is entered, then the canal may be punctured and the instrument emerges through the side.

The external os may be badly injured by repeated, clumsy attempts to introduce too thick an object into the undilated canal. If successfully passed into the cavity of the uterus, it may be pushed right up through the fundus, again to damage the contents of the peritoneal cavity.

The dangers of such instrumentation are bleeding and infection. Perforation of the wall of vagina or uterus may cause severe bleeding, which may be internal or external. Sepsis can supervene in the peritoneal cavity or pelvic tissues either directly from a dirty instrument or from transfer of vaginal, skin or bowel organisms.

Another less common danger of the use of instruments (including syringes) is cervical shock. The mere act of dilating the cervix with an instrument in an unanaesthetized patient may trigger a vagal reflex, the efferent pathway being via the parasympathetic nervous system, causing a cardiac arrest. This is known to be a more potent mechanism in states of fear, apprehension and nervous tension, which obviously will apply to many candidates for a criminal abortion.

INSUFFLATION OF AIR

In Europe, this is becoming more of historical interest, but occasional cases still occur. A rubber pump, usually a Higginson enema syringe, is used to introduce fluid under pressure into the cavity of the uterus. This strips the chorionic sac from the wall of the uterus, exposing the placental bed. If sufficient detachment is achieved, then abortion will occur. It was formerly a popular method of abortion, both by women themselves and by abortionists. The main danger – part from the usual risks of bleeding and infection from damage to the tissues by the stiff nozzle – was air embolism, and in the first half of this century it was a major cause of abortion deaths. The intention was to introduce a fluid such as water–soap solution or disinfectant through the cervix by means of the syringe nozzle, the other end, which carried a one-way valve, being dipped in a receptacle of the fluid.

As the level in the receptacle dropped, the inlet tube rose above the surface and the syringe began to inject air instead of fluid, often as soapy foam. In addition to this danger, unless the bulb of the pump was primed with fluid before use, the first ejection would be the appreciable volume of air

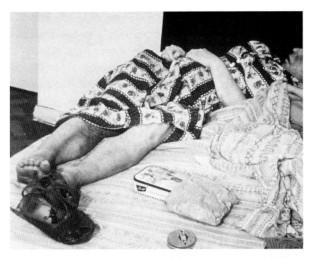

FIGURE 19.1 *The sudden unexpected death of a woman of child-bearing age should always arouse the consideration of a complication of pregnancy. This woman insufflated her uterus with a Higginson syringe and had time to clean up the equipment before collapsing with air embolism. This photograph was taken before the British Abortion Act of 1967, as such events are now uncommon.*

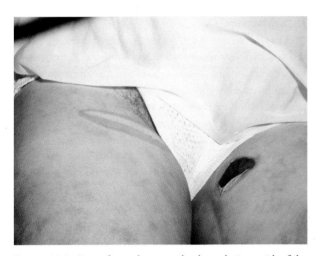

FIGURE 19.2 *Burns from a hot-water bottle on the inner side of the upper thigh in an attempt to resuscitate the victim of a criminal abortion who died from air embolism.*

contained in the empty syringe, which in itself was enough to cause a fatal embolism. Under the considerable pressure available from the instrument (as much as 28 cm of mercury according to Teare 1958), this air was forced into the exposed vascular channels of the placental bed and from there into venous sinuses and pelvic veins to cause cardiac embolism.

Though this occurred almost immediately in most instances, some delay was possible – perhaps because contained air was further squeezed by contraction of the uterus. Some victims were able to leave the premises of an abortionist and survive for up to 2 hours or more before the embolism

occurred (Simpson 1951). The addition of various substances, such as phenol, formalin, alcohol and turpentine, to the fluid introduced a toxic element, and in some cases these fluids were extruded into the peritoneal cavity through the uterine tubes, causing a chemical peritonitis.

DILATATION OF THE CERVIX

Another crude method was to introduce a 'tent' into the cervical canal. This was a strip of substance that absorbed water and became greatly enlarged, such as *Laminaria digitale* or slippery elm (*Ulmus fulva Michx*). These vegetable materials are hard and compact when dehydrated, so that a strip about 3–8 cm long could be slid into the cervix. When water was absorbed from the surrounding tissues, the cervical canal became widely dilated and abortion might take place. The risks were perforation of the cervix and also infection, especially if the strip tore into the tissues. The substances used, often crude vegetable material, could be the source of infecting micro-organisms including anaerobes.

PHYSICAL VIOLENCE

Women anxious to lose their pregnancy have resorted to extremes of physical activity and even violence in efforts to dislodge the fetus. Frenzied exercise, horse-riding and severe purging with laxatives were usually ineffective, and some unfortunate women went on to seek violent treatment from husbands or consorts. Punching and kicking of the abdomen were most common, and death from visceral rupture, such as liver, spleen or intestine, has been reported. Ironically, the uterine contents were usually undisturbed.

SYRINGE ASPIRATION

The suction method most often used in therapeutic abortion has also come to be used for illegal operations, mainly by medical or nursing personnel. A large syringe attached to a catheter or length of plastic tubing can produce suction within the uterus sufficient to rupture the chorionic sac and precipitate abortion. The method is safe as long as aseptic methods are used, though, if evacuation is incomplete, some products of conception may be left behind that can form a nidus for infection.

INTRAUTERINE INFECTION

Whatever method is used to evacuate the uterus, the risk of haemorrhage or sepsis is always present. Where an instrument, tent or syringe is used, any remaining fragments of placenta or other products of conception may form a substrate for infection. The organisms involved in sepsis are varied, the most dangerous being non-haemolytic

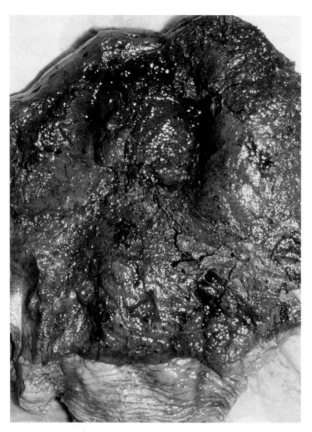

FIGURE 19.3 *Septic, necrotic uterus following an instrumental criminal abortion. The endometrium, containing some retained products of conception, is chocolate brown and foul-smelling, the predominant organism on culture being* Clostridium perfringens.

streptococci and *Clostridium perfringens*, though coliforms and staphylococci may also be responsible.

The uterus becomes swollen, spongy and discoloured. The serosal surface seen at autopsy may be brownish – especially in clostridial infections – and the endometrium may be ragged, foul-smelling and even purulent. Signs of septicaemia may develop with an enlarged, soft spleen, prominent lymph nodes and hepatorenal failure. The kidneys may show bilateral cortical necrosis in extreme cases. In clostridial septicaemias there may be a characteristic bronze coloration of the skin. This may have a mottled or 'raindrop' appearance.

THE USE OF DRUGS AND CHEMICALS

A wide variety of substances, applied locally or taken by mouth, have been used since time immemorial to induce miscarriage. Some have a sound pharmacological basis, others are dangerous, and yet more lie in the realms of folk medicine. Substances applied locally include phenols and Lysol, mercuric chloride, potassium permanganate, arsenic,

formaldehyde and oxalic acid. All have their own dangers, both from local corrosion and systemic effects if absorbed. A necrotic pseudomembrane may form in the vagina and severe damage to the cervix may also ensue.

Potassium permanganate was a substance that appeared during the last war and persisted for some years, 650 cases being reported up to 1959, though only a few were fatal. It can cause local necrosis in the vagina and, if absorbed, can have fatal systemic effects including renal failure. Permanganate can cause profuse vaginal bleeding from necrosis, which may give the impression that abortion is threatened and lead an unsuspecting doctor to carry out a curettage. 'Utus paste' is a mixture of soap, myrrh resinoid and potassium iodide, and was used earlier in the century for legitimate abortions, but soon became popular with the criminal abortionist. Another similar product containing elemental iodine, is 'Interruptin'; both were used for late abortions and the induction of labour when the fetus was dead. These pastes are squeezed into the cervical canal through an applicator and the halogen component acts as an irritant which causes eventual expulsion of the chorionic sac. Used medically, they are relatively safe (Barns 1967; Berthelsen and Ostervaard 1959), but fatalities can occur from air or fat embolism or from the toxic effects of absorption.

Substances taken by mouth or injection are legion. The old classification into 'ecbolics' and 'emmenagogues' is now quite redundant and most of the lists of substances are of historical interest only, as their efficacy is either nil or the dose needed to produce abortion is perilously near the fatal level. These include pennyroyal, tansy, rue, savin, laburnum, colocynth, aloes, castor oil, nutmeg, hellebore, cantharides, cotton root, wintergreen and turpentine. Many of these may cause purging, gastrointestinal irritation and general illness if taken in quantity, but have no specific action whatsoever on the uterus. There are other substances that have more chance of causing uterine contractions, though many of them are effective only on a late pregnancy, not at the usual time of 1–3 months when most abortions are sought.

Quinine can be dangerous, as the dosage required for any effect on the uterus is likely to cause cinchonism. Ergometrine has been known from ancient times to lead to abortion, though like most drugs its effectiveness is greater later in pregnancy. Excess dosage may cause peripheral vascular spasm and gangrene. Its availability to doctors and mid-wives is similar to pituitary extract, oestrogens, and – more recently – prostaglandins. Heavy metals, particularly lead, were used for abortion in the past. Plasters coated with a lead compound 'diachylon' were scraped to recover the metallic substances and ingested. Though abortion sometimes occurred, illness and death from acute and subacute lead poisoning was more common; this method has also become of historical interest only. It has been well said that most substances that

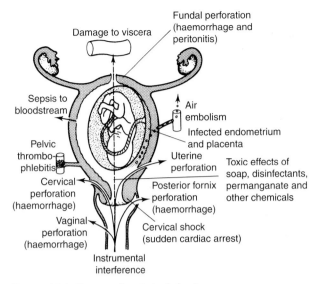

FIGURE 19.4 *Dangers of a criminal abortion.*

are successful in killing the fetus are likely to kill the mother as well.

A wide variety of medical substances have been used for abortion, including aminopterin, steroids, antimitotic drugs, such as vincristine and ergocornine, and other cytotoxic drugs used in malignant diseases. Even monoamine oxidase inhibitors have been reported as abortifacients. In all these, the autopsy findings in fatal cases will be non-specific or negative, and the history and toxicology provide virtually all the available evidence.

THE AUTOPSY IN ABORTION DEATHS

Where a death in pregnancy or the puerperium occurs, every effort should be made to obtain an autopsy, even if the death does not fall within the usual category of death reportable for medico-legal investigation. When a criminal abortion is suspected, then virtually every jurisdiction will require necropsy.

The usual full autopsy is performed, but a number of additional measures are required, varied to suit the particular circumstances. The fullest possible history is required and, where the death has taken place under medical care, a prior discussion with the clinician is vital. A careful external examination must be carried out, noting especially:

- Abnormal coloration of the skin, such as in the bronzing of clostridial septicaemia and the jaundice of liver damage.
- Signs and duration of pregnancy, such as abdominal swelling and breast changes.
- Signs of injury, including bruising or abrasion of the vulva from instrumentation, and vaginal bleeding.

Burns on the abdomen or inner sides of the upper thighs may indicate efforts at resuscitation by hot-water bottles when a woman has suddenly collapsed during an illegal abortion.

- The vagina should be examined for signs of recent or current pregnancy, and attempted or successful recent abortion. Any fluid should be removed by pipette to be examined for soap and chemicals, such as antiseptics. A swab should be taken for microbiological culture.
- Where any possibility of air embolism is considered, pre-autopsy radiology of the chest and abdomen must be performed. Some pathologists would consider this obligatory in any death associated with pregnancy, as it is the best method of detecting air embolism by visualizing air bubbles in the heart, great veins in the thorax, inferior vena cava, peritoneal cavity and – possibly – pelvic veins. In the few centres where MRI or computed tomography is available for autopsy material, this may greatly increase the chance of detecting air in the vessels.

Where radiology is not possible, air must be sought by dissection methods, which are not so reliable. The thorax is opened carefully, making sure that removal of the costal cartilages and sternum does not damage the underlying mediastinum or open any of the veins at the thoracic inlet. The cardiovascular system is first examined for the presence of air. The classic method, discussed elsewhere in this book, is to open the heart chambers *in situ* under water poured into the pericardial sac. Escaping bubbles are then said to be indicative of air embolism, though the technique is by no means as reliable as past authors have claimed. In fact, if the post-mortem interval is short, in terms of a few hours, then any fatal air embolism will almost always be quite apparent from the frothy contents of the right ventricle when it is opened in the usual way. Appreciable delay allows absorption of air, as can be proved by the failure to find air in the heart on dissection, even after radiology has clearly indicated its presence. Of course, where any degree of decomposition has set in, which may be on the first day after death in hot countries, gases of putrefaction completely negate any chances of proving air embolism.

Before the organs are disturbed, the great veins of the abdomen should be inspected for bubbles, then the pelvic veins. The uterus itself may be crepitant and bubbles may be seen under the serosal surface or even under the parietal peritoneum of the pelvis. On opening the uterus, gas bubbles may be evident in the wall or placental bed, but this is later in the examination. The usual instructions in most forensic textbooks for opening the head first, carefully removing the calvarium and minutely inspecting the cerebral veins for air bubbles, can be totally disregarded, as this is yet another

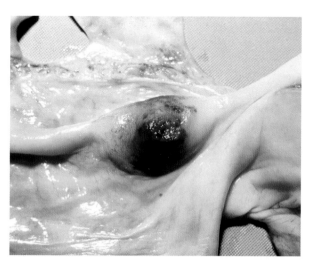

FIGURE 19.5 *Ruptured tuba in (ectopic) pregnancy. Death due to massive intraperitoneal haemorrhage. (Reproduced by kind permission of Professor E Lignitz.)*

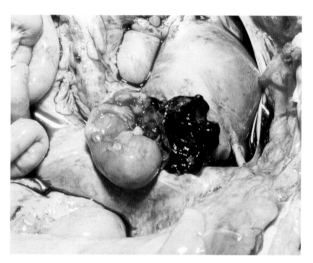

FIGURE 19.6 *Fetus and placenta in the abdominal cavity after ruptured tubal (ectopic) pregnany. Death due to massive intraperitoneal haemorrhage. (Reproduced by kind permission of Professor E Lignitz.)*

example of forensic mythology repeated from one book to the next, without critical evaluation. As discussed in Chapter 13, air embolism cannot occur in the cerebral veins and it was proved many years ago that air bubbles in those veins are artefacts caused by removing the calvarium.

The thorax and upper abdomen should be examined as usual, with particular attention to signs of infection. Blood cultures, and peritoneal and other swabs should be taken as indicated by the circumstances.

The pelvic organs should be removed *en bloc*, as in the examination of fatal rape victims. The lower end of the

abdominal incision is carried on each side around the labia and into the cleft of the buttocks to meet beyond the anus. The dissection is taken along the superior pubic rami, which are then carefully sawn through a few centimetres laterally to the symphysis on each side, the cuts being continued down through the inferior rami. The central block of bone is removed and the perineal incision dissected deeply, so that the vagina, rectum and anus, uterus, tubes and ovaries can be lifted out in continuity, and removed for detailed dissection. The vagina is carefully opened along one side to avoid over-running any midline injuries. Abrasions, bruises, lacerations and any foreign material are noted in the vagina, and any samples kept for chemical or microbiological testing. Any abnormality of the cervix is noted, especially instrument marks, such as forceps or volsellum teeth. The state of dilatation of the cervical canal is noted and the uterus opened, again keeping away from the midline if possible. The colour, size and texture of the uterus is noted, and the state of the interior is naturally vital. If the chorionic sac is still present, its integrity and the attachment to the deciduae are noted. If a fetus is present, this is examined separately for maturity and damage.

If no fetus is present, products of conception are sought and the state of the placental bed noted. Infection, bleeding and air crepitancy are all sought, and the appropriate ancillary investigations made. The tubes are then opened and any foreign fluid collected. The ovaries are examined and the state of any corpus luteum recorded. Finally, extensive histological specimens are taken from all organs and special stains employed where necessary, such as those for seeking amniotic squames in lungs and other organs. Blood, urine, liver and stomach contents are retained for analysis, should this be indicated.

AMNIOTIC FLUID EMBOLISM

Some deaths associated with childbirth or pregnancy are caused by the entry of amniotic fluid into the maternal circulation. The fluid contains fetal squames, lanugo, lipoid from the vernix, meconium, cells from chorion and amnion, and other cellular detritus. The solid elements are usually impacted in the lung capillaries, but rarely have been found in the systemic circulation, including embolization into the kidney, liver and brain. In addition to the solids, the actual fluid itself (which is naturally undetectable histologically) is blamed for the 'allergic' response that may cause such profound collapse, leading to death. Amniotic fluid embolism is also one of the most potent causes of disseminated intravascular coagulopathy, mentioned also in Chapter 13.

A variety of causes exist apart from the pelvic trauma of parturition, including rupture of the uterus, but instrumental interference late in pregnancy may also allow opening of the sinuses in the placental bed with consequent escape of amniotic fluid. Further details of the causes and mechanisms must be sought in obstetric works, but from the autopsy point of view, it is important both to bear the possibility in mind and to have techniques that will reveal the embolism after autopsy. The diagnosis is histological and depends upon identifying the squames detached from the fetal epidermis, which float freely in amniotic fluid. These can be seen in ordinary haematoxylin and eosin stained sections of the lung, but are much better visualized and a greater yield obtained if special staining methods are used, as described in Appendix 1. Fibrin deposition in many organs may occur as a result of the disseminated intravascular coagulation and careful search for this must be made, using fibrin stains. Immunohistochemical techniques have also been used in the lung sections to demonstrate human keratin-, meconium- and amniotic fluid-derived mucin as well as isolated trophoblastic cells in deaths due to AFE (amniotic fluid embolism) syndrome.

REFERENCES AND FURTHER READING

Adebahr G. 1969. [The forensic value of findings in the cadaver.] *Beitr Gerichtl Med* **25**:44–50.

Anonymous. 1999. Abortion in fact: levels, trend and patterns. In: *Sharing responsibility: women, society and abortion worldwide.* Alan Guttmecher Institute, New York, pp. 25–31.

Attwood HD. 1956. Fatal pulmonary embolism by amniotic fluid. *J Clin Pathol* **9**:38–46.

Baekgaard T. 1969. [Penalties for criminal abortion.] *Ugeskr Laeger* **131**:1069–70.

Barns H. 1967. Therapeutic abortion by means of soft soap pastes. *Lancet* **2**:825.

Benson MD, Kobayashi H, Silver RK, *et al.* 2001. Immunologic studies in presumed amniotic fluid embolism. *Obstet Gynecol* **97**:510–14.

Berthelsen H, Ostervaard E. 1959. Techniques and complications in therapeutic abortion. *Dan Med Bull* **6**:105–10.

Bowen DA. 1967. Medical investigation in cases of sudden death. *Br Med J* **2**:33–6.

Bowen DA. 1980. Criminal abortion. Fact or fiction? *Am J Forensic Med Pathol* **1**:219–21.

Breitenecker L, Husslein H. 1968. [Expert testimony as proof of previous pregnancies.] *Wien Klin Wochenschr* **80**:937–42.

Cameron J, Dayan A. 1960. Association of brain damage with therapeutic abortion induced by amniotic fluid replacement; report of two cases. *Br Med J* **1**:1010.

Cera G, Fruttero A, Rua S, *et al.* 1992. Flow cytometric studies in spontaneous abortions. Applications in the medico-legal practice. *Forensic Sci Int* **54**:167–75.

Cimbura G. 1967. Studies of criminal abortion cases in Ontario. *J Forensic Sci* **12**:223–9.

Davies S. 2001. Amniotic fluid embolus: a review of the literature. *Can J Anaesth* **48**:88–98.

Dayan AD, Cameron JM, Phillipp E. 1967. Fatal brain damage associated with therapeutic abortion induced by amniocentesis: report of one case. *Med Sci Law* **7**:70–2.

De Gennaro F. 1969. [Criminal abortion. A clinical case and medicolegal aspects.] *Minerva Ginecol* **21**:1002–5.

Demol R, Vandekerckhove D, Thiery M. 1968. [Various 'traps' in diagnosing pregnancy reactions.] *Med Leg Dommage Corp* **1**:282–9.

Eckert WG. 1985. The writings of Sir Bernard Spilsbury: Part II. *Am J Forensic Med Pathol* **6**:31–7.

Eliakis E, Coutselinis A. 1971. [Identification of meconium by the determination of acid phosphatase and spectrophotometric analysis.] *Med Leg Dommage Corp* **4**:163–8.

Fineschi V, Gambassi R, Gherardi M, *et al.* 1998. The diagnosis of amniotic fluid embolism: an immunohistochemical study for the quantification of pulmonary mast cell tryptase. *Int J Legal Med* **111**:238–43.

Garland IW, Thompson WD. 1983. Diagnosis of amniotic fluid embolism using an antiserum to human keratin. *J Clin Pathol* **36**:625–7.

Gastmeier G, Klein A, Falk H. 1969. [Contribution to inverse soap poisoning.] *Dtsch Z Gesamte Gerichtl Med* **65**:96–102.

Gerchow J, Schewe G. 1970. [Legal theory of value assessment and medical aspects of the need to protect the beginning of life.] *Beitr Gerichtl Med* **27**:61–71.

Holzer FJ. 1973. [Abortion using a bicycle pump on the mistress and unusual suicide of a blind man.] *Beitr Gerichtl Med* **30**:187–96.

Hunt AC. 1960. Amniotic fluid embolism. *J Forensic Med* **7**:74–7.

Huntington K. 1976. Forensic gynaecology. *Practitioner* **216**:519–28.

Huxley AK, Sibley MA. 1998. Alleged forgery of sonography report leads to elective abortion of late 23 week-old fetus. *J Forensic Sci* **43**:218–21.

Inoue H, Takabe F, Maeno Y, *et al.* 1989. Identification of fetal hemoglobin in blood stains by high performance liquid chromatography. *Z Rechtsmed* **102**:437–44.

Janssen W. 1967. [On the pathogenesis and forensic evaluation of brain hemorrhages following cerebral air embolism.] *Dtsch Z Gesamte Gerichtl Med* **61**:62–80.

Kenyeres I. 1976. [Various problems concerning maternal mortality during pregnancy.] *Morphol Igazsagugyi Orv Sz* **16**:120–5.

Khong TY. 1998. Expression of endothelin-1 in amniotic fluid embolism and possible pathophysiological mechanism. *Br J Obstet Gynaecol* **105**:802–4.

Kobayashi H, Ooi H, Hayakawa H, *et al.* 1997. Histological diagnosis of amniotic fluid embolism by monoclonal antibody TKH-2 that recognizes neuac alpha 2–6galnac epitope. *Hum Pathol* **28**:428–33.

Kocsis I, Argay I, Toth G. 1972. [Course of disease in an unconscious patient causing several problems.] *Morphol Igazsagugyi Orv Sz* **12**:209–11.

Kopecny J, Martincik M, Chalupa M, *et al.* 1970. [Induction of abortion using high doses of oxytocin.] *Cesk Gynekol* **35**:118–19.

Kumar GP, Kumar UK. 1994. Estimation of gestational age from hand and foot length. *Med Sci Law* **34**:48–50.

Kumar KU, Pillay VV. 1996. Estimation of fetal age by histological study of kidney. *Med Sci Law* **36**:226–30.

Kurucz E, Kosa F, Monostori E, *et al.* 1984. A new method in criminology: use of ELISA to detect AFP on different materials with monoclonal anti-alpha-fetoprotein. *Z Rechtsmed* **93**:117–21.

Lewis G. 2001. *Why mothers die. Report on confidential enquiries into maternal deaths in the United Kingdom 1997–1999.* RCOG Press, London.

Lewis G, Drife JO, Botting BJ, *et al.* 1998. *Why mothers die: report on confidential enquiries into maternal deaths in the United Kingdom 1994–1996.* TSO, London.

Lorente Acosta JA, Lorente Acosta M, Villanueva Canadas E. 1998. [The physician and medicine in the new penal code.] *Med Clin (Barc)* **111**:222–5.

Lunetta P, Penttila A. 1996. Immunohistochemical identification of syncytiotrophoblastic cells and megakaryocytes in pulmonary vessels in a fatal case of amniotic fluid embolism. *Int J Legal Med* **108**:210–14.

Mallach HJ, Pfeiffer KH. 1978. [The importance of air embolism as a primary and secondary cause of death.] *Med Welt* **29**:1391–6.

Marcinkowski T, Przybylski Z. 1968. [Teratoma as a cause of unjustified suspicion of abortion.] *Patol Pol* **19**:135–8.

Möttönen M, Isomäki AM. 1971. Amniotic fluid embolism, diagnosed by a new method. *Med Sci Law* **11**:35–7.

Nishio H, Matsui K, Miyazaki T, *et al.* 2002. A fatal case of amniotic fluid embolism with elevation of serum mast cell tryptase. *Forensic Sci Int* **126**:53–6.

Ohi H, Kobayashi H, Terao T. 1993. [A new histologic diagnosis for amniotic fluid embolism by monoclonal antibody TKH-2 that recognizes mucin-type glycoprotein.] *Nippon Sanka Fujinka Gakkai Zasshi* **45**:464–70.

Patel F. 1993. Artefact in forensic medicine. Fetal congenital abnormality. *Am J Forensic Med Pathol* **14**:212–14.

Rees PO. 1970. A case of poisoning by Epsom salt. *J Forensic Sci Soc* **10**:91–4.

Richard T, Rappolt MD, Sr. 1970. Clinical observation: apparent antagonism of ergotamine on the gravid uterus by LSD-25. *Eur J Toxicol* **3**:138–9.

Ronnau H, Wille R. 1980. [Psychological complications following abortion.] *Beitr Gerichtl Med* **38**:21–4.

Rosenzweig E, Stajduhar-Caric Z, Milicic D, *et al.* 1970. [Incidence of uterine perforations in criminal abortions.] *Rad Med Fak Zagrebu* **18**:221–4.

Russell DH. 1968. Law, medicine and minors. I. *N Engl J Med* **278**:35–6.

Schwerd W. 1965. The detection of soap abortions. In: Curry AS (ed.), *Methods of forensic science*, vol. 4. Interscience Publishers, London.

Shapiro HA. 1966. The diagnosis of death from delayed air embolism. *Acta Med Leg Soc (Liege)* **19**:207–11.

Simpson K. 1951. Air embolism. *Med Leg J* **19**:81–5.

Teare D. 1958. Death in criminal abortion. *Med Leg J* **26**:132–4.

Tesar J, Klir P, Doskocilova L. 1977. [Demonstration of neonatal blood.] *Soud Lek* **22**:9–11.

Toner PG. 1992. *The role of the histopathologist in maternal death. Maternal mortality – the way forward.* Royal College of Obstetricians and Gynecologists, London, Chapter 10.

Uszynski M, Zekanowska E, Uszynski W, *et al.* 2001. Tissue factor (TF) and tissue factor pathway inhibitor (TFPI) in amniotic fluid and blood plasma: implications for the mechanism of amniotic fluid embolism. *Eur J Obstet Gynecol Reprod Biol* **95**:163–6.

Zakharova OA, Bakshinskaia RE. 1968. [Mortality significance of acute renal insufficiency in criminal abortion.] *Sud Med Ekspert* **11**:18–20.

CHAPTER 20

Infanticide and stillbirth

Historically, infanticide has by no means always been a crime, and has been practised as a social and economic necessity since the dawn of humanity. The pathologist, however, has to deal with the practicalities of infanticide as they exist today. Though legal definitions vary among different countries, the medical concept of infanticide is uniform, being the deliberate killing of a newborn infant by the mother. In England and Wales, infanticide was not accepted as a legal entity in the criminal law until 1922. Before then all child killing was murder – and the convicted mother was liable to be sentenced to death until the Infanticide Act, which was re-enacted in a more satisfactory form in 1938 (see account by Kellett 1992).

In many other countries there is no specific infanticide legislation – even Scotland did not adopt the English statute, having a separate crime of 'child murder', but long before 1922 that country had held a more enlightened attitude towards the mentally stressed mother. In Japan, Funayama *et al.* (1994) have described cases of multiple, repeated infanticides by five mothers.

This book generally avoids territorial legal comparisons, but the foregoing facts serve to illustrate that the killing of a young child by the mother is a well-recognized medical and psychiatric phenomenon that distinguishes it from other types of homicide. The penalties should therefore be different and there is a profound responsibility laid upon the forensic pathologist called to examine such infants, to investigate the death with particular caution.

The substance of infanticide that has relevance to the pathologist is well set out in the English Infanticide Act 1938 (Section 1):

> Where a woman by any wilful act or omission causes the death of a child being under the age of 12 months, but at the time the balance of her mind was disturbed by having given birth or the effect of lactation, she may be dealt with as if she had committed manslaughter.

It should be noted that:

- Only the mother can benefit from this alternative to murder – not the father or any other person.
- The child has to be less than a year old, though in fact the majority of infanticides occur within hours or even minutes of birth.
- It has to be a 'child' – that is, a person with a separate existence living independently fully outside the mother's body.
- It must have died because of a wilful (deliberate) act of omission or commission.

All these provisos have an effect on the pathologist's task. Even in those jurisdictions where there is no formal infanticide legislation, there is usually recognition that the acts of a woman soon after childbirth, often in adverse conditions, are different from common murder.

STILLBIRTH

To clarify later definitions, a stillbirth is defined in English law and, from a medical point of view no doubt has a broadly similar description in other jurisdictions. In England and Wales, a baby is stillborn if after 24 weeks' gestation, 'it did not at any time after being completely expelled from its mother, breathe or show any other sign of life'. Theoretically, this is a medically unsatisfactory definition, as it could be alive when its head was born but die

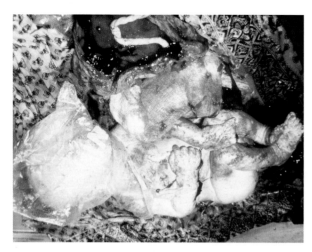

FIGURE 20.1 *Newborn baby with umbilical cord and placenta, abandoned in a car park. It was wrapped in a curtain and though the head was in a plastic bag no signs of suffocation nor of live birth could be detected. The mother was never identified.*

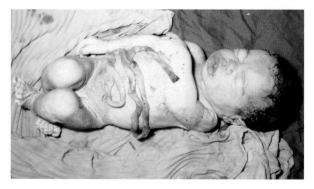

FIGURE 20.2 *Full-term newborn found wrapped in a blanket inside a shopping bag in a refuse container. The cord had been cut with a sharp instrument, but the child was not washed or fed. The lungs showed no positive evidence of respiration.*

before completion of expulsion, and therefore legally be a stillbirth. However, in practice this would be rare, as most stillbirths either die *in utero* or during the earlier stages of parturition. Stillbirths occur in about one in every 18 legitimate pregnancies in Britain, and are more frequent in illegitimate births and socially disadvantaged families.

FUNCTIONS OF THE PATHOLOGIST IN INFANTICIDE

To assist in identifying the mother, if she is unknown

Newborn infants found dead (especially in clandestine circumstances) are not necessarily the victims of infanticide. Those stillborn or dying naturally or from unintentional lack of care may be hidden or abandoned, a minor crime in Britain called 'concealment of birth'. The autopsy, as well as artefacts discovered with the body, such as bags, blankets and newspapers can assist to a greater or lesser degree in the police search for the mother.

The apparent ethnic group of the child will be disclosed and blood grouping can be performed, which may assist by eliminating or helping to confirm the consanguinity of any putative mother. In the future, DNA profiling will add greatly to identification. The appearance of the cut end and any ligation of the umbilical cord (see below) may help to decide whether the birth was one where medical, nursing or only amateur attention was available. In spite of these clues, most abandoned newborn corpses fail to be linked to

the mother, delay in discovery making both identification and evidence of live birth unattainable.

To estimate the maturity of the child

Though any newborn infant, whatever the length of gestation, can be the victim of infanticide if born alive, it is obviously relevant to this issue if the fetus is too immature to have survived birth. In another context [Infant Life (Preservation) Act 1929, concerning child destruction], the age of viability in English law was taken as 28 weeks' gestation, though this has now been reduced to 24 weeks as even younger fetuses can now survive with intensive medical support. If a child is shown to be that premature, there is a strong presumption that it would not long survive a birth away from medical attention.

To determine whether or not the child was stillborn and whether it had a separate existence

There is a presumption in English law that all infants are stillborn and, when a woman is charged with infanticide, the burden of proof is upon the prosecution to demonstrate that the child had a separate existence. Adelson (1974) states that the same legal situation exists in the USA, and gives the following useful and interesting commentary:

> Unless the pathologist has incontrovertible criteria of post-natal survival, e.g. well-expanded lungs, food in the stomach or vital reaction in the stump of the umbilical cord, he is legally bound not to diagnose live birth. Convictions for infanticide have been set aside when there has been any doubt whatsoever that the child was born alive. Many courts have pushed this proposition to the extent that the State has been given the burden of proving that the baby was born alive beyond any

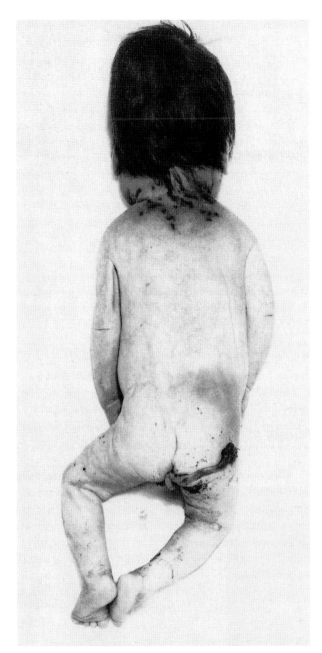

FIGURE 20.3 *A stillborn child concealed by the mother after birth. The injuries around the neck were viewed with suspicion by the police, but are the result of fingernails being used in an attempt to assist self-delivery in an unattended birth.*

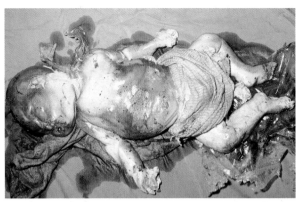

FIGURE 20.4 *A putrefied newborn infant disposed of in a plastic bag in the countryside. There is no hope of determining whether it was live or stillborn with this degree of post-mortem decomposition. There was a strip of fabric knotted around the neck, but it is impossible to decide if that was related to the death, if the child was not stillborn.*

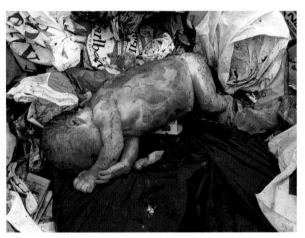

FIGURE 20.5 *A decomposed newborn infant found in a rubbish dump.*

To determine whether its death was due to natural causes or to any act of omission or commission

Where the pathologist claims to have proved separate existence (or at least, live birth), he has an additional burden in that he must show that death occurred from an act of commission or omission, The 'wilful' aspect is a matter for the lawyers, but it is for the pathologist either to demonstrate lethal injuries or to prove that some lack of care led to the death – often an impossible task. There is a considerable burden upon the investigating authorities when finding a hidden newborn infant if they wish to pursue an infanticide charge.

possible doubt rather than beyond any reasonable doubt, the latter being the general level of proof required in a criminal prosecution.

Herein lies the most difficult task for the pathologist, one which has given rise to considerable controversy in forensic pathology.

First, they must find the mother – often another impossible task. Then the pathologist must prove live birth, which is often impossible, especially in a decomposed body. To prove a separate existence is even more difficult and is rarely a purely medical decision. The firm diagnosis of death from wilful inattention is equally hard to make.

It is small wonder that only a small proportion of suspicious neonatal deaths ever reach the court – where few women are convicted, and those who are, rightly receive lenient and sympathetic treatment, usually consisting of probation and psychiatric support.

DEFINITION OF 'LIVE BIRTH' AND 'SEPARATE EXISTENCE'

There is no definition of live birth in English law, except by inference from the defined 'stillbirth', given earlier. Using the live birth as the converse of a stillbirth, the infant should have attained the gestational age of 24 weeks, but this is not a factor in 'separate existence' with which live birth is almost synonymous.

A child with a 'separate existence' would be an infant that had issued forth from its mother irrespective of its gestational age, and who breathed or showed any other signs of life after being completely expelled from the maternal passages – though the child could still be attached to the placenta within the mother. This is almost synonymous with a live birth, though medically all would agree that a child that was crying lustily, but with a foot still in the vagina, was undoubtedly live born even though it did not satisfy the legal criteria of a 'separate existence'.

Viability

Yet another medical and legal concept is that of viability, which is the potential ability of an infant to survive after birth. An immature fetus may be born alive, but be incapable of maintaining an independent existence. Naturally the stage of gestation at which this occurs varies not only with the condition of the particular fetus, but also with the state of medical knowledge and the facilities available at the relevant time and place.

In English law, a period of 24 weeks is fixed for the onset of viability, for the purposes of the Infant Life (Preservation) Act, 1929.

CONCEALMENT OF BIRTH

Mentioned earlier, this is a relatively minor crime in most jurisdictions and is basically an offence against registration,

and perhaps public decency, in that the body of an infant is neither notified to the authorities nor accorded a proper burial or other form of disposal. The crime is the hiding of the body to conceal the fact of birth. It does not depend at all on live birth, separate existence or viability, and the law is not concerned about the cause of death or whether it was stillborn. One problem is the stage of gestation at which the 'child' becomes noticed by the law – obviously an early abortion is of no concern to anyone, except the family.

Though not specified in relation to concealment of birth, English law takes no regard of products of conception under 24 weeks' gestation. In a judicial decision (*R* v *Matthews*), it was held that a charge of concealment of birth could not be sustained at an age where the law did not require the (still)birth to be registered.

Whatever the legal ramifications, the forensic pathologist is not infrequently asked to examine dead infants in which he can neither prove live birth nor a wilful act that might have caused death. The only remaining charge, if he can show an age above that of viability, is 'concealment of birth'. This is the end result of the discovery of most decomposed babies, in the minority where the mother can be traced.

THE AUTOPSY ON A SUSPICIOUS DEATH OF A NEWBORN INFANT

A number of important matters need specific attention, over and above the usual meticulous autopsy procedure on any infant.

The coverings and any other associated articles with the infant must be examined and retained. Though this is mainly police business, the pathologist usually has the task of unwrapping the baby – often in a decomposed and offensive state – from the coverings of newspaper, plastic bags, rags or blankets. He must recover any foreign material or objects that may assist in the identification of the mother when the disposal has been clandestine.

When the baby has been found in a house or other building, he may need to visit the scene, preferably with the child still *in situ*. Numerous cases are on record of the infant being in a lavatory pan and, if there are head injuries or drowning, the circumstances must be evaluated.

The external examination is, as always, important. It is vital to assess the degree of putrefaction because if it is in any way decomposed, it will almost certainly be impossible to determine whether live birth had occurred. Decomposition must be distinguished from intrauterine maceration, as the latter is definite proof of stillbirth. If death occurred within 2–3 days before expulsion from the uterus, the appearances may be fairly normal, apart from general softening and histological evidence of general cellular autolysis.

When it has been dead for many days, the macerated fetus is usually a brownish-pink, rather than the greenish hue of putrefaction. The surface is slimy, blistered, desquamating and sometimes almost jelly-like. The joints are grotesquely loose and the cranial plates may be virtually detached beneath the scalp. Their over-riding, radiologically seen as 'Spaulding's sign', is characteristic, so that the head is shapeless. Rarely, a macerated fetus – which is normally sterile – may become infected if not expelled after the membranes rupture; it will then be born in a putrefied state.

External examination will next be directed at the cord and placenta, if present. The latter must be measured and weighed to estimate the maturity and any abnormalities, such as placental infarcts, noted as possible reasons for fetal death. The cord is important as an indicator of separate existence, if survival has been for an appreciable period. Even where early putrefaction renders evaluation of breathing impossible, vital signs in the cord may indicate live birth if survival reached 24–48 hours. Until this period, no evidence of cord separation is reliable, but after a day or so, a ring of reddening appears around the base of the cord and adjacent abdominal skin. This becomes more marked in the succeeding few days as the cord dries and shrivels, detachment taking place between 5 and 9 days. As most infants die or are killed within hours of birth, however, these signs are rarely of much practical use.

The severed end of the cord should be examined, as it may indicate whether the cord had been broken or actually cut. This is occasionally important if death is the result of head injuries and the defence on behalf of the accused mother claims that the child fell to the ground head first during a precipitate delivery. The length of the cord must be measured, especially if the placental segment is available, so that the distance from the vulva to the floor can be calculated. The average cord length is about 50 cm, but more than twice this length is not uncommon, as are much shorter ones. Naturally, if a ligature is present it indicates either the attendance of a professional or at least knowledgeable person, but this is rare in these cases. The severed end may be examined in the hand, but may also be floated out in water, to better study the detail of the detachment. Morris and Hunt (1966) conducted experiments on cords and determined that they could easily be broken by hand traction. A broken cord can show a clean transverse termination, but is usually ragged. If cut by a sharp instrument such as knife or scissors the cut may be clean, but may also be ragged if the instrument is blunt.

If the baby is examined as found, either at the scene or undisturbed in wrappings, it should be noted if the cord was coiled around the neck. Although it is usually unsafe to claim that death during delivery was from pressure on the neck from the cord, the fact must be noted and evaluated along with all other findings.

The skin may still have vernix caseosa present. This is not a useful observation but, if none is present, it may indicate that the child had been washed, which suggests survival for some time after birth.

Measurements are vital for an estimate of maturity. Weight, crown–heel, crown–rump, head circumference, and foot length are required.

Abnormalities incompatible with continued life may be obvious, such as anencephaly, severe spina bifida or abdominal ectropion. It is, however, often unsafe to assume that actual live birth, as legally defined, could not have taken place.

Injuries are obviously of prime importance as evidence of the 'act of commission', though most newborns seen by the pathologist will be free of such trauma. The types of injury perpetrated by distraught mothers are numerous:

- Strangulation presents the usual features of bruises and abrasions on the neck, though these may be minimal. The classical features of facial congestion, cyanosis, oedema and petechiae may be present, but are often absent, presumably because of the ease with which the vulnerable infant dies. Abrasions on the neck, however, may also be caused by the frantic efforts of the mother to deliver herself, leaving finger-nail marks on the infant's neck. A ligature may be used, which may still be in place. Again caution must be employed, as the fact of some object around the neck, though suggestive,

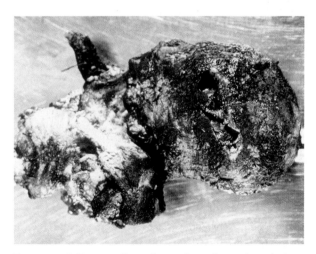

FIGURE 20.6 *Remains of a newborn infant, who was born during a weekend when the mother, a schoolgirl, was alone in her room in a boarding-school. After the birth she wrapped the child in a plastic bag. The following day she left for home and tried to burn the body in a stove but when that did not succeed she buried the partly burned body in a snowdrift where it was later found by a dog.*

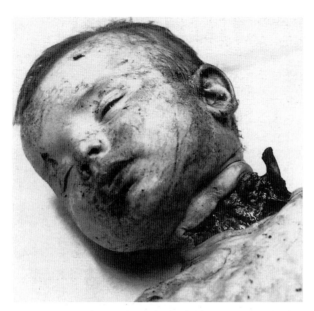

FIGURE 20.7 *Definite infanticide, the child having fully respired before having this severe incised wound of the neck made with a kitchen knife.*

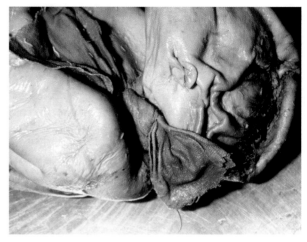

FIGURE 20.8 *A putrefied newborn infant with a scarf knotted tightly around the neck. (Reproduced by kind permission of Professor E Lignitz.)*

is not absolute proof of strangulation unless corroborative evidence of congestive and petechial signs in the face or skin, and tissue damage beneath the ligature is demonstrated. The explanation has been advanced in the past that a cloth ligature around the neck was an attempt to assist self-delivery by the woman in an obstructed labour.

▪ Smothering is almost impossible to prove, as the infant will almost never show conjunctival petechiae or other signs that may be seen in strangulation. Only if excessive pressure is applied, so that marks are left on the lips and face, can any evidence be retrieved. These must be definite intradermal or deep bruises, abrasions or marks within the lips and mouth – and not shadowy, vague variations in post-mortem staining. The arguments about criteria of suffocation in infants are further discussed in Chapter 14. Choking by the internal obstruction of the pharynx by various materials has been described in old reports, but it is excessively uncommon these days.

▪ Cutting and piercing is well known as a means of infanticide. Stabbing with scissors, either in the chest or neck, has been seen or even cutting the throat with a blade. The defence may be offered that the wounds were inflicted accidentally during frenzied efforts by the mother to cut the umbilical cord. Though not seen in Europe, deliberate infanticide has been described in India by clandestine stabbing by a long needle or pin into the spine, fontanelle, eye, or nose.

▪ Head injuries are relatively common. The mother may throw the child to the floor, or dash its head against a wall or other obstruction, sometimes by swinging it by the legs. This mode of death is similar to child abuse in older infants. The defence may be raised that the child fell to the ground, either from the mother's arms, but especially during a precipitate birth from the standing or crouching position. Though this defence sounds like a desperate excuse, the author can attest – no doubt in common with all doctors who have practical experience of childbirth – that some deliveries, especially in multiparous women, can occur with considerable speed and force. This is why the length of the cord needs to be measured, as it is obviously an effective brake on such a descent. There is no doubt, however, that cords have broken during precipitate birth, a reason for a careful inspection of the severed ends at every autopsy.

The lavatory pan has special significance in this respect, as many unexpected births have taken place whilst the woman is sitting on the toilet. A common story is that the pregnant woman, often a teenage girl – is unaware that she is pregnant and goes to the toilet under the misapprehension that she has stomach pain from constipation. There is no doubt that some naive girls are genuinely ignorant of their gravid condition, and are shocked and devastated to the point of blind panic when a baby emerges into the pan.

The question may then arise as to whether fatal head injuries on the infant can be accounted for by the descent into the lavatory. It is unlikely to produce the severe fracturing sometimes seen – and falling to the

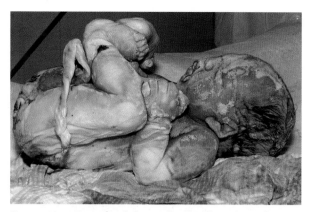

FIGURE 20.9 *Frozen newly born infant found in a freezer by the children of the family. The child and placenta were packed and frozen in separate plastic bags, the umbilical cord is still attached. The family had moved twice after the birth of the child.*

floor in a precipitate delivery is also unlikely to produce fatal damage. Much depends on the severity and nature of the scalp and skull injury, and although it cannot be said that it is impossible for a fatal head injury to be caused in this way, it must be a rare event. Minor fractures of the parietal bones may occur in natural delivery if there is excessive head moulding. These are usually unassociated with internal brain or meningeal damage, and naturally there is no associated scalp damage.

Drowning is another unusual form of infanticide, but is more often a way of disposing of an already dead child, either stillborn, a natural death or the victim of some other mode of infanticide. It may take place in any form of water, from a washbasin to the open sea. Most often the mother will use a household receptacle such as bowl, bucket or bath, but the infant may be taken out and disposed of in any source of open water, where delay in recovery may add decomposition to the pathologist's difficulties. In a recent case seen by the author (BK), the young parents admitted that the child was live born. After some hours, they wrapped the infant in a blanket with a brick and dropped it into a river. The partial remains, largely converted to adipocere, were recovered some 3 months later, there obviously being no prospect of offering any opinion upon either live birth or the cause of death. The only objective, but equivocal evidence, was the recovery of diatoms from the femoral bone marrow, which resembled those in the river water. Returning to the lavatory pan once again, cases are on record where the birth into the toilet led not to head injuries, but to drowning.

INFANTICIDE BY OMISSION TO OFFER PROPER CARE

This is both rare and almost outside the province of the pathologist's examination. If the infant is older than newborn, then deliberate starvation will leave obvious signs, but the proof of lack of care immediately after birth will be a matter of witnesses and clinical opinion. The only possible signs which the autopsy might reveal would be hypothermia (Chapter 17), and obstruction of the air passages by mucus or amniotic fluid.

PROOF OF A SEPARATE EXISTENCE

Strictly speaking, the pathologist can never demonstrate evidence of a separate existence in the English legal sense of complete expulsion from the mother, but it is usually taken to mean proof of live birth, specifically the attainment of breathing air. In the slightly older child the presence of food in the stomach would obviously prove a separate existence, but most autopsies are upon the recently newborn.

Changes in the cord have already been mentioned, but are of no use in the immediate post-partum period. Polson *et al.* (1985) make mention of the presence of 'extraneous material' in the deeper (secondary) bronchi as evidence of a stillbirth, on the grounds that, if this material, such as soil or sand, gained entry after respiration had commenced, the air in the deeper areas of the lung would prevent its ingress. The practicality of this appears suspect.

The unequivocal demonstration of breathing in a newborn infant is fraught with difficulty. Along with the estimation of the time of death, it has probably provoked more discussion, printed words and controversy than any other topic in forensic medicine. The controversy revolves around the 'hydrostatic test' on the lungs, in which it has been claimed since medieval times that, if the lungs float in water, then the infant breathed. There are modifications of technique, but this is the thrust of the claim. The authors' attitude must be stated at the outset: the test is of limited value, whatever modifications are made and it can at best be a suggestive pointer, but never a definitive test in itself.

There are too many recorded instances when control tests have shown that stillborn lungs may float and the lungs from undoubtedly live-born infants have sunk, to allow it be used in testimony in a criminal trial. Even one such failure negates the whole history of the test and the authors are saddened to contemplate the number of innocent women who were sent to the gallows in previous centuries on the testimony of doctors who had an uncritical faith in this crude technique. As this is such an important issue and one that is still contested today, the words of the late Professor Polson may be recalled from his notable textbook:

> The test was suspect even in 1900 and requires no detailed discussion, because it is now known to have no value. The lungs of the live-born, even those who have been known to live for days, may sink [Dilworth 1900; Randolph 1901] and those which float are not necessarily those of live-born infants . . . . It is therefore pointless to apply the hydrostatic test, which will impair the material for other and more important investigations.

Before dismissing the test so absolutely, there are some points both for and against its use as part of the feeble armamentarium that the pathologist has in determining this vital issue. First, the slightest degree of post-mortem decomposition immediately negates any interpretation of the flotation test. As so many potential infanticides are found hidden, buried or submerged, decomposition is more the rule rather than the exception, so the test cannot even be considered in a large proportion of cases. Even when obvious putrefaction with gas formation is not apparent, slight decomposition will still begin to produce gas on a microscopic scale from the second unrefrigerated day in temperate surroundings – and much earlier in hot climates. In recent years the advent of resuscitation attempts make the evaluation of breathing even more difficult or even impossible. The use of mouth-to-mouth revival, external cardiac massage and the administration of oxygen, completely negate any of the already fragile tests for respiration in a newborn infant.

On the positive side – assuming fresh tissue – the floating of the whole pluck of thoracic organs in water makes one tend to accept that respiration had taken place. This means that the attached heart, mediastinum and neck structures are also buoyed up by the lung – but in this case, it is almost invariable that the lungs are sufficiently aerated for this to be obvious on naked-eye inspection.

This is about the total extent of the usefulness of the hydrostatic test. The complicated instructions offered in many textbooks concerning cutting the lung into lobes and then into pieces, squeezing them with knife blades and even pressing them underfoot on the mortuary floor before floating them, all smatter of black magic and are a complete waste of time. Worse, they can simulate a false sense of scientific validity and even to an eventual miscarriage of justice.

The best way of seeking proof of respiration is to look at, to feel and to listen to the lungs. The lungs of a stillbirth are dark, small, heavy and liver-like, even though they may still float. They lie contracted against the mediastinum, though when the body is intact they must still fill the thoracic cavity, as the pliable rib cage pulls inwards and the diaphragm

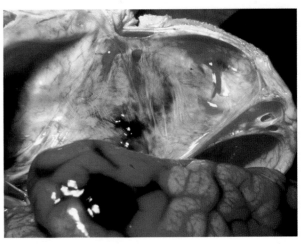

FIGURE 20.10 *A positive finding in a baby whose body was abandoned after death. Respiration had occurred but, on examination of the cranium, a tear in the tentorium was found with an adjacent meningeal haemorrhage, presumably caused by excessive moulding of the head during precipitate delivery.*

rises to eliminate the free space in the chest. Though this fact is seldom considered, it must be obvious that there can be no free space in the pleural cavities until the thorax is opened at autopsy. As soon as this is done, air enters the pleural sacs and the lungs then appear much smaller than the expanded chest cavity than is seen when the sternal plate is removed.

Unrespired lungs appear smaller than those that have breathed for a significant time, though there is a continuous range of expansion. According to Polson *et al.* (1985), unrespired lungs weigh something of the order of one-seventieth of the body weight; when aeration begins, the lung weight increases because of the increased vascular volume and become about one-thirty-fifth of the body weight. This seems at variance with actual measurements at autopsy as the combined weight of both lungs in an infant of average birth weight is about 40 g and, although there is a fairly wide variation between individuals, no combined lung weights approach 85 g, which would be one-thirty-fifth the weight of a 3000 g baby.

The texture of an unrespired lung is rubbery and uniform, with no paler, crepitant areas at the margins, which tend to be sharply angled. On slicing, the interior is uniform in colour and texture, being moist and resembling stiff strawberry jelly. On rubbing a small piece between the fingers close to one's ear, no crepitation is heard.

The lung that has respired will change quantitatively from the above appearances depending on the length of time and the depth to which breaths have been taken. Feeble or brief respiration will affect only the margins, whilst more robust or prolonged breathing may lead to total expansion. Even a single good breath can unfold some of the fetal pulmonary tissues – and of course, resuscitation, whether by mouth-to-mouth, chest compression or administration of oxygen, will actively inflate the lungs, dead or alive. Even ordinary handling of the dead baby may aspirate air into the lungs. Fully respired lungs will be obvious on inspection. The organs are pink or mottled, the medial edges overlapping the mediastinum and part of the pericardium, though not as fully as in the older neonate. The weight is greater, but not as much as recorded by Polson and colleagues, as described above. The edges of the lung, including the interlobar fissures, are more rounded by the expansion, compared with the angular margins of the unrespired organ.

The major change is in the colour and texture. It may be pink all over the surface or there may be patches of darker atelectasis under the pleura. The lung is spongy and resembles the familiar adult tissue. On cutting, the aerated texture is apparent, and on holding a piece to the ear, typical crepitance is heard on rubbing gently between the fingers.

The problem arises with the minimally respired lung, where the changes are intermediate between the two extreme states described above. The anterior margin best shows partial expansion, the areas such as the lingula, anterior diaphragmatic margin and the medial edge of the lower lobe sometimes being pinker and more expanded than the posterior parts. The most sensitive criterion is the ear crepitance test, but it is all a matter of degree as to whether the pathologist is impressed enough – having excluded any possibility of decomposition or resuscitation artefact – to consider that significant respiration has occurred.

Any doubts must be resolved in the direction of no breathing and, even in doubtful instances when the pathologist decides – on balance – that respiration has occurred, he should convey his uncertainty in the body of his report. As to the corroborative role of the flotation test, if performed, when the whole chest pluck floats, the descriptions of the lungs given above will usually indicate clearly that the lungs had breathed. A sinking lung will never correspond with a pink crepitant appearance, but what appears to be a dark, fetal lung may float. The test unfortunately tends to mislead more in one direction than the other, in that almost all lungs float irrespective of their appearance. To repeat the advice of Lester Adelson, whose experience and clarity of expression makes his voice one of the most respected in forensic pathology:

> Unless the pathologist has incontrovertible criteria of post-natal survival, e.g. well-expanded lungs, food in the stomach or vital reaction in the stump of the umbilical cord, he is legally bound not to diagnose live birth. Convictions for infanticide have been set aside where there was any

doubt whatsoever that the child was born alive. Many courts have pushed this proposition to the extent that the state has been given the burden of proving that the baby was born alive beyond any possible doubt rather than beyond any reasonable doubt, the latter being the general level of proof required in a criminal prosecution.

Histological appearances of newborn lungs

Histology is not as helpful as might be expected in the problem of demonstrating the onset of breathing. It was formerly thought that the shape of the alveoli and the height of the lining epithelium would indicate whether they had been expanded by the passage of air, but this has proved to be a disappointing exercise. According to Shapiro (1977), the height of the epithelium and the shape of the alveoli are more a measure of fetal maturity than respiration at birth. The lung parenchyma develops in the fetus as a branching ramification of the trachea and at an intermediate stage – around 800 g body weight or 4 months' gestation – appear as gland-like structures with a cuboidal or columnar cell lining. The evolution to the thin-walled adult-type alveolus is complete before full term, or when the fetal weight is about 2500 g. The alveolar spaces may be found substantially distended even in fetuses who could not have breathed air, such as the one described by Shapiro that was found free in the maternal abdomen after rupture of the uterus. No intra-alveolar epithelium was visible and the lung could not be distinguished histologically from that of a child that had breathed.

Other authors have described the maturation of the fetal lung (Kuroda *et al.* 1965; Parmentier 1962; Ham and Baldwin 1941) and it is undisputed that fully expanded alveoli can be present before full term, even in infants who have not inspired air. After the fifth month, the glandular nature of the air sacs of the lumen are filled with amniotic fluid. In fact, there is evidence that amniotic fluid may be produced by the nascent pulmonary lining, because it is present even in cases of congenital bronchotracheal atresia. When breathing starts, the alveoli further enlarge, and the fluid is partly expelled through the bronchi and partly absorbed back into the pulmonary circulation. Ham (1950) and Shapiro (1947) point out that the finding of open alveoli with no cuboidal or columnar epithelium means that the fetus has passed the two-thirds stage of its maturation process, not that it has respired air.

Further proof is found in the histological appearance of sequestrated parts of lung tissue in infants, which were not connected to the bronchial system but which still showed alveolar ducts and alveoli (Potter and Buhlender 1941; Potter 1952). Fetal lung transplanted into the anterior chamber of an animal eye also developed alveoli with terminal bronchioles (Waddell 1949). Post-mortem handling has also been incriminated for the entry of air into fetal lungs. Apparently respired alveoli have been found in lung sections from a dead infant taken from the uterus of a dead mother.

Janssen (1977) agrees that resuscitation will lead to post-mortem aeration of the lungs, but claims that such artificial respiration cannot cause the alveoli of stillborn neonates to be perfectly and uniformly aerated. Against this view, however, is the undoubted patchy appearance of the lung expansion of many infants who have undoubtedly breathed for some time, so it is difficult to see how the two situations could ever be differentiated. Janssen's statement about the histological appearances is reasonable:

> According to the present level of knowledge and possibilities for examination, ventilation of the lungs alone cannot be taken as a certain indication of a live birth. Under various circumstances, lungs originally aerated can become devoid of air: conversely, the lungs of stillborn neonates can appear aerated. It is not possible to be certain in all cases.

In general, an infant who has breathed strongly for some time – probably hours in most cases – will have lungs that histologically resemble the older child with full, uniform, expansion of alveoli. In many infants who undoubtedly have lived and breathed for an appreciable time, however, there may be only patchy expansion, which corresponds to the uneven aeration seen macroscopically under the pleural surface. The difficulty arises when paradoxical appearances are seen, examples of which are illustrated in many textbooks. Thus an undoubted stillbirth may reveal quite extensive alveolar expansion, whilst a baby that unequivocally lived for some time may show totally collapsed air sacs.

In medico-legal work, though it is quite in order to refer to the usual state of affairs, when a criminal trial is in progress, the standard of proof is 'beyond reasonable doubt' and the well-documented exceptions just mentioned (as with the flotation test) make it unsafe to be dogmatic over a histological opinion.

ESTIMATION OF MATURITY

This is a necessary part of the autopsy, both as matter of record of the size and presumed age of the infant, but also as a legal requisite in those jurisdictions that require proof of viability before either stillbirth can be recorded or a charge of infanticide brought.

First, it must be accepted that – as at any time of life – morphological measurements are by no means infallible indicators of chronological age. Personal variations are compounded by sex, race and nutritional factors to prevent

accuracy. The time of appearance of ossification centres is no longer as uniform as once thought. As with so many biological conditions, there is the typical 'bell-shaped curve' of probability, so that though most subjects will lie in the large central zone, there will be a progressively diminishing number at each extreme of the graph. It should be remembered that a female infant is usually at least 100 g less in weight at full term than the male, though individual differences in either sex can be far larger than this statistical variation. Twins, even those going to full term, are each lighter than a singleton child. The full-term singleton fetus, at **40 weeks' gestation**, will have the following vital specifications, subject to the above cautions:

- a weight of between 2550 and 3360 g
- crown–heel length of 48–52 cm
- crown–rump length of 28–32 cm
- head circumference of 33–38 cm
- the ossification centre in the lower end of the femur will almost always be present, being about 6 mm in diameter
- lanugo is absent or present only over the shoulders; head hair is about 2–3 cm long
- the testes are palpable in the scrotum; the vulval labia closes the vaginal opening
- the umbilicus is midway between xiphisternum and pubis
- there is dark meconium in the large intestine
- an ossification centre in the upper end of the tibia will be present in 80 per cent of full-term infants. The length of finger and toenails is an unreliable guide. More detailed information may be obtained from obstetric and paediatric texts.

At 36 weeks, the crown–heel length is about 45 cm and the weight around 2200 g. There will probably be ossification centres in the cuboid and capitate bones, often in the lower end of the femur and perhaps also in the upper end of the tibia.

At 28 weeks, the fetus is likely to be about 900–1100 g in weight, have a crown–heel length of 35 cm, a crown–rump length of 23 cm, and a foot length of 8 cm.

The old Haase rule-of-thumb for fetal age and size was that, up to the twentieth week, the length in centimetres was the square of the gestation period in (lunar) months. Beyond the twentieth week, the length in centimetres divided by five represents the age in months.

Examination of the ossification centres may be performed radiographically, which requires the advice of a radiologist, as the time of appearance may not be synchronous with visual identification of the centres. At autopsy it is usual to seek them directly, as follows: at the knee, the leg is flexed and a lengthwise cut made over the patella. The bones are pushed forwards through the cut, and transverse

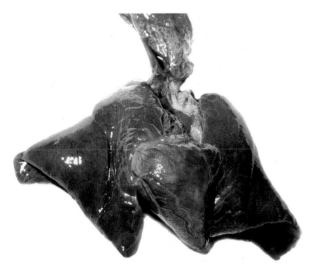

FIGURE 20.11 *The pluck of thoracic organs from a known stillbirth in hospital. The lungs are firm and heavy with no crepitation when squeezed. Margin portions of lung floated in water, however, demonstrating the fallacy of the 'flotation test'.*

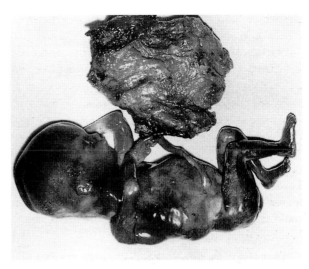

FIGURE 20.13 *Fetal maturity: by Haase's rule this 18 cm crown–heel fetus is about 4.5 months old.*

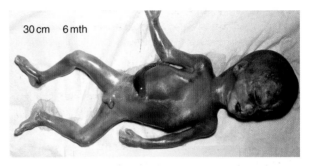

FIGURE 20.14 *Fetal maturity: this infant is 30 cm crown–heel length, which is approximately 6 months' gestation, as the length in centimetres beyond the fifth month is about five times the age in months.*

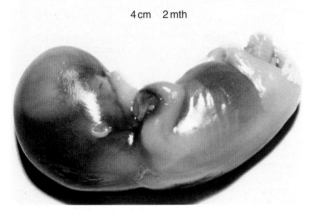

4 cm   2 mth

FIGURE 20.12 *Fetal maturity: up to the twentieth week the length of the fetus in centimetres is approximately the square of the age in months (Haase's rule).*

slices made with a knife through the cartilage of the lower end of the femur. If the ossification centre is revealed, the cuts should continue through plain cartilage above it until the diaphyseal centre is reached. This is to avoid mistaking the lower margin of the diaphyseal bone for the separate epiphyseal centre. The upper end of the tibia is then dealt with in a similar way.

In the foot, a cut is made in the axis of the limb up between the third and fourth toes into the ankle joint, to seek the cuboid bone. The talus and calcaneum can be entered by cuts across the upper dorsum of the foot when the latter is plantar-flexed. The centre in the calcaneum appears at about 7 months' gestation, that in the talus at about 7 months', and the cuboid at full term.

In assessing skeletal age in the fetus, the reference book of Fazekas and Kosa (1978) is invaluable. Other non-osseous methods of estimating maturity exist, such as the progressive development of surfactant-producing alveolar type II cells in fetal lungs (Betz *et al.* 1992).

REFERENCES AND FURTHER READING

Adelson L. 1974. *Pathology of homicide.* Thomas, Springfield.

American Academy of Pediatrics. 2001. Distinguishing sudden infant death syndrome from child abuse fatalities. *Pediatrics* **107**:437–41.

Betz P, Nerlich A, Wilske J, *et al.* 1992. Determination of fetal age by immunohistochemical estimation of surfactant-producing alveolar type II cells. *Forensic Sci Int* **53**:193–202.

Buris L, Torocsik I, Poczkodi S. 1979. Is the aeration of the lungs a reliable sign of live birth? *Z Rechtsmed* **83**:303–12.

Byard RW, James RA, Zuccollo J. 2001. Potential confusion arising from materials presenting as possible human remains. *Am J Forensic Med Pathol* **22**:391–4.

Castellana C, Kosa F. 1999. Morphology of the cervical vertebrae in the fetal-neonatal human skeleton. *J Anat* **194**:147–52.

Dilworth T. 1900. The flotation test. *Br Med J* **2**:1567.

Driever F, Dettmeyer R, Madea B. 2001. [Forensically relevant unexpected delivery after unrecognized or denied pregnancy.] *Arch Kriminol* **208**:174–81.

Fazekas G, Kosa F. 1978. *Forensic fetal osteology.* Akademiai Kiado, Budapest.

Ferreira GF, Rega RM, Mandarim-De-Lacerda CA. 1990. Allometry of hepatic weight growth in human staged fetuses. *Arch Ital Anat Embriol* **95**:223–8.

Funayama M, Ikeda T, Tabata N, *et al.* 1994. Case report: repeated neonaticides in Hokkaido. *Forensic Sci Int* **64**:147–50.

Gordon I, Shapiro H, Berson S (eds). 1988. *Forensic medicine: a guide to principles*, 3rd edn. Churchill Livingstone, London.

Ham A. 1950. *Histology*. Lippincott, Philadelphia, pp. 448–96.

Ham A, Baldwin K. 1941. A histological study of the development of the lung with particular reference to the development of the alveoli. *Anat Rec* **81**:369–79.

Janssen W. 1977. *Forensic histopathology*. Springer, Heidelberg.

Kellett RJ. 1992. Infanticide and child destruction – the historical, legal and pathological aspects. *Forensic Sci Int* **53**:1–28.

Kuroda S, Nagamori H, Ebe M, *et al.* 1965. Medicolegal studies on the fetus and infant with special reference to the histological characteristics of the lungs of liveborn and stillborn infants. *Tohoku J Exp Med* **85**:40–54.

Kuroki Y, Dempo K, Akino T. 1986. Immunohistochemical study of human pulmonary surfactant apoproteins with monoclonal antibodies. Pathologic application for hyaline membrane disease. *Am J Pathol* **124**:25–33.

Morris JF, Hunt AC. 1966. Breaking strength of the umbilical cord. *J Forensic Sci* **11**:43–9.

Oehmichen M, Gerling I, Meissner C. 2000. Petechiae of the baby's skin as differentiation

symptom of infanticide versus sids. *J Forensic Sci* **45**:602–7.

Parmentier R. 1962. L'aeration neonatale due poumon. *Rev Belg Path Med Exp* **29**:121–244.

Perdekamp MG, Bohnert M, Ropohl D. 2000. [Discovery of externally unremarkable case of homicide of an infant.] *Arch Kriminol* **206**:160–7.

Polson C, Gee D, Knight B. 1985. *Essentials of forensic medicine*, 3rd edn. Pergamon Press, London.

Potter E. 1952. *Pathology of the fetus and newborn.* Year Book Publishers, Chicago.

Potter E, Bohlender G. 1941. Intra-uterine respiration in relation to the development of the fetal lung. *Am J Obstet Gynecol* **42**:14–22.

Randolph C. 1901. The flotation test for live birth. *Br Med J* **1**:146.

Shapiro H. 1947. The limited value of microscopy of lung tissue in the diagnosis of live and still birth. *Clin Proc* **6**:149–58.

Shapiro HA. 1977. Microscopy of human fetal lung and the diagnosis of postnatal respiration. In: Wecht C (ed.), *Legal medicine annual 1976*. Appleton Century Crofts, New York.

Tabata N, Morita M, Azumi J. 2000. A frozen newborn infant: froth in the air-passage after thawing. *Forensic Sci Int* **108**:67–74.

Waddell W. 1949. Organoid differentiation of the fetal lung: a histologic study of the differentiation of mammalian fetal lung *in utero* and in transplants. *Arch Pathol* **47**:227–47.

Yamauchi M, Usami S, Ikeda R, *et al.* 2000. Medico-legal studies on infanticide: statistics and a case of repeated neonaticide. *Forensic Sci Int* **113**:205–8.

Zhu BL, Maeda H, Fukita K, *et al.* 1996. Immunohistochemical investigation of pulmonary surfactant in perinatal fatalities. *Forensic Sci Int* **83**:219–27.

Zhu BL, Ishida K, Fujita MQ, *et al.* 2000. Immunohistochemical investigation of a pulmonary surfactant in fatal mechanical asphyxia. *Int J Legal Med* **113**:268–71.

Zhu BL, Ishida K, Quan L, *et al.* 2000. Immunohistochemistry of pulmonary surfactant apoprotein A in forensic autopsy: reassessment in relation to the causes of death. *Forensic Sci Int* **113**:193–7.

CHAPTER 21

Sudden death in infancy

This distressing condition has a variety of names and abbreviations. The one now most generally accepted is the 'sudden death in infancy syndrome', often shortened to (and pronounced as) 'SIDS'. An older title was 'SUD', standing for 'sudden unexpected death', but this in itself did not denote the infant connotations. Colloquially, SIDS is known as 'cot death' in Britain and 'crib death' in North America.

DEFINITION OF THE SUDDEN INFANT DEATH SYNDROME (SIDS)

Following one of the international conferences on the condition (held in Seattle in 1969) the following useful definition of the syndrome was proposed by Beckwith and is now generally accepted: 'the sudden death of any infant or young child which is unexpected by history and in whom a thorough necropsy fails to demonstrate an adequate cause of death'. Other definitions have been proposed later, e.g. the definition by the National Institute of Child Health and Human Development (NICHD) in 1989 emphasizing the necessity of the scene of death examination, and a three-tiered definition by Beckwith 1992 in Sydney, during the Second SIDS International Conference, dividing the SIDS into three different categories according to the age, the occurrence of similar deaths in siblings or other close relatives, and the presence of petechial haemorrhages and inflammatory lesions or other abnormalities found during the autopsy. The 'Stavanger definition', proposed during the

Third SIDS International Conference in Stavanger, Norway 1994, lays stress on the importance of the investigation of the circumstances of death: sudden death in infancy unexplained after review of the clinical history, examination of the circumstances of death and post-mortem examination. However, when put to the vote during a subsequent SIDS Global Strategy Meeting in Stavanger, the original definition from 1969 received the most votes.

INCIDENCE OF SUDDEN INFANT DEATH

Until recent years, national death statistics were totally unreliable in providing data on the incidence of SIDS, as the nomenclature was confused, and the certifying habits of different pathologists and clinicians were extremely variable. According to a recent review by Rognum (1999), the percentage of sudden deaths in infancy that are diagnosed by various authors as pure SIDS varied between 2.5% and 70%. This situation still applies in many countries, especially those where high infant mortality from many causes overshadows sudden infant deaths. In advanced countries, the progressive and often dramatic reduction in total infant mortality since the beginning of the century has eliminated many infective, nutritional and congenital diseases to the point where the 'law of diminishing returns' has flattened out the mortality curve to a low level. Until 1990, there was little evidence that the SIDS rate had changed significantly for centuries or even millennia, so the pre-1990 straight-line incidence of SIDS became a far greater proportion of the total infant deaths compared with the early years of this century. In many advanced countries, SIDS is still the most common single cause of infant mortality after the perinatal period.

Until about 1990, Britain had a SIDS rate of about 2 per 1000 live births, but the risk varied considerably in various sections of the population. Golding *et al.* (1985) give a comprehensive table in their book of known variations in worldwide incidence before the recent dramatic decline. For example, in the USA there was an overall rate of 2.3/1000, though again this varies considerably from place to place, and among different ethnic and social groups. In Chicago the rate in 1969 was 3.4 compared with 1.4 in upstate New York in 1974. There is far more variation amongst ethnic groups in the USA, the rate being much higher among non-White infants. In Nebraska, for instance, the rate was 1.9/1000 Whites and 5.9/1000 in non-Whites. There is other evidence, however, that social differences are the predominant factor rather than any intrinsically ethnic cause.

As noted above, in Britain and several other European countries the SIDS rate has dropped remarkably in the past few years. In France there was a stagnation for post-neonatal mortality between 1979 and 1993 followed by a sharp decrease to 2/100 in 1995. In England and Wales there was a 69% fall in the sudden infant death rate between 1988 and 1992 from 2.01 to 0.63 and further down to 0.3 in 2000 (see Table 21.1).

The cause for this is obscure. It almost coincides with a vigorous publicity campaign by the Department of Health and the Foundation for the Study of Infant Deaths, which advocated sleeping babies on their back, not on the face and in avoiding overheating and smoking near the baby, as well as exhortations to seek medical advice whenever the infant was unwell.

However, the fall slightly antedated this campaign, so that the contribution of sleeping position, etc., to the decline

is not fully understood, though there is other evidence from The Netherlands that recommendations about sleeping supine favourably affects the death rate. However, these same years have shown a series of very mild winters, which may also be a factor.

FACTORS INFLUENCING THE RISK OF SIDS

Age

The age range in which sudden infant death occurs follows the usual 'bell-shaped curve' of most biological phenomena. As the Seattle definition stated, the ends of the curve lie at 2 weeks and 2 years, but these boundaries are far too wide for the great majority of victims. The peak incidence occurs at around 3 months and the time bracket of 2–7 months will encompass most cases. It is rare after 9 months, but deaths can occur well into the second year which, by all the criteria, can only be called 'cot deaths'.

Similarly, a few small infants die unexpectedly and inexplicably before the first month, but it must be accepted that true SIDS is not a condition of the neonatal period. There is almost always a gap between the deaths that must be attributed as being a sequel to birth, and those that suddenly occur subsequently in babies who have apparently weathered that dangerous period successfully. It is obvious, however, that such an absolute distinction cannot be made, as premature and underweight infants have a higher risk of SIDS, and some perinatal deaths are indistinguishable from SIDS in that autopsy may reveal the same negative findings.

Sex

There is a slight but definite sex bias in the syndrome, showing the usual slight weighting against the male infant, which is a common feature of many conditions and at all ages. Most surveys have shown a ratio of 1:1.3 or thereabouts, with an excess of male infants. Some other investigations, however, have indicated equal numbers and one survey actually showed a slight excess of girls.

Twinning

There is a marked excess of deaths in a member of a twin pair as opposed to singletons. Figures have varied in different surveys, but the risk is at least twofold. In the author's (BK) own hospital district (South Glamorgan), where a total birth survey is maintained, some years ago the increased risk was five times that for single babies. The reason for the excess among twins lies partly in the fact that physically disadvantaged

TABLE 21.1 *Infant mortality rates (per 1000 live births) in England and Wales in 1996–2000*

Infant mortality	1996	1997	1998	1999	2000	No.
Stillbirth	5.4	5.3	5.3	5.3	5.3	3203
Infant (under 1 year)	6.1	5.9	5.7	5.8	5.6	3399
Early neonatal (under 1 week)	8.6	8.3	8.2	8.2	8.2	1760
Neonatal (under 4 weeks)	4.1	3.9	3.8	3.9	3.9	2335
Post-neonatal (4 weeks–1 year)	2.0	3.0	1.9	1.9	1.8	1064
SIDS underlying cause (4 weeks–1 year)	0.6	0.5	0.4	0.4	0.3	203

Source: Office for National Statistics, Health Statistics Quarterly 05, Spring 2000.

infants, such as premature births and those of low birth weight are at greater risk; these two factors are often present in twins. There is no difference in incidence between identical or binovular twins. There have been at least ten reports of both twins having died of SIDS on the same day, and obviously reported cases are but a small fraction of those occurring. Some pathologists, almost exclusively in the USA, claim that simultaneous death in twins is indicative of homicide, but this view is not generally accepted.

Seasonal incidence

There is a marked seasonal variation in SIDS, the excess occurring in the colder, wetter months in temperate zones. In Europe and North America, most SIDS die between October and April, whilst in Australasia the monthly incidence is reversed. In tropical and subtropical zones, no clear pattern emerges, partly because many of the countries in these latitudes are relatively underdeveloped so have both high infant mortality, and often death certification and statistical records of lesser accuracy. SIDS undoubtedly occurs in the tropics, however, but the incidence is often swamped by that of more obvious disease. Returning to temperate zones, many efforts have been made to relate SIDS to changes of temperature and the incidence of respiratory infections in the community. The results are conflicting, but there seems little doubt that respiratory infections are a precipitating trigger in SIDS.

Social class and housing

This is not the place to expand upon the social epidemiology of cot death, but there is ample evidence that lower levels of social disadvantage, as measured by occupation and housing quality, are strongly related to the incidence of SIDS. It is difficult to reconcile these epidemiological factors with the numerous pathological theories and the few facts concerning the aetiology of sudden infant death.

THE CASE HISTORY IN SUDDEN INFANT DEATH

The history is usually brief and remarkably similar from case to case. The infant is either quite well on the preceding day or (in about half the victims) has trivial symptoms, usually of upper respiratory infection or a bowel upset. Even these symptoms may be overstated, as the history is of necessity taken retrospectively from distraught parents trying to rationalize the tragedy.

The story usually records that the infant was put to sleep in the evening and was found dead in the morning when a parent first visited it. Alternatively, the baby was given an early morning feed when it appeared well, but was later found dead in its sleeping place. Most infants are found dead in the first half of the day, before mid-morning. A minority die (or are found dead) in the afternoon and evening. Death can be rapid and silent. Though most victims die unobserved, the author's (BK) experience can confirm that a number of cases indicate that an infant observed to be quite well at a given moment can be found dead within 5 minutes, and cases are on record of SIDS occurring in hospital and even in a physician's arms.

THE SCENE OF DEATH AND EXTERNAL FINDINGS

The scene of the death is rarely available for examination in its original state. When found, the child is naturally either rushed to a doctor or a hospital, or an ambulance team arrives and attempts resuscitation, again usually hurrying to a hospital casualty department.

When found, a few children have slight oedema fluid exuding from the mouth. This may sometimes be blood-tinged, and frank bleeding – apparently from a congested mouth or pharyngeal vessel – is occasionally seen.

Stomach contents may be present in the mouth, nostrils or on the face, but this must not be assumed to be a cause of death (from aspiration), as is discussed below. The hands of the child are often found to be clenched around fibres from the bedclothes, as if there were spasmodic agonal grasping movements.

Some children are found under the bedclothes, even huddled upside down at the foot of the cot. Again, this has no significance, as thousands of healthy infants habitually sleep in this way without suffering SIDS.

A number of infants have been found moist with sweat and even with a raised body temperature. The significance of this is not known, but part of the recent preventative advice given in Britain, is to avoid overwrapping and overheating.

There are no external findings of significance. The face may be pale or slightly cyanosed or congested: there are no petechial haemorrhages in the face or eyes. The posture at death is not necessarily relevant, even if the initial sleeping position is important in the aetiology – some are found face down and may have a pallid area around the mouth and nose where pressure has prevented post-mortem hypostasis from settling. This develops after death and on no account must be misinterpreted as a pressure mark indicating suffocation.

AUTOPSY APPEARANCES

These have given rise to much controversy over the years. Essentially the gross findings are nil, almost by definition. If any significant pathological lesion is found on naked-eye examination, the death ceases to be a true SIDS, and is categorized as whatever lesion was discovered. The proportion of 'explained' cot deaths varies greatly with the pathologist, though this variation is more in relation to microscopic than gross findings. Of all babies found dead in their sleeping place, that is, 'cot deaths', most will be true SIDS, but a few will have a significant pathological condition. The relative proportions of these two subsets varies from pathologist to pathologist. Many would accept that about 15 per cent reveal some pathological lesions at autopsy, though this is not to say that those lesions – sometimes slight – were a factor in the death. For example, some mild congenital heart lesion or the presence of Down's syndrome is occasionally revealed, but this is not to say that they were causative. Thus almost all SIDS are cot deaths, but not all cot deaths are SIDS.

The external appearances have already been discussed and are essentially negative, apart from inconstant froth at the lips and nostrils, and fibres sometimes clenched in the fists. The length, weight and other physical measurements are of no direct relevance, though naturally they must always be carefully recorded as in any other infant autopsy, for it may transpire that the death was not a typical SIDS.

Internally, the findings are again non-specific in a typical SIDS. A large number of reports now exist on the microscopy, microbiology and biochemistry of the syndrome, but no diagnostic criteria have yet been confirmed. The following naked-eye features may be present at autopsy:

- Petechial haemorrhages on the visceral pleura.
- Petechial haemorrhages in the thymus gland.
- Petechiae or larger ecchymoses on the epicardial surface of the heart, especially posteriorly. These petechiae have been the subject of intense controversy since they were first described in infant deaths by Tardieu in 1855, but they are almost certainly agonal in origin. One explanation suggests that they are the result of forced inspiratory efforts against a closed airway, the latter being either from laryngeal spasm or from a collapsed pharynx in hypotonic infants, but neither of these hypotheses has been substantiated. Petechiae in the thorax are found in about 70 per cent of true SIDS infants. Thymic haemorrhages are often prominent, the organ being studded with both petechiae and larger ecchymoses: it has been claimed recently that in SIDS as opposed to mechanical suffocation, the haemorrhages are in the thymic cortex, rather than the medulla, but few pathologists accept this.

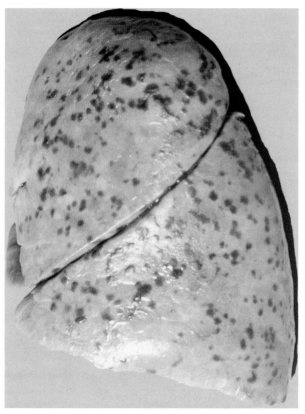

FIGURE 21.1 *Subpleural haemorrhages – the original 'Tardieu spots'. These are far more pronounced than those seen in adult lungs, being taken from a case of SIDS, in which 70 per cent of cases exhibit these lesions.*

- Gastric contents, usually milk-curds, in the air passages. All too often this has been used by some pathologists as the definite cause of death, but there is no evidence that it is the reason for the death. It is either an agonal regurgitation or even a post-mortem phenomenon. In a series of 100 consecutive autopsies, including adults and children, the author (BK) found gastric contents in greater or lesser amount in no less than 25 per cent of cadavers, almost all of which had quite satisfactory pathological lesions to account for death. This aspect is discussed in more detail in Chapter 14.
- Respiratory infections in the form of inflamed laryngeal or tracheobronchial mucosa are not common, but are macroscopically evident in some SIDS victims. If the infection is severe enough to produce pus and especially if there are obvious inflammatory changes in the lung parenchyma, then the death is removed from the SIDS category into a fatal chest infection group. The finding of minimal 'inflammatory' cells on microscopy must be viewed with caution. Some pathologists undoubtedly lay too much emphasis on sparse or small collections of leucocytes in the peribronchial zones. In control infants, small foci of lymphocytes are common and can

be disregarded. It is usually the lung histology that causes the variations in the proportions of 'cot deaths' that are classified as true 'SIDS'.

■ Pulmonary oedema is common, though usually moderate in intensity. The surface of the lungs often shows patchy sublobular partial collapse, with areas of blue lung alternating with better-aerated pink zones.

In some infants dying unexpectedly, abnormalities such as Down's syndrome, congenital heart disease or other chronic systemic disease are found. The problem then is to decide whether the death should be ascribed to 'SIDS' or to the obvious disease, even though there is no evidence that such a disease should have suddenly caused death. There is a natural temptation to use an established lesion to explain the death, especially as both doctors and parents tend to be less unhappy with a specific disease process than with the rather nebulous diagnosis of 'SIDS'.

In most cases, however, there is no real reason why an infant with Down's syndrome, perfectly well one night, should be found dead the following morning – and many relatively mild (and often previously undiagnosed) congenital defects similarly are unlikely to cause death in such an abrupt manner. It is probably more logical to assume that SIDS has occurred in a child with Down's or a septal defect, or whatever. It may be accepted that this defect may be one factor among the many involved in SIDS, and therefore it is probably reasonable to enter 'SIDS' in Part I of the certificate and add the other lesion in Part II, as a contributory cause.

HISTOLOGICAL FINDINGS IN SIDS

Again a huge and controversial topic, there have been numerous papers on the microscopic appearances in SIDS. Much of this is pure research material and is often irreproducible by other workers.

Most interest has focused on the lung changes and especially evidence of pulmonary inflammation. The frequency with which positive findings are made depends upon the criteria threshold of the observer, as mentioned earlier. Peribronchiolar cell infiltration is the main finding and some workers claim to find an abnormal cellular response in the majority of SIDS material. Others, more used to the less equivocal appearances in adults, fail to attach significance to marginal increases in cell population in the peribronchial zone.

Many of the other findings are inconstant and claimed by a variety of researchers. For example, Richard Naeye (1973) supported his hypothesis of chronic hypoxia by finding thickened pulmonary artery walls, gliosis in the brainstem, retention of brown fat in the adrenals and abnormalities in the carotid body. Changes in the myocardium, adrenals,

parathyroids and liver have all been described, but have either not survived critical assessment, appear incompatible with clinical and epidemiological data, or fail to be reproducible in subsequent investigations.

THEORIES OF CAUSATION

Since the mid-1970s more than 5000 articles have appeared concerning sudden infant death and one now needs review papers, such as those published by Valdes-Dapena, merely to keep up with mainstream research. Theories include allergy to cow's-milk proteins, house-mite allergy, deliberate suffocation, spinal haemorrhages, botulism, calcium deficiency, selenium deficiency, biotin deficiency, vitamin E deficiency, vitamin C deficiency, vitamin D deficiency, thiamine deficiency, hypoglycaemia, hypothyroidism, magnesium deficiency, carbon monoxide poisoning, carbon dioxide poisoning, overlaying, pharyngeal hypotonia, nasal obstruction, tracheobronchitis, respiratory syncytial virus, prolonged sleep apnoea, deficient or abnormal pulmonary surfactant, cardiac conduction defects, sodium overload in feeds, narrow foramen magnum, hyperthermia, hypothermia, influenza infection, metabolic enzyme defects, immunodeficiency, hypogammaglobulinaemia and many others.

In 1989 and again in 1994, press publicity in the UK drew considerable attention to claims that fungal growth on certain antiflammable chemicals used on cot mattress covers produced gases containing arsenic and antimony, and some chemical analyses showed that antimony could be demonstrated in some SIDS tissues. However, a causative link has not been proven and the theory fails to fit the epidemiology – especially as SIDS has been occurring for hundreds and probably thousands of years before mattress covers existed. Reports of cot deaths can be found in sources as ancient as the Old Testament and twelfth century Welsh literature.

In the 1970s and early 1980s, one hypothesis gained widespread favour and was beginning to gain general acceptance. This was the claim that some infants, with poor respiratory drive, suffered from exaggeration of the normal periods of apnoea that all infants have during sleep. A complex mechanism was built up in which progressive hypoxia and failure to respond adequately to hypercapnia and hypoxia drove the sleeping infant into a descending spiral of hypoxia–apnoea–hypoxia, which ended in bradycardia and cardiac arrest. Respiratory infections, sleep, and nasal obstruction contributed to an acute-on-chronic state of hypoxia, which histological findings claimed to substantiate.

This attractive theory was largely deflated, however, when prospective studies of infants with sleep apnoea and other respiratory problems were found to have no greater risk of SIDS than normal controls. The theory led to a great popularity of apnoea alarms, which parents of subsequent children following a SIDS loss have insisted on using. There is no evidence that they have any beneficial effect, other than reassurance of the parents; indeed, in some instances, the stress of waiting for the alarm to sound and the many false alarms, have led to marital problems.

In the present state of knowledge, it seems that SIDS is the final common pathway that leads to death in infants who have been compromised by a number of deleterious factors, which have to come together in one baby at one time in order to summate to a fatal outcome. The factors may be quite different in each case, but all manifest themselves in terminal acute cardiorespiratory failure.

Some of the factors are known such as sleep, which depresses the brainstem, and virus infections – especially of the respiratory tract – which provide a viraemia, reduce oxygenation and may narrow the effective airway lumen by mucus and exudate. Other factors are 'constitutional', in that many SIDS victims are physically compromised in some way, often since fetal life, being premature and of low birth weight (though most SIDS are neither of these). Other factors from the long list given above may operate in certain circumstances, such as botulism which may be relevant in some 5 per cent of SIDS in California.

It is thus futile to search for 'the cause' of cot death, as there is no single cause, but a galaxy of factors that vary from death to death, though the mediating terminal mechanism appears to be the same.

One of the most difficult aspects is the failure of pathological explanations to be compatible with epidemiological findings. It has been shown that non-specific health-care improvements reduce the incidence of SIDS, such as in the excellent ante-natal and post-natal services of countries such as Finland and Holland, which have the lowest SIDS rates – and the Sheffield project, where it was shown that the strongest factor in reducing incidence was the use the family made of the health services.

As far as the pathologist is concerned, his function is to perform a meticulous autopsy, to exclude any overt natural disease or injuries, and to offer sympathetic advice to those parents who want an explanation of the syndrome in comprehensible lay terms. There are several highly proficient counselling charities in Britain, the USA and other countries, who can provide literature and direct help to parents – and who also usually support most of the ambitious research schemes now operating.

THE SIDS AUTOPSY

The routine for an autopsy on a sudden infant death follows that for any infant and is little different from that in suspected child abuse. Indeed, exclusion of child abuse is a prime consideration as, although there is no aetiological connection between the two conditions, sometimes occult abuse – or sometimes genuine accident – may present as a 'cot death'. Some pathologists, both forensic and paediatric, insist on a whole-body radiological survey before commencing the autopsy and, where such facilities exist, this is a wise precaution. Full measurements of the infant are essential, as in all paediatric autopsies, to monitor the size-for-age of the child and to compare it with centile graphs, provided the birth weight is known.

The gross examination is the standard meticulous scrutiny of all external surfaces, orifices and organs. A full histological survey is vital, with even more blocks being taken than may be the norm for many forensic pathologists. The lungs in particular should be extensively sampled and six blocks is a bare minimum for these organs. In addition to histology, swabs should be taken from the major air passages and the lung parenchyma for microbiological culture, and heart blood may also be cultured. The middle ears should always be opened and a swab taken if infection is suspected. A separate piece of lung should be sent for virological culture. Where there has been any history of gut upset before death, a sample of ileal contents should be cultured. It has to be said that the return on such microbiological and virological studies is poor in terms of positive findings, both because of the post-mortem interval and because many of the micro-organisms found may be indistinguishable from commensals or post-mortem contaminants.

Similarly, by the very definition of SIDS, significant histological findings are absent. If a definite pathological lesion capable of causing death is discovered, the case is removed from the SIDS category and classified according to the disease process discovered. The problem arises when 'significant' or 'definite' has to be defined, as the criteria threshold of different pathologists varies considerably, especially where the diagnosis of an inflammatory condition in the lungs is concerned.

MEDICO-LEGAL PROBLEMS IN COT DEATHS

Differentiating SIDS from external suffocation

This is the oldest problem in cot death and one that is virtually insoluble on purely pathological grounds. The signs of infant suffocation are usually nil and the signs of SIDS are nil, so in a completely negative autopsy no reliable criteria exist. The presence of intrathoracic petechiae has little or no diagnostic value, in spite of one recent report that claims to distinguish SIDS from mechanical suffocation by the confinement of petechiae to the thymic cortex in SIDS. In any event, they are usually absent in known suffocation, such as those caused by a plastic bag over the head, yet some 70 per cent of SIDS have serosal petechiae.

In Britain, there are about 1000 cot deaths each year and probably up to 10 000 in the USA. The majority of these were found dead with the face uncovered, and in a posture where the mouth and nose are not obstructed. No one believes that all these children have been smothered by their parents; therefore, as petechiae are valueless for differentiation, it is not possible for an autopsy to state or even suggest that any particular child has been suffocated. This naturally presupposes the absence of facial bruising, scratching or other positive signs that would immediately remove the case from the SIDS category.

It is possible for circumstantial or other non-medical history to suggest or confirm deliberate suffocation, though this is extremely rare and not the concern of the pathologist. A caution must be offered about maternal confessions of smothering, however, as several instances are known where such a confession has proved totally false, the desperately bereaved woman in her grief and recrimination deluding herself in order to rationalize an inexplicable tragedy.

Multiple sudden infant deaths

Again, these pose a formidable problem for pathologist, paediatrician and investigating authority. Statistically, a mother will suffer a second cot death in her family every quarter of a million births, but a number of families are reported where three or even four siblings have died inexplicably. There is always the possibility of foul play in such circumstances, though some familial metabolic or other genetic disease – albeit obscure – is more likely. Even where no trace of the latter can be detected by the most exhaustive medical investigations, if the autopsies reveal no positive evidence of mechanical suffocation or other demonstrable cause of death, the pathologist cannot then substantiate any allegation of mechanical suffocation. He can – and should – express his concern to the investigating authorities but, if their investigations produce no corroborative evidence, it is pointless for him to continue to support a hypothesis that cannot be substantiated by any pathological evidence.

Counselling of parents

Many families, primarily the mother, have an intense desire to know why their baby died, a need that is often unfulfilled by any official contacts, such as with a coroner. Once any legal processes are complete, there is no reason why a pathologist should not meet and offer explanations to the parents of a child upon whom he has performed an autopsy. Often an earlier line of counselling is provided by a paediatrician, but some mothers wish to talk to the pathologist. Both Adelson (1974) and Knight (1983) have advocated that the pathologist should make himself readily available for this purpose, though some pathologists shelter behind an imaginary legal barrier to avoid what should be an ethical obligation.

ADDRESSES OF COUNSELLING ORGANIZATIONS

■ The Foundation for the Study of Infant Deaths, Artillery House, 11–19 Artillery Row, London, SW1P 1RT, UK (Tel.: General enquiries: +44 020 7222 8001; 24-hour helpline: +44 020 7233 2090; Fax: +44 020 7222 8002). http://www.sids.org.uk/
■ National Sudden Infant Death Syndrome Resource Center (NSRC), 2070 Chain Bridge Road, Suite 450, Vienna, VA 22182, USA (Tel.: (703) 821 8955; Fax: (703) 821 2098). sids@circlesolutions.com
■ SIDS International (SIDSI). http://www.sidsinternational.minerva.com.au/

REFERENCES AND FURTHER READING

Adelson L. 1974. *The pathology of homicide: a vade mecum for pathologist, prosecutor and defense counsel.* W. B. Saunders, Philadelphia.

Althoff H. 1980. *Sudden infant death syndrome.* Gustav Fischer Verlag, Stuttgart.

American Academy of Pediatrics. 2001. Distinguishing sudden infant death syndrome from child abuse fatalities. *Pediatrics* **107**:437–41.

Arnestad M, Andersen M, Vege A, *et al.* 2001. Changes in the epidemiological pattern of sudden infant death syndrome in southeast Norway, 1984–1998: implications for future prevention and research. *Arch Dis Child* **85**:108–15.

Arnestad M, Vege A, Rognum TO. 2002. Evaluation of diagnostic tools applied in the examination of sudden unexpected deaths in infancy and early childhood. *Forensic Sci Int* **125**:262–8.

Bartholomew SE, MacArthur BA, Bain AD. 1987. Sudden infant death syndrome in south east Scotland. *Arch Dis Child* **62**:951–6.

Bass M, Kravath RE, Glass L. 1986. Death-scene investigation in sudden infant death. *N Engl J Med* **315**:100–5.

Bergman AB. 1972. Unexplained sudden infant death. *N Engl J Med* **287**:254–5.

Bergman AB, Beckwith RE, Rae CO (eds). 1969. *Sudden infant death syndrome. Proceedings of the Second International Conference, Seattle 1969*. University of Washington Press, Seattle.

Bergman AB, Ray CG, Pomeroy MA, *et al.* 1972. Studies of the sudden infant death syndrome in King County, Washington. 3. Epidemiology. *Pediatrics* **49**:860–70.

Betz P, Hausmann R, Eisenmenger W. 1998. A contribution to a possible differentiation between sids and asphyxiation. *Forensic Sci Int* **91**:147–52.

Bonser RS, Knight BH, West RR. 1978. Sudden infant death syndrome in Cardiff, association with epidemic influenza and with temperature – 1955–1974. *Int J Epidemiol* **7**:335–40.

Boulloche J, Mallet E, Basuyau JP, *et al.* 1986. The value of serum IgE assay in milk aspiration and the sudden infant death syndrome. *Acta Paediatr Scand* **75**:530–3.

Bowden KS. 1953. Sudden or unexpexted deaths in infancy. *J Forensic Med* **1**:19–27.

Byard R, Krous H. 1999. Suffocation, shaking or sudden infant death syndrome: can we tell the difference? *J Paediatr Child Health* **35**:432–3.

Byard RW, Beal SM. 2000. Gastric aspiration and sleeping position in infancy and early childhood. *J Paediatr Child Health* **36**:403–5.

Byard RW, Krous HF (eds). 2001. *Sudden infant death syndrome: problems, progress and possibilities*. Arnold, London.

Camps FE, Carpenter RJ (eds). 1972. *Sudden and unexpected deaths in infancy. Proceedings of the Cambridge Symposium*. John Wright, Bristol.

Cecchi R, Bajanowski T, Kahl B, *et al.* 1995. CMV-DNA detection in parenchymatous organs in cases of SIDS. *Int J Legal Med* **107**:291–5.

Coombs RR, McLaughlan P. 1982. The enigma of cot death: is the modified-anaphylaxis hypothesis an explanation for some cases? *Lancet* **1**:1388–9.

DeSa DJ. 1986. Isolated myocarditis as a cause of sudden death in the first year of life. *Forensic Sci Int* **30**:113–17.

Dettmeyer R, Kandolf R, Schmidt P, *et al.* 2001. Lympho-monocytic enteroviral myocarditis: traditional, immunohistological and molecular pathological methods for diagnosis in a case of suspected sudden infant death syndrome (SIDS). *Forensic Sci Int* **119**:141–4.

Durigon M, Caroff J, Derobert L. 1971. [Pulmonary histology in 123 suspicious or sudden deaths in infants under one year of age.] *Med Leg Dommage Corp* **4**:287–93.

Emery JL. 1983. The necropsy and cot death [editorial]. *Br Med J Clin Res Ed* **287**:77–8.

Emery JL. 1986. Families in which two or more cot deaths have occurred. *Lancet* **1**:313–15.

Ferris JA. 1972. The heart in sudden infant death. *J Forensic Sci Soc* **12**:591–4.

Ferris JA. 1973. Hypoxic changes in conducting tissue of the heart in sudden death in infancy syndrome. *Br Med J* **2**:23–5.

Ferris JA, Aherne WA, Locke WS, *et al.* 1973. Sudden and unexpected deaths in infants: histology and virology. *Br Med J* **2**:439–42.

Fleming PJ, Gilbert R, Azaz Y, *et al.* 1990. Interaction between bedding and sleeping position in the sudden infant death syndrome: a population based case-control study [see comments]. *Br Med J* **301**:85–9.

Forsyth KD, Weeks SC, Koh L, *et al.* 1989. Lung immunoglobulins in the sudden infant death syndrome. *Br Med J* **298**:23–6.

Freed GE, Meny R, Glomb WB, *et al.* 2002. Effect of home monitoring on a high-risk population. *J Perinatol* **22**:165–7.

Froggatt P, James TN. 1973. Sudden unexpected death in infants. Evidence on a lethal cardiac arrhythmia. *Ulster Med J* **42**:136–52.

Froggatt P, Lynas MA, Marshall TK. 1971. Sudden unexpected death in infants ('cot death'). Report of a collaborative study in Northern Ireland. *Ulster Med J* **40**:116–35.

Gardner PS. 1972. Viruses and the respiratory tract in sudden infant deaths. *J Forensic Sci Soc* **12**:587–9.

Golding J, Limerick S, McFarlane A. 1985. *Sudden infant death*. Open Books, Shepton Mallet.

Gruenwald P, Hoang NM. 1960. Evaluation of body and organ weights in perinatal pathology. I. Normal standards derived from autopsies. *Am Clin Pathol* **34**:247–53.

Guilleminault C, Heldt G, Powell N, *et al.* 1986. Small upper airway in near-miss sudden infant death syndrome infants and their families. *Lancet* **1**:402–7.

Guntheroth WG. 1973. The significance of pulmonary petechiae in crib death. *Pediatrics* **52**:601–3.

Hanzlick R. 2001. Pulmonary hemorrhage in deceased infants: baseline data for further study of infant mortality. *Am J Forensic Med Pathol* **22**:188–92.

Harrington C, Kirjavainen T, Teng A, *et al.* 2002. Altered autonomic function and reduced arousability in apparent life-threatening event infants with obstructive sleep apnea. *Am J Respir Crit Care Med* **165**:1048–54.

Hatton F, Bouvier-Colle MH, Blondel B, *et al.* 2000. [Trends in infant mortality in France: frequency and causes from 1950 to 1997.] *Arch Pediatr* **7**:489–500.

Hollander N. 1988. Beta-endorphin in the brainstem, pituitary, and spinal fluid of infants at autopsy: relation to sudden infant death syndrome. *Forensic Sci Int* **38**:67–74.

Iwadate K, Doy M, Ito Y. 2001. Screening of milk aspiration in 105 infant death cases by immunostaining with anti-human alpha-lactalbumin antibody. *Forensic Sci Int* **122**:95–100.

James TN. 1968. Sudden death in babies: new observations in the heart. *Am J Cardiol* **22**:479–506.

Kariks J. 1988. Cardiac lesions in sudden infant death syndrome. *Forensic Sci Int* **39**:211–25.

Kato I, Groswasser J, Franco P, *et al.* 2001. Developmental characteristics of apnea in infants who succumb to sudden infant death syndrome. *Am J Respir Crit Care Med* **164**:1464–9.

Kelly DH, Shannon DC. 1982. Sudden infant death syndrome and near sudden infant death syndrome: a review of the literature, 1964 to 1982. *Pediatr Clin North Am* **29**:1241–61.

Knight B. 1972. Legal and administrative problems in the 'cot death syndrome'. *J Forensic Sci Soc* **12**:581–3.

Knight B. 1983. *Sudden death in infancy: the cot death syndrome.* Faber and Faber, London.

Koch LE, Biedermann H, Saternus KS. 1998. High cervical stress and apnoea. *Forensic Sci Int* **97**:1–9.

Koehler SA, Ladham S, Shakir A, *et al.* 2001. Simultaneous sudden infant death syndrome: a proposed definition and worldwide review of cases. *Am J Forensic Med Pathol* **22**:23–32.

Krous HF, Nadeau JM, Silva PD, *et al.* 2002. Infanticide: is its incidence among postneonatal infant deaths increasing? An 18-year population-based analysis in California. *Am J Forensic Med Pathol* **23**:127–31.

Ladham S, Koehler SA, Shakir A, *et al.* 2001. Simultaneous sudden infant death syndrome: a case report. *Am J Forensic Med Pathol* **22**:33–7.

Langlois NE, Ellis PS, Little D, *et al.* 2002. Toxicologic analysis in cases of possible sudden infant death

syndrome: a worthwhile exercise? *Am J Forensic Med Pathol* **23**:162–6.

Lie TJ, Rosenberg H, Erikson E. 1976. Histopathology of the conduction system in the sudden death syndrome. *Circulation* **53**:3–8.

Lundemose JB, Lundemose AG, Gregersen M, *et al.* 1990. Chlamydia and sudden infant death syndrome. A study of 166 SIDS and 30 control cases. *Int J Legal Med* **104**:3–7.

Maron BJ, Fisher RS. 1977. Sudden infant death syndrome (SIDS): cardiac pathologic observations in infants with SIDS. *Am Heart J* **93**:762–6.

Marshall TK. 1972. Epidemiology of cot deaths: the Northern Ireland study. *J Forensic Sci Soc* **12**:575–9.

Mitchell EA, Thompson JM. 2001. Parental reported apnoea, admissions to hospital and sudden infant death syndrome. *Acta Paediatr* **90**:417–22.

Naeye RL. 1973. Pulmonary arterial abnormalities in the sudden-infant-death syndrome. *N Engl J Med* **289**:1167–70.

Naeye RL. 1980. Sudden infant death. *Sci Am* **242**:56–62.

Norvenius SG. 1987. Sudden infant death syndrome in Sweden in 1973–1977 and 1979. *Acta Paediatr Scand Suppl* **333**:1–138.

Oehmichen M, Gerling I, Meissner C. 2000. Petechiae of the baby's skin as differentiation symptom of infanticide versus sids. *J Forensic Sci* **45**:602–7.

Ogbuihi S, Zink P. 1988. Pulmonary lymphatics in SIDS – a comparative morphometric study. *Forensic Sci Int* **39**:197–206.

Opdal SH, Rognum TO, Torgersen H, *et al.* 1999. Mitochondrial DNA point mutations detected in four cases of sudden infant death syndrome. *Acta Paediatr* **88**:957–60.

Oyen N, Markestad T, Skaerven R, *et al.* 1997. Combined effects of sleeping position and prenatal risk factors in sudden infant death syndrome: the Nordic Epidemiological SIDS Study. *Pediatrics* **100**:613–21.

Parish WE, Barrett AM, Coombs RR, *et al.* 1960. Hypersensitivity to milk and sudden death in infancy. *Lancet* **2**:1106–10.

Peterson DR, Beckwith JB. 1973. Magnesium deprivation in sudden unexpected infant death. *Lancet* **2**:330.

Polak JM, Wigglesworth JS. 1976. Letter: Islet-cell hyperplasia and sudden infant death. *Lancet* **2**:570–1.

Protestos CD, Carpenter RG, McWeeny PM, *et al.* 1973. Obstetric and perinatal histories of children who died unexpectedly (cot death). *Arch Dis Child* **48**:835–41.

Rasten-Almqvist P, Eksborg S, Rajs J. 2000. Heart weight in infants – a comparison between sudden infant death syndrome and other causes of death. *Acta Paediatr* **89**:1062–7.

Raven C, Maverakis NH, Eveland WC, *et al.* 1978. The sudden infant death syndrome: a possible hypersensitivity reaction determined by distribution of IgG in lungs. *J Forensic Sci* **23**:116–28.

Richards ID, McIntosh HT. 1972. Confidential inquiry into 226 consecutive infant deaths. *Arch Dis Child* **47**:697–706.

Rintahaka PJ, Hirvonen J. 1986. The epidemiology of sudden infant death syndrome in Finland in 1969–1980. *Forensic Sci Int* **30**:219–33.

Rognum TO (ed.). 1995. *Sudden infant death syndrome, new trends in the nineties.* Scandinavian University Press (Universitetsforlaget AS), Oslo.

Rognum TO. 1999. [Crib death or cot death in the nordic countries. A forensic pathologist's point of view.] *Ugeskr Laeger* **161**:6612–18.

Sadler DW. 1998. The value of a thorough protocol in the investigation of sudden infant deaths. *J Clin Pathol* **51**:689–94.

Saternus KS, Koebke J, von Tamaska L. 1986. Neck extension as a cause of SIDS. *Forensic Sci Int* **31**:167–74.

Sawaguchi T, Fujita T, Sawaguchi A, *et al.* 2000. The epidemiological study on registered cases of sudden infant death syndrome (SIDS) in Tokyo: examination of the effect of autopsy on diagnosis of SIDS and the mortality statistics in Japan. *Forensic Sci Int* **109**:65–74.

Simson LR, Jr, Brantley RE. 1977. Postural asphyxia as a cause of death in sudden infant death syndrome. *J Forensic Sci* **22**:178–87.

Sinclair-Smith C, Dinsdale F, Emery J. 1976. Evidence of duration and type of illness in children found unexpectedly dead. *Arch Dis Child* **51**:424–9.

Southall DP. 1983. Identification of infants destined to die unexpectedly during infancy: evaluation of predictive importance of prolonged apnea and disorders of cardiac rhythm or conduction. *Br Med J* **286**:1092–6.

Steinschneider A. 1972. Prolonged apnea and the sudden infant death syndrome: clinical and laboratory observations. *Pediatrics* **50**:646–54.

Steinschneider A, Weinstein SL, Diamond E. 1982. The sudden infant death syndrome and apnea/obstruction during neonatal sleep and feeding. *Pediatrics* **70**:858–63.

Sturner WQ. 1971. Some perspectives in 'cot death'. *J Forensic Med* **18**:96–107.

Sturner WQ, Dempsey JL. 1973. Sudden infant death: chemical analysis of vitreous humor. *J Forensic Sci* **18**:12–19.

Summers CG, Parker JC, Jr. 1981. The brain stem in sudden infant death syndrome. A postmortem survey. *Am J Forensic Med Pathol* **2**:121–7.

Sunderland R, Emery JL. 1981. Febrile convulsions and cot death. *Lancet* **2**:176–8.

Urquhart GE, Grist NR. 1972. Virological studies of sudden, unexplained infant deaths in Glasgow 1967–70. *J Clin Pathol* **25**:443–6.

Urquhart GE, Logan RW, Izatt MM. 1971. Sudden unexplained death in infancy and hyperimmunization. *J Clin Pathol* **24**:736–9.

Urquhart GE, Izatt MM, Logan RW. 1972. Cot death: an immune-complex disease? *Lancet* **1**:210.

Valdes-Dapena M. 1977. Sudden unexplained infant death, 1970 through 1975 an evolution in understanding. *Pathol Annu* **12**(Pt 1):117–45.

Valdes-Dapena M. 1982. The pathologist and the sudden infant death syndrome. *Am J Pathol* **106**:118–31.

Valdes-Dapena M. 1985. Are some crib deaths sudden cardiac deaths? *J Am Coll Cardiol* **5**:113B–17B.

Valdes-Dapena M. 1986. Sudden infant death syndrome. Morphology update for forensic pathologists – 1985. *Forensic Sci Int* **30**:177–86.

Valdes-Dapena MA. 1973. Editorial: Sudden, unexpected and unexplained death in infancy – a status report – 1973. *N Engl J Med* **289**:1195–7.

Valdes-Dapena MA. 1980. Sudden infant death syndrome: a review of the medical literature 1974–1979. *Pediatrics* **66**:597–614.

Variend S, Pearse RG. 1986. Sudden infant death and cytomegalovirus inclusion disease. *J Clin Pathol* **39**:383–6.

Vawter GF, McGraw CA, Hug G, *et al.* 1986. An hepatic metabolic profile in sudden infant death (SIDS). *Forensic Sci Int* **30**:93–8.

Wedgwood RJ, Benditt EP (eds). 1963. *Sudden death in infancy. Proceedings of the 1963 Seattle Conference.* United States Department of Health and Welfare, Bethesda.

CHAPTER **22**

Fatal child abuse

There is now a vast collection of publications on the child abuse syndrome, including international journals devoted to the topic. Most of this interest concerns the clinician, as child abuse is now a major concern in paediatrics. When no intervention is offered, an abused child has up to a 10 per cent risk of having eventually fatal injuries, so unfortunately the forensic pathologist will be involved in this tragic problem from time to time. This chapter will deal solely with the physical manifestations of the child abuse syndrome as seen at autopsy, though naturally these will in large measure coincide with the non-fatal injuries seen by clinicians.

GENERAL ASPECTS OF CHILD ABUSE

Though the modern phase of recognition of the syndrome dates only from the middle decades of this century, almost all the classical features were described by Tardieu in 1860 (see Knight 1986). In 1946, Caffey published his well-known first paper and, from then on, an avalanche of articles led to the present intense awareness of the problem that throws into stark contrast the apparent unawareness of the medical profession during the previous century.

Though definitions are variable, it can be said that the 'child abuse syndrome' (also known as the 'battered baby' or 'non-accidental injury in childhood') exists when an infant or child suffers repetitive physical injuries inflicted by a parent or guardian, in circumstances that exclude accident. Most of the fatal victims are young, more than two-thirds being under 3 years of age (Kempe *et al.* 1963; Lauer *et al.* 1974; Brown 1976; Helfer *et al.* 1977).

The syndrome includes, of course, psychological and sexual abuse, but the forensic pathologist can only be concerned with physical damage, some aspect of which has led to death. Though all homicides of children are 'child abuse' in the broad sense, the term is usually reserved for a fatal outcome in those who have suffered repetitive ill-treatment, though admittedly some cases span the borderline between chronic injuries and a single episode of trauma.

The definition of 'child abuse' is itself controversial, as what is unacceptable now may well have been considered valid and even desirable discipline in Victorian times. However, serious physical injury must be wrong, irrespective of societal attitudes.

Even so, for a pathologist to label an injury as 'child abuse' or 'non-accidental injury (NAI)' is to be rather pejorative and judgemental, so perhaps 'adult-induced injury' might be a more neutral description, which leaves decisions as to motivation to those who possess a wider picture of the whole circumstances. Having said that, the more gross forms of injury are self-evidently 'abuse' but, in lesser degrees of trauma, it may be impossible to differentiate deliberate battering from inexpert rough handling, albeit contributed to by exasperation, panic or even attempts at resuscitation.

Though it is vital to recognize non-fatal child abuse, because of the need for intervention to prevent the 60 per cent recurrence rate and 10 per cent mortality rate, it can be almost as tragic to falsely accuse and/or convict parents or guardians where the injuries were non-culpable.

There has sometimes been perhaps some excess of zeal on the part of paediatricians, radiologists, accident surgeons and pathologists to overinterpret injuries and scenarios that had an alternative and less sinister explanation. Though it is natural and vital for doctors to protect children and their siblings, medical opinion has to remain free from emotive bias and be confined within the bounds of what can be proved in each individual case, or injustice may be done. Some years ago, a situation developed where even innocent parents were afraid to take their accidentally injured child to a doctor, for fear of the euphemism 'non-accidental injury' being applied.

MODES OF DEATH IN CHILD ABUSE

The majority of deaths are caused manually, either by hitting or beating with the hands, shaking, throwing, dropping and – less often – by burning or suffocation. It is exceptional for death to be caused by the impact of a blunt instrument, though non-fatal bruises from beating with a strap, for instance, are sometimes seen. Shooting, strangling and stabbing are characteristic of classical homicide, which is distinct from the child abuse syndrome.

The most common mode of death is head injury. Next in frequency is rupture of an abdominal viscus, leaving a wide range of miscellaneous injuries to account for the small remainder.

THE RANGE OF INJURIES IN CHILD ABUSE

Concentrating on autopsy findings, the various types of trauma will be described, though many will not in themselves have caused or even contributed to death. Their recognition is none the less vital as, at the end of the examination, they may well be the decisive factors that may distinguish an accident from deliberate maltreatment.

SURFACE BRUISING

One of the classic aphorisms in the study of child abuse was stated by the forensic pathologists, Cameron, Johnson and

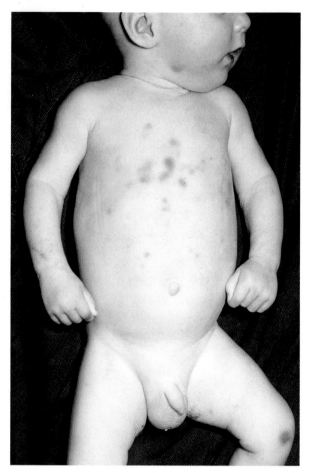

FIGURE 22.1 *Multiple fingertip bruises on the chest and abdominal wall of an infant left with a male babysitter. The child was ill on the mother's return and died during admission to a hospital casualty department (see also Figures 22.4 and 22.5).*

Camps (1966), who said: 'The skin and bones tell a story which the child is either too young or too frightened to tell.'

Skin bruising is the most common injury and may be seen almost anywhere on the child's body. There are, however, certain sites of predilection which help to strengthen the diagnosis of abuse:

■ Bruising around the limbs, especially the wrist and forearms, upper arms, thighs and – in small infants – around the ankles. These places form convenient 'handles' for an adult to grip the child. In the small infant the lower leg bruises may indicate that the child has been held by the leg or ankle in order to swing it – and may be associated with head injuries. The older child, as an adult, may be gripped by the upper arms in order to be shaken.
■ The buttocks are a frequent site of bruising from hand smacks or beating with a strap. Bruises on the thigh are less common, but on the outer side may signify slaps and on the inner, possible sexual interference.

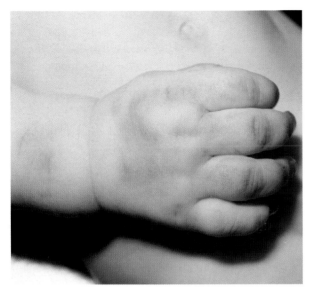

FIGURE 22.2 *Bruising of wrist and back of the hand after maltreatment by mentally ill mother (see also Figures 22.3 and 22.6).*

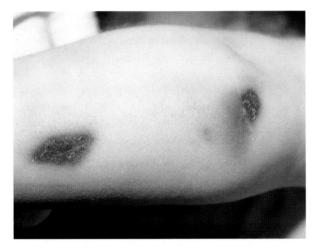

FIGURE 22.3 *Bruising of upper extremity after maltreatment by mentally ill mother (see also Figures 22.2 and 22.6).*

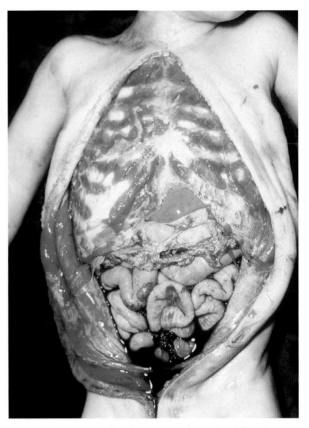

FIGURE 22.4 *Injuries found at autopsy of an infant left with a male babysitter showing a generalized haemoperitoneum.*

- The face is often bruised, especially the cheeks and mouth area, from slaps, which may also be present on the forehead and ears. Associated damage to the mouth and eyes is common. Bruising of the scalp is harder to see because of the hair, but is often part of deeper head injury.
- Bruises on the chest, abdomen and neck are usually from finger pressure rather than slaps or blows. Those on the abdomen and lower chest may be associated with deep visceral injury. Bruises may be of any size or type, but a common variety in child abuse is the small discoid lesion about 1–2 cm in diameter; these were once called

'sixpenny bruises' from the size of coinage at that time. These are caused by impact or pressure from the finger-pads of adults, and may be seen in groups around the limbs and on the neck, chest or abdomen.

Bruises from slapping or punching may be larger and irregular. Occasionally, a partial or even almost whole handprint may be seen outlined in bruises on the buttocks or trunk.

The age of bruises is an important issue in child abuse because:

- The observed age may be at variance with the history given by a parent, so increasing the suspicion of a non-accidental event.
- Bruises of different ages indicate episodes of injury at different times, one of the hallmarks of child abuse that usually continues over a period.

Though it is impossible to be accurate about the absolute age of a bruise, those of markedly different colours cannot have been inflicted during the same episode. The interpretation of patterns and the ageing of bruises are more fully considered in Chapter 4, but any bruise with yellow coloration must be more than 18 hours since infliction.

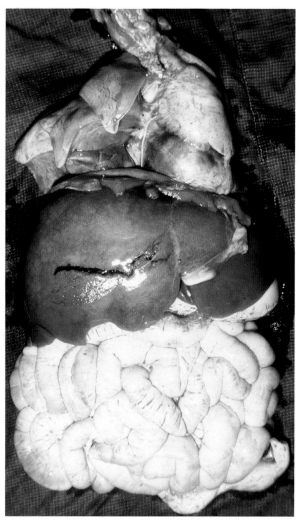

FIGURE 22.5 *The infant shown in Figures 22.1 and 22.4 showing a full-thickness tear extending through the liver. Rupture of an abdominal viscus is the second most common mode of death in child abuse, head injury being the most frequent.*

SKELETAL DAMAGE IN CHILD ABUSE

This is the second part of the aphorism about battered children as, both clinically and pathologically, diagnosis is largely a radiological matter. Just as a whole-body survey is needed in the live victim, so it is essential before an autopsy on a suspected fatal case of child abuse. Some pathologists would recommend a radiological skeletal survey on all infants prior to autopsy if they had not been under constant clinical care for some well-recognized natural disease. This would include all sudden infant deaths but, because of lack of facilities and finance, many pathologists have to confine their requests for such extensive radiology to those deaths

in which there was some possibility of abuse, though this decision may lead to injuries being missed.

The range of skeletal injuries seen in child abuse is wide and there are very extensive publications on the subject, including at least one textbook by Cameron and Rae (1975) and a section on the radiology by Evans and Knight (1981).

Worlock *et al.* (1986) compared fractures in 35 abused children with 826 controls and found that the abused were all under 5 years old, whereas 85 per cent of the others were more than 5 years. The abused infants were more likely to have multiple fractures, and to have bruising of the head and neck. Rib fractures were almost confined to abused children, when major chest trauma was excluded. Spiral fractures of the humeral shaft were more common, though classical chipped metaphyses were uncommon. They concluded that one in eight infants under 18 months of age with a fracture had been abused.

The following is a summary of the more important bony lesions.

Fractures of the skull

Skull fractures are common in fatal child abuse, often in association with intracranial haemorrhage, usually subdural, though numerically less than half of infants with subdural haematomata have skull fractures (Harwood-Nash *et al.*). He found that of 4465 childhood head injuries, 1187 had skull fractures, but that there was little correlation with neurological signs and intracranial damage, subdural haemorrhage (SDH) being twice as frequent in the non-fracture cases.

Fractures have been discussed in relation to head injuries in Chapter 5, but some particular features in child abuse must be mentioned, as it is a controversial subject, especially when such cases come to trial.

The most common fracture lies in the occipitoparietal area, but the differentiation from accidental falls is impossible on anatomical or radiological grounds alone, in spite of the dogmatic claims of some radiologists. An infant's skull is more flexible than that of an adult and may absorb some impacts without fracturing. Occasionally, a parietal bone may 'dimple' inwards without cracking, much as a table-tennis ball may be dented with a thumb. The skull of a child is much thinner than that of an adult, even though the brain size and weight is greater relative to the postcranial mass. This means that there are two opposing factors operating:

■ Because of the thin skull, less force is required for fracturing.
■ Because of the elasticity or 'springiness' of the skull, recovery from distortion caused by impact is greater, so

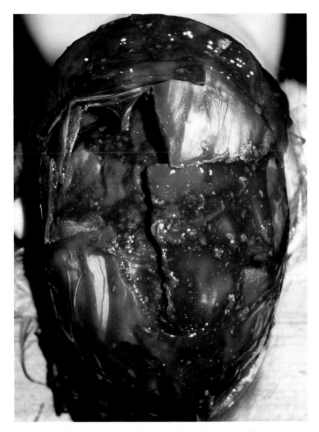

FIGURE 22.6 *Fractured skull of an infant after repeated blows against the floor by mentally ill mother (see also Figures 22.2 and 22.3).*

more force is needed to fracture the pliable bone, relative to its thickness.

Notwithstanding the flexibility, however, it remains a fact that an infant skull will fracture with the application of much less mechanical force than would be needed to fracture a mature skull. In addition, because the cranium is more easily deformed, a momentary depression of the skull can impinge upon the underlying brain (including membranes), damage it and return to its original shape so that, even in the absence of a fracture, brain damage is more likely to occur.

There is now a large literature on infant fractures (especially of the skull) in relation to child abuse, some of it contradictory.

One aspect that arouses much controversy is the height of a passive fall which can (a) fracture a child's skull and (b) cause brain damage. The two injuries are certainly not synonymous, as it is clear that most fractures, both in infants and adults, are not accompanied by any brain damage or neurological effects. However, forces that can cause a skull fracture certainly **can** – though not **must** – cause brain or meningeal lesions, and it is impossible to forecast what will happen following a fall of even minor magnitude.

Though many paediatricians will deny that a passive fall from adult waist level – or even higher – can cause either skull fracture or intracranial damage, there is experimental proof and witnessed cases on record where this has occurred.

In respect of skull fractures, Weber (1984) experimentally dropped dead infants from a horizontal position at only 'table height' (82 cm, 34 inches) onto a variety of surfaces and found that fractures were common. Fifteen infants less than 8 months old were dropped passively from a horizontal position onto concrete, carpet and linoleum; all developed cranial vault fractures in various positions. Though most fractures were in the parietal bones, some extended into the occipital bone. In 1985, Weber again dropped dead infants from 82 cm (34 inches) onto soft cushioning, such as 10 cm (4 inches) thick foam mat and 8 cm (3.2 inches) thick double blanket. Fractures were much less frequent, as was to be expected, but still one occurred on the thick foam and four out of 25 drops onto the folded blanket, all from only 82 cm (34 inches).

Reichelderfer *et al.* (1979) indicated that serious head injuries in playgrounds can occur when the impact force exceeds 50 G; a fall of only 7.5 cm (3 inches) onto concrete can generate 100–200 G and one of 0.3 m (a foot) no less than 475–500 G.

In 246 falls of infants under 5 years from bed or low structures less than 90 cm (36 inches) high, Helfer *et al.* (1977) found no serious injuries or deaths. Of these, 161 occurred at home and 175 had some injury, including two skull fractures. In 85 hospital falls, there were 28 injuries, with one skull fracture. Nimityongskul and Anderson (1987) investigated 76 childhood falls in hospital, 75 of which were younger than 5 years. The height of fall was between 30 and 91 cm (1 and 3 feet), and only one doubtful skull fracture occurred.

Of 398 falls studied by Williams (1991), 106 were observed by independent witnesses. There were 14 severe injuries in falls between 4.5 and 12.20 m (15 and 40 feet), but below 3 m (10 feet), there were no life-threatening injuries, though three skull fractures were detected. Similarly, Reiber (1993) found three skull fractures in infants who had died after witnessed short falls of less than 1 m (3 feet). This was from a series of coroners' cases where all had intracranial bleeding. One 21-month infant fell 1.5–1.8 m (5–6 feet) and had a subdural haemorrhage, but no skull fracture. Another 17-month child fell only 0.6–0.9 m (2–3 feet), but suffered a sub-dural and cerebral contusion. Reiber gives a good short survey of the competing literature, indicating that opinions fall into two groups – the 'major injury–major fall' set and the 'major injury–minor fall' camp.

Hall *et al.*'s (1989) series confirms that severe or fatal damage can occasionally arise from low falls. In a 4-year study, there were 18 deaths following falls from less than 0.9 m (3 feet). Two of these were witnessed by medical care persons, excluding abuse as a covert reason. Sixteen other similar deaths were not so witnessed, but abuse was not corroborated as a cause.

Chadwick *et al.* (1991), analysing 317 childhood falls, saw seven deaths in 100 falls from less than 1.20 m (4 feet), but doubted the veracity of the histories, as there was only one death in those who fell between 3 and 13.7 m (10 and 45 feet). Hobbs (1984) studied 89 children with skull fractures, 29 thought to have been abused. Of 20 deaths, 19 were abused. The characteristics of the battered infant fractures were multiplicity or complex configuration; depressed, wide and 'growing' fractures, the latter meaning widening of the fracture line after infliction; accidental fractures were felt to be narrow, linear and single, usually in the parietal area.

Leventhal *et al.* (1993) investigated 104 infant skull fractures and concluded that abuse was the cause in 34 per cent, accident in 62 per cent, the rest being doubtful. Billmire and Myers (1985) claimed that 64 per cent of all infant head injuries, excluding simple fractures, were caused by abuse and that of serious intracranial damage, 95 per cent were from abuse. These varying figures emphasize the lack of consensus in the literature.

Though the immature skull has more flexibility, once its elastic limit is exceeded during deformation, it will fracture. The pattern of fracturing is similar to that in the adult, but there are some variations because of the presence of open sutures and fontanelles. Fracture lines tend to end at sutures, but if they cross them there is frequently a lateral displacement so that the two limbs of the fracture are not in line. Most instances where what appears to be a fracture line crossing a suture with a 'side-step' are really two independent fractures either approaching or receding from each other, the origins or terminations being slightly offset. The most common example is seen in a child who has been dropped on the vertex of the head. Both parietal bones may then deform and crack transversely from the vertex anterior to the point of impact, the bilateral fracture lines running downwards towards the parietal bosses. The upper ends of both fractures terminate in the sagittal suture, but may be 'staggered' by a centimetre or so.

Another common fracture is a horizontal crack running backwards from the frontoparietal suture, which courses across the parietal bone, often turning down towards the base of the skull. This can be caused by a blow or fall on the side or top of the head. Such fractures can occur bilaterally, which is then an indication of an impact on the vertex of the skull, which causes marked depression of the top of the skull with crack fractures along the lines of maximum stress. These are then more marked on the outer aspect than the inner table – though the diploë of infants' skulls are absent or only partially formed, according to the age. Of course, such bilateral fractures can also be caused by two separate impacts on each side of the head; here multiple bruises on or under the scalp may assist in interpretation.

The frontal bone is less often involved than the parieto-temporal area, the frontal suture that is still present in young infants giving more flexibility than in the fused older bone. Occipital fractures may occur from falls onto the back of the head, but again these are much less common than cracks at the vertex or sides of the cranium, though, as the experiments of Weber showed, occipital bone cracks can occur from simple low-level falls in small infants. Wherever the vault fractures, if it is severe enough, extension lines may run down into the base of the skull, but this is not a frequent finding in child abuse injuries.

Sutural 'diastasis' (separation) may occur with or without fractures, the loosely knit skull plates being easily parted by distortion of the calvarium when struck. As mentioned above, some fractures widen after infliction (sometimes due to rising intracranial pressure). These so-called 'growing fractures' are thought by some writers to be more likely to be associated with abuse, though logic would relate it more to severity of impact rather than to motivation.

Limb fractures

These provide some of the most characteristic signs of child abuse, as injuries are common around the metaphyses and epiphyses of growing bones, as well as being the cause of periosteal lesions. Most of the limb injuries are indirect, that is, the bone damage is caused by stresses from abnormal angulation, torsion or traction, rather than from a direct impact upon the bone. Swinging the child by the wrists or ankles, dragging it by an arm or shin and violent shaking using the limbs as 'handles', are the usual mechanisms.

Avulsion of the metaphysis or chipping of the edges of the metaphyses or epiphyses may occur, with small fragments seen isolated on radiographs. Swinging, wrenching or twisting actions can fragment the metaphysis. Small pieces of the adjacent cortex and parts of the provisional zone of calcification may be avulsed from the shaft. The epiphysis may even separate from the metaphysis. Cameron and Rae (1975) suggested that metaphyseal fragments are virtually pathognomonic of child abuse.

The periosteum in infants is only loosely attached to the bone and easily lifts where there is shearing or traction injury. Blood accumulates under the raised periosteum and this rapidly calcifies (usually within 7–14 days) to give a characteristic radiological picture of a bony shell extending along the shaft, often thicker at the extremity, having a lumpy, irregular profile (Evans and Knight 1981). In almost half the cases, this may be seen radiographically within one week (Cameron 1970). The calcified rim may extend around the end of the metaphysis and epiphysis, or between the two, giving a 'bucket-handle' loop effect around the end of the bone, especially the lower end of the femur.

In early infancy it must be appreciated that some breech deliveries have legs that radiologically show long, smooth periosteal thickening secondary to subperiosteal bleeding caused by handling during delivery. It is also accepted that mere growth can produce faint subperiosteal calcification, but this is symmetrical and limited to the central parts of the shaft, keeping clear of the metaphyses.

A spiral fracture of the diaphysis of a long bone must be considered a suspicious injury in infants, as such a lesion is likely to be the result of a twisting strain, unlikely to occur in accidental circumstances.

The lower end of the shaft of a long bone may be 'squared-off', as described by Caffey (1946), by metaphyseal fragments reuniting. Damage to the epiphyseal cartilage may cause permanent growth defects, sometimes with increased growth from hyperaemia following injury. The axis of growth may be deviated and cupping of the metaphysis may occur because of retarded longitudinal growth in the centre.

Although the metaphyseal and epiphyseal lesions described above are classically those seen in child abuse, transverse and spiral fractures of the diaphysis are also common. In a series of 100 cases reported by Kogutt et al. (1974), these fractures were more common than the injuries to ends of the bones.

Damage to the chest cage

Apart from occasional perinatal fractures during delivery (Polson, Gee and Knight 1985), accidental fractures of ribs are very uncommon in infants, though the incidence is a matter of considerable controversy. Once again paediatricians, radiologists and pathologists may have differing views and experience.

In child abuse, ribs are commonly fractured, often several consecutive bones being affected on one or both sides. The damage may be fresh or old, giving different radiological appearances. The most characteristic picture of old fractures is of sequential callus formation seen in a vertical line down one or both paravertebral gutters. These form a 'string-of-beads' appearance on X-ray (Figure 22.7), where the ribs have been fractured near their angles, a sufficient time previously for new bone formation to occur – probably a minimum of 10 days, though dating is notoriously variable, and even the claims by experienced radiologists to date fractures have been confounded by a knowledge of the actual time of breakage.

These multiple posterior fractures are more common in small infants who have been picked up by adult hands under the armpits and squeezed from side to side. Whether or not such fractures can be caused by innocent handling, albeit rough or robust, as opposed to angry or impatient violence, is again a matter of dispute, beyond the competence

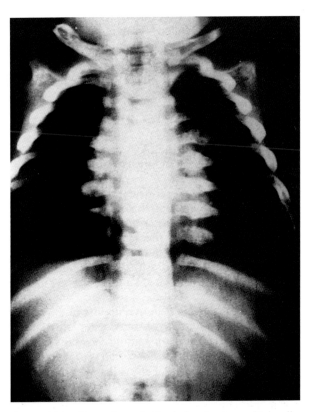

FIGURE 22.7 *Chest radiograph of an infant showing multiple callus formation on the necks of the ribs, giving a 'string of beads' appearance down the paravertebral gutter. These indicate previous multiple fractures caused by lateral squeezing by adult hands.*

of doctors to resolve – although this does not deter some from expressing strong opinions based on weak facts.

These fractures, a centimetre or so from the head of the ribs, are due to the rib being levered against the transverse process until breaking point is reached. They may be very difficult or impossible to see as fresh lesions on radiographs, if the fracture line is not exactly in line with the X-ray beam. This explains the occasional discrepancy between the radiologist's and the pathologist's report; the fractures are much more visible after a week or two, when callus is present.

If such injuries are recent (probably less than 10 days) no visible callus is formed, but the fractures may be seen on X-ray and confirmed at autopsy. However, as with fractures elsewhere – and perhaps more often in ribs than skull – the radiological and dissection diagnosis sometimes does not concur. Fractures seen at autopsy may not be visible radiologically – and conversely, alleged fractures seen on films may not be discoverable at autopsy, even after the most diligent dissection.

Rib fractures in the axillary line are likely to be the result of anteroposterior pressure, rather than side-to-side squeezing, but this mechanism is not exclusive. With fresh fractures found at autopsy, the possibility of chest compression

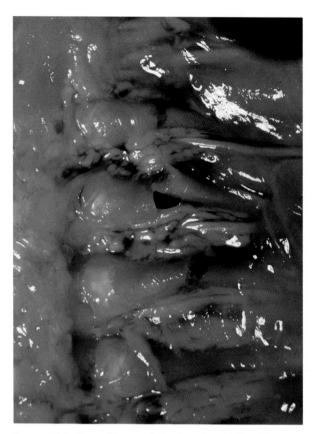

FIGURE 22.8 *Recent fractures of ribs of an abused infant. These breaks are near the necks of the ribs in the paravertebral gutter, caused by side-to-side squeezing of the chest.*

during cardiopulmonary resuscitation must always be considered, even though some paediatricians and radiologists will strenuously deny the possibility of this happening. The literature has different opinions on this matter, though it is admittedly very uncommon. As with other aspects of child abuse, the published material seems to flow more from those who lean towards abuse in the majority of injured children, rather from those who retain a more cautious approach and admit to the possibility of an innocent explanation.

It must be conceded that pliable infant ribs are unlikely to be broken by proper cardiac massage, which in infants should be performed with finger pressure; however, lay persons, especially in the panic of apparent collapse and death, may forcibly pump the small chest using techniques intended for adult resuscitation.

Fractures elsewhere are more likely to arise from direct impact such as a fist blow or kick. The clavicle is sometimes broken, usually from indirect stress from swinging by an arm. Fractures of the scapula or sternum are rare and arouse the probability of 'parental infliction' if some obvious trauma such as a traffic accident can be excluded.

Wherever the site of bony injury, the cardinal features that arouse suspicion are multiplicity and variation in fracture age. Though children often sustain accidental fractures, these are usually single lesions, unless some pathological bone disease is present. Similarly, the radiological demonstration of multiple fractures of varying ages must be accepted as evidence of abuse until proved otherwise.

Dating of fractures

As in the case of skin bruises, though the absolute dating of healing fractures by the state of callus formation is far from accurate (Evans and Knight 1981), marked differences in appearance on radiology usually indicate that the injuries were not sustained at the same time. As it can be shown, however, in control material, that the same person reveals callus of different extent and maturity in different but similar bones fractured contemporaneously, it becomes impossible to be dogmatic about radiological healing rates. Bone healing is rapid in healthy children and within months the abnormalities may have completely resolved, depending on the severity of the original damage.

Histological appearances are also very unreliable in placing an absolute date on fractures, in spite of assertions that this can be done with accuracy.

BONE DISEASES AND INFANT FRACTURES

Both in the differential diagnosis of childhood fractures and in the defence of allegations of child abuse, the several 'brittle bone diseases' that can cause abnormal skeletal fragility must be considered, on the grounds that lesser force, within normal parental handling or even spontaneous movements of the infant, could give rise to the observed fractures.

It has to be said at the outset that only a small minority of injured infants can be shown to have such abnormalities. When this possibility is being run as a defence in a criminal trial or child protection proceedings, it is essential to have an opinion from a radiologist or paediatrician with specialist knowledge of these conditions.

It is also important to have original radiographs, not copies, as the latter may not show marginal, indistinct abnormalities visible on the originals.

Osteogenesis imperfecta

This is a bone dysplasia with four types, numbered I, II, III and IV, of which there are several subgroups. The disease is an inherited disorder of connective tissue, with abnormal collagen, resulting in varying degrees of bone fragility, ligamentous laxity, skin fragility, sometimes blue sclera, hearing defects and dental abnormalities.

Types II and III have obvious bone disease and can hardly be confused with child abuse lesions.

Type I forms 70 per cent of cases and is the classical variety with a family history, blue sclera, Wormian bones and often dental changes, which again is hardly likely to be confused with abuse. It is type IV (only about 5 per cent of the overall disease incidence) that may cause difficulties in diagnosis, though it must be said that of all the medico-legal occasions in which this disease is postulated as a reason for brittle bones as a defence against allegations of abuse, the times upon which it can be proven are few indeed.

Type IVB, the larger subgroup, has dentinogenesis imperfecta. Type IVA has no family history of the disease, no osteoporosis, a high incidence of skull fractures and metaphyseal fractures and normal sclera. Subgroup IVA has Wormian bones, like IVB, but it has been postulated that some alleged cases of type IVA were really abuse.

It has been calculated that the incidence of type IV osteogenesis imperfecta in infants under one year, with fractures, no family history, no Wormian bones or dentinogenesis imperfecta is one in 1–3 million. A case would occur in a city of half a million population only once every 100–300 years.

Recent techniques of fibroblast culture and collagen analysis can provide evidence of defective connective tissue in the absence of overt clinical signs, but this is not necessarily synonymous with brittle bones. The case report by Ojima *et al.* (1994) gives a useful survey of the problem. Bone strength in otherwise normal SIDS infants has been measured by Morild *et al.* (1993) to obtain a baseline for comparison with alleged osteogenesis where this is raised as a defence against child abuse.

Infantile cortical hyperostosis ('Caffey's disease')

Here there is extensive new periosteal bone laid down around the diaphyses, the bones most involved being the ribs, ulnae, clavicles and especially the mandible. The condition is rarely seen over the age of 3 years.

Congenital syphilis

This can mimic the changes seen in child abuse, though the condition is extremely rare in most Western communities. The periosteal thickening is similar to that of trauma, but tends to be symmetrical. The metaphysis may be fractured and even separated, the shaft adjacent to the metaphysis being porotic.

Copper deficiency

Again rare, this condition has radiological features in which periosteal thickening of the shafts of the long bones may be accompanied by symmetrical spurring of the metaphyses, osteoporosis, fractures and cupping of the metaphyses. Abnormalities of the hair may be present in this deficiency disease that is caused by lack of copper impairing the enzyme lysyl oxidase. The radiological appearances may cause confusion with child abuse. Other clinical features include psychomotor retardation, hypotonia, pallor, hypopigmentation of the skin and hair, prominent scalp veins, sideroblastic anaemia and neutropenia.

Menke's syndrome ('kinky hair' syndrome)

This is another rare condition also associated with copper deficiency in which there are abnormal metaphyses. It affects males only, with abnormal hair, Wormian bones in the skull and mental retardation.

HEAD INJURY IN CHILD ABUSE

The most common cause of death in abused children is intracranial damage, with or without skull fracture. As well as being the most frequent fatal condition, brain trauma is responsible for the common tragedy of severe, and often permanent, neurological impairment.

The classic head injury associated with battered children is subdural haemorrhage, which formed part of 'Caffey's syndrome' that he described five decades ago. It was also noted in Tardieu's famous publication of 1860, when he described bleeding on the side of the cerebrum and other classical features (Knight 1986). Subdural haemorrhage is most common at the extremes of life, the topic being discussed fully in Chapter 5. In infants, it most often occurs from direct impact on the skull – as in a blow or fall. For some years, it has been held that vigorous shaking, without an impact, is also a common cause of subdural bleeding. This is a view strongly held by many paediatricians, who may prefer this mode as a first choice over a blow or fall, but recent research has thrown doubt on the common acceptance of this mechanism.

For example, the excellent textbook of DiMaio and DiMaio (1989) observes:

Many forensic pathologists have doubted that the shaken baby syndrome exists [Norton 1983]. Most have felt that the injuries to the brain, including the retinal haemorrhages, are due to undetected direct impact injuries. In all cases seen by the authors in which there has been retinal haemorrhage associated with subdural or subarachnoid bleeding, or some other brain trauma, direct impact injury to the head has been identified.

The forces generated in the cranial cavity by shaking have been shown to be of the order of 50 times less than in the deceleration stresses of an impact (Gennarelli and Thibault 1982; Duhaime *et al.* 1987). These authors investigated 13 fatalities alleged to have occurred from shaking, but though 7 showed no external head injury, all 13 revealed evidence of impact at autopsy. In infant models, they then compared impact with violent shaking; the mean tangential acceleration for 69 shaken babies was less than 10 G, whereas for 60 impacts, the mean was 428 G, some 50 times greater. The mean time for shakes was 106 milliseconds, but for impacts was only 20 milliseconds.

It is the rate of change and the duration of deceleration – the 'strain rate' – that is most damaging, rather than a steady deceleration. A head impacting on an immovable surface after a fall is an example of a high strain-rate injury, whereas low strain-rate injuries are those where the head decelerates over a longer period of time. Non-impact shaking of the head is a low strain-rate mechanical insult. Subdural bleeding from bridging veins is likely to occur from high strain-rate injury, even though this may be a low-energy injury, insufficient to cause cerebral tissue disruption. By contrast, low strain-rate injuries are more likely to cause cerebral contusion, with vascular damage only if concomitant high energy is generated (Howard *et al.* 1993).

Geddes and Whitwell (2004) have recently pointed out that there have been no formal systematic neuropathological studies of infant head injury and the evidence base for diffuse axonal injury (DAI) being a common finding in infant head injury is poor. In fact the idea of the presence of DAI in these cases was widely accepted before the advent of the modern diagnostic methods and before the diagnostic criteria for DAI had been established. Moreover, the findings of Shannon *et al.* (1998), the first formal study of microscopic damage in non-accidental injury (NAI), suggesting that axonal injury in such cases had been ischaemic or vascular in origin, had been largely ignored or misunderstood. In their recent series of 53 fatally injured infants (Geddes *et al.* 2001a, b), diffuse axonal injury was present in only two children, both of whom had multiple skull fractures and severe head injury, whereas the most frequent histological finding was global hypoxic damage in 84 per cent of the cases. In 11 of these cases (21 per cent), however, there was gross and microscopic evidence of injury to the craniocervical junction and concomitant axonal damage in the caudal brainstem long tracts in 8 subjects. This finding is in keeping with cervical hyperflexion/hyperextension injury pattern in adults and suggests as a possible mechanism of

death: brainstem injury, apnoea and hypoxic brain swelling. In another systematic study of dural bleeding in 50 paediatric cases, including intrauterine deaths up to infants of 5 months of age, but without head injury, Geddes *et al.* (2003) found fresh haemorrhage into the layers of dura in a majority (36/50) of cases. The authors believe that this is a manifestation of severe hypoxia similar to the haemorrhages found in internal organs in birth asphyxia or prematurity, rather than being caused by trauma, and postulate that hypoxia is sufficient to cause extravasation of significant amounts of venous blood both in and under the dura.

Although shaking presumably may cause subdural haemorrhage (SDH), it is likely that it is a relatively uncommon cause, compared with impact. This situation may well have arisen because a blunt impact upon the head of infant, if spread over a wide area following contact with a flat surface, can leave no external scalp mark, no subscalp bleeding and no fracture of the skull – yet the transmitted forces can still be sufficient to cause high strain-shearing stresses within the cranium leading to subdural bleeding. In addition, as has been discussed elsewhere in this book, death is often not due to the irritative or space-occupying effects of the subdural, but is due to the intrinsic brain damage beneath, even if this is occult. Diffuse axonal injury, cerebral oedema and consequent circulatory disturbances are likely to be the fatal consequences, but detecting neuronal damage may be difficult or impossible histologically, due to the relatively rapid death of the child within 12–24 hours. Also, the microscopic features of diffuse axonal injury seem to be less common and less distinct in infants compared with adults, though the use of immunocytochemical methods, such as the demonstration of β-amyloid precursor protein (βAPP), described in Chapter 5, may provide a marker of use within the first few hours after injury. These factors combine to negate any proof of an impact injury and thus the shaking theory, which requires none of these criteria to be demonstrated, is an easier option.

Howard *et al.* (1993) looked at 28 instances of SDH in infants under 18 months of age. All had a history more consistent with an impact rather than shaking. Six Caucasian infants fell less than 0.9 m (3 feet), such as from a chair or standing adult. Eight non-Caucasians fell from a sitting or standing position or rolled off a bed onto a carpeted floor. There was a history of shaking in three, but these also had signs of impact, the shaking being resuscitation attempts after falling. Of these, 47 per cent of the Caucasians and 20 per cent of the non-Caucasians had a skull fracture. The authors state: 'Our findings do not support shaking as the only cause of SDH and also suggest that non-accidental injury is a less common cause of SDH than it is believed to be.'

There is a suggestion in several papers that Asian children are more susceptible to SDH from minor trauma;

Japanese infants have been reported with SDH after falling from only a sitting position (Aoki and Masuzawa 1984; Rekate 1985).

Most direct impacts in child abuse are caused by the moving head striking a fixed object, rather than the fixed head being struck. The latter certainly occurs, but is usually from an open-handed slap, albeit often of considerable force. It is unusual for the child's head to be struck with a weapon or for a direct punch to be given with the clenched fist. The moving head injury either arises from a fall in circumstances which are non-accidental, or by deliberate swinging or throwing of the child against a hard surface, often with added momentum being gained by holding the infant's ankles or wrist. For example, one such case seen by the author (BK) was a month-old baby whose father grasped it by the ankles to dash its head against stones at the edge of a canal, after which it was stripped so that its clothing could be sold in a street market, the body then being thrown into the canal.

Several other mechanisms of head injury have been described, including some seen by the author (BK) in which fathers were throwing their baby up in the air in a catching game called 'up-and-away', but for some reason missed the child on the downward return, allowing it to fall to the floor. When unwitnessed, this situation can give rise to accusations of deliberate malice, which are difficult to disprove.

Presumably, as vigorous shaking can sometimes rupture vessels in the subdural space, this must still be accepted as an alternative to impact in the causation of subdural haemorrhage. In an infant, the head is relatively large and heavy and the neck musculature undeveloped and often hypotonic. Thus repetitive shaking of the body – often attained by grasping under the armpits – can lead to unrestrained flexion and extension movements of the head with rotational movements of the heavy cerebral hemispheres relative to the skull.

Extradural haemorrhage is uncommon in child abuse, perhaps because the meningeal arteries do not run in deep grooves or even tunnels in the immature skull, as they do in the adult. Subarachnoid haemorrhage is, as always, an inevitable accompaniment of cerebral cortical contusion.

Brain damage may be of any type, as catalogued in Chapter 5, but as in any childhood head injury, cerebral oedema is more common than in the adult. Indeed, a significant proportion of deaths after a head injury in a child are caused by raised intracranial pressure without skull fracture, meningeal haemorrhage or visible brain injury. The typical autopsy indications may be found consisting of a heavy brain, flattened gyri, obliterated sulci and slit-like ventricles. The more florid signs seen in adults, such as herniation of the hippocampal gyrus through the tentorial gap, secondary brainstem haemorrhages and coning of the cerebellar tonsils are seen less frequently in children.

When there has been a severe head injury, with or without a fractured skull, cerebral contusion or laceration may occur. The position of this damage is usually related to the site of external impact. Although many episodes of child abuse involve dropping or throwing to the floor, classical contrecoup lesions are not as common as in similar adult injuries. They certainly do occur, but are often absent when the circumstances would indicate that contralateral contusion might be expected. The smoother internal profile of the infant skull may be a factor.

The distance of a fall sufficient to cause head injury has been mentioned earlier and is a matter of considerable controversy in the literature and amongst expert medical witnesses. There is no doubt, both from reliable anecdotal evidence and from experimental data, such as that by Weber, that skull fractures can occur in infant skulls from very low passive falls, including heights not exceeding chair or table level (Weber 1984: 82 cm; 34 inches). However, as catalogued above, skulls often fracture without any significant internal brain damage – although the reverse is also true. The evidence that low falls may cause brain or meningeal lesions is much less convincing than that proving skull fractures – but the possibility exists and cannot be dismissed by inflexible, dogmatic opinion. The problem with assessing the mechanical basis of head injury is that human experimentation is virtually impossible – Weber's work on dead infants probably could not be repeated in the present ethical climate – and obviously no data can be derived from the living. Animal models are useless, so the frequent difficulties for pathologist, lawyers and the courts have to rest on available statistical evidence – which can never give a definitive answer in any one case. If a phenomenon has definitely occurred once, then it can occur again, whatever the statistical weight is against its frequency, as a precedent has been established which cannot be gainsaid as a possibility.

One of the problems is the 'standard of proof', as in the criminal courts, it is 'beyond reasonable doubt', whereas in civil matters, it only has to pass the test of 'balance of probabilities', where statistical evidence is far more persuasive.

To rely on the 'experience' of medical witnesses is also fraught with difficulty, as their anecdotal memories of previous cases will provide unsatisfactory data in respect of the causation of the injury. Where adults are accused of malice or neglect, they are very likely to fabricate or distort the circumstances of the injury, and claim that the infant fell from the chair, the arms or the bed. Even in genuine accidents, feelings of guilt, clouded recollection from grief and panic, will often lead to an inaccurate account of the circumstances, so the doctor's past experience is often of lesser value than the accused adults, the lawyers and the court imagine, due to inadequate or false knowledge of the true circumstances of previous cases.

VISCERAL INJURY IN CHILD ABUSE

Damage to internal organs is almost always confined to the abdomen, as the heart and lungs are rarely injured. As stated earlier, rupture of an abdominal viscus is the second most common cause of death in child abuse after head injury. Forcible impacts on either the lower chest or the abdominal wall are responsible. Direct punching or heavy 'prodding' are the usual mechanisms rather than being dropped or thrown, which is a common cause of head injury. Often there will be an excuse that the child fell or tripped upon some protruding obstruction, such as a toy or piece of furniture; occasionally this may be true and it is a matter of fact and interpretation as to whether the circumstantial evidence is compatible with the medical findings. The liver is frequently injured, the most common lesion being a deep tear in either lobe, sometimes being a complete penetration or, more rarely, actual detachment of hepatic tissue. A haemoperitoneum results and in fatalities, may be the proximate cause of death. A heavy blow over the lower ribs or xiphisternal area is the most likely site of impact.

The small intestine is the other common target organ, the duodenum or jejunum being the most frequent site of damage. The second part of the duodenum is vulnerable to blows in the central abdomen, as beneath this area, the duodenum crosses the midline and is liable to be 'sandwiched' between the compressed anterior abdominal wall and the promontory of the lumbar spine. As the tissue thickness is small in a child, the gut can be virtually 'guillotined' at this point and may be completely transected, appearing almost as clean-cut as if it had been done with a surgical knife. Alternatively the gut wall may be damaged and, though it may not leak or rupture at the time of impact, ischaemic and necrotic changes over the next few hours or even days may lead to a delayed rupture, with the later onset of peritonitis.

The same lesions, though rarely as sharply cut, can occur in the jejunum, often accompanied by laceration of the mesentery and haemorrhage into the peritoneal cavity instead of – or in addition to – leakage of intestinal contents.

Rupture of the stomach can occur, but must be carefully differentiated from gastric rupture from non-traumatic causes and (these days) especially from external cardiac massage, which produces linear tears in the mucosa and even rupture of the complete wall.

DAMAGE TO EYES, EARS AND MOUTH

As part of general facial damage, black eyes, and scleral and conjunctival haemorrhages are often seen, but damage to the interior of the globe is much less apparent at autopsy. Some considerable time after the general recognition of the child abuse syndrome, it was discovered that a considerable proportion of victims, both live and dead, had significant internal damage to the eyes. Direct violence to the head and allegedly shaking, can cause bleeding into the vitreous humour, dislocation of the lens, retinal detachment and retinal haemorrhages (Gilliland *et al.* 1994).

The latter can also be caused by cardiopulmonary resuscitation, where vigorous compression of the chest has been applied; the literature on this topic is controversial, but numerous references confirm this mechanism, yet others,

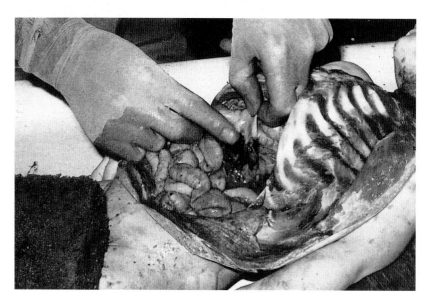

FIGURE 22.9 *A ruptured duodenum in an abused child who suffered a blow in the central abdomen. This relatively common mode of death in fatal child abuse is caused by the duodenum being guillotined against the lumbar spine by an impact that indents the thin anterior abdominal wall. The gut may be severed immediately or may become infarcted because of damaged blood supply over the ensuing few days, then rupture into the peritoneal cavity.*

such as Gilliland and Luckenbach (1993), deny it. Once again, there are hotly contested viewpoints in the position taken by different doctors over the aetiology of various lesions in child abuse, both by clinicians and pathologists. They are also, of course, often secondary to raised intracranial pressure from head injuries, rather than due to primary direct violence. During life, these can be diagnosed by ophthalmoscopy, but at autopsy they must be sought by dissection. As disfigurement of the body of a child must be avoided wherever possible, examination for eye lesions may be achieved either by enucleation and replacement with glass prostheses – or by opening the orbits from the anterior cranial fossae and removing the posterior two-thirds of the globes.

Injury to the external ear is frequent, as abuse of a child is often directed at the obvious targets, such as face, head, arms, buttocks and ears. The pinnae may be bruised or even lacerated, usually by an open-handed slap. Damage to the internal ear from heavy impacts on the head may be diagnosed clinically, though often in retrospect from later deafness. At autopsy, damage to such minute structures is rarely visible, though sometimes haemorrhage into the petrous temporal bone may be found when routinely examining this area for middle-ear sepsis.

Injury to the lips and mouth is so common as to be one of the prime diagnostic signs of the battered child. Infants and older children are commonly slapped across the mouth, the swipe usually having a tangential component that moves the tissues laterally. This causes the most reliable indicator of child abuse, the torn frenulum (or 'frenum') beneath the upper lip. This small median band of mucosa that joins the upper gum to the upper lip is ripped as the lip is jerked sideways, and is virtually pathognomonic of battering. The other possible cause of a ruptured frenulum is the forcible entry of a feeding bottle teat into the mouth of a reluctant infant. Instead of entering between the gums, the teat is rammed up between the gum and lip, causing a tear. The lesion heals rapidly, as do all injuries in the mouth and, within a few days, nothing may be seen except perhaps a loose mucosal tag or an absent frenulum, or both.

Damage to the lips themselves is common, the type of injury varying somewhat according to whether or not the child is old enough to have teeth. In any event, bruising, swelling, abrasion and sometimes external laceration may be seen. The inner mucosal aspect of the lips may be bruised even if the child has no teeth and, if the blow is hard enough, laceration can occur. This is far more likely to happen if the lips are forced against the teeth, especially the cutting edge of the incisors.

The teeth themselves may be damaged, especially in older children. Total avulsion from the sockets, loosening and breakage may occur. In small infants, developing teeth may be forced back into the sockets, like pegs into holes. Expert dental advice should be sought wherever possible when injuries to teeth and jaws are found, both in live children and at autopsy.

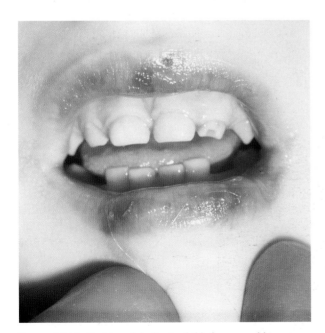

FIGURE 22.10 *Bruising of the lips in child abuse caused by smacking in the mouth. When the child is old enough to have teeth, lacerations may occur inside the lips. The frenulum behind the midline of the upper lip (not shown) was ruptured in this child, a strong pointer to a blow across the upper lip.*

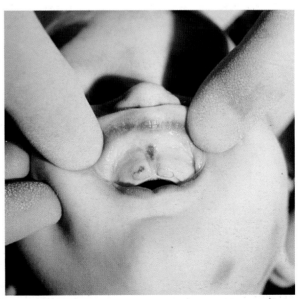

FIGURE 22.11 *Tearing of the frenulum of the upper lip of a child, a classical injury from a tangential slap across the mouth.*

BURNS IN CHILD ABUSE

Unfortunately, thermal injuries are by no means uncommon in abused infants. These may be moist scalds, dry burns or, exceptionally, electrical injuries.

Scalds result from dipping in hot fluid and often involve over-hot bath water. The line between accident and abuse may be blurred in some cases, but it can occur as a form of chastisement. In one case, a child was deliberately held in water at over 80°C as a punishment for persistently complaining about being cold. Other scalds may be from boiling water from a kettle or saucepan deliberately being poured over the child.

Dry burns can be inflicted in innumerable ways as a deliberate and sadistic act. Children have been forcibly sat on electric cooking rings and hotplates, branded with hot shovels and electric soldering-irons, or pressed against the bars of a fire. A particular type of burn seen relatively often in abused children is never the cause of death but may be found incidentally. This is the cigarette burn, seen most often on skin not normally covered by clothing, such as the hands, arms, neck and head. Such burns are usually circular, but not always; if the cigarette has been held obliquely against the skin, the mark may be triangular. The regular shape and size usually indicate the nature of the burn, though some skin diseases may simulate an old burn, such as a small patch of impetigo. Fresh cigarette burns are red, sometimes with a narrow rim of a deeper red. When healing, they become pink and later have a silvery sheen on the surface.

BITE MARKS IN CHILD ABUSE

Most bites on the skin surface are seen either in sexual offences or in child abuse. In the author's own experience, all bitten infants have had these inflicted by the mother, though published reports indicate that both male and female guardians can bite their infant charges. The topic is discussed in more detail in Chapter 26, but as they are relatively common in child abuse, a summary is repeated here.

Bites may be seen anywhere on the child's body. The arms, back of the hands, cheeks, shoulders, buttocks and abdomen are favoured sites. A bite mark usually consists of two opposing semicircles, which may be incomplete. Individual teeth marks may be visible or the dental arch may be represented by a continuous line. The mark is either an abrasion or a bruise, or a combination of both. There may be confluent petechiae in the centre caused by suction, but this is much more common in sexual assaults – the so-called 'love bite'. In child abuse, the centre is more often undamaged. The size of the dental arch should be carefully measured to determine

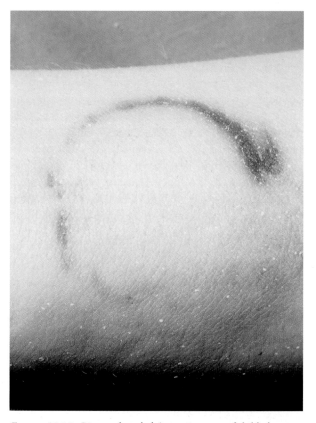

FIGURE 22.12 *Bite mark on baby's arm in a case of child abuse. The culprit was the mother. The teeth marks are deficient over one quadrant, the gap on the other side being smaller than usual.*

whether it was formed by an adult, another child or even an animal, as is sometimes alleged in defence.

In older children, the possibility of self-biting must be borne in mind – the author has seen multiple self-bites all the way up one arm in a young person.

As with all dental matters, the advice of a dentist experienced in forensic problems is highly desirable. Not only can he confirm or exclude doubtful lesions, but he can identify individual teeth marks, make casts of any residual impression in the skin and take swabs for saliva identification. He can also examine any suspects to compare their dentition with the marks – a common excuse of the parents is that another child or even the family dog caused the bite. If no forensic odontologist is available, however, the pathologist must make the best examination possible and details are given in Chapter 26.

OTHER INJURIES IN CHILD ABUSE

A variety of injuries, some bizarre and sadistic, occur from time to time in battered children. The hair may be pulled out in clumps (epilation), leaving pseudoalopecia on the

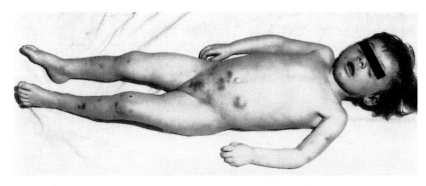

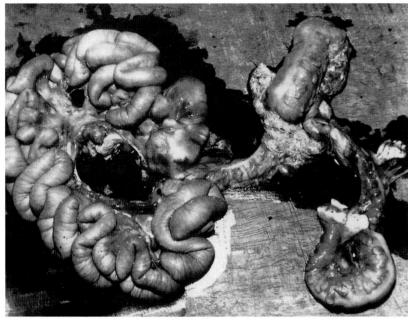

FIGURE 22.13 *A child with numerous bruises on the body, totalling 80 on the face, neck, abdomen, back and legs. The male adult in the house claimed that she had 'slipped while being bathed'. At autopsy, there was a massive haemoperitoneum arising from multiple ruptures of the mesentery.*

scalp. Fingers may be broken by hyperextension and finger-tips crushed by blows or other means. Patterned marks from straps and ropes may be seen on the skin, usually on buttocks, thighs and abdomen. 'Pinch' or 'tweaking' marks are not uncommon, made by the skin being nipped between adult fingernails. These appear as two small opposing semi-circular or triangular bruises, often with a clear zone between them.

THE AUTOPSY IN CHILD ABUSE

This follows the usual routine for any forensic autopsy, but certain additional matters must be given close attention. Because of the emotive nature of child abuse, especially where a fatality is concerned, the pathologist must pay meticulous attention to all aspects of his examination and report. A full description of the autopsy in child abuse may be found in the chapter by Knight in *Paediatric Forensic*

Pathology (Knight 1989). The following matters must be borne in mind:

- The scene should be visited wherever possible, though usually the child will already have been removed, usually to a hospital accident department. Even a retrospective visit can be helpful, however, to assess such matters as the nature of the floor and its coverings, where falls are alleged, the height of settees and chairs, and the general size and space between walls, doors and furniture, as claims of colliding with household structures are a constant line of defence – and may well be true in some instances.
- The child should be examined in its original clothing where possible.
- The appearances before washing and other cosmetic manoeuvres should be recorded; when children die in hospital accident departments, such compassionate acts may remove useful evidence, and the balance between

- sympathy and justice can sometimes be hard to reconcile.
- Careful enquiries should be made about any resuscitatory attempts, as these can introduce a number of artefacts.
- Where any suspicion of abuse is present, a full radiological skeletal survey should be carried out before the autopsy is begun.
- Full physical measurements must be made including weight, crown–heel length, crown–rump length, foot length and head diameter.
- A meticulous external examination must be made, covering every square centimetre of the body, including all body orifices. The interior of the mouth and lips must be searched.
- A full photographic record must be made of any abnormality discovered. Where bruising is suspected, but not definitely apparent, the use of both infrared- and ultraviolet-sensitive film has been advocated, though experience is required in their interpretation, as artefacts are common.
- Extensive dissection of subcutaneous tissues is required wherever bruising is seen or suspected. Incisions must be made into doubtful areas or the skin flayed away to reach such areas, if disfigurement is to be avoided.
- Full sampling of blood, urine, stomach contents, liver, ocular fluid and cerebrospinal fluid must be taken, according to the circumstances. It is best to be liberal with the range of samples – it is easy to discard unwanted samples, but difficult or impossible to obtain them at a later date.
- Where appropriate, skin samples for fibroblast culture and swabs for microbiological culture are taken. Blood samples for grouping and other blood characteristics may be needed and a sufficient amount for DNA testing.
- Bite marks may need to be swabbed for saliva and casts made of tooth indentations. The cooperation of a forensic odontologist is then vital (see Chapter 26).
- A full internal dissection of all organs is required, with full sampling for histological purposes. Further radiographs may need to be taken on isolated bones or on the chest cage. The latter can be removed entirely by careful dissection if multiple rib fractures are present. X-rays can then be taken of the detached thoracic cage free of soft tissue and further histological blocks taken for decalcification in an attempt to date the lesions.
- If there is obvious or suspected brain damage, the brain should be removed carefully and suspended in formalin until firmly fixed. On no account should 'wet cutting' take place if intracranial damage or cerebral oedema is present.
- The globes of both eyes should be removed for histological examination: they can be taken entire and false eyes replaced for cosmetic purposes – or the posterior three-quarters of the globes can be removed via a superior approach through the base of the anterior fossa.

REFERENCES AND FURTHER READING

Ablin DS, Greenspan A, Reinhart M, et al. 1990. Differentiation of child abuse from osteogenesis imperfecta [see comments]. *AJR Am J Roentgenol* **154**:1035–46.

Adams PC, Strand RD, Bresnan MJ, et al. 1974. Kinky hair syndrome: serial study of radiological findings with emphasis on the similarity to the battered child syndrome. *Radiology* **112**:401–7.

Aoki N, Masuzawa H. 1984. Infantile acute subdural hematoma. Clinical analysis of 26 cases. *J Neurosurg* **61**:273–80.

Bacon CJ, Sayer GC, Howe JW. 1978. Extensive retinal haemorrhages in infancy – an innocent cause. *Br Med J* **1**:281.

Barlow B, Niemirska M, Gandhi RP, et al. 1983. Ten years of experience with falls from a height in children. *J Pediatr Surg* **18**:509–11.

Billmire ME, Myers PA. 1985. Serious head injury in infants: accident or abuse? *Pediatrics* **75**:340–2.

Brown RH. 1976. The battered child syndrome. *J Forensic Sci* **21**:65–70.

Bush CM, Jones JS, Cohle SD, et al. 1996. Pediatric injuries from cardiopulmonary resuscitation. *Ann Emerg Med* **28**:40–4.

Caffey J. 1946. Multiple fractures in the long bones of infants suffering from chronic subdural hematoma. *Am J Roentgenol* **56**:163–72.

Caffey J. 1972. On the theory and practice of shaking infants. Its potential residual effects of permanent brain damage and mental retardation. *Am J Dis Child* **124**:161–9.

Caffey J. 1974. The whiplash shaken infant syndrome: manual shaking by the extremities with whiplash-induced intracranial and intraocular bleedings, linked with residual permanent brain damage and mental retardation. *Pediatrics* **54**:396–403.

Cameron JM. 1970. The battered baby. *Br J Hosp Med* **4**:769–74.

Cameron JM, Rae LJ. 1975. *Atlas of the battered child syndrome.* Churchill Livingstone, Edinburgh.

Cameron JM, Johnson HR, Camps FE. 1966. The battered child syndrome. *Med Sci Law* **6**:2–21.

Carty H. 1988. Brittle or battered. *Arch Dis Child* **63**:350–2.

Case ME, Graham MA, Handy TC, *et al.* 2001. Position paper on fatal abusive head injuries in infants and young children. *Am J Forensic Med Pathol* **22**:112–22.

Chadwick DL, Chin S, Salerno C, *et al.* 1991. Deaths from falls in children: how far is fatal? *J Trauma* **31**:1353–5.

Chapman S. 1990. Radiological aspects of non-accidental injury. *J R Soc Med* **83**:67–71.

Cohle SD, Hawley DA, Berg KK, *et al.* 1995. Homicidal cardiac lacerations in children. *J Forensic Sci* **40**:212–18.

Cumming WA. 1979. Neonatal skeletal fractures. Birth trauma or child abuse? *J Can Assoc Radiol* **30**:30–3.

Department of Health and Social Security. 1988. *Diagnosis of child sexual abuse.* HMSO, London.

DiMaio D, DiMaio V. 1989. *Forensic pathology.* Elsevier, New York.

Duhaime AC, Gennarelli TA, Thibault LE, *et al.* 1987. The shaken baby syndrome. A clinical, pathological, and biomechanical study. *J Neurosurg* **66**:409–15.

Duhaime AC, Alario AJ, Lewander WJ, *et al.* 1992. Head injury in very young children: mechanisms, injury types, and ophthalmologic findings in 100 hospitalized patients younger than 2 years of age. *Pediatrics* **90**:179–85.

Eisenbrey AB. 1979. Retinal hemorrhage in the battered child. *Child's Brain* **5**:40–4.

Evans KT, Knight B. 1981. *Forensic radiology.* Blackwell Scientific Publications, Oxford.

Feldman KW, Brewer DK. 1984. Child abuse, cardiopulmonary resuscitation, and rib fractures. *Pediatrics* **73**:339–42.

Fontana VI. 1964. The neglect and abuse of children. *NY State J Med* **64**:215–20.

Friendly D. 1971. Ocular manifestations of physical child abuse. *Trans Am Acad Ophthalmol Otolaryntol* **75**:318–32.

Geddes JF. 1997. What's new in the diagnosis of head injury? *J Clin Pathol* **50**:271–4.

Geddes JF, Whitwell HL. 2001. Head injury in routine and forensic pathological practice. *Curr Top Pathol* **95**:101–24.

Geddes JF, Whitwell HL. 2004. New thoughts on inflicted head injury in infants. *Forensic Sci Int* accepted for publication.

Geddes JF, Whitwell HL, Graham DI. 2000a. Traumatic axonal injury: practical issues for diagnosis in medicolegal cases. *Neuropathol Appl Neurobiol* **26**:105–16.

Geddes JF, Whitwell HL, Graham DI. 2000b. Traumatic or diffuse axonal injury? Author's response. *Neuropathol Appl Neurobiol* **26**:491.

Geddes JF, Hackshaw AK, Vowles GH, *et al.* 2001a. Neuropathology of inflicted head injury in children. I. Patterns of brain damage. *Brain* **124**:1290–8.

Geddes JF, Vowles GH, Hackshaw AK, *et al.* 2001b. Neuropathology of inflicted head injury in children. II. Microscopic brain injury in infants. *Brain* **124**:1299–306.

Geddes JF, Tasker RC, Hackshaw AK, *et al.* 2003. Dural haemorrhage in non-traumatic infant deaths: does it explain the bleeding in 'shaken baby syndrome'? *Neuropathol Appl Neurobiol* **29**:14–22.

Gennarelli TA, Thibault LE. 1982. Biomechanics of acute subdural hematoma. *J Trauma* **22**:680–6.

Gilliland MG, Folberg R. 1992. Retinal hemorrhages: replicating the clinician's view of the eye. *Forensic Sci Int* **56**:77–80.

Gilliland MG, Luckenbach MW. 1993. Are retinal hemorrhages found after resuscitation attempts? A study of the eyes of 169 children. *Am J Forensic Med Pathol* **14**:187–92.

Gilliland MG, Luckenbach MW, Chenier TC. 1994. Systemic and ocular findings in 169 prospectively studied child deaths: retinal hemorrhages usually mean child abuse. *Forensic Sci Int* **68**:117–32.

Goetting MG, Sowa B. 1990. Retinal hemorrhage after cardiopulmonary resuscitation in children: an etiologic reevaluation [see comments]. *Pediatrics* **85**:585–8.

Goldstein B, Kelly MM, Bruton D, *et al.* 1993. Inflicted versus accidental head injury in critically injured children. *Crit Care Med* **21**:1328–32.

Gornall P, Ahmed S, Jolleys A, *et al.* 1972. Intra-abdominal injuries in the battered baby syndrome. *Arch Dis Child* **47**:211–4.

Grunebaum M, Horodniceanu C, Steinherz R. 1980. The radiographic manifestations of bone changes in copper deficiency. *Pediatr Radiol* **9**:101–4.

Hahn YS, Raimondi AJ, McLone DG, *et al.* 1983. Traumatic mechanisms of head injury in child abuse. *Child's Brain* **10**:229–41.

Hall C, Shaw D. 1991. Non-accidental injury. *Curr Imaging* **3**:88–93.

Hall JR, Reyes HM, Horvat M, *et al.* 1989. The mortality of childhood falls [see comments]. *J Trauma* **29**:1273–5.

Harcourt B, Hopkins D. 1971. Ophthalmic manifestations of the battered-baby syndrome. *Br Med J* **3**:398–401.

Harwood-Nash CE, Hendrick EB, Hudson AR. 1971. The significance of skull fractures in children. A study of 1,187 patients. *Radiology* **101**:151–6.

Helfer RE, Slovis TL, Black M. 1977. Injuries resulting when small children fall out of bed. *Pediatrics* **60**:533–5.

Hobbs CJ. 1984. Skull fracture and the diagnosis of abuse. *Arch Dis Child* **59**:246–52.

Hood I, Ryan D, Spitz WU. 1988. Resuscitation and petechiae. *Am J Forensic Med Pathol* **9**:35–7.

Howard MA, Bell BA, Uttley D. 1993. The pathophysiology of infant subdural haematomas. *Br J Neurosurg* **7**:355–65.

Ingraham F, Heyl L. 1939. Subdural haematoma in infancy and childhood. *JAMA* **112**:198–204.

Ingram DM, Everett VD, Ingram DL. 2001. The relationship between the transverse hymenal orifice diameter by the separation technique and other possible markers of sexual abuse. *Child Abuse Negl* **25**:1109–20.

Kanter RK. 1986. Retinal hemorrhage after cardiopulmonary resuscitation or child abuse. *J Pediatr* **108**:430–2.

Kaur B, Taylor D. 1990. Retinal haemorrhages [see comments]. *Arch Dis Child* **65**:1369–72.

Kaur B, Taylor D. 1992. Fundus hemorrhages in infancy. *Surv Ophthalmol* **37**:1–17.

Kempe CH. 1971. Paediatric implications of the battered baby syndrome. *Arch Dis Child* **46**:28–37.

Kempe CH, Silverman FN, Steele BF, *et al.* 1963. Battered child syndrome. *JAMA* **181**:17–20.

Kiffney G. 1964. The eye of the battered child. *Arch Ophthalmol* **72**:231–3.

Kirschner RH, Stein RJ. 1985. The mistaken diagnosis of child abuse. A form of medical abuse? *Am J Dis Child* **139**:873–5.

Kleinman P. 1987. *Diagnostic imaging of child abuse.* Williams and Wilkins, Baltimore.

Kleinman PK, Marks SC, Blackbourne B. 1986. The metaphyseal lesion in abused infants: a radiologic-histopathologic study. *AJR Am J Roentgenol* **146**:895–905.

Kleinman PK, Marks SC, Adams VI, *et al.* 1988. Factors affecting visualization of posterior rib fractures in abused infants. *AJR Am J Roentgenol* **150**:635–8.

Knight B. 1986. The history of child abuse. *Forensic Sci Int* **30**:135–41.

Knight B. 1989. *The autopsy in child abuse.* In: Mason JK (ed.), *Paediatric forensic pathology.* Chapman and Hall, London.

Kobayashi M. 2001. Infant abuse in Osaka: health center activities from 1988 to 1999. *Pediatr Int* **43**:197–201.

Kogutt MS, Swischuk LE, Fagan CJ. 1974. Patterns of injury and significance of uncommon fractures in the battered child syndrome. *Am J Roentgenol Radium Ther Nucl Med* **121**:143–9.

Kravitz H, Driessen G, Gomberg R, *et al.* 1969. Accidental falls from elevated surfaces in infants from birth to one year of age. *Pediatrics* **44**(Suppl):869–76.

Lauer B, ten Broeck E, Grossman M. 1974. Battered child syndrome: review of 130 patients with controls. *Pediatrics* **54**:67–70.

Leventhal JM, Thomas SA, Rosenfield NS, *et al.* 1993. Fractures in young children. Distinguishing child abuse from unintentional injuries. *Am J Dis Child* **147**:87–92.

Mann K, Chan K, Yue C. 1986. Skull fractures in children: their assessment in relation to developmental skull changes and acute intracranial haematomas. *Child's Nerv Syst* **2**:258–61.

Mason JE. 1990. *Paediatric forensic medicine and pathology.* Chapman and Hall, London.

Maxeiner H. 2001. Demonstration and interpretation of bridging vein ruptures in cases of infantile subdural bleedings. *J Forensic Sci* **46**:85–93.

McClelland CQ, Rekate H, Kaufman B, *et al.* 1980. Cerebral injury in child abuse: a changing profile. *Child's Brain* **7**:225–35.

McCort J, Vaudagna J. 1964. Visceral injuries in battered children. *Radiology* **124**:681–4.

Milroy CM. 1999. Munchausen syndrome by proxy and intra-alveolar haemosiderin. *Int J Legal Med* **112**:309–12.

Morild I, Gjerdet NR, Giertsen JC. 1993. Bone strength in infants. *Forensic Sci Int* **60**:111–19.

Mushin AS. 1971. Ocular damage in the battered-baby syndrome. *Br Med J* **3**:402–4.

Nimityongskul P, Anderson LD. 1987. The likelihood of injuries when children fall out of bed. *J Pediatr Orthop* **7**:184–6.

Nokes L, Roberts A, Knight B. 1995. The use of the gadd severity index in forensic medicine: a case study. *Forensic Sci Int* **76**:85–90.

Norman MG, Smialek JE, Newman DE, *et al.* 1984. The postmortem examination on the abused child.

Pathological, radiographic, and legal aspects. *Perspect Pediatr Pathol* **8**:313–43.

Norton L. 1983. Child abuse. *Clin Lab Med* **3**:321–42.

O'Connor J, Cohen J. 1987. Dating of fractures. In: Kleinman P (ed.), *Diagnostic imaging of child abuse*. Williams and Wilkins, Baltimore.

Ogata M, Tsuganezawa O. 1995. An isolated perforation of the jejunum caused by child abuse. A case report. *Am J Forensic Med Pathol* **16**:17–20.

Ojima K, Matsumoto H, Hayase T, *et al.* 1994. An autopsy case of osteogenesis imperfecta initially suspected as child abuse. *Forensic Sci Int* **65**:97–104.

Parsons MA, Start RD. 2001. Acp best practice no. 164: necropsy techniques in ophthalmic pathology. *J Clin Pathol* **54**:417–27.

Pearn J. 1990. Physical abuse of children. In: Mason JK (ed.), *Paediatric forensic medicine and pathology*. Chapman and Hall, London, pp. 204–20.

Pena SD, Medovy H. 1973. Child abuse and traumatic pseudocyst of the pancreas. *J Pediatr* **83**:1026–8.

Pollanen MS, Smith CR, Chiasson DA, *et al.* 2002. Fatal child abuse – maltreatment syndrome. A retrospective study in Ontario, Canada, 1990–1995. *Forensic Sci Int* **126**:101–4.

Polson CJ, Gee D, Knight B. 1985. *Essentials of forensic medicine*, 4th edn. Pergamon Press, Oxford.

Rao N, Smith RE, Choi JH, *et al.* 1988. Autopsy findings in the eyes of fourteen fatally abused children. *Forensic Sci Int* **39**:293–9.

Reiber GD. 1993. Fatal falls in childhood. How far must children fall to sustain fatal head injury? Report of cases and review of the literature. *Am J Forensic Med Pathol* **14**:201–7.

Reichelderfer TE, Overbach A, Greensher J. 1979. Unsafe playgrounds. *Pediatrics* **64**:962–3.

Rekate HL. 1985. Subdural hematomas in infants [letter]. *J Neurosurg* **62**:316–17.

Rivara FP, Kamitsuka MD, Quan L. 1988. Injuries to children younger than 1 year of age. *Pediatrics* **81**:93–7.

Root I. 1992. Head injuries from short distance falls [see comments]. *Am J Forensic Med Pathol* **13**:85–7.

Sezen F. 1971. Retinal haemorrhages in newborn infants. *Br J Ophthalmol* **55**:248–53.

Shannon P, Smith CR, Deck J, *et al.* 1998. Axonal injury and the neuropathology of shaken baby syndrome. *Acta Neuropathol (Berl)* **95**:625–31.

Silverman FN. 1972. Unrecognized trauma in infants, the battered child syndrome, and the syndrome of

Ambroise Tardieu. Rigler lecture. *Radiology* **104**:337–53.

Smith FW, Gilday DL, Ash JM, *et al.* 1980. Unsuspected costo-vertebral fractures demonstrated by bone scanning in the child abuse syndrome. *Pediatr Radiol* **10**:103–6.

Spevak MR, Kleinman PK, Belanger PL, *et al.* 1994. Cardiopulmonary resuscitation and rib fractures in infants. A postmortem radiologic-pathologic study. *JAMA* **272**:617–18.

Tardieu A. 1860. Etude medico-legale sur les services et mauvais traiments exerces sur les enfants. *Ann Hyg Pub Med Leg* **13**:361–98.

Thomas PS. 1977. Rib fractures in infancy. *Ann Radiol Paris* **20**:115–22.

Thomas SA, Rosenfield NS, Leventhal JM, *et al.* 1991. Long-bone fractures in young children: distinguishing accidental injuries from child abuse. *Pediatrics* **88**:471–6.

Tomasi LG, Rosman NP. 1975. Purtscher retinopathy in the battered child syndrome. *Am J Dis Child* **129**:1335–7.

Touloukian RJ. 1968. Abdominal visceral injuries in battered children. *Pediatrics* **42**:642–6.

Vowles GH, Scholtz CL, Cameron JM. 1987. Diffuse axonal injury in early infancy. *J Clin Pathol* **40**:185–9.

Wagner GN. 1986. Crime scene investigation in child-abuse cases. *Am J Forensic Med Pathol* **7**:94–9.

Weber W. 1984. [Experimental studies of skull fractures in infants.] *Z Rechtsmed* **92**:87–94.

Weber W. 1985. [Biomechanical fragility of the infant skull.] *Z Rechtsmed* **94**:93–101.

Weedn VW, Mansour AM, Nichols MM. 1990. Retinal hemorrhage in an infant after cardiopulmonary resuscitation. *Am J Forensic Med Pathol* **11**:79–82.

Williams RA. 1991. Injuries in infants and small children resulting from witnessed and corroborated free falls. *J Trauma* **31**:1350–2.

Wilson E. 1977. Estimation of the age of cutaneous contusions in child abuse. *Pediatrics* **60**:750–5.

Wooley PV, Evand WA. 1955. Significance of skeletal lesions in infants resembling those of traumatic origin. *JAMA* **158**:539–43.

Worlock P, Stower M, Barbor P. 1986. Patterns of fractures in accidental and non-accidental injury in children: a comparative study. *Br Med J Clin Res Ed* **293**:100–2.

Yukawa N, Carter N, Rutty G, *et al.* 1999. Intra-alveolar haemorrhage in sudden infant death syndrome: a cause for concern? *J Clin Pathol* **52**:581–7.

CHAPTER 23

Deaths associated with surgical procedures

In most jurisdictions, deaths that occur during or within a short time after surgical operation, invasive diagnostic procedure or an anaesthetic, become the subject of a medicolegal investigation. Similarly, any death thought to be caused or contributed to, by any of these procedures – irrespective of the interval – may be enquired into if the medical attendants or the relatives consider that a causal relationship exists. To be effective such investigations must include an autopsy, and the pathologist involved in these has a difficult and often professionally sensitive task.

The pathologist should, wherever possible, be independent of the institution in which either the death occurred or which carried out the procedure. This is partly why the services of a forensic pathologist should be retained by the investigating authority, rather than a clinical or histopathologist belonging to the hospital, or associated institution. It is important that a separation should exist – and be seen to exist – between the loyalties of these two elements, not because there is any substantial likelihood of collusion, but because the public and private interest is best served by displaying the independence of the pathologist. In addition, there may be professional embarrassment when a close colleague of a surgeon or anaesthetist is placed in a potentially critical position within the same institution.

It is also sometimes useful to have the technical advice and expert opinion of an independent clinical consultant who is unconnected with the hospital, and who is not a colleague of the team involved in incident.

THE AUTOPSY ON DEATHS ASSOCIATED WITH SURGERY AND ANAESTHESIA

A number of difficulties exist, that are peculiar to this type of death. The following matters need particular attention:

■ The morphological findings, especially in so-called 'anaesthetic deaths', may be minimal or even absent so, more than in any other type of case, expert advice and full clinical information are essential.

■ Technically the autopsy on a post-operative death may be difficult as a result of the surgical intervention and its sequelae, especially in abdominal and thoracic procedures. Exudate, sepsis, adhesions, haemorrhage, oedema and distortion of the normal anatomy may make the dissection difficult, especially if the details of the surgical procedure are not fully known. Post-mortem changes can further complicate the appearances: for example, recent suture lines in the intestine or stomach may appear to be leaking, but this may be caused by autolysis, and even handling the tissues at autopsy may tear devitalized and autolytic structures even further.

■ Numerous surgical and anaesthetic devices may have been introduced into the patient during the procedure, such as airways, endotracheal tubes, indwelling needles, intravascular cannulae, self-retaining catheters, wound drains, chest tubes, monitoring electrodes, and metal or plastic prostheses. It is essential that none of these be removed before autopsy, as their proper placement and patency may need to be checked. Standing orders should be issued to hospitals within the jurisdiction of any coroner or medical examiner to the effect that no post-mortem interference with the body be made by members of the medical, nursing, technical or portering staff, as it has happened in the past that the single vital piece of evidence about some technical mishap has been discarded by some well-meaning person.

▨ Before any further disturbance of the body is made (for instance, by turning it over to look at the back) and certainly before a knife is picked up, the position of any endotracheal tube that may remain after anaesthesia must be checked. If the clinical information raises any doubt whatsoever about its malposition, then a pre-autopsy radiograph should be obtained, both anteroposterior and lateral.

Oesophageal intubation is not all that uncommon in anaesthetic mishaps and should be investigated carefully. The tube may be palpable through the skin if properly in the trachea – if there is doubt, a small primary incision in the midline of the neck with a further careful cut into the trachea can resolve the matter. Sometimes the intubation has been into the oesophagus, then been rectified after the damage has been done. Here the pathologist may find a ring of oedematous oesophageal mucosa still present at a level equal to that of the tube in the trachea. When nitrous oxide or other anaesthetic gas has previously been passed down a tube in the oesophagus there may be

distension of the stomach and intestines. A sample of the contained gas may reveal the agent on analysis.

▨ The hospital laboratory should be requested to retain any ante-mortem blood or body-fluid samples sent to them so that they remain available for analytical checks, such as blood grouping in transfusion mishaps, or creatine phosphokinase activity in malignant hyperthermia.

▨ Even more than usual, the fullest information is needed before beginning the autopsy. The patient's notes are essential, together with any other relevant information. Sometimes the nursing records may be more helpful

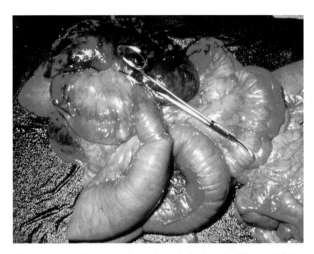

FIGURE 23.2 *Gut strangulated through the handle of forceps left in the abdomen during surgery and detected during an unrelated autopsy six weeks later for pneumoconiosis assessment.*

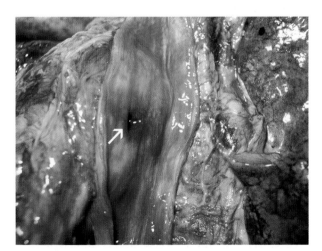

FIGURE 23.1 *Aorto-oesophageal fistula (arrow) due to ruptured anastomosis causing fatal haematemesis 18 days after replacement of the thoracic aorta with a prosthesis.*

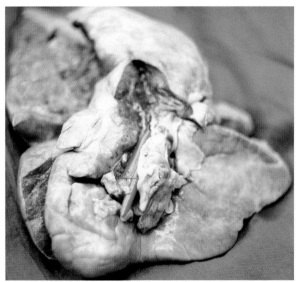

FIGURE 23.3 *Bronchial obstruction by the cover of a ballpoint pen, used by a midwife to hold down the tongue of a pregnant woman, who died days after childbirth from pneumonia.*

than the medical notes, as they are frequently more detailed and recorded at shorter intervals.

Equally important is the attendance of clinicians at the autopsy. Indeed, in deaths associated with anaesthesia, this is usually more useful than the post-mortem dissection, which frequently reveals little or no morphological evidence. Sadly, attendance at autopsies has declined markedly in recent years, as have requests for clinical autopsies, but every effort should be made to secure the presence of someone who knows the circumstances of the case well and who can point out to the pathologist the procedures that were carried out. A discussion across the autopsy table is of paramount importance and it is of little use if a junior doctor is delegated to attend, especially if he confesses to knowing little or nothing about the patient.

Especially in anaesthetic-related deaths, this dialogue with a clinician – in this case, the anaesthetist – may provide virtually all the data upon which to base a cause of death. Discussion between pathologist, surgeon and anaesthetist may arrive at an amicable conclusion that will be the best consensus of opinion to offer the investigating authority in cases where a bare autopsy might reveal little or nothing upon which to base any interpretation of the fatal processes.

■ During the autopsy, care must be taken to detect any surgical emphysema, pneumothorax or air embolism. When surgical operations have been conducted with the patient in the sitting position, as in posterior fossa neurosurgery or some thyroidectomies, the possibility of air aspiration into open veins or venous sinuses always exists.

Where infusion or transfusion mishaps may be a possibility, especially where gas pressure has been used to hasten the infusion rate, the possibility of air embolism must always be borne in mind.

THE MODE AND CAUSE OF DEATH AFTER SURGERY AND ANAESTHESIA

The rather loose terms 'operative deaths' and 'anaesthetic deaths' are usually inaccurate descriptions. When used without due consideration, they may lead to medico-legal enquiries and even civil litigation, which is not justified by the actual circumstances.

Fatalities associated with surgical intervention or invasive diagnostic procedures can be separated into several categories:

■ those directly caused by the disease or injury for which the operation or anaesthetic was being carried out

■ those caused by a disease or abnormality other than that for which the procedure was being carried out
■ those resulting from a mishap during, or a complication of, the surgical or diagnostic procedure
■ those resulting from a mishap during, or a complication of, the anaesthetic being administered.

These groups must be considered in more detail.

Deaths directly caused by disease or injury for which surgery is performed

Many deaths during a surgical or diagnostic procedure or an anaesthetic are caused by the disease process or injury for which the procedure was being performed. The death may be virtually inevitable in some 'heroic' operations where urgent intervention is the only hope of saving life. Presumably there must have been some chance of success or even palliation, otherwise the intervention would not have been justified, but the decision not to operate may be difficult. When death occurs from the effects of such disease or injury, some medico-legal systems will certify the original condition as the cause of death and omit any reference to the intervention.

The American Society of Anesthesiologists have a classification system for deaths during surgical procedures, as follows:

■ ASA 1: those with no serious disease
■ ASA 2: those who may have a serious disease, but have no limitations on their activities
■ ASA 3: those with serious disease and some limitation of their activities
■ ASA 4: those with a serious disease that is a constant threat to their health and that limits their activities
■ ASA 5: those with such serious disease that their death can be expected within 24 hours, with or without treatment.

The Society recommended that classes 1–3 require full investigation, as they were expected to survive; those in class 4 that were elective and not emergency procedures, with no expectation of death, are also included. The general principle is that unexpected deaths are investigated, though in the British coroner and Procurator Fiscal system there are no exceptions to such investigations, once reported by doctors to the appropriate legal authority.

Pathologists in some jurisdictions have problems in the nomenclature of certification following an autopsy. The strict test to be applied should be: 'Would death have occurred when it did, if the operation had not taken place?' Sometimes this is impossible to answer and the balance of probabilities may be evenly poised. If a patient has a leaking aortic aneurysm, which catastrophically ruptures whilst the surgeon is still making his skin incision, most would agree that the original disease process was the primary cause of death. Even here, however, it may be argued that the added disturbance of preparation and anaesthesia contributed something to a possible slight rise in blood pressure that further split the aneurysm wall.

Where a person dies of a pulmonary embolus 7 days after an elective gastrectomy for peptic ulcer, the connection between the operation and the death can hardly be denied, even though in up to a fifth of fatal pulmonary embolisms, depending on the study, no predisposing factors have been found (see Chapter 13).

When both trauma and surgical operation have taken place, then it can be impossible to separate the relative contributions of each to a death. A common example would be death a few days after the pinning of a fractured neck or femur in an old person. A fatal bronchopneumonia, pulmonary embolism or acute cardiac failure might all be caused either by the original trauma, by the stress of operation or by the subsequent immobilization in bed.

Death due to a disease or disability other than that for which surgery is performed

Where death is due to a disease or disability other than that for which the operation was performed, a distinction has to be drawn between those conditions that were known before the operation and those which were unsuspected.

When some disease is known beforehand, it must be evaluated in deciding whether or not the operative procedure is justified. For example, a patient with a non-obstructing hernia who has chronic obstructive airways disease might be thought to be too poor a risk for an elective, prophylactic operation. If that same patient's hernia becomes strangulated and he develops potentially fatal intestinal obstruction, however, the risk:benefit ratio dramatically changes and the danger of a perioperative death may have to be accepted. Naturally, operative and anaesthetic techniques may have to be modified to take account of the known adverse conditions.

It is different when an occult disease process is not suspected by the clinicians. It may be that they had no diagnostic means of appreciating the risk – such as an unsuspected phaeochromocytoma – but a medico-legal problem can arise if they took no reasonable precautions in detecting common risk factors, such as hypertension, lung disease or ischaemic heart disease, which in retrospect could have been diagnosed.

Death as a result of failure of surgical technique

Exceptionally, death is the result of a failure of surgical technique. This may be inadvertent, from a true 'accident', sometimes caused by unusually difficult operative circumstances, to anatomical abnormalities or even failure of equipment. When it is the result of error or incompetence, then a legal action for negligence may ensue and the pathologist must be even more meticulous than usual in producing a detailed, objective and impartial report. In all these cases, the presence of the surgeon is essential, so that agreement can be reached on what actually was found at autopsy.

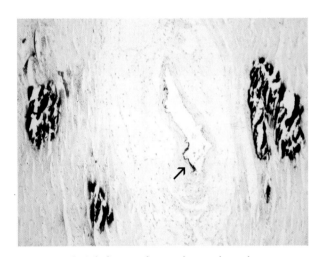

FIGURE 23.4 *Calcification of myocardium and vascular endothelium (arrow) due to postoperative rhabdomyolytic myoglobinuria and acute renal failure after reconstructive hand surgery and the interruption of blood circulation to the corresponding arm for the time of a nerve reconstruction. (Von Kossa staining, original magnification ×100.)*

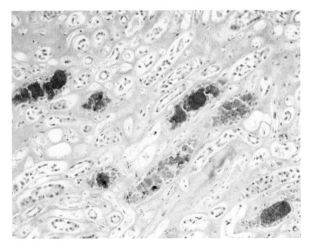

FIGURE 23.5 *Immunohistochemical demonstration of myoglobin in the renal tubuli with Anti-Human Myoglobin (Dakopatts a/s, Denmark).*

When a failure of equipment may be responsible, then expert examination and advice is essential. Anaesthetic machines, gas supply, compatibility of connections and all the sophisticated hardware of operating theatres must be subjected to the most rigorous inspection if a malfunction is suspected. This is no part of the pathologist's concern but, as he is responsible for the eventual decision about the cause of death, any conclusions about an equipment failure must be communicated to him.

Deaths due to anaesthetic administration

The foregoing categories account for most perioperative deaths and fatalities following surgery, even if delayed. True 'anaesthetic deaths' are comparatively rare, but have such potential medicolegal importance that they must be discussed in more detail.

DEATHS ASSOCIATED WITH ANAESTHESIA

Even more than is the case with surgeons, any autopsy on an anaesthetic-related death must be a cooperative process with the anaesthetist. Not only are the objective autopsy findings in true anaesthetic deaths meagre or absent, but the pathologist's training and experience of the complex techniques of modern anaesthesia is insufficient for him to appreciate, analyse and criticise constructively without the expert knowledge of the anaesthetist.

Most anaesthetic-related deaths are not caused by the anaesthetic agent itself, but due to other aspects of the procedure. Patients have anaesthetics because they have some significant – often very serious – disease or injury and, as has already been discussed, it is more likely that the fatality was the result of these or of some co-existent condition rather than the anaesthetic. There is a tendency on the part of relatives – and sometimes their lawyers – to assume that because someone died 'under' an anaesthetic, then this must be the major or even sole factor in the death because it was so closely related in time.

When factors other than anaesthesia can be excluded, certain features can be identified. A survey was conducted by Lunn and Mushin (1982) for the Association of Anaesthetists. This indicated that, although 1 in every 166 patients died within 6 days of a surgical operation, only 1 in 10 000 die solely as a consequence of the anaesthetic. Anaesthesia contributed to (but not totally caused) the death of 1 in every 1700 patients, many of these deaths being potentially avoidable.

The survey also showed that the causes have not changed significantly during the last 30 years, in spite of marked changes in anaesthetic technology and that anaesthesia may contribute to deaths that occur more than 24 hours after the administration. Many patients suffer from intercurrent disease unrelated to their surgical condition, but the implications for the anaesthetist are all too often ignored. The major causes of true anaesthetic fatalities include inexperienced and insufficiently supervised junior staff. Allowing periods of hypoxia to occur appears to be one of the common faults leading to a fatal outcome.

As far as the pathologist is concerned, the survey complained that the autopsy is of limited value in investigating the death. All too often irrelevant findings are offered, such as 'bronchitis'. Ischaemic heart disease was recorded in 39 per cent of the series. It was emphasized that the investigation of such deaths cannot be the sole province of the pathologist, but must rely heavily upon clinical data and cooperation with other doctors. Earlier investigations indicated that acute cardiovascular failure was the most common cause of unexpected death during anaesthesia. Lahey and Ruzicka in 1950 measured the risk of death during anaesthesia as about 1/1000, from all causes. Cardiac arrest was the most common single mode of death, being seen on average once or twice a year in most busy operating suites even under the most careful surgical and anaesthetic regimens. The autopsy is usually unhelpful in determining the cause, if coronary insufficiency can be excluded. Most cardiac arrest occurs under relative light anaesthesia and thus tends to occur at either the start or finish of the surgical procedure.

Reid and Brace (1940) showed that the arrest is mainly neurogenic and that any irritation of the respiratory tract, such as laryngoscopy or intubation, may cause a lightly anaesthetized patient to have a cardiac arrest. Inexperienced anaesthetists may not keep the patient at a level of unconsciousness appropriate to the manipulations of the surgeon, as it has been shown that such procedures can also precipitate arrest during light anaesthesia.

Hypoxia is also a potent precipitating factor in cardiac arrest. Deaths from respiratory failure also occur, and hypoxia is again a prime example – either from faults in the apparatus or more commonly to inexperience of the anaesthetist, especially in handling equipment with which he is not familiar. An overdose of the anaesthetic agent may depress the respiratory centres and begin a descending spiral of hypoxia. Excessive premedication and the use of muscle paralysing agents may also predispose towards respiratory failure unless appropriate measures are taken, such as assisted respiration.

Airway obstruction is another danger – from blood, teeth, dentures, faults in the connecting tubing, laryngeal spasm, swabs and an abnormal posture of the neck. Though regurgitation of gastric contents is a real danger, the use of

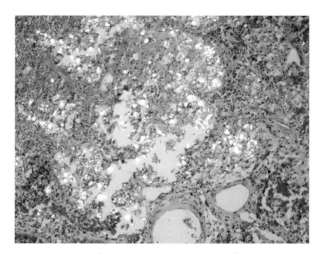

FIGURE 23.6 *Birefringent material in the alveoli due to contrast medium aspiration (barium sulphate).*

cuffed endotracheal tubes has greatly reduced the hazard. From the pathologist's point of view, the finding of gastric contents in the airways must be backed up by some clinical evidence of its ante-mortem origins, as a quarter of bodies have some gastric contents in some part of the air passages at autopsy, mostly as a result of agonal or even post-mortem transfer that is a consequence of the dying process, not a cause (Chapter 14).

Rarely, some physical fault in the anaesthetic equipment may cause death. Mention has been made of faults in the connecting tubing, which may be internal delamination, not visible from outside. Flow-meter errors occur, but a more common one is the confusion of bottled or piped gas supplies, and the inadvertent use of the wrong substance or the connection of an empty cylinder. Two such fatalities, where the wrong gas was introduced into the theatre piped supply, occurred in Hong Kong in recent years.

Fires are not uncommon, the most frequent danger being the ignition of spirit-based skin antiseptics ignited by cautery. Any electrical apparatus is potentially dangerous, and defective cauteries, defibrillators and diathermy equipment have all caused death.

Explosions from inflammable gases and vapours, such as cyclopropane and ether, have been catastrophic on occasions.

Hazards of local and epidural anaesthesia

Local anaesthetics rarely cause death, though the overall rate of complications is about 1/2000. Hypersensitivity and escape of contained adrenergic drugs form the major fatal hazards. It is said that most cases of 'hypersensitivity' are really overdosage, but there are undoubtedly some patients who have an abnormal sensitivity to the cocaine-like active constituents. Legal actions have been brought against doctors for

failure to give a test skin dose before injecting the major quantity. Diffusion away from the operative site of adrenaline-like substances used to vasoconstrict the area and thus retain the anaesthetic effect may cause a sudden cardiac arrest.

Epidural and spinal anaesthesia has returned to favour, especially in obstetrics, after a period in which spinal injection of anaesthetic agents fell into disrepute because of a number of lawsuits brought because of spinal cord damage as a result of contaminants or excessive dosage.

The upwards diffusion of the active agents may cause paralysis, and the effect upon the vasomotor system may lead to a precipitous fall in blood pressure. Total spinal anaesthesia from upward diffusion blocks all sympathetic efferent impulses so, if the concentration of the anaesthetic agent in the upper thoracic and cervical spinal fluid level is high enough, efferent transmission to all motor fibres of the respiratory muscles will be blocked.

Epidural anaesthesia has now replaced intrathecal administration, but even this has occasional tragedies, and is said to have a 1/10 000 incidence of permanent nerve paralysis. This usually comes about either from an overdose or from puncture of the theca, instead of the anaesthetic solution remaining in the epidural space. In the rare autopsies on such deaths, a sample of cerebrospinal fluid should be taken for analysis to ascertain the concentration of anaesthetic substance. An attempt should be made to find the puncture in the dura, which is easier said than done. If an epidural catheter is still in place for continuous administration of the active agent, dye or Indian ink can be injected to see if it enters the subdural space.

MALIGNANT HYPERTHERMIA

This is a familial condition in which certain agents, including some anaesthetics and muscle relaxants, precipitate a metabolic change in skeletal muscle with the production of energy, and hence a rapid and sometimes fatal rise in temperature. The basic condition is an autosomal dominantly inherited trait associated with sudden uncoupling of oxidative phosphorylation, accompanied by massive energy production from the muscles with consequent overheating.

When malignant hyperthermia is diagnosed, the family members should be investigated, preferably by muscle biopsy, to assess the risk of their suffering a similar crisis if subjected to anaesthesia. In 70 per cent of carriers, the creatine phosphokinase and aldolase activities are elevated, though the basic abnormality appears to be a defect in calcium transfer and phosphorylation within the muscle fibres. This is one reason why hospital laboratories should be asked to retain any pre-mortem blood samples, as the creatine phosphokinase activity can be estimated retrospectively.

Suxamethonium and halogenated anaesthetic agents seem particularly prone to precipitate the condition. Halothane is one of the agents associated with malignant hyperthermia, either alone or in combination with suxamethonium. The condition occurs about once in every 10 000 anaesthetics, with various estimates ranging from 1/5000 to 1/70 000. There are virtually no autopsy features of any significance and the diagnosis is made on clinical grounds. The features of malignant hyperthermia include a sudden rise in temperature, sometimes reaching 43°C, with stiffening of the skeletal muscles, rapid heart rate and respiratory distress.

Halothane anaesthesia has acquired the reputation for causing liver injury known as halothane hepatitis and, rarely, a fulminant hepatic failure. Its incidence varies between 1/35 000 and 1/600 000 and if halothane anaesthesia is repeated within one month, 1/6000–1:22 000. It is a typical example of immune-mediated adverse drug reactions. Other drugs used in anaesthesia are occasionally responsible for death. Barbiturates used in induction, such as thiopentone, may give rise to cardiorespiratory failure, often because the quantity used has been excessive. Trichlorethylene and atropine have been involved in fatalities, the usual mode being sudden circulatory failure.

AUTOPSY PROCEDURE

In most autopsies on deaths during anaesthesia, toxicological investigations are generally unrewarding, except where overdose with specific drugs such as barbiturate or adrenaline is involved. It is usually impossible to make any quantitative assessment of the amount of volatile agents present, such as nitrous oxide, halothane or cyclopropane, even though some American writers advocate clamping a main bronchus and retaining a lung in a plastic – or preferably nylon – bag, so that head-space gas can be analysed. Neither is it practical to try to prove hypoxia by post-mortem measurement of blood gases. Usually the function of the autopsy is to discover or exclude natural disease, and mechanical blockages, as the pharmacological aspects are usually beyond investigation. Even when it seems obvious that a surgical error has taken place, one should be careful and not jump to conclusions nor let this distract from a thorough investigation. A full range of specimens for histological examination should be taken to exclude occult conditions such as a lymphoma or myocarditis, as well as to investigate the severity of the disease for which the surgical procedure was being performed. This includes also the investigation of any surgical specimens taken during the operation and sent to the histopathologist. Histological examination of the brain (fixed before cutting wherever possible) must be carried out. Though most mishaps will have occurred too quickly for much hope of any stigmata of cerebral hypoxia to

be seen, changes can classically occur in Sommer's area of the hippocampal gyrus. Perhaps an even better marker is the distal parts of the cerebellar folia, where pallor and rapid loss of Purkinje cells can be seen within a few hours.

The work of Plum (Plum and Posner 1984) is relevant in this respect, as he found morphological changes in the brains of victims of only slight hypoxic periods who survived for long periods after an anaesthetic. At autopsy he recorded diffuse, severe leucoencephalopathy of the cerebral hemispheres, with sparing of the immediate subcortical connecting fibres and – usually – of the brainstem. Demyelination and obliteration of axons was observed and sometimes infarction of the basal ganglia. The cortical neurones were spared, however, and the damage appeared confined to the white matter. Plum attributed this damage to greater glycolysis in the white matter during hypoxia, compared with the grey.

Some new immunohistochemical techniques have been used in animal experiment to demonstrate structures of the cytoskeleton, e.g. in detecting ischaemic/hypoxic damage. Great caution must be exercised, however, when using these methods in autopsy material and it is therefore crucial to examine alterations occurring in the cytoskeleton as a result of post-mortem delay before conclusions can be drawn from the possible changes observed. Irving *et al.* (1997) investigated the post-mortem distribution of microtubule-associated proteins (MAP) in various regions of rat brain using immunohistochemistry. They showed that each MAP underwent unique changes that were dependent both on post-mortem interval and the brain region examined. Following long post-mortem delays, some of the changes in these proteins were similar to those seen in rodent models of cerebral ischaemia.

REFERENCES AND FURTHER READING

Adelstein A, Loy P. 1979. Fatal adverse effects of medicines and surgery. *Popul Trends* **17**:17–21.

Beecher HK, Todd DP. 1954. A study of deaths associated with anesthesia and surgery: based on a study of 599 548 anesthesias in ten institutions 1948–1952. *Ann Surg* **140**:2–12.

Briely JB. 1963. Cerebral injury following cardiac operations. *Thorax* **19**:291–6.

Britt BA, Locher WG, Kalow W. 1969. Hereditary aspects of malignant hyperthermia. *Can Anaesth Soc J* **16**:89–98.

Campling EA, Devlin HB, Lum JN. 1990. Gynaecology and the national confidential enquiry into perioperative deaths. *Br J Obstet Gynaecol* **97**:466–7.

Campling EA, Devlin HB, Lunn JN. 1989, 1990, 1992. *The report of the National Confidential Enquiry into*

Perioperative Deaths, 1989, 1990, 1992. Royal College of Surgeons, London.

Campling EA, Devlin HB, Lunn JN. 1992. Reporting to NCEPOD. *Br Med J* **305**:252.

Caplan RA, Ward RJ, Posner K, *et al.* 1988. Unexpected cardiac arrest during spinal anesthesia: a closed claims analysis of predisposing factors [see comments]. *Anesthesiology* **68**:5–11.

Carr NJ, Burke MM, Corbishley CM, *et al.* 2002. The autopsy: lessons from the national confidential enquiry into perioperative deaths. *J R Soc Med* **95**:328–30.

Corby C, Camps FE. 1960. Therapeutic accidents during the administration of barium enemas. *J Forensic Med* **7**:206–20.

Denborough MA, Lovell RR. 1960. Anaesthetic deaths in a family. *Lancet* **2**:45–6.

Dinnick OP. 1964. Deaths associated with anaesthesia: a report on 600 cases. *Anaesthesia* **19**:536–44.

Edelstein JM. 1988. Sudden death following administration of radio contrast media. *J Forensic Sci* **33**:734–7.

Edwards G, Morton HJ, Pask EA, *et al.* 1957. Deaths associated with anaesthesia: a report on 1000 cases. *Anaesthesia* **11**:194–202.

Ermenc B. 2000. Comparison of the clinical and post mortem diagnoses of the causes of death. *Forensic Sci Int* **114**:117–19.

Falk E, Simonsen J. 1979. The histology of myocardium in malignant hyperthermia: a preliminary report of 11 cases. *Forensic Sci Int* **13**:211–20.

Hunt AC. 1958. Anaesthetic causes of death on the table. *J Forensic Med* **5**:141–5.

Irving EA, McCulloch J, Dewar D. 1997. The effect of postmortem delay on the distribution of microtubule-associated proteins tau, map2, and map5 in the rat. *Mol Chem Neuropathol* **30**:253–71.

Isaacs H, Barlow MB. 1970. The genetic background to malignant hyperpyrexia revealed by serum creatine phosphokinase estimations in asymptomatic relatives. *Br J Anaesth* **42**:1077–84.

Keats AS. 1988. Anesthesia mortality – a new mechanism [editorial]. *Anesthesiology* **68**:2–4.

Lau G. 1996. Perioperative deaths: a comparative study of coroner's autopsies between the periods of 1989–1991 and 1992–1994. *Ann Acad Med Singapore* **25**:509–15.

Lau G. 2000. Perioperative deaths: a further comparative review of coroner's autopsies with particular reference to the occurrence of fatal iatrogenic injury. *Ann Acad Med Singapore* **29**:486–97.

Leading article. 1964. Halothane re-examined. *Br Med J* **3**:325.

Loghmanee F, Tobak M. 1986. Fatal malignant hyperthermia associated with recreational cocaine and ethanol abuse. *Am J Forensic Med Pathol* **7**:246–8.

Lunn J, Mushin W. 1982. *Mortality associated with anaesthesia.* Nuffield Provincial Hospital Trust, London.

Lunn JN. 1994. The national confidential enquiry into perioperative deaths. *J Clin Monit* **10**:426–8.

Lunn JN, Devlin HB, Hoile RW, *et al.* 1993. Editorial. II – The National Confidential Enquiry into Perioperative Deaths. *Br J Anaesth* **70**:382.

Macrae WA, Miller KM, Watson AA. 1979. Malignant hyperpyrexia. *Med Sci Law* **19**:261–4.

Mazzia VD, Simon A. 1979. Another look at malignant hyperthermia. In: Wecht C (ed.), *Legal medicine annual 1978.* Appleton Century Crofts, New York.

National Confidential Enquiry into Early Post-operative Deaths (NCEEPOD): various reports 1989–95. Royal College of Surgeons, London.

Plum F, Posner JB. 1984. *Diagnosis of stupor and coma,* 3rd edn. F. Davis & Co., Philadelphia.

Ranklev E, Fletcher R, Krantz P. 1985. Malignant hyperpyrexia and sudden death. *Am J Forensic Med Pathol* **6**:149–50.

Reid L, Brace D. 1940. Irritation of the respiratory tract and its reflex effect upon the heart. *Surg Gynecol Obstet* **70**:157–62.

Relton JE, Britt BA, Steward DJ. 1973. Malignant hyperpyrexia. *Br J Anaesth* **45**:269–75.

Rognum TO, Vege A. 1997. [Forensic autopsy after possible medical malpractice. A 3-year material from the institute of forensic medicine in Oslo, 1993–95.] *Tidsskr Nor Laegeforen* **117**:2969–73.

Shanks JH, McCluggage G, Anderson NH, *et al.* 1990. Value of the necropsy in perioperative deaths. *J Clin Pathol* **43**:193–5.

Start RD, Cross SS. 1999. Acp. Best practice no. 155. Pathological investigation of deaths following surgery, anaesthesia, and medical procedures. *J Clin Pathol* **52**:640–52.

Truemner KM, White S, Vanlaudingham H. 1960. Fatal embolization of pulmonary capillaries. Report of a case associated with routine barium enema. *JAMA* **173**:1089–90.

Warden JC, Horan BF, Holland R. 1997. Morbidity and mortality associated with anaesthesia. *Acta Anaesthesiol Scand* **41**:949.

CHAPTER 24

Dysbarism and barotrauma

Damage to the body from changes in external pressure usually lies in the province of specialized occupational or armed services medicine, rather than that of the forensic pathologist. The major exception is recreational and sporting diving, using SCUBA (self-contained underwater breathing apparatus) equipment. When death occurs in such circumstances, however, though criminality is rarely a factor, there is usually some form of official enquiry, be it quasi-judicial or an internal investigation. Civil suits for compensation may arise and in these circumstances a forensic pathologist may well become involved as the expert witness providing the autopsy evidence.

Injurious pressure effects are virtually always the result of a decrease in atmospheric pressure from a previous level. This can occur either from a decrease of high pressure to normal atmospheric pressure or a decrease from normal to a low pressure. An example of the first is the decompression of a diver ascending to the surface, while the second is seen in depressurization of an aircraft at high altitude. The first is by far the most common as a source of injury and death, mainly because of the great increase in recent years of diving activity associated with the offshore oil industry, which in Britain now forms the most dangerous type of commercial employment.

Dysbarism is a term that covers all adverse effects of pressure, while barotrauma describes the mechanical damage from gas released into the tissues.

In diving, each 10 m depth of water increases the pressure on the body by one atmosphere – 101 kiloPascals (kPa) – so that, in a non-rigid diving suit, the air supply has to be provided at the appropriate pressure relative to the working depth. This depth depends on the equipment used and is limited by legal constraints – for example, in Britain, dives of more than 50 m (164 ft) are not permitted using a nitrogen/oxygen mixture, a gas such as helium being mandatory. Similarly, surface decompression is only allowed at less than this depth of 50 m (164 ft).

When air is supplied at increased pressure, the contained nitrogen (and, to a much lesser extent, carbon dioxide) will progressively dissolve in the plasma and tissue fluids, the amount being governed by Henry's law (the solubility of a gas in a liquid is proportional to its partial pressure). This itself can produce nitrogen narcosis, a state resembling drunkenness in which orientation, judgement and rational behaviour may be diminished. This can occur at depths greater than 30 m. A more physical danger, however, is when a diver who has been at high pressure for long enough to have appreciable nitrogen dissolved in his tissues is returned too quickly to normal atmospheric pressure. The dissolved gas will then come out of solution, almost as champagne effervesces when the cork is released. Gas bubbles appear in the circulation, tissues and joint cavities, and can cause 'decompression sickness' with a wide range of clinical signs and symptoms.

Bubbles in the circulation can cause gas emboli that block small vessels and give rise to infarction, especially in the central nervous system, such as the spinal cord. In addition, such bubbles can interfere with the coagulation system, causing platelet aggregation and disseminated intravascular coagulation. Subcutaneous emphysema can appear as a result of gas under the skin.

PHYSICAL DAMAGE

When sudden, or too rapid, decompression occurs, there may also be physical damage from volume changes. The gas in body cavities expands markedly as the diver rises and, unless these can be progressively vented to the exterior, pressure effects from the contained gas will occur. Such effects may develop in the paranasal sinuses, if blocked, and even in the teeth, if small vacuoles of gas are trapped in the pulp cavities. The middle ear may also be involved and ruptures of the drum can occur. None of these lesions in themselves is likely to be fatal, however, unless the pain and disability interfere with performance – then drowning is the usual cause of death.

A more serious volume effect is in the thorax because, if the air in the lungs is not vented as the diver rises, the alveolar walls may be ruptured by the gas pressure. This leads to interstitial emphysema – air bursting through the respiratory membranes into the interalveolar, interlobular and interlobar septa. Bullae may appear on the pleural surface and, if these rupture, a pneumothorax is formed. Air may reach the mediastinum and track up the tissues to appear in the neck. Apart from a disabling pneumothorax, air can break into the lung capillaries and veins with the danger of air embolism to the left side of the heart, as it cannot move back down the pulmonary arteries. The filling of the left atrium and ventricle interrupts cardiac pump function and, if the volume is sufficient, can be fatal in itself.

Even though this does not occur in most cases of air entry, smaller volumes will be swept into the systemic arterial circulation and impact in the arterioles and capillaries of target organs, especially the myocardium, spinal cord and brain, causing microinfarcts, haemorrhagic necrosis and loss of function of vital tissues. This pulmonary barotrauma is not necessarily confined to deep diving, and may occur in only 2 or 3 m of water.

Many incidents occur to sporting divers, rather than to professionals, in relatively shallow water. The SCUBA diver is now a ubiquitous user of the seas, especially in the warmer, clearer waters of many parts of the world. It is estimated that there are about 80 000 recreational divers in the UK who complete more than two million dives each year. In 1987 there were 600 000 dives, which produced 162 incidents serious enough to be reported. Of these, 115 were of a 'medical' nature and included 8 deaths. There were 6 instances of air embolism, 69 of decompression sickness, 4 of hypothermia, 4 of nitrogen narcosis and 4 cases of ear damage. The incidence of medical incidents was 1/5000 dives, with 1 death in every 75 000 dives.

THE AUTOPSY IN DYSBARISM AND BAROTRAUMA DEATHS

Many of the vast quantity of reports on this subject deal with the clinical effects. Most deaths associated with diving are caused by drowning, though dysbaric disablement may have caused or contributed to the drowning. The autopsy must be directed to investigating the drowning aspect (Chapter 16), and to excluding or confirming any evidence of dysbarism or barotrauma.

The autopsy should not begin until some expert advisers are present, including someone with detailed knowledge of the equipment. If the victim has died in hospital or in a decompression chamber, then obviously much original information will be lost, as no *in situ* examination of the suit and breathing apparatus is possible. In any event, as few forensic pathologists are likely to be expert in this specialized field, every effort should be made to have the attendance of a naval or commercial person who is an authority on the equipment being used at the time of the death.

It has been recommended that the autopsy itself should be conducted in a decompression chamber in order to prevent the post-mortem dissipation of gas that must take place if the body is brought into atmospheric pressure. This is hardly likely to be a practical procedure except where the autopsy takes place under the aegis of armed-service or specialized commercial facilities, who have expert medical staff who are well versed in such procedures.

However, it must be recognized that the very act of decompression is likely to allow bubbles to form within the body, even if they were not there when death took place. This is an insurmountable difficulty for the pathologist unless, as just mentioned, the autopsy itself can be performed under pressure. Thus the finding of gas in the vessels and tissues has to be interpreted in the knowledge that they may be an artefact; part of the differentiation is quantitative, as a mass of froth distending the heart is unlikely to have accumulated post-mortem merely from the static fluid and tissues in the immediate vicinity, and is therefore more likely to have been brought there to form an 'airlock' by a vital circulation.

The autopsy should not begin – nor the body be undressed – until all necessary examination is made of the diving apparatus by an expert. Full photography at every stage, and radiology of the chest and major joints is essential before any dissection is attempted. It has been recommended that air samples should be taken by external lung puncture using a greased syringe so that chemical analysis can be performed to determine the oxygen:nitrogen ratio. This should only be performed under expert guidance. Externally, attention should be paid to the skin colour, as hypothermia is sometimes an associated hazard of diving. Unfortunately, many bodies recovered from water have a bright pink colour that may be post-mortem in origin, much as refrigerated bodies often have a pink hue. Red linear marks may be seen in those who have suffered 'squeezes' inside a neoprene drysuit when the external pressure has become excessive. Crepitance of the skin – usually of the head, neck and thorax – is an indication of barotrauma. The eardrums should be examined with an otoscope to detect any recent ruptures.

The brain should be removed before opening the body cavities, using a special technique to detect air in the cerebral arteries. Artery forceps should be placed on the middle cerebral, basilar and vertebral arteries before they are cut through; the brain should then be placed under water and the clamps removed to observe whether air bubbles escape from the cut ends of the vessels. The detection of air bubbles in the cerebral veins is of no significance, always being an artefact, as it is impossible to remove the calvarium without aspirating some air into the pial vessels. In any case, there is no way in which air in the arterial side of the cerebral circulation can penetrate the brain capillaries in sufficient volume to be visible in the cortical veins.

In the central nervous system, petechial haemorrhages may be seen in any part of the system, including the spinal cord. If the victim survives for a day or more, early infarcts may be seen. Histologically, ring-shaped haemorrhages around vessels may be seen in the white matter. In long-term survivors, living for some weeks, softening of the lateral and dorsal columns of the thoracic spinal cord may be seen if air emboli have impacted there.

Subcutaneous, mediastinal, retroperitoneal and subpleural emphysema must be sought. In the lungs, rupture of alveolar membranes allows air to track through the interstices from where it either enters the circulation or reaches the periphery of the lung to form subpleural bullae, or both. It can cross to the other lung via the hilum; in addition, local bronchial stenosis may trap air in a single lobe, causing a local distension.

The chest should be examined for pneumothorax, first by radiology and then by puncturing an intercostal space under a pool of water held in the lateral skin flap. Similarly, the heart should be examined radiologically for the presence of bubbles. If the air has emerged from the general tissue mass, it will have been conducted centrally by the venous drainage and so more air will be found in the right chambers than in the left side of the heart. If lung damage has occurred, then entry into the pulmonary venous system will bring it to the left side. It is hardly worth attempting to open the heart under a pericardium full of water, as froth in the chambers will be readily apparent if in sufficient volume to have caused death. Some authorities, however, advocate placing clamps on all the major thoracic vessels and the trachea before removing the thoracic pluck of organs. This is then placed under water and the clamps released to see if and from where air bubbles emerge.

Histologically, there are no particularly specific changes in spite of some claims. Lipoid-containing tissues, such as adipose tissue and adrenal cortex, may show microbubbles with a foamy appearance. There may be fatty change in the liver, possibly from air emboli. In lungs in which barotrauma has taken place, oedema, patchy haemorrhage, torn alveoli and focal emphysema confirm the macroscopic findings. The myocardium may show small foci of necrosis.

Fat embolism may occur, both in post-descent shock and in decompression in both water and high altitude. Not only fat, but cellular bone marrow may be found in target organs such as lung, myocardium, brain and kidney. There is controversy over the origin of fat emboli in decompression states, some claiming that it is caused by air-bubble disruption of fat depot tissues, while others favour a more complex genesis involving a redistribution of blood lipids, inter-relating with fibrin production and disseminated intravascular coagulation.

FURTHER READING

Brown CD, Kime W, Sherrer EL, Jr. 1978. Postmortem intravascular bubbling: a decompression artifact? *J Forensic Sci* **23**:511–18.

Busuttil A, Obafunwa J. 1995. A review of the forensic investigation of scuba diving deaths. *Sci Justice* **35**:87–95.

Calder IM. 1985. Autopsy and experimental observations on factors leading to barotrauma in man. *Undersea Biomed Res* **12**:165–82.

Calder IM. 1985. A method for investigating specialised accidents with special reference to diving. *Forensic Sci Int* **27**:119–27.

Calder IM. 1986. Dysbarism. A review. *Forensic Sci Int* **30**:237–66.

Calder IM. 1987. Use of postmortem radiographs for the investigation of underwater and hyperbaric deaths. *Undersea Biomed Res* **14**:113–32.

Davis OD. 1961. Physiological hazards of skin diving. *Med J Aust* **2**:1035–41.

Elliott D, Davis J. 1982. The causes of underwater accidents. In: Bennett PB, Elliott D (eds), *Physiology and medicine of diving*. Baillière Tindall, London.

Fryer DI. 1962. Pathological findings in fatal subatmospheric decompression sickness. *Med Sci Law* **2**:110–14.

Giertsen JC, Halvorsen JF. 1972. [Fatal scuba diving accidents. A discussion of 8 fatal cases.] *Tidsskr Nor Laegeforen* **12**:924–8.

Giertsen JC, Sandstad E, Morild I, *et al.* 1988. An explosive decompression accident. *Am J Forensic Med Pathol* **9**:94–101.

Goldhahn RT. 1976. Scuba diving deaths: a review and approach for pathologists. In: Wecht C (ed.), *Legal medicine annual 1976*. Appleton Century Crofts, New York.

Hart AJ, White SA, Conboy PJ, *et al.* 1999. Open water scuba diving accidents at Leicester: five years' experience. *J Accid Emerg Med* **16**:198–200.

Hayman J. 1985. Autopsy method for investigation of fatal diving accidents. *South Pacific Underwater Med Soc J* **15**:8–16.

Morild I, Mork SJ. 1994. A neuropathologic study of the ependymoventricular surface in diver brains. *Undersea Hyperb Med* **21**:43–51.

Obafunwa JO, Busuttil A, Purdue B. 1994. Deaths of amateur scuba divers. *Med Sci Law* **34**:123–9.

Smith N. 1995. Scuba diving: how high the risk? *J Insur Med* **27**:15–24.

Williamson JA, King GK, Callanan VI, *et al.* 1990. Fatal arterial gas embolism: detection by chest radiography and imaging before autopsy [see comments]. *Med J Aust* **153**:97–100.

CHAPTER 25

The pathology of sudden death

Virtually all forensic pathologists deal not only with criminal, suspicious, accidental and suicidal deaths, but with a wide range of deaths from natural causes. Many of these are sudden, unexpected, clinically unexplained or otherwise obscure, even though there need be no unnatural element in their causation.

It is good that such a large substrate of natural deaths is available to most forensic pathologists: the situation where they deal exclusively with trauma and crime is professionally unhealthy, as they become progressively more out of touch with morbid anatomy, and lose daily contact with disease processes and uninjured tissues and organs. Involvement with natural death means frequent professional intercourse with clinicians and non-forensic pathologists, with all the consequent benefits of cross-fertilization of knowledge and ideas. To work in a totally forensic vacuum is to lose touch with pathological and clinical reality, which is essential for a medico-legal expert to retain a sense of proportion and an awareness of contemporary medical advances.

Another indispensable benefit of sustained experience in natural disease is the fact that some of the most difficult

problems in criminal and litigious cases arise not out of gross, rapidly fatal, trauma, but in deaths where concurrent natural disease or complications after trauma lead to a fatal outcome. The assaulted victim that dies later from a stroke or the negligent minor accident that has a fatal pulmonary embolism – these can pose far greater difficulties over causation than a gunshot wound or a stabbing.

In this chapter no attempt is made to duplicate the detailed descriptions of disease processes provided in a score of illustrious textbooks of pathology, but a survey will be offered of the spectrum of causes of sudden or unexpected death as commonly encountered by forensic and 'coroner's' pathologists.

SUDDEN OR UNEXPECTED DEATHS

The definition of a sudden death varies according to authority and convention. The World Health Organization definition is of death within 24 hours from the onset of symptoms, but this is much too long for many clinicians and pathologists; some will only accept death within one hour from the onset of illness. We have to also bear in mind that a death may appear sudden and unexpected to an outsider but need not have been so from the point of the pathological disease process. The deceased may have been symptomless and utterly unaware of his chronic disease or he may have had symptoms but interpreted them as harmless. Also, fear, lack of human contact or his own disposition may have prevented him mentioning symptoms to anyone, including a doctor.

In many jurisdictions, deaths may only be certified by an attending physician if he has seen the patient recently and is satisfied that the death was caused by a potentially lethal disease from which he was aware the patient suffered. The fact that, without autopsy, this physician is wrong in his belief in between 25 and 50 per cent of cases cannot concern us at the moment, but the relevance is that, where a clinical doctor cannot so certify, the death is usually reported for medico-legal investigation. In many countries such notifications form by far the largest proportion of medico-legal autopsies, and in England and Wales they account for some 80 per cent of coroner's autopsies, the remainder being suicide, accident and homicide.

The description 'sudden' or 'unexpected' is not always accurate, as 'unexplained' is an equally common reason for medico-legal investigation. Here the clinician is unable to offer a cause for the death, though the patient was under medical care. Even after autopsy, the cause of death may still not be revealed and this problem of the obscure autopsy is discussed elsewhere.

In sudden death, the immediate cause is almost always to be found in the cardiovascular system, even though topographically the lesion is not in the heart or great vessels. Massive cerebral haemorrhage, subarachnoid bleeding, ruptured ectopic pregnancy, haemoptysis, haematemesis and pulmonary embolism, for example, join with heart disease and aortic aneurysms to contribute most of the vascular system reasons for sudden, unexpected death.

SUDDEN DEATH FROM CARDIAC DISEASE

Ischaemic heart disease is easily the most common cause of sudden death in Western nations. The term is employed rather loosely and inaccurately, often being used as if it was synonymous with 'coronary atherosclerosis'. Certainly the latter is the largest contributor to ischaemic heart disease, but not to the exclusion of other conditions.

As a further complication of nomenclature, 'coronary atherosclerosis' or 'coronary atheroma' is the proper title of the common degenerative disease that causes most deaths, but the term 'coronary artery disease' is so ingrained into popular usage that it is accepted as synonymous with coronary atherosclerosis, even though there are other coronary diseases.

Ischaemic heart disease comprises:

- coronary atherosclerosis
- hypertensive heart disease
- aortic valve disease
- anomalies of the coronary circulation
- other coronary artery diseases, such as polyarteritis
- cardiomyopathic enlargement
- some congenital heart disease.

CORONARY ATHEROSCLEROSIS

Sometimes called 'the Captain of the Men of Death', this is certainly the most frequent cause of sudden death in Western societies. The basic mechanism is stenosis or occlusion of one or more major branches of the coronary arteries by atheromatous lesions, or one of the complications of such a lesion. The severity of stenosis before death occurs is debatable: cardiac pathologists claim that at least 80 per cent of the normal lumen must be lost before myocardial necrosis occurs. Most forensic pathologists would admit to blaming coronary atheroma for death in autopsies where a significantly smaller percentage of the lumen was lost, when the symptomatology and circumstances were strongly suggestive. Areas of myocardial fibrosis and – rarely – even recent infarcts, may be seen in the presence of relatively small degrees of coronary atheroma. Part of the problem lies in quantifying the amount of stenosis at autopsy. Because of the empty vessels lacking the normal intraluminal blood pressure, the walls are lax, collapsed and unstretched. During life, the same lumen will be larger and only fixation at arterial pressure will retain a semblance of the original size. The pathologist sees all coronary arteries in the dead state, however, so the relative degree of stenosis is still a reliable observation, as both normal and diseased vessels can be compared, even if their absolute luminal size is incorrect.

Coronary atheroma may be focal, with irregular plaques that vary both in size and in stenosing effect from place to place. They may be few and localized, with a virtually normal lumen in the rest of the system. This means that every part of the major vessels must be examined at autopsy, with transverse cuts at no more than 3 mm intervals. It is unjustifiable to make a few cuts at wide intervals and claim that this provides a reliable estimate of the state of the coronary system. A coronary artery is like a chain – just as the latter is only as good as its weakest link, so a vessel is only as good as its narrowest point.

Two cuts, if even half a centimetre apart, may pass either side of a grossly stenosing plaque or a thrombus. Opening the vessels lengthwise obviates this danger, but this is outweighed by the disadvantage of not being able to measure accurately the degree of stenosis by making frequent crosscuts. A compromise is the best answer to this dilemma, as described in Chapter 1.

Plaques are often eccentric, leaving a crescentic residual lumen, but another variety of coronary atheroma is a more diffuse lesion, where the vessel is concentrically narrowed by a more longitudinal degeneration, forming a tube-like segment with a narrow, sometimes 'pin-hole' central lumen. The author (BK) has the impression that this is more common in younger victims and that such lesions seem less likely to be ulcerated and calcified. Both types of lesion are often found in the same patient and there is presumably no fundamental difference in their pathogenesis.

Complications in coronary atheromatous lesions

ULCERATED PLAQUES

The simple endothelial thickening develops to involve the media and usually becomes infiltrated with lipids. Whilst the covering endothelium remains intact, the danger to life is confined to the luminal reduction from the bulge of the enlarging plaque. When the fibroendothelial cap begins to break down under the pressure and erosion of the central necrosing process, the plaque may rupture into the lumen. This has several consequences, which may precipitate acute symptoms or even death.

First, a large plaque may suddenly disgorge its pultaceous contents into the lumen. This can mechanically block the vessel or seriously stenose it. Thrombosis may be precipitated at that spot by the slowed blood flow plus thrombogenic tissue elements. The cap of the plaque may be projected across the lumen, forming a sudden and perhaps complete occlusion. This will be more dangerous if the open end of the ruptured plaque faces 'upstream' into the direction of the blood flow, so that the intimal cap is lifted up, causing a valve-like obstruction. When the blood flow sweeps across the cap in the opposite direction, the cap will not be displaced, though the soft, grumous contents of the plaque will be washed downstream. Sometimes the flap can be seen in histological sections, though it is difficult to know if this is a processing artefact. It is best demonstrated directly at autopsy, when two cuts are joined longitudinally and the intima examined with a lens or low-power microscope.

The contents of the plaque may be washed downstream by the blood flow, eventually impacting in small branches and occluding them. These can be seen histologically using lipid stains and the multiple small infarcts that often ensue can be seen either in classical histological sections or, more readily, by enzyme or fluorescent techniques. They are probably responsible for many of the small fibrotic areas commonly seen in the myocardia of sufferers from long-standing coronary disease.

HAEMORRHAGE

Haemorrhage often occurs within an atheromatous plaque, usually into the softened, necrotic centre. This 'subintimal haemorrhage' may give rise to a sudden reduction in the blood-carrying capacity of a coronary artery and cause sudden death. The source of the bleeding is somewhat controversial, but the best explanation is that it comes from rupture of small blood vessels in the periphery of a plaque. A normal coronary artery does not have a blood supply to the intima but, in the disorganization frequently associated with the distorted microanatomy of a diseased coronary artery, such vessels may lie within the intima and be eroded by extension of the degenerative process.

Haemorrhages, both fresh and old, can often be demonstrated in histological sections of atheromatous plaques. It is reasonable to presume that such a bleed may be precipitated by some sudden rise in blood pressure from exertion or emotion, though, if a vessel is sufficiently eroded by atheroma, such a precipitation is not strictly necessary for such an event to take place.

The sudden release of blood into an atheromatous lesion can rapidly enlarge it and may raise the cap of the plaque towards the other side of the already stenosed lumen. It may even rupture the plaque: some subintimal haemorrhages may track circumferentially, causing a 'minidissection'. Subintimal haemorrhage as a factor in acute coronary occlusion was investigated many years ago by Patterson (1938), who believed that they played a major part in coronary thrombosis. In the same year, Wartmann demonstrated occlusion by subintimal haemorrhage without rupture of the overlying intima. Though English and Williams (1943) doubted if haemorrhage could compress the lumen against arterial pressure, other authors, including Davies and Pomerance (1975) believe that the haemodynamics within the coronary vessels are such that the pressure varies markedly from place to place, and that there may even be a contributing factor to subintimal haemorrhage by a suction effect in certain conditions. Other authors, such as Drury (1954), consider that the blood within the plaque is not caused by haemorrhage from mural vessels, but from blood percolating from the lumen of the coronary artery at the time of rupture of a plaque. This seems a minority opinion, however, as many haemorrhages can be seen (some older ones containing haemosiderin) within plaques which have a perfectly intact overlying intima.

Whatever the precise origin of the blood, it is clear that subintimal haemorrhage is a potent factor in rapidly reducing the available lumen of a coronary artery – and sometimes precipitating thrombosis by further stretching and damaging the overlying intimal cap.

CORONARY THROMBOSIS

The atheromatous plaque may not undergo these more dramatic changes, but progressive internal necrosis may erode the luminal surface and expose the fibrofatty contents. This loss of normal covering endothelium then forms a nidus for thrombus formation, which may gradually accrete in layers so further reducing the lumen or even occluding it, especially if a combination of lesions causes the plaque to expand at the same time as roughening the surface. Thus mural thrombus may completely block or severely narrow the residual lumen, with all the consequences of reduced blood flow to the distal myocardium.

A narrow lumen is by no means essential to the formation of thrombosis, as it may occur in the abnormally wide, virtually aneurysmal, coronary arteries sometimes seen in aged people. The lumen may be up to a centimetre wide yet be firmly thrombosed, presumably solely because of damage to the intima. Thrombosis often occurs in recanalized vessels, secondary thrombosis taking place after organization and re-establishment of a lumen through the previous block. Multiple coronary thromboses are by no means unusual. Many are post-infarct, the original thrombus causing myocardial necrosis and the resulting stasis in circulation, together with the thrombogenic effect of tissue damage leading to sluggish flow of readily coagulable blood.

It has also been noted that coronary thrombosis may be accompanied by thrombotic lesions elsewhere in the body. For example, a coronary thrombosis may be followed by a pulmonary embolus from thrombosed leg vein – and the converse may also occur in non-fatal pulmonary embolism. The coagulability of the blood, together with circulatory stasis, aided by immobility in bed, are obvious factors.

SITES OF CORONARY STENOSIS AND OCCLUSION

The whole length of the coronary arterial system is not uniformly vulnerable to atheromatous lesions. First, the major trunks are most affected where they lie subepicardially, often in the fatty surface tissue. Once the arteries dip down into the myocardium, these more distal intramuscular branches become much less prone to significant atheroma, especially of the grumous, degenerative type, though intimal thickening may still be seen.

Second, there are sites of predilection in the three major arteries. The most common site of occlusion is in the first 2 cm of the anterior descending branch of the left coronary artery, which is more frequent than in the common trunk. The next most frequent site is in the right coronary artery, but here the thrombosis is more distal than in the left vessel, usually seen as the vessel courses around the right margin of the heart in the atrioventricular groove part-way between aorta and the beginning of the posterior descending branch.

The third most common place is the proximal part of the left circumflex artery, soon after the bifurcation from the common trunk. The latter is then the next most frequent site, in the short segment (sometimes absent) between the aorta and the birfucation into descending and circumflex branches. At autopsy, it is always necessary to transect the proximal part of both coronary arteries right up to the coronary ostia, as occlusion can sometimes be present in the first few millimetres.

MYOCARDIAL INFARCTION

There is a different emphasis laid upon myocardial infarction by the forensic pathologist and by the clinician. To the latter, the clinical signs of chest pain and shock mean an infarct and certainly, a much higher proportion of patients who reach hospital beds do have myocardial infarcts compared with those who are taken straight to the mortuary. Recently the Joint European Society of Cardiology/American College of Cardiology Committee for the Redefinition of Myocardial Infarction produced a consensus document examining the scientific and societal implications of a new definition for myocardial infarction from seven points of view: pathology, biochemistry, electrocardiography, imaging, clinical trials, epidemiology and public policy.

In the pathology of sudden death, overt infarcts are the exception, rather than the rule. The incidence in autopsy material from sudden deaths varies considerably, partly because of the different methods of demonstrating the muscle necrosis, but speaking of obvious naked-eye infarcts, the author (BK) would estimate that, in his material considerably less than a quarter of deaths attributable to coronary atherosclerotic disease have myocardial infarction. In Finnish autopsy material of the author (PS) the 5-year average (1987–1991) of infarcts among deaths due to coronary atherosclerotic disease was 13.5 per cent. The relevance of this observation in relation to the mechanism of sudden cardiac death is discussed later.

Almost all myocardial infarcts are caused by atheromatous lesions and their complications. A few are the result of other types of coronary obstruction, such as polyarteritis, other vasculitides, embolism of various types, ostial occlusion by syphilis, severe aortic stenosis, some congenital anomalies of the coronary arteries or great vessels, dissecting aneurysms at the aortic root, and tumour or sarcoidosis affecting the coronary vessels.

Most infarcts are caused by super-added coronary thrombosis, but even this statement needs further analysis. A proportion of infarcts have no demonstrable thrombus in the supplying vessel, but this proportion can be reduced by a more careful search. There is no doubt, however, that muscle necrosis can follow severe narrowing of the supplying vessel by subintimal haemorrhage, a ruptured plaque or simple severe stenosis from atheroma. In addition, grumous debris from a ruptured plaque can produce embolic occlusions with 'microinfarcts' in the distal myocardium. The fact that some thromboses are post-infarct has already been mentioned.

It is said that the original lumen must be reduced to 20 per cent or less before the ischaemia in the distribution zone is sufficient to cause myocardial necrosis. Most pathologists with considerable experience of sudden death autopsies will, however, have numerous experiences of undoubted infarction in the absence of an 80 per cent stenosis. The embarrassing situation occasionally occurs where an infarct exists with virtually normal coronary arteries.

The contrary is much more common: the finding of complete thrombosis of a major vessel with no sign of infarction. In this case, either an effective collateral circulation provided an alternative blood supply – or the victim died before signs of infarction had time to develop.

There are several types of myocardial infarct recognizable at autopsy:

- A laminar infarct in which the subendocardial region of much – or even all – of the left ventricle is involved, sometimes extending through half or more of the thickness of the wall. This is due to a reduction in perfusion pressure to the inner zones, as all the coronary supply comes from the epicardial surface. Laminar infarcts are the result of generalized stenosis in the major branches of the coronary vessels, but there is usually a second factor, in that a drop in blood pressure or the oxygenation of the blood compromises the already poor supply so that the outer zones of the ventricular wall consume the available oxygen and nutrients, leaving little for the inner zone. This is discussed further under hypertension and aortic stenosis.
- A regional or focal infarct is more common in pure coronary artery disease, and is caused by a localized occlusion or severe stenosis in a coronary artery. These are true myocardial infarcts, as the definition of an infarct requires occlusion of the vascular supply, which strictly excludes some laminar infarcts when perfusion pressure or relative insufficiency is caused by hypertension, or

aortic valve disease. The regional infarct is a topographically demarcated zone of muscle necrosis, the size and position depending on the site of vascular occlusion, though any collateral supply may modify these. Almost all infarcts are in the left ventricle. Wartmann and Hellerstein (1948) found that between 6 and 9 per cent involved the right ventricle and that 7 per cent involved the atria, though Cushing's (1942) figure was 17 per cent for atria. Most of these infarcts, however, were overlapping from infarcts in the left ventricle.

The relative immunity of the right ventricle and atria is presumably because of the relatively thin walls, which do not require so much blood, do not have the perfusion gradient of the thick left ventricle and which can more easily obtain oxygen and other constituents from the blood in the lumen of the ventricle. The presence of a conus artery, small branches to foci, such as to the sinus node, and the presence of anastomotic channels between the left circumflex and right coronary arteries must all contribute to the better survival of these areas. The site of a left ventricular infarct does not always correspond strictly to the site of the coronary occlusion or thrombus because of the presence of a collateral circulation.

It was also shown by Wartmann and Souders (1950) that many infarcts involve only certain layers of muscle, which cannot be supplied by a particular vessel. There is obviously no simple explanation for the topography of a myocardial infarct – this is further confirmed by the patchy nature of myocardial damage on microscopic study, as the alternate necrosis and survival of adjacent fibres or even segments of the same fibre cannot be explained solely by coronary perfusion.

The autopsy diagnosis of early myocardial injury and infarction

The autopsy demonstration of an acute lesion in the heart, such as an early myocardial infarct, can have profound medico-legal implications. In a fatal traffic accident, or even rail or air crash, the proof of an acute disabling myocardial lesion in the driver may be vital in the investigation of the event and the apportionment of legal liability. In potentially criminal deaths, the presence of a recent infarct again may be relevant in causation or as a contribution to the death. It is thus important to make a full histological search for evidence of myocardial fibre damage, using all the methods available, including histochemical and fluorescent techniques.

The macroscopic appearances of myocardial infarction are described with a considerable lack of uniformity in most pathology texts, partly because of the varying ages of infarct that the authors depict. The age of an infarct is notoriously difficult to establish in the human, as the onset of clinical symptoms, however dramatically abrupt, are often much later than the onset of the pathological lesion precipitated by a coronary occlusion. In animal experiments, a coronary vessel can be ligated at zero time and serial sacrifices made at different intervals to gain an accurate estimate of the age of the infarct.

In the human, the time of chest pain and shock cannot be used in a similar fashion. When a victim of coronary disease dies say, 8 hours after the onset of acute symptoms, though one might expect an early infarct to be visible histologically or histochemically, not infrequently a demarcated yellow or tigroid area of necrosis is present, which must be several days old. The following appearances are typical of the stages of myocardial infarction, though marked divergences from this time scale are not uncommon:

■ For the first 12–18 or even 24 hours, no definite naked-eye changes are visible. The first sign towards the end of this variable period is oedema of the affected area of muscles, which causes pallor as the swollen fibres squeeze the blood from the vessels that lie between them. The normal moist lustre of the cut surface becomes more granular and dull when cut by a sharp knife. Caution must be used with this feature, because if the scissors are used to cut even normal muscle, the crushed edges of the fibres will give a similar dry, matt appearance.

■ From about the end of the first day progressively through the second and third, the area becomes better demarcated and turns yellow. With breakdown of the myocytes, streaks of red appear, being both dilated vascular channels and areas of interfibre haemorrhage. This gives a 'tigroid' appearance suggestive of tiger stripes across the area, though sometimes the yellow element is virtually uniform or the red streaks may fade after a few days.

Demarcation becomes more sharply apparent and there may be a red zone in the less damaged muscle around the periphery. The size of the infarct depends on the means with which it is visualized; the naked-eye size is less than the area detectable by classical histology and this in turn is smaller than that demonstrable by enzyme studies, where the more peripheral fibres are sick but potentially recoverable.

■ After a few days, progressing through weeks, the infarct becomes softer and more friable, justifying the old name 'myomalacia cordis'. It is at this stage, from about the second or third day onwards, that ruptures occur into the pericardial sac. Some pathology textbooks are in error in stating that such cardiac rupture occurs in early infarcts.

■ From the third week and later, the centre of the infarct becomes gelatinous, the colour fading to a translucent grey that often subsides below the level of the cut surface. This rather mucoid stage may still have old haemorrhage within it, but the stage of healing slowly develops and, during the next month or two, depending upon the size of the infarct, fibrosis replaces the dead muscle to form a scar. Even after this stage, there is often a narrow zone around the young fibrous tissue that shows muscle necrosis, though special staining or enzyme techniques may be needed to demonstrate this.

The laminar infarct goes through the same cycle of changes, but this is often less intense. Eventual fibrosis may be widespread but remains thin, often subendocardial, especially on the left ventricular aspect of the interventricular septum where a wide glistening sheet may obscure the underlying muscle. The apex also may show widespread fibrosis and all muscle may be replaced in this region, sometimes leading to a cardiac aneurysm on the free wall. Infarcts may be transmural, extending from epicardium to endocardium, or they may be confined to the inner zone. It is almost impossible to have an infarcted area confined to the outer subepicardial zone because of the topography of the coronary supply. The papillary muscles are usually involved, being particularly vulnerable to ischaemia as they are at the end of the line of coronary supply. The central part of the muscle may necrose and even rupture. Infarction usually spares the immediate subendocardial zone, the three or four most superficial layers of fibres surviving, even though they may show ischaemic damage. They presumably receive enough oxygen and nutrients from the ventricular blood to survive, though this does not seem to prevent deposition of mural thrombus over the infarcted area.

Microscopical appearances of myocardial injury and infarction

There are a vast number of publications on this subject dealing with morphological changes, classical histological methods, enzyme histochemistry, fluorescent studies, immunohistochemical methods and transmission and scanning electron microscopy. Only a brief summary can be offered here, though some of the methods of detecting very early infarction are detailed in Appendix 1.

MORPHOLOGICAL CHANGES

There is marked variation from case to case, just as in the gross appearances. The same difficulties exist about assessing the time of onset and hence the age of the infarct. This may sometimes have considerable medico-legal importance,

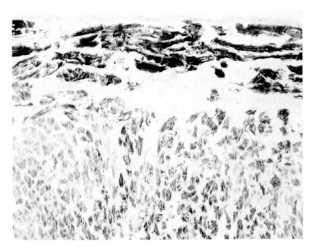

FIGURE 25.1 *Enzyme histochemistry of early myocardial damage. This photomicrograph shows strong succinate dehydrogenase reaction in the myofibres adjacent to the endocardium and moderate decrease of reaction elsewhere suggesting early injury. (Original magnification ×100.)*

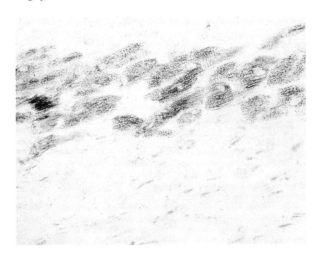

FIGURE 25.2 *Fresh myocardial infarction with β-hydroxybutyrate dehydrogenase staining showing positive reaction in the myofibres adjacent to a larger vessel seen above as an empty space. The lower part of the picture shows infarcted myofibres with some lipofuscin but no enzyme reaction. (Original magnification ×160.)*

especially when cardiac disease may have caused a traffic or other transportation accident – and is sometimes relevant in criminal circumstances. In animal experiments, changes in myocardial fibres become apparent within 30 seconds of coronary ligation, the first change being a loss of glycogen as the cell shifts from aerobic to anaerobic respiration. This cannot be observed in human material, for obvious reasons. The first observable change is subjective and different pathologists given the same material will offer different opinions on whether or not ischaemic damage is visible. Some of the earliest changes are mimicked by autolysis, especially granularity of the cytoplasm. The infarcted area becomes swollen, so that

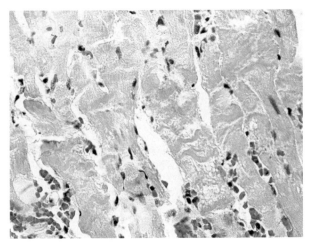

FIGURE 25.3 *Contraction bands in myocardium. (HE, original magnification ×500.)*

the interfibre clefts become obliterated, and the overall appearance is pinker and more solid in routine sections. Care must be taken to assess sections of uniform thickness, as material from other laboratories may not conform to the observer's usual quality. Along with swelling, the cytoplasm becomes granular, the 'cloudy swelling' of the old texts.

Early morphological changes seen in light microscopy are unspecific: interstitial oedema, congestion and small haemorrhages. An overstretching of myofibres with a sarcomere length of about 2.51 μm is possible only when the fibre is injured. In experimental infarction in the rat and the dog sarcomere, overstretching has been observed 15 minutes after coronary ligation. Cellular infiltration is variable and neutrophil infiltration is seen in most infarcts during the first few days being replaced by a mononuclear response within a week or so.

Contraction bands, known also as myofibrillar degeneration, and coagulative myocytolysis, are commonly described in connection with different pathological conditions. The change signifies irreversible myocyte injury. Contraction bands are irregular, dense and in haematoxylin and eosin (HE) staining eosinophilic transverse bands alternate with lighter staining granular zones in the myocyte, possibly firstly described by Smith (1904) in the periphery of myocardial infarction. These lesions have been observed in various forms of experimental heart muscle injury and have been also seen, e.g. in association with potassium deficiency, magnesium deficiency, in cases of malignant hyperthermia, in the hearts of drug addicts and in cases of sudden cardiac death.

They may also be seen after blunt trauma to the chest or even cardiopulmonary resuscitation, both where mechanical massage has been applied and especially where cardiac stimulants like noradrenaline have been injected. In fact, catecholamines seem able to cause this fibre disruption, which may also appear during electrocution and other conditions

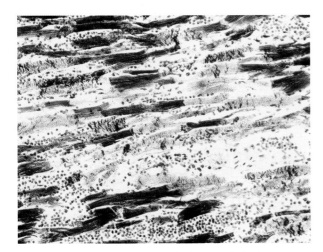

FIGURE 25.4 *Contraction bands in fresh myocardial infarction. (PTAH, original magnification ×250.)*

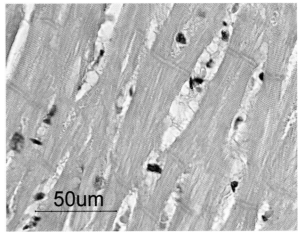

FIGURE 25.5 *Zonal lesions in haemorrhagic shock (HE).*

of cardiac stress. In sections stained with haematoxylin and eosin, pale areas in the fibre are common as a result of fibrocytolysis and the sarcolemma is often seen to be deficient at these sites. Although the change signifies fresh and irreversible myocyte injury and is more frequently observed in cardiac deaths, it is not specific to the cardiac death.

Contraction bands are best seen by phosphotungstic acid haematoxylin stain and all myocardial sections should be stained in this way as well as – or even in preference to – haematoxylin and eosin. Phosphotungstic acid haematoxylin stain does not reveal ischaemic damage at an earlier stage, but renders it far more obvious. Large areas can be scanned under low power of the microscope and the danger of missing abnormal areas is far less than with haematoxylin and eosin. The striations become distorted and break up, forming either a general 'sandy' appearance or the striking 'contraction bands' where fragmentation occurs in transverse lines across the fibre. The contractile material aggregates into thicker, darker masses, sometimes like 'Chinese writing', at first within an intact sarcolemma, but later the cell membrane ruptures and the basophilic contents scatter extracellularly.

Zonal lesions occur as a region of supercontraction of myocytes at the intercalated discs. These lesions have been observed both in the dog and in humans after haemorrhagic shock and the changes have been considered ubiquitous in and pathognomonic for hypovolaemic shock. These possibly reversible changes have been observed in experimentally induced shock in animals 15 minutes after the induction. The presence of catecholamines is also considered necessary.

Fragmentation of myocardial fibres is, at least to some extent, practically always present in adult hearts and more frequently in the wall of the left ventricle. Although it has generally been associated with post-mortem changes, it has also been shown to be more frequently seen in myocardial samples from sudden cardiac death victims. Early injury

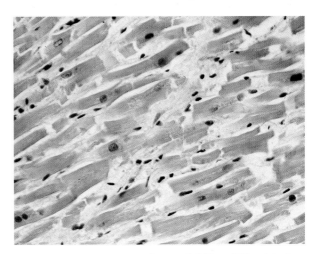

FIGURE 25.6 *Fragmentation of myocardial fibres. (HE, original magnification ×250.)*

possibly increases the brittleness of myocardium, resulting in increased fragmentation of myofibres after the fixation and cutting process. This phenomenon has, however, no value as a positive marker of myocardial injury.

Waviness of fibres was noted by Glogner (1903), who saw corkscrew-shaped myofibres in the heart and skeletal muscle in some cases of beri-beri. Similar patchy deformation of myofibres in a wavelike fashion was seen in association with fatty degeneration of the myocardium and in early and also more advanced human myocardial infarction. Both in cardiac deaths and non-cardiac deaths it can be observed more frequently in the wall of the right ventricle. It has no diagnostic significance as to the cause of death and it signifies only agonal injury.

LATER STAGES

The later stage of infarction follows the 18–24-hour period and, as by now macroscopic changes will be apparent, the histology is merely a confirmatory procedure. Even here, there is great variation in appearances, especially in cellular infiltration. There is a progressive degeneration of the fibres, best seen in longitudinal section. Eosinophila becomes stronger for a time until the internal architecture breaks down. The cellular oedema subsides and interfibre oedema takes over, separating the myofibres, a process that becomes more marked as the latter shrink and fragment.

Loss of nuclei is not an early phenomenon but, by the second to fourth days, the nuclei become hollow, shadowy and eventually ghost-like, though nuclear remnants can sometimes still be seen in completely necrotic infarcts. Cellular infiltration is variable and sometimes does not occur at all, again in contradiction to the established descriptions in most textbooks. In general, however, there is a neutrophil infiltration in most infarcts during the first few days, which subsides gradually and is replaced by a mononuclear response within a week or so. These are mainly macrophages clearing up the debris and fibroblasts coming in to lay down new collagen during repair.

By the end of the first week, disintegration of muscle fibres is well under way, and new capillaries and fibroblasts are appearing, though there are many exceptions to this timetable. In general, infarcts are older than most observers think, so that their age is usually underestimated. By the fourth week, depending upon the total size of the infarct – early fibrosis is evident but still with lacunae of necrotic, unrepaired muscle, which heals unevenly and slowly. From this point on there is a variable population of cells, leucocytes diminishing in favour of fibroblasts, macrophages and new vessels.

It is difficult, if not impossible, to date such an infarct even within weeks, and different parts of the same infarct may show quite different appearances. Only when sufficient time has elapsed for all the lesions to catch up with the end stages of firm fibrosis can one say that probably a minimum of about 3 months has elapsed – though again this is dependent on the size and other more imponderable factors, such as age and other concomitant disease.

HISTOCHEMICAL METHODS

In haematoxylin and eosin (HE) staining, increased cytoplasmic eosinophilia is an early form of cellular injury partially resulting from increased binding of eosin by cytoplasmic proteins. At the pH conventionally used in staining, eosin is negatively charged. The binding may increase because of greater exposure of positively charged reactive sites along polypeptide chains after their denaturation. The loss of cytoplasmic basophilia usually reflecting detachment and scattering of polysomes from rough-surfaced endoplasmic cisternae is considered as another cause for the increased eosinophilia.

The intensity of eosinophilia increases, sometimes uniformly, but often in patches with advancing injury. It is earlier and more distinctly seen in HE-stained cryosections and can be enhanced by placing a green filter in the light path of the microscope. Patchy hyperchromasia can be observed in all kinds of deaths and therefore it is of limited diagnostic value. Care must be taken to exclude the occasional thickened areas made by cutting artefacts, which look pinker because of a greater depth of cytoplasm. These early changes are not usually visible in the first 8–12 hours after the (presumed) onset of infarction.

Acid fuchsin (AF) was suggested to be useful for demonstration of early myocardial infarction in man or in animal experiments, but was found to be inconsistent and misleading.

Haematoxylin/basic fuchsin/picric acid stain (HBFP) was claimed to demonstrate early myocardial ischaemia and to be unaffected by post-mortem autolysis. In experiments with isolated cardiac myocytes in suspension made anoxic by complete oxygen deprivation, basic fuchsin was taken up by contracted or damaged myocytes, which, according to their morphology in suspension, revealed irregular contractions, but neither by undamaged nor necrotic myocytes. However, after the first promising reports, contradictory results started to accumulate and the method has been shown to produce inconsistent results and to be unreliable and non-specific and without value for diagnostic purposes.

FLUORESCENT METHODS

Fluorescent methods have been applied to demonstrate early myocardial infarctions and myocardial degeneration in animal experiments as well as in human heart either by using a fluorescent dye, e.g. acridin orange to stain unfixed cryostat sections or paraffin sections or utilizing the fluorescent properties of eosin in the HE-stained myocardium. Intravenously or intraperitoneally injected tetracycline has also been used in experimental infarction for demonstration of the perfused region in myocardium. Carle (1981) claimed that only hypereosinophilic cells autofluoresced, but Badir and Knight (1987) found that myocardium that had normal eosinophilic staining also fluoresced yellow in ultraviolet light; this has been confirmed by Saukko and Knight (1989).

Acridin orange stained cryosections of intact myocardium show golden brown fluorescence which turns into greenish fluorescence with increasing ischaemia time whereas eosin fluorescence of normal myocardium in paraffin-embedded samples show olive-green fluorescence which turns into yellow in injured tissue. Post-mortem autolysis does not seem to have any significant effect on the fluorescence but the high percentage of wrong positive samples indicates that at least eosin fluorescence is obviously too sensitive injury marker capable of demonstrating agonal ischaemic changes.

A major handicap common to all classical histochemical staining methods is that the basis of these colour reactions is poorly understood. Considering the possible legal implications, it is not reasonable to use such diagnostic methods for medico-legal purposes, when their diagnostic significance, to say the least, is questionable and one does not know for sure what the methods are actually measuring.

ENZYME HISTOCHEMISTRY

After Rutenburg *et al.* (1953) had found large amounts of succinate dehydrogenase in the myocardium of various species

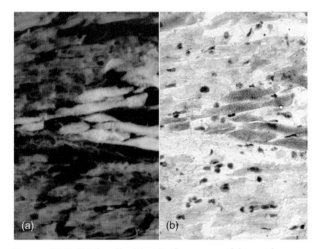

FIGURE 25.7 *Bright yellowish eosin fluorescence of damaged myofibres (a) corresponding exactly with eosinophilia as seen in the HE-stained cryosection (b) of a fresh myocardial infarction.*

using blue tetrazolium as hydrogen acceptor, this method was also applied to autopsy material and the inactivation of histochemically demonstrable succinate dehydrogenase was observed in human myocardial infarction. The enzyme histochemical methods became soon widely applied in animal experiments and also to diagnose early human myocardial infarction in autopsy material. Various oxidative enzymes were demonstrated either by incubating thick myocardial slices in a medium containing a tetrazolium salt with or without exogenous substrate and coenzyme (macromethods) or to stain cryosections observed under the microscope (micromethods). It was assumed that enzyme histochemistry might be, at least, a 'semi-quantitative' indicator of the actual biochemical activity of a given enzyme and, therefore, a scientifically more solid biochemical indicator of myocardial metabolism and injury than the previously discussed traditional histochemical methods. In all, the results between individual authors and laboratories have been extremely variable, suggesting that the situation is not that simple. Hiltunen *et al.* (1985) assessed the enzyme histochemical methods, used by the author (PS) in autopsy material, comparing the enzyme histochemical reaction with the actual biochemical acitivity of the enzymes in a global ischaemia model in an animal experiment. The results pointed out that, although the enzyme histochemical methods have been named after the enzymes, the enzyme histochemical reactivity need not necessarily correlate with the actual biochemical activity of the enzyme at all, suggesting that other factors, such as the presence of auxiliary enzyme systems or other co-factors of the histochemical reaction, may be rate-limiting. This brings about the same dilemma as with the conventional histochemistry: unless the biochemical basis of any given enzyme

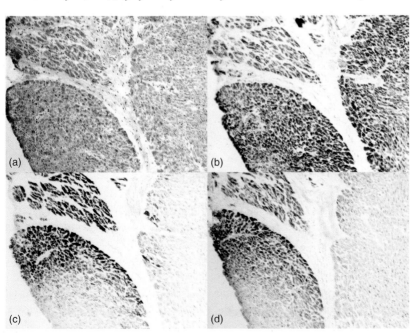

FIGURE 25.8 *The size of a myocardial injury depends upon the method used to display it. These are four serial sections of a heart from autopsy, stained in different ways. Haematoxylin and eosin stained cryosection (a) does not reveal any damage; the adjacent section (b) is stained for malate dehydrogenase activity, and shows strong and uniform reaction. Section (c) is stained for succinic dehydrogenase and reveals a varying degree of enzyme loss in almost all the section, the section (d) on the right stained for β-hydroxybutyrate dehydrogenase activity reveals slightly larger area of damage. (Original magnification ×100.)*

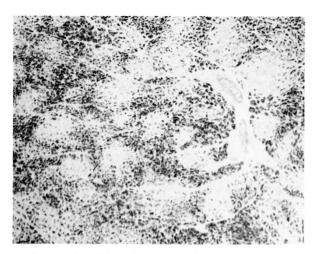

FIGURE 25.9 *Patchy loss of malate dehydrogenase reaction simulating early injury. In fact, the injury was caused by artificially prolonged agonal period due to respiratory treatment and cardiac pacing. It was equally well visible in HE staining emphasizing the necessity of control staining with conventional methods always when more sensitive methods are used.*

histochemical method is thoroughly understood, it is precarious to use it for medico-legal purposes.

IMMUNOHISTOCHEMICAL METHODS

The advances in immunohistochemistry and good results in clinical pathology as well as the availability of a great number of new antibodies have resulted in numerous publications reporting on potential markers of early myocardial injury in both animal experiments and autopsy material. As it has been shown that ischaemia damages cell membrane, contractile proteins, cytoskeleton and subcellular organelles of the myocardium relatively quickly, the search for better diagnostic methods has been directed to various components of the myofibre, e.g. basement membrane (collagen IV, fibronectin, laminin), cytoskeletal proteins (actin, desmin, alpha- and beta-tubulin), cell-matrix focal adhesion molecules (vinculin, talin), membrane-associated proteins (dystrophin, spectrin), terminal complement complex (C5b-9) and fatty acid binding protein (FABP), among many others. In spite of the plethora of publications, the results have been rather contradictory and/or their practicability difficult to assess due to shortcomings in test material or design.

In spite of better insights into the pathophysiology of myocardial injury, the practical problem as to its diagnostic significance as a cause of death has not changed: whenever myocardial injury has been detected, either macroscopically or by using whatever conventional or more sophisticated methods, **it does not necessarily prove that the injury is the cause of death, unless other causes of death have been excluded**. The rule-of-thumb is that the more sensitive

methods are used the greater the probability that agonal period and autolytic changes may be difficult to differentiate from intravital changes.

COMPLICATIONS OF MYOCARDIAL INFARCTION

Ruptured heart

Ruptured heart is the most common cause of a haemopericardium and cardiac tamponade, the rupture always occurring through an infarct. The softened, necrotic muscle gives way from the internal pressure of the ventricular blood during systole, there being no equalizing rise in external pressure. Hypertension will increase the risk, but a more potent factor is a senile, soft myocardium, so that the elderly woman is a common victim of a ruptured heart. This by no means excludes younger men if the infarct is extensive and transmural. The most common area for rupture is the more distal part of the free wall of the left ventricle. The septum occasionally ruptures and the consequent left–right shunt, whilst the patient survives, provides a classical diagnostic sign for the stethoscopes of clinicians.

The rupture does not take place in the early stages of a new infarct, but after a day or two when necrotic softening is well established. The blood usually tracks through tortuous channels between muscle bundles, rather than bursting a direct fistula from ventricle to pericardial sac. The infarcted area may not always be obvious, as the haemorrhagic patch may obscure it, but histologically the ragged tissues and the periphery may be seen to be necrosed.

Haemopericardium is the pathological condition found at autopsy and is not quite synonymous with 'cardiac tamponade', which is a clinical state caused by the progressive accumulation of blood within the closed pericardial sac. As the external pressure rises, the heart cannot fully expand in diastole to allow filling from the great veins. As input volume falls, so does stroke output. The venous drainage is dammed back so that congestion and cyanosis of the face and neck occur, until a fatal endpoint is reached.

Mural thrombosis

Mural thrombosis almost inevitably occurs when an infarct is based upon the endocardium of the left ventricle. Though there is usually a thin layer of viable (though sick) cells immediately beneath the endocardium, they do not seem to prevent deposition of platelets and fibrin.

The thrombus is often entwined between the muscular bands lining the distal ventricle, which aids its adherence. When extensive, the thrombus may fill the entire apical area of the ventricle. The layers nearest the endocardium are naturally the oldest, and visible strata (lines of Zahn) are often visible. The youngest layers on the surface are less organized and more friable, so fragments tend to break off and form emboli that enter the arterial circulation, and can cause infarcts in kidney, brain, spleen and even the myocardium itself.

Pericarditis

Pericarditis occurs with full-thickness (transmural) infarcts that form the most common cause of pericarditis in Western communities. The visceral pericardium becomes purple–red as a result of the infarct beneath, with a vascular blush on the surface. Granular fibrin deposit causes the surface to lose its glistening sheen, and strands of fibrin may link the visceral and parietal layers together. When healed, fibrous adhesions may form which can obliterate part or even all of the pericardial sac.

Myocardial fibrosis

Myocardial fibrosis has already been described, healed infarcts being replaced by dense collagen, as new muscle cannot be formed. Large plaques from healed infarcts can be anywhere in the left ventricle, depending on the vessel(s) that were occluded. The septum and the posterior wall are more common sites than the anterolateral wall, though the latter is by no means exempt. Often the fibrotic plaques are multiple or irregular, being scattered throughout the ventricular wall.

Diffuse fibrosis is common in elderly people, even when there is negligible coronary narrowing. This may be in part the result of ventricular hypertrophy in hypertension, which causes a relative ischaemia, but many old hearts with no enlargement (indeed, atrophy) reveal patchy fibrosis, either macroscopically or microscopically. In the latter case, the fibrosis is often perivascular in situation.

Cardiac aneurysms

Cardiac aneurysms occur where a large area of fibrosis replaces a previous transmural infarct, usually on the distal part of the free wall of the left ventricle. During systole, the cavity blood presses outwards onto the unsupported area and gradually herniates it into the pericardial sac. A saccular aneurysm develops and may undergo various changes, including calcification of the wall, adherence to the parietal pericardium, or filling with laminated thrombus. The aneurysm wall is tough and fibrous and, though lacking in elasticity, almost never ruptures – again contradicting some of the dicta of pathology textbooks.

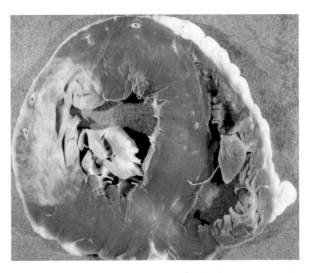

FIGURE 25.10 *An infarct of the lateral wall of the left ventricle of between 5 and 10 hours' duration. It has been rendered visible by staining the heart slice with triphenyltetrazolium chloride, which colours the normal myocardium red by the activity of tissue dehydrogenases. The infarcted area remains unstained. The infarct is virtually transmural, though some subepicardial fibres survive; the papillary muscle is particularly vulnerable, being at the distal end of the coronary supply.*

CAUSE OF DEATH IN CORONARY INSUFFICIENCY

Most sudden deaths from coronary insufficiency do not have myocardial infarction, even when the most sophisticated techniques are employed for its detection. Neither do the majority have a coronary thrombosis, though severe coronary stenosis is by definition present.

The rare case of myocardial infarction with only moderate or even minimal coronary atheroma has to be relegated to the realms of mystery in the present state of knowledge, unless some embolic cause can be found. Some pathologists invoke 'spasm' of the coronary arteries when the vessels show minimal atheromatous stenosis, but this is a hazardous diagnosis for a pathologist to make. Though spasm is certainly seen by clinicians when performing cardiac catheterizations or cardiac operations, it can never be a morphological diagnosis at autopsy, for obvious reasons.

In most sudden 'coronary' deaths, the usual autopsy finding is of severe, long-standing stenosis sometimes with foci of complete occlusion from a ruptured plaque or a subintimal haemorrhage. There may often be partial thrombosis, in that a plaque or narrow segment may have mural thrombus that further narrows the lumen, though does not totally occlude it.

There is macroscopic and microscopic evidence of myocardial fibrosis in many of these cases. This may either be a large plaque of scar tissue at the site of a previous focal infarct or more diffuse fibrosis. There may be fibrosis subendocardially and in the papillary muscles. In many of these sudden deaths there is no naked-eye or even microscopic evidence of any new lesion in the coronary system or myocardium, so why do they die?

Death must be ascribed to a rhythmical defect, rather than loss of mechanical pumping power. Myocardium and especially the pacemaking and conducting system, is vulnerable to ischaemia and hypoxia. Disturbances of rhythm, from ectopic beats to atrial fibrillation through to ventricular fibrillation and cardiac arrest, may occur, as well as heart block and the many other clinical manifestations of ischaemic heart disease from whatever cause. In addition, many victims are hypertensive and left ventricular hypertrophy exacerbates their relative coronary insufficiency. Anyone with a heart weighing more than 450 g is a candidate for sudden death, with or without coronary artery stenosis. The mechanism of this sudden type of death, where there is no large infarct, seems to be a state of electrical instability from chronic hypoxia, so that sudden stresses (such as exercise or emotion) can suddenly cause the arrhythmias mentioned above, though it must be said that death can occur without any of these factors while the victim is asleep or at rest. It is known that the myocardium is sensitive to catecholamines, this being a physiological response to intrinsic adrenergic hormones. Excess catecholamines given parenterally can cause arrhythmias and even contraction-band damage to the myofibrils. Certain other drugs, such as organic solvents, can sensitize the myocardium to even physiological amounts of noradrenaline, leading to ventricular fibrillation and sudden death.

Those with fibrosis in the myocardium may have the additional risk of interruption of the conducting system, which may give some degree of heart block or defect in the spread of the contraction impulse, rendering them more prone to arrhythmias and arrest. This is especially so where a large fibrotic plaque occupies the interventricular septum, as here the left bundle branch penetrates to supply the apical region and may be strangled by dense fibrosis.

Where there is a recent coronary thrombosis, the absence of an infarct may mean that insufficient time has elapsed for it to become apparent, but of course the pumping efficiency will be compromised and the risks of electrical disturbance will already be operating, so that all the problems listed above exist. The other reason for lack of an infarct is an adequate collateral circulation but, even though necrosis is avoided, a new coronary occlusion can only further worsen the ischaemic and hypoxic state of the myocardium, with all the potential consequences of electrical instability.

If there is an infarct, then again all the above dangers exist, but there is the added liability of a loss of mechanical pumping function, which, with a large infarct, may be a substantial

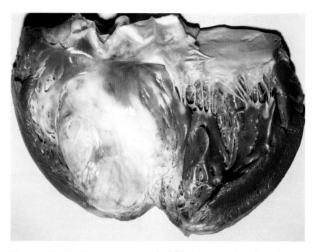

FIGURE 25.11 *Extensive myocardial fibrosis occupying the interventricular septum and apex of the heart with severe occlusive disease of the anterior descending branch of the left coronary artery. Near the apex all the muscle has been replaced by scar tissue. This type of lesion is particularly prone to cause sudden death, as well as clinically apparent dysrhythmias, as the septal fibrosis interrupts the left bundle branch of the cardiac conducting system.*

proportion of the whole cardiac output, leading to overt low-output failure during which sudden death can supervene at any time. In addition, the risks of sequelae of myocardial infarction, such as rupture and embolism, are ever present.

The role of the conducting system in sudden cardiac deaths is one which is attracting increasing interest, especially as new histological and immunohistochemical techniques are becoming available. A revised sampling technique, described by Song *et al.* (1997), uses longitudinal sectioning, reduces the workload and allows observation of continuity between different components of the cardiac conduction tissue. It demonstrates the sino-atrial (SA) node, the atrio-ventricular (AV) node and the distal part of the His bundle and the bundle branches of the cardiac conduction system in 4–5 blocks. However, although a significant number of abnormalities can be recognized, it is usually difficult or impossible to relate morphology to function. The fact that an AV or SA node, or the bundle of His or its branches shows fibrosis or some other lesion, does not necessarily mean that this played any part in the death. It has been shown that the conducting system is remodelled with advancing age – and many deaths from obvious extracardiac causes reveal lesions in the conducting system when studied at autopsy. Nevertheless, new knowledge now being accumulated about the conducting system may become useful in investigated sudden cardiac deaths, as it is obvious that a high proportion of these fatalities, which have no recent acute lesion demonstrable in the coronary arteries or myocardium, are due to arrhythmias and functional arrest, in which abnormalities of the propagation of the pacing impulse may be important. James (1996) has suggested that apoptosis, the programmed cell death, might be a logical explanation and responsible for histological abnormalities of the cardiac conduction system in sudden deaths due to progressive development of complete heart block and various arrhythmias.

HYPERTENSIVE HEART DISEASE

Hypertension may kill in a number of ways, such as by renal failure, ruptured aneurysm or cerebral haemorrhage, but here we are concerned with primary heart failure, a quite common cause of death. During life, the clinical syndrome of 'cardiac asthma' or 'paraoxysmal nocturnal dyspnoea' is caused by pulmonary oedema from hypertensive left ventricular failure. The same oedema is a marked feature of the autopsy on fatal hypertensive heart disease.

Because there is an aetiological connection between hypertension and coronary atheroma, the two conditions are often present together in a victim of sudden death, making it difficult to separate the myocardial consequences of each component. Sufficient 'pure' deaths from hypertensive heart disease are available where there is no concurrent coronary disease, however, to establish the effect of the former on the myocardium. When the left ventricle has to work against a higher pressure in the systemic arteries, the muscle fibres hypertrophy. They cannot increase in number, but they increase in length and thickness, with irregularity and enlargement of nuclei. This fibre enlargement leads to increase in the mass of the left ventricle, the well-known 'concentric hypertrophy' of hypertension.

If 360–380 g is taken as the upper limit of heart weight for an average size man, then hypertensive disease may produce hearts of 500–700 g. Hearts larger than this usually have some other cause, such as valvular disease or a cardiomyopathy. Though it is sometimes denied that hypertension can cause sudden death, most forensic pathologists would strongly disagree, all having performed numerous autopsies where no other reasonable explanation existed. The usual picture is of marked pulmonary oedema fluid running freely from the cut surfaces of the lungs because of a terminal failure of the left ventricle slightly prior to right ventricular arrest. This causes a rapid rise in pulmonary artery pressure and consequent transudation across the pulmonary alveolar membranes.

There may not always be evidence of hypertension in the often sparse history available at sudden death, but the presence of concentric hypertrophy in the absence of valve disease or a cardiomyopathy – together with characteristic changes in other vessels and organs, such as the kidney – is strong

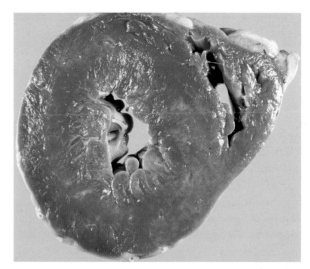

FIGURE 25.12 *Concentric hypertrophy of the left ventricle in a person with cardiomegaly from hypertension. The slice has been stained with triphenyltetrazolium chloride to reveal dehydrogenase activity; some mottled areas, especially in the septum, show pallor from reduced enzyme activity as a result of relative ischaemia of the increased muscle mass.*

evidence of raised blood pressure. Sometimes the overall weight of the heart may be normal, yet there is relative left ventricular thickening; this again suggests hypertension. In the hearts of aged people, the usual atrophy – with tortuous surface vessels – may be concealed by a left ventricular hypertrophy, keeping the heart at normal weight.

The existence of hypertensive heart disease as a specific entity was strengthened by some investigations published by the author (BK) in 1973, in which it was shown that gross enzyme deficiencies exist in the inner part of the wall of the hypertrophied left ventricle. This lesion is not specific to hypertension, but is seen whenever the left ventricle is enlarged, notably in aortic valve disease. In severe instances, the defect in dehydrogenase activity extends from endocardium almost to the epicardium, there being only a narrow zone of normal activity. In some ways this defect is similar to the 'laminar infarct' of coronary artery disease.

In pure hypertension and aortic valve disease, the cause is a relative ischaemia of the inner zone of the ventricular wall caused by insufficiency of coronary blood supply compared with the demands of the thickened ventricular mass. The reason for the laminar distribution is the anatomy of the coronary supply, graphically described by Farrer-Brown (1968, 1977). The various levels or strata of the ventricular wall have different arterial patterns. The subendocardial zone is supplied by arteries with many branching terminations that provide a profuse and concentrated blood supply. A second set of vessels passes straight through the ventricular wall without division – all the coronary supply coming, of course, from the epicardial surface. This set serves the papillary muscles and trabeculae carnae, while a third group tends to run circumferentially parallel and below the epicardium, giving branches both outwards and inwards.

Farrer-Brown found that the termination of these vessels were of two types, as they divided into arterioles and then capillaries. The direction of the tree-like branching in the subendocardial zone continued in the general line of the main artery. The area of myocardium supplied by these branches was small. This was in contrast to the pattern in the midzone of the wall, where the branches turned at an angle to the main artery and then divided to supply a much wider area of myocardium that was supplied by the terminal branch in the subendocardial zone. These anatomical differences suggest that the vessels in the mid-zone each have to supply a larger volume of muscle than in the other layers. This might well explain the greater vulnerability of this central zone to hypoxic changes, as indicated by reduced enzyme activity and the occurrence of laminar necrosis. In actual practice, the inner zone also suffers, apart from the immediate subendocardial layers, but the superficial subepicardial zone is almost always spared. The rationale of damage to the myocardium in hypertensive heart disease, as in aortic stenosis, would appear to be a relative coronary insufficiency. In pure coronary artery disease, part of a normal-sized myocardial mass is rendered ischaemic by localized reduction of blood flow by a coronary stenosis or occlusion, the resulting necrosis being distributed in a focal pattern according to the location of the block.

In hypertensive heart disease, normal coronary arteries attempt to supply a much larger muscle mass, so that there is the same imbalance between supply and demand. As there is no focal blockage, however, the resulting lesion is diffuse and the areas that suffer most are those in the mid- and inner zones, probably because of the microanatomy of the vessels described above. The same type of lesion may be seen in any severe sustained hypotensive episode of extracardiac cause, though the early onset of death in many of these will preclude the development of morphological evidence of laminar myocardial damage.

SUDDEN DEATH IN AORTIC VALVE DISEASE

A similar situation exists with aortic valve disease in which stenosis rather than incompetence can lead to sudden death. Most of the lesions are primarily degenerative, the commonest being 'idiopathic calcific aortic stenosis', most often seen in elderly men. Aortic stenosis of rheumatic origin always affects the mitral valve before the aortic, so a solitary aortic lesion cannot be ascribed to rheumatism and is therefore of

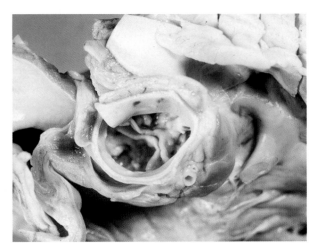

FIGURE 25.13 *Calcific aortic stenosis, a common cause of sudden unexpected death especially in older men. Though the stenosed valves are often biscuspid, the stenosis often deforms normal valves, as in this illustration. Marked left ventricular hypertrophy usually ensues, the large muscle mass becoming ischaemic, especially in the inner layers.*

the primary degenerative type. Rheumatic valve disease is becoming rare, both with the decline in rheumatic fever and the frequency with which valve lesions are treated surgically at an earlier stage, before marked ventricular hypertrophy and its myocardial lesions are evident.

In the common calcific disease, the valve is thickened and rigid, with fusion of the commissures in most cases. There may be large, irregular excrescences on the cusps and in the sinuses behind. At a later stage, the whole valve may be an almost unrecognizable, chalky mass, with a lumen barely wide enough to admit a pencil. This type of valve may have been biscuspid from birth, a condition that undoubtedly encourages calcific degeneration. Many stenotic and apparently bicuspid valves are not truly bicuspid, however, but appear so because the degenerative process has destroyed or obliterated one of the commissures between the cusps. This may often be demonstrated by the fact that a trace of the commissure may still be seen, or by the fact that the two surviving cusps are not equal in size, the commissures being placed at 120° rather than 180°.

A tight aortic valve, from whatever cause, obstructs the outflow tract of the left ventricle and causes the muscle to hypertrophy in order to eject the same stroke volume through a narrower orifice. In addition, if there is associated regurgitation, further extra work has to be performed to attempt to throw out the refluxed blood.

The effect of a severe aortic stenosis in relation to sudden death is to enlarge the left ventricle to sizes even greater than those seen in hypertension. Some of the biggest hearts (excepting some cardiomyopathies) are seen in aortic valve disease, going up to 800 g or – exceptionally – 1000 g.

Another effect of a tight valve is to lower the perfusion pressure in the coronary arteries, which is made worse if there is also an element of regurgitation. It is the diastolic pressure in the proximal aorta that feeds the coronary supply, as during systole the contraction of the heart prevents flow in the intramural arteries. A less common effect may be the distortion of the coronary ostia by calcific masses in the sinuses of Valsalva and the wall of the root of the aorta, which can partly block the entry into the coronary vessels. The combination of a large myocardial mass and decreased coronary flow is often made worse by concomitant coronary atherosclerosis, so the propensity of victims of aortic valve disease to drop dead is considerable. Elderly men are the most frequent victims. Lesions of other heart valves seldom cause sudden death as an isolated cause, though the more chronic cardiac dysfunction – mainly congestive cardiac failure – caused by them may end life rather abruptly on occasions. Rheumatic mitral stenosis is one such lesion, but perhaps a more direct mitral cause of sudden death is the 'floppy' valve usually seen in old age.

SUDDEN DEATH FROM THE CARDIOMYOPATHIES

There is a heterogenous group of diseases of myocardium associated with cardiac dysfunction known as the 'cardiomyopathies', which, though of mixed and often uncertain aetiology, have sufficient in common pathologically to merit a special identity. As they account for the second largest number of sudden deaths after coronary artery disease, i.e. about 10–15 per cent of all sudden deaths of cardiac origin, they are briefly described here, though specialized texts and papers on cardiac pathology should be consulted for details. The outstanding feature is a large heart in the absence of hypertension or valve lesions. The victims are usually young adults, partly because in older groups in which there is atherosclerotic coronary disease and also hypertension, these overlay the cardiomyopathy and make the diagnosis difficult or impossible. The only exception is if there is definite histological evidence or if the heart weight is excessive (over 700 g) in the absence of a valve defect. Cardiomyopathies are the most common cause of heart failure and are an important cause of death in children and adults. According to the Report of the 1995 World Health Organization/International Society and Federation of Cardiology Task Force on the Definition and Classification of Cardiomyopathies, they are classified into the following main types: dilated, hypertrophic, restrictive and arrhythmogenic right ventricular cardiomyopathy.

Dilated cardiomyopathy (DCM) is the most common cause of congestive heart failure. The annual incidence varies, depending on the diagnostic criteria, from two to

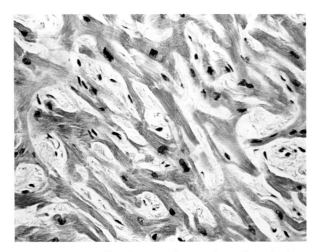

FIGURE 25.14 *Myofibre disarray in hypertrophic cardiomyopathy.*

eight cases per 100 000. Around 30–40 per cent of them are familial (FDCM), but it may also be idiopathic, viral, immune or toxic, e.g. alcoholic. Idiopathic dilated cardiomyopathy (IDCM) is characterized by dilated ventricular chamber and reduced contractility without coronary, valvular or pericardial disease. Histology is non-specific; however, viral genome has been identified in 10–34 per cent of patients with dilated cardiomyopathy.

Hypertrophic (obstructive) cardiomyopathy was first described in medicolegal autopsy material by a London forensic pathologist, Donald Teare, in 1958. Although he noted and described asymmetrical hypertrophy of the interventricular septum, so that a bulging pad of myocardium partly obstructed the left ventricular outflow tract, this cardiomyopathy is predominantly (75 per cent) a non-obstructive disease and, hence, hypertrophic cardiomyopathy (HCM) is now the preferred name. It is a primary sarcomere disorder characterized by left and/or right ventricular hypertrophy and, in most cases, inherited as a predominantly autosomal disease. It is caused by mutations of any of the genes encoding the proteins of the cardiac sarcomere.

Between 20 and 30 per cent are familial, and the condition may occur at any age from infancy to senility, though the majority of deaths occur in early middle age. The weight of the heart may range from a high normal at 400 g, to 800 g or even a kilogram. More striking than the total weight is the left ventricular preponderance, which is often maximum in the proximal septum, as described above.

Histologically the myocardium shows irregular-sized, large fibres with nuclear pleomorphism. Though once thought to be a rhabdomyoma or a hamartoma, or aberrant adrenergic tissue, the septal bulge usually shows a bizarre pattern of fibres, with loss of the orderly strata and replacement by a criss-crossing, confused architecture of muscle bundles. Interstitial fibrosis is common, and – though there may be an increase in interstitial cellularity – inflammatory infiltrate is not seen, as it would be in an active myocarditis.

Restrictive cardiomyopathy is, according to the WHO report, 'characterized by restrictive filling and reduced diastolic volume of either or both ventricles with normal or near-normal systolic function and wall thickness. Increased interstitial fibrosis may be present'. It may be idiopathic or associated with other diseases such as cardiac amyloidosis, cardiac haemochromatosis or endocardial fibroelastosis with or without hypereosinophilia.

Arrhythmogenic right ventricular cardiomyopathy (ARVC) is a primary myocardial disorder characterized by progressive fibrofatty degeneration of right ventricular myocardium, arrhythmias and risk of sudden death. In addition to familial autosomal-dominant disease with variable penetrance and polymorphic phenotype, two autosomal-recessive forms of ARVC are known.

The WHO classification includes further two groups of cardiomyopathies:

- specific cardiomyopathies that are associated with specific cardiac or systemic (ischaemic, valvular, hypertensive, inflammatory, metabolic, general systemic e.g. connective tissue or neuromuscular disorders) and
- unclassified cardiomyopathies, which do not fit readily in any group, e.g. fibroelastosis or isolated non-compaction of the ventricular myocardium (INVM), a rare disorder characterized by excessively prominent trabecular meshwork, ventricular arrhythmia and systemic embolism.

Myocarditis

Many infective diseases produce an acute myocarditis, which may be the immediate cause of death. A prime example is diphtheria, but this has virtually no forensic relevance. More important is 'isolated myocarditis', where the condition is primary and usually of unknown aetiology. It was formerly [and some recent results from an ongoing study by the author (PS) suggest, that it still is] a much-used and overused autopsy diagnosis, especially where no gross lesions could be found. Known by a variety of names, such as 'Fiedler's' or 'Saphir's' myocarditis, its incidence was said to be appreciable in victims of sudden death – and it was incriminated as the cause of accidents on the road and in the air that had been attributed to driver or pilot incapacity. In forensic pathology some 20–30 years ago, it became a 'fashionable' diagnosis on rather equivocal histological criteria. It was then found that many victims of trauma where death was rapid and where cardiac incapacity could not possibly be a causative factor in the accident, also had foci of mononuclear cells in the myocardium.

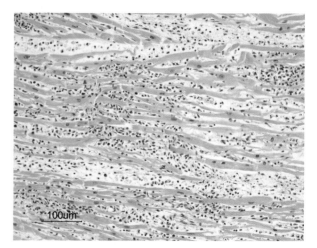

FIGURE 25.15 *Severe diffuse lymphocytic myocarditis with destruction of myocytes. (HE, original magnification ×10.)*

Stevens and Ground (1970), after finding six cases of myocarditis in 263 air pilots, when none of them could have been affected by a cardiac event, looked at a considerable number of other accident victims in circumstances in which disease was obviously unrelated to the trauma. They found about 5 per cent of young men had lesions otherwise histologically acceptable as 'myocarditis' and concluded that it was an unsafe diagnosis to use for the cause of death. Their histological minimum criteria for acceptance was one focus of 100 or more cells or many foci of half that size. Groups of lymphocytes, especially subepicardial of 40 or fewer cells, were disregarded.

In Australia, Tongue *et al.* (1972, 1977) did similar studies, but used whole transverse sections of ventricles at up to 18 levels in each heart. Their results showed that the more extensive the search, the greater the number of foci discovered in deaths that had no circumstantial relation to a sudden cardiac death. Using 18 full sections, they found that 90 per cent of the accident victims had 'myocarditis' lesions and suggested that, if the search was extensive enough, it could probably be brought up to 100 per cent.

The Dallas Classification System was proposed by eight cardiac pathologists in an attempt to provide the practicing pathologists with easily applicable and uniform criteria for the diagnosis of myocarditis in endomyocardial biopsies (Aretz *et al.* 1987). By this definition, the diagnosis of myocarditis can be made only if myocyte necrosis or degeneration or both are associated with an inflammatory infiltrate adjacent to the degenerating or necrotic myocytes. A semiquantitation of the amount of inflammatory infiltrate was suggested as mild, moderate, or severe and its distribution characterized as focal, confluent, or diffuse. The composition of inflammatory infiltrate, i.e. the presence of lymphocytes, neutrophils, eosinophils or giant cells was suggested for differential diagnosis of the aetiology. According to Feldman and McNamara (2000) the Dallas criteria probably underestimate the true incidence of myocarditis.

Among the great variety of infectious agents, viruses have been considered as important cause of myocarditis. The molecular biological techniques such as polymerase chain reaction (PCR) and *in situ* hybridization have provided new diagnostic possibilities and viral genome has been detected both in myocardial biopsies as well as in autopsy material. However, the detection rate and the viruses identified have varied markedly according to the study. In addition, drugs may cause myocarditis, either through direct toxic or immune-mediated mechanism.

Probably, the position now to be accepted is that unless multiple, florid foci are found, with myofibril necrosis seen, using special stains if necessary, bland mononuclear foci that are purely interstitial and not involving muscle fibres must be disregarded. The presence of myofibre necrosis, however localized, would appear the most important confirmatory criterion. Where stenotic coronary artery disease exists, it can be difficult or impossible to differentiate the resulting cellularity, fibrosis and fibre necrosis from that of a myocarditis.

A disease process that may well have been underestimated in the pathology of sudden death is cardiac sarcoidosis. Unless routine histology is carried out on every sudden death, this diagnosis will be missed (Fleming 1988) as will a considerable number of myocardial amyloidoses, which need special stains.

DEATH IN OLD AGE – THE SENILE MYOCARDIUM

In many autopsies on old persons, no specific lesions can be discovered that provide a clear cause of death. In the increasingly aged population of the developed nations, this problem becomes a more frequent task for the pathologist. The history of the mode of death then becomes particularly important, as it may give some clue as to which area of the indeterminate lesions should be given priority in deciding on a cause of death. For instance, if there is moderate coronary artery disease, then if the person died with sudden breathlessness or chest pain, rather than slowly fading away, more credence would be given to the coronary lesions. Many old people have good, patent coronary arteries, however, even if the walls may be calcified – if they did not have such good vessels, they probably would not have lived to 88 or 95 years, anyway.

Where nothing other than general senile atrophy of most organs is found and the history is unhelpful as to a specific mode of death, as long as the pathologist can exclude any unnatural cause, then it is quite legitimate to ascribe the death to 'myocardial degeneration due to senility'. The WHO's ICD-10 (International Statistical Classification of Diseases and Related Health Problems, Tenth Revision, Geneva 1992) provides a code for such a disease even though many cardiac pathologists seem reluctant to agree to its existence, wishing always to find some more specific disease process. In the authors' view, senile myocardial degeneration is quite acceptable, given exclusion of other causes. Senile hearts are usually small, but hypertension may have enlarged the ventricles long ago and the residual effect of this may be to sustain the heart at a normal weight. More important is the appearance of the heart, which is brown on the surface and in the muscle and is flabby and soft. The thumb can be pushed into such muscle at autopsy without difficulty. The weight may be down to 300 g or even 250 g, if no previous hypertrophy has existed. A good indication of cardiac atrophy is the presence of tortuous coronary vessels on the epicardial surface, especially the anterior descending branches. These may meander markedly, as the myocardium has shrunk, the apex has contracted nearer the base and so the vessels have to corrugate to fit into the diminished space.

Microscopically, the myocardial fibres are uneven in size, there may be a fine, diffuse fibrosis, which is not ischaemic in origin and the nuclei of the myocytes have prominent clumps of lipofuscin pigment at their poles. Unfortunately, none of these features is diagnostic of the cause of death, as other old persons dying of quite unrelated causes, such as trauma, might have equally poor heart muscle.

The justification for considering that senile myocardial degeneration is a valid cause of death comes from the species life span of different animals. Even without lethal specific disease, each species has a fairly uniform life span, the human being some 70–90 years. No one lives to 150 years, so there must be some limiting factor; as cardiac function is the most immediate arbiter of survival, it seems reasonable to indict heart contractibility as the primary factor. All tissues age, but senility of the spleen or thumbs does not have the immediacy for life support possessed by the myocardium.

SUDDEN DEATH FROM RUPTURE OF AN ANEURYSM

The most frequent extracardiac cause for sudden death arising in the cardiovascular system is a rupture of an aneurysm, almost always of the aorta or a cerebral vessel. Aortic aneurysms are of three types, all capable of catastrophic rupture.

The atheromatous aneurysm

The atheromatous aneurysm is the most common and is seen mainly in the abdominal segment of the aorta. Though atherosclerosis affects the whole length of the aorta, it is usually worse below the diaphragm, probably because of the haemodynamic effects of the larger branches that come off in this segment. Turbulence and 'Venturi' effects are known to localize the development of fatty streaks and atheromatous plaques, as they are seen first around the ostia of the intercostal vessels and become particularly severe at the major bifurcation into common iliac arteries. Though aneurysms can develop at any point in the aorta, most are below the diaphragm. Excepting dissecting aneurysms, however, any aneurysm in the thoracic segment is still more likely to be atheromatous than syphilitic, even though syphilis is virtually confined to the aortic arch. Most atheromatous aneurysms are fusiform or saccular, the bulge being either symmetrical about the axis of the vessel or more commonly bulging out more on one side than the other. Progressive destruction of the media by the fibrolipid degenerative processes of atherosclerosis leads to weakening of the aortic wall. Bulging caused by the continuous internal blood pressure begins, aided by the hypertensive tendencies of later life. The damage or complete destruction of the intima leads to platelet and fibrin deposition, so that mural thrombosis is laid down in the expanding aneurysm. This may partly or wholly fill the sac, being many centimetres thick in some instances, with well-marked stratification called the 'lines of Zahn'. The wall of the aneurysm may contain calcific fragments similar to the adjacent artery wall.

Most aneurysms remain intact throughout life and are found as incidental findings at autopsy. Naturally the incidence of ruptured aneurysms is greater in medico-legal autopsies by reason of the selective population of sudden deaths. When rupture occurs, the weakest point of the wall is penetrated by the contained blood and this usually leaks out into the retroperitoneal tissues, rather than free bleeding into the peritoneal cavity. The blood tracks behind the root of the mesentery and around the kidney. A large perirenal haematoma may form but, more often, the obvious site of bleeding is in the centre of the back of the abdomen. The diagnosis is usually quite obvious as soon as the autopsy begins for, as soon as the abdomen is opened and the intestine moved aside, a dark red mound may be seen projecting forwards over the lumbar spine, bulging at the root of the mesentery.

The development of a successful technique for the repair of many such arterial defects has reduced the death rate, though there is a substantial perioperative mortality, often because the patient is virtually moribund when the operation begins, or because gross calcification and degeneration of the remaining aortic wall makes it technically impracticable.

The dissecting aneurysm

Rupture of a dissecting aneurysm of the aorta is much less common than the atheromatous variety and seems to have

decreased even more during the past decade. It is still by no means an uncommon cause of sudden death, however, and is the second most frequent cause of a haemopericardium and cardiac tamponade. Whereas atheromatous aneurysms are usually in the abdomen, the dissecting aneurysm can span the whole length of the vessel from iliac artery to aortic valve, though the main effects are usually manifest in the thoracic segment.

The basic lesion is a degeneration of the aortic media, the so-called 'medionecrosis'. The thick elastic media becomes degenerate and cystic in the central layers, producing a vessel wall like a sandwich with a soft cleavage plane in the middle. This defect is of unknown aetiology and affects both the elastic and muscular elements of the media. It is relatively common over the age of 50, especially in men. Many aortas seen at autopsy have this degeneration, but no aneurysms, as they never develop because the blood fails to enter the potential cleavage space from the lumen of the aorta.

In most cases where a dissecting aneurysm has caused death, the blood has broken through from the lumen through a tear in an atheromatous plaque, which is a quite separate disease process existing in parallel with the medionecrosis. When blood enters the medial cleft under high arterial pressure, the two layers of the media are split apart and the dissection may rapidly travel both upwards and downwards in the aortic wall. The upper component may split its way around the arch and beyond the attachment of the pericardium. Here, just above the aortic ring, the dissecting haemorrhage often bursts through the remaining outer media and adventitia into the pericardial sac. This causes a massive haemopericardium and the cardiac tamponade described earlier in relation to ruptured myocardial infarct. The distal extension may travel down to the iliac and even femoral arteries, sheathing them in blood. Rarely, in a patient who survives a dissection, the secondary lumen formed in the cleavage plane may rupture back into the main aortic lumen, thus forming a 'double-barrelled' aorta, a curiosity occasionally found at autopsy. Death usually occurs from cardiac tamponade, but some dissections do not burst into the pericardium. Here death is by a less obvious mechanism, which may be partly the sudden narrowing of the aortic lumen and pressure on the coronary ostia and roots of the coronary arteries. In persons under 50 years of age, there is a much less common alternative cause of medionecrosis, known as Erdheim's degeneration. This is sometimes called 'mucoid medial degeneration' and is associated with Marfan's syndrome, an inherited condition characterized by arachnodactyly and optic, aural and bony lesions.

The syphilitic aneurysm

Syphilitic aneurysms are now uncommon, because of the relative rarity of tertiary lesions as treatment is available for the

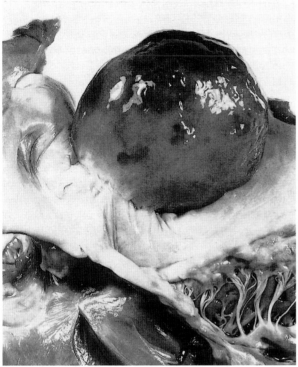

FIGURE 25.16 *Sudden unexpected death caused by a myxoma of the left atrium. The ball-shaped mucoid tumour impacted in the mitral valve during a postural change. No other cause of death was discernible.*

earlier stages of the disease. In some areas of the world, however, tertiary syphilis is not the rarity it has become in Europe and America.

The syphilitic aneurysm of the aorta is almost always in the thoracic segment and usually in the arch. Syphilitic aortitis, which precedes an aneurysm, may be recognized in the lining of the thoracic and abdominal aorta by its irregular corrugated pattern, though admixture with atheroma can obscure the classical appearances. There tend to be sinuous linear folds, like coarse wrinkles, which have been likened to the bark of an oak tree. If the aorta dissected free of adherent connective tissue is held up to a strong light, 'Gough's test' may be applied, in which translucent windows can be seen in the media. When confluent, these weak patches allow the internal blood pressure to blow out an aneurysm and the syphilitic bulge can be the largest of all, sometimes almost filling the upper part of the chest. The wall is thin and fragile, and there may be several separate bulges from overlapping aneurysms.

Pressure may erode bronchi, oesophagus, pulmonary vessels, lung and even the thoracic cage. The latter may allow the aneurysm to become subcutaneous and, in former years,

the external bursting of a pulsating chest tumour must have been a dramatic event. The usual mode of rupture is into the pleural cavity or into the oesophagus or bronchus, giving rise to a sudden, massive haematemesis or haemoptysis. Histologically, it may be impossible to confirm syphilitic aortitis, as the reactive phase of the disease may have been long burnt out, but the gross pathological appearances are diagnostic in themselves.

Fatal aneurysms of other vessels

Fatal aneurysms of other vessels are rare, apart from the cerebral arteries. Atheromatous bulges can occur on the iliac and femoral vessels, and sometimes in the mesenteric arteries. Polyarteritis nodosa can produce mini-aneurysms from the inflammatory process eroding the wall, but death is not caused by the direct effects of rupture, but by vascular problems in the coronary, renal and other arteries. Infective mycotic aneurysms are rare in civilian practice, as are traumatic arteriovenous fistulae, but are not uncommon in war casualties.

Sudden death from ruptured cerebral aneurysm

The relationship of head and neck injury to subarachnoid haemorrhage is discussed in Chapter 5, but here we are concerned solely with spontaneous rupture of an aneurysm of the circle of Willis at the base of the brain. This is one of the most common causes of death in young to middle-aged adults, if coronary disease is excluded. In women, who are relatively immune from coronary occlusion up to the fifth decade of life, ruptured berry aneurysm is proportionately much more common than in men. It is a useful rule-of-thumb, when presented with the sudden death of a woman of child-bearing age, to consider a complication of pregnancy, self-poisoning, pulmonary embolism and subarachnoid haemorrhage as the first choices.

Subarachnoid bleeding can cause virtually instantaneous death, even though the mechanism is obscure. Numerous cases have been described where a previously fit person was seen to collapse and was apparently already dead when attended by onlookers. There must be an element of cardiac arrest in these examples, caused by the sudden bathing of the brainstem in blood from a jet of arterial blood impinging on the base of the brain. As with coronary disease, arterial spasm has been invoked as a cause of the sudden death in ruptured berry aneurysm, without any proof. Most cases of subarachnoid haemorrhage have a much longer course, with clinical symptoms and signs allowing either surgical intervention or, often, spontaneous resolution.

We are by definition here, however, concerned with sudden or rapid fatalities. In the usual coroner's case, the victim is either found dead with no available history, or has died rapidly and inexplicably, or has expired after suggestive symptoms like severe headache and rapid coma. Many die after physical or emotional exertion, especially sexual intercourse or strenuous sporting activity. Those that occur during or soon after some assault or altercation are dealt with in the chapter on head injuries (Chapter 5), and can pose a major forensic problem concerning causation.

At autopsy, the diagnosis of subarachnoid haemorrhage is self-evident. As the usual point of bleeding is in the circle of Willis, the most dense haemorrhage will be over the base of the brain, especially in the basal cisterns. The blood usually spreads laterally and may cover the whole surface of the cerebral hemispheres, the hindbrain and down into the spinal canal. This will be bright red in a fresh bleed; if survival lasts a week or so, a brownish tinge will appear as the haemoglobin undergoes changes. Haemosiderin can be detected by Perl's stain after about 3 days.

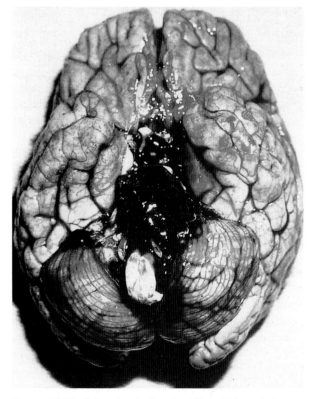

FIGURE 25.17 *A dense basal subarachnoid haemorrhage that caused rapid death. The blood clot filling the basal cisterns conceals a ruptured berry aneurysm of the circle of Willis; at autopsy, this must be removed under a stream of water, using careful blunt dissection to avoid further damage to the vessels.*

The detection of the source of the haemorrhage is sometimes difficult. An aneurysm is present in about 85 per cent of spontaneous subarachnoid haemorrhages, but the remainder reveal no aneurysm, even after an exhaustive search. This may be because of destruction of a small aneurysm at the time of rupture, but it is just as likely to be a leak from a vessel without an aneurysm, as a result of the existence of a point of weakness as described below.

A relatively rare cause of bleeding, especially in children, is the presence of a vascular malformation in the arterial system, such as an angioma, an arteriovenous anastomosis, or an aberrant vessel in the meninges. Post-mortem angiography may be of assistance in tracing intracranial bleeding from natural lesions, as in trauma. Karhunen *et al.* (1990) describe the techniques required.

Though berry aneurysms are often called 'congenital', they are not themselves present at birth, but a defect in the wall of a cerebral artery is probably present from late fetal life. The circle of Willis condenses out of an irregular embryonic meshwork of arteries over the base of the brain by unwanted vessels undergoing atrophy. Where these redundant vessels originally joined the surviving main arteries, a 'window' in the elastic and collagenous coat is left, usually at the junction of two vessels. This window is a weak point where rising blood pressure in adult life may begin to form a 'blow-out', a thin-walled aneurysm, which may be single or multiple. At a certain stage, any sudden extra rise in blood pressure or flow rate may rip the already tense sac, and cause extravasation of blood at full arterial pressure into the subarachnoid space. Where there is no aneurysm, it must be assumed that a weak point in a vessel wall has given way *ab initio*, without the prior formation of a sac.

The search for a small aneurysm at autopsy may be difficult because of the thick layer of blood clot that is trapped in the meninges and vessels. Blunt dissection should be used, employing the handle of a scalpel or the nose of a pair of forceps. The blood should be constantly washed away in a continuous stream of water. It is possible to inject water into one of the cut ends of a vertebral artery, having carefully tied or clamped the other vessel and the two cut terminations of the carotid arteries, to see where the water leaks from. The leaks are often multiple, however, from artefactual tearing of small vessels during autopsy removal of the brain. The search for an aneurysm is best carried out on the fresh unfixed brain, as formalin fixation hardens the blood clot so much that it cannot be removed without the danger of tearing the underlying vessel and any aneurysm. It is essential to carry out blunt dissection progressively in a continuous stream of water. Aneurysms are most often found at the bifurcation of the middle cerebral and posterior communicating arteries, at the bifurcation of the basilar arteries, on the middle cerebral in the Sylvian fissure, on the anterior communicating artery, or where the posterior communicating artery joins the posterior cerebral vessels. An aneurysm is sometimes on the cortical aspect of the artery and may be part-buried in the cerebral surface, making it hard to find. If the swelling (which may be completely collapsed at autopsy, especially when ruptured) is not seen on superficial examination of the circle of Willis, the vessels should be gently lifted away from the brain surface with a blunt elevator so that the underside can be inspected. Sometimes a buried aneurysm will rupture mainly into the cortex, causing a lesion that may be mistaken for an intracerebral haemorrhage. Berry aneurysms are frequently multiple and of

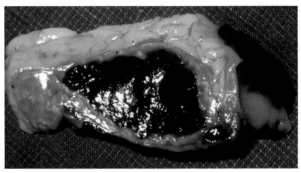

FIGURE 25.18 *Adrenal haemorrhage occurring several days after multiple injuries sustained in a traffic accident. There was no apparent abdominal injury. The haemorrhage is fresh and occupies the medulla, with the cortex stretched around the periphery.*

varying size, from a few millimetres to several centimetres, though the usual diameter is of the order of 3–8 mm.

PULMONARY THROMBO-EMBOLISM

This is discussed fully in Chapter 13, but here it is sufficient to emphasize that pulmonary embolism is the most under-diagnosed cause of death, according to Cameron and McGoogan (1981). Their figures show that less than half the deaths shown at autopsy to have been caused by a pulmonary embolism were so diagnosed by the attending clinician. Paradoxically, many other presumed deaths from this condition were found at autopsy not to have been embolic. Thus the overall statistics are not so much in error – but in relation to the wrong victims!

Pulmonary embolism is more common with advancing age, with obese subjects and in the majority of instances there is a predisposing factor such as trauma, surgical operation, confinement to bed or immobility from another cause. Even prolonged sitting can lead to deep vein thrombosis, as was seen in persons sleeping in deckchairs in air-raid shelters in the last war and, more recently, it has been described as a hazard of long air flights.

A significant proportion, however, estimated by the author (BK) at up to 20 per cent, occur unexpectedly in the absence of any of these usual factors, making the legal problem of causation difficult. This is especially so in criminal cases where a high standard of proof has to be

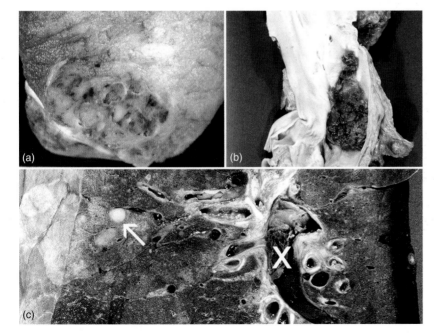

FIGURE 25.19 *A rare cause of pulmonary embolism. Metastasizing embryonal carcinoma + seminoma of the testis (a) and thrombosis attached to the wall of inferior vena cava due to metastases of the local lymph nodes (b) and (c) pulmonary metastasis (white arrow) and massive pulmonary embolism (white X).*

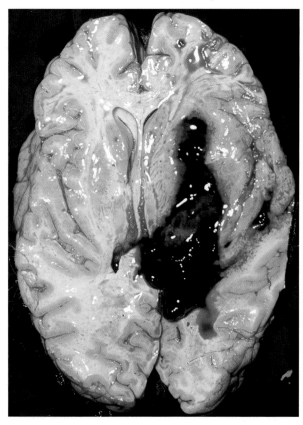

FIGURE 25.20 *A large recent intracerebral haemorrhage in a person with hypertension. The bleeding has originated in the region of the external capsule from a lenticulostriate branch of the middle cerebral artery then broken through into the posterior horn of the lateral ventricle.*

attained, rather than the balance of probabilities required for a civil action.

SUDDEN DEATH IN EPILEPSY

Every coroner's pathologist or the equivalent in other jurisdictions, has experience of sudden deaths in epileptics, when no morphological lesion can be found at autopsy. Epileptics can die unexpectedly without being in status epilepticus – or indeed, not even in a typical fit. It is true that many such deaths are not witnessed to prove that no such fit occurred, but sufficient evidence exists to indicate that a rapid sudden death can certainly occur.

There are, of course, many deaths in epileptics where the mode is apparent, such as asphyxia during a fit in bed when the face is pressed into the pillow, and saliva and mucus form an airtight seal against the fabric around the nose and mouth. Epileptics also drown in the bathtub and suffer other traumatic deaths because of fits occurring when they are in some vulnerable position.

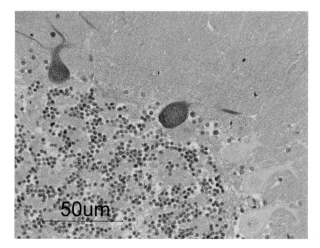

FIGURE 25.21 *Two fibrinogen-positive Purkinje cells and three negative cells in a sudden unexpected death with a history of epilepsy. (Peroxidase-DAB immunostaining, original magnification ×20.)*

These causes apart, the victim of epilepsy seems to be able to die with no apparent immediate cause and the mechanism is obscure. It has been suggested that some massive cerebral electric discharge or neurone storm occurs, leading to cardiac arrest, but this is mere hypothesis. When all investigations have been completed (including toxicological screening for antiepileptic drug overdose), after an essentially negative autopsy, then the pathologist is justified in recording 'epilepsy' as an acceptable cause of death.

The autopsy should always include a search for bites on the tip and distal sides of the tongue, which suggest a fit. A careful examination of the brain is essential, to search for any cause of post-traumatic epilepsy. In some epileptics, without coronary stenosis, patchy myocardial fibrosis has been recorded (Falconer and Rajs 1976), said to be the result of episodic hypoxia from apnoea during fits. Based on the observation of Sokrab *et al.* (1988) that Purkinje cells become labelled by plasma proteins in experimental blood–brain-barrier (BBB) breakdown, Ikegaya *et al.* (2003) investigated immunohistochemically the presence of fibrinogen-positive Purkinje cells in 50 sudden unexpected deaths. There were 24 subjects with and 26 without known history of epilepsy. Regarding ≥30 per cent of fibrinogen-positive Purkinje cells as diagnostic limit indicating recent major BBB breakdown, they found that 22 of the 24 cases with high percentage of fibrinogen-positive Purkinje cells had a history of epilepsy. One of the two remaining high-fibrinogen subjects had unknown leuco-encephalopathy and the other had essential hypertension. Only two of the low-fibrinogen cases had a history of epilepsy. The immunopositivity of Purkinje cells is not specific for epilepsy but can occur in any conditions causing BBB breakdown, most likely due to uptake of fibrinogen

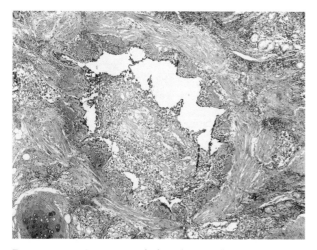

FIGURE 25.22 *Cross-section of a bronchus in sudden asthma death showing cell-laden mucus, folding of the soft tissues of the bronchial wall, thickening of the basement membrane and hypertrophy of the muscle. (HE, original magnification ×10.)*

β₂-antagonists so commonly used for the relief of bronchospasm are not so prone to cause cardiac arrhythmias, but they are by no means safe drugs in this respect. Of the 11 deaths in this Norwegian series, seven victims were found dead with a β₂-inhaler still clutched in their hands. Overdosage of the substance appears to be common. The use of theophylline derivatives combined with sympathomimetic agents tends to accentuate the cardiotoxicity of the bronchodilators.

Some of the deaths appeared to be in instances where the drug had been exhausted from the inhaler, but the propellant was still active. This may be another possible mechanism for some of these deaths, similar to the vagal inhibitory fatalities seen in butane misuse, where cold gas impinges on the pharynx.

At autopsy little or nothing is found, except confirmation of the chronic asthmatic state. On opening the chest cavity, the lungs are seen to fill the thorax, not collapsing as is usual and they have a pale spongy texture, forming stable pits when pressed with the fingers. The cut surface may reveal thick-walled prominent bronchi, often plugged with thick, clear mucus. This is not an explanation for the sudden collapse and death, however, and the mechanism remains obscure.

The topic of sudden death from asthma in childhood has been investigated by Champ and Byard (1994), who consider that it occurred only in children with significant chronic disease.

from the cerebrospinal fluid irrigating the cerebellar surface. The time interval needed for the protein accumulation in man is not known. It is probable that, in addition to fibrinogen, other plasma proteins can also be used as a marker and an auxiliary method in assessing the probability of epileptic seizures contributing to the cause of death in sudden unexpected deaths.

SUDDEN DEATH IN BRONCHIAL ASTHMA

As in epilepsy, sufferers from bronchial asthma may die suddenly and unexpectedly, without necessarily being in status asthmaticus or even in an acute asthmatic attack. The mechanism is obscure, but experience proves that such fatalities are not uncommon. About 20 years ago, there was a marked increase in sudden deaths in asthmatics, but it was recognized that this was caused by the overuse of inhalers containing bronchodilators. These adrenergic drugs, used in excess, have a direct action upon the myocardium causing tachycardia, arrhythmias and ventricular fibrillation. Awareness among prescribing doctors rapidly reduced this danger but sudden deaths still occur, even when these substances are not used to excess.

The question of sudden death in asthma was discussed by Morild and Giertsen (1989). They considered that a number of factors contributed to death. Hypoxia and respiratory acidosis occur in asthma and increase myocardial irritability. Drugs such as theophylline and sympathomimetic agents can provide ventricular fibrillation. The

RESPIRATORY OBSTRUCTION

Mechanical obstruction by foreign bodies is dealt with in Chapter 14, but some rapid – if not actually sudden – deaths can be due to fulminating natural disease.

Rupture of a retropharyngeal abscess ('quinsy'), when pus and necrotic material pour into the pharynx and larynx, is now a rare cause. Diphtheria is also virtually unknown in advanced countries so that the toxaemia, a fatal myocarditis and the possibility of laryngeal obstruction from a detached pharyngeal membrane are rarely considered by most doctors.

More common – and a cause of legal actions for negligence against doctors – is the fulminating epiglottitis caused by *Haemophilus influenzae* in children. This is a major paediatric emergency and any child with stridor of recent onset should be seen urgently by a paediatrician and anaesthetist. The gross infective oedema of the laryngeal entrance can lead to death within hours of onset of the illness, and may require rapid intubation or tracheostomy to save life.

HAEMOPTYSIS

Now that pulmonary tuberculosis is less common and treatable in advanced countries, deaths from haemoptysis are rare, as most massive respiratory haemorrhages were from this cause. However, warning signals are now evident about a revival of tuberculosis, even in 'advanced' countries. Part of the return of this scourge is due to opportunist infection in HIV-infected persons, but AIDS apart, phthisis seems to be on the march again, with worrying concerns about increasing resistance to the drugs, which revolutionized its treatment 30–40 years ago.

Bronchial tumours rarely cause fatal haemoptyses, unless a large vessel is eroded; syphilitic aortitis perforating the aorta or other large vessel is now almost a matter of history.

The bleeding rarely causes death from exsanguination except where the aorta is eroded, but smaller bleeds may fill the air passages, and cause an asphyxial-type death or a 'vagal inhibition'-type death from sudden flooding of the larynx.

GASTROINTESTINAL HAEMORRHAGE

Bleeding may take place at any point along the alimentary tract and though modern transfusion and resuscitatory methods make deaths unusual these days, some are seen in medico-legal practice when people living alone or otherwise remote from assistance, die without any medical intervention.

Bleeding from surgical operations in the mouth or pharynx, such as tooth extraction or tonsillectomy, rarely causes death, but can occasionally do so from blood and clot blocking the airways. In the oesophagus, a penetrating carcinoma may erode the aorta or other great vessel in the mediastinum, but the most frequent sources of bleeding are varices at the lower end, caused by the portal hypertension associated with hepatic fibrosis. It is often difficult to identify the varices at autopsy, as they have collapsed, but the absence of gastric or duodenal ulceration, and the congested, bluish vessels around the cardia often give away the lesion, especially in the presence of liver cirrhosis and splenomegaly.

Other causes of massive gastrointestinal bleeding are gastric and duodenal peptic ulcers, which can erode large vessels in their base. Acute erosions, though shallow, can produce considerable blood in the stomach and may require surgical resection. They are rarely the cause of lethal bleeding.

Carcinoma of the stomach can reach a large size and the crater variety may perforate a major vessel to produce severe haemorrhage. Bleeding from the small intestine is rare, except in certain haemorrhagic diatheses. More common is bleeding from colonic lesions, such as carcinomas and ulcerative colitis.

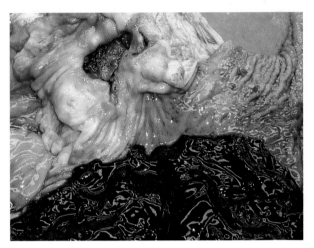

FIGURE 25.23 *Massive lethal bleeding from eroded vessels of a gastric ulcer.*

Polyps, sometimes malignant, may also give rise to melaena and even massive bleeding *per rectum*, though these are now rarely fatal unless medical intervention is delayed or absent.

FATAL ABDOMINAL CATASTROPHES

Though usually surgical emergencies, some abdominal conditions go untreated because the victim is either a solitary person living alone with no opportunity to call for help, or declines to seek medical assistance. They may well be found dead with no history to suggest a cause of death.

Mesenteric thrombosis and infarction is one such condition. The thrombosis may in fact be an embolus, rather than a thrombosis *in situ*, the most common cause of both being atherosclerosis of the aorta and its mesenteric branches. The length of small intestine supplied by the vessel becomes dark and necrotic, and may involve almost the whole length of the jejunum and ileum. Even if precipitated by an embolus, much of the rest of the arterial system may then thrombose and, on cutting into the mesentery at autopsy, the cut ends of arteries may show plugs of firm ante-mortem thrombus. The gut will be blue–red or even almost black, with loss of the serosal lustre and a friable necrotic wall.

Strangulated intestine is yet another condition that may present as sudden or rapid death, where medical attention is lacking, and even sometimes when it is negligently offered.

Hernias, both femoral and inguinal, and internal strangulation beneath fibrous bands in the peritoneal cavity, may all twist the intestine so that its blood supply is cut off, with subsequent necrosis. The gut above may develop ileus and become paralysed and dilated.

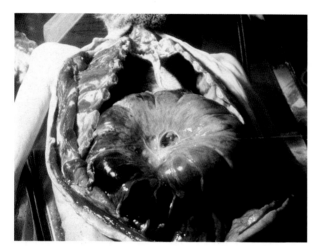

FIGURE 25.24 *Great distension of colon due to volvulus of sigmoid colon. Deceased found dead with history of abdominal pain.*

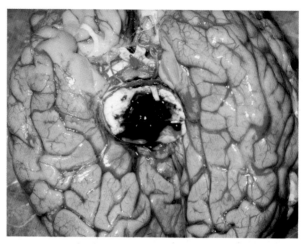

FIGURE 25.25 *A massive pontine haemorrhage in a person with hypertension. The circumstances and the irregular distribution of the bleeding within the brainstem distinguish this primary haemorrhage from the secondary lesions seen in raised intracranial pressure. Sometimes a natural intracranial haemorrhage may precipitate an accidental fall or traffic accident, however, and the resulting head injury may make it more difficult to identify the nature of the brain haemorrhage.*

Caution is needed at autopsy to differentiate the dark red colour of loops of intestine due to post-mortem hypostasis from true infarction. Hypostasis is seen to be interrupted when the gut is stretched out, due to alternate dependent loops, whereas real necrosis is usually continuous and the serosa is dull and friable.

Fulminating peritonitis may be seen in a variety of causes, again leading to death if undiagnosed or untreated. Death from acute appendicitis and appendix abscess is now uncommon, but perforation of the colon through a diverticulum, whether inflamed or merely distended and eroded by faecoliths, is common.

Tearing of the senile gut where it is adherent to other structures, such as uterus or tube, can also lead to peritonitis, and a carcinoma (often difficult to differentiate macroscopically from chronic diverticulitis) may also lead to perforation with loss of intestinal contents into the peritoneum.

A perforated peptic ulcer, usually duodenal, leads to a chemical peritonitis. The autopsy appearances are straightforward, turbid fluid being found in the peritoneal cavity, which may show early inflammatory changes, if the perforation occurred many hours previously. The perforation is most commonly found on the posterior surface of the duodenum.

GENITOURINARY SYSTEM

There is very little in the urinary system that can give rise to a sudden or rapid death, but the female genital organs certainly make up for this. Complications of pregnancy are discussed elsewhere (Chapter 19), but it should be repeated here that ectopic pregnancy, usually in the tubes, can rupture with massive intraperitoneal haemorrhage. Induced abortions, unless under reputable medical control, are another source of death

from haemorrhage, air embolism, perforation of vagina or uterus, infection and the use of toxic substances.

THE RELATIONSHIP BETWEEN TRAUMA AND DISEASE

One of the most difficult problems in forensic medicine occurs when a death takes place in a person who has suffered trauma but who has either pre-existing natural disease or where some apparently natural disease has supervened after the trauma. The relative contributions of trauma and disease may then become an acute medico-legal problem.

For example, the author (BK) conducted an autopsy on an old man of 82 years, previously in excellent health, who had been tied up and slightly injured by robbers of a sub-post office. Within 2 hours of release from his bonds the old gentleman became ill and then hemiplegic, dying of a massive cerebral haemorrhage shortly afterwards. The attackers were charged with homicide, in addition to robbery, but that charge was rejected by magistrates on the grounds that a cerebral haemorrhage could be a natural disease, unrelated to the assault. The prosecution obtained a private Bill of Indictment to circumvent the magistrates, and at the Crown Court the accused were convicted of manslaughter on the grounds that the physical and emotional stress of being assaulted and tied up probably (beyond reasonable doubt) led to an elevation of blood pressure that precipitated a cerebral haemorrhage in a previously fit person, within such a short time span.

This marginal case illustrates the problems that can occur when trauma and natural disease coexist in the same person. A common dilemma exists in relation to subarachnoid haemorrhage from a ruptured berry aneurysm when there has been a head injury.

In autopsies when an injury has been sustained by a person with substantial natural disease, the following problems must be addressed:

- whether death was caused entirely by the disease and would have occurred irrespective of the injury
- whether death was caused entirely by the injury and would have occurred whether or not the disease was present
- whether the death was caused by a combination of these two processes.

In practical terms, the most common situations involve coronary artery disease, pulmonary embolism and subarachnoid haemorrhage.

Coronary atherosclerosis

The disease has invariably been present for months or probably years before the traumatic episode, and it is therefore indisputably obvious that the trauma can have no relationship to the genesis of the disease – though relatives and some lawyers are often hard to convince on this point. Furthermore, unless there was a direct blow onto the front of the thorax, which could physically have damaged the heart surface and caused a direct traumatic lesion of the coronary system (by dislodging an atheromatous plaque – but see end of this section – causing a subintimal haemorrhage or precipitating a coronary thrombosis, a rare event), there is no way in which the injury can be accused of worsening the state of the coronary arteries. If the state of the coronary system was already poor, thus it could justifiably be claimed by the defence that death could have occurred at any time. The standard of proof in criminal cases is high and must be proved 'beyond reasonable doubt', whereas in civil disputes, only 'the balance of probabilities' must be attained.

As opposed to showing that the trauma directly worsened the physical state of the coronary vessels, it is easier to claim that the physical and emotional stress associated with the traumatic event caused increased demands upon a weakened heart and caused it to fail. Recent investigations (see end of this section) have strongly confirmed the association between acute myocardial infarction, cardiac arrest and exertion.

The adrenal response of 'fight or flight' may be invoked, it being accepted that released endogenous catecholamines such as noradrenaline can send a chronically hypoxic heart into ventricular fibrillation and arrest. There may even be morphological evidence in some cases, by the finding of contraction bands in the cardiac myofibrils, especially in the superficial subepicardial layers.

It is often an assessment of the circumstances, in addition to the autopsy findings, that decides a court's attitude to the relationship of trauma to disease. Where a man who has had no previous cardiac symptoms drops dead immediately after some assault or strenuous activity, the court is more likely to assume an association than with some cardiac cripple, who has been hovering on the brink of heart dysfunction for a long time before the traumatic event.

The average jury is likely to decide that it would be too much of a coincidence for an assault to cause a man to drop dead on the spot, even if it was shown that his coronary artery stenosis had been there for several years. Much depends upon the individual circumstances, especially where there is only a short interval between the traumatic episode and death.

The strict test is: 'Would he have died when he did die if the assault had not taken place?' This is often unanswerable on medical grounds, but the court is entitled to take a common-sense view of coincidence in terms of immediacy in time and apply the 'beyond reasonable doubt' test to it.

The fact that a person is in a parlous state of health and might die from relatively minimal trauma is no defence in law, which states that 'an assailant must take his victims as he finds them'. In other words, it is immaterial whether the attacker knows that his victim is ill or not – if death results from an illegal act against him, the charge of homicide may stand. This dictum is not adhered to slavishly by public prosecutors, however, as it is a matter of practical politics whether a criminal prosecution can be maintained with any chance of success (using public funds), against an energetic defence that can show medically that the victim had such a degree of natural disease that he might have dropped dead spontaneously at any time. The prevalence of coronary disease is so widespread that a close association in time must be shown before any causal connection can be accepted. The actual death itself need not occur very soon after the assault, however, if it can be established that the latter could have precipitated an infarct in a myocardium already compromised by coronary stenosis. It is not only a blow or some physical trauma that may precipitate a myocardial infarct or arrhythmia; as stated above, even the emotional upset that accompanies injury, or even the threat or fear of an injury, can lead to death. The blow may never actually be struck or it may fail to land, yet the threatened person may suffer a transient hypertension or tachycardia that may precipitate a subintimal haemorrhage, arrhythmia, or cerebral or subarachnoid haemorrhage that leads to death. Such an event, however, with little or no morphological evidence to be presented as evidence, has a poor chance of acceptance in court unless the circumstances are clear-cut. These cases pose a problem for police and pathologist, in that it may be difficult to decide whether to arrest and charge the potential culprit with a criminal offence.

A typical case was once seen by the author (BK) in which an elderly man was involved in an altercation with another, concerning parking a car. There was a scuffle, in which only trivial blows were exchanged, but one participant immediately developed chest pain and breathlessness, and soon died. The other man was arrested, but as autopsy showed marked cardiac enlargement, extensive myocardial fibrosis and gross occlusive coronary atherosclerosis, the prosecution decided to offer no evidence and the charge was dropped, even though the answer to the 'acid test' of whether the victim would have been likely to die at that particular time had the altercation not taken place was probably in the negative.

In civil matters, considerable sums of money may hang upon such decisions by way of damages and insurance payments. Here the standard of proof is much lower, as the plaintiff only has to show that there was a 51 per cent or better chance of the association being present, rather than the much higher standard of criminal liability.

An actual example of the civil problems was a workman who was removing a truck wheel from his employer's vehicle with a wheelbrace. Under full pressure, the threaded stud in the hub suddenly snapped and the man was thrown to the ground under the force of his own muscular effort. He was shocked and soon developed chest pain and died the next day. Autopsy revealed no fresh infarct, but there was longstanding left ventricular hypertrophy, myocardial fibrosis and stenosing coronary atheroma. The employer's liability was disputed, but eventually a compromise settlement was reached.

Recent very careful and statistically meticulous research on large cohorts, both in the USA and Germany, have shown an indisputable relationship between exertion and sudden cardiac death. Mittleman *et al.* (1993) investigated 1228 patients with acute myocardial infarcts and showed that there was a sixfold increase in the incidence of infarction during or within one hour of heavy physical exertion, such as snow shovelling, jogging or sexual activity. In Germany, Willich *et al.* (1993) researched 1194 patients with the same condition and showed a twofold increase in risk. Both surveys showed that the risk was greater in those who were otherwise sedentary and that long-term moderate exercise was undoubtedly associated with a reduced risk of infarction (Curfman 1993). Several mechanisms were proposed for the increased risk during sudden severe exertion, including the splitting and dislodgement of an atheromatous plaque. It was also claimed that increased platelet

activation occurred in sedentary people who suddenly exerted themselves. In an earlier publication, Siscovick *et al.* (1984) showed the same trend in primary cardiac arrest, exertion in otherwise sedentary persons increasing the risk, whilst habitual exercise protected.

Subarachnoid haemorrhage

Subarachnoid haemorrhage is another difficult area in which trauma and natural disease interact. When a berry aneurysm on the cerebral arteries ruptures, the allegation is often made that some traumatic occurrence precipitated that event. The matter is discussed in Chapter 5, but to recapitulate here, the problem is to decide whether the trauma itself was a mechanical factor in causing the arterial blister to burst.

A rupture is a relatively common event without external trauma, this cause of death being well-known in young to middle-aged persons who are not indulging in any strenuous activity whatsoever. It is known to occur, however, during innocent activities, such as jogging, intercourse and sporting exertion, probably because of a transient rise in blood pressure and pulse rate. Once again, a potent element may be in the adrenal response, catecholamines pushing up the blood pressure. Thus when a ruptured aneurysm occurs during or shortly after a fight or altercation, it is arguable whether a mechanical blow to the head or merely the emotional stress of a dispute is the most potent factor in causing rupture. There has been much medical argument about the role of trauma in causing the rupture, as many would maintain that the aneurysm is so deep-seated within the skull that internal pressure from hypertension is far more likely to be the reason.

Certainly, where a small aneurysm a few millimetres in size breaks, it is difficult to accept that a blow could have caused a tear, but in the more exceptional cases of a large tissue-thin globule, then it is easier to accept that intracranial stresses may have played a significant part. The role of alcoholic intoxication – another hotly disputed aspect – has been discussed in Chapter 5. The legal problem is similar in berry aneurysm deaths to that in coronary disease. The time interval is naturally important, though in most instances, bleeding occurs immediately or soon afterwards.

Autopsy is not all that helpful in assessing the relative contribution of assault versus pre-existing disease. Unless the aneurysm is found to be large and fragile, the morphological findings are mainly of use in confirming the diagnosis, evaluating any injuries and excluding any other contributory disease. It used to be the usual practice in England and Wales not to prosecute assailants when an aneurysm was demonstrated at autopsy, though in Scotland and on the continent of Europe no such reluctance was evident. Following a case in Gibraltar in 1978, however, in which a British sailor was convicted of homicide after kicking another in a drunken brawl, the latter eventually dying of subarachnoid haemorrhage from a ruptured aneurysm, such charges are now usually brought (Knight 1979).

Pulmonary embolism

The other major example of the interaction of trauma and natural disease is pulmonary embolism. This is discussed in Chapter 13, but is so important in medico-legal casework that the forensic aspects may be repeated here with advantage.

Deep vein thrombosis, almost always in the leg veins, is a common sequel to injury and consequent immobility. Virchow's triad of slowing of the circulation, local injury to vessel walls and increase in blood coagulability are the major factors, though deep vein thrombosis can occur in the absence of all three. When the leg is the site of the injury, it is more likely to occur in the ipsilateral limb, though it can occur contralaterally or bilaterally. The fact that a fatal embolus came from the contralateral limb when the other leg has been injured by no means rules out a causative element.

Pulmonary embolism typically occurs about 2 weeks after an injury or surgical operation, but the range of time during which a cause-and-effect mechanism operates can be anything from about 2 to 90 days. It becomes progressively more difficult to maintain a causative relationship, however, when the interval exceeds a few weeks.

Forensically, it is vital to show that the deep vein thrombosis post-dated the traumatic event, if an association is to be established. If a person suffers a fatal embolism a week after injury, yet histologically the deep vein thrombosis appears to be several weeks old, then obviously the injury could not have initiated the process. The embolus may, however, be much younger than the most distal part of the leg vein thrombosis (which may be as far down as the foot) as progressive proximal extension of a deep vein thrombosis undoubtedly occurs. It could still be argued, therefore, that although the original thrombosis antedated the injury, the latter encouraged extension and hence the eventual breaking off of an embolus. The case becomes weaker, however, than if the whole process was entirely subsequent to the traumatic event.

Histological dating of the embolus should always be undertaken, though it is less rewarding and more difficult than that of the leg vein thrombi, which must always be taken for microscopy with the vein wall intact. It is the thrombomural junction that gives the most information about the age of any thrombus. Thrombosis of the deep leg veins is far more common than pulmonary thromboembolism. In 100 consecutive coroner's autopsies, Knight and Zaini (1980) found 32 instances of deep vein thrombosis, but only 10 had pulmonary emboli, not all fatal.

The legal problem, outlined in Chapter 13, is that though trauma, surgery and immobility are potent factors in the development of deep vein thrombosis, the latter condition frequently occurs in the absence of all three. Thus it is difficult to maintain that any traumatic event was the cause of a subsequent fatal pulmonary embolism, as many fatal emboli occur in the absence of trauma. In a series of coroner's and hospital autopsies studied by Knight (1966), 25 per cent of fatal pulmonary emboli came 'out of the blue' in ambulant people who had no previous history of trauma or surgical operation. Later, Knight and Zaini studied 38 000 autopsy reports and found that 10 per cent of deaths due to pulmonary embolism had no history of any predisposing factors. The discrepancy in these proportions is caused by the variable standard of history reports and also by marked alterations in pathologist's reporting habits over the years – in fact, in the large series mentioned above, there was not a single fatal pulmonary embolism recorded in the 20 years from 1908 until 1928!

Even disregarding the dubious statistical value of such investigations, there can be no doubt that a significant proportion of fatal pulmonary emboli cannot be related to previous trauma. This provides a line of defence in those cases where the prosecution allege that a 'cause-and-effect' relationship exists between some criminal assault and death. It becomes a matter of law for the judge to decide whether he will let the issue go to the jury, and a matter of fact for the jury to decide whether this relationship can be 'beyond reasonable doubt' in circumstances where even conservatively, at least 10 per cent of pulmonary emboli are not related to trauma. Several court cases are within the author's (BK) experience in which quite different verdicts have been reached on essentially identical pathological evidence.

In civil cases, usually related to road traffic accidents or industrial personal injuries, the burden on the plaintiff is much lighter, as the 'balance of probabilities' test can be much more readily satisfied.

REFERENCES AND FURTHER READING

Al Rufaie HK, Florio RA, Olsen EG. 1983. Comparison of the haematoxylin basic fuchsin picric acid method and the fluorescence of haematoxylin and eosin stained sections for the identification of early myocardial infarction. *J Clin Pathol* **36**:646–9.

Anderson HN. 1964. An evaluation and comparison of macroscopic enzyme techniques for the autopsy demonstration of myocardial infarction. *J Pathol* **127**:93–8.

Ansari A, Maron BJ, Berntson DG. 2003. Drug-induced toxic myocarditis. *Tex Heart Inst J* **30**:76–9.

Aretz HT. 1987. Myocarditis: the Dallas criteria. *Hum Pathol* **18**:619–24.

Aretz HT, Billingham ME, Edwards WD, *et al.* 1987. Myocarditis. A histopathologic definition and classification. *Am J Cardiovasc Pathol* **1**:3–14.

Badir B, Knight B. 1987. Fluorescence microscopy in the detection of early myocardial infarction. *Forensic Sci Int* **34**:99–102.

Bajanowski T, Rossi L, Biondo B, *et al.* 2001. Prolonged QT interval and sudden infant death – report of two cases. *Forensic Sci Int* **115**:147–53.

Balachandra AT, O'Conner R, Bowden DH. 1987. Sudden unexpected death in asthmatics. *J Can Forensic Sci* **20**:227.

Baroldi G. 1975. Different types of myocardial necrosis in coronary heart disease: a pathophysiologic review of their functional significance. *Am Heart J* **89**:742–52.

Bateman JR, Clarke SW. 1979. Sudden death in asthma. *Thorax* **34**:40–4.

Bjork VD. 1964. *Cardiomyopathies.* Ciba Foundation Symposium. Churchill, London.

Bostrom H. 1966. Acute epiglottitis as a cause of sudden death. *Dtsch Z Gesamte Gerichtl Med* **61**:53–9.

Bouchardy B, Majno G. 1971. A new approach to the histologic diagnosis of early myocardial infarcts. *Cardiology* **56**:327–32.

Bouchardy B, Majno G. 1974. Histopathology of early myocardial infarcts. A new approach. *Am J Pathol* **74**:301–30.

Cameron HM, McGoogan E. 1981. A prospective study of 1152 hospital autopsies: I. Inaccuracies in death certification. *J Pathol* **133**:273–83.

Cardell BS, Pearson RS. 1959. Death in asthmatics. *Thorax* **14**:341–52.

Carle BN. 1981. Autofluorescence in the identification of myocardial infarcts. *Hum Pathol* **12**:643–6.

Champ CS, Byard RW. 1994. Sudden death in asthma in childhood. *Forensic Sci Int* **66**:117–27.

Chan AC, Dickens P. 1992. Tuberculous myocarditis presenting as sudden cardiac death. *Forensic Sci Int* **57**:45–50.

Clark JC. 1988. Sudden death in the chronic alcoholic. *Forensic Sci Int* **36**:105–11.

Clawson BJ. 1928. Myocarditis. *Am Heart J* **4**:1–7.

Cochrane GM, Clark JH. 1975. A survey of asthma mortality in patients between ages 35 and 64 in the greater London hospitals in 1971. *Thorax* **30**:300–5.

Copeland AR. 1986. Asthmatic deaths in the medical examiner's population. *Forensic Sci Int* **31**:7–12.

Corby C. 1960. Isolated myocarditis as a cause for sudden obscure death. *Med Sci Law* **1**:1–40.

Crawford T. 1977. *Pathology of ischaemic heart disease.* Butterworth, London.

Curfman GD. 1993. Is exercise beneficial – or hazardous – to your heart? [editorial; comment] [see comments]. *N Engl J Med* **329**:1730–1.

Cushing EH. 1942. Infarction of the cardiac auricles. *Br Heart J* **4**:17–26.

Davies M, Pomerance A. 1975. *Pathology of the heart.* Blackwell Scientific Publications, Oxford.

Davies MJ. 1981. Pathological view of sudden cardiac death. *Br Heart J* **45**:88–96.

Davies MJ, Popple A. 1979. Sudden unexpected cardiac death – a practical approach to the forensic problem. *Histopathology* **3**:255–77.

Decastello A, Remenar E, Toth J, *et al.* 1977. Post mortem detection of early myocardial infarction by determination of the tissue K^+/Na^+ ratio. *Acta Morphol Acad Sci Hung* **25**:289–96.

Derias NW, Adams CW. 1979. The non-specific nature of the myocardial wavy fibre. *Histopathology* **3**:241–5.

Derias NW, Adams CW. 1982. Macroscopic enzyme histochemistry in myocardial infarction: use of coenzyme, cyanide, and phenazine methosulphate. *J Clin Pathol* **35**:410–13.

deSa DJ. 1986. Isolated myocarditis as a cause of sudden death in the first year of life. *Forensic Sci Int* **30**:113–17.

Dettmeyer R, Schlamann M, Madea B. 1999. Immunohistochemical techniques improve the diagnosis of myocarditis in cases of suspected sudden infant death syndrome (SIDS). *Forensic Sci Int* **105**:83–94.

Dettmeyer R, Kandolf R, Schmidt P, *et al.* 2001. Lympho-monocytic enteroviral myocarditis: traditional, immunohistological and molecular pathological methods for diagnosis in a case of suspected sudden infant death syndrome (SIDS). *Forensic Sci Int* **119**:141–4.

Dettmeyer R, Reith K, Madea B. 2002. Alcoholic cardiomyopathy versus chronic myocarditis – immunohistological investigations with LCA, CD3, CD68 and tenascin. *Forensic Sci Int* **126**:57–62.

Drury RA. 1954. The role of intimal haemorrhage in coronary occlusion. *J Pathol Bacteriol* **67**:207–15.

Edston E. 1997. Evaluation of agonal artifacts in the myocardium using a combination of histological stains and immunohistochemistry. *Am J Forensic Med Pathol* **18**:163–7.

Edston E, Kawa K. 1995. Immunohistochemical detection of early myocardial infarction. An evaluation of antibodies against the terminal complement complex (C5b-9). *Int J Legal Med* **108**:27–30.

English JP, Williams FA. 1943. Haemorrhagic lesions of the coronary arteries. *Arch Intern Med* **71**:594–602.

Falconer B, Rajs J. 1976. Post-mortem findings of cardiac lesions in epileptics: a preliminary report. *Forensic Sci* **8**:63–71.

Farrer-Brown G. 1968. Normal and diseased vascular pattern of myocardium of human heart. I. Normal pattern in the left ventricular free wall. *Br Heart J* **30**:527–36.

Farrer-Brown G. 1977. *A colour atlas of cardiac pathology.* Wolfe Medical Publications, London.

Feibel JH, Campbell RG, Joynt RJ. 1976. Myocardial damage and cardiac arrhythmias in cerebral infarction and subarachnoid hemorrhage: correlation with increased systemic catecholamine output. *Trans Am Neurol Assoc* **101**:242–4.

Feldman AM, McNamara D. 2000. Myocarditis. *N Engl J Med* **343**:1388–98.

Feldman S, Glagov S, Wissler RW, *et al.* 1976. Postmortem delineation of infarcted myocardium. Coronary perfusion with nitro blue tetrazolium. *Arch Pathol Lab Med* **100**:55–8.

Ferris JA. 1974. Conducting tissue changes in sudden death. *Med Sci Law* **14**:36–9.

Ferris JA, Friesen JM. 1979. Definitions of ischaemia, infarction and necrosis. *Forensic Sci Int* **13**:253–9.

Ferris JA, MacLennan JR. 1973. A simplified method for examining the conducting tissues of the heart. *Med Sci Law* **13**:285–8.

Ferris JA, Rice J. 1979. Drug-induced myocarditis: a report of two cases. *Forensic Sci Int* **13**:261–5.

Fleming HA. 1988. Death from sarcoid heart disease: United Kingdom series 1971–1986, 300 cases with 138 deaths. In: Grassi C (ed.), *Sarcoidosis and other granulomatous disorders.* Excerpta Medica, Amsterdam, pp. 19–33.

Fleming HA, Bailey SM. 1981. Sarcoid heart disease. *J R Coll Physicians Lond* **15**:245–6, 249–53.

Fothergill DF, Bowen DA, Mason JK. 1979. Dissecting and atherosclerotic aneurysms: a survey of post-mortem examinations, 1968–77. *Med Sci Law* **19**:253–60.

Fraser PM, Speizer FE, Waters SD, *et al.* 1971. The circumstances preceding death from asthma in young people in 1968 to 1969. *Br J Dis Chest* **65**:71–84.

Fukumoto H, Naito Z, Asano G, *et al.* 1998. Immunohistochemical and morphometric evaluations of coronary atherosclerotic plaques associated with myocardial infarction and diabetes mellitus. *J Atheroscler Thromb* **5**:29–35.

Glogner. 1903. Cited by Stamer. 1907. *Virchows Arch Pathol Anat* 171.

Gore I, Saphir O. 1947. Myocarditis: a classification of 1042 cases. *Am Heart J* **34**:827–41.

Gormsen H. 1955. Sudden unexplained death due to myocarditis. *Acta Pathol Microbiol Scand* **105**(Suppl):303.

Gregersen M. 1979. Myocardial changes in sudden unexpected coronary deaths. *Forensic Sci Int* **13**:183–6.

Hansen SH, Rossen K. 1999. Evaluation of cardiac troponin I immunoreaction in autopsy hearts: a possible marker of early myocardial infarction. *Forensic Sci Int* **99**:189–96.

Hiltunen JK, Saukko P, Hirvonen J. 1985. Correlations between enzyme histochemical reactions and respective enzyme activities in global ischaemic rat hearts. *Br J Exp Pathol* **66**:743–52.

Hirvonen J, Hiltunen JK, Saukko P. 1987. Oxidative enzyme activities and respective histochemical reactions in ischemic rat myocardium. *Forensic Sci Int* **35**:231–6.

Holmbom B, Lindstrom M, Naslund U, *et al.* 1991. A method for enzyme- and immunohistochemical staining of large frozen specimens. *Histochemistry* **95**:441–7.

Hougen HP, Valenzuela A, Lachica E, *et al.* 1992. Sudden cardiac death: a comparative study of morphological, histochemical and biochemical methods. *Forensic Sci Int* **52**:161–9.

House RK. 1948. Diffuse interstitial myocarditis in children. *Am J Pathol* **24**:1235–48.

Hu BJ, Chen YC, Zhu JZ. 1996. Immunohistochemical study of fibronectin for postmortem diagnosis of early myocardial infarction. *Forensic Sci Int* **78**:209–17.

Hudson RE. 1963. The human conducting system and its examination. *J Clin Pathol* **16**:492–8.

Hudson RE. 1970. The cardiomyopathies: order from chaos. *Am J Cardiol* **25**:70–7.

Ikegaya H, Heino J, Laaksonen H, *et al.* 2003. Accumulation of fibrinogen in Purkinje cells in sudden death in epilepsy. *Forensic Sci Int* accepted for publication.

Inman WH, Adelstein AM. 1969. Rise and fall of asthma mortality in England and Wales in relation to use of pressurised aerosols. *Lancet* **2**:279–85.

Iwadate K, Tanno K, Doi M, *et al.* 2001. Two cases of right ventricular ischemic injury due to massive pulmonary embolism. *Forensic Sci Int* **116**:189–95.

Jaakkola K, Jalkanen S, Kaunismaki K, *et al.* 2000. Vascular adhesion protein-1, intercellular adhesion molecule-1 and P-selectin mediate leukocyte binding to ischemic heart in humans. *J Am Coll Cardiol* **36**:122–9.

Jääskeläinen AJ. 1968. Histochemical observations on phosphorylase, cytochrome oxidase and succinic dehydrogenase in experimental and human fresh myocardial infarcts. *Ann Univ Turku* **Series A II**(Suppl 39):1–64.

Jackson RT, Beaglehole R, Rea HH, *et al.* 1982. Mortality from asthma: a new epidemic in New Zealand. *Br Med J Clin Res Ed* **285**:771–4.

James TN. 1996. Long reflections on the QT interval: the sixth annual Gordon K. Moe lecture. *J Cardiovasc Electrophysiol* **7**:738–59.

Johnson AJ, Nunn AJ, Somner AR, *et al.* 1984. Circumstances of death from asthma. *Br Med J Clin Res Ed* **288**:1870–2.

Karhunen PJ, Penttilä A, Erkinjuntti T. 1990. Arteriovenous malformation of the brain: imaging by postmortem angiography. *Forensic Sci Int* **48**:9–19.

Kherdar A, Nevins MA. 1973. Right ventricular infarction. *Med Soc New Jersey* **70**:374–8.

Knight B. 1965. The postmortem detection of early myocardial infarction. *Med Sci Law* **5**:31–46.

Knight B. 1966. Fatal pulmonary embolism: factors of forensic interest in 400 cases. *Med Sci Law* **6**:150–4.

Knight B. 1967. Early myocardial infarction. Practical methods for its post-mortem demonstration. *J Forensic Med* **14**:101–7.

Knight B. 1971. The value of enzyme techniques in medicolegal pathology. In: Wecht C (ed.), *Legal medicine annual 1971*. Appleton Century Crofts, New York.

Knight B. 1973. The myocardium in sudden death from hypertensive heart disease or aortic stenosis. *Med Sci Law* **13**:280–4.

Knight B. 1976. Investigation of sudden deaths from myocardial ischaemia. *Forensic Sci* **8**:33–6.

Knight B. 1979. A further evaluation of the reliability of the HBFP stain in demonstrating myocardial damage. *Forensic Sci Int* **13**:179–81.

Knight B. 1979. Trauma and ruptured cerebral aneurysm. *Br Med J* **1**:1430–1.

Knight B, Zaini MR. 1980. Pulmonary embolism and venous thrombosis. A pattern of incidence and predisposing factors over 70 years. *Am J Forensic Med Pathol* **1**:227–32.

Knight BH. 1966. *The postmortem diagnosis of early myocardial infarction*. Cardiff University of Wales, Cardiff.

Lachica E, Villanueva E, Luna A. 1988. Comparison of different techniques for the postmortem diagnosis of myocardial infarction. *Forensic Sci Int* **38**:21–6.

Leadbeatter S, Stansbie D. 1984. Postmortem diagnosis of familial hypercholesterolaemia. *Br Med J Clin Res Ed* **289**:1656.

Leadbeatter S, Wawman H, Jasani B. 1989. Immuno-cytochemical diagnosis of early ischaemic/hypoxic damage in myocardium. *Acta Med Leg Soc (Liege)* **39**:187–8.

Leadbeatter S, Wawman HM, Jasani B. 1990. Further evaluation of immunocytochemical staining in the diagnosis of early myocardial ischaemic/hypoxic damage. *Forensic Sci Int* **45**:135–41.

Leestma JE, Kalelkar MB, Teas SS, *et al.* 1984. Sudden unexpected death associated with seizures: analysis of 66 cases. *Epilepsia* **25**:84–8.

Leestma JE, Hughes JR, Teas SS, *et al.* 1985. Sudden epilepsy deaths and the forensic pathologist. *Am J Forensic Med Pathol* **6**:215–18.

Lie JT, Holley KE, Kampa WR, *et al.* 1971. New histochemical method for morphologic diagnosis of early stages of myocardial ischemia. *Mayo Clin Proc* **46**:319–27.

Luke JL, Helpern M. 1968. Sudden unexpected death from natural causes in young adults. A review of 275 consecutive autopsied cases. *Arch Pathol* **85**:10–17.

Macdonald JB, Seaton A, Williams DA. 1976. Asthma deaths in Cardiff 1963–74: 90 deaths outside hospital. *Br Med J* **1**:1493–5.

Maisch B, Ristic AD, Portig I, *et al.* 2003. Human viral cardiomyopathy. *Front Biosci* **8**:S39–67.

Malik MA. 1973. Emotional stress as a precipitating factor in sudden deaths due to coronary insufficiency. *J Forensic Sci* **18**:47–52.

Malik MO. 1979. Sudden coronary deaths associated with sexual activity. *J Forensic Sci* **24**:216–20.

Mallory GK, White PD, Salcedo-Salgar J. 1939. The speed of healing of myocardial infarction. *Am Heart J* **18**:647–71.

Manion WC. 1966. Myocarditis: a review of the development of the concept. *Med Ann D C* **35**:405–13 passim.

Mann JI. 1984. Familial hypercholesterolaemia: renewed interest in an old problem [editorial]. *Br Med J Clin Res Ed* **289**:396.

Maron BJ. 1983. Myocardial disorganisation in hypertrophic cardiomyopathy. Another point of view. *Br Heart J* **50**:1–3.

Maron BJ. 2002. Hypertrophic cardiomyopathy: a systematic review. *JAMA* **287**:1308–20.

Marshall TK. 1970. Asymmetrical hypertrophy of the heart. *Med Sci Law* **10**:3–6.

Martin AB, Webber S, Fricker FJ, *et al.* 1994. Acute myocarditis. Rapid diagnosis by PCR in children. *Circulation* **90**:330–9.

Martin AM, Jr, Hackel DB. 1966. An electron microscopic study of the progression of myocardial lesions in the dog after hemorrhagic shock. *Lab Invest* **15**:243–60.

Martin AM, Jr, Hackel DB, Entman ML, *et al.* 1969. Mechanisms in the development of myocardial lesions in hemorrhagic shock. *Ann NY Acad Sci* **156**:79–90.

Mittleman MA, Maclure M, Tofler GH, *et al.* 1993. Triggering of acute myocardial infarction by heavy physical exertion. Protection against triggering by regular exertion. Determinants of myocardial infarction onset study investigators [see comments]. *N Engl J Med* **329**:1677–83.

Morild I, Giertsen JC. 1989. Sudden death from asthma. *Forensic Sci Int* **42**:145–50.

Möttönen M. 1970. Myocardial infarction and coronary atherosclerosis in forensic autopsy material. *Med Sci Law* **10**:115–19.

Nayar A, Olsen EG. 1974. The use of the basic fuchsin stain in the recognition of early myocardial ischaemia. *Cardiovasc Res* **8**:391–4.

Noren GR, Staley NA, Bandt CM, *et al.* 1977. Occurrence of myocarditis in sudden death in children. *J Forensic Sci* **22**:188–96.

Northcote RJ, Ballantyne D. 1983. Sudden cardiac death in sport. *Br Med J Clin Res Ed* **287**:1357–9.

Olsen EG. 1987. *Atlas of cardiovascular pathology.* MTP Press, Lancaster.

Osborn GR. 1963. *The incubation period of coronary thrombosis.* Butterworth, London.

Otsuka N, Hara T. 1965. Gross demonstration of the mammalian atrioventricular bundle by a periodic acid-Schiff procedure. *Stain Technol* **40**:305–8.

Park HY, Weinstein SR. 1990. Sudden unexpected nocturnal death syndrome in the Mariana islands [see comments]. *Am J Forensic Med Pathol* **11**:205–7.

Patterson JC. 1938. Capillary rupture with intimal haemorrhage as a causative factor in coronary thrombosis. *Arch Pathol* **25**:474–87.

Paul M, Schulze-Bahr E, Breithardt G, *et al.* 2003. Genetics of arrhythmogenic right ventricular cardiomyopathy – status quo and future perspectives. *Z Kardiol* **92**:128–36.

Paz Suarez-Mier M, Aguilera B. 1998. Histopathology of the conduction system in sudden infant death. *Forensic Sci Int* **93**:143–54.

Pedersen PK. 1980. Determination of potassium/sodium ratio in heart tissue. Evaluation of its use as an index of myocardial ischaemic damage. Comparison with the nitro-BT test. *Forensic Sci Int* **16**:271–80.

Penttilä A. 1980. Sudden and unexpected natural deaths of adult males. An analysis of 799 forensic autopsies in 1976. *Forensic Sci Int* **16**:249–59.

Phillips LH, Whisnant JP, Reagan TJ. 1977. Sudden death from stroke. *Stroke* **8**:392–5.

Piano MR. 2002. Alcoholic cardiomyopathy: incidence, clinical characteristics, and pathophysiology. *Chest* **121**:1638–50.

Piro FR, di Gioia CR, Gallo P, *et al.* 2000. Is apoptosis a diagnostic marker of acute myocardial infarction? *Arch Pathol Lab Med* **124**:827–31.

Plueckhahn VD, Cameron JM. 1968. Traumatic 'myocarditis' or 'myocarditis' in trauma. *Med Sci Law* **8**:177–80.

Preston HV, Bowen DA. 1987. Asthma deaths: a review. *Med Sci Law* **27**:89–94.

Priemer F, Keil W, Kandolf R. 1999. Hydrocution in a case of coxsackie virus infection. *Int J Legal Med* **112**:368–71.

Ramkissoon RA. 1966. Macroscopic identification of early myocardial infarction by dehydrogenase alterations. *J Clin Pathol* **19**:479–81.

Rammer L, Jansson O. 1976. Determination of electrolytes in the myocardium as a tool for the post-mortal diagnosis of recent infarction. *Forensic Sci* **8**:127–30.

Rampazzo A, Beffagna G, Nava A, *et al.* 2003. Arrhythmogenic right ventricular cardiomyopathy type 1 (ARVD1): confirmation of locus assignment and mutation screening of four candidate genes. *Eur J Hum Genet* **11**:69–76.

Randall B. 1980. Fatty liver and sudden death. A review. *Hum Pathol* **11**:147–53.

Reichenbach D, Benditt EP. 1970. Myofibrillar degeneration: a common form of cardiac muscle injury. *Ann NY Acad Sci* **156**:164–76.

Richardson HL, Graupner KI, Richardson ME. 1966. Intramyocardial lesions in patients dying suddenly and unexpectedly. *JAMA* **195**:254–60.

Richardson P, McKenna W, Bristow M, *et al.* 1996. Report of the 1995 World Health Organization/ International Society and Federation of Cardiology Task Force on the Definition and Classification of Cardiomyopathies. *Circulation* **93**:841–2.

Rubin E. 1979. Alcoholic myopathy in heart and skeletal muscle. *N Engl J Med* **301**:28–33.

Rump AF, Theisohn M, Klaus W. 1995. The pathophysiology of cocaine cardiotoxicity. *Forensic Sci Int* **71**:103–15.

Rus HG, Niculescu F, Vlaicu R. 1987. Presence of C5b-9 complement complex and S-protein in human myocardial areas with necrosis and sclerosis. *Immunol Lett* **16**:15–20.

Rutenburg AM, Wolman M, Seligman AM. 1953. Comparative distribution of succinic dehydrogenase in six mammals and modification in the histochemical technic. *J Histochem Cytochem* **1**:66–81.

Sahai VB, Knight B. 1976. The post-mortem detection of early myocardial infarction by a simple fluorescent method. *Med Sci Law* **16**:17–20.

Sakurai S, Inoue A, Ohwa M, *et al.* 1995. [Immunohistochemical analysis of adhesion molecules in directional coronary atherectomy specimens.] *J Cardiol* **26**:139–47.

Sandritter M, Jedstadt R. 1958. Triphenyltetrazolium (TTC) als reduktionsindikator zur makroscopischen diagnose des frischen herzinfarktes. *Zent Allg Pathol* **97**:188–9.

Saphir O. 1942. Myocarditis: general review with analysis of 240 cases. *Arch Pathol* **33**:88–99.

Saphir O, Wile SA, Reingold IM. 1944. Myocarditis in children. *Am J Dis Child* **67**:294–312.

Saraste A, Pulkki K, Kallajoki M, *et al.* 1999. Cardio-myocyte apoptosis and progression of heart failure to transplantation. *Eur J Clin Invest* **29**:380–6.

Särkioja T, Hirvonen J. 1984. Causes of sudden unexpected deaths in young and middle-aged persons. *Forensic Sci Int* **24**:247–61.

Saukko P. 1983. Evaluation of diagnostic methods for early myocardial injury in sudden cardiac deaths. *Acta Univ Oul D 107, Anat Pathol Microbiol* **17**:53.

Saukko P, Knight B. 1989. Evaluation of eosin-fluorescence in the diagnosis of sudden cardiac death. *Forensic Sci Int* **40**:285–90.

Saukko P, Lignitz E. 1990. [Sudden death caused by malignant testicular tumors.] *Z Rechtsmed* **103**:529–36.

Schwender LA, Troncoso JC. 1986. Evaluation of sudden death in epilepsy. *Am J Forensic Med Pathol* **7**:283–7.

Seligman AM, Rutenburg AM. 1951. The histochemical demonstration of succinic dehydrogenase. *Science* **113**:317–20.

Sepulchre MA, Fechner G. 1992. [Detection of ischemic myocardial damage.] *Beitr Gerichtl Med* **50**:161–7.

Siboni A, Simonsen J. 1986. Sudden unexpected natural death in young persons. *Forensic Sci Int* **31**:159–66.

Simonsen J, Falk E. 1980. A case of sudden cardiac death in connection with *Salmonella typhimurium* infection. *Forensic Sci Int* **16**:283–7.

Simpson CK. 1947. Pathology of sudden death. *Lancet* **2**:745–7.

Siscovick DS, Weiss NS, Fletcher RH, *et al.* 1984. The incidence of primary cardiac arrest during vigorous exercise. *N Engl J Med* **311**:874–7.

Smith AJ. 1904–5. On the histological behaviour of the cardiac muscle in two examples of organization of myocardial infarct. *Univ Pennsylvania Med Bull* **17**:227–34.

Sokrab TE, Johansson BB, Kalimo H, *et al.* 1988. A transient hypertensive opening of the blood-brain barrier can lead to brain damage. Extravasation of serum proteins and cellular changes in rats subjected to aortic compression. *Acta Neuropathol (Berl)* **75**:557–65.

Song Y, Zhu J, Laaksonen H, *et al.* 1997. A modified method for examining the cardiac conduction system. *Forensic Sci Int* **86**:135–8.

Song Y, Laaksonen H, Saukko P, *et al.* 2001. Histopathological findings of cardiac conduction system of 150 finns. *Forensic Sci Int* **119**:310–17.

Sopher IM. 1974. Myocarditis and the aircraft accident. *Aerosp Med* **45**:963–7.

Speizer FE, Doll R, Heaf P, *et al.* 1968. Investigation into use of drugs preceding death from asthma. *Br Med J* **1**:339–43.

Speizer FE, Doll R, Heaf P. 1982. Observations on recent increase in mortality from asthma. *Br Med J* **285**:1251–5.

Stamer A. 1907. Untersuchungen über die Fragmentation und Segmentation des Herzmuskels. *Beitr Pathol* **42**:310–53.

Stevens PJ, Ground KE. 1970. Occurrence and significance of myocarditis in trauma. *Aerosp Med* **41**:776–80.

Stolley PD, Schinnar R. 1978. Association between asthma mortality and isoproterenol aerosols: a review. *Prev Med* **7**:519–38.

Tada T, Okada H, Okada N, *et al.* 1997. Membrane attack complex of complement and 20 kDa homologous restriction factor (CD59) in myocardial infarction. *Virchows Arch* **430**:327–32.

Teare D. 1958. Asymmetrical hypertrophy of the heart in young adults. *Br Heart J* **20**:1–8.

Thomas AC, Knapman PA, Krikler DM, *et al.* 1988. Community study of the causes of 'natural' sudden death. *Br Med J* **297**:1453–6.

Thomsen H, Held H. 1994. Susceptibility of C5b-9(m) to postmortem changes. *Int J Legal Med* **106**:291–3.

Thomsen H, Held H. 1995. Immunohistochemical detection of C5b-9(m) in myocardium: an aid in distinguishing infarction-induced ischemic heart muscle necrosis from other forms of lethal myocardial injury. *Forensic Sci Int* **71**:87–95.

Tonge JI, O'Reilly MJ, Davison A, *et al.* 1972. Traffic crash fatalities. Injury patterns and other factors. *Med J Aust* **2**:5–17.

Tonge JI, O'Reilly MJ, Davison A, *et al.* 1977. Traffic-crash fatalities (1968–73): injury patterns and other factors. *Med Sci Law* **17**:9–24.

Towbin JA, Bowles NE. 2002. The failing heart. *Nature* **415**:227–33.

Varga M, Zsonda L. 1988. A simple method for postmortem detection of acute myocardial infarction. *Forensic Sci Int* **37**:259–63.

Velisheva LS, Vikhert AM, Shvalev VN, *et al.* 1981. [Sudden cardiac death in alcoholic cardiomyopathy.] *Arkh Patol* **43**:32–7.

Wartmann WB. 1938. Occlusion of the coronary arteries by hemorrhage into their walls. *Am Heart J* **15**:459–66.

Wartmann WB, Hellerstein HK. 1948. The incidence of heart disease in 2000 consecutive autopsies. *Ann Intern Med* **28**:41–50.

Wartmann WB, Souders JC. 1950. Localization of myocardial infarction with respect to the muscle bundles of the heart. *Arch Pathol* **50**:329–38.

Whitehead R. 1965. Isolated myocarditis. *Br Heart J* **27**:220–4.

Willich SN, Lewis M, Lowel H, *et al.* 1993. Physical exertion as a trigger of acute myocardial infarction. Triggers and mechanisms of myocardial infarction study group [see comments]. *N Engl J Med* **329**:1684–90.

Wilson JD, Sutherland DC, Thomas AC. 1981. Has the change to beta-agonists combined with oral theophylline increased cases of fatal asthma? *Lancet* **1**:1235–7.

Wisten A, Forsberg H, Krantz P, *et al.* 2002. Sudden cardiac death in 15–35-year olds in Sweden during 1992–99. *J Intern Med* **252**:529–36.

World Health Organization. 1985. Sudden cardiac death. Report of a WHO Scientific Group. *WHO Tech Rep Ser* **726**:5–25.

Zhang JM, Riddick L. 1996. Cytoskeleton immuno-histochemical study of early ischemic myocardium. *Forensic Sci Int* **80**:229–38.

Zugibe FT, Conley TL, Bell P, Jr, *et al.* 1972. Enzyme decay curves in normal and infarcted myocardium. *Arch Pathol* **93**:308–11.

Forensic dentistry for the pathologist

Forensic odontology – the application of dentistry to forensic problems – is a discipline in itself and requires special dental expertise not possessed by pathologists qualified only in medicine. It is therefore imperative that, wherever possible, problems involving the teeth and jaws are referred to a dentist at an early stage, preferably at the time of the original autopsy or other examination of the subject.

A number of different circumstances need to be taken into account in this respect, however. First, it has to be accepted that by no means all dentists are either interested or competent in forensic problems. It is the same with pathologists, anatomists or any other specialists, in that the lack of enough motivation and experience can make their participation in legal matters of little value. A forensic odontologist naturally provides the best expertise, as he is professionally involved in the subject and will have training or experience, or both, of dento-legal problems, even though few forensic odontologists are occupied full time in this super-speciality, most being teachers or researchers in some other branch of dental science.

In many parts of the world, there are no forensic odontologists available. In developing countries there may be no forensic dentists at all – or the only expert is in the medical school of the capital city, inaccessible to distant areas. Even in more advanced states, problems of distance and travel may make it impracticable to call an odontologist to examine the body *in situ*. Dental expertise may be made available later, if material is retained for examination for transmission to the expert. In yet other circumstances, many problems of availability, cost and the lack of perceived importance of the case may make it impossible to involve an odontologist at an early stage – or even at all. In all these instances the pathologists or

other medico-legal doctor may have no choice but to handle the dental aspects as best he can, either in the initial stages or even throughout the investigation.

This chapter is meant to be nothing more than a guide for the doctor placed in this position and is certainly not intended to encourage pathologists to attempt to replace or dispense with a good odontological opinion. It cannot be sufficiently emphasized that, where the issues are serious, every effort should be made to obtain expert forensic dental assistance. The remainder of this chapter must be looked on solely as a 'first-aid primer' for cases in which the ideal investigation cannot be attained for one reason or another. If no expert dental advice can be obtained at the outset, then the pathologist should do all he can to assemble and preserve both detailed records and physical specimens, which can be examined later by a forensic odontologist, if one can be found further along the investigative pathway.

The assistance that dentistry can render falls into two broad headings:

- the interpretation of bite marks
- personal identification, either individually or in the context of mass disasters.

BITE MARKS

One of the two major interests of forensic odontologists is one that has direct relevance to pathologists in that it concerns the interpretation of trauma to the body surface. For the sake of completeness, however, mention must first be made of bite marks on inanimate objects, usually foodstuffs.

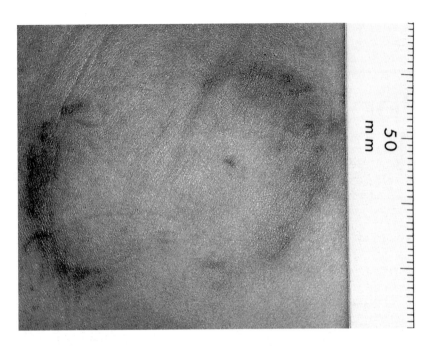

FIGURE 26.1 *Bite mark on skin. The two opposing bruises from the upper and lower dental arches are separated as usual by a gap, as only the front pans of the two arches contribute to the injury.*

This is mainly within the province of forensic science in the sense of 'criminalistics', where dental evidence is used to identify the perpetrators of a crime who happen to have left their teeth marks in some substance left at the scene. This rarely concerns forensic pathologists, except in the rare instance of their being asked by the police to examine an object, such as an apple or piece of cheese, to see if some obvious dental abnormality of a suspect could have caused the unusual bite mark.

The doctor may also be asked how the bite mark may be best preserved until the object can be examined by a forensic odontologist at a later date. Where the substance is 'plastic', such as butter, cheese, lard, wax or chocolate, for instance, it should be stored in a refrigerator to prevent melting or gradual flowing. It should not be deep frozen, as this may cause brittleness and cracking. Forensic science advice should be taken if at all available. Fruit, especially apples, seems prone to be bitten at scenes of crime, and Marshall *et al.* (1974) recommend preservation in Campden solution, a metabisulphite fluid used for fruit bottling. Alternatively, 5 per cent acetic acid in 40 per cent aqueous formaldehyde solution can be used. Ordinary histological formalin is not satisfactory – nor is refrigeration, which allows the fruit to shrivel. Whatever preservation is recommended to the police, the object should be adequately photographed with the film plane at right angles to the bite and a scale placed in the focal plane. If appropriate, swabbing for saliva traces should be carried out (see below) and then the fruit preserved for future examination.

Returning to the human body, bites are relatively common, especially in cases of child abuse and in adult sexual assault. In the former, bites may be anywhere on the infant, favourite sites being the arms, hands, shoulders, cheeks, buttocks and trunk. In the author's (BK) experience almost all bites on small children have been inflicted by the mother, but this is by no means invariable in the generality of child abuse. A common excuse from the parents is that the infant was bitten by another sibling or by the family dog – and occasionally, this explanation may be true. Others may be self-inflicted. It is therefore vital that the bite mark be properly examined to determine whether it is of a size consistent with adult dentition, or whether it is small enough to have come from another child – or is of a different shape, indicative of an animal.

The other common circumstances in which human bite marks occur are rape or other sexual offences. Here the pathologist will need to examine bites as part of the autopsy in a sexual murder – or even sometimes in live victims of an assault, if it is part of his duties to deal with clinical examinations or where no 'police surgeon' or forensic physician is available.

In this type of crime, bites may be sexually orientated or be distributed on any part of the body. Common sites are the breasts and nipples, but the neck, shoulders, thighs, abdomen, pubis and even vulva may be attacked. As noted in the chapter on sexual homicide, care must be taken to recognize that some so-called 'love bites', especially with suction petechiae, may be part of acceptable (if over-enthusiastic) sexual intercourse, but where real damage occurs, especially to breasts and nipples, then a violent or sadistic element is likely.

Bites may also be inflicted on police officers when attempting to arrest resisting offenders. They are also suffered in sporting events, especially football and some forms of wrestling, and during assaults when the victim manages to bite the assailant. In these instances bites may be

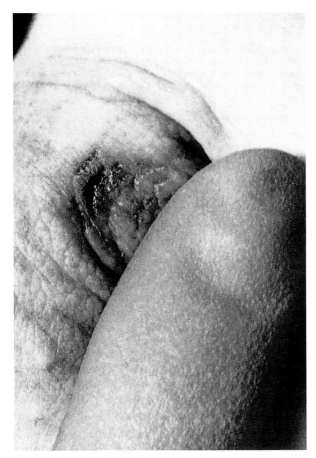

FIGURE 26.2 *Bite mark on a nipple during sexual homicide. The injury is too small for any dental matching, but a saliva sample might provide the blood group of the assailant, if he is a secretor.*

inflicted anywhere, but the hands, fingers, nose, forearms, ears and even lips may be the targets.

Some bite marks are self-inflicted; falls onto the face or a fit may cause the tongue and lips to be badly bitten. Other persons deliberately bite themselves, sometimes to fabricate injuries for a variety of motives ranging from gain to psychiatric disorder. Multiple bite marks (especially of the suction type), which are seen on accessible areas of the shoulder and arms, raise the suspicion of self-infliction, especially in older children and teenage girls.

The nature of the bite mark

Though called a 'bite mark', some of the components of the application of the mouth to skin may not be from the actual teeth. The lips can transiently mark the skin if forcibly nipped, especially on children, though the marks are short-lived and rapidly fade in life, not persisting after death unless associated with petechiae. Suction can produce a crop of punctate haemorrhages, either small petechiae or larger ecchymoses merging into a confluent central bruise.

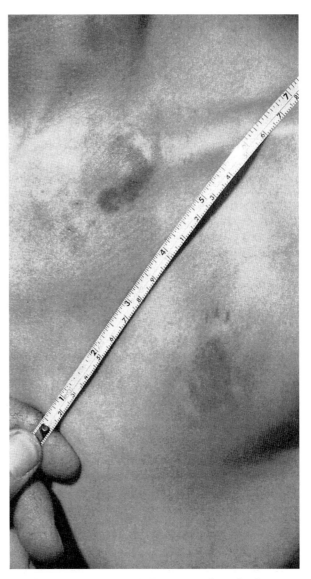

FIGURE 26.3 *Bite marks made during a sexual assault. The upper mark shows no specific features but its position is typical of a sexually orientated bite. The other shows central confluent petechiae and red bruising from suction and tongue pressure. There is a lower semi-circular pale zone corresponding with the lower lip, but the striking feature is the group of linear abrasions at the top of the mark made by the upper incisors dragging across the skin as the jaw is closed. Both bites are surrounded by zones of diffuse bruising.*

A human bite mark may present only a small part of the dental arcade, caused by the front teeth from canine to canine with an almost invariable gap at either side representing the separation of upper and lower jaw. A human bite is near circular or a shallow oval. A deep parabolic arch or a 'U-shape' can only be animal in origin. The teeth may cause clear, separate marks or they may run into each other to form a continuous or intermittently broken line. As time passes, originally clear tooth marks spread out and blur, progressively losing their definition – though abrasions on the skin surface retain their shape until scabbed healing is complete.

Teeth marks may be abrasions, bruises or laceration – or a combination of any two or three. The clarity of a bite mark depends on a number of factors. If the contour of the part bitten is irregular or markedly curved, then only part of the dental arch may contact the tissues. If the bite is forcible, then extensive subcutaneous bruising may spread laterally and blur the outline. If the bite was inflicted many days before, then healing of abrasions and lacerations, and absorption of bruising will leave progressively less detail. Where teeth have been forcibly applied, the typical appearance is of two 'bows' with their concavities facing each other and a gap at each end. Within this may sometimes be suction petechiae, which are often present without teeth marks, in the so-called 'love bite'. They are caused by the firm application of the lips, which form an airtight seal against the skin, then a sucking action reduces the air pressure over the centre. This causes a shower of petechial haemorrhages to appear from rupture of small venules in the superficial layers of the subcutaneous tissues. If forcible, the petechiae are confluent and a frank bruise, or even haematoma develops. Added to this is pressure from the tongue, pushing the tissues against the palate. This type of lesion is most often seen on the side of the neck and on the breasts of women, either in love play or after a sexual assault. They are by no means rare in child abuse, however, and are sometimes self-inflicted. Such a suction lesion must be human in origin and the claim that one is caused by a household pet can be immediately discounted.

Bites may be inflicted by the teeth closing down on a relatively flat skin surface, but there is usually an element of indrawing into the mouth, so that the teeth close down onto a parallel-sided or elliptical block of skin. In sexual bites, especially of the breast or nipple, the tissue may be actually sucked into the mouth before the jaws close upon it. This will naturally affect the shape of the resultant bite mark when the skin is released and flattens out once more.

Occasionally, the bite mark may not be two opposing arches, but more linear in pattern. This is seen especially where the upper incisors are scraped down the skin, leaving a series of parallel tracks, sometimes several centimetres long.

The lower incisors may leave either a curved line of static marks, or a straight or interrupted line below the upper incisor scrapes, as the lower teeth dig in and anchor the skin whilst the upper teeth gouge downwards towards them, during the act of closing the mouth.

The major problem with bite marks is the identification of the perpetrator and hence the problem cannot really be tackled without the expertise of a dentist fully experienced in this specialist task. Unless the dentition has some really characteristic features, especially in the incisors and canines,

then a non-dentist is a poor witness if the matter comes to a legal dispute. Some odontologists would claim that a bite mark can only be identified in a negative sense – that is, suspects can be excluded if their dentition is obviously incapable of inflicting the bite mark under investigation, but that no positive match can be claimed. Though many forensic odontologists would dispute this conservative claim, it is probably the best attitude for a pathologist involved in such a problem, unless there is some really spectacular and unique feature in the front teeth of a suspect.

Missing teeth, grossly displaced teeth and substantially damaged teeth may suggest a match with a person – or the mark may be quite inconsistent, which is helpful to the investigators if they eliminate a person or persons, especially in the restricted range of a family in which a child has been abused.

It is probably best for a pathologist to realize his limitations in this field, however, and to confine himself to taking the best physical evidence for later study by a forensic odontologist, where this is at all possible.

The investigation of a bite mark

As stated, every effort should be made to obtain the best evidence for future specialist examination. First, the bite mark should be carefully and fully photographed. If police facilities are to be used, the pathologist – as in other aspects of forensic pathology – should direct them as to the important features required on film. Often such photographers, though otherwise expert in the technical aspects of their craft, do not appreciate the problems that inadequate or inappropriate views can cause – especially at a later date, when experts reviewing the case and lawyers presenting it in court have to rely on photographs without the benefit of having seen the original lesions.

The photographs should be taken from several different angles, but especially from a directly perpendicular viewpoint, with the plane of the film at right angles to that of the lesion. Some police photographers persist in taking tangential shots that foreshorten the true shape. An accurate scale should always be adjacent to the lesion, as close as possible, but not impinging upon it or obscuring any detail.

Bites are often on a curved surface, such as the face, breast or arm, and thus can never be reproduced exactly on a flat surface, as there is bound to be slight foreshortening at the ends, but several views at slightly different angles can overcome this problem. Small lens apertures and short focal lengths will obviate the blurring that results from the lesion curving out of the focal plane. Too short a focal length will itself produce image distortion.

The lighting is important, as perpendicular lighting may lead to a flat rendering with no capture of detail. Side

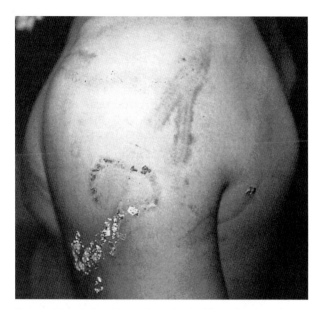

FIGURE 26.4 *A clear bite mark on the shoulder, a few days after infliction. This was from political abuse of human rights, there also being linear bruises on the shoulder and back from beating with a hose-pipe.*

lighting may throw small irregularities into relief, especially if there are tooth indentations in the skin. Both monochrome and colour photographs should be taken, with particular attention to sharp focus and correct exposure. The use of infrared-sensitive film has been recommended to reveal occult bruising, but it also appears to demonstrate artefacts. The lesion should almost fill the camera frame in some shots to capture as much detail as possible, either by short lesion-to-camera distance or the use of long-focus lenses. More general, wider shots should also be taken, however, to orientate the bite mark in relation to anatomical landmarks. During photography, care should be taken not to heat up the skin by the close proximity of high-power tungsten lamps. These should be placed at a distance or used only for short periods. Flash illumination will obviate this danger of heating the skin, which can distort the bite mark.

When photography is completed, swabs of the bite should be taken to try to recover saliva. Though not often successful, this technique can occasionally be vitally important in helping to identify or exclude the assailant, if he or she is one of the 80 per cent of people who are 'secretors', that is, who exude their blood-group substance in their saliva. Plain cotton-wool swabs are gently rubbed onto the bite – some experts recommend slightly moistening them first with water or saline. They should then be deep frozen unless sent straight to the serology laboratory.

Following photography and swabbing, there is usually little more that the pathologist can do in the absence of a dentist. If facilities are available and someone has the expertise, an impression of the bite can be made. This consists of laying a plastic substance over the bite mark, which then hardens, so as to produce a permanent negative cast of the lesion. It is usually made with a rubber- or silicone-based medium containing a catalytic hardener. Less satisfactory substances are water-based pastes, such as plaster of Paris, which are put on wet and allowed to dry before removal. These have the disadvantage of potential damage to the actual bite, if that is required for further evidential examination. Though it is unlikely that a pathologist will be able to carry out these procedures, it may be that a non-forensic dentist or a forensic scientist used to making casts of other evidence may be able to make satisfactory impressions that can then be preserved for later examination by an odontologist.

After autopsy, it is also possible for the whole area of skin carrying the bite to be removed and preserved in formalin for future examination. The shrinkage and distortion that are virtually inevitable, however, make these specimens of limited value for detailed tooth matching, though if good photographs with accurate scales are also available, they may be a useful addition to the dental evidence.

It is recommended that, as with all bruises and abrasions, the body be re-examined a few days after the first autopsy, as the appearances may be markedly enhanced. In a bite mark, faint or even absent original lesions may become more prominent, or even appear for the first time a day or two after death. The removal of skin carrying the lesion should be delayed if it is wished to see if this enhancement will occur, unless climatic conditions or lack of refrigeration would make this delay undesirable.

Matching the bite mark with the suspect's dentition

For a pathologist, this is such a specialist enterprise that it would rarely be attempted, unless there was no prospect whatsoever of a forensic dentist being available, even at a later date. As mentioned earlier, unless there is a striking dental feature in the bite mark or in the teeth of the suspect, the best that can be done is to try to exclude a limited number of potential assailants on the basis of lack of correspondence of their dentition with the bite mark. If neither mark nor teeth show any particular distinctive appearances, then even this should be avoided, without expert dental opinion. Where circumstances dictate that only the pathologist will ever be available to help the investigation, he should confine himself to the following routines:

■ The teeth of those who are either suspected by the police or who had access to the victim should be examined. In most jurisdictions it is vital that fully informed consent should be obtained from the person beforehand. The doctor must explain what he intends doing and the reason for doing it. It must be made clear that this is to be done for the purposes of a legal investigation and that any information gained might be used as evidence – and that it is not related to diagnosis or treatment for the subject's own welfare.

■ Any refusal must be a bar to any further action. Where children are concerned, usually in the setting of child abuse, the consent of the fully informed parents or guardian must be obtained. All such consent is preferably obtained in writing and many police forces have special forms for the purpose. If not written, then a dubious second best is getting oral consent; at least one witness to this must be obtained, if possible from independent persons other than relatives or police officers.

■ With consent, the dentition is then examined and the following points determined and recorded by diagram and writing. Photographs should also be taken if there is an issue of possible correspondence between the teeth and the bite – or where exclusion is legally important.

   – The presence of full or partial denture – and, if so, were they worn at the time of the incident?
   – The number of teeth in upper and lower jaw.
   – A charting of any missing teeth, especially incisors and canines.
   – An estimate of the bite overhang, or whether there is edge-to-edge occlusion or an undershoot projection of the lower teeth.
   – Recording of any broken teeth or teeth with significant individual abnormalities; these must be charted and described.
   – A record of any irregularity or marked variation in the cutting edge profile of any front teeth.
   – An evaluation of the size and prominence of any teeth, especially in the canines and incisors and any developmental abnormalities, such as an extra interposed front tooth.
   – Recording of any abnormality in the orientation of any tooth or teeth, such as twisting (rotation) in the anteroposterior tilting or double row of teeth. Gaps and irregular spacing are vital factors.

Though it is unlikely that a pathologist will have either the expertise or materials to make an impression of the bite, this might be attempted if no dental assistance of any kind is available – though the aid of a local dental practitioner would be useful in obtaining a wax or other bite registration. If this is impossible, then a bite impression into any available plastic substance might be attempted. The use of such substances as modelling clay, Plasticine, or beeswax might be

better than nothing if some unique feature required demonstration. Finally, whether it be from visual inspection of the teeth or from comparison with a cast, an attempt should be made to compare the characteristics of the bite mark with the dentition of the suspect or suspects. It is assumed that an animal bite will have already been excluded by this stage.

This comparison can be performed in various ways, different odontologists having their own techniques. Where marked abnormalities exist in the teeth, these may be present in the bite mark if the affected teeth happen to have registered in the lesion. Some forensic dentists prefer to match photographs of the mark with photographs or tracings of the teeth, the former being printed to a 1:1 magnification. Tracings can be made from positive casts of a bite impression, inking the cutting edges of the front teeth and transferring these to transparent sheets, which can then be laid over the photographs to determine correspondence. Others use a negative photograph of the teeth laid over a positive photograph of the bite, again ensuring exact correspondence of magnification.

In a bite mark it is said that a tooth impression is better evidence than an absent mark – in other words, the presence of a tooth mark means that the tooth was actually in the jaw, whereas a gap in the injury could either mean that the tooth was missing or merely that the occlusal edge had not marked the skin, perhaps because of slight shortening, unevenness or wear. In all matching procedures between a bite mark and the suspect teeth, allowance must be made for distortion of the skin surface during the biting process and the angle of attack of the teeth. Again it is emphasized that exclusion is probably a much safer exercise than an allegation of positive matching, unless there is some unique feature in the dentition. Unlike fingerprints, fewer points of definite correspondence are required to claim correspondence. This applies only in the hands of experts, where the number needed for a confident identification depends on the strength of the idiosyncratic features, but may be inferred from three or four identical points.

In practice, it is the six upper and six lower front teeth that give the most information. The canines may provide particular help when prominent and pointed. Premolars and molars are rarely useful, as might be expected from their lower profile and posterior position in the jaws.

IDENTIFICATION OF THE DEAD FROM THE DENTITION

The major contribution of forensic odontology is in the field of identification, especially in mass disasters, such as aviation and marine catastrophes. In air crashes, dental investigation is the most successful single procedure leading to identification of mutilated and burned bodies, as the passenger manifest lists provide a circumscribed population for whom dental records can be obtained in the majority of cases. In such disasters the involvement of dentists is imperative, but the size of the subject is far too large to be attempted in a book of this nature.

Apart from mass casualties, forensic odontology is frequently used in problems of individual identity that are the direct concern of the forensic pathologist, as accident, suicide and murder form the majority of such unidentified bodies.

As with skeletal remains (of which dental evidence is part), discussed in Chapter 3, there are two prime avenues of investigation:

- general or reconstructive identity, which attempts to classify the unknown person by age, sex and race
- comparative methods, which confirm or exclude the personal identity of the individual against ante-mortem dental records.

Once again, the pathologist can only act for the dentist in a 'second-best' way, when no forensic odontological expertise is available. Unlike bite marks, the material is likely to be much more permanent and, wherever possible, the pathologist should retain photographs, chartings and even the actual dentition against the time when expert dental opinion might become available. When time presses in a criminal inves-tigation, however, or where no dental help is ever likely to be forthcoming, then the pathologist has to do the best he can, though many special techniques such as radiology or tooth sections may be quite beyond his capabilities.

General or reconstructive identity

Unlike skeletal remains, the human origin of dental material is rarely in doubt. In badly decomposed or skeletalized bodies the jaws usually survive intact, though in dry skeletons, teeth may become loose and fall out, especially the single-rooted canines and incisors.

Even in fragmented bodies and skeletons, the jaw remnants and teeth are readily recognizable, even by lay persons. Where teeth have dropped out and been recovered independently of a body, they are still usually recognizable as human, as opposed to most domestic or farm animals. In countries where large primates exist, there may be some confusion, but this is a rare problem.

Having established the human origin, the next determination is sex and here teeth have a poor discriminating value, though the intact jaw is more helpful, as discussed in Chapter 3. Male teeth are usually larger, but this is generally unhelpful. The difference in size between the upper lateral

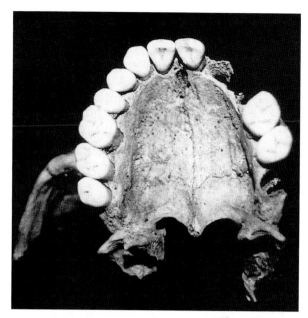

FIGURE 26.5 *Upper dental arch of a skeleton found buried on a small island in the Bristol Channel. The central incisors are 'shovel-shaped' and have a depressed groove on their posterior surface. This strongly suggests that the deceased was of mongoloid race.*

and upper central incisors is often greater in women, the male incisors being more equal in size. The female canines are usually smaller and more pointed relative to the male, more especially in the mandible than the maxilla. Girl's teeth tend to calcify and erupt earlier than boys. If the skeletal age is known, then more advanced tooth eruption in young persons is an indication of being female, though in these circumstances there are usually far better indicators of sex available elsewhere in the skeleton. The mandibular first molar often lacks a fifth cusp in the female, which is almost always present in the male. Extraction of pulp tissue from a tooth, even up to many months after extraction or death, can provide material for fluorescent staining for the female intranuclear F-body, as described in Chapter 3, but this has now been superseded by sex determination via DNA, if recoverable from the pulp.

Race is also a difficult criterion to determine from teeth. The best-known feature is the 'shovel-shaped' upper central incisors of Mongoloid races, first described in Leipzig by Muhlreiter in 1870. The posterior surfaces of these teeth have a depression centrally, with two marginal bars, causing the back of the tooth to appear like a coal shovel with turned-up edges. The feature is found mainly amongst Chinese, Mongols, Eskimos and Japanese, but is also found amongst non-Mongoloid races in lesser numbers. Some 91 per cent of Chinese, Japanese and Tibetans have such teeth, 95 per cent of Native Americans, 84 per cent of Eskimos, 46 per cent of Palestinian Arabs – and 90 per cent of Finns. It is rare amongst Negroids and Australian Aboriginals. In Caucasian races, the lateral incisors in the upper jaw are usually smaller than the central, especially in women, a feature absent or less marked in Negroid or Mongoloid races. Caucasians also have long pointed canine roots, a feature not seen in Mongoloids. Enamel pearls, small nodules of enamel on the tooth surface, are much more frequent in Mongoloid teeth. Small nodules on the lingual surface of maxillary molars, called 'Carabelli's cusp', are most common in Caucasian races and rare in the other major racial groups. The condition of bull-tooth or 'taurodontism' is most common in Mongoloid peoples: here the pulp cavity of molars is wide and deep, and the roots are fused and bent. A congenital lack of the third upper molar is most common in Mongoloids, but can occur in any race. Negroid races tend to have large teeth and often have more cusps on their molars, even up to eight, with two lingual cusps on the mandibular first premolars as an additional common finding.

The age of the person is one of the most useful findings disclosed by the teeth, especially in the first two decades of life. The sequence of deciduous or 'milk' teeth is well known, overlapping the appearance of the permanent dentition, shown in Figure 26.6. This is only an average timetable, however, and is modified by several factors, such as sex, race and climate. Again, dental expertise is needed to refine the accuracy of such estimations. The determination of age from fetal teeth is also a matter for embryologists or dentists with specialized knowledge of this period. After the third molar has erupted in the third decade of life, then age determination becomes much more difficult. Much research has been expended in forensic odontology and the name of Gustafson (see references and further reading) is well known in this respect. His criteria for age in adult life comprised six factors:

- occlusal attrition of the tip of the tooth
- secondary dentine deposition in the apex of the pulp cavity
- apical migration of the attachment of the periodontal membrane
- increase in root transparency – the best single indicator
- root resorption
- accumulation of cementum around the root.

This method, as later modified by Johanson (1971), is said to give an age accuracy within 5 years either side of the true age.

It seems pointless to rehearse these methods in advice to pathologists, however, as specialized techniques, equipment and knowledge are needed for these procedures. The standard textbooks on forensic odontology and original papers should be consulted for the details. Returning to general features of age, obvious pointers are the state of the teeth in respect

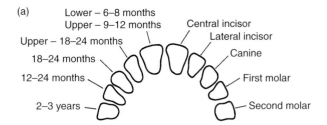

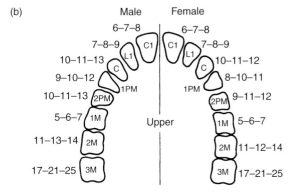

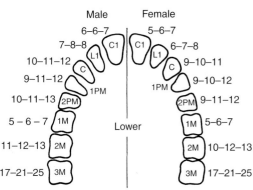

FIGURE 26.6 *(a) Dates of eruption of deciduous teeth (average times). (b) Times of eruption of permanent teeth; three dates are shown (years) for early, average and late eruption, rounded to the nearest year.*

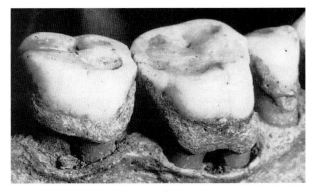

FIGURE 26.7 *Severe occlusal attrition in a jaw from the early nineteenth century. The crowns are worn down to expose the dentine by a rough diet that probably contained stone dust in the flour from contemporary milling methods.*

of wear, hygiene and colour, which may deteriorate with advancing age. Much depends upon the care with which they have been maintained, however, though marked occlusal attrition tends to go with increasing age, unless a rough diet has accelerated the wear. In Western Europe, gross occlusal attrition, sometimes down to gum level, is seen in old skeletal material. This usually indicates that the bones and teeth came from someone alive in the mid-nineteenth century or earlier, before modern milling methods removed abrasive stone dust from flour.

Edentulous jaws also suggest advancing age but, especially in former years before more conservative dentistry, even young adults often had total tooth clearances for caries. Once the teeth have gone, there is a general atrophy of the alveolar margins, but this is a poor criterion of age because of the great variability in the time when teeth are lost.

Newer techniques for age estimation include the variation with age of racemization of amino acids, especially aspartic acid, but this is a very specialized area.

Comparative identification from teeth

Establishing personal identity requires the matching of observed features with pre-existing dental records, the latter almost always obtained from previous diagnostic and therapeutic surveillance. For this method to be applied, there must be:

- Some collateral evidence to indicate either who the unknown body might be, so that records can be sought.
- Alternatively, a circumscribed population must be searched for records that may match the unknown. Such a population may be the known passengers on an aircraft or ship or a cohort of missing persons maintained on some register. It is manifestly impossible to search a large population, such as a whole country or even a city. Attempts were made in Britain to computerize dental records from the National Health Service so that a wide search could be made, but the completeness and quality of data was such that the scheme was found to be impracticable.
- The unknown person must have had dental attention in the past. The dentist or hospital must be known; the records must be traceable and, when found, must contain sufficient clinical information to provide adequate identifying features. The recovery of dental radiographs is a most useful adjunct. Unfortunately, these criteria are not always satisfied.

The dental records are needed to provide a description of the dentition and jaws at a date as late as possible before the finding of the body. Work may have been done on the deceased during life since the last record was made, if the person had been treated elsewhere and the information not recorded. Where a record does not conform to the dental state of a body who was expected to be a match, it is obvious that such discrepancies can be of two types:

1 If the record indicates some condition that is irreversible but which does not exist in the body, then that excludes matching. For example, if the record states that certain teeth have been extracted, yet they are still present in the jaws, then any hope of correspondence must be abandoned.

2 If fillings are present in the teeth, which are not shown in the records, then these may have been made later and not recorded. Of course, no discrepancies of point 1 must be present for those of point 2 to be acceptable.

Charting the teeth

In the absence of a forensic odontologist, the next best person to record the state of dentition of a dead body would naturally be a dental practitioner, to whom this task would be an everyday routine. The chart made by him could then be used for future reference in any identification procedure. This chapter is concerned with the imperfect yet sometimes inevitable circumstance where the pathologist is the only person available. Unfortunately, there are a host of different methods of charting the contents of the jaws, and, in spite of sustained efforts, no universal internationally accepted system has yet been adopted. For our purposes, any careful record of the number, position and state of the teeth made by a pathologist can be converted into whatever system of charting is required at a later stage.

Two main methods of recording data are in use: the first is a diagrammatic chart commonly used in large dental services such as the British National Health Service, seen in Figure 26.8. The other system uses a more pictorial representation of the teeth, so that all features can be recorded in a more exact topographical manner. Both systems, as well as many variants, have a notation which describes the position of the teeth, almost always in four quadrants, right upper, left upper, right lower and left lower. Unfortunately, there is considerable variation in the sequence of numeration, especially where the transition points from left to right, and from upper to lower are concerned, these being confusing and often not interchangeable. The pathologist need not concern himself too much with this problem, as his graphic representation can always be turned into whatever system of numeration is required at a later time. For example, if an unknown body has its teeth charted on one

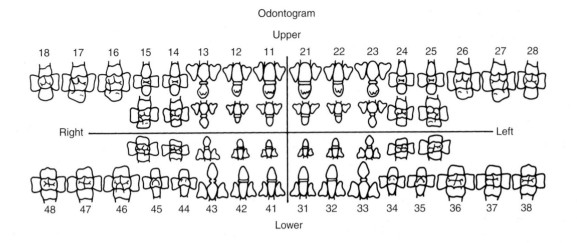

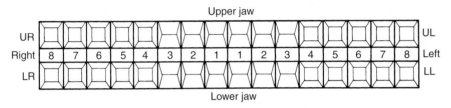

FIGURE 26.8 *Two of the many types of chart used for recording dental characteristics. The upper is the 'Odontogram' designed for Interpol. The chart displays each surface of each tooth, including the deciduous teeth. The lower chart is that used in the British National Health Service, which is a simpler design. In both charts the buccal aspects are at the top and bottom and the lingual sides of the teeth face each other centrally.*

of the common diagrams and later the dental records of a potential 'identitee' become available, the chart can be transposed into the same system as the clinical records. The notation derived from this can then be transmitted by telephone, telex, fax or other form of communication, if the records are not available at the place where the body lies. This is particularly important in transportation fatalities such as air crashes, where the home base of the victims may be far removed from the scene of death.

On the diagrammatic or anatomical charts, each tooth is represented by a pictorial symbol that provides the same number of tooth surfaces as those on the same teeth in the mouth. The incisors and canines have four surfaces represented, while the premolars and molars have an additional facet, the occlusal surface. On these diagrams, the positions of fillings, crowns, caries and damage are marked, and, of course, missing teeth are deleted.

In charting the teeth, the pathologist needs good access to the mouth and this presents the first problem. Rigor mortis in a relatively fresh cadaver may make it impossible to open the mouth without great effort. Excessive force should not be used, especially leverage with a metal instrument, because of the danger of damaging the teeth. Where the rigor cannot be

broken by sustained firm pressure on the chin – or where time prevents waiting for rigor to pass off – it may be necessary to extend the autopsy incision into a neck 'V' and dissect the skin off the lower part of the face, to gain access to the masseter and temporalis muscles, which can then be divided above their insertion into the mandible, to allow the jaw to become mobile. Care must be taken not to disfigure the face during this procedure.

When the body is decomposing, no rigor will be present. If badly rotted, then cosmetic considerations will not apply and more radical removal of the jaws may need to be performed. The same holds for badly burned bodies, where heat contraction of the facial muscles may make it impossible to open the jaws without dissecting away tissues. In both these instances, where identity is a prime consideration, both mandible and maxilla may need to be removed for retention and later examination. The mandible can be disarticulated at the temporomandibular joints and removed intact. The lower maxilla, comprising the tooth-bearing jaw, the palate and the inferior part of the facial skeleton, can be removed after the mandible has been taken. This is done by sawing horizontally across the maxilla at the level of the lower margin of the nasal aperture, taking care to saw above any tooth

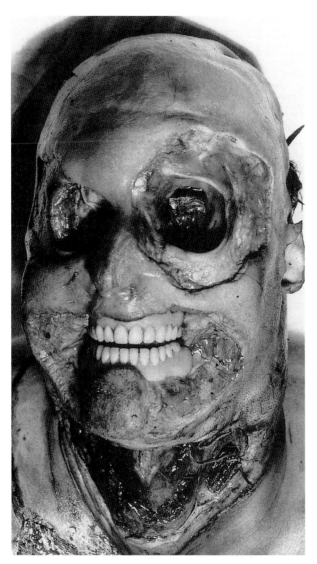

FIGURE 26.9 *Use of dentures to identify a decomposed body from the sea. Some dental prostheses carry makers' or patients' record numbers embedded in the plate material. The loss of tissue around eyes and mouth was caused by marine predators. The cut throat was made by a nylon hawser that threw this ship's officer overboard.*

roots. After photography and charting, the jaws can be preserved in formalin or a freezer. With modern serological and DNA identification techniques, the need to keep some unfixed tissue for serology and other investigations should be borne in mind. Naturally, the presence of any full or partial dentures or any other type of dental prosthesis will have been recorded and the prosthesis carefully retained for examination. Even edentulous persons may show signs of having worn dentures by the presence of pressure marks on gums or palate. Wherever possible, radiographs should be taken of the head of an unidentified body (as discussed in Chapter 3) where non-dental considerations apply, such as craniometry

or frontal sinus visualization. At the same time, the radiographs may show unexpected foreign bodies in the head and some of these may have unique dental importance, such as broken drill, broken roots or congenital abnormalities, which may be matchable with clinical films, or a note in the ante-mortem records. Radiography has a special place in forensic odontology, but specialist techniques and knowledge are likely to lie outside the abilities of a pathologist.

When, by whatever means necessary, the dental arches have been made available for examination, the following features are sought and recorded on the chart:

- Extractions – whether recent or old – should be noted from the condition of the socket.
- Fillings – their number, position and composition.
- Artificial teeth – gold, porcelain or stainless steel.
- Other prosthetic work in the mouth, such as bridgework or braces.
- Crowned teeth.
- Broken teeth.
- Pathological conditions in teeth, jaws or gums.
- Congenital defects such as enamel pearls, Carabelli's cusps or ectopic teeth.
- Malpositioned teeth – rotated or tilted for example.
- The general state of care and hygiene including caries, plaque, tobacco staining and gingivitis.
- Racial pointers, such as shovel-shaped upper central incisors or multi-cusped molars.

When all available information has been discovered and entered on the chart, the process of comparison with any ante-mortem records can be made. Much will depend on the quality and the date of these records, which are frequently less detailed and exact than the autopsy charting. Allowance must be made for the clinical records to be substantially out of date on occasions, as mentioned earlier. The process of matching is again really the work of an experienced dentist, but the major task of checking the above list against the previous records can be carried out adequately in respect of missing teeth, filling, prostheses and major trauma and other anomalies.

Anything on the clinical chart that is not represented in the actual jaws almost always excludes a matching – fillings cannot go away and extracted teeth cannot return, even though some remarkable feats of dental treatment now exist. The degree of correspondence that is acceptable for a positive match is a matter of common sense, and naturally other non-dental aspects must be taken into account – it is useless trying to claim a match on a woman's dental characteristics if other information clearly indicates that the missing person was a man. Finally, and at the risk of being over-repetitive, it must again be emphasized that, though the pathologist may be a collector of data and physical evidence, where the issues

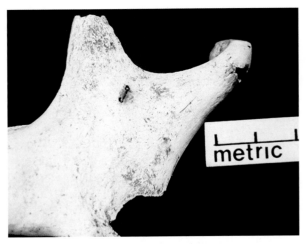

FIGURE 26.10 *A short-cut in excluding homicide. A skeleton was found buried in a suburban garden. Initial suspicions were allayed when the ramus of the mandible was seen to carry a bronze wire for attaching a spring to suspend the jaw from the skull. Police enquiries confirmed that the house had previously belonged to a member of the medical school teaching staff.*

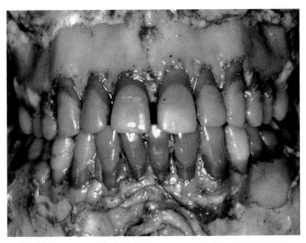

FIGURE 26.12 *Pink teeth. The jaw came from a decomposed body dumped in the countryside after death from narcotic overdose. No carbon monoxide was present in the body, the pinkness being caused by haemoglobin products staining the dentine. (Reproduced by kind permission of Professor David Whittaker.)*

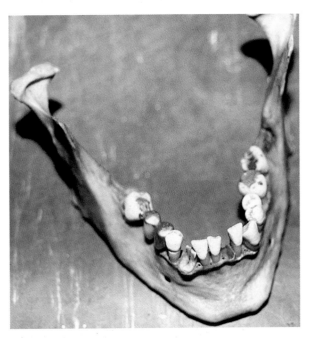

FIGURE 26.11 *A mandible from a skeletalized body found in suspicious circumstances. Identity was established solely from dental features, such as the gold bridge and acrylic tooth on the right side of the jaw and the numerous amalgam fillings. Comparison of dental radiographs obtained from a hospital confirmed the correspondence. The jaw, with the prominent square symphyseal region, is typically male.*

PINK TEETH

At autopsy on putrefied bodies, the teeth are sometimes seen to be a marked pink colour, especially near the gum line. Considerable research has been carried out into this interesting phenomenon and it is clear that the colour is the result of the dentine being stained by haemoglobin products. It was once thought that carbon monoxide played a part in the coloration, but this has been disproved. Claims that the phenomenon is a pointer to an asphyxial death can be discounted, though possibly a very 'congestive' mode of death – albeit a very non-specific condition – encourages pinkness because of retention of blood in the pulp.

REFERENCES AND FURTHER READING

Ajmal M, Mody B, Kumar G. 2001. Age estimation using three established methods. A study on Indian population. *Forensic Sci Int* **122**:150–4.

Bernitz H. 2001. Identification by means of denture marking. *SADJ* **56**:368–9.

Bernitz H, Kloppers BA. 2002. Comparison microscope identification of a cheese bitemark: a case report. *J Forensic Odontostomatol* **20**:13–16.

Borrman HI, DiZinno JA, Wasen J, *et al.* 1999. On denture marking. *J Forensic Odontostomatol* **17**:20–6.

are vital (as in a homicide investigation), every effort must be made for the material to be evaluated by a forensic odontologist, even if the details have to be sent by air mail to another country.

Bowers CM, Johansen RJ. 2002. Photographic evidence protocol: the use of digital imaging methods to rectify angular distortion and create life size reproductions of bite mark evidence. *J Forensic Sci* **47**:178–85.

Bowers CM, Johansen RJ. 2002. Digital imaging methods as an aid in dental identification of human remains. *J Forensic Sci* **47**:354–9.

Brkic H, Strinovic D, Kubat M, *et al.* 2000. Odontological identification of human remains from mass graves in Croatia. *Int J Legal Med* **114**:19–22.

Brondum N, Simonsen J. 1987. Postmortem red coloration of teeth. A retrospective investigation of 26 cases. *Am J Forensic Med Pathol* **8**:127–30.

Cameron JM, Sims BG. 1973. *Forensic dentistry.* Churchill Livingstone, Edinburgh.

Commission on Armed Forces Dental Services. 1967. *Identification by dental means,* Vol. Redaction I–IV. Federation Dentaire International, Paris.

DeVore DT. 1977. Radiology and photography in forensic dentistry. *Dent Clin North Am* **21**:69–83.

Du Chesne A, Benthaus S, Brinkmann B. 1999. Manipulated radiographic material – capability and risk for the forensic consultant? *Int J Legal Med* **112**:329–32.

English WR, Robison SF, Summitt JB, *et al.* 1988. Individuality of human palatal rugae. *J Forensic Sci* **33**:718–26.

Fearnhead RW. 1961. Facilities for forensic odontology. *Med Sci Law* **1**:273–6.

Fielding CG. 2002. Nutrient canals of the alveolar process as an anatomic feature for dental identifications. *J Forensic Sci* **47**:381–3.

Forbes G, Watson AA. 1975. *Legal aspects of dental practice.* John Wright, Bristol.

Furness J. 1976. Positive dental identification. *Int J Forensic Dent* **3**:2–5.

Furness J. 1981. A general review of bite-mark evidence. *Am J Forensic Med Pathol* **2**:49–52.

Garn SM. 1958. The sex difference in tooth calcification. *J Dent Res* **37**:561–4.

Glass RT, Jordan FB, Andrews EE. 1975. Multiple animal bite wounds: a case report. *J Forensic Sci* **20**:305–14.

Gustafson G. 1950. Age determination on teeth. *J Am Dent Assoc* **41**:45–50.

Gustafson G. 1966. *Forensic odontology.* Staples Press, London.

Haines DH. 1972. Racial characteristics in forensic dentistry. *Med Sci Law* **12**:131–8.

Hanihara K. 1967. Racial characteristics in the dentition. *J Dent Res* **46**:923–6.

Harvey W. 1976. *Dental identification and forensic odontology.* Henry Kimpton, London.

Heliman H. 1929. Racial characteristic in the human dentition. *Am Phil Soc* **67**:157–74.

Hurme VO. 1948. Standards of variation in the eruption of the first six permanent teeth. *Child Dev* **19**:213–22.

Ito S. 1976. Age determination based on tooth crown. *Int J Forensic Dent* **3**:9–14.

Jakobsen JR, Keiser Nielsen S. 1981. Bite mark lesions in human skin. *Forensic Sci Int* **18**:41–55.

Johanson G. 1971. Age determination from human teeth. *Ondontol Rev* **22**(Suppl):22–8.

Kemkes-Grottenthaler A. 2001. The reliability of forensic osteology – a case in point. Case study. *Forensic Sci Int* **117**:65–72.

Kolltveit KM, Solheim T, Kvaal SI. 1998. Methods of measuring morphological parameters in dental radiographs. Comparison between image analysis and manual measurements. *Forensic Sci Int* **94**:87–95.

Koshy S, Tandon S. 1998. Dental age assessment: the applicability of Demirjian's method in South Indian children. *Forensic Sci Int* **94**:73–85.

Lund H, Mornstad H. 1999. Gender determination by odontometrics in a swedish population. *J Forensic Odontostomatol* **17**:30–4.

Luntz L, Luntz P. 1973. *Handbook for dental identification: techniques in forensic dentistry.* Lippincott, Philadelphia.

Maples WR. 1978. An improved technique using dental histology for estimation of adult age. *J Forensic Sci* **23**:764–70.

Marshall W, Potter J, Harvey W. 1974. Bite marks in apples – forensic aspects. *Criminol* **9**:21–6.

Masters PM. 1986. Age at death determinations for autopsied remains based on aspartic acid racemization in tooth dentin: importance of postmortem conditions. *Forensic Sci Int* **32**:179–84.

McKenna CJ, Haron MI, Taylor JA. 1999. Evaluation of a bitemark using clear acrylic replicas of the suspect's dentition – a case report. *J Forensic Odontostomatol* **17**:40–3.

Meredith HV. 1946. The order and age of eruption of the deciduous dentition. *J Dent Res* **25**:43–5.

Mertz CA. 1977. Dental identification. *Dent Clin North Am* **21**:47–67.

Metzger Z, Buchner A. 1980. The application of tetracyclines in forensic dentistry. *J Forensic Sci* **25**:612–18.

Miles AEW. 1963. Dentition in the estimation of age. *J Dent Res* **42**:253–5.

Muller M, Lupi-Pegurier L, Quatrehomme G, *et al.* 2001. Odontometrical method useful in determining gender and dental alignment. *Forensic Sci Int* **121**:194–7.

Myers JC, Okoye MI, Kiple D, *et al.* 1999. Three-dimensional (3-D) imaging in post-mortem examinations: elucidation and identification of cranial and facial fractures in victims of homicide utilizing 3-D computerized imaging reconstruction techniques. *Int J Legal Med* **113**:33–7.

Nambiar P, Carson G, Taylor JA, *et al.* 2001. Identification from a bitemark in a wad of chewing gum. *J Forensic Odontostomatol* **19**:5–8.

Ogino T, Ogino H, Nagy B. 1985. Application of aspartic acid racemization to forensic odontology: postmortem designation of age at death. *Forensic Sci Int* **29**:259–67.

Ohtani S. 1994. Age estimation by aspartic acid racemization in dentin of deciduous teeth. *Forensic Sci Int* **68**:77–82.

Ohtani S, Yamada Y, Yamamoto I. 1998. Improvement of age estimation using amino acid racemization in a case of pink teeth. *Am J Forensic Med Pathol* **19**:77–9.

Pretty IA, Smith PW, Edgar WM, *et al.* 2002. The use of quantitative light-induced fluorescence (QLF) to identify composite restorations in forensic examinations. *J Forensic Sci* **47**:831–6.

Ritz-Timme S, Cattaneo C, Collins MJ, *et al.* 2000. Age estimation: the state of the art in relation to the specific demands of forensic practice. *Int J Legal Med* **113**:129–36.

Rogers SL. 1988. *The testimony of teeth: forensic aspects of human dentition.* Thomas, Springfield.

Ruddick RF. 1974. A technique for recording bite marks for forensic studies. *Med Biol Illus* **24**:128–9.

Sheasby DR, MacDonald DG. 2001. A forensic classification of distortion in human bite marks. *Forensic Sci Int* **122**:75–8.

Sims BG, Grant JH, Cameron JM. 1973. Bite-marks in the 'battered baby syndrome'. *Med Sci Law* **13**:207–10.

Sognnaes RF. 1980. Hitler and Bormann identifications compared by postmortem craniofacial and dental characteristics. *Am J Forensic Med Pathol* **1**:105–15.

Solheim T. 1980. Unusual dental forensic cases in Norway. *Am J Forensic Med Pathol* **1**:197–203.

Solheim T. 1993. A new method for dental age estimation in adults. *Forensic Sci Int* **59**:137–47.

Stevens PJ, Tarlton SW. 1966. Medical investigation in fatal aircraft accidents. The role of dental evidence. *Br Dent J* **120**:263–70.

Sweet D, Shutler GG. 1999. Analysis of salivary DNA evidence from a bite mark on a body submerged in water. *J Forensic Sci* **44**:1069–72.

Tramini P, Bonnet B, Sabatier R, *et al.* 2001. A method of age estimation using raman microspectrometry imaging of the human dentin. *Forensic Sci Int* **118**:1–9.

Valenzuela A, Martin-de las Heras S, Marques T, *et al.* 2000. The application of dental methods of identification to human burn victims in a mass disaster. *Int J Legal Med* **113**:236–9.

Whittaker D, McRonald R. 1989. *Atlas of forensic dentistry.* Wolfe Medical Publications, London.

Whittaker DK, Brickley MR, Evans L. 1998. A comparison of the ability of experts and non-experts to differentiate between adult and child human bite marks using receiver operating characteristic (ROC) analysis. *Forensic Sci Int* **92**:11–20.

Whittaker DK, Richards BH, Jones ML. 1998. Orthodontic reconstruction in a victim of murder. *Br J Orthod* **25**:11–14.

Wright FD. 1998. Photography in bite mark and patterned injury documentation – part 2: a case study. *J Forensic Sci* **43**:881–7.

Xu XH, Philipsen HP, Jablonski NG, *et al.* 1991. Preliminary report on a new method of human age estimation from single adult teeth. *Forensic Sci Int* **51**:281–8.

Yaacob H, Nambiar P, Naidu MD. 1996. Racial characteristics of human teeth with special emphasis on the mongoloid dentition. *Malays J Pathol* **18**:1–7.

CHAPTER 27

Poisoning and the pathologist

Toxicology has a number of different aspects and, in such a huge subject, various specialists have different interests. The clinical toxicologist is most concerned with diagnosis and treatment of the living patient; the analytical toxicologist has the complex task of laboratory investigation; and the pathologist is concerned with evaluating poisons as a cause or a contribution to death. Though obviously linked, these various aspects are substantially different and few people can claim to be proficient in all three. As far as the pathologist is concerned, his main task is to exclude or confirm other non-toxic factors in the death. He has then to collect suitable samples for analysis and, when the laboratory results are available, to interpret them in the light of his knowledge of the history, clinical features and autopsy appearances.

The pathologist inevitably needs the expertise of the laboratory analyst and the latter's knowledge of the therapeutic, toxic and fatal levels of the substances under consideration. Such data must, however, be evaluated in the knowledge of other pathological and physiological conditions present, so that it is the pathologist, rather than the laboratory toxicologist, who should provide the final opinion upon the proximate cause of death. This does not always happen and some laboratory report forms may be seen that unequivocally – and unwisely – state that a particular drug **caused** the death.

Where, as so often happens, the toxic levels found at post-mortem are not in a potentially fatal or even toxic range, then the pathologist should seek the advice of a **clinical** toxicologist to determine whether any of the symptoms or signs during life may assist in deciding on the cause of death. As so often happens in forensic problems, the investigation of a fatal poisoning must be a cooperative effort, especially between pathologist and laboratory analyst. Even in apparently obvious cases, such as a blood saturation of 50 per cent carboxyhaemoglobin, it is not for the analyst to declare a definite cause of death, as the victim may also have had a fractured skull – but equally, the pathologist has an obligation to provide the laboratory with the best possible samples in the best possible condition, as well as good information about the circumstances of the case.

THE CONCEPT OF THE FATAL DOSE

Many persons, including some doctors, are under the firm misapprehension that, for most toxic substances, there are relatively constant quantities that will cause death. Not only the lay public, but lawyers, police, coroners and others assume that there is a more or less linear relationship between the amount of poison that enters the body, the resulting levels in blood and tissues and the degree of disability caused – the ultimate disability being death.

In addition, it is often thought that back-calculation from blood and tissue levels can arrive at a definite assessment of how much poison was originally administered. This aspect is of particular concern to coroners and similar officers, who have to decide on motive in potential suicides, where the magnitude of any overdose may assist in distinguishing between accident and self-administration.

The pathologist has his own difficulties in respect of 'the fatal dose', as quantitative results from the laboratory have to be matched against a knowledge of published blood and tissue levels for that substance in relation to its potential toxicity. Though numerous tables of toxic levels have been published, there is considerable variation between the levels recorded. Reasons for this are explored later. It is obvious that there is no 'fatal dose' in the sense of a single threshold concentration above which a person dies and below which he survives. Instead, there is a range of levels, the upper and lower margins of which vary from one authority to another, which encompasses most deaths – but even here there are many exceptions, instances being recorded where survival occurs well above the upper limit and death occurs below the lower margin. In such cases, the task of the pathologist – which cannot always be satisfactorily discharged – is to evaluate all other non-toxicological data to see if they can modify the circumstances sufficiently to allow an acceptable explanation for the death. It is sometimes difficult to explain these concepts of great biological variation to lawyers and police officers, who expect more definite decisions, and might even feel that the pathologist is being evasive or obstructive.

The concept of the 'LD$_{50}$' is sometimes raised by the more knowledgeable lawyer, but this does not assist materially in any individual case. The LD$_{50}$ is a device used by pharmacologists and toxicologists in a statistical sense in animal experiments. Over a large number of tests, it provides a toxic level at which half the animals will be expected to die. Though the indicative value in a general sense in comparing the toxicity of one substance against another, there is no way of knowing whether the human victim of poisoning lies at the upper or lower end of the classical bell-shaped curve that characterizes most biological responses.

Far more useful is the cumulative record of actual laboratory results from toxicology centres that deal with human poisoning, which progressively build up a large database of blood and tissue levels, and correlate these with records of the clinical state, toxic effects and fatal outcome. Even here the variations are wide, as the many published tables testify, but at least general guidance can be obtained.

VARIATIONS IN PUBLISHED FATAL POISON CONCENTRATIONS

In the many publications that offer therapeutic, toxic and lethal ranges for a wide variety of poisonous substances, there is considerable variation in the quoted levels. These can be a source of confusion and sometimes dismay to the pathologist who, even with the advice of his local toxicologist, may find it difficult to decide whether a death can justifiably be attributed to a particular drug or other toxic substance. Even if he can so satisfy himself, he may be subjected to keen questioning, interrogation, doubt or criticism from colleagues, coroners, police, lawyers and others, who have access to different versions of toxic and fatal levels. The ultimate challenge may come in a criminal court, where opposing counsel may openly defy the pathologist's interpretations in cross-examination.

Dr A R W Forrest, Chemical Pathologist and Toxicologist at Sheffield's Royal Hallamshire Hospital (personal communication) points out some reasons for the variations found in such published data. He expresses the view that it is rather surprising that the order of disagreement is not greater, given the opportunities for disparity.

First, many of the published series are small, some being only individual case reports. Statistically, this is not a good foundation for establishing reference ranges, which are much better obtained from a database derived from the cumulative results of a large laboratory service, such as the British Home Office Forensic Science Service, which maintains a central computer store of all results from its laboratories.

Second, analytical techniques vary widely, both in method and accuracy. The specificity varies from laboratory to laboratory so that there may be a lack of uniformity about what is actually being measured. For example, paracetamol may be measured by a non-specific method that picks up its metabolites as well as the native drug, which will then offer a different blood level in a fatal case from that found by more specific methods. In other words, one is not comparing 'like with like'.

Third, as discussed elsewhere in this chapter, the site of sampling may introduce wide errors. With some substances, a several-fold variation in concentration may be found between femoral vein and cardiac cavity blood.

Last, errors occur because a 'fatal' level may be attributed to one substance without taking into account the level – or even the existence – of other toxic substances that the deceased may have taken, and of which the pathologist or analyst may not even have been aware. For example, the newer more potent benzodiazepines may be missed in a simple toxicological screen, but could well have contributed to the toxicological overload that caused the patient to die. In such a case, the level of the recognized drug would be blamed for the death, whereas in fact it may not have been a lethal dose in itself, though was recorded as such in any database or tables.

These facts highlight the dangers of limiting a request for analysis solely to the substance known or thought to have been taken. Often an efficient screen for other substances will reveal other unsuspected compounds, sometimes more toxic than the one originally suspected.

It has to be recognized, however, that, in many jurisdictions, the availability and expense of toxicological investigations may make it impossible to pursue a full analytical survey, especially if this is to be undertaken on a speculative basis rather than for quantification of a known or strongly suspected toxic agent. A full screen may only be practicable and justified in a suspected homicide, if laboratory facilities and fiscal support are severely restricted. In many countries homicide by poison is relatively rare and the funds to investigate accidental, suicidal and iatrogenic poisoning exhaustively may just not be available.

THE AUTOPSY IN SUSPECTED POISONING

The autopsy in these circumstances can be amongst the most difficult of problems faced by a forensic pathologist – not in the technical procedure of the examination, but in the final evaluation of all the available information.

The nature of the poisoning autopsy in Western countries has changed dramatically since the last century, when poisoning was a common method of homicide. There has been a marked change in the nature of poisons used in murder, suicide and accident. The corrosives, heavy metals and alkaloids commonly ingested in former years became relatively easy to detect, either by gross autopsy appearances or by straightforward analytical methods. Further refinements of toxicological techniques, instead of the old methods in which large samples had to be tested because of the insensitivity of laboratory tests, allow the detection of nanogram quantities.

Acids, alkalis, phenols, arsenic, antimony and strychnine, for example, became easy to detect, and in the Western world these gave way to compounds that leave little or no gross, or even histological changes in the body. Most are pharmaceutical or agrochemical substances, active in low dose compared to the old 'blockbuster' poisons. As for the majority of drugs used in legitimate medical therapy, an added problem arises when low post-mortem levels are found – is this merely a therapeutic dose or the tail-end of a declining lethal dose?

In some parts of the world, such as South-east Asia, Africa and the Indian subcontinent, poisoning remains common and more physically damaging substances continue to be seen that leave obvious autopsy lesions. Some of these are described under the appropriate headings in the succeeding chapters, but in most poisonings the major function of the autopsy is to evaluate any other conditions present, both from trauma and natural disease – but also to collect suitable material for laboratory analysis. The proper retention of optimal samples, their correct preservation and dispatch to the toxicologist are of such fundamental importance that they are discussed in detail.

POISONING DEATHS IN HOSPITAL

A considerable proportion of those who die from suspected poisoning will have died in hospital, and it is of prime importance that the medical records be obtained and studied before the autopsy begins. Even if poisoning was not confirmed or even suspected by the clinicians treating the patient, later information may have come to the pathologist to raise this possibility. Whether known or not, the results of ante-mortem investigations may be of considerable use to the pathologist. If poisoning was known or suspected before death, there may well have been toxicological analyses performed and the results of these may be of great value.

Whether poisoning was suspected or not, there may still be ante-mortem blood or urine samples (taken for biochemical or haematological tests) stored in the hospital laboratory, which may be rescued for retrospective analysis. Such ante-mortem samples are likely to be of greater use than fluids drawn off at autopsy, because of sampling defects, post-mortem changes and because toxic levels are likely to have been higher during life, representing more accurately the maximum toxic concentrations.

In addition, many patients dying in hospital from drug overdoses will have indwelling catheters in place. It is the common practice for the nursing staff to remove these at death and discard the urine. If it is possible to establish a practice in the wards where such terminal urine samples are saved, valuable material for analysis can be obtained.

THE COLLECTION OF AUTOPSY SAMPLES FOR TOXICOLOGICAL ANALYSIS

The investigation of a death from suspected poisoning may stand or fall upon the correctness or otherwise of the sampling of fluids and tissues from the body. Unsuitable samples, inadequate amounts, incorrect sampling sites, poor containers, inadequate preservation methods, and delayed or unsatisfactory storage and transport to the laboratory may frustrate or distort proper analysis. The final outcome may be wrong, either in failing to detect a poison actually present, in measuring only part of that originally present or – in some cases – even producing falsely high results that then lead to an incorrect cause of death. Not only must samples be in the optimal condition, but the accompanying information from the pathologist to the analyst needs to be as accurate and comprehensive as possible, so that the most appropriate techniques are used, and allowance made for any interfering substances that may be present.

In decomposed bodies infested with maggots, and in the absence of tissues or fluids normally taken for toxicology, Diptera and other arthropods can be used as alternative specimens for toxicological analyses. This relatively new field of forensic entomology is called entomotoxicology.

The time of sampling

It is obvious that the shorter the delay between death and the removal of samples, the better. Though some toxic substances, such as carbon monoxide, form stable compounds in the body, many others (especially volatile substances and some pharmaceutical products) will be broken down by post-mortem autolysis and decomposition. When an autopsy cannot be performed quickly after death, in terms of a few hours, then mortuary refrigeration is the first line of defence to slow up putrefactive and autolytic processes. If delay is foreseen, usually because of administrative problems in obtaining consent or authority for autopsy, it may be possible to obtain a sample of blood through the body surface, such as puncturing the femoral vein by needle and syringe. The blood can then be kept in optimal conditions, with preservative where needed, and perhaps with the serum or plasma separated from the cells to avoid haemolysis. Similarly, urine could be drawn off by catheter or even suprapubic puncture, unless strict regulations forbid this as anticipating autopsy permission.

In some jurisdictions, authority for autopsy may be particularly hard to obtain, from religious, financial or administrative reluctance. Where poisoning is suspected, permission may be granted only for external examination and sampling; here venous blood, urine and perhaps vitreous humour may have to suffice for all investigations.

Information supplied to the laboratory

When samples are submitted to the toxicologist, they should be accompanied by the best possible information relevant to the case. It is both counterproductive and an unprofessional discourtesy merely to record the personal details of the deceased and list the samples, with a terse demand such as 'Any poisons?' on the request form. Such a demand could legitimately be refused by the toxicologist, as it is quite inadequate information upon which he can be expected to function effectively and safely. The following information should be supplied and where necessary, supplemented by direct discussion either in person or by telephone:

- The personal details of the deceased, including age, sex and where thought relevant, the occupation (especially if in agriculture or industry).

- Brief details of symptoms, if any, and length of illness.
- The post-mortem interval before samples were obtained, and the actual date and time of sampling.
- The name, address and telephone number of the pathologist.
- A list of all samples provided, with an indication of the sampling site for each.
- The nature of any preservative in each of the samples.
- If there has been a delay in submitting or transporting the samples, a note of the condition under which they have been stored (for example, refrigeration or deep-freeze).
- Any special risk associated with the samples **must** be communicated to the laboratory. The most obvious are infective conditions, especially hepatitis B or C virus or HIV infection in the deceased, though other diseases such as tuberculosis, tetanus, anthrax, gas gangrene or any other bacterial or viral condition must also be specifically reported. In relation to hepatitis and HIV, even if these are not definitely confirmed, the toxicology laboratory must be told if the deceased was in a high-risk group, such as a drug addict or a homosexual. In many areas, including Britain, some toxicology laboratories will not accept samples from such high-risk groups until a blood sample has been screened for hepatitis B and HIV antibodies; if positive, they may decline to carry out the analysis or perform it only under strictly controlled conditions.

  Similar warnings must be given to the analyst if there is any possibility of certain harmful substances, such as radioactive isotopes or certain war gases, being present in the samples.
- When a death has criminal aspects, such as a murder or manslaughter, then the usual strict precautions must be taken for continuity of evidence. Each container must be carefully labelled and preferably countersigned by the pathologist. Some jurisdictions will require actual seals on the containers themselves or the package into which they are placed for transport, or both. Accompanying signed 'exhibit labels' with serial numbers corresponding exactly with numbers on the jars may be required. The containers must be given by the pathologist to a named person, usually the 'exhibits officer' of the police investigating team (or to forensic scientists if they attend the autopsy). The police officer must hand the samples personally to a member of the laboratory staff and a record of this chain of evidence must be kept, so that there can be no criticism levelled at anyone when the matter comes to court, raising doubts about the correct identity of the sample.

CONTAINERS FOR TOXICOLOGY SAMPLES

There will be considerable local variation in the type of containers used for the collection and transmission of samples to the laboratory. Some laboratories will issue their own kits, an example being those provided by the Home Office Forensic Science Service in England and Wales. These consist of a plastic bag containing a sheet of instructions about the most suitable samples, together with a large plastic pot with tightly self-sealing lid for liver, a smaller one for stomach contents, several plastic or glass 30 ml universal containers for blood and urine, a small vial containing fluoride for blood-alcohol estimation and a sterile syringe and several needles. Variations of such kits may be provided by different laboratories, but the general nature of the containers is the same. In other areas, the pathologist will provide the containers himself and they should conform to the following general specifications:

■ They should either be new or, if previously used for other samples, have been rigorously cleaned and sterilized. Even when they are new, it is preferable for containers to be washed and sterilized before use unless the manufacturer's specifications clearly make this unnecessary. All containers must be chemically clean, not just apparently clean to the naked eye. This applies particularly to any rubber, plastic or other seal within the lid or cap, which may be a trap for any debris or even residue from a previous sample.

■ Blood should be collected in screw-capped universal containers of about 30 ml or, where less will suffice, in plastic-capped tubes of about 5 ml. Urine is best held in 30 ml universal containers, as is bile. Stomach contents may be retained in glass or plastic jars with a volume of at least 250 ml, the lid being either a tight screw-thread with a cardboard or plastic liner, and a self-sealing plastic top. Some laboratories require the stomach wall as well as the contents, as toxic substances may be held in higher concentrations in the rugae and crypts of the mucosa, or even in the blood in the actual stomach wall. The size of the container may need to be larger if the organ itself is retained. Liver is usually required, preferably a piece weighing a few hundred grams, rather than the whole organ. The total weight of the liver should be communicated to the laboratory if only part is sent. It may be preserved in a larger glass or plastic container. When the laboratory wishes the whole organ, this container needs to be large enough to hold about 3 litres. If only small samples are needed, such as vitreous humour or cerebrospinal fluid, bijou bottles

of 5 ml capacity or small tubes of similar size, are needed.

In Britain, the government forensic laboratories provide special bottles for blood-alcohol estimations, for use in both drink–driving offences in the living and for autopsy samples. These are short, wide bottles of about 10 ml capacity, with a fixed top consisting of a plastic diaphragm secured by a metal flange with a central aperture. They are filled by syringe, the needle being pierced through the diaphragm, but have the disadvantage of building up pressure when the blood is injected, so that, when the needle is removed, blood may spurt back and even contaminate the operator – the reverse of the intention of these vials to be safe. The danger can be avoided by either inserting a second needle through the diaphragm to equalize the pressure, or to suck out air from the bottle with the empty syringe and needle before taking the sample so that the introduced blood replaces the lost air. Intestinal contents, with or without the gut itself, can be placed in large jars or plastic pots, similar to those used for liver.

Plastic containers, especially polypropylene, are increasingly used and have the advantage of not smashing when dropped. Some analyses, however, may be affected by the plasticizer in either the container wall or the cap – cocaine is an example. The advice of the toxicologist with whom each pathologist normally collaborates should be sought in respect of his individual preferences for containers. Where lungs or other tissues are to be submitted for analysis for volatile substances, as in solvent abuse, ordinary polythene bags are not suitable containers. Nylon bags (such as those used by arson investigators) should be used, as they are not permeable to such substances.

PRESERVATIVES IN SAMPLES

Though many samples for analysis are best sent in their original state, others require additives to maintain them in optimum condition until they reach the laboratory. In addition to such preservatives, some require anticoagulants to keep the blood fluid. The prime example of sample preservations is that for blood alcohol, as improper care of samples may distort the original alcohol level in either an upward or downward direction. The usual preservative is sodium or potassium fluoride, which is essential if the sample is not to be analysed within a few hours of withdrawal from the body.

Errors caused by post-mortem changes before the sample is removed cannot be avoided. These are variable, depending partly on the conditions of the post-mortem environment and partly on the microbiological population of the corpse. In warm conditions, fermentation by yeasts and other alcohol-producing flora can produce appreciable quantities of alcohol: it has been reported that as much as 150 mg/100 ml have been generated within 24 hours after death.

Once the blood or urine has been withdrawn from the body, however, further changes can be arrested by preservatives. Much has been published on this subject and a variety of concentrations of fluoride have been recommended by different authors. Glendening and Waugh (1965) used 100 mg of sodium fluoride/10 ml blood and found no change in the alcohol content when samples were kept at room temperature for up to 3 months. Plueckhahn (1968) found that at least 5 mg/ml of sodium fluoride was required to inhibit alcohol dehydrogenase activity, which destroys alcohol. He found, however, that this concentration failed to inhibit alcohol-forming organisms completely, such as when yeasts were introduced into the samples. Together with Ballard, he investigated the use of mercuric chloride as a preservative (Plueckhahn and Ballard 1968). This substance was also used by Bradford (1966) who added 0.5 mg of sodium citrate and 0.1 mg of mercuric chloride/ml of blood to ensure that the samples remained liquid and sterile. When he replaced the mercury by fluoride, significant changes occurred, usually a loss of alcohol, though occasionally it increased.

In most cases the delay before analysis is relatively short, being measured in days – often with refrigerated storage – so the long-term experiments mentioned here do not apply. When the ambient temperature is high, much more caution needs to be used. It would seem that for general use, a concentration of 10 mg/ml of sodium or potassium fluoride is satisfactory. Fluoride should also be added to urine and vitreous humour if alcohol estimations are required. Cocaine and its metabolites are also labile *in vitro*, and fluoride should be added to samples submitted for analysis for this drug.

Cyanide may be formed in considerable quantities in plain blood samples, which are of little use for cyanide estimation. Fluoride should be added to such specimens, as well as for carbon monoxide (carboxyhaemoglobin) if the analysis is to be delayed. In all analyses for pharmaceutical drugs, two samples of blood should be submitted, one plain in large volume of at least 25 ml and another smaller sample in fluoride.

When insulin assay is required on a blood sample, special precautions should be taken. Haemolysis of the red cells releases enzymes which will reduce the S–S bonds in insulin and destroy its immunoreactivity, so the sample should be centrifuged as soon as it is obtained to separate the serum. A heparinized sample should also be taken for glycosylated haemoglobin estimation and fructosamine assay. Vitreous humour, blood and urine samples should be placed in fluoride and sent for glucose estimation, as well as tissue samples from around any putative injection site, together with a control tissue sample from a site elsewhere on the body where insulin is unlikely to have been recently injected.

THE SITE OF SAMPLING FOR TOXICOLOGICAL ANALYSIS

It is now obvious that, in the past, serious errors were made in toxicological analyses from lack of care or consideration concerning the source of body-fluid samples. Significant variation can be found in the concentration of many substances depending on the place from which sampling was carried out. In life there may be variations when arterial as opposed to venous blood is used, as tissues may take up the compound from the arterial supply, the concentration then being lower in the venous return. Similarly, portal blood may have a substantially higher concentration of a substance that is being absorbed from the intestine, before it is extracted by passage through the liver. After death, most variation is caused by uneven destruction by enzymatic and microbiological activity – and by diffusion from sites of higher concentration. The barriers formed by living cell membranes break down after death and small molecules in particular may move easily through the tissues into vascular channels.

Post-mortem levels of many substances are unreliable because of this diffusion effect, making the interpretation of physiological components, such as sodium, potassium, calcium, glucose, urea and many others extremely difficult, if not impossible. Applying these facts to toxic compounds, the concentrations may vary considerably according to the sampling site. As an illustration, the Moorgate Tube disaster in London showed that blood-alcohol levels may vary widely between different sampling points. The driver of an underground train was killed, along with a number of passengers, but his body could not be recovered from the warm environment for several days. As it was obviously vital to know if drink had contributed to the accident, four samples were taken from various sites in the body. On analysis, a fourfold variation from between 20 and 80 mg/100 ml was obtained, presumably because of variable rates of putrefactive alcohol production, as there was no evidence to show that the driver had imbibed alcohol before death.

Most research in respect of sampling variation has been directed at alcohol. One point of dispute, which is relevant even when post-mortem changes are minimal, is whether alcohol in the stomach can diffuse after death to neighbouring organs and produce a falsely elevated alcohol concentration in blood at those sites.

The relevance is clear, in that, if a person drinks alcohol immediately before death, there will be insufficient time for it to be absorbed. Thus ethanol remaining in the stomach after death cannot have contributed to his ante-mortem blood-alcohol level, and hence his cerebral function and consequent behaviour. If however, analysis of a sample of blood taken from the heart cavities is contaminated by post-mortem diffusion from the adjacent stomach, then a falsely high reading will be obtained, which may have serious legal implications, if the error is not appreciated.

Several workers have investigated this problem, with conflicting results. Gifford and Turkel (1956) introduced alcohol into the stomachs of cadavers and found that subsequent heart blood levels increased by 25 up to 106 mg/100 ml. They then compared femoral vein blood with heart blood voided into the pericardial sac in alcohol-positive autopsies and found that the concentration in the latter was higher. Plueckhahn and Ballard (1968), however, criticized this work on the grounds that pericardial fluid alcohol was usually about 20 mg/100 ml higher than that in the heart or peripheral vessels. Plueckhahn went on to instil alcohol into the stomach of cadavers, taking multiple site samples at times from 6 to 50 hours later. His results indicated that there was a significant diffusion of alcohol to the pericardial and pleural fluids, but that the increase was minimal in intraventricular heart blood.

Pounder and Yonemitsu (1991) carried out experiments with dead bodies in which they introduced a slurry containing alcohol, dextropropoxyphene and paracetamol into the trachea to simulate aspiration of stomach contents. After a delay of 48 hours, an autopsy was carried out and drug concentrations measured in samples taken from various sites. Whilst femoral vein blood remained clear of these substances, samples from vessels in the thorax showed up to 130 mg/100 ml of alcohol with a mean of 58 in a pulmonary vein – and up to 1934 mg/l of paracetamol (mean 969), both obviously spurious due to post-mortem diffusion. This situation could have occurred from agonal regurgitation of stomach contents with recently swallowed drugs back into the air passages and shows the dangers of inappropriate sampling sites, with the femoral the place of choice.

Winek et al. (1995) have shown that, in the sampling practice of transthoracic needling, especially in cases of trauma where the gastrointestinal tract has been damaged, false elevations of blood alcohol can occur. These workers used heart blood as their control, which itself seems suspect as a satisfactory autopsy sample.

For the reasons given above, **peripheral** vein blood should be used whenever possible, avoiding heart blood as a potential source of error for alcohol and presumably other easily diffusible substances.

THE TECHNIQUE OF OBTAINING AUTOPSY SAMPLES

Blood

There are several ways of obtaining blood samples at autopsy and perhaps the most useful advice is what **not** to take. Blood should never be obtained from body cavities after evisceration, as it is almost certain to be contaminated with other body substances. The practice of scooping 'blood' – or more accurately, bloody fluid – from the paravertebral gutters or the pelvis is always unacceptable, as urine, intestinal contents, gastric contents, lymph, pleural and ascitic fluid and general tissue ooze will always find their way into such a sample and negate the reliability of analysis.

When a large haemothorax or haemopericardium is present, it may be grudgingly acceptable to use such blood or clot, if a clean sample is taken immediately on opening the chest, before any dissection or disturbance of organs is made. This is only second best to obtaining intravascular blood – and, in the case of alcohol and other diffusible substances, the results cannot be relied upon, as the sample may be contaminated by post-mortem diffusion from the stomach, as discussed in the preceding section. Carbon monoxide estimations may also be made on clean cavity blood, if nothing else is available, as sometimes happens in a badly incinerated body. As it is absorbed through the lungs, it cannot diffuse from the gastro-intestinal tract to give a false result. Even so, it is a rare autopsy that cannot provide a small sample of blood from some peripheral vein, if enough care and persistence is used.

To return to the general state of affairs, the most satisfactory way of obtaining a venous blood sample is venepuncture of the femoral vein by direct puncture in the groin before the autopsy begins. Practice is required as, unlike a living patient, the vein is not usually palpable. Once the lumen is entered, 25 ml can usually be drawn off without trouble, though a slow flow may be improved by massaging the leg to drive blood proximally or the leg may be raised, if rigor allows. Though less satisfactory than a leg vein, for reasons discussed earlier, a neck vein can also be punctured through the skin, and even after death the jugular may sometimes be both visible and palpable, especially in congestive deaths. The subclavian vein can also be tapped.

When collecting blood samples by percutaneous puncture, some pathologists prefer to use a needle designed for aspirating samples from rubber-capped vials, rather than a needle meant for clinical aspiration or injection. The same needles can be used for collecting vitreous humour. An example of this type of needle is the Becton Dickinson purple-hubbed 16 gauge one-inch or a similar American equivalent.

In some jurisdictions, especially in countries where the system allows only a low autopsy rate, transcutaneous sampling is virtually the only post-mortem investigation possible and the doctors in these areas become adept at cadaver venepuncture. Many pathologists, the authors included, have been brought up to obtain blood samples during the actual performance of autopsy and this can be as satisfactory as external venepuncture, as well as saving the expense of a new syringe and needle every time. A common procedure after evisceration is to hold a container (such as the 30 ml universal) under the severed end of the subclavian vein, within the upper part of the empty thorax. The arm is then elevated and massaged if necessary, to express blood into the container. Similarly, and perhaps preferably, the femoral or external iliac vein may be transected near the brim of the pelvis, and a container held under the cut while the leg is elevated, or massaged, or both. Either of these methods will provide ample, clean, peripheral venous blood, though care must be taken to avoid any contamination from the body cavities. This initial collection should be transferred into one or more new tubes, with preservative added if appropriate, as the first receptacle will be soiled externally during the collection process.

An alternative method of collecting a venous sample, which always gives a copious flow of blood, is to incise the internal jugular vein during the initial stages of the autopsy. As soon as the main autopsy incision is made, the flaps of the neck skin can be dissected aside and the jugular exposed, if necessary by dividing the sternocleidomastoid muscle. As in the previous technique, a bottle can be held against the vein as it is transected and the flow collected directly into it. The blood may overflow into the pouch formed laterally by the reflected skin, which forms a reservoir where a considerable volume may collect. If the flow is scanty, it can be improved by raising and lowering the head, which will cause blood to return from the upper venous drainage areas.

Even more can be expressed by pressing on the chest, but here there is the potential disadvantage of forcing up blood through the superior vena cava from the heart, which may distort the value of alcohol and other drugs that may have diffused port-mortem from the stomach. Blood should not be taken from the heart cavities, the inferior vena cava, or the portal or hepatic veins, as these may also give concentrations that are at variance with those in the peripheral vascular system. A full 30 ml of blood should be submitted to the laboratory wherever possible, together with a 5 or 10 ml fluorided sample.

Urine

Prior to, or in the absence of, an autopsy, urine can be obtained by catheter or suprapubic puncture with syringe and long needle. At autopsy it is usual to wait until evisceration has been carried out before dealing with the bladder. A sample can be obtained by puncturing the fundus with syringe and needle. Alternatively, the bladder can be stretched by pulling the fundus upwards with the fingers, then a sagittal incision made with a knife on the ventral surface, which must be free from blood soiling. The urine that wells out can be collected directly into a small container such as a 30 ml universal. If only a small amount is present, then the incision may have to be enlarged and the residual urine sucked out under direct vision, using a syringe without a needle.

Bile

This can be useful for some analyses, such as those for morphine and chlorpromazine, which are concentrated by the liver and excreted into the gallbladder. Direct collection into a bottle is advised, as bile is usually too viscous to be sucked through a needle.

Cerebrospinal fluid

This is not often required for toxicological analysis, though it may be needed for microbiological and virological studies. If needed, it should be collected by lumbar or cisternal puncture, as in the living patient. It can be difficult or impossible to obtain in this way because of the lack of any intrathecal pressure.

The body should be turned on to its side before the autopsy begins and flexed as much as possible by an assistant. If an infant, it should be sat up and again flexed forwards to curve the spine as much as possible. A needle on a syringe should then be passed between two lumbar or lower thoracic spines, and stopped as soon as any penetration of the theca is felt. Moderate suction should be maintained on the syringe piston to compensate for the lack of internal pressure. Alternatively, the needle should be passed into the midline just below the occiput and advanced upwards until the skull is contacted just posterior to the foramen magnum. The needle is slightly withdrawn and re-advanced until it slips through the posterior part of the atlanto-occipital membrane into the basal cistern when cerebrospinal fluid may be aspirated. It is of little use taking cerebrospinal fluid from the bowl of the posterior fossa after the brain has been removed as the concentration of many substances is different in blood compared with the fluid, so blood contamination distorts any results. Clear cerebrospinal fluid may, however, sometimes be obtained from the lateral ventricles, either by needle puncture or cutting down through the cortex.

Vitreous humour

This is sometimes useful, especially in bodies with appreciable post-mortem decomposition, as the fluid in the eye resists putrefaction longer than other body liquids. Vitreous fluid is also used for estimating the time since death (see Chapter 2).

A puncture should be made through the sclera at the outer canthus with a fine-gauge needle. This should be placed as far laterally as possible, pulling the lid out, so that when released it returns to cover up the puncture mark for cosmetic reasons. The fluid should be sucked out by syringe, but it will often come only slowly because of its viscosity. If the best restoration is needed, water should be reinjected through the same needle to reinflate the globe, which tends to collapse on suction.

Stomach contents

As stated earlier, these can be collected directly into wide-mouth glass or plastic pot of at least 250 ml volume. To collect them, the exterior of the stomach should be washed clean of blood and other contamination, and pulled with attached organs to the edge of the dissecting board or sink. The greater curvature should be opened cautiously with large scissors, and the jar held underneath so that the contents flow directly into it. When most have been expressed, the greater curvature can be opened up fully and the gastric lining examined. Any further contents are scraped out and any powder, capsule or tablets picked off, and either added to the main jar or placed in a separate small container. Such focal deposits form a more concentrated sample for the laboratory. Any undissolved tablets or capsules should be carefully preserved, as the laboratory or a pharmacist may be able to identify them by their appearance and colour. After the mucosa has been examined, including that of the duodenum, the stomach wall can be dissected off. Some laboratories require this for their analysis, either added to the jar of contents or sent separately. The wishes of each individual toxicologist should be discovered in advance.

Intestinal contents

These are not routinely required for analysis unless some particular gastrointestinal poison is suspected, such as one of the heavy metals. Again, the toxicologist should be consulted. If required, both ends of the small gut should be ligated by string sutures at duodenum and ileum. The intestine is cut through at these points and stripped out by cutting through the mesentery in the usual way. The intact gut can be sent to the laboratory in a large container (such as that used for liver) or – if the mucosa needs to be examined first – it should be opened in a large clean tray. One suture can be cut and the contents milked from one end to the other into a suitable jar, the gut then being opened and sent with the contents to the laboratory. The large intestine and contents are rarely required, as most toxicology laboratories are not keen on handling and storing large volumes of faeculent material. In heavy-metal poisoning, such as arsenic and antimony, however, some analysis may be required.

Vomit

This is rarely collected at autopsy, unless a large quantity has been found in the air passages. However, vomit is not infrequently collected by ambulance crews and police at the scene of the illness or agonal event, and brought with the deceased to hospital or the mortuary. If thought relevant in a case of suspected poisoning, it should be properly contained, labelled and forwarded with other samples for toxicological examination.

Other fluids

Other fluids are rarely collected, but on occasions may be useful, especially if clean blood cannot be obtained. Pericardial fluid, synovial fluid, pleural effusion and ascitic fluid can be used for qualitative analysis to identify a range of substances, though these levels can rarely be related to established ranges of blood concentrations. They may be collected and transported in the same type of container and with the same preservatives as vitreous humour.

Analysis for volatile substances

In solvent abuse and deaths from gaseous or volatile substances, the toxic material may be isolated from a whole lung. As soon as the thorax is opened at autopsy, a lung is mobilized and the main bronchus tied off tightly with a string ligature. The hilum is then divided and the lung placed immediately into a nylon bag, which is sealed and sent as soon as possible to the laboratory. Ordinary plastic (polythene) bags are not suitable for this task, as they are permeable to volatile substances. Nylon bags, as used by arson investigators to collect samples that may have volatile accelerants, do not suffer from this defect.

In collecting blood samples for volatile substances, plastic tubes or tube/syringe combinations of the 'monovette' type are unsuitable, as the concentration of such compounds as toluene or other solvents will decrease considerably over a few days in storage. Vials with a rubber septum as a seal are also unsuitable, as the volatile substance can escape through the rubber. Suitable tubes are made of glass with an aluminium foil-lined cap or a polytetrafluorethylene (Teflon) liner. This type of tube is often used in laboratories for scin-tillation counting and can be employed for the collection of solvent samples. Such tubes should be available in any busy autopsy room where solvent abuse deaths may be handled. The tubes should be filled to the top to avoid loss of vola-tile substances into the head space and should be stored at 4°C, rather than being frozen solid.

Body tissues

Body tissues may be needed for some toxicological analyses. Liver is the most usual, as it concentrates many substances and their metabolites, which may then be recoverable long after the blood and urine levels have declined. Either the whole organ is saved or an aliquot of 50–100 g, according to the wishes of the particular laboratory. If only a part is retained, it should be taken from the periphery, away from major vessels and bile ducts.

Brain and kidney may sometimes be required and again a 50–100 g aliquot is usually sufficient. As with liver, the total original weight of the organ should be recorded and notified to the toxicologist.

Where a toxic substance may have been injected into the subcutaneous tissue or muscle, these tissues should be excised and submitted to the laboratory. The usual method of iden-tifying the site is from a needle puncture mark, and a zone of skin and tissue should be removed circumferentially around this or an ellipse cut away, so that the defect can be sewn up on the body. A few centimetres in diameter around the mark is usually sufficient. The depth of the sampling depends on how deeply the needle track extends and may need to go into the underlying muscle. Radiography may assist in rare cases, as in the George Markov murder in London, where a political assassination was carried out by the introduction of a tiny sphere, presumably injected from an air weapon concealed in an umbrella. The sphere, drilled out to carry a potent toxin, probably ricin, was located by X-ray at autopsy after a small skin puncture was found. Where an injection site is sampled, it is essential that a con-trol area from a remote part of the body is also sent to the laboratory. It is usual to take this from a symmetrical zone on the contralateral side, but caution must be used, as in both drug dependence and insulin usage, alternate sides may be used at frequent intervals for injection, so another more remote site might be preferable.

The substances which may have been injected are numer-ous, but insulin, morphine, heroin, cocaine and other illicit drugs are most common. In the notorious Coppolino case in the USA, products of succinylcholine (suxamethonium) were identified from around a needle track in the buttock of an exhumed body of a woman, leading to the conviction of her anaesthetist husband for murder.

REFERENCES AND FURTHER READING

Baselt RC. 2000. *Disposition of toxic drugs and chemicals in man*, 5th edn. Chemical Toxicology Institute, Foster City, CA.

Bourel B, Fleurisse L, Hedouin V, *et al.* 2001. Immunohistochemical contribution to the study of morphine metabolism in Calliphoridae larvae and implications in forensic entomotoxicology. *J Forensic Sci* **46**:596–9.

Bradford LW. 1966. Changing attitudes in drinking driver enforcement as reflected by the actions of researchers, courts, prosecutors and society. *J Forensic Sci Soc* **6**:204–8.

Cordonnier J, Heyndricks A, Piette M. 1986. Drug levels in plasma, vitreous humor, bone marrow, liver and bile. *Police Surg* **30**:60–7.

Drummer OH, Gerostamoulos J. 2002. Postmortem drug analysis: analytical and toxicological aspects. *Ther Drug Monit* **24**:199–209.

Fermer RE. 1995. *Forensic pharmacology*. Oxford University Press, Oxford.

Gagliano-Candela R, Aventaggiato L. 2001. The detection of toxic substances in entomological specimens. *Int J Legal Med* **114**:197–203.

Gifford A, Turkel M. 1956. Diffusion of alcohol through stomach wall after death. *JAMA* **161**:866–8.

Glendening BL, Waugh TC. 1965. The stability of ordinary blood alcohol samples held at various periods of time under different conditions. *J Forensic Sci* **10**:192–200.

Goff ML, Lord WD. 1994. Entomotoxicology. A new area for forensic investigation. *Am J Forensic Med Pathol* **15**:51–7.

Grellner W, Glenewinkel F. 1997. Exhumations: synopsis of morphological and toxicological findings in relation to the postmortem interval. Survey on a 20-year period and review of the literature. *Forensic Sci Int* **90**:139–59.

Hilberg T, Rogde S, Morland J. 1999. Postmortem drug redistribution – human cases related to results in experimental animals. *J Forensic Sci* **44**:3–9.

Introna F, Campobasso CP, Goff ML. 2001. Entomotoxicology. *Forensic Sci Int* **120**:42–7.

Jenkins AJ, Levine BS, Smialek JE. 1995. Distribution of ethanol in postmortem liver. *J Forensic Sci* **40**:611–13.

Jones AW, Lofgren A, Eklund A, *et al.* 1992. Two fatalities from ingestion of acetonitrile: limited specificity of analysis by headspace gas chromatography. *J Anal Toxicol* **16**:104–6.

Klatt EC, Beatie C, Noguchi TT. 1988. Evaluation of death from hypoglycemia. *Am J Forensic Med Pathol* **9**:122–5.

Langford AM, Pounder DJ. 1997. Possible markers for postmortem drug redistribution. *J Forensic Sci* **42**:88–92.

Levine BS, Smith ML, Froede RC. 1990. Postmortem forensic toxicology. *Clin Lab Med* **10**:571–89.

McCurdy WC. 1987. Postmortem specimen collection. *Forensic Sci Int* **35**:61–5.

O'Neal CL, Poklis A. 1996. Postmortem production of ethanol and factors that influence interpretation: a critical review. *Am J Forensic Med Pathol* **17**:8–20.

Palmeri A, Pichini S, Pacifici R, *et al.* 2000. Drugs in nails: physiology, pharmacokinetics and forensic toxicology. *Clin Pharmacokinet* **38**:95–110.

Paterson SC. 1985. Drug levels found in cases of fatal self-poisoning. *Forensic Sci Int* **27**:129–33.

Plueckhahn VD. 1968. Alcohol levels in autopsy heart blood. *J Forensic Med* **15**:12–21.

Plueckhahn VD, Ballard B. 1968. Factors influencing the significance of alcohol concentrations in autopsy blood samples. *Med J Aust* **1**:939–43.

Polson CJ, Green MA, Lee MR. 1983. *Clinical toxicology*, 3rd edn. Pitman, London.

Pounder DJ, Jones GR. 1990. Post-mortem drug redistribution – a toxicological nightmare. *Forensic Sci Int* **45**:253–63.

Pounder DJ, Yonemitsu K. 1991. Postmortem absorption of drugs and ethanol from aspirated vomitus – an experimental model. *Forensic Sci Int* **51**:189–95.

Prouty RW, Anderson WH. 1990. The forensic science implications of site and temporal influences on postmortem blood-drug concentrations. *J Forensic Sci* **35**:243–70.

Shapiro HA. 1953. The concept of the fatal dose. *J Forensic Med* **1**:129–31.

Sperhake J, Tsokos M, Sperhake K. 1999. Perimortem fixation of the gastric and duodenal mucosa: a diagnostic indication for oral poisoning. *Int J Legal Med* **112**:317–20.

Stead AH, Moffat AC. 1983. A collection of therapeutic, toxic and fatal blood drug concentrations in man. *Hum Toxicol* **2**:437–64.

Wennig R. 2000. Threshold values in toxicology – useful or not? *Forensic Sci Int* **113**:323–30.

Winek CL, Jr, Winek CL, Wahba WW. 1995. The role of trauma in postmortem blood alcohol determination. *Forensic Sci Int* **71**:1–8.

CHAPTER 28

Forensic aspects of alcohol

Ethyl alcohol is the most commonly used drug in the world and has such numerous points of contact with medico-legal pathology that it has to be considered separately from all other substances. Its abuse is a prime factor in many accidents – transport, domestic and industrial – and the majority of homicides are catalysed by alcohol intake. It acts as an adjuvant to many other toxic substances, combining to cause a fatal outcome where often the other drug alone would not have caused death. The chronic abuse of alcohol leads not only to definite pathological changes in a number of target organs, but also contributes to deaths from neglect, hypothermia and burns.

This central role in forensic practice makes it imperative that a comprehensive knowledge of its metabolism and effects is held by every forensic pathologist, not only for an understanding of autopsy appearances, but to be able to assist investigative authorities to place the death into its alcoholic context.

MODE OF ACTION OF ALCOHOL

Ethanol is a small molecule that is easily miscible with water and therefore quickly diffuses through the whole of the aqueous compartment of the body.

There are slight variations in the intracellular concentration in different tissues – for instance, the red blood cells contain somewhat less alcohol than plasma, so that a whole-blood concentration is slightly less than that in separated plasma or serum. Most serous fluids are in equilibrium, however, though Plueckhahn (1968) claims that pleural and pericardial fluids have a higher concentration

than that of plasma. The aqueous humour of the eye is in equilibrium with blood, as is cerebrospinal fluid, given sufficient time for equilibration.

It is said above that alcohol disperses rapidly through the aqueous compartment and this excludes the adipose tissues, as ethanol is almost insoluble in fat. This fact has important practical significance, as people with large fat stores will produce a higher blood-alcohol level for a given intake of alcohol than persons of the same weight who are lean, as the aqueous compartment is smaller. This is particularly relevant to women, who, by virtue of their **panniculus adiposus**, may develop blood-alcohol concentrations at least 25 per cent higher than men of the same body weight after similar drinks. This must be allowed for in all calculations that attempt to relate blood-alcohol levels to intake of drink.

The behavioural effect of alcohol is caused by its action on brain cells and is a function of the concentration in the blood, the alcohol readily passing the 'blood–brain barrier' to bathe neurones via the cerebral extracellular fluid. The action of alcohol is entirely depressant, a fact not always appreciated by those who observe the apparent excitant effect of drinking. Alcohol acts on neural cells in a way similar to hypoxia, reducing their activity. In lower concentrations, this action is confined to the more specialized and sensitive cells of the cerebral cortex, leaving lower brain functions relatively unaffected. The consequent depression of these higher areas releases their inhibitory tone and thus 'takes the brakes off' more primitive and unrestrained behaviour. This was aptly described by Thomas de Quincey (1785–1859) when he wrote that 'sobriety disguiseth man'!

With increasing concentrations of ethanol, progressively lower levels of brain function are depressed and, when the vital centres in the midbrain and medulla are affected, there is a danger of fatal cardiorespiratory failure. Alcohol also causes changes in the heat regulatory mechanism, both centrally and by a vasomotor effect. Generalized vasodilatation occurs, especially in the skin, which may lead to marked heat loss and dangerous hypothermia. There is an increase in heart rate with low concentrations but, when alcohol levels approach the dangerous ranges in excess of 300 mg/100 ml, bradycardia may develop. A slight and inconstant increase in blood pressure may occur, more often in the systolic level, which increases the pulse pressure between systolic and diastolic. There is no evidence to support the contention that alcohol dilates the coronary arteries and claims that it causes dilatation of cerebral arteries (and thus worsens intracranial haemorrhage) are also equivocal. Alcohol also has a diuretic effect and, when combined with large quantities of fluid, as in excessive beer drinking, may lead to electrolyte disturbances. In healthy test subjects short-term alcohol administration causes transitory hypoparathyroidism, accounting, at least in part, for the transient hypocalcaemia, hypercalciuria and hypermagnesiuria. In alcoholic patients especially hypomagnesaemia is common.

ABSORPTION OF ALCOHOL

For all practical purposes, it may be assumed that the only route of absorption of alcohol is by mouth as, although it can be inhaled, situations where this occurs must be rare indeed. One case is known to the author (PS), in which a man suffering from a tumour of the base of the tongue, probably causing difficulties in swallowing, had instilled fruit brandy rectally via a plastic tube using a pump, and dying as the result of acute alcohol poisoning.

Almost as soon as the alcohol is swallowed, it begins to be absorbed into the blood – and as soon as that blood reaches the liver, the alcohol begins to be eliminated. Therefore the blood level (and hence the brain concentration) is a dynamic balance between absorption and elimination, the peak determining the maximum behaviour effect. Such a balance is often represented graphically by the 'blood-alcohol curve' (BAC), which indicates the intensity and duration of physiological effects.

Ethanol is capable of being absorbed by any part of the gastrointestinal canal, but in practice this is confined to the stomach and upper small intestine, as only a little alcohol remains to pass through the wall of the ileum or colon. When alcohol is taken with food, however, there seems to be a deficit in the amount absorbed, as some never appears in the bloodstream. Some of this lost alcohol may be excreted in the faeces, but when absorption is slow, more may be destroyed by the liver directly from the portal blood, never surviving to enter the systemic circulation. Nickolls (1956) estimated this lost alcohol taken with food to be between 17 and 20 per cent and Alha (1951) gave the range as 10–20 per cent. Recent studies suggest that it is probably much less, around 5 per cent.

Owing to a thinner mucosa, a better blood supply and a larger surface area, the upper small intestine – the duodenum and jejunum – has the maximum capacity for absorption, compared with the gastric mucosa. This has practical implications, as drink taken by mouth will be absorbed more quickly when:

- a gastrectomy or gastroenterostomy has been carried out previously, as the drink will pass rapidly through to the upper small intestine
- the stomach is empty, as fluid will pass through the pylorus with almost no delay.

Conversely, when the stomach contains food, the drink will be held up until digestion has proceeded sufficiently for the contents to be released into the duodenum. A fatty meal will slow this process down even more and milk feed also has a marked delaying effect. Obviously some absorption will still occur in the interim via the gastric mucosa, but not at the same high rate as in the duodenum and jejunum. As well as delaying emptying, a full stomach will retard absorption by mixing with the alcohol and physically reducing its access to the gastric lining where transit into the blood takes place.

Another factor in the speed of absorption is the concentration of the alcohol. A strength of about 20 per cent is optimum for rapid absorption, which is met (in an empty stomach) by sherry or port wine, or spirits diluted with a 'mixer', such as gin and tonic or whisky and soda. It is also said that carbonated drinks (those containing dissolved carbon dioxide, such as champagne, tonic or soda water, or lemonade) hasten absorption, perhaps because the bubbles greatly increase the surface area carrying alcohol.

Dilute drinks, such as beer (with a concentration of about 4 per cent alcohol) will be absorbed much more slowly – probably because the large volume impedes access of the alcohol molecules to the stomach lining. Beer may take twice as long to absorb as stronger drinks, though part of the delay is caused by contained carbohydrates, which is another factor that slows absorption. For example, when whisky is diluted to the same strength as beer, absorption is more rapid and the peak is higher than drinking the same amount of alcohol in the form of beer.

Very strong drink slows the rate of transfer into the bloodstream. Neat spirits or liqueurs, which may be in excess of 40 per cent alcohol, cause:

- pyloric spasm and hence retarded emptying into the duodenum

- irritation of the gastric lining, forming a barrier of mucus, which slows absorption
- reduced gastric motility, which also retards emptying.

Given an empty stomach and an optimum concentration of alcohol, most of the drug will have entered the bloodstream between 30 and 90 minutes after drinking. According to research by Wilkinson *et al.* (1977), the average times to reach peak blood concentration were 22, 40, 55 and 60 minutes after drinking 11, 22, 36 and 45 g of alcohol in a bolus of similar volumes.

It has been calculated that 98 per cent of alcohol drunk would be absorbed within 10 minutes if it went straight into the small intestine – most of the delay is due to hold-up in the stomach. Rates vary greatly among different people and even in the same person at different times, irrespective of food being taken, but an acceptable mean time would be that 60 per cent of the imbibed alcohol would be absorbed within 60 minutes and 90 per cent within 90 minutes.

Food in the stomach can, however, at least double these times and a large fatty meal can delay total absorption for a number of hours. This has an important effect on the dynamic state between absorption and elimination, as the rate of the latter is relatively constant (see below) and can therefore deal with the slow delivery of alcohol from the portal blood so effectively that the peak of the blood-alcohol curve is low – indeed the curve becomes a long shallow curve instead of a sharp hillock. Where there is a legal threshold for blood alcohol in relation to driving, the taking of food can easily cause one person who has had a large meal to remain well under this limit, whereas another person who drank the same amount at the same time may rapidly exceed the threshold if he drank on an empty stomach. Incidentally, the same effect can occur, notwithstanding food, where a man and woman drink the same amount, as described earlier.

Some drugs will affect absorption rates, by modifying the speed of stomach emptying. Atropine, chlorpromazine, tricyclic antidepressants, procyclidine, amphetamines, morphine, antidiarrhoea compounds (e.g. Lomotil), codeine, methadone, heroin, pethidine, etc., will delay gastric transit, whilst the antiemetics cisapride and metoclopramide, as well as the antibiotic erythromycin, will hasten stomach emptying.

ELIMINATION OF ETHANOL

Almost all alcohol is detoxified by the liver, only 2–10 per cent being excreted unchanged. This means that a heavy drinking session places a great metabolic burden upon the liver and is the cause of hepatic damage after long-standing drinking. The elimination mechanism is an oxidation of alcohol by liver enzymes, through acetaldehyde to acetate. The first stage is performed by the enzyme alcohol dehydrogenase but, as the second stage is much more rapid, little acetaldehyde has time to accumulate. The acetic acid is rapidly oxidized further to carbon dioxide and water. Some may also be broken down by a microsomal oxidase system.

The rate of elimination is of crucial importance to the shape of the blood-alcohol curve, the height of its peak and to the duration of the alcoholaemia. It is also central to any attempts at retrospective calculations of blood, breath or urine levels, as discussed later. Whereas the rate of absorption is variable and is affected by a number of factors, the speed of detoxification in the liver is much more constant and relatively independent of external influences. This is not to say that it is fixed and immutable, even in the same person at different times, but it is capable of reasonable approximation. Much experiment and research has been devoted to this topic and the results, though variable, lie within a fairly narrow band.

Holford (1987) reviewed 11 different studies and found average rates varying between 12.6 and 26.8 mg/100 ml/hour. Neuteboom and Jones (1990) looked at levels in 1300 drivers stopped by the police, and calculated rates between 12 and 38 mg/100 ml/hour in 95 per cent of subjects. Several had rates over 48 mg/100 ml/hour. The elimination rate appeared to increase as the net blood concentration increased, for which several explanations are possible.

As a generalization, it has traditionally been assumed that blood alcohol declines, after the peak is reached, at a rate of around 15 mg/100 ml/hour, but more recent research, especially that of Holford, indicates that this should be raised to 18.7. This applies to healthy adults who are not habituated drinkers, and includes light to moderate drinkers and those 'binge drinkers' who may indulge heavily but intermittently. The enormous number of publications on alcohol must be consulted for details of the range of variation, but basically, elimination can vary from about 12 to 27 mg/100 ml/hour.

Taking the mean as around 18 mg, a man of average size can therefore destroy about 9 g alcohol/hour, with a range variation of between 7 and 16 g. This is about the same as the 'unit' of alcohol, a concept devised for convenience in estimating the daily or weekly intake of drinkers. A 'unit' is of 10 g and is contained (approximately) in half a pint of beer, one single measure of spirits, or a standard glass of table wine.

The habituated drinker, the 'chronic alcoholic', can eliminate far faster than the average person, at least until he suffers severe liver damage in the later stages of his addiction. Though there is some controversy about the experimental evidence, workers such as Bonnichsen (1966) have shown that the rate is greater in older people, at higher blood-alcohol levels, and in habituated drinkers. The rate in the latter may be in excess of 40 mg/100 ml/hour and work at

Lion Laboratories in Wales, who manufacture equipment for breath testing, have found rates over 50 mg/100 ml/hour in chronic alcoholics.

Between 90 and 98 per cent of ingested alcohol is removed from the blood by the liver, leaving a small residue to be excreted unchanged by the kidneys, lungs, sweat, salivary and mammary glands. The ethanol in glomerular filtrate is in equilibrium with plasma, but as water is absorbed in the renal tubules, the urine concentration is higher than the blood level at the time of filtration, the ratio being approximately 123:100. This means, for example, that the legal limit for driving in Britain of 80 mg/100 ml blood is taken to be 107 mg/100 ml in urine.

Unfortunately, it is obvious that, except in the highly unlikely circumstances of ureteric catheterization, the urine concentration can never accurately represent the blood concentration at any given time. The blood concentration is almost never static, but is either rising or falling, so the amount of alcohol in the glomerular filtrate is also constantly varying. It is being mixed in the bladder, however, with previously filtered urine and will also have that which is filtered later added to it, until the bladder is emptied – so it can only provide an average concentration for the time between two micturitions. An added error is that urine produced before drinking began (and which was therefore alcohol-free) may have already been in the bladder and will dilute the alcoholic urine. In many countries, where urine is used for drink-driving testing, the subject is instructed by the police to empty his or her bladder before collection is made over the subsequent hour, in order to avoid the dilution factor.

Breath is now used by many jurisdictions to measure alcohol intake, either as a screening test before blood is taken for analysis, or as an evidential method instead of blood or urine. There is still some controversy over the scientific accuracy of this method, but usually the results are so high that errors are immaterial – or in marginal results, more accurate blood testing is indicated.

Alveolar air at 37°C is in equilibrium with the pulmonary capillary plasma alcohol, the ratio being about 2300:1, volume to volume, for blood as against breath. There is some dispute as to the true ratio, which lies somewhere between 2100 and 2400. If sufficiently deep exhalation is made to drive out dead-space air, then the collected sample can be analysed to give a measure of the blood alcohol, though slight errors occur if there is incomplete elimination of dead-space air and a drop in temperature as the air travels through the dead space. In most countries using evidential breath testing, however, the offence is not in having a breath-alcohol level in excess of an equivalent blood level, but in having excess alcohol in the breath. This obviates defence ploys that would attempt to throw scientific doubt on the relationship between the two concentrations.

ALCOHOL CONCENTRATIONS: UNITS AND VARIOUS DRINKS

The concentration (often called the 'level') of alcohol in blood, urine and breath is expressed by a variety of metric units, which may lead to some confusion. The index most widely used for blood, urine and other body fluids is the weight of alcohol per volume of diluent – for example, milligrams per hundred millilitres (mg/100 ml). The expression 'decilitre' may be used instead of 100 ml (mg/dl). In some countries in continental Europe, alcohol concentration is expressed as 'pro mille', which is grams per litre (g/l), equivalent to milligrams per millilitre (mg/ml). Elsewhere, especially in the USA, a 'percentage' system is common, but can be ambiguous as it does not intrinsically state whether the percentage is volume/volume, volume/weight, weight/weight or weight/volume. Unless otherwise stated, it is assumed to be a weight/volume.

Breath is almost universally measured as micrograms per hundred millilitres (μg/100 ml). The matter of weight and volume is important in respect of alcohol concentrations. The specific gravity of alcohol is 0.79, the compound being appreciably lighter than water. In alcoholic drinks, the manufacturer's description and labelling is almost always 'volume/volume' (v/v), but physiological calculations are made via the weight of alcohol in a given volume of body fluid (w/v). Therefore, especially for stronger alcoholic drinks, a conversion has to be made. For example, many spirits, such as whisky, may be labelled as 40 per cent v/v, but this would be only about 32 per cent weight/volume. For weak drinks, such as beer, it is hardly worth correcting the 4 per cent v/v, as calculations have a far greater intrinsic error from other factors.

Approximate strengths of common drinks are as follows (all v/v):

- beer, lager, stout: 3–5 per cent
- cider (variable): 5 per cent
- table wines (unfortified): 9–12 per cent
- fortified wines (sherry, port, vermouth): 18–20 per cent
- spirits (brandy, gin, whisky, rum, vodka): 37–42 per cent
- liqueurs (variable): 15–55 per cent.

The practice of using 'units of alcohol' has become popular in recent years, not so much for calculating concentrations, but for approximate estimates of intake, in relation to excessive drinking and the long-term medical consequences of alcohol consumption. A 'unit' is of the order of 10 per cent ethanol and very approximately delivered by 'one drink', where this is either a half pint of beer, one glass of table wine or one small measure of spirits. For example, it has been recommended that men should not exceed about 20 units per week and women 14, to avoid the risk of liver damage. It has recently been claimed that from statistical analysis of forensic autopsy material, the risk of coronary heart disease can be reduced by drinking 2 units a day (Thomsen 1995).

Calculation of blood levels from drink taken and the converse

The most important statement in this respect is to stress the utter unreliability and inaccuracy of attempting back-calculations in either direction. Only gross approximations can be achieved and no pretence at accuracy must be offered. In this book, we are not concerned with the controversial problems of trying to estimate blood or breath levels in living vehicle drivers at some time prior to an accident or other event, but with similar problems that can arise in fatal cases, especially in relation to drink and driving. In both criminal and civil disputes, evidence is often sought as to the alcoholic state of the deceased at some material time, based on calculations made from blood or urine alcohol analyses taken at autopsy. Less often, aviation, railway, diving and industrial fatalities may present the same potential problem. Criminal proceedings may arise because of alleged reckless driving on the part of another, when the drunken state of the deceased victim may offer some defence. In civil matters, often involving insurance companies, a significant blood-alcohol level may be used as contributory negligence.

Whatever the reason, the pathologist must offer interpretations of alcohol levels found at autopsy with caution, especially where retrospective calculations are requested. Less often, the pathologist may be asked what blood or urine levels might be expected at a certain time (for example, at the time of death) given a description and timetable of alcoholic drinks taken by the deceased. The same cautions against overprecise calculations must be offered here. In calculating approximate blood levels from a knowledge of the drink taken, there are several methods in use: either the well-known 'Widmark factor' or other calculations, which are really modifications or simplifications of the Widmark technique.

Widmark, in 1932, produced his well-known formula for calculating the total amount of alcohol in the body, from which knowing the body weight and assuming equilibration throughout the water compartment, the blood-alcohol level could be derived.

The Widmark equation is: $A = R \times P \times C$, where A is the total body alcohol, C the blood concentration, P the body weight in kilograms and R a factor, which is 0.68 in

men and 0.55 in women. The sex difference is due to the different fat:water ratios, men having about 54 per cent and women 44 per cent water partition by weight.

Much research and modification of Widmark's factors has been carried out. Hume and Fitzgerald (1985) claimed that the use of body water distribution was too complex. Gullberg and Jones (1994) have published data on a re-evaluation of the Widmark equation, in which they claim to be able to estimate from a single blood-alcohol determination, the amount of alcohol consumed, within an error of ±20 per cent. Pounder and Kuroda (1994) claim that the use of vitreous fluid (which is sometimes used in decomposed or damaged bodies in place of blood) to predict the blood-alcohol concentration, is too variable to be of practical use.

A useful approximate calculation, derived from Widmark, is that an intake of 0.2 g of alcohol per kilogram body weight is likely to result in a blood-alcohol concentration in men of about 25 mg/100 ml.

The following facts are of use:

- The average rate of decline of blood alcohol after the peak of the curve is reached, may be taken as about 15 mg/100 ml/hour, though recent research suggests 18 as more accurate.
- The weight of alcohol imbibed may be calculated from knowledge of the v/v strength of the liquor and the amount taken. For example, if a 'double' British measure of 40 per cent v/v whisky is drunk, then 15 ml will contain (40 × 0.8) = 32 per cent alcohol w/v in 15 ml = 4.8 g.
- The weight of alcohol/kg body weight is calculated.
- A ratio of 0.2 g alcohol/kg body weight will produce a blood level of approximately 25 mg/100 ml in a man, assuming an empty stomach.
- In women, the level so produced may be 20–25 per cent higher.
- If only beer is drunk, the peak will be considerably less, sometimes only 50 per cent that produced from wine or spirits.
- Drinking during or after a meal markedly flattens the blood–alcohol curve.

PHYSIOLOGICAL EFFECTS OF ALCOHOL

The pathologist is frequently asked in either written opinions or in court testimony to give an estimate of the behavioural state of a victim at a certain level of blood alcohol or after having taken a specified amount of drink. Though he is usually not qualified as an expert on alcoholism in any

TABLE 28.1 *General spectrum of behaviour (mg/100 ml of alcohol in blood)*

Above 30	Impairment of complex skills such as driving
30–50	Definite deterioration in driving ability
50–100	Objective signs such as loquaciousness, progressive loss of inhibitions, laughter and some sensory disturbance
100–150	Slurred speech, unsteadiness, possible nausea
150–200	Obvious drunkenness, nausea, staggering gait
200–300	Stupor, vomiting, possibly coma
300–350	Stupor or coma, danger of aspirating vomit
Over 350	Progressive danger of death from respiratory centre paralysis

clinical sense, he will be a medical practitioner with general knowledge and some personal experience of alcoholic behaviour, from his pre-pathology years. He thus can give a general opinion to assist the court, but unless he has special experience of the matter, he should not extend himself into detailed clinical expositions, which are the province of the psychiatrist with an interest in alcoholism, a police surgeon or a casualty officer, all of whom deal frequently with drunken patients. A general level of knowledge can be offered to the lawyer, police or court, however, especially in respect of the usual level of capability and consciousness at different blood-alcohol levels (Table 28.1).

The list in Table 28.1 is probably 'worst case' in nature, as many people show less effects at given blood levels. Women are usually more affected at lower levels, though the 'world record' for survival may be a woman who survived a blood alcohol of 1510 mg/100 ml (Johnson *et al.* 1982). Many drivers stopped by the police at random road blocks in Australia had blood levels over 500 mg/100 ml.

MODES OF DEATH IN ACUTE ALCOHOLISM

Death from alcoholic poisoning is not uncommon and can occur at blood levels in excess of about 300 mg/100 ml. Johnson *et al.* (1982) claimed that some deaths could be attributed to alcohol at even lower concentrations. Death can be caused either by the direct depressive effects upon the brainstem, mediated via the respiratory centres – or through secondary events such as aspiration of vomit. As discussed in Chapter 14, the use of 'aspiration of vomit' as a cause of death must be used with great caution unless there is ante-mortem eyewitness evidence. The major exception to this proviso is in acute alcoholism, where if copious inhalation of stomach contents right down to the secondary bronchi is confirmed, then in the absence of significant natural disease, injury or other toxicity, a high blood-alcohol

level may reasonably be incriminated as the probable cause. Many such fatalities occur during police custody, when considerable outcry, publicity and disciplinary investigations are the usual outcome.

Drunken persons are often involved in fatal trauma, which may be of many types. The majority of homicides are triggered by the aggressive behaviour engendered by alcohol. Road accidents, either caused by drunken drivers (often upon themselves) or by drunken pedestrians walking into traffic, are commonly related to alcoholic vulnerability. Falls are extremely frequent and often fatal. Drunken persons may fall down stairs or steps and suffer head injuries. Falls from high places are less common, but do occur from drunken carelessness or unsteady gait – exemplified by the notorious inquest on Helen Smith in Leeds in 1982.

Death from burns or carbon monoxide poisoning may occur in drunken persons who smoke when intoxicated. A common scenario is for a drunk to go to bed and fall asleep whilst smoking, the cigarette igniting the bedclothes. Sometimes, a gas, electric or kerosene heater may be knocked over during drunken staggering, which again starts a fatal fire.

Drowning is seen occasionally, especially in river or dockland areas. A typical happening is for a drunken sailor to return to his ship late at night, and fall from a bridge or gangway into the water. Death is sometimes not caused by drowning, but by sudden vagal cardiac arrest from the shock of hitting cold water or having cold water suddenly flood the pharynx and larynx. The drunken state seems to sensitize the victim to such vasovagal shock, perhaps because of the marked cutaneous vasodilatation encouraged by alcohol. The author (BK) has seen a number of such tragedies in Cardiff dockland, including a sailor and his woman companion, who both fell off the ship after carousing.

CHRONIC ALCOHOLISM

The pathological features of this condition are extensive and can only be surveyed briefly here. In this context, chronic alcoholism refers to the steady, regular abuse of drink, rather than intermittent 'binge' drinking, which gives the tissues time to recover between bouts of acute alcoholism.

At autopsy, there may be signs of general neglect and malnutrition, but many chronic alcoholics are obese or even oedematous, the latter because of chronic heart failure. The specific lesions are in the liver, heart and brain, though they may be difficult to identify as unequivocally caused by alcohol. The early stages of liver damage cause fatty change, usually with enlargement. The normal weight, according to the sex and build, is between 1300 and 1600 g, but a fatty liver may be well in excess of 2000 g.

The surface is pale and greasy, though this may not be a uniform change, especially in early or less severe cases. Patchy yellowish areas may be visible within normal hepatic parenchyma.

If the abuse continues, then the fatty change may eventually give way to fibrosis, the liver surface becoming rippled beneath its capsule. Such cirrhosis is fairly fine, with nodules of the order of 5–10 mm in diameter. In the later stages the liver becomes smaller and contracts to a hard, greyish-yellow block of only 800–1200 g.

Without a history of long-term alcohol abuse, it is difficult or impossible to be definite about the aetiology purely on autopsy appearances, though suspicion may be strong. A similar liver may develop as a sequel to hepatitis – and less often as an end result of certain dietary or metabolic defects. The spleen may be enlarged and firm, and portal varices may be present at the gastro-oesophageal junction, but these are both manifestations of portal hypertension and do not assist in determining the precise aetiology of the hepatic fibrosis. A useful index of liver damage and the progression or remission of alcoholic impairment is the level of the enzyme γ-glutamyl transpeptidase in the serum. Normal levels are less than 36 units, whereas liver damage can elevate this by a factor of many times. Alcoholic cardiomyopathy is certainly a real entity and can be diagnosed clinically. Whether it can be definitely identified on histological appearances alone is a matter of dispute. The heart is enlarged and shows patchy fibrosis with a variable mixed cellular infiltrate, hypertrophy of muscle fibres, patchy necrosis, hyalinization, oedema and vacuolization. Nuclear enlargement and polymorphism complete the range of changes, but none of these are specific, being found in hypertensive heart disease, coronary stenosis and other types of myocarditis. Combined with a definite history of chronic alcoholism, however, these relatively non-specific changes can be ascribed to alcohol if other causes can be excluded (see also Chapter 25). More specific myocardial damage has been caused by cobalt added to commercial beers and several outbreaks are on record. Systemic fat embolism has also been recorded in victims of alcoholic fatty liver. Microinfarcts in myocardium and brain are possible, though this aspect has so far been rather neglected in research. Fat stains are not usually employed in routine investigations and it is not known how the victims of a fatty liver compare with control subjects in respect of diffuse target organ embolism.

REFERENCES AND FURTHER READING

Al Lanqawi Y, Moreland TA, McEwen J, et al. 1992. Ethanol kinetics: extent of error in back extrapolation procedures [see comments]. Br J Clin Pharmacol 34:316–21.

Alha A. 1951. Blood alcohol and inebriation in Finnish men. Am Acad Sci (Fen Series A) V:Medica.

Bonnichsen R. 1966. Oxidation of alcohol. Q J Stud Alcohol 27:554–60.

Brownlie AR, Walls HJ. 1985. Drink, drugs and driving, 2nd edn. Sweet and Maxwell, London.

Buono MJ. 1999. Sweat ethanol concentrations are highly correlated with co-existing blood values in humans. Exp Physiol 84:401–4.

Chikasue F, Yashiki M, Miyazaki T, et al. 1988. Abnormally high alcohol concentration in the heart blood. Forensic Sci Int 39:189–95.

Dick GL, Stone HM. 1987. Alcohol loss arising from microbial contamination of drivers' blood specimens. Forensic Sci Int 34:17–27.

Freireich AW, Bidanset JH, Lukash L. 1975. Alcohol levels in intracranial blood clots. J Forensic Sci 20:83–5.

Gibson AG. 1975. Alcohol can be absorbed through the respiratory tract (a case report). Med Sci Law 15:64.

Grant SA, Millar K, Kenny GN. 2000. Blood alcohol concentration and psychomotor effects. Br J Anaesth 85:401–6.

Gullberg RG, Jones AW. 1994. Guidelines for estimating the amount of alcohol consumed from a single measurement of blood alcohol concentration: Re-evaluation of Widmark's equation. Forensic Sci Int 69:119–30.

Helander A, Jones AW. 2002. [5-HTOL – a new biochemical alcohol marker with forensic applications.] Lakartidningen 99:3950–4.

Holford NH. 1987. Clinical pharmacokinetics of ethanol. Clin Pharmacokinet 13:273–92.

Hume DN, Fitzgerald EF. 1985. Chemical tests for intoxication: what do the numbers really mean? Anal Chem 57:876A–878A, 882A, 884A passim.

Johnson RA, Noll EC, Rodney WM. 1982. Survival after a serum ethanol concentration of 1½% [letter]. Lancet 2:1394.

Jones AW. 2000. Aspects of in-vivo pharmacokinetics of ethanol. Alcohol Clin Exp Res 24:400–2.

Jones AW, Jonsson KA, Kechagias S. 1997. Effect of high-fat, high-protein, and high-carbohydrate meals on the pharmacokinetics of a small dose of ethanol. Br J Clin Pharmacol 44:521–6.

Kalant H. 2000. Effects of food and body composition on blood alcohol curves. Alcohol Clin Exp Res 24:413–14.

King LA. 1983. Nomograms for relating blood and urine alcohol concentrations with quantity of alcohol consumed. *J Forensic Sci Soc* **23**:213–17.

Kubo S, Dankwarth G, Püschel K. 1991. Blood alcohol concentrations of sudden unexpected deaths and non-natural deaths. *Forensic Sci Int* **52**:77–84.

Lahti RA, Vuori E. 2002. Fatal alcohol poisoning: medico-legal practices and mortality statistics. *Forensic Sci Int* **126**:203–9.

Lieber CS. 2000. Ethnic and gender differences in ethanol metabolism. *Alcohol Clin Exp Res* **24**:417–18.

Lieber CS, Davidson CS. 1962. Some metabolic effects of ethyl alcohol. *Am J Med* **33**:319–27.

Logan BK, Case GA, Distefano S. 1999. Alcohol content of beer and malt beverages: forensic consideration. *J Forensic Sci* **44**:1292–5.

Mason JK, Blackmore DJ. 1972. Experimental inhalation of ethanol vapour. *Med Sci Law* **12**:205–8.

Neuteboom W, Jones AW. 1990. Disappearance rate of alcohol from the blood of drunk drivers calculated from two consecutive samples; what do the results really mean? *Forensic Sci Int* **45**:107–15.

Nickolls LC. 1956. *The scientific investigation of crime.* Butterworths, London.

Paton A. 1988. *ABC of alcohol.* British Medical Journal publication, London.

Piette M, Timperman J, Vanheule A. 1986. Is zinc a reliable biochemical marker of chronic alcoholism in the overall context of a medico-legal autopsy? *Forensic Sci Int* **31**:213–23.

Plueckhahn VD. 1968. Alcohol levels in autopsy heart blood. *J Forensic Med* **15**:12–21.

Plueckhahn VD, Ballard B. 1968. Factors influencing the significance of alcohol concentrations in autopsy blood samples. *Med J Aust* **1**:939–43.

Pounder DJ, Kuroda N. 1994. Vitreous alcohol is of limited value in predicting blood alcohol [see comments]. *Forensic Sci Int* **65**:73–80.

Roine R. 2000. Interaction of prandial state and beverage concentration on alcohol absorption. *Alcohol Clin Exp Res* **24**:411–12.

Sunter JP, Heath AB, Ranasinghe H. 1978. Alcohol associated mortality in Newcastle upon Tyne. *Med Sci Law* **18**:84–9.

Thomsen JL. 1995. Atherosclerosis in alcoholics. *Forensic Sci Int* **75**:121–31.

Thomsen JL, Felby S, Theilade P, *et al.* 1995. Alcoholic ketoacidosis as a cause of death in forensic cases. *Forensic Sci Int* **75**:163–71.

Wilkinson PK, Sedman AJ, Sakmar E, *et al.* 1977. Pharmacokinetics of ethanol after oral administration in the fasting state. *J Pharmacokinet Biopharm* **5**:207–24.

Winek CL, Eastly P. 1976. Factors affecting contamination of blood samples for ethanol determination. In: Wecht C (ed.), *Legal medicine annual 1976.* Appleton Century Crofts, New York.

Winek CL, Esposito FM. 1985. Blood alcohol concentrations; factors affecting predictions. In: Wecht C (ed.), *Legal medicine annual 1985.* Praeger Scientific, New York.

Winek CL, Jr, Winek CL, Wahba WW. 1995. The role of trauma in postmortem blood alcohol determination [see comments]. *Forensic Sci Int* **71**:1–8.

Carbon monoxide poisoning

CAUSES OF CARBON MONOXIDE POISONING

After alcohol and some pharmaceutical drugs, carbon monoxide poisoning is probably the most common toxic condition to be met with in routine forensic pathology. The widespread introduction of natural gas (which contains no carbon monoxide) as a replacement for 'coal gas' as a heating fuel has removed a major source of the poison. Monoxide still provides lethal dangers in many other ways, however. It is produced whenever fossil fuels are incompletely oxidized to carbon dioxide and, because of its great affinity for haemoglobin, even low concentrations can be cumulative.

There are a vast number of publications on carbon monoxide toxicity, both in an environmental and industrial context. Once again, this discussion is confined to the pathologist's involvement in fatalities. A body coming to autopsy with suspected (or sometimes unsuspected) carbon monoxide poisoning, will have suffered that toxic condition by the following means.

Motor vehicle exhaust gases

Since the replacement of coal gas (containing up to 7 per cent monoxide) with natural gas, a major means of suicide has been removed. 'Putting the head in the gas oven' was the most common form of self-destruction in Britain and many other countries until this changeover. In 1961 in the UK, for example, there were 2711 suicides and 1014 accidental deaths from carbon monoxide. Since then, suicides have obtained carbon monoxide to kill themselves from the internal combustion engine. Petrol (gasoline) engines produce up to 5–7 per cent carbon monoxide in their exhaust fumes,

and more if the engine is idling, defective or improperly tuned. Diesels produce far less monoxide than petrol engines. Normally, the exhaust pipe vents the gases into the atmosphere, where it may contribute to considerable low-level monoxide contamination in large cities, such that policemen on traffic duty may have up to 10 per cent saturation of their haemoglobin. When the exhaust fumes are confined to a small space, then a dangerous or lethal level can build up in a short space of time. It is calculated that a 1.5 litre petrol engine, idling in a closed single garage, can produce a lethal concentration in the atmosphere within 10 minutes.

Some suicides will merely sit in the garaged car with a window open and allow the gas to overtake them. More commonly, some device is fitted to pipe the gas into the interior of the car and this may be done outside a garage, often in a remote parking spot. The flexible tube from a vacuum cleaner seems a favourite means, though ordinary hose-pipe, pushed inside the tail-pipe and led in through a window, is a common alternative. Apart from suicide, accidental poisoning sometimes occurs in relation to internal combustion engines. A mechanic or car owner may work on a vehicle in a closed garage, especially in cold weather, and be overcome by monoxide before he is able to remove himself from the danger. The insidious nature of the toxic effects may make him unaware of the supervening stupor and coma.

Carbon monoxide can also affect drivers of a moving vehicle, usually because of a defective exhaust system, which allows gas to percolate through the floor or engine bulkhead into the interior. Rarely, a strong following wind blows the external exhaust gas into the open doors of a van or truck. Another motoring cause is a leak in the heat exchanger in those vehicles that use a direct air supply from around the exhaust manifold to provide passenger heating.

In aircraft – usually light planes with the engine immediately adjacent to the cockpit – a leakage of exhaust gas from the motor compartment can lead to disablement of the pilot and death from a crash rather than from fatal toxicity. The same applies to those road-vehicle drivers who are overcome by the gas to an extent that makes them incapable of driving safely. The differential diagnosis in survivors is between carbon monoxide and alcohol, as the clinical symptoms of both are quite similar at one stage of the toxic process.

Deaths have also been reported in 'scuba' divers, whose air cylinders have been contaminated with carbon monoxide during refilling from faulty petrol-driven compressors.

Domestic appliances

Domestic heating appliances can produce carbon monoxide in addition to the usual dioxide from a restriction of their air supply, so that incomplete combustion of the fuel takes place. The fuel can be natural gas, which, though itself free from monoxide, is only partially oxidized from some defect of design, maintenance, or patency of the exhaust flue. Solid-fuel boilers used for central heating may have some restriction of air entry or a partial blockage of the chimney system. Paraffin (kerosene) heaters may burn with inadequate oxygen ingress and any other form of hydrocarbon fuel appliance can malfunction so that part of the products of combustion are monoxide.

The author (BK) has dealt with several deaths that occurred because the faulty installation of natural-gas fires led to absent or inadequate ventilation, causing monoxide to back-diffuse into living rooms. Gas appliances, especially water heaters, are one reason why the bathroom is such a dangerous place. Apart from the extra hazards of electricity, a bath for drowning, wet surfaces for slipping, tablets in the cabinet and sharp instruments such as razor blades, the small-sized room and the frequent installation of a gas water heater or 'geyser' makes this room a frequent locus for unnatural death. Blockage of the exit or 'flue' pipe is a common fault, sometimes from bad installation or because it becomes blocked by soot or by birds' nests.

Structural fires

A common cause of monoxide deaths arises from structural fires in houses and other buildings. As described in Chapter 11, the majority of deaths in house conflagrations are caused not by burns, but by inhalation of smoke. These fatalities are largely caused by carbon monoxide poisoning, though other lethal gases such as cyanide, phosgene and acroleins are partly responsible. Many victims of house fires die remote from the flames, and may be overcome in different rooms or even on different floors, the monoxide percolating considerable distances and killing persons either asleep or trapped elsewhere in the building.

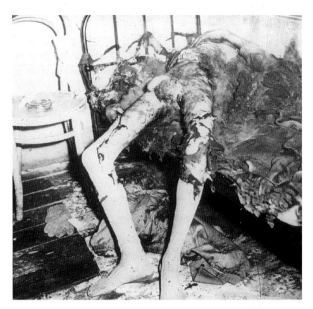

FIGURE 29.1 *Carbon monoxide poisoning in a chronic alcoholic. This is a relatively common event when a drunken person collapses with a lit cigarette across his bed (note the ashtray and cigarette packet). The burns are post-mortem, death being caused by a high level of carboxyhaemoglobin generated by the smouldering bed coverings.*

Industrial processes

Many industrial processes may lead to monoxide poisoning, especially in iron and steel works, where producer gas and water gas are deliberately formed and stored as part of the manufacturing process. Water gas can contain up to 40 per cent carbon monoxide and in former days was added to town gas for the domestic supply, which greatly enhanced the monoxide content of some 7 per cent from coal gas. Many other industrial processes, such as the Mond method of nickel production, use carbon monoxide, as well as the universal danger of any heating process producing the gas during combustion. In coal-mining, carbon monoxide is one of the gases that presents a constant threat; it escapes from the coal seams themselves but is also produced from the frequent small fires that smoulder in the recesses of the mines.

Incomplete combustion

Incomplete combustion of a gas flame from any gaseous fuel can produce carbon monoxide. Where such a flame impinges on a cold metal surface or where that surface is coated with soot, partial oxidation of the fuel supply leads to monoxide production. In appliances fuelled from the common butane or propane cylinder sources, as in caravans, campers and boats, maladjustment or restriction of ventilation can lead to slow but insidious production of monoxide. Deaths of whole families have occurred under such circumstances, as they are exposed overnight to slow accumulation of carbon monoxide from refrigerators and other appliances.

THE AUTOPSY IN CARBON MONOXIDE POISONING

As always, an adequate history may give the clue to the cause of death. Where the circumstances are obvious, such as a death in a car with a tube leading from the exhaust, the pathologist's attention will be directed towards carbon monoxide from the outset. There are many other circumstances, however, in which the history may be obscure, and only the vigilance of the pathologist and his staff will pick up the possibility of this type of toxicity. In fact, many a case has first been recognized by the mortuary technician who commented on the colour of the skin or tissues. A number of fatal monoxide poisonings have already been certified as 'natural causes' by uncritical clinicians (especially in general practice) when in fact carbon monoxide poisoning, either suicidal or accidental, was the true reason for the death. Failure to examine the body fully is the usual cause, as the pink coloration may only be noticeable in the areas of postural hypostasis not normally visible in a body in bed, though the sides and back of the neck are reasonably accessible even to cursory examination. The author (BK) recollects at least one suicide where the relatives placed the body back in bed and had it certified as 'coronary thrombosis' by an unsuspecting family doctor.

At autopsy the most striking appearance of the body is the colour of the skin, especially in areas of post-mortem hypostasis. The classical 'cherry-pink' colour of carboxyhaemoglobin is usually evident if the saturation of the blood exceeds about 30 per cent. Below this, familiarity and good lighting are needed and below 20 per cent, no coloration is visible. As these low concentrations are rarely fatal, however, little is lost. Sometimes, darker cyanosis tends to mask the skin colour, but the margins of the hypostasis and the internal tints are usually apparent.

When the victim is anaemic, the colour may be faint or even absent because insufficient haemoglobin is present to display the colour. In racially pigmented victims the colour may obviously be masked, though may still be seen on the inner aspect of the lips, the nail-beds, tongue, and palms and soles of the hands and feet. It is also seen inside the eyelids, but rarely in the sclera.

Rarely, there may be blistering of the skin of dependent areas, such as the calves and buttocks, and around wrists and knees, similar to the so-called 'barbiturate blisters'. These are not specific to carbon monoxide toxicity and are the result of

cutaneous oedema in any profound coma where there is total immobility and lack of venous return from muscle movement. As most carbon monoxide deaths are relatively rapid, such blisters are rare. Internally the most noticeable feature is again the colour. Blood and muscle will be pink as a result of carboxyhaemoglobin and carboxymyoglobin. In relatively low concentrations, in poor light and in some artificial lighting in autopsy rooms, the cherry-pink colour may be difficult to see. It can be enhanced by diluting the blood with water against a white background, as in a porcelain sink or an enamel scale-pan, when the pinkness will be more evident. The pinkness of hypothermia or refrigeration is a different colour. Unfortunately, some pathologists have a red-colour visual impairment, which makes it difficult for them to differentiate between subtle changes in redness, so laboratory analysis is always required for objective confirmation and quantification of the monoxide concentration. Other suggestive indications of carbon monoxide are that, when tissues are placed in formol saline for preservation of histology, they do not decolourize as quickly as normal tissues and remain pink for a long period. If carbon monoxide poisoning is suspected at autopsy, a quick test is to add a few drops of blood to some 10 per cent sodium hydroxide solution on a white tile or in a tube against a white background. The normal blood will immediately become brownish-green but, if significant monoxide is present, the colour will remain pink, as no methaemoglobin is formed. One has to bear in mind though, that unlike adult blood, fetal blood up to the age of 6 months is more resistant to alkali and the colour change can take hours to develop. Another simple test, mentioned in 1857 by Hoppe, is to take 3 ml blood into a test tube and dilute it with 6 ml tap water and to heat it for a short while with care in a water bath. Carbon monoxide blood turns brick red whereas control blood becomes greyish-brown. However, these crude tests are not recommended as an alternative to proper analysis.

Other signs at autopsy are non-specific. Pulmonary oedema is usually present. The author (BK) has the impression that the white matter of the brain remains unusually firm and that the whole brain after removal from the skull keeps its shape better, being rather stiff and rigid. This may be caused either by oedema or by some minimal fixation change in the brain tissue.

None of these rather idiosyncratic tests can replace proper laboratory investigation, however. Blood should be taken for analysis in the usual way, preferably from a peripheral vein. In contrast to most toxicological investigations, even foul samples can still be useful for carboxyhaemoglobin estimations. Heart blood, blood from body cavities and even from bone marrow when the bones are split open, can still provide valid material for estimating the percentage of haemoglobin converted to carboxyhaemoglobin. It is the

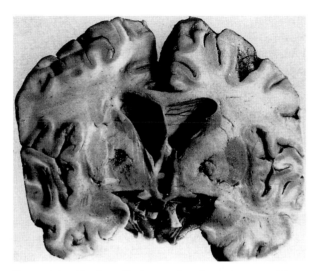

FIGURE 29.2 *Basal ganglia degeneration after carbon monoxide poisoning. The patient survived for a number of weeks, but succumbed to bronchopneumonia. There are cystic lesions in the globus area of both cerebral hemispheres.*

BLOOD ANALYSIS

Carbon monoxide has an affinity for haemoglobin that is between 200 and 300 times greater than oxygen. Therefore even small concentrations of monoxide in the inspired air will progressively displace oxygen from the erythrocytes and this will lower the oxygen-carrying capacity of the blood. It was formerly thought that all the toxic properties of carbon monoxide lay in this hypoxic action, but more recently it has been shown to interfere with other ferroproteins such as myoglobin and various enzymes including members of the cytochrome family.

The major effect is undoubtedly the reduction in oxygen transport and, for this reason, it is the percentage saturation of the total available haemoglobin that is important rather than an absolute quantity of carboxyhaemoglobin in the blood. Anaemic persons will not show the external cherry-pink colour if insufficient haemoglobin is available for the monoxide component to become visible. It is the residual non-combined haemoglobin still available for oxygen transport that is important in maintaining life. For example, an anaemic person with only 8 g/100 ml of haemoglobin having four of those occupied with carbon monoxide (50 per cent saturation) is in much worse a state than a person with a total of 14 g of which four are monoxide-occupied. There are many tables available that relate saturation levels to the clinical symptoms. There is a wide margin of variation in these, as there is with lethal levels.

Broadly speaking, the saturation levels found in fatal cases reflect both the physical state of the victim and the rapidity with which the poisoning took place. Robust, healthy adults under 60 years of age rarely die at saturation level under 50–60 per cent unless the concentration of carbon monoxide in the inspired air was so great that death occurred before gas exchange in the lungs was able to progress sufficiently to enter all available monoxide into the red cells. Death may then supervene with post-mortem saturation levels of as low as 40 per cent. Where absorption is slow and life persists longer (for there seems to be a relationship between air concentration of monoxide and length of survival), autopsy samples may show 80 per cent saturation.

Old people may die at relatively low concentrations, such as 30 per cent and, in some cases, no other cause can be found when the carboxyhaemoglobin level is only 25 per cent. This may be the result of anaemia, so that there is less reserve for oxygen carrying when part of the haemoglobin is occupied by monoxide. In many cases, the senile myocardium is already in a fragile state and any extra hypoxia will cause it to fail. Infants also seem to die at relatively low levels, perhaps because their higher respiration rate allows a more rapid absorption. The variation in fatal concentrations is

ratio of haemoglobin to the carboxy-type that is required, rather than an absolute concentration in the blood, so virtually any blood-containing fluid will provide this answer. When a body has been badly damaged by fire, fluid blood may be hard to obtain, so that any sanguineous body fluid or bone marrow can provide material for analysis. If analysis is to be delayed more than a day, it is recommended that fluoride be added as a preservative.

There are no other autopsy features in acute deaths, which form the majority seen by forensic pathologists. Where survival occurs there are a number of neurological lesions that follow severe carbon monoxide exposure. Necrosis and cavitation of the basal ganglia in the brain, notably the putamen and globus pallidus, has been known for well over a century. Within about 5 days, histological changes occur here, with 'gitterzellen' scavenging cellular debris, the foam cells and microglia presenting an appearance characteristic of tissue breakdown in the central nervous system. There may also be damage in the substantia nigra of the brainstem. In delayed deaths, petechiae and ring-shaped haemorrhages may occur in the cerebral white matter. All these changes, together with the clinical symptomatology, are exhaustively described in neurological publications.

There are also tiny focal necroses in the myocardium in delayed deaths from this cause, and similar lesions were described by Korb and David (1962) even in acute deaths. Frank myocardial infarction has often been reported after severe monoxide exposure and relative hypoxia, usually in the presence of pre-existing coronary disease, is probably the reason.

wide and quite irregular. This is best exemplified when two or more victims have died together in the same environment. The carboxyhaemoglobin concentrations of bodies lying alongside each other can sometimes be totally different, even in persons of the same age group and physical health. Any disease process can contribute to death at lower monoxide concentrations. Coronary artery disease, respiratory insufficiency and other debilitating conditions allow death to occur earlier, when the toxic level is still relatively low. Conditions that are worsened by hypoxia, such as myocardial insufficiency or obstructive airway disease, are particularly potent. In addition to disease, any separate toxic state is additive, such as hypnotic drugs or alcohol.

The method of analysis has traditionally been by reversion spectroscopy, but this is a crude technique in which accuracy cannot be attained to within 10 per cent of the true value. For most purposes related to fatalities, this is good enough, as more exact results do not add anything to the investigation. The only problem can be at the lower end of the scale, when it is difficult to be certain about positivity under about 15 per cent. Modern analytical methods include non-dispersive infrared spectrophotometry and gas chromatography. Carboxyhaemoglobin is stable and can be detected even in putrefied bodies a long time after death, as long as sophisticated laboratory techniques are used. Monoxide cannot enter a body post-mortem to any significant extent. Bodies burnt after death do not absorb any monoxide and thus a significant level (more than 10 per cent) in a body from a fire means that respiration must have been proceeding whilst the conflagration was in progress. As emphasized in Chapter 11, the converse is often not true, in that deaths from rapid fires, especially flash fires caused by petrol, for example, may have no carboxyhaemoglobin in the blood. The possibility of carboxhaemoglobin being formed in the blood post-mortem has been investigated as a possible source of error (Kojima *et al.* 1982) and fluorided samples are recommended.

A minor source of local carboxyhaemoglobin and myohaemoglobin is gunshot wounds, where the propellant gases (which are rich in the compound) are blown into the wound from contact or short-range discharges. The tissues absorb monoxide, especially around the entrance wound. It has been claimed that this is a way of differentiating the entrance from the exit wound, but in fact the whole track of the missile(s) may be sheathed in a zone of monoxide transfer into blood and muscle from a near-discharge, though theoretically there should be a gradient of concentration from one end of the track to the other (see Chapter 8).

Many other war, military and terrorist circumstances are associated with exposure to carbon monoxide. Large quantities are released from the firing of guns and, in enclosed spaces, can become a hazard. Detonation of explosives in places where there is little ventilation also allows monoxide to accumulate and it may persist long after the physical dangers of the explosion have passed.

REFERENCES AND FURTHER READING

Annotation. 1962. Carbon monoxide from paraffin stoves. *Br Med J* **1**:312.

Bohnert M, Weinmann W, Pollak S. 1999. Spectrophotometric evaluation of postmortem lividity. *Forensic Sci Int* **99**:149–58.

Bowen DAL. 1986. Acute renal failure in carbon monoxide poisoning. *J Forensic Med* **7**:78–82.

Chang MY, Lin JL. 2001. Central diabetes insipidus following carbon monoxide poisoning. *Am J Nephrol* **21**:145–9.

Chaturvedi AK, Smith DR, Canfield DV. 2001. Blood carbon monoxide and hydrogen cyanide concentrations in the fatalities of fire and non-fire associated civil aviation accidents, 1991–1998. *Forensic Sci Int* **121**:183–8.

Garland H, Pearce J. 1967. Neurological complications of carbon monoxide poisoning. *Q J Med* **36**:445–55.

Goldbaum LR. 1977. Is carboxyhaemoglobin concentration the indicator of carbon monoxide toxicity? In: Wecht C (ed.), *Legal medicine annual 1976*. Appleton Century Crofts, New York.

Goldsmith JR, Landaw SA. 1968. Carbon monoxide and human health. *Science* **162**:1352–9.

Gottfried JA, Chatterjee A. 2001. Carbon monoxide-mediated hippocampal injury. *Neurology* **57**:17.

Helpern M, Strassman G. 1943. Differentiation of fetal and adult human hemoglobin. *Arch Pathol* **35**:776.

Hoppe F. 1857. Über die Einwirkung des Kohlenoxydgases auf das Hämatoglobin. *Virchows Arch* **11**:228.

King LA. 1983. Effect of ethanol in fatal carbon monoxide poisonings. *Hum Toxicol* **2**:155–7.

Kojima T, Nishiyama Y, Yashiki M, *et al.* 1982. Postmortem formation of carbon monoxide. *Forensic Sci Int* **19**:243–8.

Kojima T, Okamoto I, Yashiki M, *et al.* 1986. Production of carbon monoxide in cadavers. *Forensic Sci Int* **32**:67–77.

Korb A, David K. 1962. Fluorescenzmikroskopische und elektronmikroskopische Untersuchungen am

Herzmuskel der Ratte nach Leuchtgasvergiftungen. *Deutsch Z Gesamt Gericht Med* **52**:549–55.

Kunsman GW, Presses CL, Rodriguez P. 2000. Carbon monoxide stability in stored postmortem blood samples. *J Anal Toxicol* **24**:572–8.

Lee CW, Yim LK, Chan DT, *et al.* 2002. Sample pre-treatment for co-oximetric determination of carboxyhaemoglobin in putrefied blood and cavity fluid. *Forensic Sci Int* **126**:162–6.

Levine B, Moore KA, Fowler D. 2001. Interaction between carbon monoxide and ethanol in fire fatalities. *Forensic Sci Int* **124**:115–16.

Lo Menzo G. 1966. Il comportomento dell'attivita citrocromossidasica a succinodeidrogenase di taluni organi nell'avvelenamento acute da co. *Folia Med* **8**:607–12.

Mant AK. 1960. Accidental carbon monoxide poisoning: A review of 100 consecutive cases. *Med Leg J* **28**:30–6.

Miro O, Casademont J, Barrientos A, *et al.* 1998. Mitochondrial cytochrome *c* oxidase inhibition during acute carbon monoxide poisoning. *Pharmacol Toxicol* **82**:199–202.

O'Donnell P, Buxton PJ, Pitkin A, *et al.* 2000. The magnetic resonance imaging appearances of the brain in acute carbon monoxide poisoning. *Clin Radiol* **55**:273–80.

Pearce J. 1968. Coal gas and the brain [leading article]. *Br Med J* **1**:767.

Petelenz T. 1972. Badania doswiadczaine dzilania. *Arch Med Sadowej Kryminol* **12**:219–25.

Seto Y, Kataoka M, Tsuge K. 2001. Stability of blood carbon monoxide and hemoglobins during heating. *Forensic Sci Int* **121**:144–50.

Simpson K. 1955. Carbon monoxide poisoning. *J Forensic Med* **2**:5–13.

Somogyi E, Balogh I, Rubanyi G, *et al.* 1981. New findings concerning the pathogenesis of acute carbon monoxide (CO) poisoning. *Am J Forensic Med Pathol* **2**:31–9.

Thom SR. 1993. Leukocytes in carbon monoxide-mediated brain oxidative injury. *Toxicol Appl Pharmacol* **123**:234–47.

Thomsen JL, Kardel T. 1988. Intoxication at home due to carbon monoxide production from gas water heaters. *Forensic Sci Int* **36**:69–72.

Uemura K, Harada K, Sadamitsu D, *et al.* 2001. Apoptotic and necrotic brain lesions in a fatal case of carbon monoxide poisoning. *Forensic Sci Int* **116**:213–19.

Walker E, Hay A. 1999. Carbon monoxide poisoning. *Br Med J* **319**:1082–3.

CHAPTER 30

Agrochemical poisoning

In the last half century there has been a technological revolution in farming methods, which has spread to almost all parts of the world. The developing nations (who in terms of area of land usage and proportion of the population who work on that land, are numerically greatest at risk) suffer most and this is sometimes exacerbated by the less stringent controls and less safe working methods that exist in those countries.

The potent chemicals used in agriculture may harm persons by accidental exposure, either during their application to crops, or due to incorrect or careless storage. Another major source of human poisoning is through self-administration, when the easily available substances are used for suicide. For example, in Sri Lanka many thousands of hospital admissions each year are for agrochemical poisoning (16 649 in 1983) with over a thousand deaths annually (1521 in 1983). Of these, about three-quarters were self-administered, the remainder being accidental and occupational.

The main dangers from agricultural chemicals lie in the pesticides, especially organophosphorus compounds, such as parathion and herbicides, such as paraquat.

PARAQUAT POISONING

Paraquat is a herbicide that is sprayed on unwanted weeds and other vegetation before planting crops. It is absorbed by the foliage and rapidly kills the plant, but is inactivated when in contact with the soil, so cannot harm the seeds or young plants that are placed in the same ground a short time later. Paraquat (and the less popular diquat) are dipyridyl compounds, paraquat chemically being 1,1'-dimethyl-4,4'-bipyridyldiylium. It is produced commercially as a brownish concentrated liquid of the dichloride salt at 10–30 per cent strength, under the trade name Gramoxone and, for horticultural use, as brown granules called Weedol at about 5 per cent concentration.

Toxicity occurs almost exclusively through ingestion, though some cases are reported where inhalation through spraying has led to a fatal outcome. A suicide from intravenous injection of paraquat has been reported by Fernandez *et al.* (1991).

Only about 5 per cent of the substance is absorbed orally. Poisoning usually occurs either by deliberate self-ingestion of the liquid concentrate, or by accidental drinking from unmarked or incorrectly marked bottles. It is said that one swallowed mouthful of Gramoxone will almost always be fatal and certainly 5 ml has caused death. The decanting of the concentrate from the original manufacturer's containers leads to many accidental deaths. Because of the relatively high cost, paraquat is often taken from the large containers and kept in lemonade or other soft drink bottles. Such decanting is illegal in some countries such as the Republic of Ireland, because of the dangers of unlabelled bottles. Unsuspecting people, especially children, then take a drink from such bottles and immediately suffer the effects of the potent toxin.

Paraquat in concentrated form, is irritant to all epithelial tissues. The lips, mouth, pharynx and oesophagus are superficially eroded, though there is nothing like the dangerous structural damage of strong acids or alkalis. The major danger of paraquat is to the lungs and liver. The lungs are affected mainly by direct aspiration, either as the irritative substance is swallowed or by regurgitation from the stomach during vomiting.

Of that absorbed through the gastrointestinal tract, the major danger is to the liver, where paraquat causes a centrilobular necrosis, with giant mitochondria and crystalline inclusion bodies seen on electron microscopy. In the kidney, renal failure may develop within 2 or 3 days from diffuse tubular damage.

The striking lesion, almost characteristic of paraquat, is in the proliferative damage to the lungs. If rapid death from acute hepatorenal failure does not occur, either because of low dosage or energetic clearance of the residual poison, then progressive lung damage may still lead to death within the next 2 weeks. When paraquat reaches the distal air spaces, diffuse pulmonary oedema and haemorrhages occur, followed by stimulation of the alveolar lining cells. Prior to this, in the first day or two, there is damage to the pneumocytes with vacuolation, desquamation and necrosis. A hyaline membrane is often visible. The mechanism appears to be that paraquat reacts with tissue elements to produce peroxides, including hydrogen peroxide, which is responsible for the damage, which can be worsened by oxygen therapy.

Within a few days repair begins, the mesenchymal interstitial cells and the alveolar lining cells dividing rapidly and filling the alveoli. Both granular and membranous pneumocytes (types I and II) are involved. Within the first week, gas exchange begins to suffer as the air spaces become occluded by mononuclear cells forming rounded-up 'fibroblasts'. If survival continues, the alveoli begin to fibrose, with reticulin and collagen being laid down to form a rigid, stiff lung.

The autopsy in paraquat poisoning

There may be ulceration around the lips and mouth from escape of paraquat concentrate. The mucosa of the mouth may be reddened or desquamated, and the oesophagus may show worse changes, including casts of shed epithelium. None of these changes is by any means inevitable, however, and the upper gastrointestinal tract may be normal.

Similarly, the stomach may show erosion and patchy haemorrhages, or may be unremarkable. The liver may show pallor or mottled fatty change to the naked eye. It is unusual for any gross charges to be visible. Other organs show no specific changes, apart from the lungs; the kidneys may reveal cortical pallor if there is renal failure.

If the victim has lived a week or more, then the lungs may reveal typical changes in that they are large and stiff, keeping their shape when removed from the chest. There may be a fibrinous pleurisy and sometimes slight bloody pleural effusions. The cut surface reveals oedema and patchy haemorrhage, though this may have subsided in cases that survive for some time. The main appearances are microscopic and, unless the history is known, the lung may be mistaken for a diffuse pneumonia. The author (BK) saw a homicide by paraquat, in which the victim was in hospital for 2 weeks with a presumptive diagnosis of 'virus pneumonia', until a confession revealed the true cause of the lung changes. Samples required at autopsy, apart from full histology, include the usual blood samples, urine, stomach contents, lung and liver.

In most instances, the relative slowness of the death allows the diagnosis to be made on history and clinical grounds, so that ante-mortem toxicology is usually well documented.

Toxicology interpretation

Blood levels of paraquat of 0.2 mg/l are sufficient to cause lung damage. Survival has been recorded, however, with plasma levels of up to 1.6 mg/l. Paraquat is excreted over a long period and can be detected in urine at autopsy many days after ingestion. Concentrations in excess of 0.07 mg/l have been found 26 days later.

The concentrations found on analysis after autopsy naturally depend upon the dose taken and the time that has elapsed since ingestion. On the first day, ranges from 0 to 63 mg/l (average 15) have been found in the blood, with urine levels of 20–1210 mg/l (average 462). Seven days later, the blood level comes down to an average of 0.8 mg/l with 4.5 in the urine. Two to three weeks after ingestion, the blood concentration averages 0.5 and the urine level 0.6 mg/l.

ORGANOPHOSPHORUS PESTICIDES

Used in huge quantities throughout the world, these substances cause thousands of deaths in southern Asia, Africa and elsewhere. The major example is parathion, with malathion and dichlorvos used far less extensively. These chemicals act on insects and other arthropods by inhibiting cholinesterase and their toxic effects on man are caused by the same mechanism.

Parathion (nitrostigmine) is extremely toxic and can be absorbed through the skin, conjunctivae, lungs and gut. Because of the inhibitory effect on plasma and erythrocyte cholinesterases, acetylcholine builds up at neuromuscular junctions and other neurotransmitter sites, resulting in hyperexcitability of both voluntary and involuntary muscle.

Other organophosphorus compounds include malathion, which is much less toxic than parathion and is used more in horticulture: dithion, diazinon, hexaethyltetraphosphate (HETP), tetraethylpyrophosphate (TEPP), octamethylpyrophosphamide (OMPA) and demeton are other pesticides of this group.

Toxic signs and symptoms appear when the cholinesterase level drops to 30 per cent of its normal activity. Fatalities begin to occur after the ingestion of 125–175 mg, though ingestion of much larger amounts can be survived. Death can occur in less than an hour after ingestion, though usually several hours elapse in those who are not going to survive.

Autopsy appearances are more helpful than with many other compounds, in that parathion is dissolved in a kerosene base, which can often be detected by its smell. A greenish colouring agent is often added to the commercial products. The stomach therefore may be seen to contain an oily, greenish scum. The gastric mucosa may be haemorrhagic, though this is too non-specific to be of much use, as is the common finding of haemorrhagic pulmonary oedema.

The author (BK), when practising pathology in Southeast Asia, noted a useful diagnostic sign in some less modern mortuaries that were infested with flies and bluebottles. When these insects alighted on an opened cadaver at autopsy, many fell dead or dying onto the autopsy table when the case in progress was a parathion poisoning.

Toxicology interpretation

Post-mortem toxicology is usually conclusive in acute poisoning. The substance resists post-mortem autolysis well and can be recovered from putrefied bodies. The range of blood parathion concentrations in fatal cases may be from 0.5 to 34 mg/l with an average of 9.0. Urinary excretion ranges from 0.4 to 78 mg/l with an average of 10 mg/l. The liver may contain from 0.1 to 120 mg/kg, averaging 11.

Malathion is much less toxic but deaths certainly occur given a greater dose. Blood levels in fatalities ingesting from 25 to 70 g malathion ranged from 100 to 1880 mg/l with a mean of 815. The liver contained from 200 to 1700 mg/kg, with an average of 1300.

Other pesticides and insecticides include chlorinated compounds such as aldrin, DDI (dicophane), lindane (Gammaxane) and dieldrin. Other types include the carbamates (opxymyl, landrin and aldicarb), dinitrophenols, pyrethrum and derris. The phenolic pesticides include DNOC (dinitro-orthocresylphosphate) and dinitrobutylphenol. None of these has any specific autopsy features and the diagnosis rests upon the history, circumstances, and post-mortem analysis of blood, urine and liver.

REFERENCES AND FURTHER READING

Baselt RC. 2002. *Disposition of toxic drugs and chemicals in man*, 6th edn. Biomedical Publications, Foster City, CA.

Beebeejaun AR, Beevers G, Rogers WN. 1971. Paraquat poisoning-prolonged excretion. *Clin Toxicol* **4**:397–407.

Carson DJ, Carson ED. 1976. The increasing use of paraquat as a suicidal agent. *Forensic Sci* **7**:151–60.

Copeland AR. 1988. Organophosphate related fatalities – a violitional biohazard? *Forensic Sci Int* **39**:155–62.

Cravey RH. 1979. Poisoning by paraquat. *Clin Toxicol* **14**:195–8.

Crowley WJ, Jr, Johns TR. 1966. Accidental malathion poisoning. *Arch Neurol* **14**:611–16.

Davies DS. 1987. Paraquat poisoning: The rationale for current treatment regimes. *Hum Toxicol* **6**:37–40.

Davies DS, Hawksworth GM, Bennett PN. 1977. Paraquat poisoning. *Proc Eur Soc Tox* **18**:21–6.

De Alwis LB, Salgado MS. 1988. Agrochemical poisoning in Sri Lanka. *Forensic Sci Int* **36**:81–9.

Dearden LC, Fairshter RD, McRae DM, *et al.* 1978. Pulmonary ultrastructure of the late aspects of human paraquat poisoning. *Am J Pathol* **93**:667–80.

Fernandez P, Bermejo AM, Lopez Rivadulla M, *et al.* 1991. A fatal case of parenteral paraquat poisoning. *Forensic Sci Int* **49**:215–24.

Fernando R. 1989. *Pesticides in Sri Lanka*. Friedrich-Ebert Stifting, Colombo.

Gage JC. 1960. The detection of organic phosphorus compounds. *Med Sci Law* **1**:137–44.

Grant H, Lantos PL, Parkinson C. 1980. Cerebral damage in paraquat poisoning. *Histopathology* **4**:185–95.

Harsanyi L, Nemeth A, Lang A. 1987. Paraquat (gramoxone) poisoning in south-west Hungary, 1977–1984. Toxicological and histopathological aspects of group intoxication cases. *Am J Forensic Med Pathol* **8**:131–4.

Karalliedde L, Senanayake N. 1988. Acute organophosphorus insecticide poisoning in Sri Lanka. *Forensic Sci Int* **36**:97–100.

Klein-Schwartz W, Smith GS. 1997. Agricultural and horticultural chemical poisonings: mortality and morbidity in the United States. *Ann Emerg Med* **29**:232–8.

Kuo TL, Kuo CY. 1988. Determination of paraquat from formalin-fixed tissue. *Forensic Sci Int* **38**:243–9.

Neoral L, Dusek J, Smysl B. 1977. [A contribution to the pathogenesis of lethal paraquat poisoning (author's transl)]. *Z Rechtsmed* **80**:1–7.

Parkinson C. 1980. The changing pattern of paraquat poisoning in man. *Histopathology* **4**:171–83.

Peiris JB, Fernando R, De Abrew K. 1988. Respiratory failure from severe organophosphate toxicity due to absorption through the skin. *Forensic Sci Int* **36**:251–3.

Petty CS. 1958. Organic phosphate insecticide poisoning. *Am J Med* **23**:467–70.

Przybylska A. 1999. [Intoxications caused by plant protection chemicals in 1997.] *Przegl Epidemiol* **53**:121–8.

Rebello G, Mason JK. 1978. Pulmonary histological appearances in fatal paraquat poisoning. *Histopathology* **2**:53–66.

Reif RM, Lewinsohn G. 1983. Paraquat myocarditis and adrenal cortical necrosis. *J Forensic Sci* **28**:505–9.

Russell LA, Stone BE, Rooney PA. 1981. Paraquat poisoning: toxicologic and pathologic findings in three fatal cases. *Clin Toxicol* **18**:915–28.

Stewart MJ, Moar JJ, Mwesigwa J, *et al.* 2000. Forensic toxicology in urban South Africa. *J Toxicol Clin Toxicol* **38**:415–19.

Teare RD. 1976. Poisoning by paraquat. *Med Sci Law* **16**:9–12.

Tompsett SL. 1970. Paraquat poisoning. *Acta Pharmacol Toxicol (Copenh)* **28**:346–58.

Vercruysse A. 1964. Acute parathion poisoning; forensic problems. *J Forensic Med* **11**:107–19.

Wesseling C, van Wendel de Joode B, Monge P. 2001. Pesticide-related illness and injuries among banana workers in Costa Rica: a comparison between 1993 and 1996. *Int J Occup Environ Health* **7**:90–7.

Zivot U, Castorena JL, Garriott JC. 1993. A case of fatal ingestion of malathion. *Am J Forensic Med Pathol* **14**:51–3.

CHAPTER 31

Poisoning by medicines

GENERAL CONSIDERATIONS

In most countries, especially those with advanced economies and relatively sophisticated medical services, poisoning with medicinal compounds is common. In many such countries, poisoning with therapeutic substances exceeds deaths from other types of toxic agents, especially in suicidal and accidental poisoning.

This is explained by the ease of access of such substances, whether they are obtainable from a doctor on prescription or on demand across the counter of a pharmacy. Where state-sponsored health services exist, the cost to the recipient may be minimal or absent and this ease of access contributes to opportunities for self-poisoning, whether it be deliberate self-destruction, suicidal gestures or accidental ingestion – the latter especially in children. Unfortunately, overprescribing or the supply of too great a quantity of drugs at one time allows excessive stocks of drugs to be easily available to the public.

Though only a minority of victims of medicinal poisoning fail to recover, there are still an appreciable number of deaths. These come to the attention of the investigative authorities and hence to pathologists. The autopsy investigation of a fatality from a therapeutic substance can be difficult, for a number of reasons:

- The nature of the substance may be uncertain or unknown.
- There may be more than one such substance involved.
- There may be a delay between ingestion and death sufficient to allow blood, urine and tissue concentrations to decline below fatal, toxic or even therapeutic levels.
- Analysis may be difficult to arrange because of lack of facilities.
- Information about fatal levels may be unobtainable.
- Most medicinal poisons leave virtually no characteristic features at autopsy, so diagnosis depends upon laboratory findings.
- Post-mortem changes may make analysis difficult, inaccurate or impossible.
- Where death is delayed after taking the substance, none may be recoverable from the stomach (which has emptied) or even from the intestine.
- The original substance may be rapidly metabolized into one or more breakdown products, adding to difficulties in identification and interpretation.

AUTOPSY APPEARANCES

The lack of characteristic autopsy appearances is often very frustrating for the pathologist. Unless there is an indicative or suggestive history as to which drug was taken – a matter for the investigators in respect of circumstances and recovery of containers – then an autopsy may have to be performed 'blind'. Where no significant morphological lesions can be discovered, then a full toxicology screen must be considered, which in some jurisdictions may be difficult or impossible to obtain, or be extremely expensive.

The majority of modern medicinal substances are, by design, bland and non-irritant to the tissues and gastro-intestinal tract. Most of those met with in forensic practice are taken orally and, though the active constituents may be potent in their pharmacological effect on target organs and tissues, the medicine will cause no erosion or damage to the alimentary tract. Thus little or no physical evidence can be obtained from a gross or even microscopic examination of the gastrointestinal tract or other organs. Much of the physical bulk of modern tablets or capsules is merely the vehicle for introducing the active component into the body and is thus unlikely to have any adverse effect.

When a medicinal compound causes death, the mode of death is most often some form of cardiorespiratory failure, often secondary to depressive effects on the central nervous system. This mode of death causes only non-specific changes discernible at autopsy, which are usually of no use in indicating the basic reason for the death. Acute congestive cardiac failure, pulmonary oedema, sometimes cerebral oedema, generalized organ congestion, scattered petechiae on serous membranes – none of these is of any real use to the pathologist, who has to rely on the results of toxicological analysis for a definitive answer.

There are some therapeutic substances, which, though not the cause of specific lesions, may suggest themselves from their autopsy appearances. An example is the widespread membrane ecchymoses sometimes seen in aspirin poisoning. This could not in any way be sufficient to provide a legally acceptable cause of death, however, unless absolutely reliable circumstantial evidence existed, together with the finding of a large bolus of undissolved tablet remnants in the stomach. Even then it might be contested that the substance was not aspirin – or not aspirin alone – unless analytical confirmation was obtained.

RESULTS OF LABORATORY TESTS

As discussed in Chapter 27, the investigation of fatal poisoning is a collaborative investigation between pathologist and toxicologist. The autopsy excludes, confirms or evaluates any trauma or natural disease, and provides suitable material for analysis. The toxicology laboratory conducts the technical assays, and produces qualitative and quantitative results. The toxicologist/analyst interprets those results to the pathologist, by providing an indication of the therapeutic, toxic and fatal ranges of concentrations in various body fluids and tissues, and by pointing out problems such as decline from post-ingestion survival, conversion to metabolites and many others. The pathologist then collates this information with his own knowledge of the history and autopsy findings to offer the best interpretation of the investigation for judicial

authorities. Most problems arise either because the information about the medicine (especially if it is newly developed or where its toxicity is low) is incomplete in terms of toxic blood and tissue levels – because post-ingestion survival has allowed the originally lethal levels to have subsided to therapeutic or even lower limits. What is offered in the remainder of this chapter is a digest of information about such potentially lethal levels, culled from a variety of sources. The ranges are often wide as most of the data are of necessity derived anecdotally, and the problems of uncertainty of dosage, variation in post-ingestion survivals and wide individual biological variation make it impossible to lay down strict thresholds between therapeutic, toxic and fatal concentrations.

Wherever possible, the advice of the analytical toxicologist should be taken about each case – but where this is impracticable, then the following data and similar material, which is constantly being updated in forensic and toxicological publications, may be of assistance. The choice of substances is arbitrary, but represents the most common medicines seen in suicidal and accidental poisoning.

ANALGESICS

Aspirin (acetylsalicylic acid) and salicylates

Aspirin is the most widely used therapeutic drug, being analgesic, antipyretic and anti-inflammatory. It was formerly very common as an agent of self-poisoning, both accidental in children and suicidal in adults. In Britain in the last two decades, its use as a self-poisoning agent has declined remarkably, so that fatalities are now rarely seen.

The therapeutic dose is usually 325–975 mg, that is, 1–3 tablets. Rarely, persons with an aspirin hypersensitivity may become ill or even die after therapeutic doses, suffering urticaria, angioneurotic oedema, hypotension, vasomotor disturbances and laryngeal and glottal oedema.

Patients on long-term salicylate therapy for arthritic or rheumatic diseases may take 3–5 g/day and slowly reach blood concentrations which would be in the lethal range if caused by acute overdoses. Those on 3 g/day have blood levels varying between 44 and 330 mg/l.

Apart from deaths caused by hypersensitivity, death in an adult is unlikely with the ingestion of fewer than about 50 tablets, that is, about 16 g. The blood concentration (measured as total salicylate), from a medicinal dose of 975 mg, ranges from about 30 to 100 mg/l (with a mean of 77) 2 hours after ingestion. There is a rapid fall to around 25 mg/l some 8 hours later.

At autopsy, aspirin is one of the few medicines that may cause some gross abnormalities, though they are not particularly specific. Externally there is nothing to see, unless vomiting has taken place, when dark or even red, bloody gastric contents may be expelled. Rarely, there may be some haemorrhagic manifestations in the form of skin petechiae.

Internally, the stomach may still contain a mass of fused, unabsorbed tablets. These tend to start dissolving and then aggregate into a grey or dirty-white mass if a large number (several hundred) have been swallowed. The gastric mucosa may be eroded by the irritative, acidic substance. This may be localized in the stomach or spread widely across the fundus and cardia. The lining may be dotted with acute erosions, sometimes causing bleeding that may amount to a frank haematemesis. Black altered blood may lie in the stomach and pass into the intestine to form a melaena if survival is long enough. Mucosal petechiae and ecchymoses in the stomach, without actual erosive destruction, may be seen as part of a haemorrhagic result of the anticoagulant action of aspirin. Similar petechiae may be spread through other organs and especially serous membranes, particularly on the parietal pleura and epicardium. Even single tablets may cause a small ulcer if they stick to the stomach lining – this is sometimes seen incidentally at autopsy in non-poisoning cases, where a tablet has been swallowed shortly before death.

Post-mortem toxicology requires the usual samples of blood, urine, stomach contents and liver. The mass of aspirin in the stomach may remain for several days in life, forming a partly insoluble concretion that may retard the absorption of the drug. This is why it is always worth washing out the stomach of a live victim, as a large proportion of the aspirin may be removed before it can cause systemic effects. With the advent of soluble aspirin or effervescent preparations, this aspect is lost as no such insoluble bolus forms. At autopsy, part of such a mass can be sent for analysis, whilst quick 'spot' tests can be carried out on another part. Such quick chemical confirmation may be performed in the autopsy room itself, by using a 10 per cent solution of ferric chloride. If a small quantity is added to a urine sample or to the surface of the tablet mass, an immediate purple–blue colour suggests aspirin. This is by no means specific, but is merely suggestive. If negative, however, then aspirin can be virtually discounted. These are only rapid screening methods and by no means replace proper laboratory analysis.

Toxic blood levels (measured as total salicylate) begin at about 300–500 mg/l, though both death and survival are consistent with far higher or lower levels. Blood concentrations in fatal cases may range from about 60 to 7300 mg/l, some authorities suggesting that 500 mg/l is an average minimum level. The liver concentration in fatalities varies from 2.5 to 1000 mg/kg and urine salicylate from 20 to 1350 mg/l, emphasizing the wide levels that are compatible with life. Salicylate has a rather slow clearance rate from the blood, the half-life being up to a day in some massive overdoses.

Aspirin poisoning is dangerous in that sudden cardiac arrest can occur in the absence of any toxic symptoms. This accounts for the deaths that take place after patients have been discharged fit from the emergency departments of hospitals. They may have seemed quite well and symptom free, but suffer a fatal collapse up to a day or so later. Fatal cardiac arrhythmias can supervene without warning and make it advisable, where possible, to admit patients with aspirin overdoses for observation for a day or so.

PARACETAMOL

Paracetamol is also known as acetominophen, N-acetyl-p-aminophenol or 4'-hydroxyacetanilide. It is an analgesic and antipyretic, without the anti-inflammatory properties of aspirin, for which it is often used as an alternative because of the lack of gastric irritation.

In wide use, especially in combination with other drugs such as codeine and dextropropoxyphene, paracetamol is one of the most common agents in self-induced poisoning by medicinal products. It is used alone in therapeutic doses of up to 500 mg. Overdoses of 20 g or more are potentially lethal, but much less is needed in combination with other drugs, such as propoxyphene. Paracetamol is a potent liver poison, as a small proportion is converted by the liver enzyme 'P450' (microsomal mixed function oxidase) into a toxic compound, probably N-acetyl-p-benzoquinone. Normally, glutathione and other sulphydryl compounds detoxify this substance, but in overdose, these are exhausted and the toxic agent causes a profound centrilobular hepatic necrosis. The concurrent administration of other drugs, such as phenobarbitone or phenytoin in epileptics or chronic alcoholism, activate the P450 enzyme and worsen the toxicity through this mechanism.

At autopsy there is nothing specific to observe in the gastrointestinal tract. In massive overdosage, there can rarely be rapid death from a direct depressive action on the central nervous system, but most deaths are delayed 2–4 days whilst liver failure develops. At autopsy, the liver may be enlarged, but is often under the normal weight of 1500 g. It may be pale yellow or tan, or the damage may be only visible histologically, when a centrilobular necrosis is seen. Renal changes in the form of tubular necrosis may also be present and occasionally myocardial fibre damage may be visible histologically.

Analytically, the therapeutic range of plasma concentrations 6 hours after a 324 mg dose is 2–6 mg/l, though some

TABLE 31.1 *Fatal concentrations of some antidepressants (mg/l or mg/kg)*

	Blood (average)	Urine (average)	Liver (average)
Amitriptyline	2.7–4.7 (3.7)	0.4–7.9 (3.4)	13–317 (130)
Dothiepin	0.3–2.5 (1.5)	0.4–5.1 (3.2)	2.0–14 (8)
Imipramine	6–8.5 (7.3)	0.6–54 (20)	33–381 (166)
Tranylcypromine	3.7	25.0	7.3

TABLE 31.2 *Fatal concentrations of three benzodiazepines (mg/l or mg/kg)*

	Blood	Urine	Liver
Chlordiazepoxide	20	8	10
Diazepam	5–19	3	16
Nitrazepam	1.2–9.0	1–10	0.7–4.0

TABLE 31.3 *Fatal concentrations of two phenothiazines (mg/l or mg/kg)*

	Blood (average)	Urine (average)	Liver (average)
Chlormethiazole	10–214 (55)	5–114 (43)	42–190 (94)
Chlorpromazine	6.6	1.2	84

records claim peak levels of up to 25 mg/l. The plasma half-life is a guide to hepatotoxicity, it being dangerous to have a half-life of more than 2 hours at a level of 300 mg/l at 4 hours after ingestion. Typical blood levels in overdoses when at least 10–15 g have been taken are 100–400 mg/l, with an average around 250. The urine may contain 150–800 mg/l, but all levels depend on dose and survival time. Paracetamol may exhibit post-mortem redistribution.

The inclusion of other drugs, especially dextro-propoxyphene (and, of course, alcohol), may markedly reduce the level needed for a fatal outcome. Paracetamol was the most frequently detected substance in a compilation of post-mortem femoral blood concentrations of drugs (Druid and Holmgren 1997) based on a selection of 15 800 samples sent to the Department of Forensic Chemistry in Linköping, Sweden, during 1992–95. In their series of 139 fatal intoxications with paracetamol in combination with other drugs and/or alcohol, the median concentration of paracetamol was 170 mg/l (range 90–320).

ANTIDEPRESSANT DRUGS

The tricyclic antidepressants are frequently involved in self-poisoning, partly associated with the type of patient for whom they are prescribed.

Amitriptyline, dothiepin, doxepin and trimipramine have additional sedative properties. Those with little or no sedating action include protriptyline, nortriptyline, imipramine, clomipramine, iprindole, lofepramine, desipramine and butriptyline.

Tetracyclic antidepressants include maprotiline and mianserin. Other types include the monoamine oxidase inhibitors, which are well known to have dangers related to the concurrent ingestion of other drugs and foods, especially those with sympathomimetic action and tyramine content, such as rich cheese, yeast extracts, red wine and beans. Dangerous hypertension may ensue with the risk of cerebrovascular haemorrhage. Drugs of this class include phenoxypropazine, tranylcypromine, isocarboxazid and phenelzine.

THE BENZODIAZEPINES

These widely used drugs are employed for their sedative and tranquillizing effects. A large number of both 1,4- and 1,5-benzodiazepines are available, divided into short-acting, intermediate-acting and long-acting compounds.

Long-acting benzodiazepines include: flurazepam, nitrazepam, diazepam, ketazalam, chlordiazepoxide, clobazam, chlorazepate, medazepam and alprazolam. Intermediate-acting benzodiazepines include: loprazolam, lormetazepam, temazepam, flunitrazepam, lorazepam, bromazepam and oxazepam. A short-acting benzodiazepine is triazolam.

THE PHENOTHIAZINES

This group of tranquillizer drugs includes: haloperidol (butyrophenone), chlormethiazole, chlorpromazine, fluphenazine, diphenylbutylpiperidine, promazine, trifluoperazine and prochlorperazine.

The autopsy appearances are non-specific and toxicology may resolve any diagnostic problems if the death has occurred fairly soon after ingestion – which may often not be the case, when history and ante-mortem investigations can provide the only answer.

THE BARBITURATES

The massive problem posed by therapeutic administration of barbiturates until about 20 years ago has largely abated in countries with a responsible medical profession, which voluntarily refrained from the prescription of these drugs except where specifically indicated. Their use as sleeping tablets and general soporific sedative agents led to widespread abuse, so that at one time they were easily the most common agent of drug addiction. The development of non-barbiturate hypnotics, such as the benzodiazepines, helped to remove the need for the older and more lethal compounds. Unfortunately, barbiturates are still widely available on the illicit market, either alone or in combination with other substances such as amphetamines.

Barbiturates exist in many forms, the best classification (which relates to their degree of toxicity) being their speed of action:

- Long-acting barbiturates: barbitone, phenobarbitone and phenytoin, which is still prescribed for epilepsy.
- Intermediate-acting barbiturates: amylobarbitone, sodium amytal, pentobarbitone, allobarbitone, butobarbitone and pentobarbitone.
- Short-acting barbiturates: hexobarbitone, cyclobarbitone, secobarbital and thiopentone.

Much lower blood levels will be found in fatal poisonings in the short-acting group as death may occur more quickly from the usual mode of action, a central depression of the respiratory centres. The author (BK) has knowledge of a death within 20 minutes of taking a massive overdose of 'Seconal'.

At autopsy, the signs are of general cardiorespiratory failure, with often a cyanotic, congestive appearance. Though non-specific, probably the congested lungs in acute barbiturate poisoning are more intense than in any other condition. These organs may be almost black and the whole venous system is engorged with dark, deoxygenated blood. There may be 'barbiturate blisters' on dependent parts of the skin surface, especially buttocks, backs of thighs, calves and forearms, though as discussed in the chapter on carbon monoxide poisoning, these blisters are common to all states of deep coma.

Internally there may be local signs of erosion from the drug itself. The gastric mucosa may be badly damaged from the alkaline attack of drugs such as sodium amytal which, being the sodium salt of a weak organic acid, hydrolyses in the stomach. The fundus may be thickened, granular and haemorrhagic. The cardia and lower oesophagus may be eroded from reflux and, if the victim regurgitates, then black, altered blood may appear at the nose and mouth.

The capsules of certain barbiturates also leave characteristic traces in the mouth, oesophagus and stomach. The colour varies with the manufacturer, but the turquoise–blue of sodium amytal capsules may stain the stomach contents and even be visible through the wall of the intestine when the abdomen is opened. Other pigmented gelatine capsules can be red, yellow or blue. As with so many

TABLE 31.4 *Fatal concentrations of barbiturates (mg/l or mg/kg)*

	Blood	Urine	Liver
Phenobarbitone	55–144	–	–
Amylobarbitone	29–68	210	106–580
Secobarbitone (or quinal barbitone)	5–52	–	15–330

other drugs, combination with alcohol greatly increases the dangers of a fatality.

INSULIN POISONING

Formerly a rarity, death from parenteral administration of insulin is now not uncommon. The Beverley Allitt case in Britain in recent years showed that multiple deaths can occur, especially where medical or nursing staff are concerned, as well as those in proximity to diabetics, as both groups may have access to insulin.

Another change is the relative ease with which analysis of body fluids and tissue can be carried out now, compared with the great technical difficulties of only a few years ago, so that fewer such deaths may be missed from lack of reliable insulin assays.

Fatal insulin toxicity may be accidental, suicidal or homicidal. The accidental fatalities are usually examples of medical error, mostly from misreading the label on the box or ampoule. A former student of the author (BK), on the fourth day of her first intern post, gave ten times the dose of insulin to a patient during a pituitary function test, by wrongly assuming that the stated number of units written on the box were the total ampoule contents, instead of being the strength per millilitre.

Suicide by insulin is not uncommon; the author (BK) has seen it given into a saline drip by a doctor and also injected into the abdominal wall by a non-diabetic who stole it from her diabetic neighbour's refrigerator.

As stated, homicide and attempted homicide have given rise to some notorious cases, both in UK and the USA. In one case known to the author (PS), a previously healthy 48-year-old man was delivered unconscious to the emergency unit because of a suspicion of decompression sickness. The treatment was aborted as the patient was found to be hypoglycaemic (nadir serum glucose 0.3 mmol/l) and treatment and diagnostics of hypoglycaemia commenced. Serum samples drawn at admittance were stored frozen, whereby it was possible to show retrospectively that, while the concentration of insulin in serum was high (75 mU/l, increasing further to over 240 mU/l in the next few hours), concentration of C-peptide was low (below detection limit of 0.1 nmol/l) at the hypoglycaemic stage, suggesting that the patient had received exogenous insulin somehow, and the police were informed. Due to severe hypoglycaemic brain damage, the patient remained in a vegetative state for 2 months before dying of multiorgan failure. Circumstantial evidence obtained during the ensuing criminal investigation was considered by the court to prove the patient's wife (a nurse) guilty of murder (Koskinen *et al.* 1999).

Insulin is, of course, inactive orally and has to be given by injection to perform its hypoglycaemic effect. At autopsy, where either from the circumstances or the finding of needle marks, insulin is a possibility, peripheral blood samples and skin and underlying tissue from the injection site should be carefully preserved, together with control skin from another site.

The fine needles usually used by diabetics may leave virtually no mark on the skin. The author (BK) has tested some such needles on cadaver skin and found that, often, the mark cannot be seen immediately after withdrawal, unless a small vessel has been damaged.

Although insulin has been recovered many days, even weeks, after death, the sooner the better as far as collecting samples is concerned. Serum should be separated from red cells and the former frozen until sent to the analysts, unless whole blood can be sent straight away. Skin and tissue samples should either be frozen or kept in the refrigerator – not fixed. Porcine or bovine insulin can be detected as such but, if therapeutic insulin is of human origin, then it cannot be distinguished on analysis from the patient's own insulin. As well as immunoassay of the insulin itself, the measurement of C-peptide, produced on a one-to-one basis by the pancreas, assists in distinguishing endogenous from exogenous insulin. All such interpretations are a matter for specialists in this field, upon whose advice the pathologist must rely.

Attempting to prove insulin-induced hypoglycaemia by measuring glucose levels in human post-mortem fluids is impracticable, due to the unreliability of such estimations after death.

Very low vitreous humour glucose levels may strongly suggest hypoglycaemia, but are not absolutely acceptable.

REFERENCES AND FURTHER READING

Baselt RC. 2002. *Disposition of toxic drugs and chemicals in man*, 6th edn. Biomedical Publications, Foster City, CA.

Bauman WA, Yalow RS. 1981. Insulin as a lethal weapon. *J Forensic Sci* **26**:594–8.

Beastall GH, Gibson IH, Martin J. 1995. Successful suicide by insulin injection in a non-diabetic. *Med Sci Law* **35**:79–85.

Brodsgaard I, Hansen AC, Vesterby A. 1995. Two cases of lethal nitrazepam poisoning. *Am J Forensic Med Pathol* **16**:151–3.

Cardauns H, Iffland R. 1973. [Fatal intoxication of a young drug addict with diazepam (author's transl).] *Arch Toxikol* **31**:147–51.

Chaturvedi AK, Hidding JT, Rao NG, *et al.* 1987. Two tricyclic antidepressant poisonings: levels of amitriptyline, nortriptyline and desipramine in post-mortem biological samples. *Forensic Sci Int* **33**:93–101.

Crifasi J, Long C. 1997. The GCMS analysis of tranylcypromine (parnate) in a suspected overdose. *Forensic Sci Int* **86**:103–8.

Druid H, Holmgren P. 1997. A compilation of fatal and control concentrations of drugs in postmortem femoral blood. *J Forensic Sci* **42**:79–87.

Engelmann L, Kohler H. 1971. [Clinical aspects of chlordiazepoxide poisoning.] *Dtsch Gesundheitsw* **26**:435–9.

Fatteh A, Blanke R, Mann GT. 1968. Death from imipramine poisoning. *J Forensic Sci* **13**:124–8.

Fermer R. 1995. *Forensic pharmacology*. Oxford University Press, Oxford.

Finkle BS, McCloskey KL, Goodman LS. 1979. Diazepam and drug-associated deaths. A survey in the United States and Canada. *JAMA* **242**:429–34.

Fletcher SM. 1983. Insulin. A forensic primer. *J Forensic Sci Soc* **23**:5–17.

Forbes G, Pollock Weir W, Smith H, *et al.* 1965. Amitriptyline poisoning. *J Forensic Sci Soc* **5**:183–7.

Giusti GV, Chiarotti M. 1979. Lethal nitrazepam intoxications, report of two cases. *Z Rechtsmed* **84**:75–8.

Griffiths GJ. 1973. Overdose of parstelin (tranylcypromine). *Med Sci Law* **13**:93–4.

Haibach H, Dix JD, Shah JH. 1987. Homicide by insulin administration. *J Forensic Sci* **32**:208–16.

Iwase H, Kobayashi M, Nakajima M, *et al.* 2001. The ratio of insulin to C-peptide can be used to make a forensic diagnosis of exogenous insulin overdosage. *Forensic Sci Int* **115**:123–7.

Junge M, Tsokos M, Puschel K. 2000. Suicide by insulin injection in combination with beta-blocker application. *Forensic Sci Int* **113**:457–60.

Kanto J, Sellman R, Haataja M, *et al.* 1978. Plasma and urine concentrations of diazepam and its metabolites in children, adults and in diazepam-intoxicated patients. *Int J Clin Pharmacol Biopharm* **16**:258–64.

Kernbach-Wighton G, Puschel K. 1998. On the phenomenology of lethal applications of insulin. *Forensic Sci Int* **93**:61–73.

Koskinen PJ, Nuutinen HM, Laaksonen H, *et al.* 1999. Importance of storing emergency serum samples for uncovering murder with insulin. *Forensic Sci Int* **105**:61–6.

Langford AM, Taylor KK, Pounder DJ. 1998. Drug concentration in selected skeletal muscles. *J Forensic Sci* **43**:22–7.

Ledda F. 1968. [Acute chlordiazepoxide poisoning in a drug addict, followed by withdrawal syndrome.] *Clin Ter* **44**:167–71.

Levy WJ, Gardner D, Moseley J, *et al.* 1985. Unusual problems for the physician in managing a hospital patient who received a malicious insulin overdose. *Neurosurgery* **17**:992–6.

Lutz R, Pedal I, Wetzel C, *et al.* 1997. Insulin injection sites: morphology and immunohistochemistry. *Forensic Sci Int* **90**:93–101.

Mackell MA, Case ME, Poklis A. 1979. Fatal intoxication due to tranylcypromine. *Med Sci Law* **19**:66–8.

Marks V. 1995. Hypoglycaemia – real and unreal, lawful and unlawful: the 1994 Banting lecture. *Diabet Med* **12**:850–64.

Marks V, Teale JD. 1999. Hypoglycemia: factitious and felonious. *Endocrinol Metab Clin North Am* **28**:579–601.

Mirchandani H, Reich LE. 1985. Fatal malignant hyperthermia as a result of ingestion of tranylcypromine (parnate) combined with white wine and cheese. *J Forensic Sci* **30**:217–20.

Noirfalise A, Dodinval P, Quiriny J, *et al.* 1987. Death through injection of barbiturates. *Forensic Sci Int* **35**:141–4.

Patel F. 1992. Fatal self-induced hyperinsulinaemia: a delayed post-mortem analytical detection. *Med Sci Law* **32**:151–9.

Patel F. 1995. Successful suicide by insulin injection in a non-diabetic. *Med Sci Law* **35**:181–2.

Phillips AP, Webb B, Curry AS. 1972. The detection of insulin in postmortem tissues. *J Forensic Sci* **17**:460–3.

Polson C, Green M, Lee M. 1983. *Clinical toxicology*, 3rd edn. Pitman, London.

Pounder DJ, Owen V, Quigley C. 1994. Postmortem changes in blood amitriptyline concentration. *Am J Forensic Med Pathol* **15**:224–30.

Price LM, Poklis A, Johnson DE. 1991. Fatal acetaminophen poisoning with evidence of subendocardial necrosis of the heart. *J Forensic Sci* **36**:930–5.

Schneider V, Dulce HJ. 1979. [Suicidal poisonings with insulin and their demonstration on the corpse (radioimmunoassay).] *Arch Kriminol* **164**:142–52.

Sticht G, Kaferstein H. 1980. [Results of toxicological investigations on vesparax-poisonings (author's transl).] *Z Rechtsmed* **85**:169–75.

Sturner WQ, Putnam RS. 1972. Suicidal insulin poisoning with nine day survival: recovery in bile at autopsy by radioimmunoassay. *J Forensic Sci* **17**:514–21.

Williams KR, Pounder DJ. 1997. Site-to-site variability of drug concentrations in skeletal muscle. *Am J Forensic Med Pathol* **18**:246–50.

Wilson Z, Hubbard S, Pounder DJ. 1993. Drug analysis in fly larvae. *Am J Forensic Med Pathol* **14**:118–20.

Winston DC. 2000. Suicide via insulin overdose in nondiabetics: the New Mexico experience. *Am J Forensic Med Pathol* **21**:237–40.

Yacoub M, Cau G, Faure J, *et al.* 1968. [Medico-legal diagnosis of fatal imipramine poisoning.] *Med Leg Dommage Corp* **1**:211–13.

Yonemitsu K, Pounder DJ. 1993. Postmortem changes in blood tranylcypromine concentration: Competing redistribution and degradation effects. *Forensic Sci Int* **59**:177–84.

CHAPTER 32

Death from narcotic and hallucinogenic drugs

These substances are discussed solely from the point of view of the pathologist dealing with fatal cases.

Drugs of dependence may be absorbed orally, by intravenous, subcutaneous or – rarely – intramuscular injection, by smoking, or by nasal sniffing. The routine at autopsy, in respect of obtaining samples for toxicological analysis, is altered according to the route of administration. As mixing of drugs and addition of non-narcotic drugs is common, it is the usual practice to take a wide range of samples even if the primary route is known with some degree of certainty. For example, an addict dying 'on the needle' where intravenous injection is obvious, will still have stomach contents taken for investigation. The standard samples should be taken, as described in a previous chapter, comprising several samples of venous blood (one with fluoride), stomach and contents, liver and urine. In some circumstances, additional samples such as bile, cerebrospinal fluid and vitreous humour may be taken, as well as brain or kidney. The great advances in the analytical techniques allow the analysis of drugs also in other biological samples, such as saliva, sweat and hair. Hair analysis can also provide evidence of long-term exposure to drugs (weeks, months or years), because most drugs, if not all, incorporate in hair and are relatively stable. At least 50 mg of hair should be collected, cutting about a pencil thickness of strands of hair as close to the skin as possible from the back of the head, dried and stored in a sealed plastic bag or tube at room temperature.

When the drug has been injected, then an ellipse of skin around the injection mark, extending down through the subcutaneous tissue to the muscle, should be excised, along with a control area of skin from another non-injected site. These should be refrigerated, not fixed in formalin, until delivery to the laboratory can be arranged. Full histology should always be taken, especially if drugs have been injected, as foreign substances may be discovered as embolic particles, especially in the lungs. Pulmonary granulomata are well-known histological features of 'mainlining' addicts taking impure drugs intravenously, as the lung capillaries filter out coarse particulate matter used to dilute the active narcotic. Talc is particularly prone to form granulomata, sometimes with foreign body giant cells. Under polarized light, doubly refractile particles may be seen in the centre of the reactive nodules. Sometimes, strands of cotton may form foreign bodies, derived from the cloth strainer used to filter particles crudely from the drug solution before injection.

Siderophages were also claimed to be increased in these lungs, compared with healthy young adult controls. However, Lockemann and Püschel (1993), studying lungs stained for iron with Perl's reaction, found conflicting results in two large series and conclude that the pathognomonic value of these cells in drug takers is uncertain.

If drugs may have been taken by the nasal route, such as cocaine and heroin, then dry swabs from each nostril should be taken.

MORPHINE AND OTHER OPIOID DRUGS

Morphine is the major representative of the general group of opioids, which comprise natural opium and a whole series of chemically related derivatives. They may be taken orally or injected and several, such as crude opium and heroin – may be absorbed by inhaling smoke. Morphine itself is poorly absorbed from the gastrointestinal tract; heroin can be taken via the nasal mucosa.

The group consists of opium, morphine, heroin (diacetyl morphine), codeine (dimethyl morphine), dihydrocodeine (DF 118), etorphine (Immobilon), methadone, papaverine, pethidine, dipipanone, dextromoramide, dextropropoxyphene, pentazocine, cyclazocine, diphenoxylate, buprenorphine, tramadol, fentanyl and many more.

Autopsy appearances

The autopsy findings in deaths from all these drugs are relatively non-specific. Toxicological analysis and expert interpretation of the results are necessary for the proper elucidation of the deaths, but certain features can be useful pointers. The first is the presence of injection marks. When fresh, they look just like any other needle mark commonly seen from therapeutic or diagnostic procedures. They are commonly on the arms, either in the classical position in the antecubital fossa on the front of the elbow, or into one of the prominent veins of the forearms or dorsum of the hand. The left side is favourite as most people are right-handed, but in habitual users, sclerosis of the veins may lead to the arms being used randomly. The veins of the dorsum of the foot may be used when the hands and arms have become unusable because of thrombosis and scarring. Less common sites are in the thighs but here, as with the abdominal wall, the injections may be subcutaneous, rather than intravenous. This mode of injection is known as 'skin-popping' and can lead to areas of subcutaneous sclerosis, fat necrosis, abscesses and, if the injections are deeper into the muscle, to chronic myositis.

Other external signs may be tattoos, often bizarre and connected with the drug subculture. One specific type is tattooing, often of numerals, such as '13', on the buccal (inner) surface of the lower lip. Where chronic addiction has taken its toll, the body may be emaciated, dirty and show signs of infection, especially in the form of skin ulceration. Rarely, there may be necrosis or even loss of phalanges from thrombotic or septic emboli. Old injection marks, sometimes with associated bruising, may be found, the bruising undergoing the usual spectrum of colour changes if not recent. The veins may show overlying fibrosis where phlebitis has occurred, or old venous thrombosis with firm cord-like vessels under the skin.

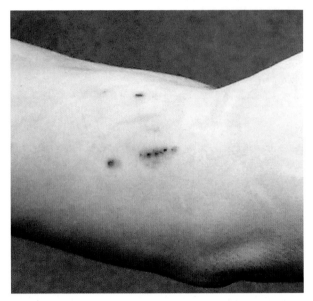

FIGURE 32.1 *Fresh injections marks on the arm of a drug addict.*

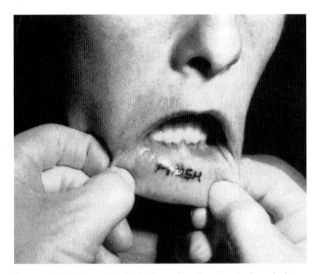

FIGURE 32.2 *Tattoo inside the lower lip of a narcotic drug dealer.*

Where sudden death has occurred in habituated addicts, there may be gross pulmonary oedema, with a plume of froth exuding from the mouth or nostrils, suggestive of drowning. As Polson *et al.* (1983) point out, this may cause some confusion when the victim is found dead in a bathroom, a common venue (along with toilets) for drug administration. This pulmonary oedema is sometimes a striking feature of rapid death in those who are habituated to opioid drugs, especially heroin. It does not seem to occur in novices to the habit, who tend to die in a different way, from a sudden primary cardiac arrest. The oedema may be blood-tinged, again causing confusion with drowning. The cause is not known, but is often attributed to some 'allergic' phenomenon, a rather unsatisfactory explanation. It has been claimed that it sometimes may be caused by adulterants in the drugs, such as quinine, but this is doubtful.

The death may be so rapid that the needle may still be found in the vein when the body is discovered, often in a public lavatory or sometimes in the presence of other addicts, who may then be charged with criminal offences in relation to the death as well as with possessing and using illicit drugs.

There are no other more specific autopsy appearances. Though clinically, a constricted pupil is a prominent sign of morphine administration, after death, any kind of pupil alteration may occur. They may remain small, dilate, or become quite unequal – this applies to any form of death, so no specificity exists for opioid poisoning.

Among new recruits to drug dependence, some die at the first injection of a parenteral dose of heroin or morphine. The mode of death appears to be a cardiac arrest following an arrhythmia and ventricular fibrillation, but no morphological signs can be found. It may be related to sensitization of the myocardium to catecholamines by the drug, the excitement and apprehension being similar to the triggers that seem to cause sudden death from falling into cold water or having a criminal abortion.

The other aspect of autopsies on drug-dependent victims is the risk of infection to pathologist and mortuary staff. Addicts form a high-risk group for both hepatitis B and C, HIV and AIDS. The way in which such autopsies are dealt with in different jurisdictions must vary widely, but it is common practice for HIV and hepatitis testing to be carried out prior to autopsy, unless the policy of the particular autopsy service is to accept all cases with appropriate safety techniques. The analytical laboratory must be informed of any high-risk samples being sent to them, and some will be reluctant to handle blood or tissue samples with positive serology. The pathologist may well refuse to carry out an autopsy on a suspect body until a negative result has been returned on a sample of blood taken (with adequate precautions) from the femoral vein. If positive for hepatitis B or C virus, and especially if the victim shows any signs of hepatic involvement such as jaundice, then many pathologists would decline to carry out a full autopsy unless there are pressing reasons. In that case, scrupulous safety precautions must be taken (see Chapter 1).

In relation to AIDS and HIV positivity, opinions and practices vary widely in the present state of knowledge. It seems obvious that the HIV virus is not in the same category of infectivity as hepatitis. Though autopsies on patients dying of clinical AIDS are routinely performed, there is a difference in the potential risk of a literally 'cold' autopsy being performed on a hospital death after a day or two in the mortuary refrigerator, compared with the urgent activities of a forensic pathologist who may be called upon to conduct an autopsy on a still-warm corpse within a few hours of a suspicious death. However, as mentioned in Chapter 1, HIV may remain viable for many days after death.

TOXICOLOGICAL RESULTS

As with all deaths from toxic substances, the interpretation of laboratory analytical results may present considerable difficulties. There may be a long delay between the administration of the drug and death, during which time the blood, urine and even tissue levels may decline, or even disappear. Many drugs break down rapidly in the body and their metabolites may be the only recognizable products of their administration. In some cases, data on lethal blood levels may be imperfectly known and great variations in personal susceptibility may make the range of concentrations found in a series of deaths so wide as to be rather unhelpful.

As mentioned above, some persons die rapidly after the first episode of taking a 'normal' dose of a drug because of some ill-understood personal idiosyncrasy and here quantitative analysis may not assist.

Where habituation and tolerance has developed, drug users may have concentrations in their body fluids and tissues far higher than lethal levels published for non-habitués. In general, the great usefulness of toxicological analysis is both qualitative and quantitative. The former will show what drugs have been taken in the recent past; the length of time that drugs or their metabolites – persist in different fluids and tissues varies widely.

The quantitative analysis can be useful, especially when the results reveal high levels – into the toxic or lethal ranges. These ranges are usually obtained anecdotally from surveys of large numbers of deaths but, as stated, can differ in terms of minimum and maximum values from different laboratories. The problems of idiosyncratic sensitivity and tolerance cause such published ranges to act only as a general yardstick and deaths that occur outside the ranges (usually off the lower end) cannot be excluded from having been caused by the drug in question if other factors may have been involved. Such factors include the presence of other drugs or alcohol, or both, delayed death and abnormal sensitivity.

Thus the analysis is not the final arbiter of the cause of death, although it is a highly important component of the whole range of investigation. The pathologist has the duty to correlate and interpret all known facts. He must fit the circumstances, the presence of natural disease, trauma and other toxic substances with the laboratory findings, to arrive at the most reasonable cause of death.

The advice of the toxicology laboratory is vital in this process, especially in relation to known lethal ranges and the significance of metabolites, but the analysts should not become the sole arbiter of the cause of death.

METHADONE

Methadone has come to be used primarily as a treatment for established heroin dependency, but unfortunately appears to substitute one form of addiction for another, albeit somewhat less lethal, though recent experience in Scotland (1995) has shown that deaths from methadone may exceed those from heroin, whose use it was intended to supplant. Its clinical uses are as an analgesic more powerful than morphine, with the advantage that it is almost as potent by oral administration as by injection. It has strong and often undesirable sedative properties, however, and is virtually as addictive as the other opioids.

Many deaths occur from its misuse, when obtained either legitimately for the replacement of heroin dependency or on the large illegal market. Most deaths follow oral administration and appear to be due to lack of tolerance, in the absence of which even 50 mg may be lethal, though some recipients appear to die at the outset of the replacement treatment (Drummer *et al.* 1992).

In post-mortem samples, the liver has the highest concentration. The fatal levels found on analysis overlap those found in persons on maintenance doses for heroin replacement, making interpretation difficult. The blood levels published by Manning in 10 fatal cases showed: blood – mean 1.0 mg/l (range 0.1–1.8); liver – mean 3.8 mg/l (range 1.8–7.5); bile – mean 7.5 mg/l (range 2.9–18.0); and brain – mean 1.0 mg/l (range 0.5–1.4).

HALLUCINOGENS

Few of the hallucinogenic drugs are primary causes of death, but some may lead to traumatic deaths because of the abnormal behaviour of the person who is under their influence. For example, the victim of a lysergic acid diethylamide (LSD) 'trip' may be under the impression that he can fly and thus project himself from a high window. Some drugs, however, may have direct toxic effects, though, as with so many drugs of dependence, the autopsy findings are negative or totally non-specific.

Phencyclidine

Chemically this is 1-(1-phenylcyclohexyl) piperidine hydrochloride, known as PCP or 'angel dust' among many

TABLE 32.1 *Blood and tissue concentrations (mg/l or kg) of narcotic drugs from various series of fatalities (Baselt et al. 1975; Stead and Moffat 1983)*

	Baselt *et al.*		
	Range	Mean	Stead and Moffat
Heroin			
Blood	0.05–3.0	0.3–0.4	>0.1 (mean 0.43)
Urine	0.7–86	5–18	
Bile	3.2–119	32	
Morphine			
Blood	0.2–2.3	0.7	>0.2 (mean 0.7)
Urine	14–18	3.0	
Liver	0.4–18	52	
Cocaine			
Blood	0.9–21	5.2	3.1 (one case)
Urine	1.4–215	47	
Liver	0.1–20	4.3	
Amphetamine			
Blood	0.5–41	8.6	>0.5
Urine	25–700	237	
Liver	4.3–74	30	
Phencyclidine			
Blood	0.3–25	4.8	>0.3 (mean 2.9)
Urine	0.4–120	35	
Liver	0.9–170	23	
Pethidine (meperidine), orally			
Blood	8–20	12	>2 (mean 14)
Urine	150	150	
Liver	5–10	7	

other nicknames. It is often used in combination with other drugs of addiction. A number of deaths have been reported from its use, a variety of modes including hyperthermia, intracranial haemorrhage and high output cardiac failure.

Phencyclidine is excreted in the urine for a long time after ingestion and autopsy samples may be positive for up to a week.

Lysergic acid diethylamide (LSD)

The well-known LSD, which takes its acronym from the German 'Lysergsäurediäthylamid', is a powerful hallucinogenic which is not fatal in itself, as mentioned above. It is an indole alkaloid derivative, of which other members are psilocybin and psieocin, contained in the Mexican mushroom (*Psilocybe mexicana*).

Mescaline, obtained from the cactus *Lophophora williamsii* of central America, is chemically trimethoxyphenethylamine, again not in itself a lethal substance.

CANNABIS

Cannabis, with all its various names in different parts of the world, has at least six active chemical constitutents, the most important of which is one of the tetrahydrocannabinols. Though its effects are a matter of controversy, there seems to be general agreement that used alone, it cannot be blamed for a single death. Proof of the intake of cannabis can be obtained from analysis of urine, blood, and swabs from lips and fingers.

THE AMPHETAMINES

Now rarely used in reputable medical practice because of the undesirable side effects, the amphetamine group of drugs was formerly employed for the abolition of fatigue and for the suppression of appetite. Methylamphetamine sulphate and dexamphetamine were the commonest analogues of amphetamine itself and are still widely available on the illicit market. Death is uncommon from overuse of the amphetamines alone. At autopsy there are no specific findings, apart from the rare possibility of a cerebral or subarachnoid haemorrhage from the induced hypertension.

Toxicology data suggests that after a therapeutic dose of 10 mg, the blood concentration at 2 hours is about 0.035 mg/l. After 30 mg, a peak plasma level of about 0.11 mg/l was observed at 2–5 hours, declining to 0.084 mg/l at 4.5 hours. Chronic abusers consuming large amounts may have blood levels of up to 2–3 mg/l. In the rare fatalities, there is a wider range of blood levels at autopsy, from 0.5 to 41 mg/l (average 8.6), depending on the size of the overdose and the time until death. Liver levels of 474 mg/kg (average 30) and high urine excretion, ranging from 25 to 700 mg/l, with an average of 237 mg/l, are common.

Methylenedioxymethamphetamine (MDMA) or 'ecstasy'

In recent years, new derivatives of amphetamine have appeared in the drug abuser's pharmacopoeia, though the substances have been available for medical use for many years. The most commonly encountered is MDMA (3,4-methylenedioxymethamphetamine), known as 'ecstasy', 'XTC' or 'ADAM'. Others of the groups are MDA (methyl 3,4-methylenedioxyamphetamine) and MDM (*n*-methyl-MDA). MDMA or 'ecstasy' was developed as long ago as 1914 and for some time had a role in psychotherapy as a consciousness-altering agent. It is now widely used as an illegal hallucinogenic drug, and though deaths have been few,

they are now being reported from both the USA and Britain. The author (BK) conducted an autopsy on the first fatality in the British Isles, in a man who swallowed a considerable supply on being challenged by the police. There were no autopsy signs apart from a marked generalized cyanotic congestive state and the diagnosis was made purely on toxicological evidence.

Since the first edition of this book, MDMA deaths have increased markedly due to its ubiquitous availability to young people, especially at 'rave' parties: hyperthermia, dehydration and myocytolysis are some of the potentially fatal consequences.

COCAINE

Along with heroin, cocaine and its associated drugs like 'crack' form the core of the hard-drug problem, from which fatalities are likely to arise. As cocaine is rapidly destroyed when given orally, it is usually taken by injection or sniffed. Recently, a fatality has been reported from absorption from administration via the rectum. This is in addition to some deaths in which cocaine smugglers have died after packets of the drug hidden in their alimentary tract have broken, causing a massive overdose. In India, cocaine has been used by means of urethral instillation and may also be used in the vagina by prostitutes.

In areas where cocaine usage is common, a significant proportion of fetal deaths are associated with the narcotic. In a series reported in New York by Morild and Stajic in 1990, of 103 fetal deaths, toxicology revealed cocaine in 64. The study suggested that fetal death, *abruptio placentae* and abortion were caused by maternal use of the drug.

Death has been recorded by as little as 20–30 mg being applied to the nasal mucosa, but a gram taken by mouth may not be lethal. As with other narcotics, marked habituation and tolerance occurs in chronic users, making estimates of dangerous dose levels difficult to forecast. Intravenous doses are of the order of 100 mg, a common lethal dose being 10 times greater, though far larger amounts can be tolerated by habitual users. Absorption via the nasal mucosa is less effective and larger doses are needed for the same effect than when used parenterally. Though ulceration and even perforation, of the nasal septum in chronic users is mentioned in most standard texts, they are extremely rare lesions.

Death may occur with considerable rapidity in cocaine overdose or hypersensitivity. It may be quite sudden, from cardiac arrest, in first-time users.

At autopsy, there are no specific features. The pulmonary oedema often seen in heroin deaths is not present with cocaine, though the mode of death is also a dysrhythmia.

The diluent used in 'cutting' the drug for street sale may be found in the injection sites, the regional lymph nodes, in the lungs and in other organs. Adulterants may be similar to those used with heroin and include talc, starch, quinine, lactose and dextrose. Particles of cocaine itself may also be found as microemboli. Strychnine has been used because of its bitter taste, like quinine. Deliberate poisoning by a supplier has been known by either increasing the strychnine content or by supplying pure cocaine or heroin, leading to a massive overdose.

Cocaine is an excitant and stimulator of the autonomic nervous system. Sudden dramatic rises in blood pressure can occur, sometimes to over 300 mmHg and cerebral haemorrhage is a possible complication of this acute hypertension.

As with the opioids, autopsy may reveal complications of the septic methods used for injection, apart from the already stated risks of virus infection, such as hepatitis and HIV. In former years, in New York and California, transmission of malaria was a well-known problem amongst those who shared syringes and needles – indeed, one suggestion for the use of quinine as a diluent, was as a treatment for the *Plasmodium*.

Pyogenic infections are most common, with phlebitis and distant embolic abscesses occurring. The injection sites may ulcerate, there can be regional lymphadenitis, but more serious sequelae that may be fatal include endocarditis. This can affect any heart valve, including those on the right side, which are not usually affected in post-rheumatic endocarditis. Many organisms are involved, mainly haemolytic and non-haemolytic streptococci, *Streptococcus faecalis*, *Staphylococcus aureus* and *Pseudomonas aeruginosa* and some fungi. Post-mortem blood cultures frequently show such a mixed flora from contamination that isolation of the true causative organism may be difficult, but a heavy predominant growth may be significant. The advice of a microbiologist should be enlisted in assessing the relevance of a positive blood culture.

Any drug used intravenously, if it has particulate matter admixed, such as starch or talc, may cause foreign-body granulomata in the lungs, when the undissolved components are filtered out in the pulmonary capillary bed. Such granulomata are characteristic of intravenous drug abusers – when viewed under a polarizing microscope, refractile elements may be easily visualized.

As cocaine is so commonly used by sniffing, swabs should always be taken from each nostril using a plain cotton-wool swab. An unused swab should be sent to the laboratory as a control. The full range of blood, urine, stomach contents, liver and vitreous samples should routinely be taken at autopsy. Blood levels in fatal cases vary widely, but typical ranges extend from 1 to 21 mg/l, with a mean of 5.2 mg/l according to Baselt *et al.* (1975).

REFERENCES AND FURTHER READING

Baden MM. 1972. Narcotic abuse: a medical examiner's view. *N Y State J Med* **72**:834–40.

Baden MM. 1972. Homicide, suicide, and accidental death among narcotic addicts. *Hum Pathol* **3**:91–5.

Baselt RC, Allison DJ, Wright JA, *et al.* 1975. Acute heroin fatalities in San Francisco. Demographic and toxicologic characteristics. *West J Med* **122**:455–8.

Billman GE. 1995. Cocaine: a review of its toxic actions on cardiac function. *Crit Rev Toxicol* **25**:113–32.

Burgess C, O'Donohoe A, Gill M. 2000. Agony and ecstasy: a review of MDMA effects and toxicity. *Eur Psychiatry* **15**:287–94.

Carter N, Rutty GN, Milroy CM, *et al.* 2000. Deaths associated with MBDB misuse. *Int J Legal Med* **113**:168–70.

Chakko S, Myerburg RJ. 1995. Cardiac complications of cocaine abuse. *Clin Cardiol* **18**:67–72.

Davis WM, Hatoum HT, Waters IW. 1987. Toxicity of MDA (3,4-methylenedioxyamphetamine) considered for relevance to hazards of MDMA (ecstasy) abuse. *Alcohol Drug Res* **7**:123–34.

Doss PL, Gowitt GT. 1988. Investigation of a death caused by rectal insertion of cocaine. *Am J Forensic Med Pathol* **9**:336–8.

Dowling GP, McDonough ET, Bost RO. 1987. 'Eve' and 'ecstasy'. A report of five deaths associated with the use of MDEA and MDMA. *JAMA* **257**:1615–17.

Drummer OH, Opeskin K, Syrjänen M, *et al.* 1992. Methadone toxicity causing death in ten subjects starting on a methadone maintenance program. *Am J Forensic Med Pathol* **13**:346–50.

Edland JF. 1972. Liver disease in heroin addicts. *Hum Pathol* **3**:75–84.

Finkle BS, McCloskey KL. 1978. The forensic toxicology of cocaine (1971–1976). *J Forensic Sci* **23**:173–89.

Garriot JC, Sturner WQ. 1973. Morphine concentrations and survival periods in acute heroin fatalities. *N Engl J Med* **289**:127–8.

Gill JR, Hayes JA, deSouza IS, *et al.* 2002. Ecstasy (MDMA) deaths in New York city: a case series and review of the literature. *J Forensic Sci* **47**:121–6.

Giroud C, Menetrey A, Augsburger M, *et al.* 2001. Delta(9)-THC, 11-OH-delta(9)-THC and delta(9)-THCCOOH plasma or serum to whole blood concentrations distribution ratios in blood samples taken from living and dead people. *Forensic Sci Int* **123**:159–64.

Gowing LR, Henry-Edwards SM, Irvine RJ, *et al.* 2002. The health effects of ecstasy: a literature review. *Drug Alcohol Rev* **21**:53–63.

Greene MH, Luke JL, Dupont RL. 1974. Opiate 'overdose' deaths in the District of Columbia. I. Heroin-related fatalities. *Med Ann D C* **43**:175–81.

Hayner GN, McKinney H. 1986. MDMA. The dark side of ecstasy. *J Psychoactive Drugs* **18**:341–7.

Helpern M, Rho YM. 1966. Deaths from narcotism in New York city. Incidence, circumstances, and post-mortem findings. *N Y State J Med* **66**:2391–408.

Henry JA. 2000. Metabolic consequences of drug misuse. *Br J Anaesth* **85**:136–42.

Huestis MA, Henningfield JE, Cone EJ. 1992. Blood cannabinoids. II. Models for the prediction of time of marijuana exposure from plasma concentrations of Δ^9-tetrahydrocannabinol (THC) and 11-nor-9-carboxy-Δ^9-tetrahydrocannabinol (THCCOOH). *J Anal Toxicol* **16**:283–90.

Isner JM, Estes NA, Thompson PD, *et al.* 1986. Acute cardiac events temporally related to cocaine abuse. *N Engl J Med* **315**:1438–43.

Karch SB, Billingham ME. 1988. The pathology and etiology of cocaine-induced heart disease. *Arch Pathol Lab Med* **112**:225–30.

Karch SB, Stephens B, Ho CH. 1998. Relating cocaine blood concentrations to toxicity – an autopsy study of 99 cases. *J Forensic Sci* **43**:41–5.

Katsumata S, Sato K, Kashiwade H, *et al.* 1993. Sudden death due presumably to internal use of methamphetamine. *Forensic Sci Int* **62**:209–15.

Kringsholm B. 1988. Deaths among drug addicts in Denmark in 1968–1986. *Forensic Sci Int* **38**:139–49.

Kringsholm B, Christoffersen P. 1987. Lung and heart pathology in fatal drug addiction. A consecutive autopsy study. *Forensic Sci Int* **34**:39–51.

Kringsholm B, Christoffersen P. 1987. Lymph-node and thymus pathology in fatal drug addiction. *Forensic Sci Int* **34**:245–54.

Kringsholm B, Voigt J, Dalgaard JB, *et al.* 1981. Deaths among narcotic addicts in Denmark in 1978 and 1979. *Forensic Sci Int* **18**:19–30.

Laposata EA, Mayo GL. 1993. A review of pulmonary pathology and mechanisms associated with inhalation of freebase cocaine ('crack'). *Am J Forensic Med Pathol* **14**:1–9.

Ling LH, Marchant C, Buckley NA, *et al.* 2001. Poisoning with the recreational drug paramethoxyamphetamine ('death'). *Med J Aust* **174**:453–5.

Lockemann U, Püschel K. 1993. Siderophages in the lung of drug addicts. *Forensic Sci Int* **59**:169–75.

Manno JE, Manno BR, Kemp PM, *et al.* 2001. Temporal indication of marijuana use can be estimated from plasma and urine concentrations of Δ^9-tetra-hydrocannabinol, 11-hydroxy-Δ^9-tetra-hydrocannabinol, and 11-nor- Δ^9-tetra-hydrocannabinol-9-carboxylic acid. *J Anal Toxicol* **25**:538–49.

Martin TL. 2001. Three cases of fatal paramethoxy-amphetamine overdose. *J Anal Toxicol* **25**:649–51.

Mirchandani HG, Rorke LB, Sekula Perlman A, *et al.* 1994. Cocaine-induced agitated delirium, forceful struggle, and minor head injury. A further definition of sudden death during restraint. *Am J Forensic Med Pathol* **15**:95–9.

Moore C, Negrusz A, Lewis D. 1998. Determination of drugs of abuse in meconium. *J Chromatogr B Biomed Sci Appl* **713**:137–46.

Morild I, Stajic M. 1990. Cocaine and fetal death. *Forensic Sci Int* **47**:181–9.

O'Connor A, Cluroe A, Couch R, *et al.* 1999. Death from hyponatraemia-induced cerebral oedema associated with MDMA ('ecstasy') use. *N Z Med J* **112**:255–6.

Parr MJ, Low HM, Botterill P. 1997. Hyponatraemia and death after 'ecstasy' ingestion. *Med J Aust* **166**:136–7.

Paties C, Peveri V, Falzi G. 1987. Liver histopathology in autopsied drug-addicts. *Forensic Sci Int* **35**:11–26.

Polson CJ, Green MA, Lee M. 1983. *Clinical toxicology*, 3rd edn. Pitman, London.

Price KR. 1974. Fatal cocaine poisoning. *J Forensic Sci Soc* **14**:329–33.

Ramcharan S, Meenhorst PL, Otten JM, *et al.* 1998. Survival after massive ecstasy overdose. *J Toxicol Clin Toxicol* **36**:727–31.

Rammer L, Holmgren P, Sandler H. 1988. Fatal intoxication by dextromethorphan: a report on two cases. *Forensic Sci Int* **37**:233–6.

Richards RG, Reed D, Cravey RH. 1976. Death from intravenously administered narcotics: a study of 114 cases. *J Forensic Sci* **21**:467–82.

Siegel H, Helpern M, Ehrenreich T. 1966. The diagnosis of death from intravenous narcotism. With emphasis on the pathologic aspects. *J Forensic Sci* **11**:1–16.

Stead AH, Moffat AC. 1983. A collection of therapeutic, toxic and fatal blood drug concentrations in man. *Hum Toxicol* **2**:437–64.

Steentoft A, Worm K, Christensen H. 1988. Morphine concentrations in autopsy material from fatal cases after intake of morphine and/or heroin. *J Forensic Sci Soc* **28**:87–94.

Stevens BC. 1978. Deaths of drug addicts in London during 1970–4: toxicological, legal and demographic findings. *Med Sci Law* **18**:128–37.

Suarez RV, Riemersma R. 1988. 'Ecstasy' and sudden cardiac death. *Am J Forensic Med Pathol* **9**:339–41.

Watling R. 1983. Hallucinogenic mushrooms. *J Forensic Sci Soc* **23**:53–66.

Weinmann W, Bohnert M. 1998. Lethal monointoxication by overdosage of MDEA. *Forensic Sci Int* **91**:91–101.

Wetli CV. 1987. Fatal cocaine intoxication. A review. *Am J Forensic Med Pathol* **8**:1–2.

CHAPTER 33

Corrosive and metallic poisoning

Toxicology is a vast subject, most of it concerned with the nature, occurrence, symptomatology, biochemistry, mode of action and treatment of a wide range of poisonous substances. Many forensic medicine textbooks, especially those from Asia, devote a major part of their text to all these aspects of hundreds of toxic substances, many of which are seldom – if ever – encountered by a pathologist in most parts of the world. As the autopsy appearances of most poisons are non-specific, it seems fruitless to offer a repetitive catalogue, and therefore the descriptions selected here refer to some of those that either have specific features or are encountered more often. This chapter describes the autopsy appearances in a range of poisons that can broadly be classed as 'corrosive', even if this is not necessarily their main lethal mode of action. In addition, several toxic heavy metals will be discussed, again from the point of view of autopsy findings and relevant toxicological laboratory findings.

CYANIDE

Cyanide is a relatively common poison, both in suicide, accident and, occasionally, homicide. It forms part of lethal toxicity of many fires in buildings, where smoke inhalation kills the majority of victims, rather than burns (Chapter 11). Although the autopsy diagnosis of acute cyanide poisoning is rarely in doubt, toxicological analysis may be difficult to interpret because of both the destruction and production of cyanide in the dead body and even in stored blood samples awaiting analysis. Acute cyanide poisoning is most often self-administered (70 per cent in one series), in which case usually the sodium or potassium salt is swallowed. It may be accidental or industrial, in which case either salts may be involved, or it may be the free gas liberated from some commercial process.

Homicidal poisoning is rare, except for the mass homicides which still occur, such as the Jonesville tragedy in Guyana, or the use of cyanide as a weapon of war against civilians in the Middle East. It has also been used for judicial execution in parts of the USA, a practice which seems to be reviving in recent years.

Cyanide acts only as free hydrogen cyanide and therefore swallowed salts need to meet either water or gastric acid before liberating hydrocyanic acid, a process that takes only a few seconds. The fatal dose of cyanide is small, of the order of 150–300 mg, which allowed it to be used as hidden suicide pills by prominent Nazis at the end of the last war. Recovery has been recorded from far greater doses, however, such as 2–4 g of potassium cyanide. Much depends on the purity of cyanides, as they tend to decompose in storage and old samples may contain only half the weight as active cyanide.

Autopsy findings in cyanide poisoning

Cyanide acts by linking with the ferric iron atom of cytochrome oxidase, preventing the uptake of oxygen for cellular respiration. Cyanide cannot combine directly with haemoglobin, but can do so through the intermediary

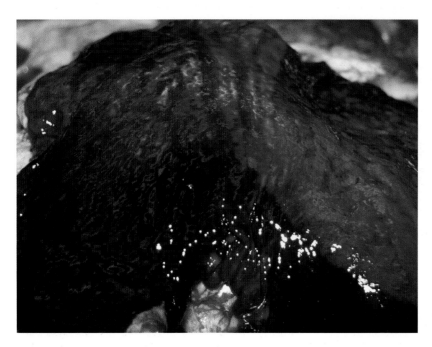

FIGURE 33.1 *Haemorrhagic gastric mucosa in cyanide poisoning.*

compound methaemoglobin. Cyanides are moderately corrosive through their alkaline nature, causing local tissue damage that is unrelated to their more general toxicity via enzyme inhibition.

Externally there can be wide variations in the appearance. Traditionally, the hypostasis is said to be brick-red, due to excess oxyhaemoglobin (because the tissues are prevented from using oxygen) and to the presence of cyanmethaemoglobin. Many descriptions refer to a dark pink or even bright red skin, especially in the dependent areas, which can be confused with carboxyhaemoglobin. The few cases seen by the authors have shown a marked dark cyanotic hypostasis, perhaps caused by lack of oxygenation of the red cells by paralysis of the respiratory muscles. There may be no other external signs apart from the colour of the skin and possibly black vomit around the lips.

There may be a smell of cyanide about the body, though it is well known that many persons cannot detect this, the ability being a sex-linked genetic trait. This may be of importance to pathologists and mortuary staff, as corpses dead of cyanide poisoning can present a health hazard. A former colleague of the author (BK) became ill and was temporarily disabled shortly after conducting an autopsy on a suicide who had swallowed a massive amount of potassium cyanide. Presumably he had inhaled hydrogen cyanide from the stomach contents when examining the viscera.

Internally the tissues may also be bright pink caused by the oxyhaemoglobin that cannot be utilized by the tissues – which is probably more common than the presence of cyanmethaemoglobin. The stomach lining may be badly damaged and can present a blackened, eroded surface, by altered blood staining the stripped mucosa. This is mainly because

of the strongly alkaline nature of the hydrolysed sodium or potassium salts of cyanide; hydrogen cyanide itself causes no such damage. In less severe cases, the stomach lining will be streaked with dark red striae, where the rugae have been eroded while leaving the intervening folds relatively unharmed. The stomach may contain frank or altered blood from the erosions and haemorrhages in the walls. If the cyanide was in dilute solution, there may be little damage to the stomach, apart from pinkness of the mucosa and perhaps some petechial haemorrhages. There may also be undissolved white crystals or powder, with the almond-like smell of cyanide mentioned above.

As death is usually rapid, little of the contents will have passed into the intestine. The oesophagus may be damaged, especially the mucosa of the lower third, though some of this may be a post-mortem change from regurgitation of the stomach contents through the relaxed cardiac sphincter after death. The other organs show no specific changes and the diagnosis is made by history, smell and the reddish colour of the internal tissues, and often skin.

Toxicological analysis

The usual blood, stomach contents, urine and any vomit should be submitted to the laboratory, taking particular care that the samples present no hazard to those packing, transporting or unpacking them. The laboratory should be warned in advance that a possible cyanide case is coming their way.

If death was possibly caused by the inhalation of hydrogen cyanide fumes, a lung should be sent intact, sealed in a nylon (not polyvinylchloride) bag.

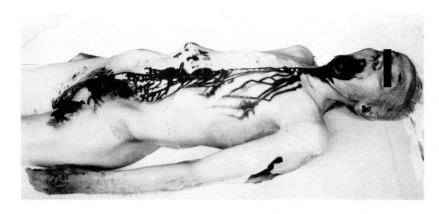

FIGURE 33.2 *Skin burns on a victim of lysol suicide. The trickle pattern makes it obvious that the man was either standing or sitting erect when he drank the fluid. Lysol burns are usually leathery and brownish-purple.*

It is important to get the samples to the laboratory as soon as possible (in terms of days) to avoid the spurious formation of cyanide in stored blood samples. This usually occurs at room temperature so, if there is to be a delay, refrigeration is essential. By contrast, some positive samples may actually decrease on storage, as described by Curry (1969). Up to 70 per cent of the cyanide content may be lost after some weeks, from reaction with tissue components and conversion to thiocyanate.

The amount found on analysis naturally depends on the amount taken and the time between administration and death. Though the latter is usually measured in minutes, low dosage – or treatment – may allow survival for hours or even days.

Assuming that no spurious cyanide is formed, any significant amount found is evidence of cyanide ingestion, which in itself is abnormal and presumably confirmatory evidence of poisoning. However, Karhunen *et al.* (1991) have reported a case in which post-mortem burning of a homicide victim led to a blood cyanide level of 10 mg/l, presumably due to passive diffusion of cyanide through body cavities opened by the fire.

Typical blood levels in one series of fatal cases following ingestion of the poison range from 1 to 53 mg/l, with an average of 12 mg/l. The spleen always has the highest tissue concentration, presumably because it contains so many red cells; in the same series, the spleen level was between 0.5 and 398 mg/l, with a mean of 44 mg/l. In another series, mean blood levels were 37 mg/l.

CORROSIVE ACIDS, ALKALIS AND PHENOLS

Corrosive poisons were formerly common suicidal agents, though they are now relatively rare in Western countries, probably because of the ease of obtaining less painful substances. In some parts of the world, mineral acids are still often used for homicide, assault ('vitriol-throwing') and suicide. In Malaya, reagents used in rubber production, such as formic and acetic acids, were often taken as a means of self-destruction by young women, especially Tamil rubber workers.

In Britain, acids and alkalis are now almost unknown as agents of death. Even the occasional use of sulphuric 'battery acid' as a weapon of assault rarely causes death. The phenolic corrosives, however, such as carbolic acid and lysol, are occasionally encountered as suicidal agents. Toxicologically, none of these presents much problem, as the damage is often structural rather than poisonous, unless the victim survives long enough to have complications such as renal failure or chest infections. All the corrosive substances have the following features in common:

- There may be spillage of the fluid on the exterior of the body, corroding the skin in a pattern which may be helpful in reconstructing the posture of the victim at the time of drinking the substance. The lips may be burnt, and trickle and splash marks may run from the mouth down the chin, neck and chest. The pattern of burns at the mouth may sometimes indicate the shape of the container from which the poison was drunk, as the wide brim of a cup may mark the cheeks, while a bottleneck may sit more cleanly in the mouth. If the person was standing or sitting, then these runnels of fluid may pass down the chin onto chest and abdomen. If lying, then they may run across the face and cheeks and pass to the back of the neck. Further spillage may come from the nostrils due to spluttering and gagging. The hands may also be affected if the hands are instinctively brought up to the face.

- The interior of the mouth may be eroded, and the tongue swollen or shrivelled, according to the nature of the corrosive agent. The pharynx, larynx and oesophagus are all eroded, and if survival lasts more than a few minutes the glottis area may become oedematous. Spillage into the larynx and air passages may allow the respiratory mucosa to be damaged, and aspiration of liquid or vapour into the lungs can cause rapid pulmonary oedema and haemorrhages.

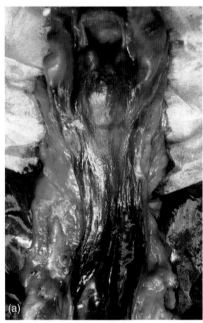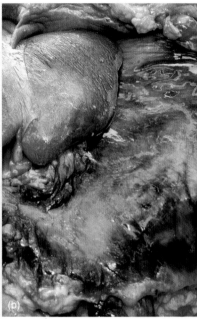

FIGURE 33.3 *Corrosion of larynx, oesophagus (a) and stomach (b) in suicidal ingestion of concentrated hydrochloride acid with alcohol.*

■ The lower oesophagus and stomach rapidly become damaged, with discoloration, desquamation and sometimes perforation. Attempts at passing a stomach tube may themselves penetrate the softened wall of the oesophagus or stomach. If survival lasts long enough, some corrosive may pass through to damage the small intestine, but this is rare because of the time factor and spasm of the pylorus.

■ All may cause death by pulmonary oedema from spillage into the lungs: if survival lasts a day or more, then a fulminating bronchopneumonia may be the terminal event.

The different corrosive agents have different actions on soft tissues, which can sometimes be differentiated by appearance and smell, though the mineral acids are not all that different. The phenolic compounds can usually be detected by smell alone. Strong acids act by dehydrating the tissues, coagulating the proteins and converting haemoglobin to haematin.

Sulphuric acid, in concentrated form, is extremely corrosive and produces great heat in contact with water or tissues. The tissues are grey to black, rather dry and dehydrated. They may actually be charred into a blackened crust by the generated heat. The gastric lining may be grey, dark brown or black, or mixtures of all colours, depending upon the amount of altered blood in each part. Perforation may occur.

The oesophagus and stomach may be grey and swollen, depending on the amount of acid and the amount of food already in the stomach. The tongue may be grey or black and distorted.

Nitric acid is similar, but has a brownish-yellow cast to its mucosal damage. There may be yellow or brown sharp-edged patterns on the skin burns of the face, with the usual trickle marks coming down from the corners of the mouth. Yellow fumes may arise from the stomach contents if a considerable quantity is present. The internal appearances are of yellowish-brown sloughing, though perforation seems less common than with sulphuric acid.

Hydrochloric acid has similar effects, especially on mucous membranes, but is not so injurious to intact skin as sulphuric and nitric acids. The stomach may be converted into a slimy, softened mass and can perforate. The colour is greyish to black, depending on the amount of altered blood.

Sodium hydroxide in concentrated form is also a corrosive, but soft, slippery slime is the characteristic appearance and feel to tissues damaged by caustic soda. The colour is dirty white to grey.

Phenol and lysol are also damaging and affect the tissues in much the same way as acids and alkalis. Carbolic acid (pure phenol) tends to stiffen the tissues and bleach them so that hard, cracked, whitish surfaces are seen on the face and skin. Internally, the same stiffness is noted in the oesophagus and stomach. Lysol is a soapy solution of phenol and cresols. It discolours the tissues a brownish purple, but is otherwise similar to phenol in its action.

OXALIC ACID AND OXALATE SALTS

These are not so corrosive as the mineral acids, but are poisonous and often act quickly, death occurring within minutes or the hour, from shock or hypocalcaemia. The acid is locally corrosive, but also has a systemic effect that may well be fatal even if the local damage is non-lethal.

At autopsy, if an appreciable amount of either the white crystals or a strong solution has been swallowed, the local effect is a bleaching, the mucosa of mouth, pharynx and oesophagus being white, though local haemorrhage can streak this with red. The stomach contains altered blood from the damaged mucosa and is dark brown or black from acid haematin, the wall studded with acute erosions. Calcium oxalate crystals may be seen in the stomach contents or in scrapings from the mucosa.

In those who have survived the acute phase, death may be caused by abnormalities of the muscle function (including the myocardium) from the hypocalcaemia, caused by the precipitation of body calcium as insoluble calcium oxalate. More common is renal failure, death occurring 2–10 days later. The renal tubules suffer necrosis, primarily in the proximal convoluted tubules. This is not caused by the presence of calcium oxalate crystals, though these can be demonstrated histologically in the kidney.

ETHYLENE GLYCOL POISONING

Though in no sense a corrosive poison, ethylene glycol has certain features in common with oxalate poisoning and is so common relative to death from mineral acids that it cannot be omitted. The glycols are used widely as antifreeze agents in motor engines and as solvents in industry, so they are easily available. Because of their chemical inclusion in the alcohol group, they are abused as a source of intoxication, as well as being accidental and suicidal agents. At least 40–60 deaths a year are reported and this is probably an underestimate. The compounds involved are ethylene, diethylene, propylene and hexylene glycols. These do not have the same toxic effects (in fact, propylene glycol is virtually non-toxic), but ethylene glycol is the most commonly encountered. When drunk in excess of 100–200 ml, it is almost certain to be fatal unless specific treatment is given, such as dialysis and competition with alcohol.

The first effects resemble drunkenness, but this passes into coma and death often within the first day. The glycol is metabolized in the body, a small but significant amount (about 1 per cent) being converted to oxalic acid, via the process glycol–glyoxal–glycolic acid–formic acid–glyoxylic acid–oxalic acid. It is not clear which of these compounds causes the most damage to the tissues.

At autopsy there is no local damage, but widespread precipitation of the sheaf-like doubly refractile crystals of calcium oxalate into the tissues can be rendered visible microscopically by the use of polarized light. It is a matter of controversy whether this crystal deposition is the cause or

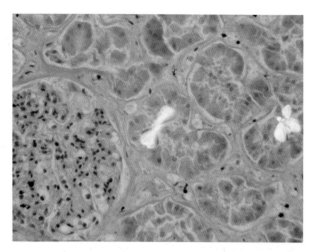

FIGURE 33.4 *Birefringent calcium oxalate crystals in kidney in ethylene glycol poisoning as seen in polarized light under a microscope.*

merely a side effect of the lethal action of glycols. There may be cerebral oedema and a chemical meningoencephalitis. In the kidney there is a tubular necrosis similar to that in oxalate poisoning, and the crystals can be seen in the interstitial tissues and the tubules. Diffuse liver damage can also occur.

Laboratory analysis in ethylene glycol poisoning

The blood levels naturally depend on the time that has elapsed since ingestion. It is usually greater than 300 mg/l and the mean is as high as 2400 mg/l in samples taken before the second day. The brain may contain from 300 to 4000 mg/kg and the urine from 600 to 10 000 mg/l, with a mean of 5700 mg/l.

METALLIC POISONS

There is a whole range of metallic poisons, most of them from the upper reaches of the Periodic Table, accounting for their usual description as 'heavy metals'. The vast majority of toxic effects come from environmental and occupational poisoning, both chronic and acute. Acute poisoning by suicide, accident and homicide is becoming much less common, both because of the availability of other toxic agents, and because of greater awareness and controls on the environmental and industrial hazards of heavy metals. In former years, especially the nineteenth century, heavy-metal poisoning was common in homicide, but is now rarely seen in Western countries, mainly because they are now known to be easily detectable.

As the subject is dealt with in great detail by so many textbooks and monographs, only one such poison – arsenic – will be discussed, together with a mention of any significant differences with other metals.

Arsenic

A constituent of all animal tissue, arsenic is the twelfth most abundant element on earth. This emphasizes the need for strict controls when making analysis for arsenic in human fluids or tissues, as the excretion of a healthy person on a diet rich in fish (especially shellfish) can exceed that seen in chronic arsenical poisoning. Similarly, where an exhumation is performed after allegations of poisoning, full control samples of soil and grave water must be taken to ensure that arsenic found in the body could not have arisen from local contamination (Chapter 1).

Arsenic metal is not poisonous, only its compounds. These interfere with cellular respiration by combining with the sulphydryl groups of mitochondrial enzymes, especially pyruvate oxidase and certain phosphatases. Arsenic has a particular target in vascular endothelium, accounting for the many lesions caused by increased permeability, tissue oedema and haemorrhage, especially in the alimentary canal.

Arsenical poisoning may arise from the ingestion of arsenious oxide, a tasteless white powder – from copper, sodium and potassium arsenites, arsenates of lead and calcium, arsenic sulphides and gaseous arsine (confined to industry). In forensic practice, the rare cases of arsenic poisoning are now usually from arsenious oxide or one of the arsenites.

Arsenical poisoning may be acute or chronic, the latter being the presentation of most environmental and occupational toxicity. Suicides are obviously invariably acute, whereas the uncommon homicidal cases may be either acute or chronic.

FATAL DOSAGES IN ARSENICAL POISONING

If taken on an empty stomach, especially in solution, only about 150 mg may be fatal, but usually some 250–300 mg are needed as a minimum lethal dose. Much larger quantities have been survived and there is some evidence that tolerance to arsenic can be attained. With large doses, much may be vomited. Death can be rapid – within hours from 'shock' and cardiorespiratory failure – or may be delayed for many days, when hepatorenal failure is the mode of death. In chronic poisoning, no lethal dosage can be indicated, as if the ingestion exceeds the small normal excretion rate, then a cumulative build-up of arsenic will occur.

Autopsy findings

In acute poisoning the findings may be minimal, if death occurs within hours. There may be some mild irritation of the upper gastrointestinal tract, such as reddening of the gastric mucosa, especially along the top edges of the rugae. The description of 'red velvet' has been applied to some stomach linings in acute arsenic poisoning. There may be mucus coating and granules of the poisonous agent may be trapped on the lining – a reason for sending both contents and stomach wall for analysis, as in most suspected poisonings of any type. The intestines are usually normal in acute poisoning.

The only other lesion commonly seen is subendocardial haemorrhage on the left ventricular wall. This, of course, is a common finding in any severe shock condition when sudden hypotension occurs. It is seen in any gross injury, with loss of blood volume, blood pressure and neurogenic shock. Head injuries and raised intracranial pressure are other conditions in which these lesions are prominent (Chapter 13). The phenomenon can be rapid, the author (BK) having seen them in the victims of military air crashes where the heart was avulsed from its base at the moment of impact. One of the best descriptions of subendocardial haemorrhages was given by Sheehan in 1940 in obstetrical catastrophes. The haemorrhages are situated on the upper part of the interventricular septum and on the opposing papillary muscles. The most severe the author (BK) has ever seen was in a massive suicidal overdose of arsenious oxide, where the haemorrhages were actually raised blood-filled blisters under the endocardium. These suggested the true diagnosis before analysis was carried out, albeit with an element of speculative good luck.

In chronic arsenical poisoning, the picture is quite different, though unless some suggestive history or circumstantial evidence is available, the diagnosis may be extremely difficult. As many a clinician has discovered to his chagrin in the past years, many a chronic arsenical poisoning has been misdiagnosed as a gastroenteritis.

Part of forensic mythology surrounds the alleged preservation of corpses dying from arsenic poisoning. This has been endlessly discussed, but there is no real evidence that it is true. A more likely explanation is that the dehydration from diarrhoea in chronic poisoning retards the usual moist putrefaction.

Externally there may be a diffuse abnormality of the skin, with a dry, scaly, hyperkeratotic surface. Clinically, there is a 'rain-drop' punctate pigmentation, but this may not be apparent after death unless really marked. It is more common in skin flexures and over the forehead and neck. There may be some hair loss. Puffy thickening and oedema of the face has been described, suggestive of myxoedema.

Internally the stomach may be normal or may show a chronic gastritis with thickening of the mucosa and subserous coats. Mucus formation may be noticeable and there may be a patchy inflammatory redness of some of the rugae. Sometimes there is a haemorrhagic gastritis with acute and chronic erosions. The small intestine is dilated and generally reddened, with thickened mucosa, the whole picture being of a non-specific congestion oedema so commonly seen in any enteritis.

There is rarely any mucosal ulceration. The contents may be copious and fluid, the usual description of 'rice-water' being applied. The large intestine may show minimal changes or be normal: the contents may be fluid and similar to the small bowel. The liver may reveal fatty change or more severe necrosis, sometimes at the periphery of the lobule. Severe liver damage may be associated with externally apparent jaundice. The kidney is damaged in chronic toxicity, there being non-specific tubular necrosis. The myocardium may also show myofibril damage, interstitial collection of cells and sometimes fatty degeneration.

TOXICOLOGY SAMPLING AND ANALYTICAL RESULTS

In acute poisoning, the major requirement is the stomach and contents, and preferably the small intestine, tied off at each end. Blood, urine and liver should also be taken.

In chronic poisoning, especially if the diagnosis is not firmly established from circumstantial and gross autopsy findings, a much wider range of samples is needed:

■ blood from peripheral veins
■ stomach and contents
■ small intestine and contents
■ sample of large bowel contents
■ urine
■ bile
■ whole liver
■ one kidney
■ nail clippings or whole nails
■ hair samples – whole length of at least 20 hairs, including roots.

Arsenic levels in blood are elevated only for a short time following absorption, unless exposure is continuous. The highest concentrations of arsenic are found tissues rich in sulphydryl (SH-) groups, such as skin, hair and nails. Typical levels of arsenic found in healthy persons unexposed to extra amounts over and above that normally (but variably) present in their environment are as follows: urine, <2–$20\,\mu g/l$; blood, <0.5–$4\,\mu g/l$; liver, $<60\,\mu g/kg$ (dry weight); nails, $<10^3\,\mu g/kg$ (dry weight).

It was formerly thought that it took a week or two for ingested arsenic to find its way into the keratinized tissues such as hair and nails. More sensitive analytical techniques have, however, shown that it can appear there within hours

TABLE 33.1 *Levels in acute arsenious oxide poisoning from 49 fatalities (Rehling 1967)*

	Range	Average
Blood (mg/l)	0.6–9.3	3.3
Liver (mg/kg)	2.0–120	29.0
Kidney (mg/kg)	0.2–70	15.0
Spleen (mg/kg)	0.5–62	8.8
Brain (mg/kg)	0.2–4.0	1.7

of ingestion by mouth. The explanation was originally offered that arsenic was rapidly secreted into sweat, and spread to the hair and nails by surface diffusion. This has recently been disproved by neutron activation analysis and the mechanism remains obscure. The test for estimating the timing and duration of arsenic administration by analysing different lengths of the hair shaft has thus been vindicated. Arsenic can remain stored in keratin for several years after administration ceases.

Antimony

Antimony is similar to arsenic in many respects. Apart from industrial exposure, the usual vehicle of poisoning is 'tartar emetic', antimony potassium tartrate. This has been used suicidally and homicidally, as well as in some accidental deaths. The pathology and toxicology are similar to that of arsenic, the minimum fatal dose of the tartrate being about 150 mg, though this was formerly the normal intravenous dose in the treatment of bilharzia. Vastly greater amounts of tartar emetic have been survived, so the minimal lethal dose is not a particularly useful concept, as with many other poisons.

Occupationally unexposed people have either zero or not more than 0.01 mg/l of antimony in their blood and a tenth of this concentration in their urine.

Baselt (2002) quotes a case of acute poisoning from antimony trichloride where the following concentrations (in mg/l or mg/kg) were found on analysis: blood, 4–6; liver, 45; kidney, 32; bile, 404.

Thallium

Though other heavy metals have declined in forensic importance over the past century, thallium has several times been used homicidally in recent years, sometimes for multiple poisonings. Thallium is used as a rat killer and widely employed in industry, especially in glass manufacture. It has curious aspects in relation to forensic pathology, in that it can be seen radiologically in the intestine and deposited in the liver, so in the rare event of a pathologist suspecting thallium poisoning,

TABLE 33.2 *Fatal thallium concentrations (mg/l or mg/kg) collected by Baselt (2002)*

	Range	Average
Blood	0.5–11	4.0
Urine	1.7–11	5.2
Kidney	6–20	11.0
Liver	5–29	15.0

X-rays of the body should be taken before autopsy. The other unique aspect is that it is probably the only homicidal agent to be confirmed after cremation. In the Young case in Britain in 1971, where two people died and several others were non-fatally poisoned by Young, thallium was detected retrospectively in the ashes of one of his victims.

The fatal dose is somewhere about 1 g, depending upon the type of thallium compound employed, as there are several different salts available, such as the acetate, sulphate or nitrate. The estimates vary from 6 to 40 mg/kg body weight, with an average of about 12 mg/kg.

Autopsy appearances are variable and non-specific, but pallor and streaking of a pale, degenerate myocardium have been recorded. Hair loss is one of the clinical signs that arouses suspicion of thallium poisoning, as it was formerly used as a depilatory. This effect begins about a week after administration, but may not be noticeable for twice that time. Large tufts tend to come away, rather than a general thinning. Loss of the outer third of the eyebrows is said to be a significant sign, though these are also the areas that are lost in hypothyroidism.

Examination of the roots of surviving hairs may show a black coating, caused not by the thallium itself, but by an excess of melanin. Liver necrosis and renal tubular necrosis are non-specific findings in those who survive for some time.

REFERENCES AND FURTHER READING

Ballantyne B. 1976. Changes in blood cyanide as a function of storage time and temperature. *J Forensic Sci Soc* **16**:305–10.

Barillo DJ, Goode R, Esch V. 1994. Cyanide poisoning in victims of fire: analysis of 364 cases and review of the literature. *J Burn Care Rehabil* **15**:46–57.

Baselt RC. 2002. *Disposition of toxic drugs and chemicals in man*, 6th edn. Biomedical Publications, Foster City, CA.

Baud FJ, Barriot P, Toffis V, *et al.* 1991. Elevated blood cyanide concentrations in victims of smoke inhalation. *N Engl J Med* **325**:1761–6.

Blackwell M, Robbins A. 1979. Arsine (arsenic hydride) poisoning in the workplace. *Am Ind Hyg Assoc J* **40**:A56–61.

Bogusz M. 1980. Vitreous humour as reliable material for ethylene glycol determination. *Forensic Sci Int* **16**:75–6.

Bowen DA, Minty PS, Sengupta A. 1978. Two fatal cases of ethylene glycol poisoning. *Med Sci Law* **18**:101–7.

Broor SL, Kumar A, Chari ST, *et al.* 1989. Corrosive oesophageal strictures following acid ingestion: clinical profile and results of endoscopic dilatation. *J Gastroenterol Hepatol* **4**:55–61.

Chaturvedi AK, Smith DR, Canfield DV. 2001. A fatality caused by accidental production of hydrogen sulfide. *Forensic Sci Int* **123**:211–14.

Cheng JT, Beysolow TD, Kaul B, *et al.* 1987. Clearance of ethylene glycol by kidneys and hemodialysis. *J Toxicol Clin Toxicol* **25**:95–108.

Chikasue F, Yashiki M, Kojima T, *et al.* 1988. Cyanide distribution in five fatal cyanide poisonings and the effect of storage conditions on cyanide concentration in tissue. *Forensic Sci Int* **38**:173–83.

Christesen HB. 1995. Prediction of complications following caustic ingestion in adults. *Clin Otolaryngol* **20**:272–8.

Curry A. 1969. *Poison detection in human organs.* Thomas, Springfield, IL.

Curry AS. 1963. Cyanide poisoning. *Acta Pharmacol Toxicol* **20**:291–4.

Curry AS, Price DE, Rutter ER. 1967. The production of cyanide in post mortem material. *Acta Pharmacol Toxicol (Copenh)* **25**:339–44.

Davis LE, Standefer JC, Kornfeld M, *et al.* 1981. Acute thallium poisoning: toxicological and morphological studies of the nervous system. *Ann Neurol* **10**:38–44.

Dilawari JB, Singh S, Rao PN, *et al.* 1984. Corrosive acid ingestion in man – a clinical and endoscopic study. *Gut* **25**:183–7.

Erkens M, Kellner H. 1981. [Toxicologic course studies in thallium poisoning.] *Beitr Gerichtl Med* **39**:157–61.

Fernando GC, Busuttil A. 1991. Cyanide ingestion. Case studies of four suicides [published erratum appears in *Am J Forensic Med Pathol* 1993 Dec;**14**(4):353]. *Am J Forensic Med Pathol* **12**:241–6.

Ferrari LA, Arado MG, Giannuzzi L, *et al.* 2001. Hydrogen cyanide and carbon monoxide in blood of convicted dead in a polyurethane combustion: a proposition for the data analysis. *Forensic Sci Int* **121**:140–3.

Galvan-Arzate S, Santamaria A. 1998. Thallium toxicity. *Toxicol Lett* **99**:1–13.

Gebel T. 2000. Confounding variables in the environmental toxicology of arsenic. *Toxicology* **144**:155–62.

Hawley CK, Harsch HH. 1999. Gastric outlet obstruction as a late complication of formaldehyde ingestion: a case report. *Am J Gastroenterol* **94**:2289–91.

Herrero F, Fernandez E, Gomez J, *et al.* 1995. Thallium poisoning presenting with abdominal colic, paresthesia, and irritability. *J Toxicol Clin Toxicol* **33**:261–4.

Hoffman RS. 2000. Thallium poisoning during pregnancy: a case report and comprehensive literature review. *J Toxicol Clin Toxicol* **38**:767–75.

Howell JM. 1986. Alkaline ingestions. *Ann Emerg Med* **15**:820–5.

Ikegaya H, Iwase H, Hatanaka K, *et al.* 2000. Postmortem changes in cytochrome *c* oxidase activity in various organs of the rat and in human heart. *Forensic Sci Int* **108**:181–6.

Ikegaya H, Iwase H, Hatanaka K, *et al.* 2001. Diagnosis of cyanide intoxication by measurement of cytochrome *c* oxidase activity. *Toxicol Lett* **119**:117–23.

Jacobsen D, Akesson I, Shefter E. 1982. Urinary calcium oxalate monohydrate crystals in ethylene glycol poisoning. *Scand J Clin Lab Invest* **42**:231–4.

Jacobsen D, Ostby N, Bredesen JE. 1982. Studies on ethylene glycol poisoning. *Acta Med Scand* **212**:11–15.

Kamijo Y, Soma K, Asari Y, *et al.* 1998. Survival after massive arsenic poisoning self-treated by high fluid intake. *J Toxicol Clin Toxicol* **36**:27–9.

Karhunen PJ, Lukkari I, Vuori E. 1991. High cyanide level in a homicide victim burned after death: evidence of post-mortem diffusion. *Forensic Sci Int* **49**:179–83.

Kazsuba A, Vitez A, Gall J, *et al.* 2000. Gastric hyalinization as a possible consequence of corrosive injury. *Endoscopy* **32**:356–8.

Lander H, Hodge PR, Crisp CS. 1965. Arsenic in hair and nails: its significance in acute arsenical poisoning. *J Forensic Med* **12**:52–67.

Lokan RJ, James RA, Dymock RB. 1987. Apparent post-mortem production of high levels of cyanide in blood. *J Forensic Sci Soc* **27**:253–9.

Makela JT, Laitinen S. 1997. Corrosive oesophageal injury. A study of four cases. *Ann Chir Gynaecol* **86**:360–3.

Marquet P, Clement S, Lotfi H, *et al.* 1996. Analytical findings in a suicide involving sodium azide. *J Anal Toxicol* **20**:134–8.

McCallum R. 1989. The industrial toxicology of antimony. The Ernestine Henry lecture 1987. *J R Coll Physicians Lond* **23**:28–32.

Meggs WJ, Hoffman RS, Shih RD, *et al.* 1994. Thallium poisoning from maliciously contaminated food. *J Toxicol Clin Toxicol* **32**:723–30.

Metter D, Vock R. 1984. [Structure of the hair in thallium poisoning.] *Z Rechtsmed* **91**:201–14.

Mollhoff G, Schmidt G, Bosche J. 1979. ['Thallium poisoning' – neurologic and forensic aspects.] *Arch Kriminol* **163**:1–13.

Moore D, House I, Dixon A. 1993. Thallium poisoning. Diagnosis may be elusive but alopecia is the clue. *Br Med J* **306**:1527–9.

Naon H, Shaul D, Mahnovski V, *et al.* 1996. Fibroproliferative disorder of the antrum after an alkali ingestion. *Am J Gastroenterol* **91**:383–4.

Neil MW. 1957. Immune to cyanide? *J Forensic Med* **4**:17–19.

Nolte KB, Dasgupta A. 1996. Prevention of occupational cyanide exposure in autopsy prosectors. *J Forensic Sci* **41**:146–7.

Pense SC, Wood WJ, Stempel TK, *et al.* 1988. Tracheoesophageal fistula secondary to muriatic acid ingestion. *Burns Incl Therm Inj* **14**:35–8.

Peterson CD, Collins AJ, Himes JM, *et al.* 1981. Ethylene glycol poisoning: pharmacokinetics during therapy with ethanol and hemodialysis. *N Engl J Med* **304**:21–3.

Poklis A, Saady JJ. 1990. Arsenic poisoning: acute or chronic? Suicide or murder? *Am J Forensic Med Pathol* **11**:226–32.

Questel F, Dugarin J, Dally S. 1996. Thallium-contaminated heroin. *Ann Intern Med* **124**:616.

Raekallio J, Jääskeläinen AJ, Mäkinen PL. 1967. The simple demonstration of calcium oxalate crystals in kidneys of victims of ethylene glycol poisoning. *J Forensic Sci* **12**:238–40.

Rehling CJ. 1967. Poison residues in human tissues. *Prog Chem Toxicol* **3**:363–86.

Saha JC, Dikshit AK, Bandyopadhyay MK, *et al.* 1999. A review of arsenic poisoning and its effects on human health. *Crit Rev Environ Sci Technol* **29**:281–313.

Shabalina LP, Spiridonova VS. 1979. Thallium as an industrial poison (review of literature). *J Hyg Epidemiol Microbiol Immunol* **23**:247–55.

Sheehan HL. 1940. Subendocardial haemorrhages in shock. *Lancet* **1**:831–2.

Stajduhar-Caric Z. 1968. Acute phenol poisoning. Singular findings in a lethal case. *J Forensic Med* **15**:41–2.

Stoeppler M, Vahter M. 1994. Arsenic. In: Herber RFM, Stoeppler M (eds), *Techniques and instrumentation in analytical chemistry*, vol. 15, *Trace element analysis in biological specimens*. Elsevier, Amsterdam, London, New York, Tokyo, pp. 291–320.

Tromme I, Van Neste D, Dobbelaere F, *et al.* 1998. Skin signs in the diagnosis of thallium poisoning. *Br J Dermatol* **138**:321–5.

Villanueva E, Hernandez-Cueto C, Lachica E, *et al.* 1990. Poisoning by thallium. A study of five cases. *Drug Saf* **5**:384–9.

Walton EW. 1978. An epidemic of antifreeze poisoning. *Med Sci Law* **18**:231–7.

Weinig E, Schmidt G. 1966. [On the distribution of thallium in the organism in fatal thallium poisoning.] *Arch Toxikol* **21**:199–215.

Westveer AE, Trestrail JH, Pinizzotto AJ. 1996. Homicidal poisoning in the United States: an analysis of the uniform crime reports from 1980 through 1989. *Am J Forensic Med Pathol* **17**:282–8.

Winek CL, Fusia E, Collom WD, *et al.* 1978. Cyanide poisoning as a mode of suicide. *Forensic Sci* **11**:51–5.

Winek CL, Bricker JD, Fochtman FW. 1980. Lithium intoxication. A case study. *Forensic Sci Int* **15**:227–31.

Winek CL, Esposito FM, Cinicola DP. 1990. The stability of several compounds in formalin fixed tissues and formalin-blood solutions. *Forensic Sci Int* **44**:159–68.

Winek CL, Rozin L, Wahba WW, *et al.* 1995. Ingestion of lye. *Forensic Sci Int* **73**:143–7.

Wormald PJ, Wilson DA. 1993. Battery acid burns of the upper gastro-intestinal tract. *Clin Otolaryngol* **18**:112–14.

Wu ML, Tsai WJ, Yang CC, *et al.* 1998. Concentrated cresol intoxication. *Vet Hum Toxicol* **40**:341–3.

Zamir O, Hod G, Lernau OZ, *et al.* 1985. Corrosive injury to the stomach due to acid ingestion. *Am Surg* **51**:170–2.

C H A P T E R **34**

Deaths from organic solvents

A wide range of organic compounds used in industry and in the home as solvents may cause injury or death, especially when used carelessly or for improper purposes. Other organic substances, often gaseous, can also be fatal when used or abused in the same circumstances.

SOLVENT ABUSE

This phenomenon arose, spontaneously and independently, in several parts of the world in the 1960s. It consists of deliberately inhaling a variety of substances, especially organic solvents, in order to achieve a distortion of consciousness. The effects vary from a state resembling alcoholic intoxication through euphoria (sometimes of an erotic nature) and distortion of perception, to actual hallucinations. The practitioners of this activity are predominantly, though by no means exclusively, male and most are between the ages of about 14 and 22 years, though again there are a few beyond either end of this age range. The majority of deaths occur in solitary users, some 70 per cent being reported by Anderson *et al.* (1985) as having happened when the young person was alone. Sniffing can certainly be a group activity, however, as is seen in schools and even the streets of some cities.

At first, the most common substance inhaled was a toluene-based adhesive and therefore the name 'glue-sniffing' soon became attached to the habit, though in fact many substances now used are not adhesives. The more accurate title of 'solvent abuse' has now been applied to this widespread and dangerous habit. Although (like the sexual asphyxias, with which there is some cross-relationship) the ratio of deaths to non-fatal escapades is relatively small, the large number of children and young people who indulge in the habit means that a considerable death toll occurs annually.

The usual method of abuse is for a quantity of the solvent or other chemical to be placed in a plastic bag – which may be any kind from a large black polythene garbage sack to a used potato-crisp packet. The open end is then placed against the nose and mouth, and the air inside re-breathed. The warmth of the hand holding the bag, as well as the warm breath, encourages vaporization of the solvent, which enters the tidal air stream and is absorbed through the pulmonary membranes into the blood. When the substance is not a viscous glue, it may be placed on a handkerchief or rag, and inhaled direct as a pad over the nose and mouth.

When gaseous substances are abused, they may be introduced directly into the mouth or nose. A common variety is butane or propane, taken from either a large cylinder used for camping, heating and cooking, or from the small ampoule cylinders sold for refilling gas cigarette lighters. Others are used directly from pressurized aerosol cans, including pain-relieving sprays used for the relief of muscular conditions. Yet again, sniffing may be attained by merely inhaling directly from the neck of a container. Tins, jerry-cans and the petrol-fillers of motor vehicles may be used in this way. Some fire extinguishers contain an organic bromine derivative which is also abused for inhalation. This has a particular propensity for sensitizing the myocardium to catecholamines.

Dangers of solvent abuse

SUDDEN DEATH

The major cause of death appears to be sudden cardiac arrest, following an arrhythmia. Any of the solvents appears to have the ability to sensitize the myocardium to the action of catecholamines, such as noradrenaline. Any sudden 'flight-or-fight' stimulus, even some considerable time after sniffing solvents, has the ability to precipitate ventricular fibrillation and hence sudden death. A recent instance seen by the author (BK) involved a youth whose habit was to steal fire extinguishers from trains parked in sidings and inhale the bromine-based contents. Having been in trouble with the police before, he took fright on seeing a constable approaching, though in fact the officer was merely walking his dog. The boy ran from his group of friends and did not reappear, being found dead in some bushes some time later, though he had not 'sniffed' that day. The autopsy and toxicology were negative, apart from residual traces of organic substance in his blood.

In addition to this physiological mechanism, actual myocarditis can occasionally occur, as in a 15-year-old girl who dropped dead whilst inhaling from the petrol tanks of vehicles. At autopsy all that the author (BK) could find was a florid, diffuse interstitial myocarditis with minimal myofibril necrosis.

CHEMICAL EFFECTS

The mechanical means of obtaining concentrated solvent vapour is in itself dangerous. Persistent rebreathing can produce hypoxia and hypercapnia, which is additive to the toxic effects of the solvent itself. When large plastic bags are used, the abuser sometimes places his head within the bag and this risks the dangers of rapid death from plastic bag asphyxia (Chapter 14). It is difficult to know if some of these cases are at least partially instances of erotic hypoxia, the effects of both oxygen lack and the hallucinogenic effect of the solvent combining to give both sexual pleasure and a heightened risk of death.

Another potent risk is vomiting while the effects of the solvent incapacitate the victim sufficiently to prevent his reflexes from protecting or clearing his glottis or air passages. The usual warning must be given, however, about uncritically accepting the finding of gastric contents in the air passages at autopsy. This may well have been an agonal regurgitation in a victim who was dying of the common cardiac (ventricular fibrillation) effect of solvents on the myocardium. This has medico-legal relevance in that a fellow abuser or even some other bystander may be accused of failing to render assistance in clearing the air passages, when in fact this was the effect, rather than the cause of death. This is not to say that aspiration of vomit cannot be the cause of death, as in alcoholic intoxication, but the autopsy finding should be backed up with some circumstantial evidence that it occurred before the agonal period.

PHYSICAL DANGER

When gaseous substances are used, such as butane or propane from cylinders, or propellants from aerosol cans, a physical danger is added to the chemical effects. The gases are commonly directed or sprayed into the open mouth while inhalation is performed. The release of high-pressure gas causes rapid cooling by the 'refrigerator effect' and the impact of this on the palate, pharynx and larynx may cause a reflex cardiac arrest. The author (BK) has dealt with two such cases, one in a school yard, where the users of small propane refuellers virtually dropped dead in the presence of other youths. The mechanism of this phenomenon is disputed, but freezing of the sensitive pharyngolaryngeal area is surely a parallel to the sudden deaths seen when cold water enters the nasopharynx in sudden immersion deaths.

DANGER TO LONG-TERM USERS

Long-term users can suffer liver damage, typical of halogenated hydrocarbon exposure, with fatty change in the liver and sometimes associated renal damage.

SUBSTANCES USED IN ABUSE

Toluene

Toluene was one of the first substances recognized as giving rise to 'glue-sniffing', as it is the solvent for many adhesives, such as the proprietary glue 'Evostick'. It is an aromatic petrol hydrocarbon used widely in industry as a solvent and thinner for adhesives and paints. It resembles benzene in many of its properties, another substance that can be used in solvent inhalation. Toluene can cause acute and chronic intoxication in industrial situations. Exposure to relatively high concentrations in the air, between 10 000 and 30 000 p.p.m. can cause drunkenness, mental confusion and coma within a few minutes.

In non-fatal toluene abuse, blood levels of 0.3–7.0 mg/l were measured by Bonnichsen *et al.* (1966), with urine excretion of up to 5 mg/l. Those with blood concentrations of 1.0–2.5 mg/l showed some sign of intoxication, while half of those between 2.5 and 10 mg/l were admitted to hospital with marked symptoms. Those who were unconscious or dead had blood levels in excess of 19 mg/l. Nomiyama and Nomiyama (1979) found blood levels of between 50 and 80 mg/l in three fatalities. Baselt (2002) quotes a fatal range of between 10 and 48 mg/l with an average of 22 mg/ml for fatalities, the average in the lung being 12 mg/l and in the brain 47 mg/l. Brain damage has been reported in long-term abusers, with electroencephalographic changes, encephalopathy and occasional cerebral atrophy.

Petrol (gasoline), xylene and benzene

These closely resemble toluene in behaviour, though benzene is said to be more potent in causing intoxication. As with toluene and most other solvents, they can burn the skin if left in contact with it for some time. The odour threshold for benzene has been reported as 1–5 p.p.m. in air. In chronic exposure, benzene can cause bone-marrow depression and fatal aplastic anaemia, but this is not a feature of the shorter exposures in solvent abuse.

Methylene chloride and ethylene dizchloride

These are found in paint strippers and, as these solvents, in many other products. One used for abuse is the solvent for typewriter correction fluids, such as Tippex.

Butane and propane

These have been mentioned earlier, being used direct from pressurized containers. They are light hydrocarbons, being the upper fractions of oil distillation.

Fluorocarbons

These are the substances now blamed for having the worst effect on the ozone layers of the upper atmosphere. They are widely used as refrigerants and propellants in aerosol containers. It is in this latter role that they are widely abused for euphoric and hallucinatory effects. The various compounds are numbered, rather than named, two fluorine atoms being incorporated into molecules that otherwise resemble carbon tetrachloride. Those used for propellants are FC-11 and FC-12.

A similar compound incorporating bromine instead of fluorine is used as a fire extinguisher, as is carbon tetrachloride itself. As long ago as 1970, Bass published a series of 110 sudden deaths, including many from fluorocarbons. As mentioned earlier, these substances sensitize the myocardium to circulating catecholamines. The range of blood concentrations in fatal cases in respect of FC-12 is 0.6–12 mg/l, with a mean of 3.0 mg/l and for FC-11, 1.2–32 mg/l, with a mean of 12 mg/l. In the lung, FC-12 may be present at levels of 0.9–134 mg/kg, with a mean of 33 mg/kg; for FC-11 the corresponding figures are 5.8–94 mg/kg, with a mean of 43 mg/kg.

Carbon tetrachloride

Used as a degreaser, dry-cleaner and fire extinguisher, carbon tetrachloride is easily available from retail outlets as a spot remover. It is quite toxic, though it (unwisely) used to be used in human pharmacy to treat intestinal worms. As little as 3–5 ml can be fatal. Much of its toxicity is industrial, but it has also been used in suicide and solvent abuse. Chronic exposure can cause liver and renal damage, worsened by the simultaneous use of alcohol. Addiction can occur, even from initial exposure during industrial use.

As with most halogenated hydrocarbons, the liver suffers from exposure to tetrachloride. There is a centrilobular necrosis, usually preceded by fatty change if the poisoning is low level and lasting. In fatal cases there may well be virtually total acute yellow atrophy. The liver damage is markedly worsened by a high alcohol intake. Renal changes consist of a tubular necrosis and diffuse fatty degeneration in the cortex.

Post-mortem blood levels vary greatly, but a fatal case has been recorded with a concentration of 260 mg/l. Korenke and Pribilla (1969) found tissue levels at autopsy a week after inhalation as being 142 mg/kg in the liver and 39 mg/kg in the lung.

Other halogenated hydrocarbons

Other halogenated hydrocarbons have similar effects to carbon tetrachloride, but the level of toxicity varies with the number of chlorine atoms in the molecule. The ascending order of danger is methyl chloride, trichlormethane, chloroform and carbon tetrachloride. Others include trichlorethylene, used widely in both anaesthesia (Trilene) and in dry-cleaning. Several other similar compounds have been the cause of fatalities in industry as well as in solvent abuse. The pathological features are similar in most of them, the effects being on the central nervous system in acute massive overdose, whether by ingestion or inhalation, and upon the liver and kidneys in more chronic intoxications.

THE AUTOPSY ON FATAL SOLVENT-ABUSE VICTIMS

The scene should be visited if possible, though it is rare to find the body there, as strenuous resuscitation and removal by ambulance is always a prime consideration in children and young persons found apparently dead. The paraphernalia of sniffing may be seen in its original state.

At autopsy, the clothing should be examined, even though it has almost always been removed for resuscitation attempts. Any soiling with adhesive or solvent stains should be detected and, though volatile, should be kept for forensic science investigation. The best means is to pack them as soon as possible in a nylon bag to retain any vapour; these solvents will penetrate a polyvinylchloride bag and be lost.

Externally, the face should be inspected for any signs of chronic or recent solvent abuse. The act of holding a bag against the lower face, often contaminating it with glue or solvent, may leave skin lesions. These can be red erythematous pimples or actual excoriations from the irritant action of the solvent. The lesions may become infected or scratched, becoming crusted. The rest of the autopsy may be unrewarding from the point of view of gross pathology. Rarely, there may be a fatty liver from long-standing damage from the solvent, especially the halogenated hydrocarbons. Full samples for histological examination should be taken to determine the state of the myocardium, liver and brain. More immediate is the need to obtain samples for analysis.

Vigorous resuscitation, including mouth-to-mouth and chest compression, together with mechanical ventilation and oxygen administration, will obviously blow off much of the solvent in the lungs. If it has already been absorbed, however, some will come back into alveolar air from the lung tissue and the sensitivity of the head-space gas chromatography used for its detection is often sufficient to identify the substance, which can also be detected in blood and tissues.

Blood samples should be taken in the usual manner, including a tube with fluoride for alcohol, which is sometimes also present. A lung should be taken intact for the laboratory. It was formerly the practice to aspirate air from the trachea before removal of viscera, using a 50 ml syringe, which was then sealed and sent to the laboratory. This is impracticable, and the best method is to open the pleural cavity and pass a string ligature round the hilum of a lung, pulling it tight to occlude the main bronchus. This is then drawn tight and the hilum transected. In actual fact, little is lost if the lung is cut off without this procedure, as long as it is put straight into a nylon bag without delay and without squeezing out the contained air. The nylon bags are those that arson investigators use to save material for fire-accelerant examination, as they are impervious to organic solvents.

A urine sample, and unfixed tissue from liver and brain should also be supplied to the toxicology laboratory, though local discussion should be made to determine the requirements of each laboratory.

REFERENCES AND FURTHER READING

al-Alousi LM. 1989. Pathology of volatile substance abuse: a case report and a literature review. *Med Sci Law* **29**:189–208.

Anderson HR, Macnair RS, Ramsey JD. 1985. Deaths from abuse of volatile substances: a national epidemiological study. *Br Med J Clin Res Ed* **290**:304–7.

Backer RC, Pisano RV. 1978. Gas chromatography-mass spectrometry of fluorocarbons 11 and 12 in biologic specimens. *Clin Toxicol* **12**:69–75.

Barrowcliff DF. 1978. Chronic carbon monoxide poisoning caused by methylene chloride paintstripper. *Med Sci Law* **18**:238.

Baselt RC. 2002. *Disposition of toxic drugs and chemicals in man*, 6th edn. Biomedical Publications, Foster City, CA.

Bass M. 1970. Sudden sniffing death. *JAMA* **212**:2075–9.

Bonnichsen R, Maehly AC, Moeller M. 1966. Poisoning by volatile compounds. I. Aromatic hydrocarbons. *J Forensic Sci* **11**:186–204.

Chao TC, Lo DS, Koh J, *et al.* 1993. Glue sniffing deaths in Singapore – volatile aromatic hydrocarbons in post-mortem blood by headspace gas chromatography. *Med Sci Law* **33**:253–60.

Clark MA, Jones JW, Robinson JJ, *et al.* 1985. Multiple deaths resulting from shipboard exposure to trichlorotrifluoroethane. *J Forensic Sci* **30**:1256–9.

Claydon SM. 1988. Myocardial degeneration in chronic solvent abuse. *Med Sci Law* **28**:217–18.

Editorial. 1982. Solvent abuse. *Lancet* **2**:1139–40.

Escobar A, Aruffo C. 1980. Chronic thinner intoxication: clinico-pathologic report of a human case. *J Neurol Neurosurg Psychiatry* **43**:986–94.

Fuke C, Berry CL, Pounder DJ. 1996. Postmortem diffusion of ingested and aspirated paint thinner. *Forensic Sci Int* **78**:199–207.

Garriott J, Petty CS. 1980. Death from inhalant abuse: Toxicological and pathological evaluation of 34 cases. *Clin Toxicol* **16**:305–15.

George B. 1960. Kerosene poisoning. *Med Sci Law* **1**:14–52.

Harada K, Ichiyama T, Ikeda H, *et al.* 1999. A fatal case of oral ingestion of benzine. *Am J Forensic Med Pathol* **20**:84–9.

Harrer G, Kisser W, Pilz P, *et al.* 1973. [Three cases of trichloroethylene resp. Carbon tetrachloride 'sniffing' with fatal outcome.] *Nervenarzt* **44**:645–7.

Heath MJ. 1986. Solvent abuse using bromochlorodifluoromethane from a fire extinguisher. *Med Sci Law* **26**:33–4.

Inoue H, Iwasa M, Maeno Y, *et al.* 1996. Detection of toluene in an adipoceratous body. *Forensic Sci Int* **78**:119–24.

Isenschmid DS, Cassin BJ, Hepler BR, *et al.* 1998. Tetrachloroethylene intoxication in an autoerotic fatality. *J Forensic Sci* **43**:231–4.

Kamijo Y, Soma K, Hasegawa I, *et al.* 1998. Fatal bilateral adrenal hemorrhage following acute toluene poisoning: a case report. *J Toxicol Clin Toxicol* **36**:365–8.

Kim NY, Park SW. 2000. The comparison of toluene determination between headspace-solid phase microextraction and headspace methods in glue-sniffer's blood and urine samples. *J Forensic Sci* **45**:702–7.

Kimura K, Nagata T, Hara K, *et al.* 1988. Gasoline and kerosene components in blood – a forensic analysis. *Hum Toxicol* **7**:299–305.

King MD, Day RE, Oliver JS, *et al.* 1981. Solvent encephalopathy. *Br Med J Clin Res Ed* **283**:663–5.

Korenke HD, Pribilla O. 1969. [Suicide by single inhalation of carbon tetrachloride (CCl_4), with resulting leukoencephalopathy.] *Arch Toxikol* **25**:109–26.

Kringsholm B. 1980. Sniffing-associated deaths in Denmark. *Forensic Sci Int* **15**:215–25.

Levine B, Fierro MF, Goza SW, *et al.* 1981. A tetrachloroethylene fatality. *J Forensic Sci* **26**:206–9.

Morinaga M, Kashimura S, Hara K, *et al.* 1996. The utility of volatile hydrocarbon analysis in cases of carbon monoxide poisoning. *Int J Legal Med* **109**:75–9.

Nomiyama K, Nomiyama H. 1979. [Health effects of trichloroethylene in human subjects (author's transl).] *Sangyo Igaku* **21**:311–34.

Park SW, Kim N, Yang Y, *et al.* 1998. Toluene distribution of glue sniffers' biological fluid samples in Korea. *J Forensic Sci* **43**:888–90.

Poklis A. 1975. Determination of fluorocarbon 11 and fluorocarbon 12 in post-mortem tissues: a case report. *Forensic Sci* **5**:53–9.

Ramsey JD, Flanagan RJ. 1982. The role of the laboratory in the investigation of solvent abuse. *Hum Toxicol* **1**:299–311.

Reed BJ, May PA. 1984. Inhalant abuse and juvenile delinquency: a control study in Albuquerque, New Mexico. *Int J Addict* **19**:789–803.

Ridgway P, Nixon TE, Leach JP. 2003. Occupational exposure to organic solvents and long-term nervous system damage detectable by brain imaging, neurophysiology or histopathology. *Food Chem Toxicol* **41**:153–87.

Sourindrhin I. 1985. Solvent misuse [editorial]. *Br Med J Clin Res Ed* **290**:94–5.

Standefer JC. 1975. Death associated with fluorocarbon inhalation: report of a case. *J Forensic Sci* **20**:548–51.

Suwaki H. 1983. A follow-up study of adolescent glue-sniffers in Japan. *Br J Addict* **78**:409–13.

Tranthim-Fryer DJ, Hansson RC, Norman KW. 2001. Headspace/solid-phase microextraction/gas chromatography-mass spectrometry: a screening technique for the recovery and identification of volatile organic compounds (VOC's) in postmortem blood and viscera samples. *J Forensic Sci* **46**:934–46.

Trochimowicz HJ, Azar A, Terrill JB, *et al.* 1974. Blood levels of fluorocarbon related to cardiac sensitization: II. *Am Ind Hyg Assoc J* **35**:632–9.

Wang CC, Irons SV. 1961. Acute gasoline intoxication. *Arch Environ Health* **2**:715–20.

Watson JM. 1977. 'Glue-sniffing' in profile. *Practitioner* **218**:255–9.

Watson JM. 1979. Morbidity and mortality statistics on solvent abuse. *Med Sci Law* **19**:246–52.

Winek CL, Collom WD. 1971. Benzene and toluene fatalities. *J Occup Med* **13**:259–61.

Winek CL, Wahba WW, Huston R, *et al.* 1997. Fatal inhalation of 1,1,1-trichloroethane. *Forensic Sci Int* **87**:161–5.

APPENDIX 1

Technical methods

STAINING TECHNIQUES

Periodic acid–Schiff (PAS) for myocardium

In established early infarcts of probably at least 28–24 hours' duration, damaged myofibres stain a pale purple-blue with PAS, compared with the pinker colour of healthy fibres. This stainable material is diastase resistant and is probably a mucoprotein.

(a) Bring sections to water.
(b) Immerse in 1 per cent periodic acid for 5 minutes.
(c) Wash in water for 5 minutes.
(d) Rinse in distilled water.
(e) Immerse in Schiff's reagent for 10 minutes.
(f) Wash in water for 10 minutes.
(g) Stain in haematoxylin for 30 seconds.
(h) Blue in tap water and mount in usual way.

Malic acid dehydrogenase (MDH)

Enzyme histochemistry is the most reliable method of detecting early myocardial infarction. Succinic, lactic, malic, β-hydroxybutyric dehydrogenases and cytochrome oxidase are among those used by many workers and each has its advocates. The author (BK) prefers malate dehydrogenase, though β-hydroxybutyrate is also recommended. Fixed tissue cannot be used, as frozen cryostat sections are required. The method for malate dehydrogenase is given, though the technique for other enzymes is similar, using different substrates; details are found in standard histochemistry texts.

MALATE DEHYDROGENASE METHOD FOR MYOCARDIUM

Normal myocardium stains dark blue–black, mostly concentrated on intracellular mitochondria, with some staining of the cytoplasm. Fibres damaged by anoxia or ischaemia progressively lose their staining properties and may be completely devoid of colour when totally infarcted. There is almost always perivascular survival of a few layers of cells and the subendocardial and subepicardial layers usually also survive: this acts as a built-in control for the staining reaction.

Stock solutions

Buffer
0.2 M for pH 7.0 (store at 0–4°C).

Solution A: 2.4 g trometamol (TRIS) in 100 ml distilled water	25 ml
Solution B: 0.1 M hydrochloric acid	45 ml
(Use ANALAR concentrated HC1 diluted 1/12 for molar, then dilute further 10 times for 0.1 M)	
Distilled water	30 ml

Malic acid substrate
L-Malic acid 6.7 g in 50 ml distilled water.
Add 12 g TRIS to buffer to pH 7.0.
Store frozen.

Sodium cyanide
0.1 M solution: weigh out 0.25 g sodium cyanide in 100 ml distilled water.
Add 8–8.5 ml M hydrochloric acid to buffer at pH 7.2.
Store at 0–4°C.

Tetrazolium salt
Make up nitroblue tetrazolium at 1 mg/ml strength in distilled water. Keep frozen.
Nicotinamide adenine dinucleotide (NAD) – keep solid desiccated in freezer.

Method
Cut cryostat sections from myocardium frozen either in liquid nitrogen or in isopentane/solid carbon dioxide slush.

(a) Place slides carrying sections in 37°C incubator.
(b) Make up incubating medium as follows:

Sodium cyanide solution (0.1 M at pH 7.2)	0.1 ml
NAD coenzyme	6 mg
Nitroblue tetrazolium solution	0.25 ml
TRIS buffer pH 7.0	0.55 ml
Malic acid substrate (1 M at pH 7.0)	0.1 ml

  (Check pH and adjust with a small amount of TRIS)
(c) Warm the incubating medium to 37°C and place sufficient on each section with a pipette, covering the section completely. Leave for 30 minutes, mount in glycerine jelly or an aqueous mountant. A negative control can be set up as required by omitting the malate substrate from the incubating medium.

Haematoxylin–eosin (H and E) autofluorescence

Routine formalin-fixed H and E sections can be examined under ultraviolet light for autofluorescence of those fibres that have anoxic or ischaemic damage. Fibres with early infarction show a shift of their secondary emission towards the yellow, away from the usual olive-green of healthy fibres. It has been said that only fibres that reveal increased eosinophilia in ordinary tungsten light will fluoresce in this way, but the authors and co-workers have noted yellow shift in fibres that cannot be detected in tungsten light as being eosinophilic.

Acridine-orange fluorescent stain for myocardium

Either formalin-fixed paraffin sections or unfixed frozen sections can be stained by this technique. The former must be brought to water first. After staining and mounting in water (no other mountant can be used, not even Fluormount), the sections are examined immediately under ultraviolet light. They can be photographed if required.

If the cover-slip is removed and the sections allowed to dry, however, they can be retained indefinitely. To review, they need only be wetted and a cover-slip replaced. Normal myocardium is a golden brown or sometimes yellowish brown depending on the optical system used. Damaged fibres show a colour shift to green when viewed under ultraviolet light.

Method
A stock solution of 1 per cent acridine-orange in water is kept refrigerated. This lasts for several months. For use, it is diluted 1/10 with distilled water.

(a) Bring sections to water.
(b) Agitate in the 0.1 per cent stain for approximately 5 seconds, though the time is not critical.
(c) Briefly wash, wipe off the excess water from around the section.
(d) Apply a cover-slip.

They are then ready for immediate examination. The pH of the washing water is not critical and tap water can be used if the pH range is between 6.0 and 7.0.

Martius scarlet blue (MSB) stain for fibrin

This trichrome stain is useful for examining thrombi and emboli and for seeking fibrin in disseminated intravascular coagulation.

(a) Bring sections to water.
(b) Stain with celestine blue for 3 minutes and Mayer's haematoxylin for 1 minute.
(c) Blue in water.
(d) Rinse in 95 per cent ethanol and then stain for 2 minutes with 0.5 per cent Martius yellow in 95 per cent ethanol containing 2 per cent phosphotungstic acid.
(e) Rinse in water and stain with 1 per cent brilliant crystal scarlet in 2.5 per cent glacial acetic acid for 10 minutes.
(f) Rinse in water and treat with 1 per cent aqueous phosphotungstic acid for 5 minutes.
(g) Rinse in water and stain with 0.5 per cent soluble blue (Acid Blue 93) in 10 per cent aqueous acetic acid for 10 minutes.
(h) Rinse and mount.

This method stains fibrin red, erythrocytes yellow and collagen blue.

Lendrum's stain (phloxine-tartrazine)

Though this stain has a number of applications, such as the demonstration of viral inclusion bodies, its major forensic use is in the detection of amniotic fluid embolism deaths associated with pregnancy. The fetal squames are rendered visible much more readily than in haematoxylin–eosin stain.

(a) Stain with Mayer's haematoxylin for 6 minutes and rinse in running water for 5 minutes.

(b) Stain with 0.5 per cent phloxine in 0.5 per cent calcium chloride solution for 20 minutes in a Coplin jar.

(c) Rinse in water and drain almost dry.

(d) Flood with a saturated solution of tartrazine in cellusolve ($C_4H_{10}O_2$; ethylene glycol monomethyl ether), which differentiates counterstain. This takes about 7 minutes and should be monitored microscopically so that red cells appear red–brown.

(e) Rinse by two changes in 95 per cent ethanol and two changes in absolute ethanol.

(f) Transfer straight to xylol and mount.

The keratin of amniotic squames is stained red; nuclei blue and cytoplasm yellow.

The 'WHO' method

The 'WHO' method is similar for demonstrating keratin and mucin-like substances in amniotic fluid embolism.

(a) Bring sections to water.

(b) Stain with celestine blue/Mayer's sequence, rinse.

(c) Differentiate quickly in 0.5 per cent acid–alcohol, then blue.

(d) Stain with erythrosin (1 per cent) for 5 minutes and rinse.

(e) Differentiate quickly in 95 per cent alcohol, rinse.

(f) Stain, with alcian green solution for 5 minutes.

(g) Rinse – the section should now be slightly pink.

(h) Rinse and treat with 95 per cent alcohol.

(i) Stain with ethanolic saffron for 5 minutes.

(j) Mount without going through water.

The alcian green is made by mixing 50 ml of 1 per cent aqueous solution of alcian green with 50 ml of 1 per cent acetic acid then adding 20 mg of thymol and filtering. Ethanolic saffron is made by cutting up strands of saffron and warming in 95 per cent alcohol until no more will elute. This should be a deep yellow solution.

DIATOM TECHNIQUE IN SUSPECTED DROWNING

There are several versions of this method, each with its own advocates. More recent methods have used suction of the filtrate through a millipore membrane to trap the diatoms, but the author (BK) has encountered early clogging of the membrane by debris and prefers the older centrifugation. References to the published methods will be found in Chapter 16.

Take a sample of water from the site where the body was recovered or where the immersion was first thought to have occurred. Several litres should be collected in a clean container and allowed to settle overnight. The top 90 per cent volume is then carefully decanted and the remainder centrifuged. The deposit should be examined under phase-contrast or dark-ground microscopy to see if any diatoms are present. If not, it is pointless to examine the autopsy tissues. If present, they should be retained for species comparison.

If the water contains diatoms, then the material retained at autopsy can be processed. The following procedure should have been followed:

(a) The sternum or a long bone such as the femur, or both, should be removed from the body in the usual way. It should be taken to a part of the mortuary or a side room distant from the cadaver and well-washed externally in a clean bowl or sink. Tap water can be used, if it is checked at intervals to ensure that it is diatom-free. Some water supplies at irregular times contain a few diatoms, though these are rarely numerous enough to cause problems in interpretation.

When the exterior of the bone has been well washed to remove any contamination from the exterior of the body, a clean saw (not used in that autopsy) is employed to open the marrow cavity of femur or sternum. With a clean scalpel or gouge, several grams of marrow are removed into a glass universal (30 ml) container. Obtain red marrow if possible, as fatty yellow marrow causes problems during digestion.

(b) Whole kidney, lung, liver or brain is also washed in this way and 1×1 cm cubes (several from each organ) cut with a clean scalpel from the deeper tissue. The organs can then be returned to the autopsy area for the usual gross examination.

(c) Each container, holding its separate tissue, is placed in a fume cupboard and covered with five times the volume of concentrated nitric acid. If metal caps are used on the containers, they may need to be shielded by polythene sheet to prevent dissolution. Digestion is allowed to proceed at room temperature for 1–2 days or, if the matter is urgent, they can be heated in a water-bath for a number of hours or overnight. When the solid cubes have dissolved into a slurry the containers are gently centrifuged, the supernatant acid poured off and replaced with distilled water. This process is repeated twice more to dilute the acid, knocking up the deposit, and recentrifuging, the final spin being as hard as possible to produce a small button of deposit. This may require transferring to a smaller conical centrifuge tube.

(d) A portion of this is transferred by pipette or loop to a slide and covered with a cover-slip to examination under phase-contrast or dark-ground illumination.

A prolonged search under medium power of the microscope is required before the sample is declared negative. The lung sample should be examined first, as if it is negative it is unlikely that other organs can be truly positive, for diatom-containing water can percolate passively down the air-passages even after death.

Opinion is divided about how many diatoms can be accepted as presumptive evidence of drowning when found in distant organs like brain, bone marrow and kidney. One solitary organism is certainly insufficient and the author (BK) requires five as a minimum under one coverslip before acceptance. The tissue examined may make a difference to the yield. Peabody strongly recommends brain as the choice and condemns femoral marrow, but bone marrow was the tissue used by the pioneers of the technique and seems to the authors to be satisfactory. The type of diatom found in the tissues should correspond to those found in the water sample, though it must be admitted that most diatoms seem to the non-botanical eye to be ovoid or boat-shaped. Expert advice from a suitable biologist should be sought if the issue is important.

USEFUL CONVERSION TABLES

TABLE A1.0 *Conversion factors*

To convert from	To	Multiply by
Centimetres	Inches	0.394
Inches	Centimetres	2.540
Grams	Pounds	0.002
Pounds	Grams	453.592

To convert Centigrade to Fahrenheit, multiply by 1.8 and add 32.
To convert Fahrenheit to Centigrade, subtract 32 and divide by 1.8.

TABLE A1.1 *Approximate weight of bodies*

Stones	Pounds	Kilograms
1	14	6.3
2	28	12.7
3	42	19.0
4	56	25.4
5	70	31.7
6	84	38.1
7	98	44.4
8	112	51.0
9	126	57.0
10	140	63.0
11	154	70.0
12	168	76.0
13	182	82.0
14	196	89.0
15	203	92.0
18	252	114.0

TABLE A1.2 *Height of bodies*

Feet and inches	Inches	Centimetres
4'10"	58"	145.0
4'11"	59"	147.5
5'	60"	150.0
5'1"	61"	152.5
5'2"	62"	155.0
5'3"	63"	157.5
5'4"	64"	160.0
5'5"	65"	162.5
5'6"	66"	165.0
5'7"	67"	167.5
5'8"	68"	170.0
5'9"	69"	172.5
5'10"	70"	175.0
5'11"	71"	177.5
6'	72"	180.0
6'1"	73"	182.5
6'2"	74"	185.0

TABLE A1.3 *Approximate breath–blood-alcohol equivalents*

μg/100 ml breath	mg/100 ml blood
10	23
20	45
30	68
40	91
50	114
60	137
70	160
80	182
90	205
100	228

1 μg/100 ml in breath = 2.28 mg/100 ml in blood.
1 mg/100 ml in blood = 0.43 μg/100 ml in breath.

TABLE A1.4 *Length conversion of wounds, etc.*

Inches	Centimetres
0.25	0.63
0.5	1.27
1.0	2.54
1.5	3.81
2.0	5.08
2.5	6.35
3.0	7.62
4.0	10.16
5.0	12.70

TABLE A1.5 *Normal ranges of biochemical blood analyses*

Sodium	133–147 mmol/l
Potassium	3.4–5.0 mmol/l
Urea	2.5–7.5 mmol/l
Calcium	2.2–2.6 mmol/l
Chloride	95–106 mmol/l
Bicarbonate	22–28 mmol/l
Glucose (fasting)	3.6–5.6 mmol/l
Lactate	0.8–2.0 mmol/l
Phosphate (inorganic)	0.8–1.4 mmol/l
Magnesium	0.6–1.0 mmol/l
Serum protein (total)	60–80 g/l
Albumin	35–48 g/l
Bilirubin	up to 17 µmol/l
Alkaline phosphatase	30–90 IU/l
Amylase	70–300 IU/l
Creatinine	50–100 µmol/l
Creatine kinase (CPK)	Up to 240 IU/l

TABLE A1.6 *Body weight and length 15–30 years.* In this table, three weights (without clothing) are given for each body length: (1) weight for persons of average build = middle entry; (2) weight for lightly built persons = top entry; (3) weight for heavily built persons = bottom entry*

Women

Body length (cm)	Weight (kg) 15 yrs	20 yrs	25 yrs	30 yrs
142.5	40.8	43.0	44.0	45.3
	45.3	47.6	49.0	50.3
	51.2	53.0	55.3	56.6
145	41.2	43.5	44.8	46.2
	45.8	48.5	49.8	51.2
	51.6	53.9	56.2	57.5
147.5	41.7	44.4	45.8	47.1
	46.2	49.4	50.7	52.1
	52.1	55.7	57.1	58.4
150	42.6	45.3	46.7	47.6
	47.1	50.3	51.6	53.0
	53.0	56.6	58.0	59.8
152.5	43.5	46.7	47.1	48.5
	48.5	51.6	52.6	53.9
	54.4	58.0	59.3	60.7
155	44.8	47.6	48.5	49.8
	49.8	53.0	53.9	55.3
	55.3	59.8	60.7	62.1
157.5	46.2	48.9	50.3	51.2
	51.2	54.4	55.7	56.6
	57.5	61.2	62.5	63.9

Men

Body length (cm)	Weight (kg) 15 yrs	20 yrs	25 yrs	30 yrs
150	41.7	45.8	47.6	49.4
	46.2	50.7	53.0	54.8
	51.6	57.1	59.3	61.6
152.5	42.6	46.7	48.5	50.3
	47.1	51.6	53.9	55.7
	53.0	58.0	60.7	62.5
155	43.5	47.6	49.4	51.2
	48.5	53.0	54.8	56.6
	54.4	59.3	61.6	63.4
157.5	44.9	48.9	50.7	52.1
	49.8	54.4	56.2	58.0
	56.2	61.2	63.0	65.2
160	46.2	50.3	52.1	53.5
	51.2	55.7	58.0	59.3
	57.5	62.5	65.2	66.6
162.5	47.6	51.6	53.9	55.3
	53.0	57.5	59.8	61.2
	59.3	64.8	67.0	68.9
165	49.4	53.5	55.7	56.6
	54.8	59.3	61.6	63.0
	61.6	66.6	69.3	70.7

(continued)

TABLE A1.6 *Body weight and length 15–30 years.* (continued)*

Women					Men				
	Weight (kg)					**Weight (kg)**			
Body length (cm)	**15 yrs**	**20 yrs**	**25 yrs**	**30 yrs[†]**	**Body length (cm)**	**15 yrs**	**20 yrs**	**25 yrs**	**30 yrs[†]**
160	47.1	50.3	51.2	52.5	167.5	51.2	55.3	57.1	58.4
	52.5	55.9	57.1	58.4		56.6	61.2	63.4	64.8
	59.3	62.5	6.43	65.7		63.4	68.9	71.1	72.9
162.5	48.9	51.2	52.5	53.9	170	52.5	56.6	58.9	59.8
	54.4	57.1	58.4	59.8		58.4	63.0	56.2	66.6
	61.2	64.3	65.7	67.5		65.7	70.7	73.4	74.7
165	50.7	53.0	54.4	55.7	172.5	54.4	58.4	60.2	61.6
	56.2	58.9	60.2	61.6		60.2	64.8	67.0	68.4
	63.4	66.1	67.5	69.3		67.5	73.0	75.2	77.0
167.5	52.1	54.9	55.7	57.1	175	55.7	59.8	62.1	63.9
	58.0	60.7	62.1	63.4		62.1	66.6	68.9	70.7
	65.2	68.4	69.8	71.6		69.8	74.7	77.5	79.3
170	53.9	56.2	57.5	58.9	177.5	58.0	61.6	63.9	65.7
	59.8	62.5	63.9	65.2		64.3	68.4	71.1	72.9
	67.5	70.2	71.6	73.4		72.0	77.0	79.7	82.0
172.5	55.3	57.5	59.3	60.2	180	59.8	63.9	66.1	68.0
	61.6	63.9	65.7	67.0		66.6	70.7	73.4	75.7
	69.3	72.0	73.8	75.7		74.7	79.3	82.4	85.2
175	57.1	59.3	60.7	61.6	183	62.1	65.7	68.4	70.7
	63.4	65.7	67.5	68.4		68.9	72.9	76.1	78.4
	71.6	73.8	75.7	77.0		77.5	82.0	85.6	87.9
178	59.3	60.7	62.1	63.4	185.5	63.9	68.0	71.1	72.9
	65.7	67.5	68.9	70.2		71.1	75.2	78.8	81.1
	73.9	76.1	77.5	78.9		79.7	84.3	88.3	91.1
180	61.2	63.0	63.4	64.8	188	66.1	69.8	73.0	75.7
	68.0	69.8	70.7	72.0		73.4	77.5	81.1	83.8
	76.1	78.4	79.7	81.1		82.4	87.0	91.1	94.2

* From Basel JR, Geigy AG. 1953. *Wissenschaftliche Tabellen*, p. 199. By permission.
[†] Fourth decade weight should be maintained throughout life.

TABLE A1.7 *Weight of fetus (g) in relation to age (month)* *

Lunar month	Streeter	Scammon and Calkins
Second	1.1	3.5
Third	14.2	14.3
Fourth	108.0	86.8
Fifth	316.0	260.9
Sixth	630.0	551.6
Seventh	1045.0	971.4
Eighth	1680.0	1519.0
Ninth	2378.0	2196.1
Tenth	3405.0	2998.8

* From Potter EL. 1961. *Pathology of the fetus and infant*, 2nd edn. Chicago, Year Book Medical Publishers. By permission.

TABLE A1.8 *Length (cm) of fetus in relation to age (month)* *

	Crown–rump length		Crown–heel length	
Lunar month	**Streeter**	**Scammon and Calkins**	**Dietrich**	**Scammon and Calkins**
Second	2.3	–	3.0	–
Third	7.4	5.1	9.8	7.0
Fourth	11.6	10.7	18.0	15.5
Fifth	26.4	15.5	25.0	22.7
Sixth	20.8	19.7	31.5	29.2
Seventh	24.7	23.6	37.1	35.0
Eighth	28.3	27.1	42.5	40.4
Ninth	32.1	30.5	47.0	45.4
Tenth	36.2	33.6	50.0	50.2

* From Potter EL. 1961. *Pathology of the fetus and infant*, 2nd edn. Chicago, Year Book Medical Publishers. By permission.

TABLE A1.9 *Weights of the organs at various ages (in grams)**

	Lungs		Brain		Heart		Kidneys		Liver		Spleen	
	Men	Women	Men	Women	Men	Women	Men	Women	Men	Women	Men	Women
New born	51.7	50.9	353	347	19	20	24	24	124	125	8	6
0–3 mth	68.8	63.6	435	411	–	–	–	–	–	–	–	–
3–6 mth	94.1	93.3	600	534	–	–	–	–	–	–	–	–
6–9 mth	128.5	114.7 }	877	726	41	36	60	52	300	240	26	25
9–12 mth	142.4	142.1 }										
1–2 yr	170.3	175.3	971	894	54	48	72	65	400	390	35	34
2–3 yr	245.9	244.3	1076	1012	63	62	85	75	460	450	42	41
3–4 yr	304.7	265.5	1179	1076	73	71	93	84	510	500	48	47
4–5 yr	314.2	311.7	1290	1156	83	80	100	93	555	550	53	52
5–6 yr	360.6	319.9	1275	1206	95	90	106	102	595	595	58	57
6–7 yr	399.5	357.5	1313	1225	103	100	112	112	630	635	62	62
7–8 yr	365.4	404.4	1338	1265	110	113	120	123	665	685	64	67
8–9 yr	405.0	382.1	1294	1208	122	126	128	135	715	745	68	71
9–10 yr	376.4	358.4	1360	1226	132	140	138	148	770	810	73	77
10–11 yr	474.5	571.2	1378	1247	144	154	150	163	850	880	82	85
11–12 yr	465.6	535.0	1348	1259	157	168	164	180	950	950	91	93
12–13 yr	458.8	681.7	1383	1256	180	188	178	195	1050	1080	101	103
13–14 yr	504.5	602.3	1382	1243	202	207	196	210	1150	1180	111	112
14–15 yr	692.8	517.0	1356	1318	238	226	212	222	1240	1270	121	120
15–16 yr	691.7	708.8	1407	1271	258	238	229	230	1315	1330	135	127
16–17 yr	747.3	626.5	1419	1300	282	243	244	236	1380	1360	145	134
17–18 yr	776.9	649.5	1409	1254	300	247	260	240	1450	1380	152	140
18–19 yr	874.7	654.9	1426	1312	310	250	270	244	1510	1395	157	146
19–20 yr	1035.6	785.2	1430	1294	318	251	282	247	1580	1405	160	151
20–21 yr	953.0	792.8	–	–	322	252	290	248	1630	1415	162	155

* Boyd E. 1962. In: Altman and Dittmer (eds), *Growth, including reproduction and morphological development.* Biological Handbooks, Federation of American Societies for Experimental Biology, Washington, pp. 346–8.

TABLE A1.10 *Heart: men and women, weight in relation to body weight by sex**

Men				Women			
Body weight		Heart weight (g)		Body weight		Heart weight (g)	
Pounds	Kilograms	Mean	Range	Pounds	Kilograms	Mean	Range
				90	40	162	135–193
				95	43	171	143–204
				100	45	180	150–215
105	47	205	165–241	105	47	189	158–226
110	50	215	173–253	110	50	198	165–237
115	52	225	181–264	115	52	207	172–248
120	54	235	190–276	120	54	215	180–259
125	56	245	198–287	125	56	225	188–268
130	58	255	206–299	130	58	234	195–277
135	60	265	213–310	135	60	244	203–286
140	63	274	221–322	140	63	253	211–295
145	65	284	229–333	145	65	262	219–304
150	68	294	237–345	150	68	272	225–313

(continued)

TABLE A1.10 *Heart: men and women, weight in relation to body weight by sex* (continued)*

Men				Women			
Body weight		Heart weight (g)		Body weight		Heart weight (g)	
Pounds	Kilograms	Mean	Range	Pounds	Kilograms	Mean	Range
155	70	304	245–356	155	70	282	233–322
160	72	313	253–368	160	72	288	240–330
165	74	323	261–370	165	74	297	247–337
170	77	333	268–371	170	77	306	255–343
175	79	343	280–372	175	79	315	283–350
180	81	353	288–373	180	81	324	301–356
185	83	363	296–382	185	83	333	309–361
190	86	373	304–392	190	86	342	317–366
195	88	382	312–402	195	88	351	325–371
200	90	392	320–412				

Average weight of adult male heart: 294 g

Average weight of adult female heart: 250 g

* Data from Smith HL. 1928. The relation of the weight of the heart to the weight of the body and of the weight of the heart to age. *Am Heart J* **4**:79–93.
NB There is considerable variation in published tables of heart weights: probably hypertensive hearts account for some of the upper ranges of 'normal'. However, the authoritative publication of Hangartner *et al.* gives considerably higher normal maximum weights. (Hangartner J, Marley N, Whitehead A, Thomas A, Davies M. 1985. The assessment of cardiac hypertrophy at autopsy. *Histopathology* **9**:1295–306.)

TABLE A1.11 *Heart: normal weight in relation to body length*

Body length (cm)	Heart weight (g)		Body length (cm)	Heart weight (g)		Body length (cm)	Heart weight (g)	
	Males	Females		Males	Females		Males	Females
	$\sigma = \pm 40$	$\sigma = \pm 30$		$\sigma = \pm 40$	$\sigma = \pm 30$		$\sigma = \pm 40$	$\sigma = \pm 30$
135	254	219	157	296	258	179	338	297
136	256	220	158	298	259	180	340	299
137	258	222	159	300	261	181	342	300
138	260	224	160	302	263	182	344	302
139	262	226	161	304	265	183	346	304
140	264	227	162	306	267	184	348	306
141	266	229	163	308	268	185	349	307
142	268	231	164	310	270	186	351	309
143	270	233	165	311	272	187	353	311
144	272	235	166	313	274	188	355	313
145	273	236	167	315	275	189	357	315
146	275	238	168	317	277	190	359	316
147	277	240	169	319	279	191	361	318
148	279	242	170	321	281	192	363	320
149	281	243	171	323	283	193	365	322
150	283	245	172	325	284	194	367	323
151	285	247	173	327	286	195	368	325
152	287	249	174	329	288	196	370	327
153	289	251	175	330	290	197	372	329
154	291	252	176	332	291	198	374	331
155	292	254	177	334	293	199	376	332
156	294	256	178	336	295	200	378	334

σ = standard deviation.
From Zeek PM. 1942. Heart weight. I. The weight of the normal heart. *Arch Pathol* **34**:820–32.
Copyright 1942, American Medical Association.
NB But see also Hangartner *et al.* 1985 (details above).

TABLE A1.12 *Brain: adults**

Age (years)	Brain weight (g)			
	Men		Women	
	Mean	Range	Mean	Range
17–19	1340	1170–1527	1242	1120–1420
20–29	1396	1158–1620	1234	1057–1565
30–39	1365	1075–1685	1233	1038–1440
40–49	1366	1069–1605	1240	995–1543
50–69	1375	1113–1665	1200	820–1477
60–69	1323	1018–1610	1178	920–1372
70–85	1279	1039–1485	1121	832–1370

* Data from Sunderman FW, Boerner F. 1949. *Normal values in clinical medicine.* W. B. Saunders Company, Philadelphia.

TABLE A1.13 *Brain: children**

Age	Body length (cm)	Brain weight (g)
Birth–3 days	49	335
3–7 days	49	358
1–3 wks	52	382
3–5 wks	52	413
5–7 wks	53	422
7–9 wks	55	489
3 mths	56	516
4 mths	59	540
5 mths	61	644
6 mths	62	660
7 mths	65	691
8 mths	65	714
9 mths	67	750
10 mths	69	809
11 mths	70	852
12 mths	73	925
14 mths	74	944
16 mths	77	1010
18 mths	78	1042
20 mths	79	1050
22 mths	82	1059
24 mths	84	1064
3 yrs	88	1141
4 yrs	99	1191
5 yrs	106	1237
6 yrs	109	1243
7 yrs	113	1263
8 yrs	119	1273
9 yrs	125	1275
10 yrs	130	1290
11 yrs	135	1320
12 yrs	139	1351

* Data from Sunderman FW, Boerner F. 1949. *Normal values in clinical medicine.* W. B. Saunders Company, Philadelphia.

SAMPLES AND CONTROLS NEEDED FOR DNA PROFILING

The essence of DNA profiling in forensic work is comparison between two samples. One is the 'test' sample from the living or dead subject (or objects with which he or she has been in contact, such as clothing) and the other the 'control', a somewhat inaccurate term for the samples obtained from a suspect, a group of suspects or a screening programme which may have hundreds or even thousands of items.

Since the beginning of the DNA analysis, significant advances have been made in methodology allowing forensic identification of individuals from minute amounts of DNA. Microgram amounts of relatively undegraded DNA is required for multi-locus typing of the restriction fragment length polymorphism (RFLP) analysis and hundreds of nanograms for single-locus typing. Polymorphic DNA sequences can be detected from the root of shed or freshly plucked single human hairs using the polymerase chain reaction (PCR). Mitochondrial DNA (mtDNA) has been detected even in a sample from a single hair shaft.

Blood

As red cells have no nuclear DNA, sufficient blood must be obtained to extract DNA from the much sparser leucocytes. At least 1 ml and preferably 5 ml are taken into an EDTA tube, which extracts metallic ions and not only prevents clotting, but inhibits enzymes in blood or micro-organisms, which may break down DNA during storage.

The blood sample, in a plastic (not glass) tube, should be frozen solid in a deep-freeze or the ice-making compartment of an ordinary refrigerator. As frozen blood is useless for some other forensic investigations, the DNA sample should be clearly marked as such. Other samples, for grouping and many other serological and toxicological tests, must be taken and stored at only 4°C.

If a blood sample is to be taken directly to the laboratory for DNA profiling, then freezing is not necessary, but wherever there is delay, either freezing or, at second best, effective cooling should be carried out.

Most of the laboratories are using nowadays FTA paper for the collection of blood samples. FTA paper is an absorbent cellulose-based paper that contains chemical substances to protect DNA molecules from nuclease degradation and preserve the paper from bacterial growth (Seah and Burgoyne 2000). As a result, DNA on FTA paper is stable at room temperature over a period of several years. The use of FTA paper simply involves adding a spot of blood to the paper and allowing the stain to dry.

Blood stains, as opposed to liquid blood, should either be sent intact on surfaces, kept as cool as possible before and during transit to the laboratory – or rubbed with a cotton-wool swab moistened with water. This swab is then air-dried without heat and frozen. Although not required for DNA testing, always provide the laboratory with control swabs for conventional blood grouping, including swabs rubbed on an area of the fabric away from obvious stains, as well as an unused swab.

Dried blood stains on hard surfaces can be scraped off with a scalpel into a small plastic container and sent as they are, kept as cool as possible.

Buccal cells

A disposable toothbrush may also be used for collecting buccal cells in a non-threatening manner. This method can be very helpful when samples need to be collected from children and this is the method actually used for most of paternity testing labs. After the buccal cells have been collected by gently rubbing a wet toothbrush across the buccal surface, the brush can be tapped onto the surface of FTA paper for sample storage and preservation.

Seminal and vaginal fluids

Swabs from vagina, rectum, mouth, etc., should be air-dried as quickly as possible, but not heated. They should then be stored in deep-freeze, unless sent straight to the forensic science laboratory. Liquid semen found in the vagina or elsewhere should be recovered with a fine pipette, placed in a small plain tube and frozen solid.

Seminal stains on small items of fabric or any other small objects may be frozen or kept as cool as possible during transit. Bulk clothing cannot be frozen and should merely be kept cool, transit to the laboratory being made as soon as possible, using strong sterilized paper bags, not impervious polythene, which encourages mould formation. Alternatively, damp swabs may be taken of suspect stains, which are then dried and frozen. As with blood, suspect dried seminal stains on hard surfaces may be scraped off and transmitted dry to the laboratory.

Mouth swabs may be taken either to seek semen in suspected oral intercourse (though positive recoveries are very rare) or to obtain buccal mucosa for DNA identification. In the latter case, the yield is small, so at least three to four swabs must be rubbed hard against the inside of the cheek – or the mouth lining scraped with an instrument and then smeared

onto a swab. All such swabs should be frozen in the usual manner.

Hairs – head, pubic, etc.

Collection of hairs – head, pubic, eyebrow, axillary – from the victim or at the scene of crime is extremely important as a 2 cm piece of single hair is actually sufficient for mtDNA analysis. It is of paramount importance to avoid cross-contamination and to submit the hairs in sterilized paper bags, well identified.

Autopsy tissue samples

At least 0.5 g of tissue should be cut from the parenchyma of an organ and placed in a small plastic tube with no fixative or preservative. This should be frozen solid. Spleen is said to be one of the best organs for DNA recovery, though liver, muscle, kidney and brain may also be used. The fresher the tissue the better, and totally putrefied material was formerly of little use, as the nuclear chromatin was degraded. However, rapidly developing new techniques are allowing the recovery of recognizable DNA from old material.

For identification of skeletal remains using DNA technology, a well-preserved tooth is the tissue of election. In addition, long bones (femur) or ribs can also be used.

Other general remarks

The sensitivity of DNA technology is changing the strategy of sample collection. Very sensitive low-copy-number DNA methods are being developed allowing the detection of subnanogram amounts of DNA. For this reason, it is extremely important to avoid cross-contamination from the personnel collecting the samples.

DNA can even be obtained from personal objects, fingerprints, sweat and of course from saliva recovered from bite marks.

Finally, as for other type of forensic evidence, the chain of custody must be extremely well-preserved.

FURTHER READING

Badir B, Knight B. 1987. Fluorescence microscopy in the detection of early myocardial infarction. *Forensic Sci Int* **34**:99–102.

APPENDIX 2

Council of Europe Committee of Ministers Recommendation No. R (99) 3

RECOMMENDATION NO. R (99) 3 OF THE COMMITTEE OF MINISTERS TO MEMBER STATES ON THE HARMONISATION OF MEDICO-LEGAL AUTOPSY RULES[1]

(Adopted by the Committee of Ministers on 2 February 1999 at the 658th meeting of the Ministers' Deputies)

The Committee of Ministers, under the terms of Article 15.*b* of the Statute of the Council of Europe,

Considering that the aim of the Council of Europe is to achieve a greater unity between its members;

Having regard to the principles laid down in the Convention for the Protection of Human Rights and Fundamental Freedoms and, in particular, the prohibition of torture or inhuman or degrading treatment or punishment, and the right to life;

Conscious that it is normal practice for autopsies to be carried out in all Council of Europe member States to establish the cause and manner of death for medico-legal or other reasons or to establish the identity of the deceased;

Considering the importance of compensation for victims and families in criminal and civil proceedings;

Underlining the need for investigation, description, photographic documentation and sampling during medico-legal autopsy to follow primarily medical and scientific principles and simultaneously consider legal requirements and procedures;

Conscious that the increasing mobility of the population throughout Europe and the world, as well as the increasing internationalisation of judicial proceedings, require the adoption of uniform guidelines on the way autopsies are to be carried out and on the way autopsy reports are to be established;

Considering the Council of Europe Agreement on the Transfer of Corpses (European Treaty Series No. 80) and having regard to the difficulties often experienced by the receiving country when a dead body is repatriated from one member state to another;

Aware of the importance of proper autopsy procedures, in particular with a view to bringing to light illegal executions, and murders perpetrated by authoritarian regimes;

---

[1] When this recommendation was adopted, the Representatives of Denmark and the Netherlands, in application of Article 10.2*c* of the Rules of Procedure for the meeting of the Ministers' Deputies, reserved the right of their Governments to comply or not with paragraph 2 (scope of the recommendation) of the present recommendation.

When this recommendation was adopted, the Representative of Germany, in application of Article 10.2*c* of the Rules of Procedure for the meeting of the Ministers' Deputies, reserved the right of his Government to comply or not with paragraph 2 *f* and *h* of the present recommendation.

Underlining the need to protect the independence and impartiality of medico-legal experts, as well as to make available the necessary legal and technical facilities for them to carry out their duties in an appropriate way and to promote their training;

Considering the importance of national quality control systems to ensure the proper performance of medico-legal autopsies;

Underlining the need to strengthen international co-operation with a view to the progressive harmonisation of medico-legal autopsy procedures at a European level;

Having regard to Recommendation 1159 (1991) on the harmonisation of autopsy rules adopted, at its 43rd Ordinary Session, by the Parliamentary Assembly of the Council of Europe;

Having regard to the Model Autopsy Protocol of the United Nations, endorsed by the General Assembly of the United Nations in 1991;

Taking into account the 'guide on disaster victim identification' adopted by the International Criminal Police Organisation (Interpol) General Assembly in 1997,

1 Recommends the governments of member states:
  (i) to adopt as their internal standards the principles and rules contained in this recommendation;
  (ii) to take or reinforce, as the case may be, all appropriate measures with a view to the progressive implementation of the principles and rules contained in this recommendation;
  (iii) to set up a quality assurance programme to ensure the proper implementation of the principles and rules contained in this recommendation.
2 Invites the governments of member states to inform the Secretary General of the Council of Europe upon his or her request of the measures taken to follow up the principles and rules contained in this recommendation.

PRINCIPLES AND RULES RELATING TO MEDICO-LEGAL AUTOPSY PROCEDURES

Scope of the recommendation

1 In cases where death may be due to unnatural causes, the competent authority, accompanied by one or more medico-legal experts, should where appropriate investigate the scene, examine the body and decide whether an autopsy should be carried out.
2 Autopsies should be carried out in all obvious or suspected unnatural death, even where there is a delay between causative events and death, in particular:

a homicide or suspected homicide;
b sudden, unexpected death, including sudden infant death;
c violation of human rights such as suspicion of torture or any other form of ill treatment;
d suicide or suspected suicide;
e suspected medical malpractice;
f accidents, whether transportational, occupational or domestic;
g occupational disease and hazards;
h technological or environmental disasters;
i death in custody or death associated with police or military activities;
j unidentified or skeletalised bodies.
3 Medico-legal experts must exercise their functions with total independence and impartiality. They should not be subject to any form of pressure and they should be objective in the exercise of their functions, in particular in the presentation of their results and conclusions.

Principle I – Scene investigation

A *General principles*
  1 In case of obvious or suspected unnatural death, the physician who first attended the dead body should report to the competent authorities, the latter deciding whether an examination should be carried out by a qualified medico-legal expert or by a physician familiar with medico-legal examination.
  2 Particularly in cases of homicide or suspicious death, medico-legal experts should be informed without delay and, where appropriate, go immediately to the place where the body is found and have immediate access there. In this respect, there should be an adequate structure of co-ordination among all persons involved and, in particular, among judicial bodies, medico-legal experts and police.
B *Examination of the body*
  1 Role of the police
    The following tasks, among others, should be carried out by police officers:
    a record the identities of all persons at the scene;
    b photograph the body as it is found;
    c make sure that all relevant artifacts are noted, and that all exhibits, such as weapons and projectiles, are seized for further examination;
    d in agreement with the medico-legal expert, obtain identification of the body and other pertinent information from scene witnesses, including those who last saw the decedent alive, where available;

e protect the deceased's hands and head with paper bags, under the control of the medico-legal expert;

f preserve the integrity of the scene and surroundings;

2 Role of the medico-legal expert

The medico-legal expert should without delay:

a be informed of all relevant circumstances relating to the death;

b ensure that photographs of the body are properly taken;

c record the body position and its relation to the state of the clothing and to the distribution pattern of rigor mortis and hypostasis, as well as the state of *post-mortem* decomposition;

d examine and record the distribution and pattern of any blood stains on the body and at the scene, as well as other biological evidence;

e proceed to a preliminary examination of the body;

f except where the body is decomposed or skeletal, note the ambient temperature and deep-rectal temperature of the body, and estimate the time of death by recording the degree, location and fixation of rigor mortis and hypostasis, as well as other findings;

g make sure that the body is transported and stored in a secure and refrigerated location in an undisturbed state.

Principle II – Autopsy physicians

Medico-legal autopsies should be performed, whenever possible, by two physicians, of whom at least one should be qualified in forensic pathology.

Principle III – Identification

In order to ensure that proper identification of the body is carried out in accordance with the disaster victim identification guide adopted by the General Assembly of Interpol in 1997, the following criteria should be considered: visual recognition, personal effects, physical characteristics, dental examination, anthropological identification, fingerprints and genetic identification.

1 Visual identification

Visual identification of a body should be carried out by relatives or persons who knew and have recently seen the decedent.

2 Personal effects

A description of clothing, jewellery and pocket contents should be recorded. These may assist correct identification.

3 Physical characteristics

Physical characteristic should be recorded through an external and an internal examination.

4 Dental examination

Where appropriate, the examination of teeth and jaws should be carried out by a dentist with medico-legal experience.

5 Anthropological identification

Whenever human material is skeletised or in an advanced stage of decomposition, an anthropological identification should be carried out, if necessary.

6 Fingerprints

Where appropriate, fingerprints should be taken by police officers. A close collaboration should exist between all experts involved.

7 Genetic identification

Where appropriate, genetic identification should be carried out by an expert in forensic genetics.

It is appropriate to take biological samples from the deceased in order to assist genetic identification. Measures should be taken in order to avoid contamination and guarantee appropriate storage of biological samples.

Principle IV – General considerations

1 Medico-legal autopsies and all related measures must be carried out in a manner consistent with medical ethics and respecting the dignity of the deceased.

2 Where appropriate, the closest relatives should be given an opportunity to see the corpse.

3 Before beginning the autopsy, the following minimum rules should be applied:

a record the date, time and place of autopsy;

b record the name(s) of the medico-legal expert(s), assistant(s) and all other persons present at the autopsy with indication as to the position and role of each one in the autopsy;

c take colour photographs or video, where appropriate, of all relevant findings and of the dressed and undressed body;

d undress the body, examine and record clothing and jewellery, verify the correspondence between injuries on the body and clothing;

e where appropriate, take X-rays, particularly in cases of suspected child abuse, and for identification and location of foreign objects.

4 Where appropriate, before beginning the autopsy, body orifices should be appropriately swabbed for the recovery and identification of biological trace evidence.

5 If the decedent was hospitalised prior to death, admission blood specimens and any X-rays should be obtained as well as hospital records.

Principle V – Autopsy procedures

I EXTERNAL EXAMINATION

1 The examination of the clothing is an essential part of the external examination and all findings therein are to be clearly described. This is especially important in those cases where the clothing has been damaged or soiled: each area of recent damage must be described fully and relevant findings are to be related to the site of injuries on the corpse. Discrepancies in such findings are also to be described.

2 The description of the body following an external examination must include:

  a age, sex, build, height, ethnic group and weight, nutritional state, skin colour and special characteristics (such as scars, tattoos or amputations);

  b post-mortem changes, including details relating to rigor and post-mortem hypostasis – distribution, intensity, colour and reversibility – and putrefaction and environmentally induced changes;

  c findings on a primary external inspection and description which, if required, include sampling of stains and other trace evidence on the body surface and a reinspection after removal and cleaning of the body;

  d inspection of the skin of the posterior surfaces of the corpse;

  e description and careful investigation of the head and the facial orifices includes: colour, length, density and distribution of hair (and beard); nasal skeleton; oral mucosa, dentition and tongue; ears, retro-auricular areas and external meati; eyes: colour of irises and sclerae, regularity and appearance of pupils, sclerae, conjunctivae; skin (presence and absence of petechiae to be described); if fluids have been evacuated from facial orifices, their colour and odour;

  f neck: checking for excessive mobility, presence and absence of abrasions, other marks and bruising (including petechiae) over the entire circumference of the neck;

  g thorax: shape and stability; breasts; aspect, nipples and pigmentation;

  h abdomen: external bulging, pigmentation, scars, abnormalities and bruising;

  i anus and genitals;

  j extremities: shape and abnormal mobility, abnormalities; injection marks and scars; palmar surfaces, finger and toe nails;

  k material findings under fingernails.

3 All injuries, including abrasions, bruises, lacerations and other marks have to be described by shape, exact measurement, direction, edges, angles and location relative to anatomical landmarks. Photographs should be taken. Bite marks shall be swabbed, and casts made where necessary.

4 Signs of vital reaction around wounds, foreign particles inside wounds and in their surroundings and secondary reactions, such as discolouration, healing and infections must also be described.

5 The investigation of cutaneous and sub-cutaneous bruising may require local skin incision.

6 Where appropriate, specimens from wounds must be removed for further investigations, such as histology and histochemistry.

7 All signs of recent or old medical and surgical intervention and resuscitation must be described. Medical devices must not be removed from the body before the intervention of the medico-legal expert.

8 A decision has to be taken at this stage as to the strategies of investigation and the necessity of documentation by X-rays and other imaging procedures.

II INTERNAL EXAMINATION

A General

1 All relevant artifacts produced by the dissection and from sampling procedures, must be documented.

2 All three body cavities – head, thorax and abdomen – must be opened layer by layer. Where appropriate, the vertebral canal and joint cavities should be examined.

3 Examination and description of body cavities include: an examination for the presence of gas (pneumothorax), measurement of volume of fluids and blood, appearance of internal surfaces, intactness of anatomical boundaries, external appearance of organs and their location; adhesion and cavity obliterations, injuries and haemorrhage.

4 The demonstration and dissection of the soft tissues and musculature of the neck have to be components of all medico-legal autopsies (see the paragraph concerning special procedures).

5 All organs must be examined and sliced following established guidelines of pathological anatomy. This includes opening of all relevant vessels, for example, intracranial arteries, sinuses, carotid arteries, coronary arteries, pulmonary arteries and veins, aorta and vessels of the abdominal organs, femoral arteries and lower

limb veins. Relevant ducts have to be dissected, for example, central and peripheral airways, biliary ducts and ureters. All hollow organs have to be opened and their content described by colour, viscosity, volume (samples should be retained, where appropriate). All organs have to be sliced and the appearance of the cut surface described. If injuries are present, the dissection procedure may have to vary from the normal one: this should be appropriately described and documented.

6 All internal lesions and injuries must be precisely described by size and location. Injury tracks must be described in order to include their direction as regards the organ anatomy.

7 The weight of all major organs must be recorded.

B Detailed

1 *Head*

  a Before opening the skull, the periosteum must be scraped off in order to display or exclude any fractures.

  b The head examination procedure must allow the inspection and description of the scalp, external and internal surfaces of the skull and of the temporal muscles.

  c The thickness and appearances of the skull and sutures, the appearances of the meninges, the cerebrospinal fluid (CSF), the wall structure and contents of cerebral arteries and sinuses must be described. The description of the bones must also include an examination of their intactness, including the connection between the skull and the first two vertebrae.

  d In obvious or suspected head injury (for example, if a detailed examination is required or if autolysis or putrefaction is present) fixation of the whole brain is recommended before its dissection.

  e Middle ears must be always opened and nasal sinuses where indicated.

  f The soft tissue and skeleton of the face is dissected only in relevant cases, using a cosmetically acceptable technique.

2 *Thorax and neck*

The opening of the thorax must be performed using a technique which allows the demonstration of the presence of pneumothorax and the inspection of the thorax walls, including the postero-lateral regions. *In situ* dissection of the neck must display the details of its anatomy.

3 *Abdomen*

The opening procedure of the abdomen must allow an accurate examination of all layers of the walls, including the postero-lateral regions. *In situ* dissection is necessary in certain cases, particularly for the demonstration of injury tracks and evacuation of fluids. Dissection of organs should observe anatomical continuity of systems, where possible. The whole intestine must be dissected and its contents described.

4 *Skeleton*

  a The examination of the thoracic cage, the spine and the pelvis must be part of the autopsy procedure.

  b Where appropriate traumatic deaths need a precise dissection of the extremities, possibly complemented by X-ray examination.

5 *Special procedures*

  a If there is any suspicion of neck trauma, the brain and thoracic organs are to be removed prior to the dissection of the neck, to enable detailed dissection to take place in a bloodless field.

  b If there is a suspicion of air embolism, pre-autopsy radiology of the thorax must be performed. The first stage of the autopsy in such a case must be a careful partial opening of the thorax and dislocation of the lower three-quarters of the sternum with the subsequent opening of the heart under water, allowing the measurement and sampling of escaping air or gas.

  c For the demonstration of particular injury patterns, deviation from the normal procedure of dissection has to be accepted, provided that such procedures are specifically described in the autopsy report.

  d The dissection in traumatic deaths must include a full exposure of the soft tissues and musculature on the back of the body. The same procedure must be applied to the extremities (so called 'peel-off' procedure).

  e In suspected or overt sexual assaults, the sexual organs are to be removed *en bloc* together with the external genitalia, rectum and anus, before they are dissected. Relevant swabs of orifices and cavities must be taken prior to this procedure.

6 *Sampling*

The scope of the sampling procedure is to be case-dependent. However, the following minimum rules should be applied:

  a in all autopsies, the basic sampling scheme includes specimens from the main organs for histology and peripheral blood sampling (such as for alcohol and drug analyses and genetic identification), urine and gastric contents. All blood samples must be peripheral blood and not heart or thoracic;

  b if the cause of death cannot be established with the necessary degree of certainty, sampling includes additional specimens and fluids for metabolic studies and thorough toxicology. This includes blood, vitreous humour, CSF, bile, hair samples and further relevant tissues;

c if death is related to physical violence, sampling includes the injuries, for example to determine wound age and any foreign materials in the wounds;

d if reconstructions are desirable, the removal of bones and osseous compartments may become necessary;

e if identification is the predominant aim, the removal of jaws and other bones may be necessary;

f if strangulation or the application of physical force to the neck is suspected or diagnosed, the entire neck structures, musculature and neurovascular bundles must be preserved for histology. The hyoid bone and the laryngeal cartilages must be dissected very carefully;

g biological samples must be collected in tightly closed jars, properly preserved and placed under seal and transported to the laboratory in perfect safety;

h certain specimens and fluids need to be sampled in a special way and analysed without delay.

7 *Release of the body*
After a medico-legal autopsy has been carried out, medico-legal experts should ensure that the body is returned in a dignified condition.

Principle VI – Autopsy report

1 The autopsy report is as important as the autopsy itself, as the latter is of little value if the findings and opinions of the medico-legal expert are not communicated in a clear, accurate and permanent document. The autopsy report should be an integral part of the autopsy procedure and be drafted carefully.

2 The report should therefore be:
a full, detailed, comprehensive and objective;
b clear and comprehensible not only to other doctors, but also to non-medical readers;
c written in a logical sequence, well-structured and easy to refer to in various sections of the report;
d be in a legible and permanent form, with hard paper copy even if it is retained in electronic storage;
e be written in a discursive 'essay' style;

3 When drafting an autopsy report, the following minimum content should be included:
a legal preface to fulfil statutory requirements, if needed;
b serial number, computer retrieval coding and International Classification of Disease Code (ICD) code;

c full personal details of deceased (including name, age, sex, address and occupation) unless unidentified;
d date, place and time of death, where known;
e date, place and time of autopsy;
f name, qualifications and status of medico-legal expert(s);
g persons present at the autopsy and their function;
h name of the authority commissioning the autopsy;
i person(s) identifying the body to the medico-legal expert;
j name and address of the medical attendant of the deceased;
k a synopsis of the history and circumstances of the death, as given to the medico-legal expert by the police, judges, relatives or other persons, as well as information contained in the file, where available;
l description of the scene of death, if attended by the medico-legal expert; reference should be made to the provisions contained in Principle I above;
m external examination; reference should be made to the provisions of Principle V above;
n internal examination by anatomic systems, together with a comment on every organ. Reference should be made to the provisions of Principle V above;
o a list of all samples retained for toxicology, genetic identification, histology, microbiology and other investigations should be included; all such specimens should be identified and attested by the medico-legal expert according to the legal system of the state concerned, for continuity of evidence;
p results of ancillary investigations, such as radiology, odontology, entomology and anthropology should be included, when such results are available;
q one of the most important parts of the autopsy report is the evaluation of the significance of the accumulated results by the medico-legal expert. After termination of the autopsy, evaluation is usually provisional because later findings and later knowledge of other circumstantial facts can necessitate alteration and modification. Medico-legal experts must interpret the overall findings so that the maximum information and opinion can be offered. Also questions that have not been raised by the competent authority must be addressed if they could be of significance;
r based on the final interpretation, the cause of death (in the International Classification of Disease should be given. Where several alternatives for the cause of death exist and the facts do not allow a differentiation between them, the medico-legal expert should describe the alternatives and, if possible, rank them in order of probability. If this is

not possible, then the cause of death should be certified as 'Unascertained';

    s the report should be finally checked, dated and signed by the medico-legal expert(s).

4 The date of the autopsy and the date of the provisional report should never be more than a day or two apart. The date of the autopsy and the date of the final report should be as close together as possible.

APPENDIX TO RECOMMENDATION NO. R (99) 3

SPECIFIC PROCEDURES (SELECTED EXAMPLES)

1 *Constriction of neck (hanging, manual and ligature strangulation)*

The examination of the scene where the body was found is extremely important: for example the presence of a chair or similar platform; fastening of the strangulation device; technique of tying of the knot; adhesive taping of hands and objects for trace evidence:

– Strangulation marks: depth, width, intermediate rings, direction, suspension point, raised ridges of skin, zones of hyperaemia, presence of duplicate strangulation marks; further specific neck injuries: dried excoriations due to slippage of the implement, marks due to textile weave pattern and structure, distribution of petechiae in the skin, bruising, scratch marks, blisters in the strangulation mark.

– Bleeding from facial orifices. Differences in widths of the pupils, localization of hypostasis, presence and distribution of congestion.

– Injuries due to convulsions, defensive injuries, injuries due to being held forcibly.

Dissection of the soft tissues, of the musculature and of the organs of the neck in a bloodless field is essential.

2 *Drowning/Immersion*

Note carefully the following findings: foam at the mouth, cutis anserina, maceration, mud and algae, lesions due to water animals, injuries due to surroundings (for example rocks and ships), loss of nails, skin, localization of livor mortis.

Technique: sampling of gastric contents, precise description of the lungs (weight, measurement, extent of emphysema), sampling, lung fluid, liver and other tissues, for the possible demonstration of diatoms and other contaminants.

If required, sampling of drowning medium (for example river, bath water) should be carried out.

3 *Sexually motivated murder*

The inspection and documentation of the scene of crime, e.g. relative to the injury pattern, is especially important. All injuries must be photographed together with a scale. If required, the body surfaces must be investigated under UV light and taped. Search for and sampling of foreign biological material must include pubic hairs and secretions on the body surface as for instance originating from bites. Such material must be preserved carefully for DNA investigation and protected against contamination. 'En bloc' dissection of the genital organs is strongly recommended. It is also necessary to proceed to the careful removal and sampling of material under the fingernails and control hairs.

4 *Death from child abuse and neglect*

State of nutrition and general care, thorough description and documentation of external injuries and scars, thorough examination for bone fractures (X-ray), must be evaluated.

Consider the removal of a variety of tissues: for example all injuries, regional lymph nodes in malnutrition, endocrine organs, immuno-competent tissues, specimens from different parts of the intestine.

5 *Infanticide/still-birth*

Special techniques of dissection are necessary to expose the falx cerebri and the tentorium cerebelli; describe the site of caput succedaneum; remove all fractures 'en bloc'; investigate all bone centres of ossification (size and presence). Special care is to be applied to the thoracic organs: degree of inflation of the lungs, flotation test 'en bloc' and 'en detail'. However, the limitations of the flotation test must be appreciated. All malformations must be described. As regards abdominal organs, gas content of the intestine must be investigated. The umbilical cord and the placenta must be subject to morphological and histological examination.

6 *Sudden death*

A subdivision into three main categories relative to the further strategy after gross examination is useful:

a findings that obviously explain the sudden occurrence of death (for example haemopericardium, aortic rupture). Cases belonging to this category can usually be regarded as sufficiently solved;

b findings that could explain the death but allow other explanations. Cases belonging to this category necessitate the exclusion of , for example,. poisoning and possibly histological proof of recent or chronic alterations relative to the cause of death;

c findings are either nil/minimal or do not explain the occurrence of death. Cases belonging to this category will usually require extensive further investigations.

This is especially so with sudden infant death cases. In such cases a more comprehensive investigative scheme is essential.

7 *Shooting fatalities*
The following should be carried out:
– extensive account on the scene of the incident, of weapons involved, of types of bullets, of sites of 'environmental' damage, of cartridge cases and of relative positions of persons involved;
– thorough examination of the clothing and description of relevant damage and careful sampling;
– thorough investigation and documentation of any blood (splashes) on the body surfaces (including clothing and hands);
– precise description of bullet entry and exit wounds relative to anatomical landmarks and distances from the soles of the feet and bullet tracks within the body;
– description of any impression marks of the muzzle;
– excision of uncleaned skin specimens surrounding entry and exit wounds;
– X-ray before and/or during autopsy (where necessary);
– determination of bullet tracks and their direction(s);
– final determination of direction(s) of fire, of the succession of shots, of intra-vital occurrence, of the victim's position (s).

8 *Death caused by explosive devices*
a As well as evaluating the cause of death, autopsy is essential to assist in reconstructing the nature of the explosion and identifying the type and maker of the explosive device, especially in aircraft sabotage or other terrorist actions.
b Full X-ray of the body must be made to detect and localise any metallic objects, such as detonator components, which may lead to the identification of the explosive device.
c The pattern of injury may indicate that the dead person was a perpetrator of the explosion, for example maximum injury in the lower abdominal region suggests that he or she carried the device on his or her lap during a premature explosion.
d At autopsy, all foreign objects in the tissues, identified on X-rays, must be carefully preserved for forensic examination.
e Samples of tissues, clothing, etc., must be retained for chemical analysis to identify the type of explosive.

9 *Blunt and/or sharp force injuries*
The following should be carried out:
– examination of the weapons or objects that are possibly involved (especially their dimensions);

– extensive examination and inspection of clothing (including damage, stains);
– careful dissection and description of all tracks (layer by layer) including their dimensions and weapon-related traces, signs of vitality.

10 *Fire Deaths*
The following should be carried out:
– examination of remains of clothing, - specific types and shapes of skin combustions;
– search for heat-related alterations and peculiarities;
– demonstration/exclusion of fire accelerants.;
– search for signs of vitality: carbon monoxide, HCN, soot inhalation, skin lesions.

11 *Suspicion of intoxication (General Outlines)*
11.1 Where anatomical findings do not reveal a cause of death and/or there is vague suspicion of poisoning, basic sampling should include peripheral blood, urine, stomach contents, bile, liver and kidney.
11.2 If specific suspicion arises, sampling should be group-related as follows:
– hypnotics, sedatives, psycho-active drugs, cardiac drugs and analgesics, pesticides: as aforementioned under (11.1);
– drugs of abuse: as aforementioned under (11.1) and additionally cerebrospinal fluid, brain tissue, injection marks, hairs;
– volatile fat-soluble substances such as fire accelerant and solvents: as aforementioned under (11.1) and in addition: blood from left ventricle, brain tissue, subcutaneous fat tissue, lung tissue, clothing;
– nutritional intoxication: as aforementioned under (11.1) and in addition: intestinal contents, if possible taken from 3 different sites;
– suspicion of chronic intoxication (heavy metals, drugs, pesticides etc.) as aforementioned under (11.1) and in addition: hairs (tufts), bones, fat tissue, intestinal contents.

12 *Decomposed bodies*
The presence of decomposition does not remove the need for a full autopsy.
Radiological examination will exclude bony injury, the presence of foreign bodies, for example bullets.
Toxicological studies (particularly estimation of alcohol concentrations) should be carried out but interpreted with great caution.

Index

References to autopsy, death and homicide are limited in the index, as these are major subject of the book. Readers are advised to seek more specific references. *vs* denotes differentiation or comparison.

vulva
  examination at autopsy 16
  injuries 233
    in sexual offences 423, 424

Wales, dating skeletal remains in 126
walkers, deaths from exposure and 419
'washer-woman's skin' 395, 396
wasting conditions 414
water
  adipocere formation 70
  carbon monoxide poisoning 561
  deprivation 412
  explosions in 275
  immersion deaths and *see* immersion deaths
  in plastic bags 360
Waterhouse–Friederichsen syndrome 349
Webley veterinary pistol 273
Weedol 566
weight
  body 603
    external examination 12
  brain, at autopsy 29
  heart *see* heart, weight
wetcutting, brain, at autopsy 27
whip, multi-thonged 303
whiplash injury 215, 283, 284
whipping, torture and human rights abuse 303
WHO method, staining 602
Widmark equation/factor 556
Wilson's classification of burns 312–13, 313
World Health Organization (WHO)
  cardiomyopathies classification 508

cardiomyopathies definition 507
death certificates 55
staining method 602
sudden death definition 492–3
'undetermined death' 10
wound classification 137
wounding, survival period after 169–71
wounds
  'ante-mortem' *vs* 'post-mortem' 167–9, 170–1
  chronological histological changes 167–8
  classification and types 137
  dating 166–9, 170, 171
  defence 165–6, 167, 168
  definition 136
  gunshot/firearm *see* rifled weapons, wounds; shotgun wounds
  healing 103, 167–8
  histochemical changes 168–9
  mechanism 136–7
  negative/positive vital reactions 169
  pathology 136–73
  razors/glass and china 163–4
  scissor 164–5, 166
wrists
  slashing, scars in identification 102
  suicidal cutting 237–8

XTC (Ecstasy) 581
xylene abuse 597

Zahn, lines of 503, 510
zonal lesions 499
zygomatic process, sex determination 109